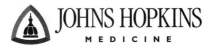
JOHNS HOPKINS
M E D I C I N E

THE JOHNS HOPKINS

ABX Guide

Diagnosis and Treatment of Infectious Diseases

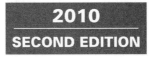
2010
SECOND EDITION

Edited by

John G. Bartlett, MD

Paul G. Auwaerter, MD, FACP, FIDSA

Paul A. Pham, PharmD

Division of Infectious Diseases

The Johns Hopkins University School of Medicine

D0003865

JONES AND BARTLETT PUBLISHERS
Sudbury, Massachusetts
BOSTON   TORONTO   LONDON   SINGAPORE

World Headquarters

Jones and Bartlett Publishers
40 Tall Pine Drive
Sudbury, MA 01776
978-443-5000
info@jbpub.com
www.jbpub.com

Jones and Bartlett Publishers Canada
6339 Ormindale Way
Mississauga, Ontario L5V 1J2
Canada

Jones and Bartlett Publishers
International
Barb House, Barb Mews
London W6 7PA
United Kingdom

Jones and Bartlett's books and products are available through most bookstores and online booksellers. To contact Jones and Bartlett Publishers directly, call 800-832-0034, fax 978-443-8000, or visit our website, www.jbpub.com.

Substantial discounts on bulk quantities of Jones and Bartlett's publications are available to corporations, professional associations, and other qualified organizations. For details and specific discount information, contact the special sales department at Jones and Bartlett via the above contact information or send an email to specialsales@jbpub.com.

The authors, editor, and publisher have made every effort to provide accurate information. However, they are not responsible for errors, omissions, or for any outcomes related to the use of the contents of this book and take no responsibility for the use of the products and procedures described. Treatments and side effects described in this book may not be applicable to all people; likewise, some people may require a dose or experience a side effect that is not described herein. Drugs and medical devices are discussed that may have limited availability controlled by the Food and Drug Administration (FDA) for use only in a research study or clinical trial. Research, clinical practice, and government regulations often change the accepted standard in this field. When consideration is being given to use of any drug in the clinical setting, the health care provider or reader is responsible for determining FDA status of the drug, reading the package insert, and reviewing prescribing information for the most up-to-date recommendations on dose, precautions, and contraindications, and determining the appropriate usage for the product. This is especially important in the case of drugs that are new or seldom used.

Our goal is to provide health professionals focused, core prescribing information in a convenient, organized, and concise fashion. The information provided in *The Johns Hopkins ABX Guide* is designed to support, not replace, the relationship that exists between a patient/site visitor and his/her physician. The guide is intended as a quick and convenient reminder of information you have already learned elsewhere; it is not meant to be a replacement for training, experience, continuing medical education, or studying the latest drug prescribing literature.

Production Credits

Executive Publisher: Christopher Davis
Senior Acquisitions Editor: Alison Hankey
Production Editor: Wendy Swanson
Senior Marketing Manager: Barb Bartoszek
V.P., Manufacturing and Inventory Control:
  Therese Connell

Text Design and Composition: diacriTech
Cover Design: Scott Moden
Cover Image: Top—© Tischenko Irina/ShutterStock,
  Inc.; Bottom—© Sybille Yates/ShutterStock, Inc.
Printing and Binding: Malloy, Inc.
Cover Printing: Malloy, Inc.

ISBN: 978-0-7637-8108-8

6048

Printed in the United States of America
14 13 12 11 10   10 9 8 7 6 5 4 3 2 1

Contributors

Editors

John G. Bartlett, MD
Professor
Division of Infectious
  Diseases
Johns Hopkins University
  School of Medicine

*Paul G. Auwaerter, MD,
  FACP, FIDSA*
Associate Professor
Clinical Director, Division
  of Infectious Diseases
Johns Hopkins University
  School of Medicine

Paul A. Pham, PharmD
Research Associate
Division of Infectious
  Diseases
Johns Hopkins University
  School of Medicine

Authors

Joel Blankson, MD, PhD
Johns Hopkins University
Assistant Professor
Director, Inpatient HIV
  Unit
Division of Infectious
  Diseases
Johns Hopkins University
  School of Medicine

Chris F. Carpenter, MD
Attending Physician
Fellowship Program
  Director, Infectious
  Diseases
Beaumont Hospital, Royal
  Oak, MI
Associate Professor of
  Medicine
Wayne State University
  School of Medicine

Sara E. Cosgrove, MD, MS
Associate Professor of
  Medicine
Division of Infectious
  Diseases
Director, Antibiotic
  Management Program
Associate Hospital
  Epidemiologist
Johns Hopkins University
  School of Medicine

James DeMaio, MD
Bradenton, FL

Susan E. Dorman, MD
Associate Professor
  of Medicine and
  International Health
Division of Infectious
  Diseases
Johns Hopkins University
  School of Medicine

Khalil G. Ghanem, MD, PhD
Assistant Professor of
  Medicine
Division of Infectious
  Diseases
Johns Hopkins University
  School of Medicine

Ophir Handzel, MD, LL.B
Fellow, Otology/Neurotology
Massachusetts Eye and Ear
  Infirmary
Harvard Medical School

*Christopher J. Hoffmann,
  MD, MPH*
Assistant Professor of
  Medicine
Johns Hopkins University
  School of Medicine

Noreen A. Hynes, MD, MPH
Assistant Professor
Director, Geographic
  Medicine Center
Division of Infectious
  Diseases
Johns Hopkins University
  School of Medicine

Daniel J. Lee, MD, FACS
Director, Wilson Auditory
  Brainstem Implant
  Program
Department of
  Otolaryngology
Massachusetts Eye and Ear
  Infirmary
Assistant Professor
Department of Otology and
  Laryngology
Harvard Medical School

Spyridon Marinopoulos, MD
Assistant Professor
General Internal
  Medicine
Johns Hopkins University
  School of Medicine

Robin McKenzie, MD
Assistant Professor of
  Medicine
Division of Infectious
  Diseases
Johns Hopkins University
  School of Medicine

Michael Melia, MD
Associate Fellowship
  Program Director
Instructor
Division of Infectious
  Diseases
Johns Hopkins University
  School of Medicine

Ralph Metson, MD
Clinical Professor of Otology
  and Laryngology
Massachusetts Eye and Ear
  Infirmary
Harvard University

Dionissis Neofytos, MD, MPH
Assistant Professor
Transplant and Oncology
  Infectious Disease
  Program
Division of Infectious
  Diseases
Johns Hopkins University
  School of Medicine

Eric Nuermburger, MD
Associate Professor
  of Medicine and
  International Health
Johns Hopkins University
  School of Medicine

*Raj Sindwani, MD, FACS,
  FRCS*
Section Head
Rhinology, Sinus, and Skull
  Base Surgery
Cleveland Clinic

Lisa Spacek, MD, PhD
Assistant Professor
Division of Infectious Diseases
Johns Hopkins University
  School of Medicine

Timothy R. Sterling, MD
Professor of Medicine
Vanderbilt University School
  of Medicine

Mark Sulkowski, MD
Associate Professor of
  Medicine
Division of Infectious
  Diseases
Johns Hopkins University
  School of Medicine

Aditi Swami, MD
Infectious Diseases Consultant
Detroit, MI

David Thomas, MD, MPH
Professor
Chief of Infectious Diseases
Johns Hopkins University

Joseph Vinetz, MD
Professor of Medicine
Division of Infectious
  Diseases
School of Medicine
University of California,
  San Diego

Aimee Zaas, MD, MHS
Associate Professor of
  Medicine
Division of Infectious
  Diseases and
  International Health
Institute of Genome Sciences
  and Policy
Duke University Medical
  Center

The POC-IT Center

*Paul G. Auwaerter, MD,
  FACP, FIDSA*
Executive Director
Chief Medical Officer

Steven A. Libowitz
Senior Director

Nicole Sokol
Information Project
  Administrator

Danielle Meinsler
Project Analyst

Contents

Diagnosis

Pathogens

Management

Drugs

Vaccines

Foreword

The Johns Hopkins POC-IT ABX Guide was initially a project and product of the Division of Infectious Diseases at Johns Hopkins University School of Medicine. It was launched in 2000 as a website and was then adapted for use with handheld devices in April 2001, and a print version was published in 2005. The idea was then, and remains, to present timely and accurate recommendations for the management of the most common infectious diseases in a format concise enough to fit the small screen of a handheld device. This approach forced extraordinary discipline in economy of language, restricting the authors to include only the most practical and important issues of clinical practice. The result is that clinicians can usually locate, access, and apply information at the point of care in under a minute. The adaptation of this material for this new print publication—*The Johns Hopkins ABX Guide: Diagnosis and Treatment of Infectious Disease, Second Edition*—captures these important features.

The online guide, and this print version of it, come at a time when the field is sizzling from our recent experiences with MRSA, Acinetobacter, influenza, *C. difficile*, and multiply resistant Gram-negative organisms, just to name a few hot topics. A great concern is the evolution of resistance—the inevitable consequence of antibiotic use and abuse. This concern is now compounded by the relative paucity of new antimicrobial agents that is sometimes referred to as the "dry pipeline." We are in a period during which physicians are challenged to be particularly careful in antibiotic use. In some instances, physicians will need to resort to antibiotics that have been used infrequently for years or decades, such as colistin, and at other times employ some relatively new agents such as telavancin, tigecycline, and peramivir.

Several features of the book are worth special emphasis.

Credibility. Each topic is written by an experienced clinician, someone who actually practices medicine and has been asked to write a monograph based on his or her experience, augmenting the piece with recommendations from authoritative and evidence-based sources, when these exist. Thus, most of the recommendations are based on guidelines from the Centers for Disease Control and Prevention, scholarly professional societies, reviews by the Cochrane Library, BMJ reviews, HCRQ reviews, and more. Once completed, these documents are reviewed by at least three other professionals in order to ensure consistency and accuracy.

Timeliness. All of medicine changes rather rapidly, but no field moves with the same velocity as infectious diseases in terms of diagnostic testing, recognition of new pathogens, surprising new pathogens and epidemics, and changes in management guidelines. Most of the monographs included here were originally written between 2000 and 2002, but all have been updated annually through November 2009.

Presentation. The method of presentation of information is the one we have found most useful for guidance in the field of infectious diseases for primary care practitioners, the professional category that writes 80% of scripts for antibiotics. Decisions on format and content are based on 12 years of experience with this guidance including external reviews, feedback from users, and extensive clinical application by the authors. Each of the five sections—diagnoses, pathogens, management, anti-infectives, and vaccines—has a standardized format designed to provide the most important information relevant to patient care in terms of management decisions, thus answering many common practitioner queries.

In sum, this book is designed as an authoritative resource dealing with virtually all important antimicrobial agents, the vast majority of infectious diseases, and commonly encountered pathogens. The recommendations are based on reliable sources, the information is timely, and the format permits easy, rapid access to clinically relevant information.

John G. Bartlett, MD
Professor of Medicine
The Johns Hopkins University School of Medicine
Editor-in-Chief, The Johns Hopkins POC-IT ABX Guide

NOTE. This book is the text edition of the web-based version of the Johns Hopkins POC-IT ABX Guide (http://hopkins-abxguide.org); however, the book required editing to accommodate the needs of a more succinct text that could be a pocket print version. These cuts were made by editing entries, eliminating more obscure topics or topics that receive very little web traffic, and eliminating all but the source documents for recommendations. The electronic version contains more information if you wish to review full references and other information.

Preface

Clinicians need accurate, concise, and easy-to-use information at point-of-care. *The Johns Hopkins ABX Guide: Diagnosis and Treatment of Infectious Diseases, Second Edition* has been designed to meet the ever more urgent needs of time-strapped clinicians by distilling complex material into need-to-know information that is easily accessible, rapidly viewable, and up to date, helping health care professionals raise the standards of care and improve patient safety.

This guide is organized into five sections—diagnoses, pathogens, management, drug therapy, and vaccines. Each section is organized alphabetically for quick reference, with each module sharing common order and structure and annotated references. The first section, Diagnosis, includes diagnostic criteria, common pathogens, prevention, and thorough treatment regimens that include adjunctive therapy. The second section, Pathogens, which is further organized by class, covers the clinical relevance of the organism, site of infections, and treatment regimens according to the infection site. New to this edition is the Management section on how to handle common syndromes with advice on differential diagnosis and treatment. Section 4, Drugs, comprises anti-infectives including antibacterials, antifungals, antiparasitics, antivirals, and biological agents. This comprehensive section consists of indications, dosing and dosing adjustments, drug interactions, information regarding use during pregnancy and breast feeding, important notes, and charts that show the available forms of the drug as well as brand names, route of administration, and estimated costs. The fifth section, Vaccines, is comprised of common vaccines, citing diagnostic criteria, treatment regimens, and important clinical points.

Also included in this guide are three appendices, the first of which includes tables and algorithms relevant to material referenced under specific modules. Appendix II contains tables of general interest as well as antibiotic sensitivity charts that show at a glance how the most commonly used antibiotics act against a wide range of pathogens. The final section of the book features a new appendix of drug-to-drug interaction tables that detail the effect of interactions and provide recommendations and comments on many of the most widely used anti-infectives.

Drug Name Abbreviations

/r	Ritonavir <400 mg/day
3TC	Lamivudine
5-FC	Flucytosine
ABC	Abacavir
ABV	Doxorubicin/Bleomycin/Vincristine
ADV	Adefovir
AMB	Amphotericin B
APV	Amprenavir
ASA	Aspirin
ATV	Atazanavir
Azithro	Azithromycin
AZT	ZidoVudine
d4T	Stavudine
ddC	Zalcitabine
ddI	Didanosine
DLV	Delavirdine
DRV	Darunavir
EFV	Efavirenz
EMB	Ethambutol
ENF (T-20)	Enfuvirtide
EPO	Erythropoietin
ETR	Etravirine
FPV	Fosamprenavir
FQ	Fluoroquinolone
FTC	Emtricitabine
FTV	*Fortovase*
G-CSF	Filgrastim
GAZT	AZT-glucuronide
GM-CSF	*Prokine*
HU	Hydroxyurea
IDV	Indinavir
INF	Interferon
INH	Isoniazid
INV	*Invirase*
IVIG	Intravenous Immune Globulin
LPV	Lopinavir
LPV/r	Lopinavir/Ritonavir
NNRTI	Non-nucleoside reverse transcriptase inhibitor
NRTI	Nucleoside reverse transcriptase inhibitor
NSAID	Nonsteroidal anti-inflammatory drud
NFV	Nelfinavir
NVP	Nevirapine
PCN	Penicillin
PEG-IFN	Peg Interferon
PI	Protease inhibitor
PZA	Pyrazinamide
RAL	Raltegravir
RBT	Rifabutin
RBV	Ribavirin
RTV	Ritonavir

SM	Streptomycin
SMX	Sulfamethoxazole
TDF	Tenofovir
TDF/FTC	Truvada
TMP	Trimethoprim
TMP-SMX	Trimethoprim-Sulfamethoxazole
TPV	Tipranavir
TZV	Trizivir
VZIG	Varicella Zoster Immune Globulin
ZDV	Zidovudine

DRUG ADMINISTRATION AND GENERAL ABBREVIATIONS

µL	microliter
µmol	micromole
Abnl	abnormal
Abx	antibiotic(s)
Ac	before meal
admin	administered
ADR	adverse drug reaction
All	allergy, allergic
ART	antiretroviral therapy
AUC	area under the curve
bid	twice per day
Bx, Bxp	biopsy
c	copies
ca	cancer
caps	capsule
CCR5	Chemokine Receptor 5
cg	centigram
cm	centimeter
cm^2	centimeters squared
cx	culture
CVVH	continuous veno-venous hemofiltration
d/c	discontinue, discharge
Ddx	differential diagnosis
dL	deciliter
DS	double strength
dx	diagnosis
Dz	disease
g	gram
H_2O	water
HAART	highly active antiretroviral therapy
Hg	mercury
hr, hrs	hour, hours
hs	hours of sleep
hx	history
IM	intramuscular
Infxn	infection
IU	international unit
IV	intravenous
kg	kilogram
L	liter
m	meter

m^2	meters squared
Mc	megacycle
mcg or μg	microgram
mEq	milliequivalent
mg	milligram
min, mins	minute, minutes
mL	milliliter
mm	millimeter
mm^3	millimeters cubed
mmol	millimole
mo, mos	month, months
mU	milliunits
N	normal (solution) or total sample size
ng	nanogram
nm	nanometer
OI	opportunistic infection
OTC	over-the-counter
oz	ounce
PE	physical exam
Plt	platelet
PO	by mouth
PRN or prn	as needed
PSI	pounds per square inch
Pt	patient
pt-yrs	patient-years
qd	every day
qid	four times a day
qmo	every month
qod	every other day
qwk	every week
RBC	red blood cell
r/o	rule out
Rx	treatment, prescription
rxn	reaction
s	second
sol'n	solution
SQ	subcutaneously
SS	single strength
sx	symptoms
TAMs	Thymadine Analogue Resistance Mutations
tid	three times per day
tiw	three times per week
tx	treatment
Txf	transfusion
Txp	transplant
U	unit
vol	volume
w/	with
w/i	within
w/o	without
WBC	white blood cell
wk, wks	week, weeks
wnl	within normal limits
×	times/for
yr, yrs	year, years

SECTION 1
DIAGNOSIS

Biodefense

ANTHRAX—INHALATION

John G. Bartlett, MD

PATHOGENS
- *Bacillus anthracis*

CLINICAL
- Epidemiology: exposure in time and place to airspace of case/environment. If non-biowarfare, a high density of anthrax spores are usually inhaled from infected animal fur, hide, or wool.
- Symptoms: **Stage 1** (first 3–4 days)—fever, chills, sweats, GI sx, cough, HA, malaise, chest pain, but no coryza; **Stage 2**—sepsis.
- Confirmed case (CDC): compatible clinical illness plus positive culture or 2 other tests (PCR, immunohistochemistry, serology).
- Suspected case: compatible illness plus one non-culture test or epidemiological link.
- Lab: blood, respiratory, pleural or other body fluid culture.
- CXR: wide mediastinum and bloody pleural effusion. CT scan: hyperdense mediastinal nodes + edema.

TREATMENT
Treatment: 60 days
- Ciprofloxacin 400 mg IV q8h combined with second agent: clindamycin 600 mg IV q8h or penicillin G 4MU q4–6h or meropenem 1 g IV q6–8h or rifampin 300 mg q12h.
- Clindamycin: use strongly recommended for role in preventing toxin production.
- Alt: doxycycline 100 mg IV q12h or levofloxacin 750 mg IV q24h, need to combine with second agent.
- Pregnancy: avoid doxycycline. Use ciprofloxacin and change to penicillin when sensitivities are known.
- Corticosteroids: no role known.
- Human-derived anthrax immune globulin (AIG) available from CDC 800-232-4636. Decision on use made on case by case basis—must be given early.
- Total duration of antibiotic treatment: 60 days—may often switch to oral agents at 14–21 days.

Treatment—special populations
- Pregnancy, lactation: in place of long-term doxy/cipro regimen, consider amoxicillin 0.5–1 g PO three times a day +/– rifampin 300 mg PO twice daily after >14–21 days and stable to complete 60–100 days.
- Immunosuppressed: standard treatment.
- Pediatric: cipro 10–15 mg/kg IV q12h, not to exceed 1 g/day or doxy >8 yrs >45 kg, 100 mg q12h; >8 yrs and <45 kg or <8, 2.2 mg/kg q12h.

FOLLOW UP
- Need to treat 60–100 days or longer because spores persist *in vivo* >30 days. Rx required in primate model. Ciprofloxacin, levofloxacin, and doxycycline considered equal/superior to other abx.

OTHER INFORMATION
- Keys to dx: exposure + CT chest, bloody pleural effusions and positive pretreatment blood cultures.
- Key Rx: early abx and drain pleural effusions.
- Notify local Infection Control and Public Health Dept. immediately; inhalation anthrax = bioterrorism.

BASIS FOR RECOMMENDATIONS
Inglesby TV, O'Toole T, Henderson DA, et al. Anthrax as a biological weapon, 2002: updated recommendations for management. *JAMA*, 2002; Vol. 287; pp. 2236–52.
Comments: Updated recommendations that represent a consensus among experts—prior recommendations hold except penicillin deleted as first line agent due to penicillinase production (this applies to all strains and they appear sensitive *in vitro*). Fluoroquinolone other than cipro will probably work, but only cipro is FDA approved and tested in the monkey model.

Update: Investigation of bioterrorism-related anthrax and interim guidelines for clinical evaluation of persons with possible anthrax. *MMWR Morb Mortal Wkly Rep*, 2001; Vol. 50; pp. 941–8.

Comments: Lab tests for inhalation anthrax: WBC, X-ray, blood cx. Consider—Chest CT, flu test. Lab tests for cutaneous anthrax: GS and cult lesion pre-Rx. Consider—bx if GS and cult neg.

BOTULISM

John G. Bartlett, MD

PATHOGENS
- Clostridia that produces human pathogenic neurotoxins types A, B, E, and F.
- Known botulinum toxin producing strains include: *C. botulinum*, *C. butyricum*, and *C. baratii*.

CLINICAL
- Epidemiology: U.S. average 100–150 cases/yr, infant 60–100/yr, foodborne 10–20/yr, wound and unspecified 20–40/yr.
- Highest rates: Republic of Georgia, Russia, China; highest in U.S. rates—Alaska.
- Foodborne: Usually home prepared cured meat, canned vegetables and fermented fish.
- Sx: diplopia, dysphagia, dysarthria, then symmetric descending paralysis.
- Signs: alert but with ptosis, paresis (symmetrical), hyporeflexia, afebrile.
- Differential diagnosis: Guillian-Barré, myasthenia, stroke, CNS depressants (EtOH, CO, organophosphates), Eaton Lambert (lung ca), tick paralysis.
- Clinical forms: infant, foodborne, wound, iatrogenic, bioterrorism.

MORE CLINICAL
- Major Considerations for Differential Diagnosis: Guillian Barré: ascending paralysis, hx of recent prior infection, paresthesias; obtain EMG.
- Myasthenia: recurrent paralysis, weakness; obtain EMG; observe response to anticholinesterase.
- Stroke: asymmetric paresis; obtain MRI.
- Intoxications: exposure-organophosphates, CO, nerve gas, EtOH; obtain drug/toxin/CO levels.
- Lambert-Eaton: incrementally decreased strength with sustained contraction; evidence of lung ca; EMG similar to botulism.
- Tick paralysis: paresthesias; ascending paralysis; tick history.

DIAGNOSIS
- Clinical suspicion foremost. All forms show identical sx: acute, afebrile, descending flaccid paralysis; cranial nerves always involved.
- Typical presentation: trouble with vision, speaking and swallowing, then hypotonia.
- Botulinum toxin in blood, vomiting, gastric aspirate, stool, food source (mouse assay at CDC/state labs). Usual sources are serum and stool.
- Mouse lethality assay standard and sensitive (20 pg/mL but requires 4–6 days.) EIA is fast and simple, but less sensitive.
- EMG: nerve terminal disease; CSF analysis is negative.

TREATMENT
Adults
- U.S. mortality—6.6%. Need antitoxin and respiratory support.
- Principles: consider diagnosis if alert, no fever, flaccid symmetrical paralysis + cranial nerves palsies; consider bioterrorism—treat with antitoxin (adults) + respiratory support.
- Report suspected/established cases immediately to local health dept or CDC 404-639-2888.
- Foodborne: remove toxin with gastric lavage, cathartics and enemas.
- Antitoxin to types A, B, and E—obtain from CDC 770-488-7100 or 404-639-2888.
- Skin test with antitoxin: if positive desensitize.
- Antitoxin 10 ml (5500–8500 IU each toxin) diluted 1:10 in saline—slow IV; start ASAP—does not reverse existing paralysis but stops progression.
- Antitoxin is equine serum: 5–10% of recipients get urticaria, serum sickness etc; anaphylaxis—2%.
- Heptavalent antitoxin (A, B, C, D, E, F, and G) is available from U.S. Army; may be necessary with unusual type in bioterrorism.
- May give activated charcoal while waiting for antitoxin. Efficacy not established.

Support
- Monitor for respiratory failure.
- Support measures: feeding tube or parenteral nutrition.
- Mechanical ventilation required in 20% adults.
- Antibiotics: indicated only for infectious complications; avoid aminoglycosides (may worsen neuromuscular blockade).
- Wound botulism: must debride infected site.

Prevention
- Monitor exposed pts closely and treat immediately if sx of botulism.
- Antitoxin works prophylactically, but supply scarce and hypersensitivity risk is great.
- No person-person transmission observed.
- Food-borne botulism, most prone foods: low acid content, e.g., asparagus, green beans, beets and corn. Outbreaks described from chopped garlic in oil, chile peppers, tomatoes, improperly handled baked potatoes wrapped in aluminum foil, and home-canned or fermented fish.
- Persons who do home canning should follow strict hygienic procedures to reduce contamination of foods.
- Botulism toxin destroyed by high temperatures, persons who eat home-canned foods consider boiling the food.
- Instructions on safe home canning can be obtained from county extension services or from the U.S. Department of Agriculture.
- *Clostridium botulinum* spores can be in honey and a source of infection for infants, children less than 12 mos old should not be fed honey. Honey is safe for persons 1 yr of age and older.

FOLLOW UP
- Key point: antitoxin does not reverse existing paralysis, rather prevents further progression.

OTHER INFORMATION
- Forms: infant (foodborne), adult (foodborne), wound (injected), iatrogenic (cosmetic) and inhaled (bioterrorism).
- Clues to bioterrorism: many pts w/ flaccid paralysis; unusual types (not A, B or E), common geography without common food source.
- Main concern with bioterrorism—adequate ventilator supply to support large numbers for anticipated need of 3 mos.

BASIS FOR RECOMMENDATIONS
Arnon SS, Schechter R, Inglesby TV, et al. Botulinum toxin as a biological weapon: medical and public health management. *JAMA*, 2001; Vol. 285; pp. 1059–70.
Comments: Topic reviewed in context of bioterrorism. Features that suggest bioterrorism. Outbreak of flaccid paralysis with prominent bulbar palsy; Unusual types: C, D, F, G, or E without aquatic food source; Common geography but no common food source; Multiple simultaneous outbreaks.

FRANCISELLA TULARENSIS see p. 268 in Pathogens Section

HEMORRHAGIC FEVER VIRUSES

John G. Bartlett, MD

PATHOGENS
- Ebola virus: Africa
- Marburg virus: Africa
- Lassa fever virus: West Africa
- New World Adenoviridae South America (Argentine hemorrhagic fever virus, Bolivian hemorrhagic fever virus, Junin hemorrhagic fever virus, etc.)
- Rift Valley fever virus: Africa, Saudi Arabia
- Yellow fever virus: Africa, tropical Americas
- Omsk hemorrhagic fever virus: Central Asia
- Kyasanur Forest fever virus: India

- Crimean-Congo hemorrhagic fever: Eastern Europe, Africa
- Dengue fever virus

CLINICAL

- Definition: fever + bleeding diathesis caused by infection of a virus listed above.
- Transmission: by animals (including human-human) or insects, but not known for Ebola and Marburg viruses.
- All agents are candidates for bioterrorism; some previously weaponized by U.S. and Russia.
- Clinical features: fever, severely ill, hemorrhage, and thrombocytopenia.
- Also common: myalgias, rash, encephalitis, headache, diarrhea, abdominal pain, hypotension, conjunctivitis, pharyngitis.
- Differential diagnosis: influenza, dengue, meningococcemia, malaria, salmonellosis, plague, toxic shock syndrome, hantavirus.
- Prognosis (mortality): Ebola 50–90%, Marburg 30–60%, Lassa 15–20%, Yellow fever 20%, Omsk 2%, Kyasanur 3–10%.
- Reporting: immediately to State Health Dept and CDC if case suspected: acute fever <3 wks duration, severe illness, no alternative dx + unexplained hemorrhage.

DIAGNOSIS

- Consider risk factors, travel to endemic area and contact with cases.
- Specimens require BSL-4 lab.

TREATMENT

Infection Control

- Person-person transmission: Ebola Marburg, Lassa. There is no person-person transmission with Rift Valley, yellow fever, Omsk, Kyasanur Forest.
- None ever acquired in U.S.: consider acquisition if within 21 days of travel or bioterrorism—report immediately to public health authorities.
- Enhanced barrier and airborne precautions until Marburg and Ebola ruled out.
- Barrier: double glove, impermeable gowns, face shield, goggles, leg and shoe covers.
- Airborne: N-95 mask or air-purifying respirators (PAPR).
- If available: negative pressure isolation room w/ 6–12 air exchanges/hr.
- Surveillance of those exposed for febrile disease for 21 days post contact.
- Lab: aerosol risk—essential tests only, prefer point-of-care analyzers, no pneumatic tubes. Lab techs use airborne and contact precautions, blood specimens—pretreat w/ Triton X-100.
- Environment: surfaces—household bleach 1:100; cloth—double bag and wash hot cycle w/ bleach; autoclave or incinerate.
- Cadavers: trained personnel, airborne and contact precautions, prompt burial or cremation, no embalming.

Patient Care

- Support: IV fluids, mechanical ventilation, dialysis, pressors, anti-seizure meds.
- **Avoid:** aspirin, NSAIDS.
- Ribavirin: Lassa, Rift Valley Fever (only) IV 2 g × 1, then 1 g/day × 6 days then 500 mg/day (Need treatment IND for IV form, see ribavirin module, p. 700).
- Ribavirin PO: >75 kg 600 mg twice daily; <75 kg 1000 mg/day in 2 doses.
- Ebola, Marburg, Yellow fever, Omsk, Kyasanur—no antivirals.

Contacts of Patients

- Monitor temps twice daily × 21 days post contact.
- Temp >101°F: ribavirin (above oral doses) unless known to be Ebola/Marburg/Yellow fever/Omsk/Kyasanur.
- Vaccines—Yellow fever only; not effective post exposure.

BASIS FOR RECOMMENDATIONS

Borio L, Inglesby T, Peters CJ, et al. Hemorrhagic fever viruses as biological weapons: medical and public health management. *JAMA*, 2002; Vol. 287; pp. 2391–405.

Comments: The recommendations of the Johns Hopkins Center for Biodefense which represents the basis for these guidelines.

YERSINIA PESTIS see p. 347 in Pathogens Section

Bone/Joint

ACUTE RHEUMATIC FEVER see p. 60 in Fever Section

DIABETIC FOOT INFECTION

Eric Nuermberger, MD

PATHOGENS

- *Staphylococcus aureus*
- *Streptococcal species*
- *Enterobacteriaceae*
- *Pseudomonas aeruginosa*
- *Enterococcus*
- Anaerobes
- Superficial infections (cellulitis, cellulitis involving blisters and shallow ulcers) are typically caused by *S. aureus* or beta-hemolytic streptococci.
- Infections of ulcers that are chronic or previously treated with antibiotics may be caused by aerobic Gram-negative bacilli as well as Staph or Strep.
- Deep soft tissue infections, osteomyelitis, and gangrene are more often polymicrobial, including aerobic Gram-negative bacilli and anaerobes (anaerobic streptococci, Bacteroides fragilis group, Clostridium species), but Staphyloccocus aureus is also common as single pathogen.

CLINICAL

- Common complication of diabetes (accounts for 25% of diabetic hospitalizations); poses amputation risk.
- Risk factors for development: neuropathy, existing foot deformity, peripheral arterial disease, prior infection, prior ulceration.
- Hx: cellulitis or ulcer usually painless due to diabetic neuropathy.
- PE: range of findings include a) cellulitis, b) infection of superficial ulcer, c) deep soft tissue infection, d) osteomyelitis (including ulcer penetrating to bone), e) gangrene (demarcated tissue-wet or dry).
- Evaluation should include assessment of the size/extent of the wound, severity of neuropathy, vascular supply, glycemic control and ability to off-load the wound.

DIAGNOSIS

- Deep tissue specimens (e.g., bone biopsy, abscess fluid, specimen from debrided ulcer base) give most reliable culture/susceptibility data. Superficial cultures (e.g., swabs) do not correlate reliably with deep cultures.
- Radiology: plain film insensitive for early osteo; bone scan highly sensitive, but not specific; MRI is best study (95% sens, 99% spec), but some false positives due to neuropathic osteoarthropathy.
- Tagged white cell scans have better sensitivity/specificity than bone scans.
- Ability to probe to bone at base of ulcer considered diagnostic for osteomyelitis, but some consider the test as having a low positive predicative value (e.g., 0.57) but may be better in that negative probe-to-bone test may exclude osteomyelitis.

TREATMENT

Cellulitis or mild superficial ulcer infection

- Goals to cover streptococci for cellulitis, mild ulcers may need staphylococcal +/– MRSA and Gram-negative coverage.
- Cephalexin 500 mg PO four times a day × 14 days
- Amoxicillin/clavulanate 875–1000 mg PO twice daily × 14 days
- Ampicillin/sulbactam 3 g IV q6h × 14 days
- Cefazolin 1–2 g IV q8h × 14 days
- Nafcillin or oxacillin 2 g IV q4h × 14 days

- Clindamycin 300 mg PO three times a day × 14 days (incl. MRSA)
- Trimethoprim-sulfamethoxazole 2 DS tabs PO twice daily × 14 days (incl. MRSA)
- Clindamycin 600 mg IV q6–8h × 14 days
- Linezolid 600 mg PO twice daily × 14 days
- Vancomycin 15 mg/kg IV q12h

Deep soft tissue infection or osteomyelitis

- Urgent surgical consultation recommended.
- Consider vascular evaluation.
- Modify regimen according to culture results from deep wound cultures, bone biopsy.
- Ampicillin/sulbactam 3 g IV q6h or ticarcillin/clavulanate 3.1 g IV q6h or piperacillin/tazobactam 3.375 g IV q6h.
- Alternatives: clindamycin 600 mg IV q6h + (levofloxacin 750 mg PO once daily or ciprofloxacin 750 mg PO (400 mg IV) q12h).
- Ceftriaxone 2 g IV once daily + metronidazole 500 mg IV q6–8h.
- Ertapenem 1 g IV once daily
- Add vancomycin 15 mg/kg IV q12h or linezolid 600 mg IV/PO q12h to the above regimens if suspicion of MRSA is moderate to high, or infection is severe.
- Parenteral therapy until stable, then orals for up to 4 wks in absence of osteomyelitis.
- For osteomyelitis: debridement of necrotic bone and often needing ≥2 wks of parenteral therapy and 4–6 wks total antibiotics or no debridement and 2–6 wks of parenteral therapy and ≥2 mos of oral therapy frequently required.

Limb-/Life-threatening infection

- Urgent surgical consultation, urgent vascular evaluation. Pick abx regimen based on sensitivity data (if known), likelihood of MRSA (should be considered likely in most circumstances) and host issues.
- Clindamycin 900 mg IV q8h + ciprofloxacin 400 mg IV q12h or tobramycin 2.0 mg/kg IV × 1, then 1.7 mg/kg IV q8h.
- Clindamycin 900 mg IV q8h + ceftazidime 2 g IV q8h or cefepime 2 g IV q8h or cefotaxime 2 g IV q8h or ceftriaxone 2 g IV once daily.
- Piperacillin/tazobactamagain. 3.375 g IV q4h or ticarcillin/clavulanate 3.1 g IV q4h.
- Imipenem 500 mg IV q6h or meropenem 1 g IV q8h or ertapenem 1 g IV once daily.
- Vancomycin 15 mg/kg IV q12h + aztreonam 2 g IV q8h + metronidazole 500 mg IV q6h.
- Vancomycin 15 mg/kg IV q12h + cefepime 2 g IV q12h or ceftazidime 2 g IV q8h + metronidazole 500 mg IV q6h.
- Treatment generally requires prolonged parenteral and oral therapy, duration determined by outcome and presence or absence of osteomyelitis.

Follow Up

- Antimicrobial therapy best if combined with enforced non-weight bearing status (e.g., contact casting), glycemic control, scrupulous wound care, and complete debridement or resection of infected bone.

Other Information

- Choose IV antibiotics when systemically ill w/ severe infection, unable to take orals.

Basis for Recommendations

Lipsky BA, Berendt AR, Deery HG, et al. Diagnosis and treatment of diabetic foot infections. *Clin Infect Dis*, 2004; Vol. 39; pp. 885–910.

Comments: Authoritative guidelines from IDSA with major emphasis on diagnosis of infection, classification of severity, microbiology, and management strategies, including surgical and other adjunctive modalities.

HARDWARE ASSOCIATED SEPTIC ARTHRITIS

Eric Nuermberger, MD

Pathogens

- *Staphylococcus* (coagulase-negative)
- *Staphylococcus aureus*
- Viridans streptococci
- Enterococcal species

- Gram-negative enteric bacteria
- *Pseudomonas aeruginosa*
- *Candida* species
- *Propionibacterium acnes* (especially shoulder implant infections)
- Anaerobes
- Mycobacteria (*M. tuberculosis* and non-TB mycobacteria): rare
- **Early infection (1st 3 mos):** predominantly *S. aureus*, β-hemolytic strep, Gram-negative bacilli. **Delayed (3 mos–2 yrs):** predominant pathogens are coagulase-negative Staphylococci and *S. aureus*. **Late (>2 yrs):** *S. aureus*, coag. neg. Staph, viridans streptococci, enterococci; less commonly Gram-negative rods.

CLINICAL

- Approximately 12,000 prosthetic joint infections occur/ yr in U.S.
- Risk of infection is higher for knee (0.5–2%) vs. hip (0.5–1%) vs. shoulder (0.5–1%) replacement.
- Risk factors: surgical site infection or hematoma, prolonged surgery, rheumatoid arthritis, diabetes, corticosteroid use, previous joint infxn, and staphylococcal nasal carriage or perioperative infection away from joint.
- Early-onset infections present within 2–3 mos of surgery with hx of joint pain (95%), fever (43%), swelling (38%), drainage (32%). Exam: erythema, induration, and edema at incision site +/– wound drainage.
- Late-onset infections present >3 mos. post-op with progressive joint pain and/or instability, often w/o fever or local signs of infections. Exam: findings may be minimal.

DIAGNOSIS

- Radiology: plain films may show lucencies at bone-cement interface, misalignment, cement fracture, or periosteal reaction in late-onset infection.
- Radiology: nuclear scans (triple phase bone or wbc scans) are more sensitive. Utility of PET remains controversial.
- Lab: joint aspirate typically with cloudy fluid, WBC >50,000–150,000 cells/mms cubed predominantly neutrophilic and positive Gram-stain or culture.
- ESR, CRP may be helpful but are neither sensitive (especially for indolent infections) nor specific (e.g., for pts with inflammatory arthritis).
- Operative specimens: recommend at least three separate deep swab or biopsy samples from different locations for Gram-stain, culture, histopathology.
- Gram-stain/culture of wound or sinus tract drainage may aid microbiologic diagnosis in early infection or if *S. aureus* is isolated, otherwise may just reflect colonization.
- Sonication and culture of explanted prosthesis increases microbiologic diagnoses. Not widely available but relatively simple to perform.
- Shoulder infections or *P. acnes* suspect: must alert lab to hold culture for 7–10 days as *P. acnes* grows slowly.

TREATMENT

Replacement arthroplasty (Two-stage procedure)

- Preferred strategy for management of difficult-to-treat pathogens (e.g., MRSA) and late onset infections because bacteria in device-related biofilm cannot be eradicated by abx alone.
- **Stage 1:** remove prosthesis and replace with abx-impregnated spacer, debride infected tissue.
- IV abx for 6–8 wks. For difficult-to-treat organisms (e.g., MRSA) or complicated pts, consider 2–4 wks off abx, then aspirate joint for cell count and culture. If positive, repeat irrigation/ debridement, then IV antibiotics for 6 wks, then repeat aspirate.
- **Stage 2:** When no clinical signs/sx of infxn and/or aspirate negative, replace joint with new prosthetic and abx-impregnated cement.

Alternative surgical options

- Early infections may respond to debridement and retention with 2–6 wks IV and subsequent oral abx for total of 3–6 mos if acted upon early (e.g., within 1–2 wks of symptom onset), stable joint, and infection with highly-susceptible organism (e.g., viridans strep or staph) or may be attempted in the frail elderly pt. In these pts rifampin typically used in combination with other agent (β-lactam, vancomycin, or fluoroquinolone). Infectious diseases consultation recommended.

- One-stage arthroplasty (removal and replacement of prosthesis during the same operation)—may be less successful. In U.S., usually reserved for infections with highly-abx-susceptible organisms (e.g., *streptococci*).
- Arthrodesis required when tissues inadequate for functional arthroplasty or for antibiotic-resistant organisms or prior failed replacement.
- Amputation is last resort for intractable pain, incurable infection, or heavy bone loss that prevents arthrodesis.

Suppressive antibiotic therapy

- Suppressive abx therapy appropriate if removal of prosthesis not possible, prosthesis is stable, and pathogen susceptible to oral abx.
- Success long term often not durable due to loosening of prosthesis, purulent arthritis and/or fistulization, or sepsis.
- Suppressive oral therapy is most effective after surgical irrigation and debridement and perhaps induction phase with IV antibiotics.
- Staph or GNR: ciprofloxacin (GNR only) 750 mg PO twice daily, levofloxacin 750 mg PO every day, or moxifloxacin 400 mg PO every day (+ rifampin 600 mg PO every day for Staph species).
- MSSA: cephalexin 500 mg PO four times a day or dicloxacillin 500 mg PO four times a day.
- Strep or *enterococci*: amoxicillin 0.5–1 g PO three times a day.
- Staph (incl. MRSA): minocycline 100 mg PO twice daily + rifampin 600 mg PO every day.
- Staph (incl. MRSA): trimethoprim/sulfa 1 DS tab PO twice daily + rifampin 600 mg PO every day.
- Enteric GNR or polymicrobial: amoxicillin/clavulanate 875 mg PO twice daily.
- *Candida*: fluconazole 400 mg PO every day.

OTHER INFORMATION

- No guidelines regarding PJI or management have yet been published, although IDSA may have a statement ready in Fall 2009.
- When possible, avoid antibiotics (including perioperatively) before obtaining joint aspirate or intraoperative cultures for microbiologic diagnosis of suspected PJI.
- Culture of *S. epidermidis* or other common contaminant more likely true infxn if: seen on Gram-stain, grown on agar (not broth only), and >1 culture specimen positive.
- Aspiration cultures may be falsely negative especially in late-onset infections, requiring open biopsy of synovium and/or periprosthetic tissue cultures.
- For cultures before elective revision arthroplasty, send 3 or more specimens from different sites in operative space.

BASIS FOR RECOMMENDATIONS

Pappas PG, Kauffman CA, Andes D, et al. Clinical practice guidelines for the management of candidiasis: 2009 update by the Infectious Diseases Society of America. *Clin Infect Dis*, 2009; Vol. 48; pp. 503–35.
Comments: Resection arthroplasty usually required for cure. Limited experience re: abx choice, but fluconazole deemed sufficient. Chronic suppressive therapy has been successful when resection is not feasible or desirable.
Zimmerli W, Trampuz A, Ochsner PE. Prosthetic-joint infections. *N Engl J Med*, 2004; Vol. 351; pp. 1645–54.
Comments: Recent succinct review of the subject. Optimal antibiotic therapy hinges upon identification of the infecting organism. Excellent algorithms to assist management decisions.

LYME ARTHRITIS

Eric Nuermberger, MD and Paul G. Auwaerter, MD

PATHOGENS

- *Borrelia burgdorferi*
- Other strains: *B. garinii*, *B. afzelii*

CLINICAL

- Suspect in pts with outdoor activity, history of tick bite in endemic region, or prior history of Lyme disease (e.g., erythema migrans).
- Pts with early Lyme disease may have arthralgia and/or arthritis of both large and small joints.

- **Late lyme arthritis:** recurrent attacks (wks or mos) of objective joint swelling in one or few large (usually weight bearing as an mono- or oligoarthritis: knee→shoulder→ankle →elbow→TMJ→wrist→hip) joints, generally with intercurrent remission even without therapy. Effusion→pain.
- May occur in up to 60% of untreated pts.
- Without treatment, arthritis may continue with characteristic relapsing/remitting pattern, may last > 6 yrs. Approximately 10–20% of afflicted pts per yr resolve their arthritis without therapy.
- **Persistent Lyme arthritis:** at least one episode of continual joint inflammation lasting 1 yr or longer, despite prior treatment with oral and parenteral antibiotic therapy. This culture negative process may afflict up to 5–10% of pts despite multiple antibiotic treatments.
- Pts with persistent Lyme arthritis often with certain immunogenetic backgrounds: especially HLA-DR4, HLA-DR2, or both. HLA-DR4 is associated with a lack of response to antibiotics.

Diagnosis
- Synovial fluid: WBC 10,000–100,000 cells/milliliter^3 cubedl (average 20–24,000) with predominance of PMNs.
- ESR may be normal or only mildly elevated (~30 mm/hr).
- Evidence of *B. burgdorferi* infection in synovial fluid: positive culture (<20%), PCR (depending on lab, >85%) are definitive.
- Highly supportive evidence from typical arthritis pattern and positive blood serology for *B. burgdorferi* by ELISA with Western blot IgG (≥5 of 10 bands). Serologies (EIA with WB IgG, IgM only is not acceptable) are robustly positive in these pts. A negative Lyme serology essentially rules out the diagnosis of Lyme arthritis.
- Erosions rarely observed on radiographs.
- Positive PCR synovial results can be used as a guide to determine need for antibiotic therapy.
- Synovial fluid Western blot testing is unvalidated and should not be used.

Treatment
Initial therapy: Late Lyme Arthritis
- One or 2 courses of oral therapy suggested as initial therapy in previously untreated pts.
- **Preferred:** Doxycycline 100 mg PO twice daily × 28 days.
- Amoxicillin 500 mg PO three times daily × 28 days.
- **Alt:** cefuroxime axetil 500 mg PO twice daily × 28 days.
- Constant pain usually decreases within 2–3 wks of treatment, but swelling and intermittent pain may persist to 8 wks.
- For persistent or recurrent symptoms after 2 courses of oral treatment, may opt to administer parenteral therapy (see below), but if PCR negative, unclear if approach yields improvement.
- Prolonged courses of oral antibiotics have not been shown to aid improved outcomes and such use is discouraged.

Parenteral Therapy: Late Lyme Arthritis
- Parenteral therapy is recommended if arthritis is accompanied by neurologic manifestations, including positive LP, or after failure(s) of oral therapy. Some advocate with severe initial Lyme arthritis presentations.
- Ceftriaxone 2 g IV q24h × 14–28 days.
- Cefotaxime 2 g IV q8h × 14–28 days.
- Penicillin G 18–24 million units IV divided q4h × 14–28 days.
- There is no evidence that >2 courses of parenteral drug therapy yields any additional efficacy.

Adjunctive Therapy: Persistent Lyme Arthritis
- For pts with persistent/recurrent arthritis despite 1 mo of appropriate parenteral therapy, mechanism is likely immune-mediated (pts with high levels of cytokines in joint fluid): consider rheumatology evaluation if needed to assist with use of non-antimicrobial therapies below. No trials exist to guide selection of these modalities.
- Non-steroidal anti-inflammatory drugs, e.g., ibuprofen, naproxen, etc.
- Intraarticular corticosteroid injections.
- Hydroxychloroquine (may take wks or mos to show benefit) or methotrexate (ditto).

- Arthroscopic synovectomy for persistent pain and functional limitation (usually defined as >6 mos of symptoms despite anti-inflammatory therapy).
- Some have used TNF-alpha inhibitors in severe cases, but clinical data limited.

FOLLOW UP
- Main goal of antibiotic therapy is to prevent future joint flares (except for those who ultimately prove to have persistent arthritis).
- Use objective clinical findings (inflammatory arthritis, neurologic signs), not non-specific symptoms (fatigue, arthralgia), to monitor treatment efficacy.
- Although reports exist of continued PCR positivity after antibiotic therapy, most studies find that *B. burgdorferi* PCR becomes negative with 1 or 2 mos of antibiotic therapy.
- Based upon early natural history studies of Lyme arthritis, most pts resolve symptoms over mos–yrs without long-term impact on joint function.

OTHER INFORMATION
- Because Lyme disease is primarily a clinical diagnosis, laboratory serologic testing is adjunctive. Seropositivity alone does not imply active disease or causality.
- Post-treatment Lyme disease syndrome (PTLD) is favored as a term when subjective symptoms such as fatigue, arthralgia, myalgia, neurocognitive symptoms, and sleep disturbance occur after bona-fide Lyme disease and appropriate antibiotic therapy. "Chronic Lyme disease" is discouraged as a term that blurs the distinction between PTLD and objective findings of late Lyme disease such as a monoarthritis.
- Pts with late Lyme arthritis virtually always have positive Lyme serology (EIA + IgG Western blot).
- Any associated neurologic or cognitive complaints should be pursued (consider MRI, lumbar puncture, neuropsychiatric testing) to evaluate for neuroborreliosis that may require parenteral therapy.
- Synovial fluid PCR may help differentiate cause of poor response.

MORE INFORMATION
Post-Lyme disease syndromes following appropriate abx therapy (myalgia, fatigue, etc.) do not respond to additional antibiotic therapy. We suggest trials of low impact aerobic exercise conditioning programs, NSAIDs, cognitive behavioral therapy as initial strategies. For some pts, trials of venlafaxine XR (for those with significant somatic pain titrating up to 150–225 mg once daily) or SSRI's (especially with anxiety) or tricyclics (for those with especially with disturbed sleep) may be helpful.

BASIS FOR RECOMMENDATIONS
Wormser GP, Dattwyler RJ, Shapiro ED, et al. The clinical assessment, treatment, and prevention of lyme disease, human granulocytic anaplasmosis, and babesiosis: clinical practice guidelines by the Infectious Diseases Society of America. *Clin Infect Dis*, 2006; Vol. 43; pp. 1089–134.
Comments: Authoritative literature review and practice guidelines from a panel of Lyme experts.

OSTEOMYELITIS, ACUTE

Eric Nuermberger, MD

PATHOGENS
- *Staphylococcus aureus*
- Coagulase-negative *staphylococci*
- *Streptococci*
- *Enterococcus*
- *Pseudomonas aeruginosa*
- *Escherichia coli*
- *Salmonella* species
- *Serratia* species
- Other Gram-negative enteric bacilli
- Much less common: anaerobes, fungi, mycobacteria, *brucella*
- Typical settings: hardware (Staph), IV drug use (*S. aureus, Pseudomonas, Serratia*), sickle cell (*Salmonella*), diabetes (Group B strep), nail through sneaker (*Pseudomonas*), human

bite (Eikenella), animal bite (Pasteurella), urinary tract infection or manipulation (*E.coli*, *Proteus*, other Gram-negative bacilli)

CLINICAL

- Distinction between acute and chronic osteomyelitis is vague: "acute" includes first presentation of osteomyelitis, acute symptomatology (< 2 wks), and absence of necrotic bone or sequestrum.
- Acute symptoms and signs: fever/chills/night sweats, localizing pain/tenderness, or swelling/erythema (more common with hematogenous infections).
- Exposure of bone on visual inspection or by probing is virtually diagnostic for osteomyelitis arising from a contiguous focus.
- Laboratory: elevated ESR, CRP expected; elevated WBC and platelet counts common.
- Radiology: periosteal elevation, focal osteopenia, cortical thinning or scalloping on plain film or CT; marrow edema on MRI; tracer uptake on radionuclide scans.
- Microbiology: isolation of pathogen from bone lesion (aspiration or bxp) or blood culture in setting of suggestive bony changes.
- Acute hematogenous osteo: most common in children (usually *S. aureus*) or in adults with age > 50, IV drug use, hemodialysis, diabetes, sickle cell disease, other risk factors for bacteremia.
- Typical sites: vertebra (adults > children), long bones (children > adults), axial joints (sternoclavicular, sacroiliac especially in IV drug users).
- Acute hematogenous osteo is usually monomicrobial; whereas contiguous-focus infections tend to be polymicrobial.
- Community-associated MRSA strains may cause hematogenous osteomyelitis and pathologic fracture after soft tissue infection.

DIAGNOSIS

- Suspicion based on history, physical exam, and supportive laboratory findings.
- Imaging is important for diagnosis, staging, and follow-up.
- Plain films are sufficient if typical findings are present, but are not very sensitive in early osteomyelitis.
- MRI and radionuclide scans are more sensitive in early or ambiguous cases.
- MRI is preferred for suspected vertebral osteomyelitis to exclude paravertebral abscess, cord impingement.
- In MRSA era, it's especially important to establish the microbial etiology (ideally before antibiotic initiation).
- Indications for surgery: failure to respond to abx, soft tissue abscess, joint infection, and spinal instability.

TREATMENT
Hematogenous osteomyelitis (Pathogen-directed)

- General recommendation is 2–6 wks parenteral therapy +/– subsequent oral therapy to complete 4–8 wks.
- Use susceptibility information to help guide choices (parenteral or oral).
- Staph (MSSA): nafcillin or oxacillin 2 g IV q4h or cefazolin 2 g IV q6–8h.
- Staph (MSSA): ceftriaxone 2 g IV q24h (option for outpatient).
- Staph (MSSA or MRSA): clindamycin 600 mg IV q6h or 900 mg IV q8h.
- MRSA: vancomycin 15 mg/kg IV q12h (+/– rifampin 600 mg PO once daily). Goal vancomycin trough >15 mg/L.
- MRSA: linezolid 600 mg IV or PO q12h or daptomycin 6–8 mg/kg/day IV (less experience).
- Strep: penicillin G 2–4 MU IV q4–6h or ampicillin 2 g IV q6h (+/– gentamicin 1.0 mg/kg IV q8h for *Streptococcus agalactiae*, other higher PCN MIC strep or enterococcal species)
- GNB: ampicillin/sulbactam 3 g (2 g/1 g respectively) IV q6h or ticarcillin/clavulanate 3.1 g IV q4–6h or piperacillin/tazobactam 3.375 g IV q4–6h
- GNB: ciprofloxacin 400 mg IV q12h (may make early transition to oral therapy: 750 mg PO q12h) or levofloxacin 750 mg IV/PO once daily. Other quinolones probably adequate.
- GNB: ceftriaxone 2 g IV q24h or cefotaxime 2 g IV q6–8h or ceftazidime 2 g IV q8h or cefepime 2 g IV q8h.

Contiguous focus or inoculation osteomyelitis
- Leg/foot ulcer: orthopedic consult, consider vascular evaluation if signs of insufficiency present.
- Decubitus ulcer: plastic surgery consult.
- Osteomyelitis under chronic ulcer is often polymicrobial. If vascular insufficiency present, include anaerobic coverage.
- General recommendation is 6–8 wks of abx (at least 2 wks of initial IV therapy or until clinical improvement/stability) following surgical debridement.
- Use regimens under hematogenous osteomyelitis when guided by culture data. Empiric regimens given below. Add vancomycin when MRSA risk factors present.
- Clindamycin 600 mg IV q6h or 900 mg IV q8h + ciprofloxacin 400 mg IV or 750 mg PO q12h or levofloxacin 750 mg IV or PO once daily.
- Ampicillin/sulbactam 3 g (2 g/1 g respectively) IV q6h or ticarcillin/clavulanate 3.1 g IV q4–6h or piperacillin/tazobactam 3.375 g IV q4–6h.
- Ertapenem 1 g IV q24h or imipenem 500 mg IV q6h or meropenem 1 g IV q8h.
- Ceftriaxone 2 g IV q24h or cefotaxime 2 g IV q6–8h or ceftazidime 2 g IV q8h or cefepime 2 g IV q8h + metronidazole 500 mg IV q6h.
- Human or animal bite: ampicillin/sulbactam 3 g (2 g/1 g respectively) IV q6h.

Oral regimens (to follow parenteral therapy)
- Erratic oral bioavailability of penicillins and cephalosporins, plus lower vascular penetration of bone makes these agents less desirable. However, streptococci are often highly susceptible. Use pathogen sensitivities to guide therapy.
- Staph (MSSA, MRSA) or anaerobes: clindamycin 300–450 mg PO q6h.
- Staph (MSSA, MRSA): minocycline 100 mg PO twice daily (+/– rifampin 600 mg PO once daily).
- Staph (MSSA): any fluoroquinolone (if sensitive) + rifampin 600 mg PO once daily.
- Staph (MSSA, MRSA) or GNB: trimethoprim/sulfamethoxazole DS 2 tabs PO q8–12h (+/– rifampin 600 mg PO once daily for Staph).
- GNB: ciprofloxacin 750 mg PO q12h or levofloxacin 750 mg PO twice daily.
- Anaerobes: metronidazole 500 mg PO q6–8h.
- Mixed infection: clindamycin + fluoroquinolone.
- MRSA or VRE: linezolid 600 mg PO q12h.
- Human or animal bite: amoxicillin/clavulanate 875–1000 mg PO twice daily.

FOLLOW UP
- Selected pts may be converted to oral agents after 2 wks of IV therapy, if there are good oral options based on bioavailability and susceptibility testing.
- CRP should return to normal range prior to discontinuation of therapy.
- Follow-up imaging should be interpreted with caution as bony changes are slow to resolve (especially MRI enhancement) and may initially appear worse despite appropriate therapy.

BASIS FOR RECOMMENDATIONS
Calhoun JH, Manring MM. Adult osteomyelitis. *Infect Dis Clin North Am*, 2005; Vol. 19; pp. 765–86.
Comments: Current, concise review of the pathogenesis, clinical features, diagnosis, and treatment approach, including surgical management.

OSTEOMYELITIS, CHRONIC

Eric Nuermberger, MD

PATHOGENS
- *Staphylococcus aureus*
- Coagulase-negative *staphylococci*
- *Streptococcus* species
- *Enterococcus*
- *Pseudomonas aeruginosa*
- Gram-negative enteric bacilli
- Anaerobic bacteria

DIAGNOSIS

- *Mycobacterium tuberculosis*
- Fungi

CLINICAL

- "Chronic" infection may be defined by previous failed treatment, symptom duration >3 wks, presence of bony sequestrum, persistent drainage or sinus tract; but the hallmark is necrotic bone.
- Chronic osteomyelitis may arise from hematogenous seeding, inoculation during trauma or surgery, or spread from a contiguous infection.
- Pain and constitutional symptoms may be limited compared to acute infections.

DIAGNOSIS

- Exposure of bone on visual inspection or by probing with cotton swab is diagnostic for osteomyelitis arising from a contiguous focus.
- Bony changes (necrosis, sclerosis, periosteal new bone formation, sequestra) should be present on plain x-rays or CT scan.
- Given chronic nature and wide etiologic spectrum, microbial etiology should generally be established prior to initiating abx.
- Confirmatory evidence is isolation of pathogen from bone or blood in setting of radiographic changes or acute inflammation on a pathologic specimen from bone biopsy.
- In general, superficial cultures of sinus tracts and contiguous ulcers are unreliable and should not guide therapy if bone biopsy is possible.

TREATMENT

Parenteral therapy with curative intent

- 4–6 wks of IV therapy after aggressive surgical debridement then ≥8 wks oral therapy. Use susceptibilities to guide choices.
- Staph (MSSA): nafcillin or oxacillin 2 g IV q4h or cefazolin 2 g IV q8h.
- Staph (MSSA), streptococci: ceftriaxone 2 g IV q24h (convenient for outpatient parenteral therapy).
- Staph (MSSA, MRSA), strep, anaerobes: clindamycin 600 mg IV q6h or 900 mg IV q8h.
- MRSA: vancomycin 15 mg/kg IV q12h + rifampin 600 mg IV or PO once daily. Strive for vancomycin trough level of 15–20 mg/dL.
- Strep: penicillin G 2–4 MU IV q4–6h or ampicillin 2 g IV q6h (+/– gentamicin 1.0 mg/kg IV q8h for *S. agalactiae* or enterococcal species).
- GNB/anaerobes: ampicillin/sulbactam 3 g IV q6h or ticarcillin/clavulanate 3.1 g IV q4–6h or piperacillin/tazobactam 3.375-g IV q4–6h.
- GNB: ciprofloxacin 400 mg IV q12h (may make early transition to oral therapy: 750 mg PO q12h) or levofloxacin 750 mg IV (then PO) once daily.
- GNB: ceftriaxone 2 g IV q24h or cefotaxime 2 g IV q6–8h or ceftazidime 2 g IV q8h or cefepime 2 g IV q8h.
- GNB, mixed infection: ertapenem 1 g IV q24h (convenient for outpatient parenteral therapy).
- Oral regimens (consolidative or suppressive).
- Staph (MSSA or MRSA): minocycline 100 mg PO twice daily or trimethoprim/sulfamethoxazole DS 2 tabs PO twice daily three times a day or linezolid 600 mg PO twice daily or clindamycin 300–450 mg PO four times a day (+ rifampin 600 mg PO once daily).
- Staph (MSSA), Strep, GNB, anaerobes: amoxicillin/clavulanate 500 mg PO q8h.
- Staph (MSSA), anaerobes: clindamycin 300–450 mg PO four times a day (+/– rifampin 600 mg PO once daily).
- GNB: ciprofloxacin 750 mg PO q12h or levofloxacin 500–750 mg PO qd.
- GNB: trimethoprim/sulfamethoxazole DS 2 tabs PO twice daily.
- Anaerobes: metronidazole 500 mg PO q6–8h.
- Polymicrobial infections may require combination therapy.

Adjunctive surgical therapy

- Drainage of infection and complete debridement of necrotic bone cannot be overemphasized and may be the only curative intervention.
- Management of dead space by local tissue flap, free flap, or cancellous bone graft when necessary.

- Antibiotic-impregnated beads to sterilize and temporarily fill dead space.
- Local delivery of antibiotics to dead space via impregnated acrylic beads or implantable infusion pump.
- Bone saucerization and grafting.
- Revascularization.
- Hyperbaric oxygen therapy—controversial role.
- Amputation.

FOLLOW UP
- Usual reason for failure—inadequate debridement or abx non-compliance or host problem (e.g., immune suppression).
- Rising ESR/CRP values after therapy may indicate relapse.

OTHER INFORMATION
- Identification of pathogen(s) is essential—if possible, defer treatment until after bone biopsy.
- Following any surgical debridement, the remaining tissue bed is considered contaminated and treated with abx for at least 6 wks.

BASIS FOR RECOMMENDATIONS
Calhoun JH, Manring MM. Adult osteomyelitis. *Infect Dis Clin North Am,* 2005; Vol. 19; pp. 765–86.

Comments: Current, concise review of the pathogenesis, clinical features, diagnosis, and treatment approach, including surgical management.

SEPTIC ARTHRITIS, COMMUNITY-ACQUIRED

Eric Nuermberger, MD

PATHOGENS
- *Staphylococcus aureus*
- β-hemolytic streptococci
- *Neisseria gonorrhoeae*
- *Escherichia coli*
- Other Enterobacteriaceae
- *Pseudomonas aeruginosa*
- *Kingella kingae*

CLINICAL
- Virtually every bacterial pathogen has been associated with septic arthritis.
- Most cases of septic arthritis develop from hematogenous seeding of the joint during transient or sustained bacteremic episodes, but traumatic or iatrogenic inoculation of bacteria also occurs.
- Pathogen associations: rheumatoid arthritis—*S. aureus*; IVDU—*S. aureus, P. aeruginosa*; dialysis—*S. aureus*; unpasteurized dairy products—Brucella spp.; Sickle Cell Dz—Salmonella spp.; diabetes-Grp B strep; children—*K. kingae.*
- Gonococcal arthritis no longer considered to be the most common cause of community-acquired septic arthritis in young adults.
- Suspect gonococcal arthritis in young adults, particularly if: sexually active, recent menses or childbirth, pustular skin lesions, tenosynovitis.
- Pts with gonococcal arthritis typically present 1 of 2 ways: triad of pustular skin lesions, tenosynovitis (knees, wrists, ankles, fingers), arthralgia without purulent arthritis or purulent arthritis without skin lesions.
- *Neisseria meningitidis* may mimic disseminated gonococcal infection and tenosynovitis or arthritis.

DIAGNOSIS
- Hx: fever, chills, malaise, joint pain, swelling, decreased ROM.
- Joint exam: tenderness, erythema, heat, swelling, decreased ROM (usually marked).
- Joint aspirate: + Gram-stain and/or cx, neutrophilic leukocytosis (esp. >50,000/mm^3), low glucose (<40 mg/dl), and no crystals.

- Other diagnostic considerations: negative Gram-stain/cx from joint, but + cx from blood, cervix, urethra, throat, or rectum; positive nucleic acid test on urine or joint fluid; and/or typical skin lesions suggests gonococcal arthritis
- Ddx: rheumatoid arthritis, gout, pseudogout, reactive arthritis (all cause PMN's in joint fluid); viral arthritis, Lyme disease. Consider trauma or hemorrhage if bloody.

TREATMENT
Empiric antimicrobial therapy
- Gram-positive cocci in clusters, MRSA risk factors or β-lactam allergy: vancomycin 15 mg/kg IV q12h.
- Gram-positive cocci in clusters, no MRSA risk factors: nafcillin or oxacillin 2 g IV q4h.
- Gram-positive cocci, no MRSA risk factors: cefazolin 2 g IV q8h.
- Gram-positive cocci in chains (streptococci presumed): Pen G 12–18 MU or ampicillin 2 mg IV q4h.
- Gram-negative cocci (presumptive Neisseria): ceftriaxone 1–2 g IV/IM q12–24h or cefotaxime 2 g IV q8h.
- Gram-negative rods: ceftazidime 2 g IV q8h or cefepime 2 g IV q8h.
- Negative Gram-stain, previously healthy, no MRSA risk factors: cefazolin 2 g IV q8h.
- Negative Gram-stain, health-care associated or other MRSA risk factors: vancomycin 15 mg/kg IV q12h plus ceftazidime 2 g IV q8h, cefepime 2 g IV q8h or piperacillin/tazobactam 4.5 g IV q6h.
- Human, dog or cat bite: ampicillin/sulbactam 1.5–3 g IV q4h.
- Empirical therapy should be modified by culture results.
- Risk factors for hospital-acquired strains of MRSA: recent hospitalization or nursing home admission, hemodialysis, diabetes, intravenous drug use, recent antibiotic exposure, recent incarceration, recent skin/soft tissue infection in pt or close contact. Community-acquired MRSA afflicts often without any traditional pre-existing risk factors.

Pathogen-directed antimicrobial therapy
- Staph (MSSA): nafcillin or oxacillin 2 g IV q4h × 3 wks.
- Staph (MSSA): cefazolin 2 g IV q8h × 3 wks.
- Staph (MRSA or Type I penicillin allergy): vancomycin 15 mg/kg IV q12h × 3 wks.
- Strep (including PCN-sensitive *S. pneumoniae* [MIC <4 mg/L]): PCN G 12–18 MU IV/qday divided dose or ampicillin 2 g IV q4h × 2 wks.
- *S. pneumoniae*(PCN-resistant): ceftriaxone 1–2 g IV q12h or cefotaxime 2 g IV q8h if susceptible, or vancomycin 15 mg/kg IV q12h × 2 wks.
- Enteric GNB: ceftriaxone 1–2 g IV q12h or cefotaxime 2 g IV q8h × 3 wks.
- GNB (*P. aeruginosa*): ceftazidime 2 g IV q8h or cefepime 2 g IV q8h, plus gentamicin or tobramycin 5 mg/kg IV q24h × 3 wks.
- GNB: ciprofloxacin 400 mg IV q8–12 h or 750 mg PO q12h or levofloxacin 750 mg IV or 750 mg PO qday × 3 wks.
- Polymicrobial: ampicillin/sulbactam 1.5–3 g IV q4h × 3 wks.
- Polymicrobial: clindamycin 600 mg IV q6–8h × 3 wks plus ciprofloxacin 400 mg IV or 750 mg PO q12h or levofloxacin 750 mg IV or 750 mg PO qday × 3 wks.
- Gram-positive etiology + Type I penicillin allergy: vancomycin 15 mg/kg IV q12h × 3 wks.

Therapy of gonococcal arthritis/disseminated gonococcal infection
- **Parenteral therapy (preferred):** ceftriaxone 1 g IV or IM q24h or cefotaxime 1 g IV q8h or ceftizoxime 1 g IV q8h.
- Ciprofloxacin 400 mg IV q12h or levofloxacin 500 mg IV q24h, if known susceptible.
- Spectinomycin 2 g IV or IM q12 h (β-lactam allergy but no longer available in U.S.).
- Continue parenteral therapy until clinical improvement, then switch to oral therapy to complete 1 wk of therapy (purulent arthritis may require 2 wks of antibiotic therapy).
- **Oral therapy:** Cefixime or cefpodoxime 400 mg PO twice daily.
- Ciprofloxacin 500 mg PO twice daily or ofloxacin 300 mg PO twice daily or levofloxacin 500 mg PO qday (if susceptible).
- All pts should also be empirically treated for concomitant chlamydia infection with doxycycline 100 mg or ofloxacin 300 mg PO twice daily × 7 days or, if pregnant, azithromycin 1000 mg PO once.

- Sexual partners should receive ceftriaxone 125 mg IM or cefixime 400 mg PO once plus doxycycline 100 mg PO twice daily × 7 days.
- Fluoroquinolones are an alternative option if susceptibility can be documented by culture and should not be used empirically in the U.S. for any pts, and especially for infections in men who have sex with men or infections acquired in/from Asia, Great Britain, California, and Hawaii or other areas with high prevalence of resistance; ceftriaxone is treatment of choice.

Adjunctive therapy
- Repeated aspiration: most pts are treated successfully by initial diagnostic joint aspiration and parenteral antibiotic therapy.
- Repeated closed drainage may be necessary for reaccumulation of fluid.
- Volume of synovial fluid, cell count, and percentage of PMN's should decline with consecutive taps; synovial fluid culture should become sterile within the first several days of therapy (staph may be >7 days).
- Surgical drainage: consider if failure to improve within 72 hrs, infected joint inaccessible or cannot be drained adequately by needle aspiration, soft tissue or bony extension, or infection of a prosthetic joint infected.
- Some experts advise earlier surgical intervention for Gram-negative pathogens or pts with rheumatoid arthritis.
- Intraarticular antibiotics not recommended.

OTHER INFORMATION
- Early treatment with IV abx and aspiration or surgical drainage reduces joint destruction.
- When GC suspected, culture blood, urethra, cervix, rectum, pharynx, pustules, and joint fluid. Notify microbiology laboratory to assure proper handling. Send urine nucleic acid test.
- Recommended treatment duration is 1 wk for GC; 2 wks for *streptococci, H. influenzae*; 3 wks for staph or GNB. Treatment must, however, be individualized and may require a longer duration in some pts.
- Signs, symptoms, CRP can be used to help guide duration.

BASIS FOR RECOMMENDATIONS

Centers for Disease Control and Prevention; Workowski KA, Berman SM. Sexually transmitted diseases treatment guidelines 2006. Centers for Disease Control and Prevention. *MMWR Recomm Rep*, 2006; Vol. 55; pp. 1–94.

Comments: Included are guidelines for the treatment of disseminated gonococcal infection and arthritis in an era of decreasing drug susceptibility. The impact of increasing fluoroquinolone resistance rates among urethral isolates upon the treatment of gonococcal arthritis remains unclear.

Ross JJ. Septic arthritis. *Infect Dis Clin North Am*, 2005; Vol. 19; pp. 799–817.

Comments: Detailed current review of the topic, including pathogenesis, differential diagnosis, surgical management and management of prosthetic joint infections. Few controlled studies available that address the dose and duration of antimicrobial therapy for non-gonococcal acute septic arthritis. Fortunately, most antibiotics achieve acceptable concentrations in the synovial fluid.

Cardiac

CARDIOVASCULAR DEVICE INFECTIONS

Lisa A. Spacek, MD, PhD and Khalil G. Ghanem, MD, PhD

PATHOGENS
- *Staphylococcus aureus*
- Coagulase-negative staphylococci
- *Enterococcus* species
- *Escherichia coli*
- *Klebsiella* species
- *Corynebacterium* species
- *Candida* species

CLINICAL
- Devices include permanent pacemakers (PPMs), implantable cardioverter-defibrillators (ICDs), and left ventricular assist devices (LVADs). Infection can be early (<1 yr after device placement or most recent surgical modification) or late (>1 yr after device placement or most recent surgical modification).
- Clinical presentations range from local signs at pocket site with pain, erythema, purulent drainage, and wound dehiscence to bloodstream infection with high fever, sepsis, and embolic/thrombotic events as well as indolent infection with low-grade fever and weight loss.
- Device-related infection may involve pocket infection, blood stream infection, and endocardial infection (valvular and nonvalvular).
- Majority of pts present with pocket infection (52%), 17% with pocket infection and bacteremia, and 23% with device-related endocarditis.
- Epidemiology: intraoperative contamination, hematogenous contamination, and contiguous spread.
- Pathogenesis: microbial adherence due to attachment of staphylococci to extracellular matrix proteins or formation of biofilm.
- Risk factors include: extended duration of use, multi-organ failure, extended ICU stay, diabetes mellitus, malnutrition, malignancy, postoperative hematoma, and use of a temporary electrode.
- Rates of infection for PPMs, 0.1–20%; for ICDs, 0–3%; and for LVADs, 25–70%.

DIAGNOSIS
- Diagnosis is based on clinical symptoms and blood and generator pocket cultures.
- Transesophageal echo (TEE) recommended in all pts with positive blood cultures or prior antibiotic treatment. Transthoracic echo lacks sensitivity.
- Laboratory abnormalities include leukocytosis (WBC >10K), anemia, elevated ESR, and positive blood cultures.
- Complications include endocarditis; septic arthritis; osteomyelitis; pulmonary, brain, liver, perinephric, and splenic abscesses.

TREATMENT
Overview
- Complete removal of cardiac device, if feasible, is recommended by the American Heart Association.
- Generator tissue Gram-stain and culture and lead tip culture should be obtained.
- The type of antimicrobial tx depends on culture data. Early empiric therapy should cover nosocomial-acquired Gram-positive organisms: vancomycin is a reasonable first choice, with modification based on culture data.
- Reassessment of need for cardiac device is recommended. Reimplantation of a new device may not be required in 13–52% of cases.
- Laser sheath technology allows photoablation of fibrous attachments without mechanical force and reduces the rate of complications associated w/ device removal.
- Most reports of successful eradication of infection without complete removal of the device occur with Gram-negative bacteremia.

Pacemaker/ ICD/ LVAD Infections

- Endocarditis: recommend device removal and pathogen-directed parenteral therapy for 4–6 wks. Count duration of antibiotics from day of device removal.
- Lead vegetation complicated by septic emboli/thrombosis, osteomyelitis, abscesses: recommend device removal and 4–6 wks of antibiotics.
- Bacteremia and negative TEE: recommend device removal and 2 wks of antibiotics (2–4 wks of antibiotic tx for *S. aureus*).
- Negative blood cultures w/o prior antibiotic tx: treat for pocket infection with 10–14 days of antibiotics.
- In most cases, removal of LVAD is not feasible. Long-term suppression is usually the goal until transplantation, after which time, a course of abx to cure the infection is initiated.
- If removal of cardiac device is not feasible, the addition of rifampin may be considered. Rifampin may cause abnormalities in liver function and may decrease anticoagulation effect of warfarin.
- If blood cultures persistently positive, treat with antibiotics for at least 4 wks.
- If cardiac device cannot be removed, then long-term suppressive antibiotic therapy is recommended.

Reimplantation

- Timing of reimplantation is based on clinical presentation and pathogen. Blood stream infection requires longer tx course.
- Reimplantation should occur at a new, clean site. Adequate debridement and infection control recommended prior to reimplantation.
- If endocarditis with valve vegetation, repeat blood cultures after device removal, then reimplantation 14 days after first negative blood culture.
- If lead vegetation, then reimplantation after repeat blood cultures are negative × 72 hrs.
- If no endocardial infection is present, then reimplantation after repeat blood cultures are negative × 72 hrs.

BASIS FOR RECOMMENDATIONS

Baddour LM, Bettmann MA, Bolger AF, et al. Nonvalvular cardiovascular device-related infections. *Circulation*, 2003; Vol. 108; pp. 2015–31.

Comments: This American Heart Association statement includes discussion of intracardiac device infections. Supports trans-esophageal echocardiogram as imaging modality of choice and, if feasible, removal of infected device.

Uslan DZ, Baddour LM. Cardiac device infections: getting to the heart of the matter. *Curr Opin Infect Dis*, 2006; Vol. 19; pp. 345–8.

Comments: The large majority of cardiac device infections are likely due to pocket site contamination at the time of device placement. Hematogenous seeding from a distant focus of infection, particularly due to *Staphylococcus aureus*, can account for late-onset infection. Although no prospective studies have been conducted to date, management with parenteral antibiotics and complete device removal is the current standard of care.

ENDOCARDITIS

John G. Bartlett, MD

PATHOGENS

- Frequency (based on 1779 cases 2000–03: JAMA 2005;293:3012)
- *S. aureus:* 32%
- Viridans streptococci: 18%
- Enterococcus: 11%
- Coagulase-negative staphylococcus: 11%
- Streptococcus bovis: 7%
- Streptococcus (other): 5%
- HACEK organisms: 2% [*Haemophilus parainfluenzae, Haemophilus aphrophilus, Actinobacillus actinomycetemcomitans, Cardiobacterium hominis, Eikenella corrodens, Kingella kingii*].
- Gram-negative bacilli: 2%
- Fungi: 2% [*Candida species, Aspergillus species* (blood cultures rarely positive for aspergillus)].

- Culture negative: 8% [consider HACEK organisms, nutritionally deficient *Streptococcus species* (e.g., Abiotrophia), *Coxiella burnetii* (Q fever), *Chlamydia psittaci*, *Mycoplasma* spp., *Legionella pneumophila*, *Bartonella species*, *Brucella species*, *Tropheryma whipplei*].

CLINICAL

- Symptoms include fever, malaise, chest/back pain, cough, dyspnea, arthralgias, myalgia, neurologic sx, wt loss, night sweats.
- Predisposing conditions: IDU, rheumatic heart disease, valvular insufficiency, indwelling catheters, pacemakers, prosthetic heart valves, congenital heart disease, prior endocarditis.
- PE and lab (Duke criteria) = [2 Major] or [1 Major + 3 Minor] or [5 Minor], see diagnosis section.

DIAGNOSIS

- **Duke Clinical Criteria** (See Appendix I, pp. 758–759 for definition of Duke Criteria): 2 Major or 1 Major + 3 Minor or 5 Minor.
- **Major (microbiology):** a) typical organisms × 2 blood cultures (e.g., *Strep viridans*, *S. bovis*, HACEK, *S. aureus*, or enterococcus) with no primary source, b) persistent bacteremia (>12 hrs), c) 3/3 or 3/4 positive blood cultures.
- **Major (valve):** a) echo w/ vegetation, b) new valve regurgitation.
- **Minor:** a) predisposing cardiac condition or IDU, b) fever >38°C (100.4°F), c) vascular phenomenon (arterial emboli, mycotic aneurysm, intracerebral bleed, conjunctival hemorrhage, Janeway lesions), d) immune phenomenon (glomerulonephritis, Osler nodes, Roth spots, positive rheumatoid factor), e) positive blood culture not meeting above criteria and f) echo—abnl but not diagnostic.

TREATMENT

Antibiotic Therapy: Empiric

- Empiric, acute endocarditis: [nafcillin or oxacillin 2 g IV q4h +/− gentamicin or tobramycin 1 mg/kg IV q8h] or [vancomycin 15 mg/kg IV q12h].
- Empiric, subacute endocarditis: [ampicillin/sulbactam 3 g IV q6h + gentamicin or tobramycin 1 mg/kg IV q8h] or [vancomycin 15 mg/kg q12h + ceftriaxone 2 g IV q12h or gentamicin/tobramycin 1 mg/kg IV q8h].
- Culture and sensitivity results when available will define treatment.

Cardiac Valve Replacement

- Indications for surgery: CHF, hemodynamic compromise, fungal etiology, unresolving bacteremia, continuing embolization, progressive heart block, valvular ring abscess, relapse.
- Prognosis for IDU with artificial valve depends on rehabilitative potential from IV drug abuse.
- Post-surgical antibiotic therapy: >2 wks postop. Consider full 4–6 wk abx course if micro culture of valve or blood cx is positive at time of surgery.

OTHER INFORMATION

- Special cx requirements: HACEK, *Legionella*, *Mycoplasma*, nutritionally variant strep (Abiotrophia), *Bartonella*, *Coxiella*, *Brucella*, Gonococci, *Listeria*, *Nocardia*, Corynebacteria, TB.
- Penicillin allergic pts: skin test for allergy. Consider cephalosporins. Vancomycin commonly used if documented PCN anaphylaxis. Consider PCN desensitization.
- Mycotic aneurysm: concern if focal headaches and neurologic changes, especially if also w/ meningitis. 75% occur in middle cerebral artery, 20% multiple locations.
- Mycotic aneurysm: CT scan and lumbar puncture may help determine aneurysmal rupture. Consider angiography for those with suspected hemorrhage or those with persistent focal headache and CSF pleocytosis. If possible, delay valve replacement surgery, and resultant anticoagulation if documented aneurysm, in order to allow healing. Highest risk: *S. aureus*, especially endocarditis + meningitis.
- Right-sided endocarditis in injection drug users and prosthetic valve endocarditis.

BASIS FOR RECOMMENDATIONS

Baddour LM, Wilson W, Bayer AS, et al. Infective endocarditis. *Circulation*, 2005; Vol. 11; pp. e394.
Comments: The AHA 2005 recommendations for antibiotics used here.

ENDOCARDITIS, PROPHYLAXIS

John G. Bartlett, MD

PATHOGENS
- Oral flora: Streptococcus viridans group

CLINICAL
- Indications based upon American Heart Assoc 2007. Prior indications such as mitral valve prolapse, valvular regurgitation/stenosis have been left not recommended.
- Heart conditions: prosthetic valve, previous endocarditis, congenital heart disease, heart transplant with valvulopathy.
- Dental procedures: manipulation of gingiva, periapical area of teeth or perforation of oral mucosa.
- GI and GU procedures no longer require specific prophylaxis regarding endocarditis.
- Biopsies through infected respiratory mucosa or skin/skin structure also recommended indications for prophylaxis.

TREATMENT
- Time: single dose 30–60 min before procedure.
- Oral agent: amoxicillin 2 g PO × 1 dose.
- Oral + penicillin allergy: clindamycin 600 mg or azithromycin 500 mg or clarithromycin 500 mg.
- Parenteral: ampicillin 2 g IV or IM or cefazolin 1 g IM or IV or ceftriaxone 1 g IM or IV.
- Parenteral + penicillin allergy: cefazolin or ceftriaxone 1 g IV or IM or clindamycin 600 mg IV or IM.

OTHER INFORMATION
- The 2007 guidelines for prophylaxis are dramatically different.
- Cardiac lesions are restricted mainly prior endocarditis, prosthetic valve and selected uncorrected or recently repaired congenital heart conditions.
- Dental procedures are kept but GI and GU procedures are no longer indications.
- Central issue: The relative contribution of dental work to the total microbial load with transient bacteremia from multiple sites in healthy people.
- Highest risks: prosthetic valve, prior endocarditis and surgical shunts. The 2006 British endocarditis guidelines limit prophylaxis to these 3.

MORE INFORMATION
Procedures that merit prophylaxis for endocarditis (2006 British Guidelines).
- Dental: Dento-gingival manipulation.
- GI: Esophageal sclerotherapy, dilation, laser Rx; ERCP, hepatobiliary procedures, lithotripsy, surgery on intestinal mucosa.
- GU: Cystoscopy, urethral dilatation, TURP, transrectal prostate bx.
- Gyn: Vaginal hysterectomy, C-section.

BASIS FOR RECOMMENDATIONS
Wilson W, Taubert KA, Gewitz M, et al. Prevention of infective endocarditis: guidelines from the American Heart Association: a guideline from the American Heart Association Rheumatic Fever, Endocarditis and Kawasaki Disease Committee, Council on Cardiovascular Disease in the Young, and the Council on Clinical Cardiology, Council on Cardiovascular Surgery and Anesthesia, and the Quality of Care and Outcomes Research Interdisciplinary Working Group. *J Am Dent Assoc*, 2008; Vol. 139 Suppl; pp. 3S–24S.
Comments: Both references are for the same document which is the AHA guidelines for antibiotic prophylaxis for endocarditis.

Wilson W, Taubert KA, Gewitz M, et al. Prevention of infective endocarditis: guidelines from the American Heart Association: a guideline from the American Heart Association Rheumatic Fever, Endocarditis, and Kawasaki Disease Committee, Council on Cardiovascular Disease in the Young, and the Council on Clinical Cardiology, Council on Cardiovascular Surgery and Anesthesia, and the Quality of Care and Outcomes Research Interdisciplinary Working Group. *Circulation*, 2007; Vol. 116; pp. 1736–54.
Comments: Both references are for the same document which is the AHA guidelines for antibiotic prophylaxis for endocarditis.

DIAGNOSIS

ENDOCARDITIS, PROSTHETIC VALVE

John G. Bartlett, MD

BACTERIOLOGY (Wang, et al. JAMA 2007; 297:1354)

- Early <2 mos: Coag-neg Staphylococcus (17%); *S. aureus* (40%); *Streptococci* (2%); *Enterococci* (8%); *S. bovis* (2%); fungal (9%); Gram-negative bacilli (6%)
- Late >2 mos: Coag-neg Staphylococcus (20%); *S. aureus* (18%); *Streptococci* (12%); *Enterococci* (13%); *S. bovis* (7%); fungal (11%); Gram-negative bacilli (1%)

CLINICAL

- Common sx: fever, malaise, chest/back pain, cough, dyspnea, arthralgia, neurologic sx, wt loss, night sweats. In early infection (<2 mos after surgery), CHF or shock may predominate over subtle symptoms.
- Diagnosis by Duke criteria = [2 Major] or [1 Major + 3 Minor] or [5 minor] per below
- **Major (microbiologic):** 1. typical organisms × 2 blood cx, 2. persistent bacteremia (>12 hrs), 3. 3/3 or 3/4 positive blood cx, 4. blood cx + or IgG Ab titer >1:800 for *Coxiella burnetii*.
- **Major (valve):** 1. vegetation seen on echocardiography, 2. new valvular regurgitation.
- **Minor:** 1. predisposing heart condition or IDU, 2. fever >38°C (100.4°F), 3. vascular phenomenon 4. immune phenomenon 5. positive blood cxs not meeting above criteria.
- Vascular phenomenon (arterial embolism, septic pulmonary infarct, mycotic aneurysm, intracerebral bleed, conjunctival hemorrhage, Janeway lesions). Immune phenomenon (glomerulonephritis, Osler node, Roth spot, rheumatoid factor).
- Typical Organism: *S. viridans*, *S. bovis*, HACEK, *S. aureus*, *Enterococcus* w/o other primary source.

TREATMENT

Antibiotic Therapy

- Penicillin susceptible *Strep* species (MIC <0.12 µg/ml): AQ pen G 24 mil U IV q24h continuous infusion or divided q4–6h IV or ceftriaxone 2 g IV q24h either +/− gentamicin 3 mg/kg IV q24h. Alt: vancomycin 15 mg/kg q12h IV × 6 wks.
- Penicillin resistant *Strep* species (MIC >0.12 ug/ml): Aq penicillin G or ceftriaxone as above—plus gentamicin 3 mg/kg IV or IM × 6 wks. Alt: vancomycin 15 mg/kg IV q12h × 6 wks.
- *S. aureus* (MSSA): nafcillin or oxacillin 2 g IV q4h × 6 wks + rifampin 300 mg IV/PO tid × 6 wks + gentamicin 1 mg/kg IV q8h × 2 wks.
- *S. aureus* (MRSA): vancomycin 15 mg/kg IV q12h ≥ 6 wks plus rifampin 300 mg IV/PO tid + gentamicin 1 mg/kg IV q8h × 2 wks.
- Enterococcus: ampicillin 2 g IV q4h × 4–6 wks or Aq pen G 18–30 mil U/day × 4–6 wks plus gentamicin 1 mg/kg/day q8h × 4–6 wks. Alt: vancomycin 15 mg/kg IV q12h × 6 wks plus rifampin 300 mg IV/PO tid plus gentamicin 1 mg/kg IV q8h.
- E. faecium (VRE): linezolid 600 mg IV or PO × ≥ 8 wks, daptomycin 6–10 mg/kg/day IV × ≥ 8 wks.
- HACEK: ceftriaxone 1 g q12h IV or IM, ampicillin/sulbactam 3 g IV q6h, ciprofloxacin 750 mg PO bid or 400 mg IV. Cipro regimen only recommended if intolerant of ceftriaxone of ampicillin. Levofloxacin or moxifloxacin may be substituted for ciprofloxacin.
- Culture-negative (<1 yr): vancomycin 15 mg/kg q12h × 6 wks + gentamicin 1 mg/kg q8h IV/IM × 2 wks + cefepime 2 g IV q8h + rifampin 300 mg PO/IV q8h × 6 wks.
- Culture negative (>1 yr): suspected *Bartonella*, culture negative—ceftriaxone sodium 2 g IV/IM q24h plus gentamicin 1 mg/kg IV/IM q8h IV/IM +/− doxycycline 100 mg IV/PO q12h. If documented *Bartonella*, culture positive—doxycycline 100 mg IV/PO q12h plus gentamicin 1 mg/kg IV q8h. If gentamicin cannot be given, replace with rifampin 300 mg PO/IV q8h.

Surgical Intervention

- Indications for surgery: moderate to severe CHF, unstable prosthesis, perivalvular extension, persistent bacteremia despite optimal ABX, certain organisms (fungi, *P. aeruginosa*, *S. aureus*), relapse.
- Relative surgical indications: vegetations >10 mm, culture negative PVE with unexplained fever >10 days.
- Timing of surgery depends on optimization of hemodynamic status prior to surgery, not sterilization of blood cultures or duration of ABX. Risk low of infecting new valve, some prefer bioprostheses.
- In the setting of neurologic complications, the risk of hemorrhagic transformation is decreased by delaying surgery if cardiac hemodynamics permit.

Special Considerations

- Infection <2 mos following cardiac surgery are often nosocomially linked, the microbiology of these episodes is distinct from episodes acquired later, which is more similar to native valve endocarditis.
- *Legionella pneumophila* and *Legionella dumoffii* PVE is linked to tap water exposure of postoperative (sternal) wounds or chest tubes.
- *Mycobacterium chelonae* PVE is linked to contamination of the bioprosthesis during manufacturing.
- Anticoagulation is controversial, but probably indicated with PVE involving valves that require anticoagulation when not infected (mechanical valves).
- Bioprosthetic valves that typically do not require anticoagulation do not warrant anticoagulation when infected.
- Anticoagulation must be very carefully controlled for fear of hemorrhagic infarcts.

FOLLOW UP

- Length of ABX after surgery is determined by operative findings. If there is evidence of ongoing infection then treat with a full course of standard antibiotics postoperatively.
- If there is no sign of ongoing infection at surgery, the sum of the pre- and post-operative antibiotic course should equal the recommended duration of therapy for the specific causative organism.

OTHER INFORMATION

- Vancomycin is considered inferior to oxacillin or nafcillin for methicillin-sensitive strains of *S. aureus*.
- TEE is diagnostically superior in PVE and preferred over TTE.

BASIS FOR RECOMMENDATIONS

Baddour LM, Wilson WR, Bayer AS, et al. Infective endocarditis: diagnosis, antimicrobial therapy, and management of complications: a statement for healthcare professionals from the Committee on Rheumatic Fever, Endocarditis, and Kawasaki Disease, Council on Cardiovascular Disease in the Young, and the Councils on Clinical Cardiology, Stroke, and Cardiovascular Surgery and Anesthesia, American Heart Association: endorsed by the Infectious Diseases Society of America. *Circulation*, 2005; Vol. 111; pp. e394–434.

Comments: AHA recommendations used for this module.

ENDOCARDITIS — INJECTION DRUG USERS

John G. Bartlett, MD

PATHOGENS

- *Staphylococcus aureus* (MSSA or MRSA): most common
- Streptococci viridans group
- Enterococcus
- Gram-negative bacilli (e.g., *P. aeruginosa*)
- Candida species (usually *C. albicans*)

CLINICAL

- Fever, malaise, chest/back pain, cough, dyspnea, arthralgia/myalgia, neurologic sx, wt loss, night sweats.
- Suspect endocarditis in any IDU with FUO (fever of unknown origin).
- Pathogens: *S. aureus*–60%, Streptococcal species–20%, *P. aeruginosa*–10%, Candida–5%, *S. epidermidis*–2%.
- Valve involved: tricuspid–60%.

DIAGNOSIS

- **Duke Clinical Criteria:** 2 Major or 1 Major + 3 Minor or 5 Minor.
- **Major (microbiology):** a) typical organisms × 2 blood cultures (e.g., *Streptococcus viridans*, *S. bovis*, HACEK organisms, *S. aureus*, or Enterococcus) with no primary source, b) persistent bacteremia (>12 hrs), c) 3/3 or 3/4 positive blood cultures.
- **Major (valve):** a) echo w/ vegetation, b) new valve regurgitation.
- **Minor:** a) predisposing cardiac condition or IDU, b) fever >38°C (100.4°F), c) vascular phenomenon (arterial emboli, mycotic aneurysm, intracerebral bleed, conjunctival hemorrhage, Janeway lesions), d) immune phenomenon (glomerulonephritis, Osler nodes,

Roth spots, positive rheumatoid factor), e) positive blood culture not meeting above criteria and f) echo—abnl but not diagnostic.

TREATMENT

Antibiotics: empiric

- Preferred: vancomycin 15 mg/kg q12h, strive for trough >15–20 mcg/ml × 4 or 6 wks if complicated case.
- Alt (if low MRSA prevalence): oxacillin/nafcillin 2 g IV q4h +/– gentamicin 1 mg/kg IV q8h.

Pathogen-specific recommendations

- *S. aureus* (MSSA, preferred): oxacillin or nafcillin 2 g IV q4h × 6 wks, +/– gentamicin 1 mg/kg IV q8h × 3–5 days. Alt: cefazolin 2 g IV q6h IV × 6 wks +/– gentamicin 1 mg/kg IV q8h × 3–5 days.
- *S. aureus* (MSSA, 2 wks course for tricuspid valve if: veg <2 cm, no emboli besides lung, negative blood cultures by day 4): nafcillin/oxacillin 2 g IV q4h × 2 wks + gentamicin 1 mg/kg IV q8h × 2 wks.
- *S. aureus* (MRSA or pen allergy): vancomycin 15 mg/kg q12h × 6 wks; goal trough >15–20 mcg/ml.
- *Streptococcus viridans* (pen sensitive, MIC ≤0.12): aqueous penicillin G 12–18 mil Units by continuous infusion or divided into 4–6 daily doses × 4 wks, or ceftriaxone 2 g IV q24h × 4 wks, or aqueous pen or ceftriaxone (above doses) + gentamicin 1 mg/kg IV q8h × 2 wks or if pen allergy, vancomycin 15 mg/kg IV q12h × 4 wks. Alt: ceftriaxone 2 g IV q24h plus gentamicin 3 mg/kg IV q24h × 2 wks.
- *Strep viridans* (pen MIC >0.12 µg/ml-≤0.5 µg/ml): aqueous pen G 24 mil U IV by continuous infusion or divided into 4–6 doses/day + gentamicin 1 mg/kg IV q8h × 4–6 wks or vancomycin 15 mg/kg q12h IV × 4 wks (PCN allergic).
- Strep species (pen MIC >0.5 µg/ml, also including Abiotrophia defectiva and *Granulicatella* species, Gemella species): use Enterococcal regimen.
- Enterococcus: ampicillin 2 g IV q4h or aqueous pen G 18–20 mil U/day IV continuous or divided into 4–6 doses × 4–6 wks plus gentamicin* 1 mg/kg q8h IV or IM × 4–6 wks or vancomycin 15 mg/kg q12h IV plus gentamicin* 1 mg/kg q8h IV or IM × 4–6 wks. *Substitute streptomycin 7.5 mg/kg IV or IM if gentamicin resistant. VRE (*E. faecium*): linezolid 600 mg IV or PO q12h × > 8 wks or quinupristin/dalfopristin 22.5 mg/kg/day in 3 divided doses × > 8 wks.
- *P. aeruginosa* (use *in vitro* data, preferred): tobramycin 2.5 mg/kg IV q8h IV (high dose, peak goal 15–20 mcg/ml) + piperacillin 4 g IV q4h or ceftazidime 2 g IV q8h × 4–6 wks. Alt: aztreonam, ciprofloxacin or imipenem—each given with either tobramycin, gentamicin, or amikacin depending on susceptibilities.
- Candida (preferred): amphotericin B 0.8–1 mg/kg/day IV + flucytosine 100–150 mg/kg/day divided q6h + surgery. Alternative: fluconazole 400 mg IV/day + surgery.
- HACEK: ceftriaxone 2 g q24h × 4 wks or ampicillin-sulbactam 3 g IV q6h × 4 wks or ciprofloxacin (use only if intolerant of β-lactams) 500 mg PO twice daily or 400 mg IV q12h × 4–6 wks. Culture negative: ampicillin-sulbactam 3 g IV q6h × 4–6 wks plus gentamicin 1 mg/kg q8h IV or IM or vancomycin 15 mg/kg IV q12h plus gentamicin 1 mg/kg IV q8h plus ciprofloxacin 750 mg PO twice daily or 400 mg IV q12h × 4–6 wks.

Surgery

- Indications: severe heart failure, uncontrolled infection, persistent bacteremia despite abx, fungal endocarditis, unstable prosthetic valve, periannular extension.
- Tricuspid valve: may consider valvectomy or vegetectomy + valvuloplasty. Aortic or mitral-valve: usually requires replacement.
- Issues: some heart surgeons are reluctant to operate on addicts for IE, some require assurance there will be drug rehabilitation.

OTHER INFORMATION

- Usual presentation: fever, chest × ray with septic emboli, blood culture yields *S. aureus,* echocardiogram–tricuspid valve vegetations.
- Surgery: prognosis for prosthetic valve without drug rehabilitation is poor. For tricuspid valve endocarditis–valvectomy is an option.
- Concurrent HIV infection increases mortality rate when CD4 counts <200.

BASIS FOR RECOMMENDATIONS

Baddour LM, Wilson WR, Bayer AS, et al. Infective endocarditis: diagnosis, antimicrobial therapy, and management of complications: a statement for healthcare professionals from the Committee on Rheumatic Fever, Endocarditis, and Kawasaki Disease, Council on Cardiovascular Disease in the Young, and the Councils on Clinical Cardiology, Stroke, and Cardiovascular Surgery and Anesthesia, American Heart Association: endorsed by the Infectious Diseases Society of America. *Circulation*, 2005; Vol. 111; pp. e394–434.

Comments: Latest set of AHA recommendations used for this module.

Chambers HF, Korzeniowski OM, and Sande MA. Staphylococcus aureus endocarditis: clinical manifestations in addicts and nonaddicts. *Medicine (Baltimore),* 1983; Vol. 62; pp. 170–7.

Comments: Major differences are: 1) the better prognosis in the addict population; 2) the high rate of tricuspid valve involvement; and 3) the high frequency of pulmonary complications. Finding supporting tricuspid valve endocarditis were: pleurisy 30%, pulmonary infiltrates (presumably septic embolic) 80%, signs of tricuspid valve insufficiency (gallop, large V wave, pulsatile liver) 30%.

DIAGNOSIS

MYOCARDITIS

Michael Melia, MD and Paul G. Auwaerter, MD

PATHOGENS

- **Viral:** coxsackie A or B, echoviruses, HIV, adenovirus, HHV-6, polio, mumps, rubeola, influenza A or B, parainfluenza, rabies, rubella, dengue, lymphocytic choriomeningitis, varicella zoster, CMV, EBV, vaccinia, hepatitis B or hepatitis C, RSV, parvovirus B19, yellow fever, chikungunya virus.

- **Bacterial/rickettsial:** *C. diphtheriae, C. perfringens, Mycoplasma pneumoniae, S. pyogenes* (toxin-mediated, Acute Rheumatic Fever), *N. meningitidis,* Salmonella, Brucella, *S. aureus,* Listeria, Legionella, Mycoplasma, Chlamydia spp., Rickettsia, Ehrlichia, *Vibrio cholerae, Borrelia burgdorferi.*

- **Fungi:** aspergillus, candida, cryptococcus, histoplasma, Coccidioides.

- **Parasites:** *Trypanosoma cruzi, T. gambiense, T. rhodesiense, T. spiralis, Toxoplasma gondii,* Schistosoma species, visceral larval migrans.

- **Other:** idiopathic, collagen vascular disease, thyrotoxicosis, TTP, peripartum, radiation induced, cocaine, drug-induced, heavy metals, pheochromocytoma, giant cell myocarditis, sarcoid, Kawasaki disease, inflammatory bowel disease, vaccines (especially smallpox).

CLINICAL

- Clinical symptoms may vary. Asymptomatic vs. febrile, malaise, myalgia, arthralgia, dyspnea/orthopnea/PND, edema, palpitations, precordial discomfort, upper respiratory and/or gastrointestinal tract symptoms.

- Clinical signs: prolonged elevation of CK-MB and troponin T levels, fever, cardiomegaly, mitral/tricuspid murmurs, ECG abnormalities (ST-T wave change, heart block, dysrhythmias), shock, heart failure. Implicated in 8–12% of cases of sudden cardiac death in young adults.

- Imaging studies: chest XR w/ cardiomegaly; echocardiogram w/ change over time in movement and function; MRI w/ evidence of LV dysfunction/edema; Indium 111-labelled antimyosin antibody imaging is abnormal.

DIAGNOSIS

- Creatine kinase has low predictive value. Troponins have low sensitivity but reasonable specificity (~90%) and positive predictive value (also ~90%). Echocardiographic findings are useful but overlap with those of other cardiomyopathies.

- If available, cardiac MRI can differentiate between myocarditis and other cardiomyopathies, such as those induced by ischemia and stress (a.k.a. takotsubo). MRI can also help target biopsy site(s) and follow disease activity longitudinally.

- Endomyocardial biopsy: remains the "gold standard," although expect yield in only 10–20% for specific etiology. Early biopsies may be more sensitive and serial biopsies can help diagnosis. Recommended for new onset heart failure and either hemodynamic compromise or conduction block or ventricular arrhythmias, with or without left ventricular dilation.

- Dallas criteria includes myocyte necrosis and lymphocytic infiltration. Utility in diagnosis and prognosis has been questioned.

- Isolation of organism: viral isolation can be difficult, viral serum antibody titers can aid diagnosis, as can molecular techniques.
- Lyme serology useful in endemic areas.

TREATMENT
Viral Myocarditis

- Supportive therapy: bed rest, intravascular volume control, arrhythmia management, heart failure management (initial stabilization if needed then heart failure management).
- Corticosteroids: very controversial role in treatment of viral (acute lymphocytic) myocarditis mainly as good controlled trials are lacking, and viral myocarditis usually resolves spontaneously. Some recommend in later course of illness if progressive left ventricular dysfunction exists. Myocarditis due to systemic auto-immune diseases may benefit from immunosuppressive therapy.
- Cytomegalovirus myocarditis: ganciclovir can be used for severe CMV myocarditis.
- Cardiac transplantation: may be necessary in severe cases, however, the majority of cases resolve without further sequelae.
- Experimental therapy includes hyperimmunoglobulin and interferon therapy as yet without clear therapeutic roles.
- HIV-associated myocarditis: HAART and ACE inhibitors. Steroids are controversial. Consider neoplastic or secondary infectious cause (*T. gondii, M. tuberculosis, C. neoformans*, CMV).

Lyme Carditis

- First degree heart block (most common, PR interval $>$ 0.3 seconds): doxycycline 100 mg PO twice-daily, or amoxicillin 500 mg PO three times a day, or cefuroxime 500 mg PO twice-daily.
- High degree atrio-ventricular block: ceftriaxone 2 g IV q24h $\times$ 14–28 days or Penicillin G 20 mU IV (divided q6h) $\times$ 28 days + cardiac monitoring. Many switch to oral regimen for completion of course when 2° or 3° heart block resolves.
- Complete heart block is reversible, therefore permanent pacemaker not usually recommended.
- After 24 hrs of antibiotics, if complete heart block or heart failure does not improve, some recommend corticosteroid therapy.
- Acute myocarditis is a rare complication of Lyme disease. Chronic complications or death are extremely rare. There is not clear association of dilated, chronic cardiomyopathy and Lyme disease.

OTHER INFORMATION

- Most pts with viral myocarditis recover completely. In one recent retrospective review, however, NYHA functional class III or IV heart failure and positive immunohistochemistry on endomyocardial biopsy were associated with poor prognosis. In the same review, beta-blocker use was associated with freedom from cardiac death or heart transplantation.
- Corticosteroid use is very controversial, especially in acute phase of myocarditis (possible rapid clinical deterioration). Randomized controlled trials are needed.
- NSAIDS are not effective, and may be detrimental in myocarditis.
- Vaccinia-related myocarditis: incidence after smallpox vaccination is about 1:15,000. In certain cases, steroids or vaccinia immune globulin (CDC,770-488-7100) may be useful.

BASIS FOR RECOMMENDATIONS

Wormser GP, Dattwyler RJ, Shapiro ED, et al. The clinical assessment, treatment, and prevention of lyme disease, human granulocytic anaplasmosis, and babesiosis: clinical practice guidelines by the Infectious Diseases Society of America. *Clin Infect Dis,* 2006; Vol. 43; pp. 1089–134.
Comments: Current IDSA guidelines for the treatment of **Lyme disease**.

Magnani JW, Dec GW. Myocarditis: current trends in diagnosis and treatment. *Circulation,* 2006; Vol. 113; pp. 876–90.
Comments: Overview that forms the basis for recommendations made in this module.

Hunt SA, Abraham WT, Chin MH, et al. ACC/AHA 2005 Guideline Update for the Diagnosis and Management of Chronic Heart Failure in the Adult: a report of the American College of Cardiology/American Heart Association Task Force on Practice Guidelines (Writing Committee to Update the 2001 Guidelines for the Evaluation and Management of Heart Failure): developed in collaboration with the American College of Chest Physicians and the International Society for Heart and Lung Transplantation: endorsed by the Heart Rhythm Society. *Circulation,* 2005; Vol. 112; pp. e154–235.
Comments: Current guidelines for the management of heart failure symptoms.

PERICARDITIS

Paul G. Auwaerter, MD

DIAGNOSIS

PATHOGENS

- **Bacteria:** *Staphylococcus aureus*
- *Streptococcus pneumoniae*
- *Neisseria meningitidis*
- *Haemophilus influenzae*
- *Salmonella spp*
- *Pseudomonas aeruginosa*
- Anaerobes
- **Viruses:** Enteroviruses (Coxsackie, Echovirus)
- HIV (AIDS-associated pericarditis)
- Influenza
- Mumps
- Varicella zoster virus
- Epstein Barr virus
- **Fungal:** *Coccidioides immitis*
- *Histoplasma capsulatum*
- *Candida spp.* (immunocompromised pts)
- *Aspergillus spp.* (immunocompromised pts)
- *Cryptococcus neoformans* (immunocompromised pts)

CLINICAL

- Acute pericarditis: acute fulminant onset of high fevers, shaking chills, dyspnea, chest pain/ pleuritic, arthralgia, myalgia. Can be more insidious with subacute, chronic presentations.
- PE: tachycardia, friction rub, muffled heart sounds, jugular venous distention, and pulsus paradoxus.

DIAGNOSIS

- EKG: sinus tachycardia, diffuse ST/T wave changes (elevation), or electrical alternans from tamponade.
- Radiographic: increased cardiac silhouette, +/− pleural effusion or wide mediastinum.
- Echo: pericardial effusion or cardiac tamponade (may appear near normal with constrictive pericarditis); CT- pericardial effusion or thickening.
- Cornerstone: pericardial fluid Gram-stain and culture of organism (obtain C&S, fungal, and AFB studies). Increased PMNs or pus = pyogenic purulent pericarditis.
- Ddx includes non-infectious considerations: post-MI/Dressler's syndrome, uremia, neoplasm, irradiation, dissecting aortic aneurysm, sarcoidosis, collagen vascular disease, drug-induced.

TREATMENT

Antibiotic therapy: Purulent Pericarditis

- Empiric: vancomycin 15 mg/kg IV q12h + [ceftriaxone 2 g IV q24] × 14–42 days. Aspiration/ drainage crucial to determine if purulent pericarditis exits and for therapeutic intervention with antibiotics.
- *S. pneumoniae* (pen sens): penicillin G IV, cefotaxime, or fluoroquinolone × 14–42 days.
- *S. pneumoniae* (pen resist): fluoroquinolone, vancomycin × 14–42 days.
- *S. aureus* (MSSA): nafcillin, oxacillin, cefazolin, vancomycin (PCN allergic), clindamycin × 14–42 days.
- *S. aureus* (MRSA): vancomycin, linezolid × 14–42 days.
- *N. meningitidis:* penicillin G., ceftriaxone, cefotaxime × 14–42 days. Test complement deficiency. Prophylaxis for very close contacts: rifampin 600 mg PO q12h 3 days or ciprofloxacin 500 mg PO × 1 or ceftriaxone 250 IM × 1.
- GNB: fluoroquinolone, cefepime × 14–42 days.
- Anaerobes: clindamycin, metronidazole, beta-lactam/beta-lactamase inhibitor × 14–42 days.
- Mycoplasma pneumoniae: doxycycline, macrolide × 14–42 days.
- Legionella pneumophila: fluoroquinolone, azithromycin × 14–42 days.

Surgical intervention
- Surgical drainage essential for moderate to severe tamponade or purulent pericarditis.
- Pericardiotomy with biopsy increases diagnostic yield (especially TB, fungal) compared to pericardiocentesis.
- Pericardial drain may help prevent reaccumulation.
- Pericardial window: if thick purulent drainage or reaccumulation.
- Pericardiectomy for severe constrictive pericarditis.

Special considerations, including viral pericarditis
- Intrapericardial infusion of antibiotics is unnecessary, as parenterally administered antibiotics reach high concentrations in the pericardium.
- Enteroviral (viral) pericarditis: treatment includes supportive care and NSAIDs. Avoid steroids in early disease. Unclear if steroids later in disease course prevent recurrence. This is often a clinically unproven diagnosis. Acute/convalescent serology supportive of diagnosis; stool enteroviral cx or PCR indirect evidence but only pericardial fluid/tissue secures dx.
- AIDS pericarditis: often asymptomatic. Invasive to dx, so questionable if asymptomatic. Symptomatic cases warrant aggressive dx to rule out infection and neoplasia.
- Vaccinia-related myopericarditis: incidence after smallpox vaccination is about 1:15,000. In certain cases, steroids or vaccinia immune globulin (CDC, 770-488-7100) may be useful.
- *Mycobacterium tuberculosis*: intrapericardial infusion of antibiotics is unnecessary, as parenterally or orally administered antibiotics (rifampin, pyrazinamide, isoniazid, ethambutol) reach high concentrations in the pericardium. The addition of prolonged steroids (up to 12 wks) may reduce inflammation and prevent constrictive pericarditis.

OTHER INFORMATION
- Classic symptoms and signs of pericarditis are often absent. High index of suspicion is necessary, pt with fever and ECG changes.
- Predisposing conditions: prior pericardial effusions, renal failure, thoracic surgery, diabetes, myeloproliferative disorders, local/distant infections (endocarditis/pneumonia), + PPD.
- NSAIDS and steroids should probably be avoided in those with signs of myocarditis.
- Pts with recurrent idiopathic or viral pericarditis, colchicine at 1 mg/day may be effective for reducing recurrent episodes.

BASIS FOR RECOMMENDATIONS

Lange RA, Hillis LD. Clinical practice. Acute pericarditis. *N Engl J Med,* 2004; Vol. 351; pp. 2195–202.
Comments: Practical overview of the syndrome and its management.

Maisch B, Seferovic PM, Ristic AD, et al. Guidelines on the diagnosis and management of pericardial diseases executive summary; The Task force on the diagnosis and management of pericardial diseases of the European society of cardiology. *Eur Heart J,* 2004; Vol. 25; pp. 587–610.
Comments: Thoroughly referenced diagnostic and treatment guidelines including a discussion of specific forms of infectious pericarditis.

Dermatologic

ACNE VULGARIS

Christopher J. Hoffmann MD, MPH

PATHOGENS
- Propionibacterium species
- Pathogenesis: (1) abnormal follicular keratinization and occlusion, (2) excessive oil/sebum production, (3) bacterial superinfection (*P. acnes*), (4) release of inflammatory mediators.

CLINICAL
- Hx: insidious development of multiple follicular lesions with periods of clinical improvement and exacerbation. Peak prevalence: age 17, may start as early as 8 yrs, and late as 30 or 40 yrs.
- Natural hx: most cases involute spontaneously and completely after a few years (>60%), but individuals have chronic acne through adult life.
- PE: any combination of open and closed comedones, inflammatory papules, pustules, nodules and cysts, affecting the face, neck, upper chest, back, and/or proximal extremities.
- Other associated findings: excessive oiliness of the skin, post-inflammatory hyper/hypo-pigmentation, atrophic or hypertrophic scars, excoriations; hirsutism and/or alopecia in women.
- Lab: no dx test for acne vulgaris.
- DDx: folliculitis, miliaria (heat/sweat rash), acneiform drug eruptions, acne rosacea, perioral dermatitis, follicular mucinosis (grouped papules/plaques of pilosebaceous glands w/ associated hair loss), papular urticaria, follicular eczema.

MORE CLINICAL
- 1—Additional information to be obtained in the history:
- Duration of the disease and point of maximal severity
- Current and past acne treatments
- Current and past medications
- Type and frequency of cosmetics and moisturizers used
- Environmental exposure to contactants such as oils and greases
- Personal history of other skin diseases
- Family history of acne
- Seasonal variation
- Aggravation by emotional stress
- For women: relationship to menses, increase of terminal body hair, thinning of scalp hair, excessive weight gain, use of oral contraceptives
- 2—Frequently more than 1 type of lesion is seen simultaneously, but comedones are always present.
- 3—Bacterial cultures are only indicated when atypical pathogens are suspected due to unusual clinical presentation.
- 4—Hormonal profiling is only recommended when there is clinical suggestion of hyper-androgen state.
- 5—Skin biopsy is only recommended in those rare instances when differentiation from other diseases is not possible based on clinical examination alone.

DIAGNOSIS
- Clinical based on presence of comedones, papules, pustules, nodules or cysts in characteristic locations (e.g., face, chest, shoulders, or back).

TREATMENT
General comments
- Determine the severity, predominant type of skin lesions, and response to prior therapy to choose the most appropriate type of treatment.
- Given the chronic potential of the disease, management for acute disease + chronic maintenance may be needed.

Therapeutic approach based on severity
- Mild (comedonal): topical retinoid (can use azelaic acid or salicylic acid).
- Moderate (mixed papular/pustular): topical retinoid + topical antibiotic +/– benzoyl peroxide.
- Moderate-severe (nodular): topical retinoid + topical antibiotic + benzoyl peroxide.
- Severe (nodular/conglobate): oral isotretinoin (or high dose oral antibiotic + topical retinoid + benzoyl peroxide).
- Maintenance: topical retinoid +/– benzoyl peroxide.
- *Re-assess:* q4–6 wks on therapy.

Topical therapy
- Benzoyl peroxide 2.5–10% (Acne-Aid, Ambi 10, Benoxyl 10, Benzac, Brevoxyl, Desquam, PanOxyl) lotion, liquid soap, cream or gel qday-bid.
- Erythromycin 2% (Akne-Mycin, A/T/S, Emgel, Erycette, EryDerm, Erythra-Derm, Erygel, Erymax, Staticin, Theramycin Z, T-Stat) lotion, solution, cream or gel qhs.
- Benzoyl peroxide 5%/erythromycin 3% gel (Benzamycin) qHS; Benzoyl peroxide 5%/clindamycin 1% gel (Benzaclin, Duac) qHS.
- Clindamycin solution, lotion or gel (Cleocin T, Clindagel, Clindets) qhs.
- Sodium sulfacetamide 10% lotion (Avar, Clenia, Plexion, Rosula, Rosanil, Sulfacet-R, Klaron) qday-bid.
- Tretinoin 0.025–0.1% (Retin-A, Retin-A micro, Renova, Avita, Altinac) cream, gel, solution qhs.
- Tretinoin 0.25%/clindamycin 1.2% gel (Ziana) qhs
- Azelaic acid 20% (Azelex, Finacea, Finevin) cream qday-bid.
- Adapalene 0.1% (Differin) gel qhs.
- Tazarotene 0.05%. 0.1% (Avage, Tazorac) cream or gel qhs.
- Salicylic acid 3–5% or lactic acid 12% compounded in lotion or cream base qday-bid.

Systemic therapy
- Tetracycline 250–500 mg PO once or twice daily.
- Doxycycline 50–100 mg PO once or twice daily.
- Minocycline 50–100 mg PO once or twice daily.
- Erythromycin 250–500 mg PO four times a day or 333 mg PO three times a day × 1 mo.
- TMP/SMX DS 1 tab PO once or twice daily.
- Azithromycin (Z-Pack) q15d or qmo.
- Dapsone 50–100 mg PO once daily.
- Isotretinoin (Accutane) 0.5–1 mg/kg/day × 20 wks. Female pts must be enrolled in the FDA-mandated program (IPLEDGE) for the prevention of pregnancy while on isotretinoin. Monthly participation by the physician and pt is required. For female pts who are sexually active with males, two methods of birth control are required while on this medication and for 3 mos after the treatment. Monthly serum pregnancy tests are also mandatory. For both males and females, monitoring of liver function tests, serum cholesterol and triglyceride levels are also required regularly.
- Hormonal therapy: oral contraceptives, estrogen or anti-androgen agents (spironolactone, flutamide).
- Prednisone 20–40 mg PO qd × 1–2 wks (in cases of acne fulminans, pyoderma faciale or in early association with isotretinoin).

Special situations
- For women with acne that worsens around the time of menses, a combination oral contraceptive pill may be effective to control acne.
- For women with signs of hyperandrogenism (acne in the chin/neck area, hirsutism), spironolactone is useful as well. Note: spironolactone is a teratogen, causes feminization of male fetuses.

Surgical therapy
- I+D of cysts and fistula tracts.
- Intralesional injection of nodules and cysts with triamcinolone 2.5–5 mg/cc.
- Punch excision, punch elevation, and punch grafting of depressed, "ice-pick" scars.
- Collagen injections in depressed, rolled scars.
- CO_2 laser resurfacing.

- Dermabrasion.
- Aminolevulinic acid-based photodynamic therapy for moderate to severe inflammatory acne.
- 50% TCA application to ice-pick and roiled scars.

Phototherapy
- Treatments include: visible light, specific narrow band light, intense pulsed light, pulsed dye laser, and photodynamic therapy.
- Studies limited and comparative studies lacking, however, phototherapy is reasonable second/third line option for moderate to severe acne. After completing phototherapy (with topical or systemic therapy), topical maintenance therapy with topical retinoid +/– benzoyl peroxide.

OTHER INFORMATION
- *P. acnes* secretes several extracellular products such as hyaluronidase, proteases, lipases, and chemotactic factors that may play a significant role in the inflammatory reaction seen in acne.
- Pregnancy: safety issues regarding use of erythromycin (PO or topical), benzoyl peroxide (topical), azelaic acid (topical), clindamycin (topical).
- Benzoyl peroxide has antibiotic properties and is believed to reduce the emergence of resistance to other antibiotics when used in combination.

BASIS FOR RECOMMENDATIONS
Webster GF. Acne vulgaris. *BMJ*, 2002; Vol. 325; pp. 475–9.
Comments: A summary of important points obtained through an extensive literature review.

BALANITIS

Spyridon Marinopoulos, MD

PATHOGENS
- *Candida albicans*
- *Trichomonas vaginalis*
- *Chlamydia trachomatis*
- *Neisseria gonorrhoeae*
- *Treponema pallidum* (syphilis)
- Herpes Simplex Virus
- Human papillomavirus (HPV)
- *Streptococcus species*
- *Staphylococcus aureus*

CLINICAL
- Inflamed glans penis +/– prepuce. Hx: tender glans, discharge, difficult to retract prepuce +/– impotence/difficult urination. PE: penile erythema/edema/ulcers/plaques +/– discharge +/– phimosis.
- Various types: (1) candidal: KOH prep/cx, (2) aerobic: cx for Strep/Staph/Gardnerella (r/o syphilis/trich/HSV), (3) anaerobic: foul-smelling d/c, edema + LN. GS-mixed flora, cx. (4) HPV: typical pathology.
- (5) circinate: manifestation of Reiter's. Bx—spongiform pustules, may be chlamydia probe positive. (6) irritant/allergic: ? secondary to condoms, diaphragms, lubricants/spermicides, etc. Hx atopy common. Patch testing. Bx nonspecific.
- (7) fixed drug eruptions: medication hx (tetracycline, sulfa, PCN, salicylates, phenacetin, phenolphthalein, some hypnotics), + oral/ocular mucosa lesions. Rechallenge to confirm dx.
- (8) lichen sclerosus (balanitis xerotica obliterans): dx by bx. 1% risk CA. Annual f/u needed.
- (9) Erythroplasia of Queyrat: bx shows squamous cell carcinoma in situ.
- (10) Zoon's (plasma cell): "cayenne pepper spots." May resemble #9. Dx by biopsy.
- Ddx: leukoplakia, lichen planus, psoriasis, seborrheic dermatitis, pemphigus, dermatitis artefacta, Bowen's disease, Bowenoid papulosis. If resistant to rx, consider biopsy r/o penile CA.

DIAGNOSIS
- Adult males: acceptable to assume and treat empirically most cases for probable candidal balanitis, then reassess. If no response/persistent cases: use culture to diagnose and then guide abx treatment, appropriate abx.
- Consider dermatology consultation or if resistant to treatment, consider biopsy r/o penile CA.

TREATMENT

Topical

- All cases: retract prepuce daily and soak in warm water/NS to clean glans penis and prepuce. If phimosis, refer urology to relieve surgically. Avoid soaps while inflammation present.
- Candida balanitis: clotrimazole 1% or miconazole 2% cream applied topically twice daily until resolved (recommended regimen). If marked inflammation, add 1% hydrocortisone twice daily. If azole allergy/resistance, use nystatin cream 100000 U twice daily.
- Aerobic balanitis: mupirocin 2% ointment applied tid, covers staph/strep.
- Anaerobic balanitis: clindamycin 2% cream twice daily until resolved (alternative, oral metronidazole).
- HPV balanitis: 5 FU 5% cream 1–2 ×/wk or podophyllotoxin 0.15% gel/soln twice daily tiw. Reassess in 1 mo.
- Lichen sclerosus (balanitis xerotica obliterans): clobetasol 0.05% or betamethasone 0.05% daily until remission (recommended regimen). May need to continue qwk to maintain remission.
- Zoon's (plasma cell) balanitis: topical steroids (e.g., clobetasol 0.05%) once daily to twice daily. Refractory cases: topical tacrolimus 0.1% twice daily or pimecrolimus 1% twice daily.
- Erythroplasia of queyrat: 5 FU 5% cream (alternative to surgery). Note: annual follow up required (since SCC *in situ*).
- Circinate balanitis: hydrocortisone 1% twice daily for symptomatic relief + treat underlying infection (e.g., chlamydia). Use more potent topical steroid (e.g., clobetasol 0.05%) if ineffective.
- Fixed drug eruption or irritant/allergic balanitis: 1% hydrocortisone twice daily until resolved + avoid precipitant.

Systemic

- Candida balanitis: fluconazole 150 mg PO × 1 dose, very effective (use if severe/ persistent or pt with diabetes mellitus, but some prefer as primary regimen).
- Aerobic balanitis: guide by cx and rx by organism—strep, staph, HSV, trichomonas, syphilis, gonorrhea.
- Staph/strep: cephalexin 500 mg PO four times a day or erythromycin 500 mg PO twice daily × 7 days or azithromycin 500 mg, then 250 mg × 5 days (Z-Pak) or clindamycin 300–450 mg PO three times a day × 7 days.
- Anaerobic balanitis: metronidazole 500 mg PO twice daily × 7 days (recommended regimen). Alternative: amoxicillin/clavulanate 500 mg PO three times a day × 7 days.
- HSV initial episode: acyclovir 400 mg PO three times a day or valacyclovir 1 g PO twice daily × 10 days. HSV recurrence: acyclovir 400 mg PO three times a day or famciclovir 125 mg PO three times a day × 5 days or valacyclovir 500 mg PO twice daily × 3 days.
- Trichomonas vaginalis: metronidazole 2 g PO × 1 or 500 mg PO twice daily × 7 days.
- Syphilis (primary): benzathine pen G 2.4 mU IM × 1 (preferred). Alternatives: see syphilis module p. 338.
- Gonorrhea: ceftriaxone 125 mg IM × 1 or cefixime 400 mg or ciprofloxacin 500 mg or ofloxacin 400 mg or levofloxacin 250 mg all PO × 1 single dose + treatment for *Chlamydia trachomatis*.
- Circinate balanitis (chlamydia): doxycycline 100 mg PO twice daily × 7 days or azithromycin 1 g PO × 1 + treat for gonorrhea.
- Fixed drug eruption (severe cases only): oral corticosteroids steroids, e.g., prednisone or medrol dosepack.

Surgical

- Lichen Sclerosus (in addition to topical rx): if phimosis, circumcise. If meatal stenosis, consider meatoplasty, urethroplasty or laser vaporization.
- Zoon's (plasma cell) balanitis: circumcision may lead to resolution of lesions. CO_2 laser used to treat individual lesions.
- Erythroplasia of Queyrat: local excision adequate and effective (recommended regimen). Note: annual follow up required (premalignant condition). Alternatives: laser resection or cryotherapy.

OTHER INFORMATION

- Causes/associations: infection, diabetes mellitus, poor hygiene (uncircumcised), chemical irritants (soap, petroleum jelly), anasarca, drugs, morbid obesity, penile CA.
- Screen sexual partners in any type of balanitis caused by an STD and including candida.
- High rates of fluoroquinolone-resistant GC have been reported in MSM and Asia, Pacific Basin, Hawaii, and California. Use ceftriaxone or cefixime.

BASIS FOR RECOMMENDATIONS

Buechner SA. Common skin disorders of the penis. *BJU Int,* 2002; Vol. 90; pp. 498–506.

Comments: Review highlights clinical features, dx and rx of most common dermatoses of male genitalia.

British Association of Sexual Health and HIV 2002 national guideline on the management of balanitis. *British Association of Sexual Health and HIV—Medical Specialty Society,* 1999 Aug (revised 2002); Various pagings.

Comments: Comprehensive review of the different types of balanitis and their management.

Author opinion.

DIAGNOSIS

CELLULITIS/ERYSIPELAS

John G. Bartlett, MD

PATHOGENS

- *Streptococcus* species usually group A (*S. pyogenes*, most cases).
- Other: Streptococcus groups B, C, G (especially group G).
- *Staphylococcus aureus*—MRSA now dominates both in and out of the hospital.
- Dog/cat bite: *Pasteurella multocida, Capnocytophaga* canimorsus
- Salt water exposure: *Vibrio vulnificus*
- Fresh or brackish water exposure: *Aeromonas hydrophila, Plesiomonas shigelloides.*
- Neutropenia: *P. aeruginosa,* other GNB.
- Human bite: *Eikenella corrodens,* anaerobes, *S. aureus.*
- Occasional causes (see individual pathogen modules): other *Vibrio* spp. (saltwater exposure), other *Aeromonas* spp. (freshwater exposure), *S. pneumoniae, H. influenzae, Legionella* spp., *Helicobacter cinaedi* (immunocompromised), *Erysipelothrix rhusiopathiae* (meat/fish exposure), *Staphylococcus epidermidis* (immunocompromised pts), Group B streptococci (infants), fungal.

CLINICAL

- Definition: spreading infection of skin. (1) Erysipelas—superficial, sharply demarcated nearly always group A streptococcus; (2) Cellulitis—deeper (subcutaneous)—also usually group A. streptococcus, but Group G dominates recent reports.
- Predisposing conditions: trauma, lymph stasis (prior radiation, mastectomy, saphenous vein harvest), injection drug use, ulcers, wounds, dermatophytic infections.
- Exam: red, hot, tender skin with edema ± fever and adenopathy.
- Differential diagnosis: allergy, gout, zoster, erythroderma, insect bite, panniculitis, Lyme disease (erythema migrans), Sweet's syndrome, pyoderma, fixed drug reaction, thrombophlebitis, necrotizing fasciitis.
- Lab: blood cultures are <5% positive; needle aspirates—usually negative; punch biopsy yield is 20–30%. Typically, cx not performed with presumption that most cases are due to strep or staph.
- Blood cultures indicated but usually negative. Obtain especially if: significant systemic signs and symptoms present in immunocompromised pts, unusual pathogen suspected, no response to adequate antibiotic therapy.

DIAGNOSIS

- Usually clinical diagnosis based on appearance and symptoms.
- Imaging helpful in some cases: ultrasound (to differentiate DVT), CT (if suspecting necrotizing fasciitis).

TREATMENT

Outpatients (oral antibiotics)

- Streptococci (only consider if erysipelas): penicillin Vk 500 mg PO four times a day × 10 days, amoxicillin 500 mg PO three times a day × 10 days or pen G benzathine 1.2 mil U IM × 1, cephalexin 500 mg PO four times a day × 10 days.

- Penicillin allergy: azithromycin 500 mg PO × 1 day, then 250 mg PO daily × 4 days, clarithromycin 250 mg PO twice daily × 7–10 days, clindamycin 300 mg PO three times a day × 7–10 days.
- Streptococci and *Staphylococcus aureus* (most cases of cellulitis, must presume MRSA): clindamycin 300 mg PO three times a day × 7–10 days.

Hospitalized patients
- Streptococci and *Staph aureus* (presume MRSA): clindamycin (if D test neg) 600 mg IV q8h, vancomycin 15 mg/kg IV q12h, linezolid 600 mg IV q12h or daptomycin 4 mg/kg IV q24h.
- Streptococci only (e.g., erysipelas): penicillin G 2–4 mil U IV q4–6h, cefazolin 0.5–1.5 g IV q8h, cefotaxime 1–2 g IV q8h, ceftriaxone 1–2 g IV q24h, clindamycin 600 mg q8h IV or 300 mg PO four times a day, or penicillin + clindamycin.
- Penicillin allergy: clindamycin or vancomycin (above doses).

Adjunctive therapy
- Erysipelas: consider prednisone 30 mg with taper over 8 days.
- Elevation of affected site.
- Treat associated conditions: Tinea pedis, venous stasis, lymphedema, eczema, trauma sites.
- Dermatophytic infections: topical terbinafine or clotrimazole.

Prevention
- Prevent edema (diuretics, limb elevation, compression stockings, decongestion therapy).
- Keep skin hydrated (emollients).
- Treat dermatophytic infections.
- Prevention of recurrent cellulitis especially with lymphedema: penicillin V 500 mg PO twice daily, amoxicillin 250–500 mg PO twice daily, clindamycin 150–300 mg PO daily, erythromycin 250 mg PO 1–2 ×/day.

FOLLOW UP
- Symptoms typically dissipate within first few days of antibiotic therapy or longer even though the symptoms may disappear earlier.
- Cellulitis may appear to worsen the first 24–48+ hrs despite antibiotics. This may be due to toxins and/or bacterial lysis that drive inflammation even though abx have achieved bacteriocidal effect.
- Severe cellulitis may predispose to repeat bouts; "cellulitis begets cellulitis."

OTHER INFORMATION
- (1) *S. aureus* including MRSA now the leading cause of soft tissue abscesses—easy to culture; (2) *S. pyogenes:* major cause of cellulitis and very hard to culture and (3) Gr A strep is always sensitive to penicillin which is drug of choice.
- Most common form of cellulitis—leg (tibial area) with breach in skin usually due to intertrigo.
- Usual pathogen: Gr A strep, especially if leg, perianal or buttock area; cellulitis complicating edema or lymphedema.
- Treatment—always cover Streptococci which is always sensitive to penicillins.

BASIS FOR RECOMMENDATIONS
Stevens DL, Bisno AL, Chambers HF, et al. Practice guidelines for the diagnosis and management of skin and soft-tissue infections. *Clin Infect Dis,* 2005; Vol. 41; pp. 1373–406.
Comments: Foundation for recommendations presented in this module.

FOLLICULITIS

John G. Bartlett, MD

PATHOGENS
Common pathogens:
- *S. aureus*, especially community-acquired MRSA (USA 300 strains)
- *P. aeruginosa*, associated with whirlpools, hot tubs, heated swimming pool exposures
- Pityrosporum, HIV-associated

Less common pathogens:
- Coliforms: e.g., *Klebsiella, Proteus* spp., etc.

- Demodex folliculorum, mostly HIV-associated
- Note: most HIV-associated cases of folliculitis have no clearly identified pathogen.

CLINICAL

- Exam: erythematous papules and/or pustules centered by hair follicles. Mainly on the back, buttocks, chest, neck, and thighs.
- Superficial folliculitis: superficial, fragile pustules are predominant (fewer inflammatory lesions).
- Deep folliculitis: inflammatory papules and/or nodules are predominant.
- *Staphylococcus aureus* usual cause. Usually localized and only mildly symptomatic process. Can be generalized and significantly pruritic in immunocompromised states.
- Gram-negative folliculitis: develops abruptly in individuals with acne vulgaris undergoing chronic systemic antibiotic therapy with development of very inflammatory lesions affecting the "T-zone" of the face.
- Pseudomonas folliculitis: develops 6 hrs to 3 days after swimming in inadequately chlorinated hot tubs, whirlpools and heated swimming pools.
- Drug-induced folliculitis: monomorphic lesions on head, upper trunk, and proximal upper extremities. Drugs commonly associated: corticosteroids, androgens, ACTH, lithium, isoniazid (INH), phenytoin, B-complex vitamins.
- Differential diagnosis: insect bites, papular urticaria, drug reactions, scabies, varicella, disseminated zoster, molluscum contagiosum.

DIAGNOSIS

- Usually a clinical diagnosis.
- Gram-stain, cultures, KOH prep, and saline examination recommended only when usual treatment fails, especially in immunocompromised pts.
- Eosinophilic folliculitis: histologic diagnosis where the hair follicle is permeated by multiple eosinophils. It is seen mainly in HIV-infected individuals as a very pruritic papular eruption. Its cause remains unknown and controversial. It is not the most common type of folliculitis seen in these pts.

TREATMENT

Topical therapy

- Topical route <u>preferred</u> treatment. Presumptive organism is *S. aureus.*
- Erythromycin 2% (solution, lotion, gel) twice daily.
- Clindamycin (solution, lotion, gel) twice daily.
- Mupirocin 2% cream twice daily.
- Benzoyl peroxide 2.5, 4.0, 5.0, or 10% (cream, lotion, gel, wash) daily or twice daily.
- Sodium sulfacetamide 10% lotion twice daily or Hibiclens bathing.
- Antiseptic/antibacterial soaps (e.g., Hibiclens) can be used in conjunction with above topicals. May use daily or twice daily.
- Continue treatment till complete clinical cure.
- *Pseudomonas aeruginosa* folliculitis: benzoyl peroxide cream, gel, or soap; chlorhexidine soap.

Systemic therapy

- MRSA (most common): TMP-SMX, DS PO twice daily +/– maintenance one DS tab daily or SS twice daily.
- Minocycline or doxycycline 50–100 mg PO twice daily × 2–4 wks.
- Clindamycin 300 mg PO three times a day × 7–10 days.
- Cephalexin 500 mg PO four times a day × 7–10 days (MSSA only).
- Dicloxacillin 500 mg PO four times a day × 7–10 days (MSSA only).
- Amoxicillin-clavulanate 875/125 mg PO twice daily × 7–10 days (MSSA only).
- Gram-negative rods (coliforms): TMP-SMX 1 DS PO twice daily, amoxicillin/-clavulanate 825/125 mg PO twice daily.

HIV-infected patients

- Pityrosporum: ketoconazole topical (shampoo or cream) daily or twice daily or itraconazole 100–400 mg PO daily × 2 wks.
- Demodex: permethrin topical cream qHS × 7 days or metronidazole 0.75–1% topical (lotion, cream, gel) qHS × 4–8 wks.

- Eosinophilic folliculitis: cetirizine 20–40 mg PO daily, hydroxyzine 25–50 mg PO qHS, metronidazole 250 mg PO three times a day × 3–4 wks and mid-potency (class III-IV) topical corticosteroids for inflammatory lesions.
- Phototherapy (PUVA or UVB) is effective in cases unresponsive to other treatments.

Prevention
- Cover lesions.
- Recurrent infections: mupirocin to nostrils twice daily × 5 days in *S. aureus* carriers, Hibiclens bathing daily.

FOLLOW UP

Recurrent folliculitis
- **Suggests chronic** *S. aureus* (nasal) carriage, in immunocompetent individuals.
- **Mupirocin** 2% (nasal solution or ointment) apply twice daily × 5 days. May need to repeat qmo.
- **Hibiclens topical:** use daily, bath or shower.
- **Avoid shaving.** Clean all sports equipment with disinfectant. All toweling, bedding with hot water.
- **Severe:** consider systemic therapy, e.g., TMP-SMX DS or SS PO daily. Alternative: doxycycline 100 mg PO twice daily + rifampin 300 mg PO twice daily × 7 days.

OTHER INFORMATION
- Predisposing factors: frequent shaving, occlusion (tight clothes, prosthesis), prolonged decubitus, diabetes, immunosuppression, and chronic exposure to topical corticosteroids, ointments, and greases.
- Folliculitis in HIV-infected individuals can cause intense pruritus. It usually requires a combination of multiple topical and systemic meds and recurs frequently.

BASIS FOR RECOMMENDATIONS
Author opinion.
Comments: No comprehensive guidelines exist.

FURUNCLE/CARBUNCLE

Paul G. Auwaerter, MD

PATHOGENS
- *Staphyloccocus aureus*
- Cutaneous abscesses often polymicrobial while true furuncles and carbuncles are due to *S. aureus.*

CLINICAL
- May occur in completely health individuals but risks increased with diabetes, immunocompromise, poor hygiene, elderly, staphylococcal nasal carriage, hot/tropical climate, contact with CA-MRSA carriers.
- **Furuncle:** begins at hair follicle but becomes deeper into dermis and subcutaneous tissue. Turns to a deep seated, firm, tender nodule then abscess that enlarges, becomes erythematous, painful, and fluctuant after several days.
- Most commonly affects warm, moist areas such as the neck, axillae, groin, buttocks, and thighs, but may occur anywhere on hairy skin.
- Differs from folliculitis, which remains superficial, localized to epidermis, and centered about hair follicles.
- **Carbuncle:** deeper and wider lesions with interconnecting subcutaneous abscesses arising from infection of several neighboring hair follicles. Multiple draining sinuses may develop into ulcers that heal with scarring. Carbuncles are common on the nape of the neck.
- Surrounding cellulitis and systemic symptoms including of fever and malaise may be present (more often seen with carbuncles).
- Community-acquired MRSA (CA-MRSA): now common cause of severe and recurrent furunculosis sometimes associated with cellulitis, rarely necrotizing fasciitis. Usually needs surgical drainage.
- Ddx: epidermoid ("sebaceous") cysts with cheesy material often with skin flora even if uninflamed, erythema nodosum, other forms of panniculitis, arthropod (spider) bites, hypersensitivity reactions, vasculitis, mycobacterial infections, cutaneous B- or T-cell lymphomas.

DIAGNOSIS
- Usually a clinical diagnosis, assume that entity is MRSA unless culture evidence otherwise.
- Furuncles look like a pimple or nodule that evolves into a nodule with pointing and/or draining purulent material which can be bloody. Carbuncles are larger and may have an appearance of coalescing nodules.
- Culture and sensitivity testing are usually not necessary if only routine I&D required. Obtain if planning systemic therapy (e.g., fever, associated with significant cellulitis, hospitalization), pt with significant comorbidities, occurrence on face/nose or concern for CA-MRSA outbreak.

TREATMENT
General management/topical care
- Moist heat (compresses) or hot packs used 3–4 × daily until drainage or resolution. This alone may be sufficient for small furuncles.
- Surgical incision and drainage, if possible, is MOST IMPORTANT. Necessary for large furuncles and carbuncles when fluctuation is palpable or lesions point. Evacuation of pus best with thorough probing to break loculations and remove all inflammatory material.
- Systemic antibiotics are usually unnecessary unless fever or significant surrounding cellulitis present. May consider for facial lesions or host with significant comorbidities.
- After drainage, wash area w/antiseptic/antibacterial (e.g., Hibiclens) soap. Application of Mupirocin 2% ointment twice daily may assist for resolution of superficial infection.
- Keep the area covered with gauze until wound closes.
- Topical care usually curative for single lesions not associated with cellulitis or systemic symptoms.
- CA-MRSA: most strains are sensitive to TMP-SMX, tetracyclines (minocycline, doxycycline), and clindamycin.

Systemic therapy, adult
- Indicated only in cases with associated systemic symptoms (e.g., fever), extensive cellulitis, or concern as compromised host.
- Choices often made without benefit of culture, and therefore often default to choices covering for MRSA.
- Community-acquired MRSA strains often susceptible to TMP-SMX, tetracyclines (minocycline, doxycycline), and clindamycin if oral therapy considered. Fluoroquinolone susceptibility possible but not reliable and should not be used for severe infections or without careful consideration due to potential for emergence of resistance. Oral linezolid an option, but expensive.
- **Mild-moderate (MRSA, choice provide 80–92% coverage)**: TMP-SMX DS 1–2 pills PO twice daily, doxycycline or minocycline 100 mg PO twice daily, clindamycin 300–450 mg PO q8h—follow susceptibility profile of culture and adjust if needed.
- **Severe (MRSA, providing near 100% staph coverage)**: vancomycin 15 mg/kg IV q12h, linezolid 600 mg IV/PO q12h, daptomycin 4 mg/kg IV q24 (6 mg/kg w/bacteremia), tigecycline 100 mg IV loading dose followed by 50 mg IV q12h but would avoid in bacteremia, clindamycin 600 mg IV q8h (only if known susceptible; avoid with bacteremia).
- **Mild-moderate (MSSA)**: dicloxacillin 500 mg PO four times a day, cephalexin 500 mg PO four times a day, doxycycline or minocycline 100 mg PO twice daily or clindamycin 300–450 mg PO three times a day.
- **Severe (MSSA)**: nafcillin or oxacillin 1–2 g q4h, cefazolin 1 g IV q8h, clindamycin 600 mg IV q8h.
- Unclear with mild to moderate infections (with sufficient drainage) that discordant treatment if MRSA positive leads to poor outcomes.

Recurrent furunculosis
- Treatment goal: eradicate chronic *S. aureus* carriage and potential fomite transmission. Little good clinical data to guide recommendations.
- Often described in settings of close personal contact: families, sexual partners, sports teams. Personal hygiene and contact with individuals suffering from furunculosis are important risk factors.
- Recurrent furunculosis is not thought to represent an immune deficiency in most individuals, but why some colonizers are afflicted with boils and others not is unclear. May rarely represent host immune deficiency (e.g., CGD) in some children.

- Use nasal swab to assess for *S. aureus* carriage, presence of MRSA, and guide abx selection (if necessary).
- General measures: antiseptic soaps such as chlorhexidine or hexachlorophene (apply to all intact skin, let stand for 2–5 minutes and then rinse: perform daily to several times/wk); loose-fitting clothes; frequent changes of underwear and linens; avoidance of trauma/irritation of skin, especially shaving.
- Use 10% dilute bleach to disinfect all bathroom surfaces (tub, floor, sink, toilet).
- Topical nasal carriage application: mupirocin (Bactroban) nasal, ½ tube each nares twice daily or 2% ointment twice daily × 5 days. May repeat the first 5 days of every mo. May reduce recurrence rate ~50%.
- Systemic (if above measures fail): clindamycin 150 mg PO daily × 3 mos (preferred, offers ~80% reduction in rate), TMP-SMX 1 DS PO daily × 3 mos, doxycycline 100 mg PO daily × 3 mos.
- Combination of nasal mupirocin, chlorhexidine washes, doxycycline 100 mg PO twice daily + rifampin 600 mg PO daily all for 7 days, may offer shorter course of therapy to decrease recurrent furunculosis.

OTHER INFORMATION

- Local predisposing factors (recurrent furunculosis): hyperhidrosis, poor hygiene, constant friction and pressure, ingrown hairs.
- Systemic predisposing factors (recurrent furunculosis): obesity, blood dyscrasias, malnutrition, immunodeficiency, diabetes, chronic dialysis, IV drug abuse.
- Slim data exists to guide optimal antibiotic treatment for CA-MRSA.

BASIS FOR RECOMMENDATIONS

Stevens DL, Bisno AL, Chambers HF, et al. Practice guidelines for the diagnosis and management of skin and soft-tissue infections. *Clin Infect Dis*, 2005; Vol. 41; pp. 1373–406.
Comments: IDSA recommendations that form the basis for recommendations in this module.

Author opinion.
Comments: No guidelines exist for decolonization strategies.

IMPETIGO

Paul G. Auwaerter, MD

PATHOGENS

- *Staphylococcus aureus*
- *Streptococcus pyogenes* (Group A Streptococci)

CLINICAL

- Most commonly affects children ages 2–5 yrs, but can strike at any age. Often highly contagious and associated with poor hygiene.
- *S. aureus* causes most cases followed by *S. pyogenes* sometimes in combination with *S. aureus*. Two forms: bullous and non-bullous. Bullous impetigo = almost always *S. aureus*.
- Impetigo can develop as a secondary process in lesions of eczema, scabies, herpes, etc.
- Non-bullous impetigo: single or multiple, isolated or coalescent, small, superficial pustules progressing to erosions covered by stuck-on, honey-colored crusts, surrounded by erythematous halo.
- Bullous impetigo: bullae with minimal or no inflammation. Denuded areas after the blisters rupture are covered by thin, varnish-like light brown crusts.
- Frequent regional lymphadenopathy, but impetigo usually NOT associated with systemic symptoms.
- Ddx: varicella, herpes simplex infection, atopic dermatitis, contact dermatitis, scabies, candidiasis, guttate psoriasis.
- Lab: Gram-stain of pus or base of the lesions reveal GPC. Cx and sensitivity testing indicated, especially if treatment failure, or concern for MRSA.
- Streptococcal impetigo complications: post-streptococcal acute glomerulonephritis, scarlet fever, urticaria, and erythema multiforme.

DIAGNOSIS

- Often a clinical diagnosis.
- Lab: Gram-stain and culture of pus or base of the lesions. Should reveal GPC on Gram-stain.

TREATMENT

General management

- Soften crusts with vaseline or antibiotic ointment several times/day.
- Wash individual lesions with antibacterial soap or antiseptic solution and water trying to gently remove crusts twice a day.
- Instruct the pt not to touch lesions and to wash hands frequently.
- Clip fingernails short to decrease risks of excoriation, self-inoculation, and contagion spread.
- Keep out of school until crusted lesions have healed.
- Cleanliness and prompt care of minor skin wounds such as minor cuts, abrasions, and insect bites prevents the disease.

Topical therapy

- Usually effective in treating mild and localized disease. Typically does as well as oral therapy in studies.
- Mupirocin 2% (Bactroban) ointment or cream three times a day—5 ×/day for 7 days.
- Retapamulin (Altabax) 1% ointment use twice daily to affected areas × 5 days.
- Fusidic acid another topical option, but unavailable in U.S.
- Bacitracin, neomycin compounds not recommended.
- Hydrogen peroxide ineffective.

Systemic therapy

- Indicated in cases of bullous impetigo or extensive disease +/– regional lymphadenopathy. Use antistaphylococcal penicillins or cephalosporins. May combine with topical therapy.
- Amoxicillin/clavulanate: <u>Adult</u>: 875 mg PO twice daily × 10 days. <u>Children</u>: 90 mg/kg/day in 2 divided doses × 10 days.
- Cephalexin: <u>Adult</u>: 250 mg PO four times a day. <u>Children</u>: 90 mg/kg/day divided into 2 or 4 doses PO × 10 days.
- Clindamycin: <u>Adult</u>: 300–400 mg PO three times a day. <u>Children</u>: 10–20 mg in 3 divided doses PO × 10 days.
- Erythromycin: <u>Adult</u>: 250 mg PO four times a day. <u>Children</u>: 40 mg/kg divided in 2 or 4 doses PO × 10 days.
- Dicloxacillin: <u>Adult</u>: 250 mg PO four times a day. <u>Children</u>: 12 mg/kg divided in 4 doses PO × 10 days.
- Penicillin or amoxicillin therapy is no longer recommended.

FOLLOW UP

- Cellulitis develops in approximately 10% of the cases that are not treated.
- Bullous impetigo in infants can progress to Staphylococcal scalded skin syndrome.
- In cases of frequent recurrences, suspect Staphylococcal carriage by the pt or family members.
- Improved skin hygiene most helpful for prevention.

OTHER INFORMATION

- Most common skin infection in children; highly contagious, especially w/poor hygiene and crowding (schools, day-care centers, orphanages); more common in hot and humid weather.
- Ecthyma is a form of impetigo characterized by deeper ulcer that heals with scarring.
- Unclear that therapy helps prevent streptococcal-related glomerulonephritis.

BASIS FOR RECOMMENDATIONS

Stevens DL, Bisno AL, Chambers HF, et al. Practice guidelines for the diagnosis and management of skin and soft-tissue infections. *Clin Infect Dis*, 2005; Vol. 41; pp. 1373–406.

Comments: Rationale for recommendations presented in this module.

LICE see p. 372 in Pathogen Section

MYCOBACTERIUM LEPRAE see p. 296 in Pathogen Section

ONYCHOMYCOSIS

Christopher J. Hoffmann MD, MPH

PATHOGENS
- *Trichophyton rubrum*
- *Trichophyton mentagrophytes*
- Non dermatophytes (10–20% of cases) including *Candida spp.* and soil molds

CLINICAL
- One, several, or all fingernails and/or toenails affected with fungal infection. Toenail infections are much more common.
- Separation of the nail plate(s) from the nail bed; thickening and/or destruction and/or discoloration of the nail plate(s). Accumulation of debris and keratotic material under nail(s).
- Affected nails may be tender, especially if the periungual tissue inflamed or secondarily infected by Candida (paronychia).
- Important hx: previous episodes of onychomycosis, nail trauma, tinea pedis, diabetes mellitus, HIV infection and other immunocompromised states (including medication induced and Down syndrome), hyperhidrosis, and peripheral vascular disease.
- Three common clinical presentations: (1) distal (most common, caused by fungal penetration of distal or lateral margins of nail and nail bed), (2) proximal subungual (invasion under the proximal nail fold, appearance of infection beneath nail in proximal nail bed, occurs most commonly among immunocompromised), and (3) white superficial onychomycosis (white and patchy nail discoloration of nail surface (most commonly presents in children).
- DDx: traumatic nail dystrophies (chronic trauma), psoriasis, lichen planus, contact dermatitis due to nail polish, Darier's disease (autosomal dominant disease with keratosis folliculiris, nail involvement), Reiter's syndrome, and crusted Norwegian scabies. Rare: yellow-nail syndrome, periungual squamous-cell carcinoma, and melanoma.

DIAGNOSIS
- KOH prep: subungual keratotic debris, scales from underside of affected portion of nail or nail clippings showing septated hyphae (dermatophytes) or yeasts (candida).
- Fungal cx in Sabouraud's medium of nail clippings and/or subungual scrapings is more sensitive than KOH prep.
- Nail clippings may also be submitted for histologic analysis using special stains for fungi.
- Nail biopsy should only be considered when KOH and cultures are repeatedly negative and only for obtaining additional information for ddx.
- Evidence of tinea pedis and discoloration of nails is highly predictive of onychomycosis.

TREATMENT
Systemic therapy
- Terbinafine (Lamisil) 250 mg PO qday × 6 wks (fingernails) or × 12 wks (toenails). Durable 1 yr response rate: 42–60%.
- Itraconazole (Sporanox) 100 mg PO twice daily or 200 mg PO qday × 8 wks (fingernails) or × 12 wks (toenails). <u>Pulse regimen</u>: 200 mg PO twice daily × 1 wk per mo, for 2 mos (fingernails), or 3 mos (toenails). Response rate: 32–64%.
- Fluconazole (Diflucan) 150–300 mg PO qwk × 6–12 mos (until complete normal nail growth). Response rate: 48%.
- Griseofulvin microsize caps (Grifulvin v) 750–1000 mg PO qday × 6–9 mos (fingernails) or × 12–18 mos (toenails).
- Griseofulvin ultramicrosize (Gris-PEG) 250 mg PO three times a day × 4–6 mos (fingernails) or × 8–12 mos (toenails). Response rate: 60%.

Topical therapy
- Topical medications are not usually curative. Most effective for distal onychomycosis.
- Ciclopirox 8% (Penlac) nail lacquer, apply topically twice daily × 48 wks. Response rate (1 yr): 5–20%.

- Naftifine (Naftin) gel topically twice daily.
- Urea 40% gel applied to the nails qHS in conjunction with the above topicals.

Adjuvant measures

- Clipping free and detached nail borders, filing down excessive thickness of nail plate using an emery board weekly.
- Urea 40% cream (Carmol 40) on nail under occlusion every night followed by mechanical curettage of the softened nail plate. It is important to protect the periungual tissue with tape or vaseline.
- After systemic treatment completed, pts should be encouraged to discard old shoes, especially the ones worn without socks to prevent recurrences.
- Topical antifungal powders applied to socks and shoes daily, helps decrease recurrences after successful treatment is achieved.

OTHER INFORMATION

- If using terbinafine or azoles, be wary of pre-existing liver disease and monitor for hepatoxicity (check ALT at 4–6 wks of therapy and discontinue if raised).
- More than 80% onychomycosis caused by dermatophytes, but other agents possible: *Candida albicans* and, rarely, non-dermatophyte molds such as Scopulariopsis, Acremonium, etc.
- Incidence of onychomycosis increases with old age; up to 48% of those over 70 yrs affected.
- Susceptibility to acquiring onychomycosis appears to be genetically determined. Susceptible individuals have frequent recurrences and less than optimal response to treatment.

BASIS FOR RECOMMENDATIONS

de Berker D. Clinical practice. Fungal nail disease. *N Engl J Med,* 2009; Vol. 360; pp. 2108–16.
Comments: Review of presentation, diagnosis, and management of onychomycosis.

Drake L.A., Dinehart S.M. et al. Guidelines of care for superficial mycotic infections of the skin: onychomycosis. *Guidelines of Care—Dermatology World Supplement, American Academy of Dermatology,* 1995; pp. 27–32.
Comments: Consensus of the AAD regarding diagnosis, management and follow-up of onychomycosis.

ORAL CANDIDIASIS

Paul G. Auwaerter, MD

PATHOGENS

- *Candida albicans*
- Non-albicans Candida spp [*C. parapsilosis, C. glabrata, C. tropicalis* and *C. krusei*]

CLINICAL

- Predisposing factors: age (infancy, old age), immunocompromised states (HIV, chemo Tx, corticosteroids), malignancies, head and neck radiation therapy, dentures, antibiotics, endocrine (pregnancy, diabetes), smoking, drooling, inhaled corticosteroids.
- Clinical Presentations: (1) Pseudomembranous (thrush): white curd-like plaques most commonly on the buccal mucosa, oropharynx, gingiva, and dorsum of the tongue. Easily scraped off, leaving a raw, reddish, tender patch.
- The white, curd-like material represents a mixture of yeasts, bacteria, inflammatory cells, fibrin, and desquamated epithelial cells.
- (2) Erythematous (atrophic) type: red, shiny, flat patches on the palate or dorsum of the tongue, associated with absence or decreased numbers of papillae. Also called denture stomatitis, more common in older adults.
- (3) Hyperplastic (hypertrophic) type: hard, white-yellowish plaques affecting the buccal mucosae, the sides and/or the dorsum of the tongue, resembling leukoplakia. Cannot be scrapped-off.
- (4) Angular cheilitis type (perleche): red, fissured, sometimes ulcerated crusts on the corners of the mouth. Oral mucosal involvement may or may not be seen.
- Ddx: other forms of leukoplakia (traumatic, oral hairy leukoplakia, malignant), lichen planus, geographic tongue (psoriasis), other forms of glossitis (pellagra, Moeller's).
- Risk factors associated with development of azole resistance include: non-albicans species, low CD4 counts in HIV-infected individuals, more than 5 episodes of oropharyngeal candidiasis in the past yr, chronic use of azoles.
- In HIV-infected individuals, the development of oral candidiasis is a sign of immunologic deterioration and often therapeutic failure.

DIAGNOSIS

- Esophageal candidiasis may develop with odynophagia or pain on swallowing. Esophagitis and thrush may co-exist in immunosuppressed pts, but absence of thrush does not R/O esophagitis. In HIV-infected pts *Candida* esophagitis is an AIDS defining illness.

DIAGNOSIS

- Often clinical diagnosis. If needed, KOH prep shows budding yeasts and pseudo-hyphae which are thicker and more irregularly shaped than true hyphae.
- Fungal cultures are rarely necessary for diagnosing candidal thrush, but may be needed for speciation and sensitivity testing in cases not responding to usual therapy.
- Biopsy of oral lesions may be helpful to distinguish oral leukoplakia and other erosive/ ulcerative oral lesions that may mimic some of the clinical variants of candidiasis.

TREATMENT

Topical therapy

- Preferred: clotrimazole (Mycelex) 10 mg troche, dissolve one troche slowly, without chewing 5 ×/day × 7–14 days.
- Alternatives: nystatin (Mycostatin) available as 200,000 U pastilles dosed 1 or 2 pastilles 4–5 times per day × 7–14 days or oral suspension (100,000 U/ml) 4–6 ml PO three times a day–four times a day × 7–14 days. Nystatin cream or ointment applied to inner aspects of dentures after each meal × 14 days. Bitter taste, most prefer clotrimazole.
- Angular cheilitis: nystatin/triamcinolone (Mycolog-II) cream or ointment topically qAM and qHS; clotrimazole/betamethasone (Lotrisone) cream topically qAm and qHS.
- While nystatin suspension is frequently prescribed as swish-and-swallow therapy, it is less effective than other forms of topical antifungals because the duration of tissue contact is insufficient.
- Amphotericin oral suspension no longer commercially available.
- In HIV-infected individuals without esophageal involvement and with CD4 cell counts >50, recurrences should be always be treated topically as long as this is still effective. Topical therapy should never be discontinued before 14 days.

Systemic therapy

- Recommended in cases of extensive oropharyngeal involvement with severe pain, refractory candidiasis, recurrent disease with evidence of extra oral involvement, and when compliance is a problem.
- Most data from trials in HIV-infected pts.
- Fluconazole (Diflucan) 100 mg PO once daily × 7–14 days. Some studies show superiority over topical therapy.
- Itraconazole (Sporanox) 200 mg tablet PO once daily or 200 mg suspension PO once daily × 7–14 days.
- In case the pt does not respond to systemic therapy, the first step is to repeat another 14-day course of the same medication at a higher dose (double dose is recommended). If there is still no response, culture and sensitivity testing are recommended.
- Voriconazole or posaconazole effective, but reserved for unusual cases with non-*albicans* species, suspected resistance.
- Voriconazole has not been studied for the treatment of oropharyngeal candidiasis; it has been found at least as effective as fluconazole in the treatment of Candida esophagitis (*Clin Infect Dis,* 2001 Nov 1; Vol. 33(9); pp. 1447–54.)
- Severe cases likely associated with esophageal candidiasis can be treated with azoles (fluconazole, voriconazole, posaconazole) or echinocandins (caspofungin, micafungin, anidulafungin). Amphotericin B products may be used in severe cases during pregnancy.

General comments

- Duration of treatment may range from 7 to 14 days after clinical improvement. Response can be clinical or/and mycologic. Relapse rates are lower if a mycologic cure is achieved.
- Pts who wear dentures must remove them prior to applying topical medications and must soak them in an chlorhexidine solution every night. Most commercially available denture soaking tablets are fungicidal.
- Daily oral hygiene: wash dentures with chlorhexidine 0.12% oral rinse (Peridex), allow dentures to dry completely, brush affected mucosa, oral antifungals to be used without the dentures in place.

- Angular cheilitis develops as a result of a mixed infection by Candida and Streptococci from the oral cavity. Saliva and food residues trapped in the corners of the mouth compound the problem. Pts must wash the area 2–3 ×/day after meals.

Prophylaxis
- Fluconazole works as a primary preventative measure, but not recommended due to concerns for emergence of resistance.
- If recurrences common, options for secondary prophylaxis: fluconazole 100 mg PO daily or 200 mg PO 3 ×/wk, itraconazole 200 mg PO daily or clotrimazole/nystatin daily.
- For AIDS pts, consider dapsone instead of TMP-SMX for PCP prophylaxis.

Follow Up
- Oral candidiasis is a recurring problem unless the predisposing factor is corrected.
- Immune reconstitution is highly effective at preventing recurrent thrush if secondary to AIDS.

Other Information
- Candida yeasts are part of the normal flora of certain areas of the skin, mouth, intestinal tract, and vagina. Multiple factors may cause the development of the clinical infection known as candidiasis.
- Non-albicans species of Candida have been isolated more frequently, especially in pts with advanced HIV disease. These are commonly intrinsically resistant to therapy with azole antifungals.

Basis for Recommendations
Pappas PG, Rex JH, Sobel JD, et al. Guidelines for treatment of candidiasis. *Clin Infect Dis*, 2004; Vol. 38; pp. 161–89.
Comments: IDSA recommendations, fluconazole works better in some studies but topical therapy preferred.

PARONYCHIA

Spyridon Marinopoulos, MD

Pathogens
- *Staphylococcus aureus* including community-acquired strains of MRSA (acute)
- *Streptococcus spp.* (acute)
- Anaerobes (acute)
- *Candida albicans* (chronic)
- Atypical mycobacteria (chronic)
- Gram-negative rods (chronic)

Clinical
- **Acute:** hx—tender/red perionychium +/– abscess. Rapid progression (days). PE: erythema/edema/tenderness along lateral nail fold, fluctuance (abscess). Etiology: bacterial.
- **Chronic:** hx-tenderness/edema/erythema (< than in acute), no abscess, +onycholysis. Indolent course >6 wks. PE-erythema/edema/tenderness, boggy nail fold, no fluctuance. Etiology: fungal/inflammatory/mycobacterial/GNR.
- Risk factors—**acute:** nail biting, finger sucking, mani/pedicure, hangnails, trauma/foreign body. Potential side effect of epidermal growth factor inhibitors. CHRONIC: exposure to water/irritants (bartenders, dishwashers, housekeepers), psoriasis, DM, meds.
- Ddx: felon, skin Ca (SCC/BCC/melanoma), pemphigus vulgaris, pyogenic/foreign body granuloma, wart, syphilitic chancre, Reiter's, psoriasis, herpetic whitlow, mucous cyst, subungual fibroma, leukemia cutis.

Diagnosis
- Diagnostic studies (consider for serious/refractory cases): Gram-stain, bacterial cx, KOH prep, fungal and AFB cxs, biopsy. X-ray if foreign body, trauma or suspect osteomyelitis.
- Assess for diabetes by glucose check, HgA1c.

Treatment
Topical/miscellaneous
- **All cases:** avoid irritants, manicures/pedicures, finger sucking, nail biting, exposure to moisture. Use protective gloves when necessary.
- **Acute paronychia—note:** topical abx penetrate nail plate poorly, do not use for rx of acute paronychia. Prescribe oral abx instead.

- Warm compresses/soaks w/ half-strength hydrogen peroxide or Burrow's soln (OTC aluminum acetate, Domeboro) three times a day—four times a day × 20 min may be effective.
- **Chronic paronychia—note:** topical rx first line. If ineffective, consider PO and/or surgical rx.
- Ciclopirox (Loprox) 0.77% cream to affected area twice daily × 6–12 wks (+ strict irritant avoidance) effective.
- Alternatives: betamethasone 0.05%-clotrimazole 1% (Lotrisone) cream to affected area twice daily × 2–4 wk.
- Miconazole (Monistat-Derm) 2% cream twice daily to nail folds until resolved.
- Econazole (Spectazole) 1% cream once daily to nail folds until resolved.
- **Note:** if caused by meds—(leading causes could include indinavir, lamivudine, isotretinoin)—d/c meds and reassess.

Oral antibiotics

- **Note:** mixed infections common in paronychia; cx may help determine appropriate rx.
- **Acute paronychia:** PO abx alone not sufficient if abscess present; I&D required. Most authorities support use of PO abx even w/adequate I&D.
- Preferred: amoxicillin-clavulanate 500 mg PO three times a day or 875 mg twice daily × 7 days or until infection resolves.
- Preferred (PCN allergy): clindamycin 300 mg PO q6h × 7 days or until infection resolves.
- Alternative (ineffective if anaerobes suspected): dicloxacillin 250–500 mg PO four times a day or cephalexin (Keflex) 500 mg PO q6h × 7 days or until infection resolves.
- **Acute paronychia** (CA-MRSA suspected): trimethoprim-sulfamethoxazole 1DS (160 mg/800 mg) PO q12h or clindamycin 300–450 mg PO q6h +/– rifampin 600 mg PO once daily. Alternatives: minocycline 100 mg PO q12h or doxycycline 100 mg PO q12h.
- Rx duration 10–14 days although rx for 2 or 3 wks may be needed in severe cases or vulnerable hosts. Tailor rx to c+s results.
- **Chronic paronychia** (PO second line, use topical rx first): fluconazole 100–200 mg PO qwk until normal nail anatomy restored.
- Alternatives: itraconazole (Sporanox) 200 mg PO twice daily × 1 wk × 3 consecutive mos or terbinafine (Lamisil) 250 mg PO once daily × 3 mos.
- **Chronic paronychia + suspected bacterial superinfection:** Add abx as in acute paronychia.

Surgical

- **Note:** consult hand surgeon if cellulitis, deep space infection, glomus tumor, mucous cyst, or osteomyelitis suspected.
- **Acute paronychia:** I&D necessary if abscess and no drainage w/soaks alone. Use anesthesia (digital block/ethyl chloride spray) unless skin yellow/white (infarcted nerve endings).
- Insert #11 surgical blade under affected cuticle margin and extend incision along lateral nail bed. Keep blade directed away from nail plate to avoid permanent nail growth abnormalities. (see http://jaapa.com/issues/j20021101/articles/procfamparonych.html for further details)
- Alternative (superficial abscess): run large gauge needle along nail into abscess (no need for local anesthesia).
- Continue frequent warm soaks after I&D to assist wound drainage.
- Follow up in 48 hrs to remove packing, irrigate area and reevaluate wound.
- **Note:** if **subungual abscess** (pus under nailbed), I&D alone not sufficient; must remove entire nail plate.
- **Note:** I&D not indicated for herpetic whitlow, mucous cyst, glomus tumor, osteomyelitis (all may be confused for paronychia).
- **Chronic paronychia** (conservative rx ineffective): refer hand surgeon for eponychial marsupialization (excision of 3 mm wide crescent-shaped piece of skin/thickened tissue from eponychium).
- Alternative: remove entire nail and apply antifungal-steroid ointment—i.e., betamethasone 0.05%-clotrimazole 1% (Lotrisone)—to affected area twice daily × 2–4 wks.

OTHER INFORMATION

- Recommendations are author's opinion. If no response to rx in 4–5 days, cx, bx +/– refer to hand surgeon. Complications: nail loss, osteomyelitis, flexor tendon septic tenosynovitis, felon.
- Think felon if pain/erythema/edema in pad of fingertip. Refer to hand surgeon for urgent I&D to prevent osteomyelitis, permanent nail deformity, ischemic necrosis of fingertip.

- Think CA if irregular border/surrounding tissue w/ irregular appearance. Think melanoma if brown/black nail lines and subungual pain. Refer to dermatology for bxp.
- Think mucous cyst if painless edema lateral to nail plate in pt w/ OA. Think glomus tumor if constant severe pain w/ nail plate elevation/bluish discoloration and blurring of lunula. Refer hand surgeon.
- Think herpetic whitlow if vesicles, ulceration, crusting, intense pain. Tzanck smear: multinucleated giant cells. I&D contraindicated (risks hematogenous viral dissemination). Rx HSV.

BASIS FOR RECOMMENDATIONS

Rigopoulos D, Larios G, Gregoriou S, et al. Acute and chronic paronychia. *Am Fam Physician*, 2008; Vol. 77; pp. 339–46.
Comments: Pathophysiology and treatment options for acute and chronic paronychia are presented.

SARCOPTES SCABIEI VAR. HOMINIS (SCABIES) see p. 373 in Pathogen Section

TINEA CAPITIS/TINEA BARBAE

Christopher J. Hoffmann MD, MPH

PATHOGENS
- *Trichophyton tonsurans*
- *Microsporum canis*
- *Trichophytin verrucosum*

CLINICAL
- **Tinea capitis:** single or multiple scaly and/or crusted patches and/or plaques, most often associated with alopecia affecting the scalp or beard area +/– inflammation. Either inflammatory or non-inflammatory presentation.
- Non-inflammatory: hairs may have a dull-grey color, break off easily and when close to the scalp surface, may appear as "black dots." Scaling is usually seen, but papules and pustules are rare.
- Inflammatory: erythematous edematous plaques with follicular papules, pustules, nodules, oozing, and crusting resembling a pyoderma. Hairs become loose and fall off in a patchy or matted pattern.
- Clinical patterns: gray type (circular patterns of alopecia and scaling), moth-eaten (patchy alopecia with generalized scaling), kerion (inflammatory boggy area with pustules, lymphadenopathy, usually caused by *M. canis*; can lead to permanent scarring), black dot (patches of alopecia dotted with broken hair), diffuse scale (widespread, scaling), pustular type (alopecia with scattered pustules), favus (cup-shaped yellowish crusts surround affected hairs causing matted hair loss and musty odor).
- Lymphadenopathy seen in inflammatory types of tinea, even when secondary bacterial infection is absent.
- **Tinea barbae:** similar to tinea capitis, but affects hair follicles of the beard and mustache areas. It is usually caused by zoophilic dermatophytes, commonly *Trichophyton verrucosum* and seen more commonly in farmers and animal handlers.
- Affected individuals can simultaneously develop an "id" or hypersensitivity reaction to the fungal infection characterized by inflammatory papules or an eczematous reaction at a distant site, more commonly trunk, hands or feet (can also occurs with other tinea infections).
- History: exposure to animals, contact with other persons with tinea capitis or other dermatophyte fungal infections and recent travel abroad.
- Differential diagnosis includes: seborrheic dermatitis, psoriasis of the scalp, trichotillomania (compulsive hair pulling), alopecia areata, atopic dermatitis, and bacterial scalp folliculitis.

DIAGNOSIS
- Wood's light examination may show a characteristic blue-green fluorescence depending on the fungus present. *T. tonsurans*, the most common agent in the U.S., does not fluoresce under this light.

DIAGNOSIS

45

- KOH prep performed on scales from the scalp and plucked hairs (use cytobrush or toothbrush) may show hyphae and spores of dermatophytes which can be seen inside the shaft (endothrix) or outside the hair cuticle (ectothrix).
- Fungal culture of scales (cotton swab, brush—can use cytobrush or sterile toothbrush) and plucked/clipped hairs from the affected area is more sensitive than KOH prep, but results take much longer. Speciation of the fungus is important.
- Bacterial culture is usually recommended in inflammatory lesions to rule out a secondary infection or a primary pyoderma of the scalp.
- Biopsy is only indicated when KOH prep and cultures are repeatedly negative.
- Accurate diagnosis is important prior to initiating a long-term course of systemic antifungal therapy.
- Culture is important for assessing refractory cases.

TREATMENT

Systemic therapy

- **Griseofulvin** children: 15–20 mg/kg/day 8 wks for (8–10 wks in *M. canis* infections). Adults: 375 mg (ultramicrosize) or 500 mg (Grifulvin V or microsized) PO qday × 4–6 wks.
- **Terbinafine** (Lamisil) children: 62.5 mg PO qday <20 kg, 125 mg PO qday for children 20–40 kg × 4 wks. Adults and children >40 kg: 250 mg PO qday × 4 wks.
- **Itraconazole** (Sporanox) children: 5 mg/kg PO qday or 100 mg PO qday × 2–4 wks for children. Adults: 200–300 mg PO once daily × 2–4 wks. Pulse regimen: 3–5 mg PO once daily (child) or 200 mg PO qday (adult) × 1 wk repeated × 1–2 mos.
- **Fluconazole** children: 6 mg/kg/day × 20 days or 6–8 mg/kg/wk once a wk × 4–8 wks.

Adjunctive therapy

- Ketoconazole (Nizoral) 2% shampoo: apply to scalp and rinsed off after 5–10 minutes every other day for the duration of the oral therapy.
- Selenium sulfide 2.5% shampoo or lotion: use on scalp and rinse off after 5–10 minutes every other day for the duration of the oral therapy.
- Contagion may occur through fomites, therefore special caution should be taken with brushes, combs, towels, etc.
- Asymptomatic carrier state is common among personal contacts of individuals affected by *T. tonsurans*, therefore they should be treated with shampoos such as ketoconazole 2% or selenium sulfide 2.5%.

OTHER INFORMATION

- Tinea capitis is the most common fungal infection in school-age children. It is less frequent in infants and adolescents and very rare in adults.
- Tinea capitis has a worldwide distribution. In the United States, the most common etiologic agent is *Trichophyton tonsurans*, which is responsible for >90% of the cases in urban areas.

BASIS FOR RECOMMENDATIONS

Drake L.A., Dinehart S.M et al. Guidelines of care for superficial mycotic infections of the skin: tinea capitis and tinea barbae. *American Academy of Dermatology Guidelines of Care, Dermatology World Supplement*, 1995.

Comments: Official guidelines of the American Academy of Dermatology on the diagnosis and management of tinea capitis and tinea barbae.

TINEA CORPORIS/TINEA CRURIS

Christopher J. Hoffmann MD, MPH

PATHOGENS

- Tinea corporis and tinea cruris are fungal infections of the stratum corneum and terminal hair shaft caused by certain species of dermatophytes (genera Epidermophyton, Microsporum, Trichophyton)
- *Trichophyton rubrum*
- *T. mentagrophytes*
- *T. tonsurans*
- *T. violaceum* (Africa, India)
- *Microsporum canis*
- *Epidermophyton floccosum*

CLINICAL

- Typical presentation: annular erythematous plaque with raised leading edge and scaling clearance at center of lesion with scattered nodules (note: scrotum is usually spared with tinea cruris).
- Atypical: erythematous papules, series of vesicles, ill-defined borders, papular. Zoophilic *Trichophyton verrucosum* can cause intense inflammatory reactions with pustular lesions. Atypical lesions are most common among immunocompromised pts.
- Important history: (a) current and previous topical and/or systemic treatment, (b) occupational exposure (veterinarian, zookeeper, lab worker, farmer, pet shop worker), (c) environmental exposure (gardening, pets, contact sports, locker rooms, gyms, affected family members), (d) prior hx of dermatophyte infection.
- Pruritus is usually present, especially in tinea cruris. Pain varies with intensity of inflammation or secondary bacterial infection.

DIAGNOSIS

- Ddx tinea cruris: erythrasma (caused by *Corynebacterium minutissimum*, coral fluorescence under Wood's light), Darier's disease (genetic disease), cutaneous candidiasis, figurate erythemas, contact dermatitis.
- Ddx tinea corporis: impetigo, nummular dermatitis, asteatotic eczema, psoriasis, parapsoriasis, secondary syphilis.
- Laboratory confirmation is particularly important if systemic therapy is anticipated.
- KOH prep of scales obtained from the active border is positive for septated hyphae of dermatophytes.
- Cultures in dermatophyte-specific media are more sensitive, but not as practical (may take 1–4 wks for growth).

TREATMENT

Topical

- Recommended for localized, uncomplicated non-inflammatory lesions.
- Terbinafine 1% (Lamisil) cream once daily × 3–4 wks.
- Naftifine 1% (Naftin) cream qday, gel twice daily × 2–4 wks.
- Econazole 1% (Spectazole) cream daily or twice daily × 2–4 wks.
- Ketoconazole 2% (Nizoral) cream, shampoo daily or twice daily × 2–4 wks.
- Clotrimazole 1% (Lotrimin, Mycelex) cream, lotion, solution twice daily × 2–4 wks.
- Oxiconazole 1% (Oxistat) cream, lotion four times daily × 2–4 wks.
- Miconazole 2% (Monistat-Derm, Micatin) cream, powder, spray twice daily × 2–4 wks.
- Sulconazole 1% (Exelderm) cream, solution daily or twice daily × 3–4 wks.
- Ciclopirox 1% (Loprox) cream twice daily × 2–4 wks.
- Tolnaftate 1% (Tinactin) cream, gel, powder, spray twice daily × 2–4 wks.

Topical Therapy with Corticosteroids

- Severe inflammatory lesions can be treated with a combination topical anti-fungal and steroid.
- Clotrimazole-betamethasone (Lotrisone) cream twice daily × 2–3 wks (can also use separate topical fungal and steroid creams).

Systemic

- Indications: failure of adequate topical therapy, intolerance to topical medications, extensive and/or disabling, multifocal or inflammatory disease, deeper infection with hair follicle involvement.
- Before selecting a systemic antifungal drug, make sure to check the potential drug-drug interactions.
- Periodic monitoring of liver function tests and CBC prior to and during systemic therapy if duration of treatment is longer than 4 wks.
- Combination topical corticosteroid/antifungal mixtures can be used in selected cases and for a short period of time only.
- Terbinafine (Lamisil) 250 mg PO daily × 2–4 wks.
- Itraconazole (Sporanox) 200 mg PO daily × 2–4 wks or 200 mg twice daily × 7 days.
- Fluconazole 50–100 mg PO daily or 150 mg once weekly × 2–3 wks. Alt:

DIAGNOSIS

- Alt: ketoconazole (Nizoral) 200 mg PO daily × 2–4 wks.
- Griseofulvin microsize (Grifulvin V) 500 mg PO daily, or griseofulvin ultramicrosize (Gris-Peg) 375 mg PO daily × 2–4 wks.

General measures

- Avoidance of tight fitting clothes/underwear.
- Drying agents such as aluminum acetate or diluted acetic acid solutions may be used as soaks 3–4 × daily on intertriginous areas when maceration and oozing are present.
- If secondary bacterial infection is suspected, obtain bacterial cultures and start adequate oral antibiotic coverage.
- Avoidance and proper treatment of infected animals/people.

FOLLOW UP

- Recurrences are common, especially in tinea cruris. This may be due to premature discontinuation of topical therapy when the symptoms subside after a few days.
- Recurrent, extensive and unresponsive dermatophyte infections suggest an underlying systemic disease. Ruling out HIV infection is mandatory in these cases.

OTHER INFORMATION

- Predisposition to acquiring a dermatophyte infection varies significantly. Not every exposed individual will acquire it, even in cases of prolonged and intimate contact with infected persons.
- Peak prevalence of dermatophyte infections of the skin occurs after puberty. This is especially true for Tinea pedis, tinea manuum, and tinea cruris. Tinea corporis and tinea faciei can occur in pre-pubertal populations.
- Dermatophytoses can significantly decrease quality of life of affected individuals. This is especially true in cases of tinea cruris due to the intense pruritus associated.
- Topical steroids cause decrease of inflammation and apparent clinical improvement, but if used alone or for a long period of time, it may cause the infection to spread to deeper layers and hair follicles producing granulomatous inflammation (Majocchis granuloma).

BASIS FOR RECOMMENDATIONS

Smith EB. The treatment of dermatophytosis: safety considerations. *J Am Acad Dermatol*, 2000; Vol. 43; pp. S113–9.

Comments: Hepatitis is a possible risk with all oral antifungal agents, with the highest risk noted for ketoconazole.

Lesher JL. Oral therapy of common superficial fungal infections of the skin. *J Am Acad Dermatol*, 1999; Vol. 40; pp. S31–4.

Comments: After extensive review of the available literature, it was found that tinea corporis and tinea cruris were successfully treated by 50 to 100 mg fluconazole daily or 150 mg once weekly for 2 to 3 wks, by 100 mg itraconazole daily for 2 wks or 200 mg daily for 1 wk, and by 250 mg terbinafine daily for 1–2 wks.

TINEA PEDIS

Christopher J. Hoffmann MD, MPH

PATHOGENS

- *Trichophyton rubrum*
- *Trichophyton mentagrophytes*
- Rare: *Epidermophyton floccosum, Candida, Acremonium, Fusarium*

CLINICAL

- Three general presentations: all spare the dorsum, may cause pruritis and hyperhidrosis.
- (1) Interdigital: mildly erythematous plaques with peripheral scaling and fissures, especially common in the 3rd and 4th web spaces, may be pruritic or asymptomatic (more often *T. rubrum*).
- (2) Moccasin-style: often asymptomatic, fine powdery scaling plaques with mildly erythematous base on heels, soles and lateral aspects of the feet (more often *T. rubrum*).
- (3) Vesiculobullous: vesicles/bullae, may have purulent exudate, typically on the instep, usually intensely pruritic (more often *T. mentagrophytes*).
- Can trigger an "id" reaction on the hands characterized by the appearance of multiple, very pruritic, minute deep seated vesicles on the fingers and palms. This may progress to a chronic phase resembling hand eczema.

- Gram-negative toe web infection is a common complication of macerated and fissured interdigital tinea pedis and is characterized by malodorous purulent discharge associated with significant pain.
- Complications: if left untreated, chronic tinea pedis may cause the development of onychomycosis (20% of pts with *Tinea pedis* have subclinical onychomycosis).
- Risk of lower extremity cellulitis increases approximately two-fold (especially interdigital form).

DIAGNOSIS

- Differential diagnosis: contact dermatitis, psoriasis, atopic dermatitis, erythrasma, intertrigo, palmo-plantar keratoderma.
- Lab: KOH prep of scales or vesicle roof shows septated hyphae of dermatophytes. Wood's lamp examination of the interdigital spaces may be helpful to rule out erythrasma (coral fluorescence).
- Fungal culture may be helpful in cases when KOH prep is repeatedly negative, which is not uncommon in inflammatory cases. Speciation does not influence the therapeutic decisions. Skin biopsy is only recommended when other dermatoses need to be ruled out.

TREATMENT

Topical therapy

- Preferred approach for most cases. Duration of treatment usually 2–4 wks.
- Terbinafine 1% (Lamisil) cream apply daily × 2 wks.
- Naftifine 1% (Naftin) cream daily, gel twice daily × 2 wks.
- Butenafine (Mentax) cream twice daily × 2 wks.
- Ketoconazole 2% (Nizoral), cream twice daily × 3–6 wks.
- Tolnaftate 1% (Tinactin) cream, gel, powder, spray twice daily × 3–4 wks.
- Clotrimazole 1% (Lotrimin) preparation twice daily × 2–4 wks.
- Econazole 1% (Spectazole) daily × 4 wks.
- In hyperkeratotic tinea pedis, systemic therapy may yield superior results over topical preparations.

Systemic therapy

- Consider for severe cases. Procure with culture confirmation, especially in cases of topical failure.
- In hyperkeratotic tinea pedis, systemic therapy may yield superior results over topical preparations.
- Terbinafine (Lamisil) 250 mg PO daily × 2 wks.
- Fluconazole 150 mg PO qwk × 4 wks.
- Griseofulvin ultramicrosize (Gris-Peg) 375 mg PO twice daily or griseofulvin microsize (Grifulvin V) 500 mg PO twice daily × 4–8 wks.

Adjunctive therapies

- Keratolytic agents such as urea 20–40% (Carmol cream) or salicylic acid 3–5% preparations can be used in cases with severe hyperkeratosis of the soles.
- Drying agents such as aluminum acetate, potassium permanganate or diluted acetic acid can be used as soaking solutions twice daily in cases of wet interdigital tinea and in cases of Gram-negative bacterial toe web infection.
- Topical or systemic corticosteroids may be needed in cases of extensive or severe inflammatory tinea pedis.
- Topical or systemic antibiotics are needed in cases of secondary Gram-negative toe web infection.
- Topical antifungals used in conjunction with systemic antifungals may speed mycologic cure.

Prophylaxis

- To prevent infection/recurrences consider behavioral changes.
- Correction of hyperhidrosis.
- Wearing absorbent socks.
- Thorough drying of the toes after showers.
- Use of an antifungal powder applied to feet, socks, and shoes regularly.

FOLLOW UP

- Some studies suggest that use of corticosteroids in addition to antifungals lead to higher failure rates or persistent infection [Alston, *Peds* 2003;111:201–203].

- Recurrences common, especially with immunocompromised pts.
- Long-term application may be required in pts who experience frequent recurrences.

OTHER INFORMATION
- Epidemiology: 5–50% of population has tinea pedis. Prevalence is higher among manual laborers, athletes and older ages.
- Tinea pedis caused by *T. rubrum* is more persistent, recalcitrant to therapy and recurrences occur in up to 70% of cases.
- Most tinea is caused by *T. rubrum* (75%). However, among athletes, *T. mentagrophytes* is more common.

BASIS FOR RECOMMENDATIONS
Drake L.A., Dinehart S.M. et. al. Guidelines of care for superficial mycotic infections of the skin: tinea corporis, tinea cruris, tinea faciei, tinea manuum and tinea pedis. *Dermatology World—American Academy of Dermatology, Guidelines of Care,* 1995; pp. 22–6.
Comments: Standard of care according to the guidelines from the American Academy of Dermatology Guidelines/ Outcomes Committee on the diagnosis and management of tinea pedis.

TINEA VERSICOLOR

Christopher J. Hoffmann MD, MPH

PATHOGENS
- *Malassezia furfur* (Pityrosporum ovale)
- *Malassezia globosa*
- *Malassezia symphodialis*
- *Malassezia silffiae*

CLINICAL
- Tinea versicolor is a superficial infection of the stratum corneum caused by a yeast that is part of the normal cutaneous flora in 90–100% of individuals, therefore it is not a contagious process. The pathogenesis may occur when the round yeast form changes to a mycelial form and invades the stratum corneum.
- Malassezia spp. grow in lipid-rich environments, thus the distribution in sebum-rich areas and the patterns of presentation during adolescence.
- Rash is usually asymptomatic, but may be mildly to moderately pruritic.
- Hypopigmented and/or hyperpigmented scaly patches (non-elevated or minimally elevated) affecting mainly the trunk, neck, and proximal extremities (sebum-rich areas).
- Lesions are usually multiple, small, round, or oval, in shape or coalescent into large, irregularly shaped patches.
- Differential diagnosis includes: pityriasis rosea, seborrheic dermatitis, vitiligo, pityriasis alba, secondary syphilis, hypopigmented variant of cutaneous T-cell lymphoma, and Hansens disease.
- Hyperpigmented lesions can mimic confluent and reticulated papillomatosis, which will be KOH negative and responds to minocycline
- Associations with Tinea versicolor: topical climate/warm weather, malnutrition, oral contraceptives, systemic corticosteroids and other immunosuppressants, hyperhidrosis.

DIAGNOSIS
- Woods lamp examination aids in revealing the true extent of involvement by showing yellowish fluorescence of the lesions (only some Malassezia spp fluoresce, florescence in only 1/3 of cases; thus limited sensitivity, but highly specific).
- KOH prep of scales show short, stubby, blunt-ended interlaced hyphae with clusters of spores and yeast cells ("spaghetti and meat balls" appearance).
- Fungal cultures are not required for diagnosis or management of the disease. Growth of the yeast in cultures requires special media.
- Skin biopsy is not recommended unless KOH preps are repeatedly negative and other dermatoses need to be ruled out.

TREATMENT
Topical therapy
- Topical therapy alone is indicated as first line regimen and is effective in most cases.

- Selenium sulfide 2.5% (Selsun), ketoconazole (Nizoral), or zinc pyrithione shampoo scrubbed onto the affected areas using a mildly abrasive sponge and rinsed off in 3–5 minutes daily × 1 wk or every other day × 2 wks.
- Selenium sulfide 2.5% lotion applied to the affected areas and rinsed-off after 10 minutes daily × 7 days or left overnight and rinsed off in the morning as a single application (repeat in 1 wk).
- Econazole 1% (Spectazole), ketoconazole 2% (Nizoral), clotrimazole 1% (Lotrimin), oxiconazole 1% (Oxistat), miconazole 2% (Micatin), sulconazole 1% Exelderm) cream, lotion or solution, all once daily × 1–2 wks.
- Terbinafine (Lamisil) 1% spray or cream or butenafine 1% cream (Mentax) daily × 1–2 wks.
- Ciclopirox 1% (Loprox) cream qday × 1–2 wks.
- Miscellaneous: benzoyl peroxide 5–10% lotion, gel, cream, or wash; sulfur and salicylic acid preparations; propylene glycol 50% solution; sodium thiosulfate 25% with salicylic acid 1%, all applied qday × 1–2 wks.

Systemic therapy
- Oral treatment is recommended in cases with extensive involvement, with frequent recurrences, when topical treatment failed or when pt is sensitive to or unable to apply topical medications.
- Topical medications can be used in association with systemic treatment
- Ketoconazole 400 mg PO single dose repeated in 1 wk or 200 mg PO qday × 7–10 days.
- Fluconazole 300 mg PO single dose, repeated in 1 wk.
- Itraconazole 200 mg PO qday × 7 days.
- Exercise with sweating 2 hrs after taking the oral medication improves drug delivery to the skin. Showers should be avoided for 12 hrs.

Prophylaxis
- Prophylaxis of recurrences is recommended for susceptible individuals in the spring and summer months.
- Easily accomplished by using one of the recommended shampoos as a body wash weekly.

FOLLOW UP
- Residual pigmentary changes (hypo- or hyperpigmentation) may persist even after the process is completely treated. Skin color returns to normal shade gradually after subsequent sun exposures.

OTHER INFORMATION
- Recurrences are common, especially in warmer weather—summer months.

BASIS FOR RECOMMENDATIONS
Drake LA, Dinehart SM, et al. Guidelines of care for superficial mycotic infections of the skin: pityriasis (tinea) versicolor. *Dermatology World, American Academy of Dermatology,* 1995; pp. 36–8.
Comments: Guidelines of care and recommendations from the AAD's Guidelines and Outcomes Committee for diagnosis and management of superficial fungal infections.

WARTS (NON-GENITAL)

Christopher J. Hoffmann MD, MPH

PATHOGENS
- HPV 1: palmar and plantar warts (Verruca plantaris)
- HPV 2,4: common warts (Verruca vulgaris)
- HPV 3,10: flat warts (Verruca plana)
- HPV 5: squamous cell carcinoma in EV
- HPV 3,5,8: Epidermodysplasia verruciformis (EV)
- HPV 16: digital squamous cell carcinoma

CLINICAL
- Etiology: human papillomaviruses (HPV), diverse group of non-enveloped, ds DNA tumor viruses. At least 130 genotypes have been identified. HPV typing not recommended.
- Infection occurs through personal contact or fomites.
- Common warts: exophytic, hard, rough papules; may coalesce to form larger plaques. Black dots (thrombosed capillaries) may be seen.

- Plantar warts: thick, usually flat, endophytic, yellowish colored rough plaques. Black dots may also be seen. Pain may be present. May resemble calluses.
- Other variants: flat warts (minimally elevated, usually light-colored, small papules), filiform warts (pedunculated, firm papules, often with finger-like projections; may resemble a small "horn").
- Natural hx: >60% resolve spontaneously in <2 yrs due to natural immunity, lower rates of resolution among immunocompromised.

DIAGNOSIS
- Diagnosis: clinical examination in most instances.
- Histopathology (biopsy) in atypical cases.

TREATMENT
General
- Many treatments and most RCTs of limited value. Response to placebo around 30–50%, to intervention 30–80%.

Verruca vulgaris (common warts)
- Salicylic acid (OTC 17% or higher % by prescription). File wart with pumice or emory board, soak in warm water, apply compound to wart. Repeat daily for days to weeks.
- Cryotherapy q3–4wks followed by OTC salicylic acid plasters and/or paring of lesions.
- Trichloroacetic Acid (TCA, 70–90%) applied by the physician preceded by paring of lesions qwk or q2wks.
- 5-fluorouracil cream (5%) applied under occlusion qHS; local irritation common.
- Sensitization in the office with 2% squaric Acid (SADBE) followed by application of 0.2% to warts, 2 wks later.
- Cantharidin (blister beetle extract) applied by physician q3–4wks.
- Imiquimod cream qHS × 4–6 wks.
- Intralesional injection of 1% cidofovir or bleomycin in extensive, recalcitrant cases.

Verruca palmares et plantares (plantar warts)
- Salicylic acid (OTC 17% or higher % by prescription, higher % likely more effective) File wart with pumice or emory board, soak in warm water, apply compound to wart. Repeat daily for days to weeks.
- Regular paring and use of keratolytic plasters between visits is critical to ensure treatment success.
- Combination modalities help to increase therapeutic success rates.
- Combination 1: cryotherapy followed by patient-applied imiquimod under occlusion (duct tape) qhs.
- Combination 2: cryotherapy followed by patient-applied podophyllotoxin cream or gel under occlusion (duct tape) qhs.
- Combination 3: 5 fluoro-uracil cream every other evening alternating with imiquimod cream on other evenings under occlusion (duct tape).

Peri-ungual verruca
- Verrucae around the nail are often recalcitrant to treatment and often cause nail dystrophy.
- Topical therapies often do not get under the nail fold.
- Laser therapy with Flashlamp pulsed dye (585 nm) may be effective.
- Squaric acid (SADBE) sensitization, cidofovir, or bleomycin injections are alternatives.

FOLLOW UP
- Intact cell-mediated immunity appears critical to eradication of HPV by host.
- Defects in cell-mediated immunity make treatment more difficult and strict pt compliance is required for HPV containment.

OTHER INFORMATION
- High concentrations of trichloroacetic acid may cause permanent scarring.
- Podophyllin and podophyllotoxin are **teratogenic**.

BASIS FOR RECOMMENDATIONS
Gibbs S, Harvey I. Topical treatments for cutaneous warts. *Cochrane Database Syst Rev,* 2006; Vol. 3; Vol. CD001781.
Comments: Cochrane review of RCTs for wart removal. Although cryotherapy is often thought to be the most effective method for dealing with warts (and among the most expensive), there is not enough evidence to truly support this notion as the initial treatment for cutaneous viral warts.

CONJUNCTIVITIS, ACUTE

Spyridon Marinopoulos, MD

PATHOGENS
- *Haemophilus influenzae*
- *Neisseria gonorrhoeae*
- *Chlamydophila trachomatis*
- *Staphylococcus aureus*
- Adenovirus
- HSV
- VZV
- Picornavirus

CLINICAL
- Allergic: IgE response to environment allergens. Hx: bilateral redness, watery d/c, itching (hallmark), worse with rubbing. PE: diffuse injection, watery/mucoserous discharge, indistinguishable from viral.
- Bacterial: Hx/PE: uni/bilateral redness. Thick, globular, purulent white, yellow, or green d/c at lid margin/eye corners. Eye stuck shut in AM. If tender preauricular LN, think GC/chlamydia.
- Rapidly progressive redness, hyperpurulence, tenderness, lid edema and tender preauricular LN suggest gonococcal hyperacute bacterial conjunctivitis. Lab: pus w/ Gram-negative diplococci.
- Viral: Hx: thin, watery/mucoserous rather than purulent discharge. +/– viral URI. Burning, sandy or gritty feeling common. PE: diffuse conjunctival injection and profuse tearing +/– preauricular LN. Most commonly caused by adenovirus.
- HSV: red, irritated, watery eye often accompanied by multiple vesicles on eyelid, but may also involve face. Eyelid edema and ulcers may be present. May involve cornea.
- VZV (herpes zoster ophthalmicus): severe pain and skin lesions in dermatomal pattern involving the ophthalmic division of the trigeminal nerve. Conjunctival injection, redness, and serous or purulent discharge. Preauricular adenopathy common. Constitutional sx include fever, malaise, nausea, and vomiting.
- Epidemic keratoconjunctivitis (EKC): highly contagious, fulminant-type, viral conjunctivitis. Presents w/ severe foreign-body sensation and decreased visual acuity.
- Acute hemorrhagic conjunctivitis (AHC): epidemic form of highly contagious conjunctivitis characterized by sudden onset of painful, swollen, red eyes, with conjunctival hemorrhaging and excessive tearing. Caused by picornavirus. Rx symptomatic. Disease course 5–7 days. Almost always resolves without sequelae.

DIAGNOSIS
- Conjunctival scrapings or cultures (bacterial/viral) are generally not needed except in resistant cases, hyperpurulent or fulminant cases, or recurrent disease. Gonococcal disease is most commonly diagnosed by Gram-stain which shows characteristic Gram-negative intracellular diplococci. Chlamydia is most commonly diagnosed by DFA (Direct Fluorescent Antibody) staining of conjunctival smears.
- DDx subconjunctival hemorrhage, blepharitis, eyelid disorders, scleritis, episcleritis, keratitis, pterygium, acute anterior uveitis, acute angle closure glaucoma.

TREATMENT
Topical Antibiotics
- Comment: use for bacterial conjunctivitis. All doses while awake. Ointments may blur vision × 20 min post administration. Must use systemic abx for gonorrheal/chlamydial disease.
- Trimethoprim-polymyxin B (Polytrim) sol 1 gtt q3h × 7–10 days.
- Bacitracin-polymyxin B (Polysporin) ophthalmic 1 gtt q3–4h × 7–10 days.

- Sulfacetamide (Bleph-10) 10% sol 1–2 gtt q2–3h × 7–10 days, taper to twice daily with improvement. Some staph strains may be resistant.
- Erythromycin ophthalmic oint 1/2-in four times a day inside lower lid × 5–7 days. Some staph strains may be resistant.
- Fluoroquinolones: use for more serious cases, especially if suspected Pseudomonas (contact lens wearers) or corneal ulcers exist.
- Levofloxacin (Quixin) 0.5% sol 1–2 gtt q2h × 2 days then 1–2 gtt four times a day × 5 days or ofloxacin (Ocuflox) 0.3% sol 1–2 gtt q2–4h × 2 days then 1–2 gtt four times a day × 5 days or Cipro (Ciloxan) 0.3% sol 1–2 gtt q2h × 2 days then 1–2 gtt q4h × 5 days.
- Bacitracin-neomycin-polymyxin B (Neosporin Ophthalmic) sol 1–2 gtt q4h × 7–10 days. Up to 10% pts allergic to neomycin.
- Tobramycin (Tobrex) 0.3% sol 1–2 gtt q4h × 7 days or gentamicin (Garamycin, Genoptic) 0.3% sol 1–2 gtt q4h × 7 days.
- **Avoid:** chloramphenicol (Chloroptic) 0.5% sol 1–2 gtt 4–6 ×/day × 3 days, use only if no other options avail. Bone marrow aplasia with prolonged/frequent use has resulted in death.

Systemic Antibiotics

- Comment: in pts with gonococcal disease, treat sexual partners and consider/treat chlamydial co-infection. Vice versa for pts w/ chlamydial conjunctivitis. Also consider/screen for other STDs.
- Hyperacute bacterial conjunctivitis (*Neisseria gonorrhoeae*): ceftriaxone 1 g IM × 1 dose effective. Some reports advocate Rx q24h × 7 days.
- Alternative for pen/ceph allergic pts: spectinomycin 2 g IM × 1 dose (currently unavailable in U.S.) or see *N. gonorrhoeae* module on p. 301 for alternatives.
- Cefixime 400 mg now available in U.S. as alternative PO Rx to ceftriaxone for uncomplicated GC infection, but no proof of effectiveness for conjunctival disease.
- Fluoroquinolones no longer recommended for GC secondary to the development of widespread resistance.
- Adult inclusion conjunctivitis (*chlamydia trachomatis*): azithromycin 1 g PO × 1 dose or doxycycline 100 mg PO q12h or tetracycline 250 mg PO q6h or erythromycin 250 mg PO q6h × 14 days.

Topical Antivirals

- HSV: refer all suspected cases to Ophthalmology. Rx with topical idoxuridine, vidarabine, or trifluridine.

Systemic Antivirals

- VZV: acyclovir 800 mg PO 5×/day or valacyclovir 1 g PO three times a day × 7–10 days. Refer to ophthalmologist to r/o keratitis.

Miscellaneous

- Comment: there is no role for the use of steroid eye drops or antibiotic/steroid drop combinations to rx conjunctivitis in the primary care setting. Refer to Ophthalmology if contemplating use. Steroids may worsen an underlying HSV infection.
- All pts with red eye: discontinue contact lenses and resume only when eye is white and without discharge after rx completed. Discard lens case and disinfect or replace lens.
- Use comfort measures such as cold compresses and artificial tears as needed.
- Allergic: pheniramine-naphazoline (Naphcon-A) 1–2 gtt four times a day PRN. May try lopatadine (Patanol) 0.1% sol 1 gtt twice daily or ketorolac tromethamine (Acular) 0.5% sol 1 gtt four times a day if above not effective.
- Hyperacute bacterial conjunctivitis: saline lavage to clear mucopurulent debris and dilute effects of released toxins on ocular tissues. Monitor closely for possible keratitis and perforation.
- Viral conjunctivitis: instruct pt to avoid sharing personal items (towels, sheets, pillows etc.), use meticulous hand washing and avoid close personal contact for approximately 2 wks.
- Pts with adenoviral conjunctivitis need to dispose of unclean contact lenses as adenovirus survives chemical and hydrogen peroxide disinfection.
- Epidemic keratoconjunctivitis (EKC): refer to ophthalmology. Highly contagious disease requiring implementation of isolation and infection control procedures.

OTHER INFORMATION
- Cultures not necessary for dx and rx unless recurrent, severe sx or suspected hyperacute conjunctivitis. Consider GC/Chlamydia in sexually active pts. Refer immediately.
- Advise immediate contact lens discontinuation in any pts with red eye. Refer to Ophthalmology urgently if keratitis, iritis/uveitis, scleritis, or angle closure glaucoma suspected by hx or PE.
- Think of secondary bacterial conjunctivitis or pseudomonal infection, ulcerative keratitis and have low threshold for referral in contact lens wearers. Foreign body sensation and corneal opacity on penlight exam.
- **Red flags**: severe pain/photophobia/decreased acuity. Refer ASAP if any of above present, worse after 1–2 days of rx or no better after 7 days. Exception: viral conjunctivitis sx may worsen first 3–5 days, reassure if no red flags.

BASIS FOR RECOMMENDATIONS
Sheikh A, Hurwitz B. Antibiotics versus placebo for acute bacterial conjunctivitis. *Cochrane Database Syst Rev*; 2006; Vol. CD001211.

Comments: Review of 5 randomized controlled trials with 1034 participants found that the use of antibiotics in acute bacterial conjunctivitis is associated with significantly improved rates of clinical and microbiological remission.

Leibowitz HM. The red eye. *N Engl J Med*, 2000; Vol. 343; pp. 345–51.

Comments: An excellent review of the common conditions manifesting as "the red eye" aimed at the primary care physician.

ENDOPHTHALMITIS

Aimee Zaas, MD

PATHOGENS
- *Staphylococcus aureus*
- *Propionibacterium* species
- *Enterococcus*
- *Bacillus cereus*
- *Candida* species
- *Aspergillus*
- *Fusarium*
- Gram-negative pathogens
- Gram-positive pathogens

CLINICAL
- Ocular inflammation due to introduction of an infectious agent into posterior segment of eye.
- Types: post-operative, post-traumatic (penetrating globe injury), and hematogenous spread ("endogenous endophthalmitis").
- Endophthalmitis can present mildly as painless floaters/visual change or fulminantly with pain, chemosis, visual loss, and fevers.
- Presentation: depends on pathogen virulence; range from mild irritation to profound pain, exophthalmos, periorbital extension.
- *B. cereus* is among the most aggressive cause of endophthalmitis. Seen in IDU and post-traumatic; has brown necrotic ring/hypopyon.
- Case reports of aggressive endophthalmitis during use of anti-TNF therapy may herald novel risk factor.

DIAGNOSIS
- Sampling and culture of vitreous imperative for etiology and sensitivities; 70% yield positive culture.
- PCR of vitreous samples can identify pathogen in nearly 100% of cases; use as adjunct to cx if available.
- Post op: culture if hypopyon, white plaque/ocular inflammation unresponsive to steroids, beaded opacities in anterior chamber/vitreous unresponsive to steroids, opacified bleb.
- Endogenous: culture if systemic infection with ocular inflammation, host risk factors with signs of ocular inflammation, chronic inflammation not responsive to steroids.
- Routine ocular exam for all pts with persistent fungemia recommended.

TREATMENT

Endogenous Endophthalmitis (EE)

- Bacterial (intravitreal antibiotics): ceftazidime 2.2 mg in 0.1 mL (Gram-negative coverage), vancomycin 1.0 mg in 0.1 mL (Gram-positive coverage).
- Systemic fluoroquinolones penetrate vitreous; no trials to support use.
- Repeat vitreal tap at 48–72 hrs and redose antibiotics if no improvement/worsening.
- Candida: early vitrectomy combined with systemic antifungal therapy (amphotericin B or fluconazole) recommended.
- Candida: 6–12 wks systemic therapy with voriconazole 400 mg IV/PO q12 × 2 doses then 200–300 mg IV/PO q12 or amphotericin B 0.7–1.0 mg/kg or fluconazole 400 mg/day IV/PO. AmB has renal toxicity; voriconazole has drug-drug interactions, phototoxicity, and hepatotoxicity; also causes visual changes (temporary) in up to 25%.
- Candida: intravitreal amphotericin B controversial; dose is 5–10 μg.
- Candida: caspofungin may be effective, but not well studied as yet; some references report no ocular penetration of caspofungin.
- Aspergillus: intravitreal amphotericin B 5–10 μg with dexamethasone 400 μg; repeat in 2 days post vitrectomy; no studies of voriconazole or caspofungin.
- Fusarium: successful case report of posaconazole (systemic and ocular).
- Bacillus: treat aggressively with vitrectomy, intra-vitreal vancomycin and systemic vancomycin.
- Systemic therapy guidance based upon culture, systemic infection source (e.g., endocarditis, bacteremia), etc.

Post-Operative Endophthalmitis

- Intra-vitreal antibiotics alone generally suffice, based on large randomized trial.
- Coagulase-negative staphylococci, Gram-negative rods and streptococci most common.
- Empiric therapy: intra-vitreal vancomycin plus ceftazidime.
- Gram-positive: vancomycin 1 mg/0.1 mL; may repeat at 48–72 hrs if not improving.
- Gram-negative: amikacin 0.4 mg/0.1 mL may be used; has risk of retinal microvasculitis.
- Gram-negative: ceftazidime 2.25 mg/0.1 mL is drug of choice; may repeat at 48–72 hrs if not improving.
- Oral fluoroquinolones penetrate vitreous but have not been studied in treatment trials.
- Intravitreal corticosteroids controversial.
- Despite recommendation for intra-vitreal antibiotics alone, many clinicians use systemic abx as well for severe cases.

Post-Traumatic Endophthalmitis

- Immediate vitrectomy with bacterial/fungal cultures, remove foreign bodies and necrotic tissue.
- Empiric intravitreal antibiotics: vancomycin 1 mg/0.1 ml and ceftazidime 2.25 mg/0.1 ml; consider amphotericin B 5–10 μg if rural/vegetable matter injury.
- Systemic broad-spectrum antibiotics recommended: vancomycin and ceftazidime are a good intravitreal choices.
- All intravitreal antibiotic should be mixed in normal saline.

FOLLOW UP

- In series of 114 pts with endophthalmitis, the most frequent complications were vitreous or retinal hemorrhages (n = 17, 14%), retinal detachment (n = 17, 14%), choroidal detachment (n = 3, 3%), secondary glaucoma (n = 7, 6%), and recurrent endophthalmitis (n = 3, 3%).

OTHER INFORMATION

- Post-operative: late infections (years after surgery) often due to *Propionibacterium acnes.*
- *P. acnes* often causes a white plaque on the posterior lens capsule; can be biopsied for culture.
- Post traumatic: risks are foreign body, delayed globe closure and extent of globe laceration.
- EE is result of systemic infection; risks are immune compromise, intravenous lines, hyperalimentation, IDU, malignancy; 25% bilateral.
- EE can be caused *by S. pneumoniae, H. influenza, N. meningitidis* in otherwise healthy pts.

BASIS FOR RECOMMENDATIONS
Sternberg P, Martin DF. Management of endophthalmitis in the post-endophthalmitis vitrectomy study era. *Arch Ophthalmol,* 2001; Vol. 119; pp. 754–5.
Comments: Expert opinion on endophthalmitis management; advocates aggressive approach for delayed post operative and post traumatic endophthalmitis.

OCULAR KERATITIS

Khalil G. Ghanem, MD

DIAGNOSIS

PATHOGENS
- Gram-positive cocci
- Gram-positive bacilli
- Mycobacteria
- Spirochetes
- Varicella-zoster virus
- Herpes simplex virus
- Fusarium
- Onchocerca
- Acanthamoeba
- The most common pathogens: *Streptococcus pneumoniae, Staphylococcus aureus, Pseudomonas aeruginosa,* and *Moraxella* spp. The other organisms listed above are relatively much less common.

CLINICAL
- Keratitis = inflammation of cornea. Approximately 50% of cases are infectious (of which ~80% are bacterial). Epithelium of cornea and conjunctiva continuous—same agents can cause both keratitis and conjunctivitis.
- Signs/symptoms: pain, +/– decreased vision, tearing, photophobia, blepharospasm, loss of transparency, ulcerated epithelium, stromal inflammation and keratolysis (loss of substance), and corneal scar/tear.
- Exam: topical anesthetic, slit lamp [inflammation +/– hypopyon (WBC in anterior chamber), hyphema, synechiae, and glaucoma]. With advanced disease: endophthalmitis.

DIAGNOSIS
- Corneal scrapings (multiple samples for Gram, giemsa, AFB, and GMS stains and cultures); corneal bx (in nonsuppurative cases).
- If no diagnosis, then consider therapeutic keratoplasty for dx and rx.
- Gram-stain: diagnostic accuracy is 75% if 1 organism and only ~35% if >1 organism.

TREATMENT
Antimicrobial Agents
- Routes of administration: solutions, subconjunctival, continuous lavage, hydrophilic contact lenses.
- All the following choices are ophthalmic solutions except where specifically noted.
- While awaiting cx data, and if suspect bacterial cause, start broadly (e.g., cephalosporin and aminoglycoside) and narrow spectrum later.
- Gram-positives: cephalosporin (cefazolin) or topical vancomycin (if resistance suspected) for staph.
- Gram-negatives (topicals): aminoglycosides [gentamicin (0.3%–1.5%), amikacin, tobramycin], ciprofloxacin 0.3%, norfloxacin 0.3% or ofloxacin 0.3%.
- Antifungals: AmphoB 1.5 mg/ml, fluconazole solution, chlorhexidine gluconate 0.2%, natamycin (not available in U.S.). Oral antifungals often necessary depending on infection.
- Acanthamoeba: polyhexamethylene biguanide, chlorhexidine gluconate or hexamidine + surgery. Length of antibiotic Rx: 3–4 wks.
- Onchocerciasis: oral ivermectin.
- Herpes: debridement + trifluridine or acyclovir ophth solution × 10 days + corticosteroids for stromal keratitis. Consider acyclovir 400 mg PO twice daily × 1 yr to prevent recurrence.

- Duration of therapy depends on disease, frequent slit lamp exams necessary. Early on, frequent (q30min) applications necessary. Hospitalization for moderate to severe disease strongly recommended.

Other Modalities
- Steroidal ophthalmic solutions: controversial in bacterial keratitis except in syphilis and lyme, avoid in fungal keratitis. Very effective for HSV stromal keratitis.
- Keratoplasty: adjunct in severe bacterial infection. Frequently necessary w/ acanthamoeba to remove cysts.
- Prevention: for contact lens wearers, there are specific recommendations (see http://www.fda.gov/cdrh/medicaldevicesafety/atp/041006-keratitis.html).

OTHER INFORMATION
- Infectious keratitis can lead to blindness; **immediate** ophthalmology consult is mandatory and hospitalization strongly recommended in moderate to severe cases to monitor for corneal perforation.
- Interpretation of MIC resistance patterns should take into account the **very high** concentrations of drug that can be achieved using topical ophthalmic applications.
- Contact lens associated keratitis: in addition to Pseudomonas, consider Acanthamoeba in this setting, especially if "sterile" standard cultures.
- Recent FDA/CDC warning about fungal (Fusarium) keratitis in soft contact lens wearers; it may be associated w/ a specific contact lens solution.

BASIS FOR RECOMMENDATIONS

Suwan-Apichon O, Reyes JM, Herretes S, et al. Topical corticosteroids as adjunctive therapy for bacterial keratitis. *Cochrane Database Syst Rev,* 2007; Vol. CD005430.

Comments: This comprehensive analysis revealed that there were no good quality randomized trials to guide recommendations for the use of adjunctive topical corticosteroids in bacterial keratitis.

Thomas PA, Geraldine P. Infectious keratitis. *Curr Opin Infect Dis,* 2007; Vol. 20; pp. 129–41.

Comments: The authors of this recent comprehensive paper review the latest evidence for treating infectious keratitis.

ORBITAL CELLULITIS

Khalil G. Ghanem, MD

PATHOGENS
- *Haemophilus influenzae*
- *Streptococcus pyogenes*
- *Streptococcus pneumoniae*
- Aspergillus
- Mucor, zygomycetes

CLINICAL
- **Preseptal cellulitis** = anterior to orbital septum; hyperemia of eyelids, soft tissue edema, and NO orbital congestion.
- **Postseptal cellulitis** = orbital cellulitis; acute infection of orbital contents.
- Etiology: (1) spread from ANY infected sinuses most common, (2) direct inoculation: post-trauma (or surgery), (3) acute dacryocystitis, (4) bites, (5) hematogenous (very rare).
- Symptoms: early: fever, lid edema, and rhinorrhea. Later: orbital pain, headaches and tenderness to palpation of lids, lids hyperemic, conjunctival hyperemia, chemosis, and proptosis.
- PE: limited ocular motility; decreased visual acuity (later), decreased corneal sensation, congested retinal veins.
- Lab: mild leukocytosis (~15,000), blood cx: variable yield, conjunctival cx may help.

DIAGNOSIS
- Scans: CT w/ contrast initial study of choice: best to visualize bony changes.
- CT in preseptal cellulitis is normal +/− soft tissue edema.
- MRI useful for dx of cavernous sinus thrombosis.
- **Staging and management: Stage I:** preseptal cellulitis, lid swelling; CT normal. Outpatient oral antibiotics. **Stage II:** edema, chemosis, proptosis, limitation of EOM; CT w/ mucosal

swelling but NO fluid collection. IV antibiotics (usually 10–14 days). **Stage III:** occasional visual loss, CT subperiosteal abscess, globe displacement, extraocular muscles involved. Parenteral antibiotics and consider surgical drainage if not better in 24 hrs. **Stage IV:** ophthalmoplegia with visual loss; CT with proptosis, abscess formation and periosteal rupture. Give IV antibiotics AND arrange for surgical management.

TREATMENT
Antimicrobials
- Begin immediately after cultures; do not wait for radiology results.
- Coverage for Gram-positive bacteria in addition to anaerobes as initial regimen. Can be modified based on cx data.
- **Antibacterials:** ampicillin/sulbactam (Unasyn) 3 g IV q6 (for adults). Ceftriaxone 1 g IV q12h +/– vancomycin 1 g IV q12h [Mandell: Principles and Practice of Infectious Diseases, 5th Ed., 2000].
- Other choices: clindamycin 300 mg IV q8h or Cefuroxime 750 mg–1.5 g IV q8h.
- If stage I (preorbital): can use oral amoxicillin/clavulanate 500 mg three times a day or clindamycin 300 mg four times a day for 10–14 days.
- Duration: 10–14 days usual unless bone changes suggestive of osteomyelitis; then 3–6 wks.
- Initially, rx with IV antibiotics if orbital cellulitis. Switching to oral feasible based on clinical judgment.
- Although still rare, there have been several case reports of CA-MRSA causing periorbital cellulitis.
- **Antifungals:** consider if suspicious amphotericin B for zygomycetes (mucor) or aspergillus (usually from sinus extension) in addition to mandatory and prompt surgical debridement.
- Voriconazole can be considered as first line therapy rather than amphotericin B for aspergillus (if conclusively proven) in view of its excellent activity and better toxicity profile [no prospective studies in this setting, however].
- Posaconazole now available as alternate regimen (PO) for treatment of zygomycetes.

Surgical
- Orbital cellulitis requires close consultation with ophthalmology and ENT.
- Surgical debridement is warranted with abscesses or if medical management fails to lead to an improvement in the first 24–36 hrs.
- Cultures should be obtained if surgical debridement is pursued; often have high yield.
- If fungal: surgical debridement immediately.

OTHER INFORMATION
- Periorbital cellulitis: occurs in young, with mean age 21 mos. Trauma and bacteremia are most common causes. Orbital cellulitis: mean age 12 yrs; sinusitis most common cause.
- Posterior orbital cellulitis: profound visual loss AND ophthalmalgia early and in absence of inflammatory signs!; usually sphenoid or ethmoid spread. STAT CT; consider doppler imaging.
- In pts with DKA and visual sx, rhinocerebral mucormycosis should be suspected and **immediate** surgical consultation obtained for debridement.
- Cavernous sinus thrombosis: suspect with internal and external ophthalmoplegia (CNs III, IV, V, and VI involved). Obtain MRI.

BASIS FOR RECOMMENDATIONS
Uzcátegui N, Warman R, Smith A, et al. Clinical practice guidelines for the management of orbital cellulitis. *J Pediatr Ophthalmol Strabismus*, 1998; Vol. 35; pp. 73–9; quiz 110–1.

Comments: Retrospective study on 101 pts: the incidence of orbital infection, manifested by lid swelling alone was much more common (stages I and II) than orbital infection involving postseptal findings (stages III, IV, and V); 84.16% compared with 15.84%, respectively.

Fever

ACUTE RHEUMATIC FEVER

Paul G. Auwaerter, MD

PATHOGENS
- Group A (beta-hemolytic) streptococcus

CLINICAL
- Syndromic immunologic (non-suppurative) aftermath of Group A strep (GAS) pharyngitis.
- In U.S., now rare w/ attack rate declining (likely well <0.4%) after GAS pharyngitis, but more common in developing world. Most frequent in 6–15 yrs olds.
- Average latent period following sore throat is 19 days, but range 1–5 wks.
- Carditis more common in younger children. It may be asymptomatic or cause congestive heart failure.
- Rates of arthritis tend to increase w/ age. Tends to be a migratory arthritis involving knees, elbows, ankles, and wrists but not very small joints.
- Sydenhams Chorea tends to be a late finding. Irregular, abrupt, and relatively rapid involuntary movements are seen in the face, neck, trunk, and limbs.
- SQ nodules (associated w/ severe carditis) and erythema marginatum (pink or red rings, slightly raised and non-pruritic seen on trunk and extremities) occur <10%.

MORE CLINICAL
WHO Criteria (2001–2002): Less stringent than Jones criteria
  1. Chorea and indolent carditis do not require evidence of antecedent group A streptococcus infection
  2. First episode per Jones criteria
  3. Recurrent episodes:
     - If no established RHD: as per first episode
     - If established RHD: requires two minor manifestations, plus evidence of antecedent group A streptococcus infection. Evidence of antecedent group A streptococcus infection as per Jones criteria, but with addition of recent scarlet fever.

DIAGNOSIS
- ARF likely by Am. Heart Assoc. criteria = 2 major, or 1 major and 2 minor. Recurrences of ARF unlikely to meet full criteria.
- **Major Criteria:** carditis, polyarthritis, chorea, subcutaneous nodules, erythema marginatum.
- **Minor Criteria:** fever, arthralgia, heart block, elevated ESR/CRP or wbc #.
- **Supportive:** recent positive GAS throat cx, rising ASO titer.

TREATMENT
Treatment of ARF
- Arthralgia or mild arthritis, no carditis: analgesia only, e.g., codeine or propoxyphene.
- Moderate or severe arthritis, no carditis or carditis w/o CHF: ASA 90–100 mg/kg PO in divided doses for 2–6 wks.
- Carditis w/ CHF +/– arthritis: prednisone 40–60 mg PO once daily with subsequent taper. Steroid recommendation is not based on good, prospective randomized trial data.
- If throat GAS (+), treat with benzathine PCN G 1.2 million units IM × 1.

Prevention
- Duration rather than dose believed important for GAS eradication from oropharynx.
- Parenteral: PCN benzathine 1.2 million units IM (single dose), if wt <60 lb dose 600,000 million units IM.
- Oral: PCN VK 250 mg PO three times a day (children), 500 mg PO three times a day (adolescents, adults) for full 10 days. Amoxicillin liquid often preferred w/ young children, dose 25–50 mg/kg/day PO q8h for full 10 days.
- PCN allergic: erythromycin 40 mg/kg/day 2–4 times daily (max. 1 g/day) for full 10 days.
- Treatment of strep throat even 9 days after onset is still effective in prevention of ARF.

Secondary prevention ARF
- To prevent recurrent attacks, exact role controversial.
- Benzathine PCN G 1.2 million units IM q4wk (or q3wk if high risk) or PCN VK 250 mg PO twice daily.
- Erythromycin 250 mg PO twice daily if PCN allergic.
- Duration of secondary prevention uncertain, many discontinue by late teenage/early adult years or 10 yrs after last attack if adult.

FOLLOW UP
- Hx of prior ARF significantly elevates risk of future bouts of ARF and rheumatic heart disease.
- Only long-term sequela of ARF is rheumatic heart disease (valvular). Only 6% risk if no carditis at initial ARF, climbs to 40–65% w/ murmurs or CHF at initial disease.

BASIS FOR RECOMMENDATIONS
Carapetis JR, McDonald M, Wilson NJ. Acute rheumatic fever. *Lancet,* 2005; Vol. 366; pp. 155–68.

Comments: Recent review article that serves along with the Jones criteria as the basis for recommendations in this module.

Dakamo AS. Ayoub E, Bierman EZ et al. Guidelines for the diagnosis of rheumatic fever: Jones criteria, updated 1992. *Circ,* 1993; Vol. 87; p. 302.

Comments: Basis for current diagnostic guidelines. The revision of the classic Jones criteria formulated by T. Duckett Jones has become more flexible by allowing a presumptive diagnosis of recurrent ARF by considering suggestive clinical findings along with evidence of a recent streptococcal infection. Recurrences of ARF tend to be milder and less likely to fulfill full Jones criteria.

CHRONIC FATIGUE SYNDROME

Lisa A. Spacek, MD, PhD and Khalil G. Ghanem, MD, PhD

PATHOGENS
- No causal relationship has been confirmed with any infectious agents and chronic fatigue.

CLINICAL
- Chronic fatigue syndrome (CFS): clinically evaluated, medically unexplained fatigue for >6 mos + 4 of the following: impaired memory, sore throat, tender glands, stiff/aching muscles, joint pain, new headaches, unrefreshing sleep, and post-exertional fatigue.
- Concomitant disorders that occur with CFS: fibromyalgia (35–70%), multiple chemical sensitivities, anxiety/depression, irritable bowel syndrome (IBS), Gulf War Syndrome, and TMJ disorders, etc.
- Prevalence: 0.2% in general population. Female predominance (2.9:1).
- Psychiatric, infectious, endocrine, and sleep disorders argued; but no causality established.
- Chronic fatigue may occur after well-documented infections (post-infectious fatigue syndrome): infectious mononucleosis (primary EBV), Lyme disease, Q fever, Ross River virus infection, and others.

DIAGNOSIS
- No laboratory tests are diagnostic for CFS.
- Consider alternative medical diagnoses: sleep disorders, adrenal insufficiency (unusual without weight loss), iron overload or deficiency hypothyroidism, hypogonadism, anxiety, depression, orthostatic hypotension.

TREATMENT
Non-Pharmacological
- Light aerobic exercise programs for conditioning are beneficial.
- Cognitive behavioral therapy.
- Sleep hygiene.
- Probiotics reported to decrease anxiety symptoms.

Pharmacological
- No pharmacological regimens have proven benefit in treating pts with CFS.
- Medications may be useful for treatment of specific symptoms. Clinicians may consider employing antidepressants (tricyclics such as nortriptyline, SSRIs, venlafaxine) or stimulants (modafinil, amphetamines) in severe cases.

BASIS FOR RECOMMENDATIONS

Afari N, Buchwald D. Chronic fatigue syndrome: a review. *Am J Psychiatry*, 2003; Vol. 160; pp. 221–36.

Comments: Excellent review article on CFS: authors go over CDC case definition, hypothesized pathophysiological mechanisms, all treatment controlled trials and their result.

FEVER AND NEUTROPENIA

Khalil G. Ghanem, MD

DEFINITION

- Fever: single oral temp >38.3°C (101°F) or temp >38°C (100.4°F) for >1 hr AND neutropenia: absolute neutrophil count (ANC) <500 cells/mm³ or <1000 cells/mm³ with predicted decline to <500 cells/mm³ [reference; CID 2002].

INDICATIONS

Pathogens

- Gram-negative bacilli (*Pseudomonas* spp., Enterobacteriaceae, etc); consider antibiotic resistant GNB (e.g., ESBLs)
- *Staphylococcus aureus* (including MRSA) and coagulase-negative *Staphylococci*
- *Viridans streptococci* (demonstrated to be serious pathogens especially in pts with malignancy/mucositis)
- *Enterococcus* spp.
- *Corynebacterium jeikeium* (not an infrequent cause of catheter-related infections in this pt population)
- *Bacillus* spp.
- *Propionibacterium* spp.
- Anaerobes: less commonly implicated (e.g., periodontal or perirectal abscess, intra-abdominal infection)
- *Candida* spp.
- *Aspergillus* spp. and other filamentous fungi (e.g., *Fusarium* spp.)

DIAGNOSIS

- Detailed history and PE (see below).
- Obtain 2 sets blood cxs; preferably from peripheral veins × 2 (1 minimum) + catheter lumen(s).
- UA w/ micro, CBC w/ diff; LFTs, electrolytes.
- Sputum for Gram-stain and cx; consider bronchoscopy/BAL if respiratory complaints persist and are significant.
- CXR, scans (CT, US, MRI) as per signs/symptoms.

CLINICAL RECOMMENDATIONS

Clinical

- Detailed history, recent exposures, sick contacts.
- Risk factors: degree of neutropenia (ANC severity: <100 <500 <1000), rapid decline in ANC, remission of cancer or not, duration of neutropenia., other comorbidities; existence of central lines.
- Correlate date fever onset to date of cytotoxic therapy to predict duration of neutropenia (nadir count usually 10–14 days after chemo).
- PE: exam especially periodontium, pharynx, lungs, perineum/anus, skin, eyes, vascular access sites, BM bx sites.

Approach to Treatment

- Proceed with Hx, PE, labs(cx), assess risk of pt and determine whether to use PO (low risk pt, see below) or IV therapy.
- Begin abx (mono or combo) and continue at least 3–5 days before considering any changes unless new cx data available or clinical deterioration.
- Decide if Gram-positive coverage warranted.
- Persistent fever (d3–5): clinical re-assessment including cx and scans. Decide if continue abx (if pt stable) or change/add abx (if disease progression, or vancomycin criteria met) or add antifungal.

- Antifungals routinely added after 3–5 days of febrile neutropenia despite broad antibacterial coverage and no identified cause: ampho B (or lipid formulations), voriconazole or posaconazole (although not adequately studied), caspofungin (other echinocandins anidulafungin, micafungin, but not adequately studied for febrile neutropenia; only caspofungin FDA approved).
- Prior to antifungal initiation, work-up for fungal infection should be complete: assess host and clinical factors, bx any suspicious skin lesions, CT of chest/abdomen, sinuses, nasal endoscopy (if indicated), cx's as appropriate, galactomannan enzyme immunoassay.
- If chest CT with nodular lesions +/– halo sign, amphotericin B products or voriconazole favored.
- Amphotericin B 0.5–1 mg/kg/day IV or ambisome 5 mg/kg/day, voriconazole 6 mg/kg IV q12h × 2 and then 4 mg/kg IV q12h, posaconazole 200 mg POq6h × 7 days and then 400 mg PO q12h, caspofungin 70 mg IV × 1 and then 50 mg IV q24h.
- Routine antivirals not indicated unless lesions c/w herpes/VZV lesions present (use acyclovir). CMV rare except in BMT pts (use ganciclovir).
- Colony-Stimulating Factors (G-CSF): can shorten duration of neutropenia but NOT duration of fever or decrease infection mortality; routine use NOT recommended.
- Consider use of G-CSF in severely neutropenic pts w/ documented infections that do not respond to appropriate rx or when prolonged delay in marrow recovery is anticipated.
- If central line present, remove if feasible for positive blood cxs for *S. aureus*, *Pseudomonas* spp., *Stenotrophomonas* spp., *Corynebacterium JK*, *Bacillus* spp., *Candida* spp., fast-growing atypical mycobacteria (if feasible).

Oral Antibiotic Therapy
- Adults who are low risk pts may use: ciprofloxacin + amoxicillin/clavulanate. Make sure pts observed carefully and have access to appropriate medical care 24/7.
- **Lower risk pts:** ANC >100, absolute monocytes count >100, nl CXR, nl LFTs, and creatinine, no clinical IV site tunnel/exit site infection, temp <39°C. Also no abdominal pain, evidence of impending bone marrow recovery, no comorbidities. Neutropenia expected to last <10 days.
- Oral therapy: ciprofloxacin 500 mg PO twice daily and amoxicillin/clavulanate 500 mg PO q8h.

Monotherapy and Combination Parenteral Antibacterial Therapy
- No difference between combination or monotherapy for empirical rx of uncomplicated febrile neutropenia. Monotherapy could potentially increase antibiotic resistance (especially w/ use of cephalosporins).
- Choice of empiric therapy: base upon history and exam, antibiotic allergies, historical culture data (if available), recent antibiotic exposure, institutional resistance patterns.
- **Monotherapy:** cefepime, ceftazidime or carbapenem (imipenem/meropenem) FDA approved. Carbapenems are preferred if ESBL rate is high (AVOID cephalosporins).
- **Combination:** aminoglycoside + [antipseudomonal PCN (piperacillin/tazobactam) or cefepime or ceftazidime or carbapenem]. Two antipseudomonal beta-lactams together (not favored).
- Potential advantages of combination rx: synergistic effects against GNRs and decrease in the emergence of drug-resistance. Balance with the potential for nephro- and ototoxicity.
- Ceftazidime 2 g IV q8h or cefepime 2 g IV q8h or imipenem 1 g IV q6h (caution in pts with renal insufficiency in view of seizure potential) or meropenem 2 g IV q8h.
- Addition of aminoglycoside for combination therapy: gentamicin or tobramycin 2 mg/kg q8h or 5 mg/kg q24h (once daily preferred: less toxicity) or amikacin 15 mg/kg/day or divided q8–12h.
- Vancomycin: considered if clinically suspected serious catheter-related infection, known MRSA colonization, positive BC results w/ GPC prior to final identification, or hypotension. Otherwise follow initial cx data and add vancomycin as needed. Linezolid can be an option, but not favored if suspect serious or high-grade bacteremia.
- Other drugs used: vancomycin 15 mg/kg IV q12h, linezolid 600 mg IV/PO q12h, daptomycin 6–8 mg/kg IV q24h.
- Quinolones are NOT recommended as routine initial monotherapy agents due to lack of prospective data, and use of quinolones as routine prophylaxis in many centers may predispose to resistance.

Duration of Treatment

- If an infectious source identified continue targeted abx tx for at least the standard duration of the given infection.
- If pt afebrile in 3–5 days: if ANC >500 × 2 days, may d/c abxs if no infection identified; if ANC <500, continue abx at least 7 days or ideally until ANC >500 or suspected source treated (if pt high risk). Consider switch to oral ciprofloxacin + amoxicillin/clavulanate or can D/C abxs if afebrile for >7 days (if pt low risk).
- Persistent fever: if ANC >500, d/c abx 4–5 days after ANC >500 and reassess. If ANC <500, continue × 14 days and reassess.
- The most important determinant for successful cessation of abx is neutrophil count recovery.

OTHER INFORMATION

- Less than 50% of febrile neutropenics will have an established infection and 1 of 5 pts with ANC <100 cells/mm^3 will have bacteremia.
- Signs and symptoms (induration, erythema, pustulation, CXR infiltrates, CSF pleocytosis) may be absent in pts with neutropenia.
- Median time to defervescence in adequately treated pts is 5 days (range 2–7 days). DO NOT modify initial abx choice unless clinical deterioration or new cx data dictate it.
- Sinusitis should be aggressively diagnosed and treated as neutropenia is a risk factor for invasive mould infections.

BASIS FOR RECOMMENDATIONS

Walsh, TJ, Teppler, H, Donowitz, GR, et al. Caspofungin versus liposomal amphotericin B for empirical antifungal therapy in pts with persistent fever and neutropenia. *N Engl J Med,* 2004; Vol. 351; pp. 1391.

Comments: Important study comparing caspofungin to L-AMB for empirical treatment of febrile neutropenia. This study showed similar overall success rates, breakthrough fungal infections, and resolution of fever.

Hughes WT, Armstrong D, Bodey GP, et al. 2002 guidelines for the use of antimicrobial agents in neutropenic pts with cancer. *Clin Infect Dis,* 2002; Vol. 34; pp. 730–51.

Comments: The most recent update of IDSA guidelines for the diagnosis and management of neutropenic fever.

Generalized Infections

LEPTOSPIRA INTERROGANS see p. 279 in Pathogens Section

LYME DISEASE

John G. Bartlett, MD

DIAGNOSIS

PATHOGENS

- *Borrelia burgdorferi sensu lato*
- Other strains may cause LD in regions outside the U.S., e.g., *B. garinii, B. afzelii* in Europe. May not trigger positive U.S. Lyme serologic assays.

CLINICAL

- Most common tick-borne disease in U.S. Vector = *Ixodes scapularis* (deer tick), highly endemic regions include river/costal regions of NE, MidAtlantic, and Wisc/Minn. Less common in West, transmitted by black-legged tick, *I. pacificus.*
- Early (3–30 days after tick bite): localized—erythema migrans with red ovoid lesion at tick bite site (central clearing, "bull's eye" only in minority of larger lesions)—no serology necessary; disseminated—multiple erythema migrans, typically smaller and with fever and systemic symptoms more common.
- Carditis: part of early, disseminated infection. A–V block ($1° > 2° > 3°$), but usually only third-degree block recognized clinically.
- Neurologic: usually early, disseminated (wks-mos after bite) cranial nerve palsy including Bell's palsy, lymphocytic meningitis or radiculitis w/pain, paresis or paresthesias. Late Lyme disease manifestations (rare): encephalopathy, peripheral neuropathy (sensory).
- Arthritis: early disease = polyarthralgia or polyarthritis/tendonitis. Late (mos-yrs) = joint swelling + pain, usually weight bearing joint. Knee most common. Usually a monoarthritis, but recurrent without antibiotic therapy.
- Late cutaneous (mostly seen in Europe): lymphocytoma and acrodermatitis: serology positive in 90–100% and PCR for *Borrelia* usually positive.

DIAGNOSIS

- Early, localized (erythema migrans): characteristic rash in endemic region with possibility of tick exposure. Serology unnecessary except in confusing cases, check acute (may be negative 30–70% of cases) and convalescent serology.
- Early disseminated: history of recent erythema migrans rash or positive Lyme serology (EIA + Western blot).
- Late Lyme disease: diagnosis by condition + positive blood serology (EIA + Western blot); arthritis—serology or Lyme PCR, neuroborreliosis—serology + abnl CSF or Lyme CSF index (ratio CSF Lyme ab to serum Lyme ab, normalized for protein amount, suggestive if $>1.0–1.2$).
- Note: subjective symptoms alone, e.g., fatigue, neurocognitive symptoms, fibromyalgia-like sx awre not an indication for Lyme testing.
- Lyme IgM Western blot should not be used to diagnosis any condition >1 mo duration due to high rate of false positives.

TREATMENT

Lyme Disease Regimens (IDSA Guidelines, CID 2006)

- Early disease (preferred, oral): amoxicillin 500 mg three times a day or doxycycline 100 mg twice daily or cefuroxime 500 mg twice daily × 2 wks. Doxycycline advantage is that it can treat other tick-borne infections, e.g., Ehrlichia chaffeensis or Anaplasma phagocytophilum or Rocky Mountain Spotted Fever.
- Alternative (oral): azithromycin 500 mg PO daily × 7–10 days or clarithromycin 500 mg twice daily × 14–21 days (be wary of higher treatment failure rates).
- Parenteral (preferred): ceftriaxone 2 g q24h
- Alternative: cefotaxime 2 g IV q8h or penicillin G 3–4 mil U q4h (18–24 mil units/day).

65

Regimens by Clinical Features

- Erythema migrans: oral regimen 14 days (range 14–21 days). Doxycycline 100 mg PO twice daily × 10 days equivalent in one study (Ann Intern Med 2003).
- Meningitis or radiculopathy: parenteral regimen × 14 days (range 10–28 days).
- Cranial nerve palsy: oral regimen 14 days (range 14–21 days), some use parenteral regimen especially if abnl CSF seen.
- Cardiac disease: oral or parenteral regimen 14 days (range 14–21 days).
- Arthritis (late lyme disease): oral regimen 28 days.
- Recurrent arthritis after oral regimen: repeat oral 28 days course or parenteral regimen 14–28 days.
- CNS or peripheral nervous system disease: parenteral regimen 14 days (range 14–28 days).
- Acrodermatitis chronica atrophicans (seen mostly in Europe): oral regimen 21 days (14–28 days).

Prevention

- Tick checks daily. Removal within 36 hrs is most effective prevention.
- Tick control: acaricide starting in early May.
- DEET repellants, especially Edtiar (Ultrathon) for skin.
- Permethrin applied to clothes, shoes, tents, etc.
- Prophylactic doxycycline 200 mg PO × 1 dose within 72 hrs post tick bite–87% effective, best only in highly endemic region.
- Lyme vaccine—no longer available (2002).

Not Recommended

- Avoid repeated treatment same episode or combination antibiotic therapy.
- No merit: hyperbaric oxygen, IVIG, ozone, cholestyramine, vitamins, nutritional management, magnesium, chelation therapy.
- Avoid empiric treatment for babesiosis or Bartonella.
- Prolonged courses of antibiotics beyond those recommended.

OTHER INFORMATION

- Dx based on epidemiology (endemic area +/– tick bite), POs. serology (except w/ erythema migrans or acute neurologic disease—early) and typical symptoms
- Pts with chronic fatigue, joint stiffness, and/or muscle aches should not have Lyme disease serology and should not receive Lyme disease treatment
- Serology: EIA or IFA and western blot—takes 4–6 wks for seroconversion (reliable test)
- Tick bite: coinfection risk ~1–3%; Lyme, ehrlichiosis, babesiosis, RMSF; prophylactic doxy 200 mg × 1 for Lyme risk

MORE INFORMATION

LYMErix vaccine discontinued by manufacturer March 2002 due to poor sales.

BASIS FOR RECOMMENDATIONS

Halperin JJ, Shapiro ED, Logigian E, et al. Practice parameter: treatment of nervous system Lyme disease (an evidence-based review): report of the Quality Standards Subcommittee of the American Academy of Neurology. *Neurology,* 2007; Vol. 69; pp. 91–102.
Comments: Recommendations for treatment of nervous system Lyme disease from the American Academy of Neurology. This is the source document for recommendations used here.

Wormser GP, Dattwyler RJ, Shapiro ED, et al. The clinical assessment, treatment, and prevention of lyme disease, human granulocytic anaplasmosis, and babesiosis: clinical practice guidelines by the Infectious Diseases Society of America. *Clin Infect Dis,* 2006; Vol. 43; pp. 1089–134.
Comments: IDSA guidelines: Basis for all treatment recommendations given here.

Wormser GP, Dattwyler RJ, Shapiro ED, et al. The clinical assessment, treatment, and prevention of lyme disease, human granulocytic anaplasmosis, and babesiosis: clinical practice guidelines by the Infectious Diseases Society of America. *Clin Infect Dis,* 2006; Vol. 43; pp. 1089–134.
Comments: IDSA Guidelines for management of Lyme disease. This document is basis for recommendations used here.

American College of Physicians. Guidelines for laboratory evaluation in the diagnosis of Lyme disease. American College of Physicians. *Ann Intern Med,* 1997; Vol. 127; pp. 1106–8.
Comments: The ACP provides Guidelines For *B. Burgdorferi* Serology. First, determine the probability of Lyme disease. The test should be done when the probability is 20–80%. The test is 2 stages: a screening EIA or IFA followed by a Western blot in those that are indeterminant or positive. Pts with erythema migrans or arthritis + a history of a tick bite should be treated empirically.

LYMPHADENOPATHY

Paul G. Auwaerter, MD

DIAGNOSIS

PATHOGENS

- **Acute generalized:** HIV, syphilis, EBV, CMV, Toxoplasma, Brucella, cat scratch disease, sarcoid, lymphoma, Stills, IBD, Whipple's, hypersensitivity rxn. HAART-associated immune reconstitution syndrome in HIV+ pts.
- **Acute localized:** <u>Cervical:</u> group A strep, EBV, TB, cat scratch disease, lymphoma, temporal arteritis. <u>Pre-auricular:</u> adenovirus, conjunctivitis, tularemia, cat scratch (Parinauds syndrome). <u>Epitrochlear:</u> hand infection (medial 3 fingers), syphilis. <u>Inguinal:</u> syphilis, herpes, LGV, chancroid, HIV, lymphoma, tularemia, plague.
- **Chronic generalized:** syphilis, TB, histoplasma, cryptococcosis, CGD, lymphoma, HIV, sarcoid, hyperthyroidism, chronic fatigue syndrome, posttransplant lymphoproliferative disorder.
- **Chronic localized:** TB, cryptococcus, histoplasma, cat scratch disease, lymphoma, metastatic cancer, Kikuchi-Fujimoto disease, Rosai-Dorman disease.

CLINICAL

- Palpable lymph nodes (>1 cm abnormal). Must distinguish generalized vs. localized; chronic vs. acute. See Pathogens section above for some common processes that may account for etiological explanation.
- PE: asses temperature, inspect mucus membranes, organomegaly, and genitalia.
- Painful LN = suggests inflammation, suppuration, or bleeding into necrotic area.
- Rubbery LN = suggests lymphoma.
- Stony hard LN = cancer or actinomycosis.
- LN may be single or "matted" (several nodes moveable as a group).

DIAGNOSIS

- Lab: CBC, HIV, RPR, CMV, EBV and other tests as indicated by hx. Other diagnostic considerations could include bartonella or toxoplasma serology, viral hepatitis serologies, PCR for Tropheryma whipplei, GI endoscopy.
- LN bx if unexplained nodes persist >4 wks or have malignant characteristics or rapidly enlarging. Fine needle biopsy often done as first step, but excisional biopsy always superior especially for lymphoma.
- Send bx tissue for C and S, fungal and AFB stains/cxs along with surgical pathology +/– flow cytometry.
- PPD.

TREATMENT

Diagnosis (Partial list of common considerations)

- Syphilis: RPR/FTA
- Group A streptococcus: throat culture, rapid antigen testing
- EBV: Monospot, anti-VCA IgM, IgG antibodies
- CMV: serology (IgM, IgG)
- HIV: serology, viral load RNA PCR (for detection of acute infection). Pts with CD4 <50, abdominal LN may be due to disseminated MAC.
- Cat scratch disease: LN biopsy, culture, serology (anti-*Bartonella henselae* Abs), PCR
- Brucella: serology, culture
- TB: culture, histology
- Whipple's: tissue (LN, GI) bx, PCR
- Tularemia: serology, PCR (experimental). Culture is dangerous, notify microbiology lab if suspect.
- Histoplasma: culture, histopathology, urine antigen testing (usually negative unless disseminated infection)

TREATMENT REGIMEN DETAILS

Plague (Yersinia pestis): culture, Gram-stain, Wayson stain, serology

FOLLOW UP

- Lymphadenopathy due to infection. Resolution of infection should lead to normalization of LN, although viral processes can wax and wane for up to 6 mos (e.g., EBV).

- Follow pt with chronic lymphadenopathy and negative node bx closely, re-biopsy if nodes persist or enlarge.

OTHER INFORMATION

- Watch for secondary malignancies and unusual OIs in HIV+ pts not on HAART.
- Immune reconstitution syndrome (IRIS) is a hard dx to prove, but can be clinically suspected in AIDS pts started on anti-retroviral therapy.
- Keep low threshold for proceeding with diagnostic biopsy. Some regions usually always concerning such as supraclavicular LN, target the largest node, remove entire node (including capsule), discuss with pathologist/microbiologist in advance.

BASIS FOR RECOMMENDATIONS

Author opinion.

Comments: No guidelines available for diagnostic algorithm.

TROPHERYMA WHIPPLEI see p. 342 in Pathogens Section

BACTERIAL CYSTITIS, ACUTE, UNCOMPLICATED

Noreen A. Hynes, MD, MPH

PATHOGENS

- Bug distribution: (1) *E. coli* = 80–90% in outpatients, 18–57% for in-pts. (2) *S saprophyticus* = 0–2% in outpatients, much higher in young women.
- Uropathogenic *E. coli* (UPEC) = Subset of extraintestinal *E. coli* (ExPEC) most likely to cause UTIs are groups B2 and D that have "fitness elements" providing them with advantage in extraintestinal niche.
- Uncomplicated UTI, >95% of infections due to single organism.
- Other organisms less common and include: other Enterobacteriaceae, *P. aeruginosa*, Grps B and *D streptococci*, and enterococci. Rarely *H. influenzae*, anaerobes, *salmonella*, *shigella*, *adenovirus* type 11, ureaplasma mycoplasma.
- Factors favoring bacterial persistence/colonization and infection: (1) bacterial binding via fimbriae, (2) high growth rates despite high osmolarity and urea concentrations and low pH.
- Factors favoring bacterial elimination include: (1) high urine flow rate, (2) frequent voiding, (3) bactericidal effects of secreted proteins, (4) bladder mucosa, and (5) inflammatory responses.

CLINICAL

- **Definition:** uncomplicated cystitis = urgency, frequency, dysuria in otherwise healthy, non-pregnant woman, with lab evidence of pyuria, urine cx + for uropathogen in amounts of at least 1,000 cfu/mL; no urinary sx in past 4 wks. No fever, CVA tenderness or flank pain.
- In sexually active women: dysuria without pyuria suggests an STI rather than UTI.
- Risk factors for acute uncomplicated UTI in premenopausal women: (1) coitus, (2) prior hx of UTI, (3) spermicide exposure, and (4) recent antimicrobial use.
- Risk factors for acute uncomplicated UTI in postmenopausal women: (1) coitus, (2) prior hx of UTI, (3) incontinence, and (4) diabetes mellitus.
- Risk factors for recurrent uncomplicated UTI in premenopausal women: same as above **and** (a) maternal hx of UTI or (b) hx of childhood UTI [both factors consistent with hereditary predisposition].
- UTIs common among women of all ages; uncomplicated cystitis incidence 0.5–0.7 episodes per woman/yr.
- Asymptomatic bacteriuria prevalence: 5–6% among healthy, sexually active, non-pregnant women; increases with age.

DIAGNOSIS

- 1) Dipstick positive leukocyte esterase test or positive nitrite (75% sensitive, 82% specific); 2) >100,000 CFU/mL on midstream clean-catch urine culture; 3) >9 WBCs/HPF.
- **Important:** uncomplicated UTI does not require **culture** unless apparent treatment failure noted with empiric therapy.
- Symptomatic sexually active women with dysuria without pyuria: screen for STIs including chlamydia, gonorrhea, trichomoniasis, and HSV.

TREATMENT

Short Course Therapy (Empirical Treatment)

- Resistance patterns of *E. coli* to TMP-SMX and the fluoroquinolones are highly variable across U.S. and are continuing to change. Clinicians are strongly urged to recognize resistance patterns in their community.
- Nitrofurantoin is encouraged for use (see Longer Duration Therapy) given rates of TMP-SMX *E. coli* resistance >10% in all U.S. Regions examined and as a fluoroquinolone-sparing agent for women with mild to moderate symptoms **and** allergy to TMP-SMX or prior antibiotic in previous 3 mos (except for nitrofurantoin) or live in a locality with prevalence of *E. coli* resistance of TMP-SMX >10–20% in women with uncomplicated UTI.

- Trimethoprim-sulfamethoxazole DS (Bactrim/Septra) 1 tab PO twice daily × 3 days (preferred for empiric Rx if local prevalence of *E. coli* resistance to TMP-SMX < 10–20%; if > 10–20% use fluoroquinolone)—Check with local laboratory for resistance at least once every 6 mos.
- Trimethoprim 300 mg PO once daily × 3 days (do not use if resistance to TMP-SMX is > 10–20%). Check with local laboratory for *E. coli* resistance rates every 6 mos.
- TMP-SMX and TMP alone are first line Rx because they are cheap and there is a critical need to reserve FQs for use in complicated UTIs. Overuse in acute cystitis may lead to resistance.
- Norfloxacin 400 mg PO twice daily × 3 days for women with <u>severe symptoms</u> **and** allergy to TMP-SMX or abx Rx in the last 3 mos (except a FQ) or live in locality with *E. coli* resistance ≥20% in women with acute uncomplicated UTI.
- Ciprofloxacin 250 mg PO twice daily × 3 days for women with <u>severe symptoms</u> **and** allergy to TMP-SMX or abx Rx in the last 3 mos (except a FQ) or live in locality with *E. coli* resistance >20% in women with acute uncomplicated UTI.
- Ofloxacin 200 mg PO twice daily × 3 days for women with <u>severe symptoms</u> **and** allergy to TMP-SMX or abx Rx in the last 3 mos (except a FQ) or live in locality with *E. coli* resistance >20% in women with acute uncomplicated UTI.
- Amoxicillin/clavulanate 500/125 mg PO twice daily × 3 days (higher percentage of organisms resistant to amoxicillin alone. This regimen is inferior to ciprofloxacin and if amox/clavulanate used, longer duration therapy is indicated (see Longer Duration Therapy).
- There is no single dose treatment regimens using fluoroquinolones that are FDA-approved that have equal efficacy to the 3-days regimens in terms of sterilization of urine and recurrence rate. Therefore, single dose regimens are to be avoided.

Longer Duration therapy
- Nitrofurantoin macrocrystals 50 or 100 mg four times daily PO × 7 days; Nitrofurantoin monohydrate macrocrystals 100 mg twice daily PO × 7 days
- Amoxicillin/clavulanate 500/125 mg PO twice daily × 7 days (higher percentage of organisms resistant to amoxicillin alone).
- Trimethoprim-Sulfamethoxazole DS 1 tab PO twice daily × 5–7 days (preferred for empiric Rx if prevalence of *E. coli* resistance to TMP-SMX <10–20%; if >20% use fluoroquinolone).
- Trimethoprim 100 mg PO twice daily × 7 days.
- Cephalexin 250 mg PO three times daily × 7 days.
- Norfloxacin 400 mg PO twice daily × 7 days.
- Ciprofloxacin 250 mg PO twice daily × 7 days.
- Amoxicillin 250 mg PO three times daily × 7 days.

Treatment in Women with Diabetes Mellitis
- Do **not** use short-course (3-days) Rx in diabetics.
- Treat for 7–10 days with any agent listed under "Longer Duration Rx" outlined above.

FOLLOW UP
- Older women with acute bacterial cystitis should be managed using a longer regimen; empiric therapy should never be with TMP/SMX in this age group.
- If *S. saprophyticus* is the suspected or known cause of the UTI, then the longer therapy (7 days) should be used due to increased efficacy.
- In postmenopausal women with uncomplicated recurrent UTI the major risk factors are anatomical or functional defects including a) incontinence, b) post-void residual urine, and c) cystocele. Additional factor is the relative lack of estrogen effect. This results in loss of dominance of lactobacilli among vaginal flora with subsequent increase in vaginal pH, increased colonization of the introitus with *E. coli*. This provides a setting for increased number of UTIs. Studies have shown that the use of topical estrogens reverses these changes and greatly reduces the incidence of recurrent UTI in such women not using HRT.

OTHER INFORMATION
- The *most* common bacterial infection in women. The incidence of acute, uncomplicated UTIs in young women is 0.5–0.7 episode/yr with approximately 6 associated disability-days/episode.
- 25%–40% of women who have an initial bout of acute, uncomplicated bacterial cystitis will have recurrent infections.

- Women with diabetes mellitus or other significant comorbidities should receive 7 to 10 days of therapy and should not be treated with a 3-days regimen.

BASIS FOR RECOMMENDATIONS

Grabe M, et al. *Guidelines on the Management of Urinary and Male Genital Tract Infections*, 2008.

Comments: These are the latest European Association of Urology Guidelines. These guidelines follow the IDSA recommendation of using trimethoprim-sulfamethoxazole TMP-SMX as the 1st line of therapy for acute, uncomplicated UTI in women in areas where uropathogenic *E. coli* resistance to TMP-SMX is < 20%.

BACTERIAL PROSTATITIS, ACUTE

Noreen A. Hynes, MD, MPH

PATHOGENS

- *Escherichia coli*
- Other Enterobacteriaceae
- *Enterococcus* species
- General comments: (1) *E. coli* accounts for approximately 75%; other Enterobacteriaceae— most of the rest. (2) Uncommon pathogens: *P. aeruginosa*, *S. saprophyticus*, *S. aureus*, and *E. faecalis*, *N. gonorrhoeae*, *C. trachomatis*, fungi, viruses. (3) Prostatitis due to Enterococcus spp. or Pseudomonas spp. is more difficult to treat.

CLINICAL

- Acute bacterial prostatitis (ABP) = Category I prostatitis by NIH classification. Only 5% of all prostatitis is ABP!
- Men 35–64 yrs are at highest risk. Usual mechanism is reflux of infected urine into the intraprostatic ducts. Urethral inoculation after instrumentation (including ultrasound-guided transrectal prostate needle biopsy), catheterization, or insertive anal intercourse may also be risk factors.
- ABP is a acute severe systemic illness: symptoms: (1) sx of UTI: dysuria, frequency, urgency plus (2) sx of prostatitis: low back pain, perineal/penile/rectal pain +/– (3) sx of bacteremia: fever, rigors, arthralgia, myalgia. Symptoms of systemic toxicity are commonly seen along with pain on defecation in many with lower abdominal pain or suprapubic discomfort with referral to lower lumbar region, genitalia, or thigh. Nocturia, sometimes with gross hematuria can be noted.
- ABP signs: (1) localized to prostate: extremely tender, tense, swollen gland; warm to touch [**do not massage!**] +/– (2) bacteremia: fever, tachycardia.Ceftriaxone should **not** be used as monotherapy as the beta-lactams do not penetrate the prostate well; it has been demonstrated to work well in combination with an aminoglycoside. Bladder outlet obstruction (edema of prostate) may be seen.
- Dx: bacteriuria and pyuria on midstream urine. If sterile cx, acute bacterial prostatitis unlikely. Also obtain blood cultures for bacteria and antibiotic sensitivities.
- Acute nosocomial bacterial prostatitis should be diagnosed if an indwelling catheter is present in the outpatient or inpatient setting with accompanying features of acute bacterial prostatitis; although *E. coli* is the most common organism isolated, increased risk of *Pseudomonas* sp and *S. aureus* in this pt group. Therefore, use parenteral treatment initially.
- Presents dramatically and is essentially a **clinical** diagnosis.
- Complications include: (1) prostate abscess, (2) prostatic infarction, (3) chronic bacterial prostatitis, (4) granulomatous prostatitis.

DIAGNOSIS

- Mid-stream urine sample: dipstick and for culture and sensitivity testing.
- Blood cultures.
- Do not perform prostatic massage!! This would be very painful, could induce bacteremia, and is of little benefit in establishing the diagnosis in ABP as pathogens usually found in the urine.
- The UK guidelines recommend post-cure search for structural urinary tract abnormality. In U.S. this recommendation made if prostatitis ruled out as the cause of bacteriuria with pyuria i.e when cystitis alone is suspect or the man is over the age of 64 yrs.

- Consider additional testing for gonorrhea, chlamydia, and trichomoniasis in sexually active young men with a new sex partner in the last 3 mos, multiple concurrent sex partners, or unprotected receptive anal intercourse.

TREATMENT

Outpatient Therapy

- Local uropathogenic *Escherichia coli* antimicrobial resistance patterns should be used to guide antibiotic choice as resistance to **both** ciprofloxacin (1st line) or trimethoprim-sulfamethoxazole (2nd line). Select cephalosporin-based regimens if resistance is ≥10%.
- Preferred oral regimen (UK Guidelines 2001–2): ciprofloxacin 500 mg PO twice daily × 28 days **or** ofloxacin 200 mg twice daily × 28 days.
- Allergy to quinolones: TMP-SMX 1 DS PO twice daily × 28 days **or** TMP 200 mg twice daily × 28 days.

Intravenous Therapy

- Ceftriaxone 1–2 g IV q12–24h (depending on severity) **plus** gentamicin 1.7 mg/kg q8h (depending upon renal function) until can tolerate PO regimen and afebrile for 48 hrs; then PO regimen to complete 28 days Rx.
- Cefotaxime 1–2 g q6–8h (up to 12 g/days) **plus** gentamicin 1.7 mg/kg q8h depending upon renal function) until can tolerate PO regimen and afebrile for 48 hrs; then PO regimen to complete 28 days Rx.
- Beta-lactam allergy: Although not FDA-approved for this use, ciprofloxacin 400 mg IV q12h could be used along with gentamicin 1.7 mg/kg q8h (depending on renal function) until able to tolerate PO regimen and afebrile: then to complete a full course of 28 days of treatment.

Supportive Therapies and Modalities

- Bed rest often needed.
- Antipyretics/antiinflammatory for fever, myalgia, arthralgia.
- Foley catheter may be needed to relieve bladder outlet obstruction due to prostatic edema.
- Stool softeners.
- Hydration.
- Sitz bath.

Prevention: Prophylaxis for Ultrasound Guided Transrectal Prostate Biopsy

- Local uropathogenic *Escherichia coli* antimicrobial resistance patterns should be used to guide antibiotic choice as resistance to **both** ciprofloxacin (1st line) or trimethoprim-sulfamethoxazole (2nd line). Select cephalosporin-based regimens if resistance is ≥10%.
- Outpatient procedure: ciprofloxacin 750–1000 mg orally × 1 up to 30 min—2 hrs before the time of the outpatient procedure if uropathic *E. coli* resistance to fluoroquinolones is ≤10%.
- Inpatient procedure or if uropathic *E. coli* resistance to fluoroquinolones is >10%.: Ceftriaxone 1 g IV **plus** gentamicin 1.7 mg/kg 1–2 hrs before the procedure.

FOLLOW UP

- Follow-up after 72 hrs of treatment; if not responding, consider search for prostate abscess using transrectal ultrasound.
- Duration of therapy (4 wks) guided by intent to prevent relapse.
- Continue follow-up for at least 3 mos after diagnosis as only 68% remain infection free at this time.
- After full recovery, investigate urinary tract to exclude structural cause for prostatitis.
- Properly managed acute bacterial prostatitis has a very good outcome.

OTHER INFORMATION

- Indications for hospitalization/IV RX: febrile with toxicity, concomitant illness, debilitated by age, immunosuppressed.
- Good antibiotic penetration into all areas of prostate achieved due to intense inflammation. Antibiotics should be continued or changed according to sensitivity results.
- Do not perform prostatic massage! Extremely painful and of little benefit as pathogens almost always isolated from urine.
- Persistent fever after 48 hrs of antibiotics requires transrectal U/S to look for abscess.
- In middle-aged men, Prostate Specific Antigen (PSA) levels may be elevated for 3–6 mos after acute phase of inflammation. If transurethral ultrasound done, hypoechoic areas in prostate peripheral zone may persist for many mos. Use color Doppler ultrasound to differentiate these areas from prostatic cancer.

BASIS FOR RECOMMENDATIONS

Grabe M, et al. *Guidelines on the Management of Urinary and Male Genital Tract Infections*, 2008.

Comments: The most recent guidelines on the management of acute bacterial prostatitis by the European Association of Urology. The guidelines are similar to the those issued by the U.K.'s (British Association of Sexual Health and HIV) in 2001. There remain no U.S. published treatment guideline for acute or chronic bacterial prostatitis.

Kravchick S, Cytron S, Agulansky L, et al. Acute prostatitis in middle-aged men: a prospective study. *BJU Int*, 2004; Vol. 93; pp. 93–6.

Comments: The authors conducted a prospective study of 28 men, ages 50–67 (mean 61) yrs, to examine the clinical outcome of acute prostatitis in middle-aged men focusing on the optimal time to reassess PSA level, known to increase in any inflammatory process, and the role of imaging modalities, transrectal ultrasound and color Doppler ultrasound, in characterizing prostatic changes. Only 68% remained infection free at 3 mos; 6% developed abscesses; 39% had persistent PSA elevation at 3 mos. 3 of 8 pts who underwent biopsy for persistent elevated PSA had prostate CA.

Clinical Effectiveness Group. National guideline for the management of prostatitis (British Association of Sexual Health and HIV—formerly the Association of Genitourinary Medicine and the Medical Society for the Study of Venereal Diseases). *http://www.bashh.org/guidelines.asp*, 2001.

Comments: This evidence-based guideline is a distillation of a 1966-2000 Medline search using "prostatitis," the Cochrane Database of Systematic Reviews and the Cochrane Controlled Clinical Trials Register up to 2000. Additional references were also included. Probably the best current distillation and assessment of data on prostatitis.

Lipsky BA. Prostatitis and urinary tract infection in men: what's new; what's true? *Am J Med*, 1999; Vol. 106; pp. 327–34.

Comments: A good general article which again reinforces that fluoroquinolones are preferred over SMX/TMP and that treatment should be for 4 wks.

BACTERIAL PROSTATITIS, CHRONIC

Noreen A. Hynes, MD, MPH

PATHOGENS

- *Escherichia coli*
- Other Enterobacteriaceae
- Some Gram-positive organisms such as *Enterococcus faecalis* or *Staphylococcus saprophyticus* occasionally are the etiologic agents.
- Fungal and viral causes have very rarely been identified.

CLINICAL

- Chronic bacterial prostatitis (CBP) = Category II prostatitis by NIH classification.
- There is no standardized clinical definition although the condition is well recognized in clinical practice.
- Presents with vague symptoms which are not specific to chronic bacterial prostatitis. NB: the majority of persons with these vague sx will not have CBP.
- Sx: perineal pain, lower abdominal pain, penile pain (especially at meatus), testicular pain, post-ejaculatory pain, rectal or lower back pain, dysuria. Fever, prostration, bacteremia is not a feature.
- Symptoms may be described a dull ache or pain "up inside the rectum" especially when sitting. May complain for an itching sensation "deep inside." The dysuria may be mild discomfort on voiding, with or without frequency or urgency. Very occasionally there is a minimal urethral discharge of clear, whitish fluid. Pts with condition are often very anxious prior to diagnosis expressing concerns about sterility, impotence, prostate cancer or enlarged prostate.
- Signs: few objective signs. Gland may or may not be locally or diffusely tender to palpation.

DIAGNOSIS

- Lower urinary tract localization procedure (Meares-Stamey 4-glass test) = definitive modality for dx: lab-based gold standard uses 4-glass method—sequential cx of urine and expressed prostatic secretions (see More Diagnosis section).
- Modified Meares-Stamey test (2-glass test) has been advocated by many as an acceptable alternative to the 4-glass method.
- Pt preparation for localization test: no antibiotics for 1 mo before test, no ejaculation for 2 days prior to test, full but not distended bladder at the time of test.
- Do not perform prostatic massage for localization test if there is any evidence of urethritis or UTI. Treat these first.

- Measure PSA in all men >45 yrs although may be elevated due to inflammation. If elevated and chronic bacterial prostatitis confirmed, treat prostatitis first and repeat PSA after treatment rather than proceeding directly to biopsy.
- Transrectal ultrasound may identify abscesses or cysts that could be amenable to aspiration with subsequent sx relief. This modality cannot differentiate bacterial from non-bacterial chronic prostatitis.
- In immunocompromised pts, ask laboratory to also look for fungi on the localization test specimens.

MORE DIAGNOSIS

Meares-Stamey 4-Glass Test/Prostatic Massage Procedure:

- Retract foreskin (if present).
- Clean the glans penis and meatal opening to prevent contamination.
- VB1 (Glass 1) = Collect the first 5–10 mL of the first voided urethral urine.
- Ask the pt to void further about 100–200 mL and discard this urine.
- VB2 (Glass 2) = Collect the first 5–10 mL after the above discard as the midstream urine.
- EPS = (Glass 3) Expressed prostatic secretions: by digital rectal examination, beginning at the periphery working toward the midline—perform a vigorous massage of the prostate gland for 1 minute and collect any expressed secretions in a sterile container.
- Wet Prep = prepare a wet prep of the EPS to determine the PMNs present per HPF (×400).
- pH of EPS sample: pH ≥8 is suggestive of prostatitis.
- VB3 = (Glass 4) Immediately after massage collect 5–10 mL of post massage urine.
- Send all samples for Gram-stain and quantitative cultures. NB: a **dry** prostatic massage is a common occurrence.

Interpretation of Prostatic Massage Results

- To identify an etiologic agent: prostate colony count in EPS and VB3 must be ≥10 times VB1–2.
- Prostatic inflammation = ≥10 PMN/HPF in EPS; if massage is dry, then VB3 PMN/HPF >10 PMN/hpf than VB1 and VB2 is diagnostic.
- If there is significant bacteriuria in VB2 and VB3, give (non-prostate penetrating) nitrofurantoin 50 mg PO four times a day × 3 days and then repeat the procedure.

2-Glass Modified Meares-Stamey Test

- Collect only midstream (VB2) and EPS samples.
- Conduct same tests as for standard test. Recommended Regimens

TREATMENT

Recommended Regimens

- Empiric therapy is not indicated chronic bacterial prostatitis; it is not an emergency. Treatment decision should await the results from a 4-glass or 2-glass modified Meares-Stamey test (see above More Diagnosis section) before treatment as 90% or more of prostatitis does not have a microbiological etiology.
- Ciprofloxacin 500 mg PO twice daily × 28 days.
- Norfloxacin 400 mg PO twice daily × 28 days.
- Ofloxacin 200 mg PO twice daily × 28 days.
- Some studies have looked at treatment periods of >28 days but there is no evidence that increasing duration is superior to the recommended 28 days.

Quinolone Allergy Regimens

- Doxycycline 100 mg PO twice daily × 28 days (less toxicity than minocycline regimen).
- Minocycline 100 mg PO twice daily × 28 days.
- Trimethoprim-Sulfamethoxazole 1 double-strength tablet PO twice daily × 28 days.
- Trimethoprim 200 mg PO twice daily × 28 days.
- If minocycline or doxycycline is used, antibiotic testing is very important because many uropathogens are tetracycline resistant. Many reported studies using TMP-SMX have used treatment periods of longer than 90 days.

FOLLOW UP

- All pts should receive a detailed explanation of chronic bacterial prostatitis with particular emphasis on the need for follow-up and the difficulty in realizing successful treatment due to poor penetration of antibiotics into the prostate gland.

- Pts should be followed up at 2 wks; 1 mo and monthly thereafter for up to 6 mos to determine if retreatment will be needed. 2 or 4 glass test should be repeated at 6 mos.
- If infection recurs, may need to determine if prostatic calculi are present—a known source of recurrent chronic bacterial prostatitis. Urological consultation is warranted if stones or obstruction found.
- After treatment, evaluate pt for structural or functional abnormalities using CT and measurement of residual urine voiding. The yield on these tests is 23–50% depending upon the patient's age and if he has preexisting conditions.

OTHER INFORMATION

- The 4-glass localization test, although time consuming is key to differentiating this condition from non-bacterial causes.
- Before localization test: (1) no antibiotics for at least 1 mo, (2) no ejaculation for 2 days, (3) full, non-distended bladder. Do not perform if evidence of urethritis or UTI. RX acute problem first.
- Prostatic calculi suggested as source of recurrent infection. Very common radiologic finding. Radical **turp** or total prostatectomy may be effective in carefully selected pts.

BASIS FOR RECOMMENDATIONS

Grabe M, et al. Guidelines on the management of urinary and male genital tract infections. *http://www.uroweb.org/nc/professional-resources/guidelines/online/*, 2008.

Comments: The most recent guidelines on the management of chronic bacterial prostatitis by the European Association of Urology. The guidelines are similar to the those issued by the U.K.'s (British Association of Sexual Health and HIV) in 2001. There remain no U.S. published treatment guideline for chronic bacterial prostatitis.

Clinical Effectiveness Group National guideline for the management of prostatitis (British Association of Sexual Health and HIV—formerly the Association of Genitourinary Medicine and the Medical Society for the Study of Venereal Diseases). *http://www.bashh.org/guidelines.asp*, 2001.

Comments: This evidence-based guideline is a distillation of a 1996–2000 Medline search using "prostatitis," the Cochrane Database of Systematic Reviews and the Cochrane Controlled Clinical Trials Register up to 2000. Additional references were also included. Probably the best current distillation and assessment of data on prostatitis.

EPIDIDYMITIS, ACUTE

Noreen A. Hynes, MD, MPH

PATHOGENS

- *Chlamydia trachomatis*
- *Neisseria gonorrhoeae*
- Enteric pathogens

CLINICAL

- An acute clinical syndrome. Triad = pain, swelling and inflammation of the epididymis of <6 wks duration.
- One-third will report sudden onset, two-thirds gradual onset. May have history of urethral discharge and/or dysuria, esp if an STD. Hx of urinary tract instrumentation or surgery often in non STD cases.
- Severe scrotal pain, usually **unilateral**, with or without inguinal pain.
- PE: testicle usually in normal position in scrotum; swollen, tender epididymis on palpation. Scrotum of affected side may be erythematous and edematous.
- **Rule out testicular torsion in all cases:** This is a surgical emergency. Examination of Gram-stain and urine helps differentiate epididymitis from torsion; torsion usually without white cells and/or bacteria. Ultrasound exam or urology consultation. In severe epididymitis, cases with acute swelling of spermatic cord may cause flank pain if obstruction of ureter occurs as it crosses cord.
- DDX: testicular torsion, abscess, hydrocele, spermatocele, hernia, trauma, testicular cancer, drugs, esp. amiodarone.
- Urethritis, often asymptomatic, usually found in sexually transmitted acute epididymitis. Bacteruria secondary to obstructive urinary disease seen in non-STD cases.

DIAGNOSIS

- Gram-stain for dx of urethritis (>5 WBC/oil immersion field—highly sensitive and specific for urethritis and gonococcal urethritis in men) **or**

- Positive leukocyte esterase test of unspun FVU or microscopic exam of FVU sediment with >10 WBC/hpf, cx of intraurethral exudate or (preferred) nucleic acid amplification test (NAAT) for GC/CT, syphilis serology, HIV test.

TREATMENT

Empiric Rx: When Gonorrhea or Chlamydia Most Likely Cause (Age <35 Yrs)

- Ceftriaxone 250 mg IM once **plus** doxycycline 100 mg PO twice daily × 10 days.
- Allergy to cephalosporins: *N. gonorrhoeae* resistance rates to fluoroquinolone antibiotics have increased to >25% in some U.S. cities and are no longer recommended for use in treatment of gonococcal infections at any site. For pts with a history of cephalosporin allergy consultation with a specialist is recommended for allergy testing and desensitization, if needed, prior to treatment with a cephalosporin. Spectinomycin has not been demonstrated to achieve adequate tissue penetration in treatment of gonococcal epididymitis and cannot be recommended.

Empiric Rx: Enteric Organism Most Likely (Age ≥35 Yrs)

- Ofloxacin 300 mg PO twice daily × 10 days.
- Levofloxacin 500 mg PO qday × 10 days.

Adjunctive therapy for all

- Bed rest.
- Scrotal elevation.
- Analgesics until fever and local inflammation subside.
- Reexamine **every** pt within 72 hrs to assess original DX and RX. Failure to improve by this time requires reevaluation of diagnosis and treatment.
- Swelling and tenderness persisting after completion of Abx should be evaluated comprehensively with DDx = (1) tumor, (2) abscess, (3) infarction, (4) testicular cancer, (5) TB, and (6) fungi.

Management of Sex Partners

- Suspect or confirmed cases should refer **all** sex partners (within the 60 days prior to sx onset) for evaluation and treatment.
- Avoid sexual intercourse until pt and all sex partners are cured (i.e., after completion of treatment for both).

Special Patient Populations: HIV and Immunocompromised

- HIV infected men with acute epididymitis should receive same Rx outlined for uninfected persons.
- TB and fungi are more frequent causes of acute epididymitis in HIV infected and other immunocompromised men than uninfected immunocompetent men.

OTHER INFORMATION

- **Men <35 yrs**: usual etiology is *C. trachomatis* and *N. gonorrhoeae*. In men who engage in insertive rectal intercourse, coliforms are also likely. More unusual organisms— *P. aeruginosa*.
- **Men ≥35 yrs**: the most common pathogens—coliforms and *P. aeruginosa* but CT and GC must always be considered. Also, underlying structural pathology or chronic bacterial prostatitis should be considered.
- Acute epididymitis develops in 1–5% of men with untreated gonorrhea or chlamydia.

MORE OTHER INFORMATION

Some, rare organisms can be spread hematogenously: *S. pneumoniae*, *Brucella* spp., *N. meningitidis*, *T. pallidum*, *Nocardia* spp., *H. influenzae* type B, histoplasmosis, Coccidioides, blastomycosis, cryptococcosis, candidiasis, CMV. Unless pt exam is early in course of evolving acute process, physical exam may not be able to tell epididymitis from torsion.

Epididymo-orchitis has been described in 12% to 19% of men with Behçets disease. This is non-infective and thought to be part of the disease process.

BASIS FOR RECOMMENDATIONS

Centers for Disease Control and Prevention (CDC). Update to CDC's sexually transmitted diseases treatment guidelines, 2006: fluoroquinolones no longer recommended for treatment of gonococcal infections. *MMWR Morb Mortal Wkly Rep*, 2007; Vol. 56; pp. 332–6.

Comments: Fluoroquinolones (FQ) have been used in the U.S. for the treatment of gonorrhea since 1993. Since 2000, FQ resistance among *Neisseria gonorrhoeae* isolates reported by the Centers for Disease Control and Prevention

(CDC)-sponsored sentinel surveillance system, the Gonococcal Isolate Surveillance System (GISP) has been steadily increasing. Data available from the GISP for 2005 and preliminary data from 2006 demonstrate FQ resistant gonorrhea continues to increase among heterosexuals as well as men who have sex with men. Rates among heterosexual men are now as high as 26.6% in some cities. Therefore, on 13 April 2006, the CDC revised its *2006 Sexually Transmitted Diseases Treatment Guidelines* and no longer recommend the use of any FQ for the treatment of proven or suspect gonorrhea at any site of infection.

Centers for Disease Control and Prevention. Sexually transmitted diseases treatment guidelines 2002. Centers for Disease Control and Prevention. *MMWR Recomm Rep,* 2006; Vol. 55; pp. 1–94.

Comments: The 2006 CDC treatment guidelines provide clinicians with a readily available reference for STD treatments recommended by a panel of national and international experts in STD diagnosis, treatment, prevention and control. These guidelines available electronically at: http://www.cdc.gov/std/treatment/.

GENITAL WARTS/ANOGENITAL WARTS

Noreen A. Hynes, MD, MPH

PATHOGENS

- Human papillomavirus (HPV) types associated with visible, usually benign, anogenital warts—most commonly types 6 and 11 (so-called low risk types); less common HPV types causing visible warty lesions include 16, 30, 40, 41, 42, 43, 44, 54, 55. Among visible wart associated HPVs, types 6, 11, 16, 18, and 31 are commonly associated with squamous intraepithelial lesions (SIL) and less commonly type 30. The visible wart associated types that have also been associated with carcinomas include types 16 and 54, both of which are less commonly associated with visible warts.

CLINICAL

- Most anogenital HPV infections are subclinical or asymptomatic due to one or more of approximately 40 types of non-oncogenic and oncogenic virus types. Although the seroprevalence of infection is approximately 25% for sexually active women and 20% for sexually active men, less than 5% of infections result in visible warts. In one cross sectional survey in one U.S. city only 0.8% of U.S. women aged 21–29 yrs and 0.6% of women aged 30–39 yrs had visible anogenital warts. **Most visible warts are caused by non-oncogenic ("low risk" HPV types).** Approximately 5% of adults report having ever had genital warts.
- **Modes of transmission:** genital and anogenital warts are primarily transmitted through sexual contact and approximately 65% of sexual partners of persons with visible anogenital warts will also develop visible lesions supporting concordant infections with the same HPV type(s); perinatal transmission does occur with a small number of infants born to women with genital warts developing juvenile oropharyngeal papillomatosis (JORP) and cutaneous warts developing in the first wk of life. Blood-borne transmission has not been demonstrated.
- **Natural history:** untreated anogenital warts may resolve spontaneously, remain unchanged or increase in size; highest risk for visible warts appears to be in those <25 yrs of age.
- **History:** sexual contact 4 to 6 wks prior to noting the appearance of lesions with a partner with warts at the time of sexual contact or with a recent history of penile warts.
- **Symptoms:** affected persons usually do not have associated symptoms despite visible lesions; occasionally pts report mild pruritis, burning, discomfort or bleeding (often secondary to irritation or minor trauma to the area).
- **Lesion locations:** in men, most lesions are found on the penis, scrotum, urethral meatus, perianal, or intraanal (particularly in men who have sex with men although overall prevalence of anal HPV infection was ~25% in one cohort of heterosexual only men); in uncircumcised men—85–90% located in preputial cavity; circumcised men—most lesions found on penile shaft; 1–25% involve initial 3 cm of urethral meatus. In women, locations variable including posterior introitus>>labia majora>labia minora>clitoris. Overall, perineum> vagina>anus>cervix>urethra; perianal lesions also common. HIV infected and other immunocompromised persons may have more numerous and larger warts.
- **Physical signs of the 4 warty lesion types:** condylomata acuminata—cauliflower-like lesions and found most often on moist, partially keratinized skin; papular warts—1–4 mm dome-shaped, flesh-colored papules found on fully keratinized skin; <u>flat warts</u>—macular to slightly papular lesions found on partially or fully keratinized skin; and keratotic warts—may have

an appearance similar to a seborrheic keratotic lesion, a common skin wart, or a crust like layered lesion and found only on fully keratinized skin.

- **Differential diagnosis:** accuminate lesions—skin tags, condylomata lata (of secondary syphilis); papular lesions—benign pearly penile lesions, sebaceous glands; keratotic lesions—seborrheic keratitis; flat lesions—molluscum contagiosum.
- **Treatment decisions:** should be guided by pt preference, anticipated adherence to treatment regimen selected, resource availability, experience of provider, and wart characteristics including size, location, and number. No particular treatment has been proven to be superior to another.

DIAGNOSIS

- Usually by visual inspection (use of hand-held magnifying glass may be helpful) of the anogenital skin and speculum examination for visualization of the vaginal canal and uterine cervix. Can be confirmed by biopsy when needed; nucleic acid tests to confirm the presence of HPV are not recommended for routine diagnosis or as an aid in managment. Acetic acid (3–5%) application has inadequate sensitivity or specificity and is not recommended for routine diagnosis but clinicians who routinely diagnosis and treat HPV and are experienced in diagnosing the full spectrum of lesion types, may use this agent to confirm the diagnosis of flat warts. Proctoscopy should be considered in pts who have rectal bleeding in the setting of visible perianal warts.
- **Indications for biopsy:** diagnosis is uncertain, disease does not respond or worsens on therapy, the pt is immunocompromised, warts with unique characteristics that could signal another condition including those warts that are pigmented, ulcerated, fixed, or bleeding.
- **Other diagnostic tests:** In pts with acuminate lesions, serologic testing for (secondary) syphilis should be considered as the lesions may have a similar appearance; HIV testing is indicated as well as testing for other STDs including chlamydia and gonorrhea.

TREATMENT

Patient-applied Regimens for External Anogenital Warts (Men and Non-pregnant women)

- **Podofilox 0.5% solution or gel.** Apply solution with a cotton swab or gel with a finger to the visible genital warts twice a day for 3 days, followed by no therapy for 4 days. This cycle is repeated, as needed, up to 4 times. Total treated wart area should not exceed 10 cm^2 and the total volume of podofilox should not exceed 0.5 mL per day. Ideally, the provider should apply the first treatment thereby demonstrating proper treatment to the pt.
- **Imiquimod, 5% cream.** Apply cream once daily at bedtime, 3 times per wk for up to 16 wks. Wash area of application with soap and water 6–10 hrs after application.

Provider-applied Interventions for Anogenital Warts

- **Cryotherapy with liquid nitrogen or a cryoprobe.** Repeat application every 1 to 2 wks, as needed. This method should only be used by trained personnel.
- **Podophyllin resin, 10% to 25%, in tincture of benzoin.** Once only applications by trained personnel with disposal of the container after single use to prevent nosocomial infection. Apply a small amount to each wart and allow to air dry. Limit application to <0.5 mL of podophyllin or an area <10 cm^2 per session. Do not use if there are any open lesions or wounds in the area of application. Instruct the pt to wash the application area with soap and water 1–4 hrs after the application to reduce local irritation. Repeat weekly as needed. Safety in pregnancy is **not** established.
- **Trichloroacetic acid (TCA) or bichloroacetic acid (BCA), 80% to 90%.** Apply a small amount to the warts **only** using a wooden applicator stick or plastic wand and allow to dry (the areas are dry when a white "frost" is seen on the painted lesions) before the pt is permitted to sit or stand. Excess unreacted acid should be removed with baking soda (sodium bicarbonate) or liquid soap. The treatment can be repeated weekly, as needed.
- **Surgical removal** using either a electrosurgery, curettage, tangential shave or scissor excision. This should be carried out only by trained personnel.

Provider-Applied Treatments for Cervical, Vaginal, Urethral Meatal, and Perianal Warts

- **Uterine cervical warts:** consultation with a specialist required for exophytic cervical warts.
- **Vaginal warts:** TCA or BCA, 80% to 90% applied to warts. A small amount is applied to the warts and allowed to dry until the "white frost" develops; excess acid can be neutralized with baking soda, talcum powder, or liquid soap. Treatment can be repeated weekly, if needed.

DIAGNOSIS

- **Urethral meatal warts:** cryotherapy with liquid nitrogen weekly, as needed or podophyllin 10% to 25% in tincture of benzoin applied to **dry** meatal opening. Treatment may be repeated weekly, if needed and should not be used in pregnant women.
- **Perianal warts:** cryotherapy with liquid nitrogen, as needed or TCA or BCA 80% to 90% applied to warts. A small amount should be applied only to the warts and allowed to dry to the point where "white frost" is visible. Excess acid can be neutralized with baking soda, talc or liquid soap. Treatment can be repeated weekly, if needed. **Intra-anal warts should be referred to a surgeon for removal and follow-up.**

Treatment of Anogenital Warts during Pregnancy
- No pt-applied treatments should be used.
- **Cryotherapy with liquid nitrogen or a cryoprobe.** Repeat application every 1 to 2 wks, as needed. This method should only be used by trained personnel.
- **Trichloroacetic acid (TCA) or bichloroacetic acid (BCA), 80% to 90%.** Apply a small amount to the warts *only* using a wooden applicator stick or plastic wand and allow to dry (the areas are dry when a white "frost" is seen on the painted lesions) before the pt is permitted to sit or stand. Excess unreacted acid should be removed with baking soda (sodium bicarbonate) or liquid soap. The treatment can be repeated weekly, as needed.

Treatment of Anogenital Warts in HIV-Infected Persons
- Use the same modalities as for HIV uninfected persons

FOLLOW UP

Patient Follow-up
- Pt should return for follow-up evaluation 3 mos after genital warts have cleared and cautioned that recurrence is possible, particularly in the first 3 mos after completion of treatment.
- Women should be counselled to undergo regular Pap screening as recommended for women without genital warts.
- Vaccination with the quadrivalent HPV vaccine (containing antigens to types 6, 11, 16 and 18) should be recommended for 11–12 yr-old girls (but can be administered to girls as young as 9 yrs of age) and b) 13–26 yr-old females who have not yet received or completed the vaccine series. Having genital warts is not a contraindication to vaccination as prevention of infection with the other genotypes in the vaccine is still possible.
- HIV-infected men with perianal or intra-anal warts: this group is at high-risk for squamous cell carcinoma of the anus due to oncogenic HPV types and should have an anal Pap smear taken (I was not aware there were formal recs for anal paps in men).

Management of Sex Partners
- Examination of sex partners is not needed as there are no data to indicate that reinfection plays a role in visible anogenital wart recurrence.
- Sex partners who have genital warts should be considered for counseling and examination for other STDs, including HIV.
- Female sex partners in the target age groups for quadrivalent HPV vaccine should be counselled regarding the availability of the vaccine.

OTHER INFORMATION
- **Variant lesions: Erythroplasia of Queyrat** (on the glans penis)—lesions are morphologically similar to those of Bowen's disease and occur on the glans penis and under the prepuce, almost exclusively in uncircumcised men. The histopathology is intraepithelial neoplasia. Pts with suspect BD should be referred to a dermatologist for management. HPV is suspected but not proven as the etiological agent of some or all of the cases. **Bowenoid papulosis**—usually HPV type 16-induced papules with a distinctive histopathology (called Bowen's disease when occuring outside the anogenital region and also seen in Erythroplasia of Queyrat) of focal epidermal hyperplasia and dysplasia and evidence of squamous cell carcinoma (SCC) in situ. No racial, gender preferences; found in sexually active young adults with mean age of 31 yrs. **Giant condyloma of Buschke-Lowenstein (GCBL)**—slow growing verrucous lesion that is highly destructive to contiguous tissue; most commonly found on glans penis seldom metastasizes. Most commonly located on the glans penis in (usually uncircumcised men) > other anogenital mucosal surfaces, including the vulva, vagina, rectum, scrotum, and bladder. HPV is suspect cause with types 6 and 11 commonly found and types 16 and 18 occasionally

found; type 54 rarely found. In U.S. accounts for 5–24% of penile cancers and 0.3–0.5% of all male malignancies. GCBL located outside the penis are much more infrequent. Bladder lesions have been associated with schistosomiasis (ie, *Schistosoma haematobium*). Pts with suspect GCBL should be referred for diagnosis and treatment to a dermatologist.

- Treatment goals for visible genital warts: in most cases, removal is for cosmetic purposes, reduction (not elimination) in viral load and therefore reduce infectivity (unproven).
- HPV vaccine available as cervical cancer prevention. Uncertain role regarding prevention of venereal warts.

BASIS FOR RECOMMENDATIONS

American Academy of Pediatrics Committee on Infectious Diseases. Recommended immunization schedules for children and adolescents—United States, 2007. *Pediatrics*, 2007; Vol. 119; pp. 207–8, 3 p. following 208.

Comments: The January 2007 American Academy of Pediatrics recommended immunization schedules for children and adolescents for the first time include universal immunization of all females beginning at age 12 yrs (or as early as 9 yrs in some cases) for "catch up" immunization of other girls and women who have not been vaccinated with HPV vaccine (the first was approved by the FDA in November 2006). These recommendations mirror the interim recommendations of the Advisory Committee on Immunization Practices (ACIP) outlined in a press release by CDC in November 2006. No final recommendations have been published.

Centers for Disease Control and Prevention, Workowski KA, Berman SM. Sexually transmitted diseases treatment guidelines, 2006. *MMWR Recomm Rep*, 2006; Vol. 55; pp. 1–94.

Comments: The 2006 CDC treatment guidelines for STDs clearly state that HPV DNA testing for cervical HPV infection should be limited based upon the interim screening recommendation promulgated by the American Cancer Society and others. Treatments for genital warts is clearly outlined and explained. These guidelines were published prior to licensure of the new quadrivalent HPV vaccine (late 2006).

PYELONEPHRITIS, ACUTE, UNCOMPLICATED

Noreen A. Hynes, MD, MPH

PATHOGENS

- *Escherichia coli*
- *Staphylococcus saprophyticus*
- *Proteus* spp.
- Uncomplicated acute pyelonephritis is almost always due to *E. coli* or *S. saprophyticus*. A few may be due to *Proteus* spp. Other organisms when identified, including *Klebsiella* spp., *S. aureus*, Enterococcus spp. are strongly suggestive of a complicated urinary tract infection such as the presence of an underlying structural abnormality or a compromised host. Such infections should be managed in consultation with a specialist.

CLINICAL

- **History:** may or may not have hx of symptoms of an episode of lower tract UTI (uncomplicated acute bacterial cystitis); no hx of urologic abnormalities (pyelonephritis in such pts is considered complicated and should be managed in consultation with a specialist); not common in men unless there is some anatomical abnormality of the urinary tract; other dx have been excluded. Essentially all cases in women 18–40 yrs; risk factors: sexually active, diaphragm user. In young sexually active females seek history of new sex partner.
- **Clinical:** fever, chills, flank pain; nausea/vomiting may be present; pathognomonic = tenderness to palpation/percussion over CVA unilaterally or bilaterally; hematuria (common and may be gross).
- **Atypical presentations:** common and may obscure dx—including abdominal pain, respiratory complaints, pelvic pain which may predominate.
- **Outpatient management candidates:** <60 yrs, female, not pregnant, without nausea, vomiting, dehydration, no evidence of sepsis, without high fever.
- **Criteria for hospitalization:** male sex (underlying urinary tract abnormality very common); pregnant woman; signs/symptoms of pyelonephritis with high fever ($>102.2°F/39°C$, high WBC (with left shift), vomiting, dehydration, evidence of sepsis (extremely rare in acute, uncomplicated pyelonephritis) or systemic inflammatory response syndrome (SIRS—> 1 of the following: temperature $>100.2°F/38°C$ or $<96.8°F/36°C$; heart rate >90 beats/min,

respiratory rate >20 breaths/min or $PaCO_2 <$ 32 mmHg/4.3 kPa, WBC <4,000 cells/mL or >12,000 cells/mL or >10% immature band forms).

- **Complications:** renal abscess, nephronia (focal bacterial nephritis).
- **Lab:** urine cx—>100,000 CFU/mL of etiologic agent; spun urine—>9 WBC/HPF; overall >80% due to *E. coli*, 10–20% due to *S. saprophyticus;* in women 16–35 yrs *S. saprophyticus* may cause up to 40% of acute pyelonephritis and is usually less severe that that seen due to *E. coli.*
- **DDX:** PID, appendicitis, urolithiasis, biliary tract disease, acute pancreatitis, basal pneumonia.
- *S. saprophyticus* occurrence: accounts for up 10–20% of acute pyelonephritis in women but up to 40% of those age 16 to 35 yrs. Timing: UTIs and pyelonephritis peak in late summer and early fall in temperate regions. Risk factors: recent sexual intercourse, use of spermicide-impregnated condoms, swimming, and an occupation in meat processing (up to to 7% of cattle and pigs carry in the GI tract) are identified risk factors.

DIAGNOSIS

- **Mid-stream urine (MSU):** for urinalysis and culture and sensitivity. Freshly collected urine specimens for culture need to be received in the laboratory within 1 hr or collection (or used within 18 hrs if stored at 4°C) to reduce the risk of growth/overgrowth of organisms in the urine during transport.
- **Urine culture and sensitivity:** Bacteriuria of $>10^5$ bacteria/mL in an MSU sample is usually considered diagnostic for a UTI. A count of $<10^3$ bacteria/mL is most probably due to contamination.
- **Blood culture:** although positive in 20–30%, little evidence supporting that results have influenced the clinical management or the outcome.

TREATMENT

Empiric Outpatient Treatment

- **Oral:** ciprofloxacin 500 mg PO twice daily × 14 days.
- Ofloxacin 200 mg PO twice daily × 14 days.
- Levofloxacin 500 mg PO once daily × 14 days.
- Norfloxacin 400 mg PO twice daily × 14 days.
- **Alternatives:** ceftriaxone 1 g IM × 1, then an oral fluoroquinolone to complete 14 days.
- Gentamicin 2 mg/kg IM or IV × 1, then an oral fluoroquinolone to complete 14 days.
- Ciprofloxacin 400 mg IV × 1, then an oral fluoroquinolone to complete 14 days.
- Levofloxacin 500 mg IV × 1, then an oral fluoroquinolone to complete 14 days.
- Initial empiric treatment should be modified based upon the results of urine culture and sensitivity and blood culture results. Completion of 14 days of fully effective treatment is key to resolution of infection.

Empiric Inpatient Treatment

- Ciprofloxacin 400 mg IV q12h. Treat IV × 48 hrs or after resolution of severe symptoms; then PO to complete 14 days.
- Gentamicin, tobramycin, netilmicin 2 mg/kg loading dose IV, then 1.5–3.0 mg/kg/day or divided dose, until afebrile 48 hrs or after resolution of severe symptoms, then PO treatment to complete 14 days.
- Amikacin 7.5 mg/kg IV loading dose; then 15 mg/kg/day or divided dose, until afebrile × 48 hrs or after resolution of severe symptoms, then PO treatment to complete 14 days.
- Ampicillin/sulbactam 1–2 g IV q6h until afebrile × 48 hrs or after resolution of severe symptoms, then PO cephalosporin to complete 14 days.
- Cefotaxime 1 or 2 g IV q8h until afebrile × 48 hrs or after resolution of severe symptoms, then give PO cephalosporin to complete 14 days.
- Ceftriaxone 1 g IV once daily until afebrile × 48 hrs or after resolution of severe symptoms, then give PO cephalosporin to complete 14 days.
- Ceftazidime 1–2 g IV q8–12h until afebrile × 48 hrs or after resolution of severe symptoms, then give PO cephalosporin to complete 14 days.
- Levofloxacin 500 mg IV once daily until afebrile × 48 hrs or after resolution of severe symptoms, then give PO levofloxacin to complete 14 days.
- Avoid fluoroquinolones in pregnant women.

- Initial empiric treatment should be modified based upon the results of urine culture and sensitivity and blood culture results. Completion of 14 days of fully effective treatment is key to resolution of infection.

OTHER INFORMATION

- Recommendations based on IDSA Guidelines that are also endorsed by the European Soc Clin Micro Infect Dis and Amer Urol Assn.
- High risk for complications: diabetes, pregnancy, immunocompromised, previous pyelonephritis, sx >14 days, structurally abnormal urinary tract—begin treatment for these in hospital regardless of symptoms.
- Some experienced clinicians have successfully treated mild cases with 5- to 7-days RX of aminoglycosides, beta-lactams, or fluoroquinolones.
- Route of infection is ascending: organisms enter urethra, colonize bladder, ascend to the renal pelvis and ultimately invade renal parenchyma.
- More virulent forms of *E. coli* cause are more likely to cause uncomplicated acute pyelonephritis than cause cystitis but are more susceptible to antimicrobial therapy.

BASIS FOR RECOMMENDATIONS

American College of Obstetricians and Gynecologists. ACOG Practice Bulletin No. 91: Treatment of urinary tract infections in nonpregnant women. *Obstet Gynecol*, 2008; Vol. 111; pp. 785–94.

Comments: This is the most recent update by the American College of OB/GYN of their practice guidelines on urinary tract infections, including pyelonephritis. These guidelines are consistent with those published by the Infectious Disease Society of America in 1999 and support a full 14 days of treatment, beginning with broad spectrum empiric therapy that is then narrowed based upon culture results.

Warren JW, Abrutyn E, Hebel JR, et al. Guidelines for antimicrobial treatment of uncomplicated acute bacterial cystitis and acute pyelonephritis in women. Infectious Diseases Society of America (IDSA). *Clin Infect Dis*, 1999; Vol. 29; pp. 745–58.

Comments: Provides the full IDSA guideline. Gives rationale for current RX guidelines, using evidence-based decision making. Endorsed by American Urologic Ass'n and European Soc for Clin Micro and Infect Disease.

URETHRITIS (MEN)

Noreen A. Hynes, MD, MPH

PATHOGENS

- *Chlamydia trachomatis* (CT): most frequent cause of urethritis in men accounting for 23%–55% of cases. However, the proportion of non-gonococcal urethritis (NGU) cases due to CT is declining gradually.
- *Mycoplasma genitalium*: may be the 2nd most frequent cause of urethritis in the U.S. and UK. May account for between 15% and 22% of cases of acute NGU. Also has a role in chronic NGU.
- *Neisseria gonorrhoeae*: as a cause of urethritis, gonorrhea is increasingly a geographically isolated infection in the U.S. It persists in inner-city populations, in particular.
- *Trichomonas vaginalis*: is the cause of only about 2% of cases of acute NGU but probably a higher proportion of chronic NGU.
- *Ureaplasma urealyticum*: biovar 2 is probably a more important cause of acute NGU than previously realized. In 1999 the organism was divided into 2 species: *U. parnumparnum* (Biovar 1) and *U. urealyticum* (Biovar 2). Studies suggest only the latter associated with urethritis.
- Less common causes include herpes simplex virus (rare in absence of obvious skin lesions), adenovirus, *Haemophilus* spp, yeasts, *N. meningitidis*, *Staphylococcus saprophyticus*.

CLINICAL

- **Symptoms**: urethral discharge of mucopurulent or purulent material, dysuria, penile irritation or pruritis. Asymptomatic infections are common.
- **Signs**: urethral discharge which may only be present after milking the urethra. Some may be without discharge with findings only on laboratory testing.
- Non sexually transmitted causes of NGU (ddx): UTI, bacterial prostatitis, urethral stricture, phimosis, following urethral instrumentation, cases secondary to chemical irritation.
- Complications of untreated urethritis: epididymitis, sexually acquired reactive arthritis (SARA), Reiter's syndrome (esp after chlamydia NGU).
- Urethritis has been shown to facilitate the transmission and acquisition of HIV infection.

DIAGNOSIS

- **Rapid point-of-care test of urethritis:** non-gonococcal urethritis (NGU)—Gram-stain of urethral secretions ≥5 WBCs/oil immersion averaged over 5 fields w/ greatest concentration of PMNs; gonococcal urethritis—the additional presence of Gram-negative intracellular diplococci (sensitivity = 95%). Other point of care findings include positive leukocyte esterase test on first void urine (FVU); ≥10 WBCs/HPF on microscopic exam of FVU.
- **Other general point-of-care tests:** positive leukocyte esterase test on first void urine (FVU), correlates with NGU but not as sensitive as Gram-stain of secretions; >10 WBCs/HPF on microscopic exam of FVU.
- **Chlamydia:** tissue culture has a sensitivity of 70%–80% and a specificity of 100% but is not widely available; enzyme immunoassay sensitivity is 73%–95% sensitive for cervical specimens; direct fluorescent anti body test is 50% to 81% sensitive; DNA probe is slightly more sensitive than culture; nucleic acid amplification tests (NAATs) are of urethral specimen or urine 85%–95% sensitive and 99% specific.
- **Gonorrhea:** Gram-stain is sufficient for diagnosis in men unless suspect antimicrobial resistance or collect specimens from other exposure sites (pharynx, rectum); culture on selective media has a sensitivity of 86%–96%; DNA probe has almost equivalent sensitivity to culture; nucleic acid amplifications tests (NAATs) of secretions or urine are 95%–98% sensitive.
- **Trichomoniasis:** non-microscopy based point of care diagnostics are >83% sensitive and >97% specific and include OSOM Trichomonas Rapid Test (Genezyme Diagnostics, Cambridge, MA) which takes 10 minutes (83% sensitivity, 98.8% specificity). Culture using Diamond's media and commercially available culture based tests such as the InPouch system are 90–95% sensitive and >95% specific.
- **Mycoplasma:** cx is available using mycoplasma agar; organism is very slow growing taking 2–3 wks; nucleic acid tests are available for research purposes but are not FDA cleared.
- **Ureaplasma:** cx require ureaplasma species-specific transport media with refrigeration at 4°C (39°F); can be cultured in urea-containing broth in 1 to 2 days; do not use of cotton swabs to collect specimen. Several rapid, sensitive polymerase chain reaction assays for detection have been developed but are not available routinely and are not FDA cleared. Antibody test is of limited value and should not be used for routine diagnosis.

MORE DIAGNOSIS

- The quality of the Gram-stain smear is heavily dependent on how the smear was taken.
- There is no published data on whether a cotton-tipped swab or a 5 mm plastic loop is better for collection of urethral secretions.

TREATMENT

Gonococcal Urethritis

- *N. gonorrhoeae* resistance rates to fluoroquinolone antibiotics have increased to >25% in some U.S. cities and are no longer recommended for use in treatment of gonorrhea in the U.S.
- Ceftriaxone 125 mg IM × 1 *plus* azithromycin 1 g PO × 1 or doxycycline 100 mg PO twice daily × 7 days if chlamydia infection has not been ruled out.
- Cefixime 400 mg PO × 1 *plus* azithromycin 1 g PO × 1 or doxycycline 100 mg PO twice daily × 7 days if chlamydia infection has not been ruled out.
- Alternative regimens: spectinomycin (not currently available in the U.S.) 2 g IM (do not use if oral exposure suspected).
- Cephalosporin/ penicillin allergic pts: if spectinomycin is not available, pts with a history of allergy should be referred to a specialist for possible desensitization prior to treatment with a recommended cephalosporin.

Non-Gonococcal Urethritis

- Azithromycin 1 g PO × 1.
- Doxycycline 100 mg PO twice daily × 7 days.

Recurrent or Persistent Urethritis

- Metronidazole 2 g PO or Tinidazole 2 g PO once **plus** erythromycin base 500 mg PO four times a day × 7 days.
- Metronidazole 2 g PO or Tinidazole 2 g PO once **plus** erythromycin ethylsuccinate 800 mg PO four times a day × 7 days.

FOLLOW UP
Patient care and education

- Instruct pts to return for evaluation if sx persist or recur after completion of rx. Lab confirmation of persistence or relapse needed before retreatment.
- Abstain from sexual intercourse for 7 days after treatment started, provided sx have resolved and sex partners have been adequately treated.
- Refer for additional evaluation of persistent pain, discomfort or dysuria (>3 mos)—suggest chronic prostatitis or chronic pelvic pain syndrome in men.
- If lab results indicate a new STD is present, pts should be tested for other STDs including syphilis and HIV.
- Pts should notify all sex partners within the preceding 60 days of the need for evaluation and treatment. Pathogen-specific testing of the pt is strongly urged to facilitate partner management.

OTHER INFORMATION
- Rx of HIV-infected persons is the same as for HIV-uninfected persons.

BASIS FOR RECOMMENDATIONS
Centers for Disease Control and Prevention (CDC). Update to CDC's sexually transmitted diseases treatment guidelines, 2006: fluoroquinolones no longer recommended for treatment of gonococcal infections. *MMWR Morb Mortal Wkly Rep,* 2007; Vol. 56; pp. 332–6.

Comments: Fluoroquinolones (FQ) have been used in the U.S. for the treatment of gonorrhea since 1993. Since, 2000 FQ resistance among *Neisseria gonorrhoeae* isolates reported by the Centers for Disease Control and Prevention (CDC)-sponsored sentinel surveillance system, the Gonococcal Isolate Surveillance System (GISP) has been steadily increasing. Data available from the GISP for 2005 and preliminary data from 2006 demonstrate FQ resistant gonorrhea continues to increase among heterosexuals as well as men who have sex with men. Rates among heterosexual men are now as high as 26.6% in some cities. Therefore, on 13 April 2006, the CDC revised its *2006 Sexually Transmitted Diseases Treatment Guidelines* and no longer recommend the use of any FQ for the treatment of proven or suspect gonorrhea at any site of infection.

Centers for Disease Control and Prevention, Workowski KA, Berman SM. Sexually transmitted diseases treatment guidelines, 2006. *MMWR Recomm Rep,* 2006; Vol. 55; pp. 1–94.

Comments: The CDC treatment guidelines are considered the STD practice guidelines for use in the United States. The guidelines stress the importance of partner referral in the overall STD prevention control strategy. Pts should refer for evaluation and treatment all sex partners within the preceding 60 days. Testing for GC and CT are strongly encouraged.

URINARY TRACT INFECTION, COMPLICATED (UTI)

James DeMaio, MD

PATHOGENS
- Enterobacteriaceae, *Pseudomonas aeruginosa* and *Acinetobacter* spp. are among the most common. Resistant strains frequently encountered.
- MRSA, *Enterococcus* spp. (including VRE), *Candida* spp. and fastidious organisms possible.
- Infections may be polymicrobial, especially if chronic urinary catheter or stents are present.

CLINICAL
- Complicated UTI is an infection of the lower or upper urinary tract in the presence of an anatomic abnormality, a functional abnormality or a urinary catheter (FDA definition).
- Risk factors for complicated UTIs: Structural abnormality—enlarged prostate, calculi, obstruction, catheter or stent, neurogenic bladder; Metabolic/Hormonal Disorder—pregnancy, diabetes; Immune Defect—renal transplant, neutropenia, HIV.
- Not all complicated UTIs are created equal. Metabolic and immune defect associated UTIs are usually easy to treat and may not relapse. Structural abnormality associated UTIs are often difficult to treat, frequently relapse, and may require urological intervention.
- Symptoms are highly variable. Lower tract infection classically presents with suprapubic pain, increased urinary frequency, dysuria, and foul-smelling urine. Upper tract infection associated with flank pain, fever and chills.
- Presentation often modified by host factors: Elderly may have mental status change only; catheterized pts may have fever only; quadriplegics may have fever and and increased spasticity or autonomic dysreflexia.

DIAGNOSIS

- Urinalysis: leukocyte esterase (+), nitrite (+), urine with > 10 WBC/hpf, culture >10^5 organisms per ml.
- Microbiology: urine culture and sensitivity are critical in order to optimize treatment. Gram-stain of spun urine may be useful in selecting empiric antibiotics. Note: if indwelling catheter or urinary stent, ask laboratory to identify all species since multiple isolates or "skin flora" may be discarded as contaminants.
- If pt is severely ill or not improving with therapy, then urinary tract obstruction must be ruled out. Either renal ultrasound or abd/pelvic CT are appropriate initial tests.

TREATMENT

Medical treatment (antibiotics)

- Empiric therapy must be broad spectrum with definitive therapy based on culture and sensitivity.
- If pt mild to moderately ill: levofloxacin (500 mg IV/PO q24) or ciprofloxacin (500 mg PO twice daily/400 mg q12h IV) are reasonable empiric choices if pt has not recently received a FQ, is not from a long-term care facility (LTCF), and FQ resistance is low.
- If pt severely ill or received recent FQ or from LTCF: select broad empiric coverage with either cefepime 2 g IV q12 hrs, ceftazidime 2 g IV q8hrs, imipenem 500 mg IV q6hrs, meropenem 1 g IV q8hrs, doripenem 500 mg IV q8hrs or piperacillin-tazobactam 3.375–4.5 g IV q6hrs (order of preference based on local sensitivity patterns). Note that all of the listed agents must be adjusted for renal insufficiency.
- If pt severely ill and urine Gram-stain shows Gram (+) cocci: consider adding vancomycin empirically.
- Once culture and sensitivity available, switch to narrow spectrum as much as feasible.
- Duration: most experts recommend 10–14 days of total therapy. European guidelines recommend stopping treatment 3 to 5 days after either defervescence or elimination of the complicating factor (e.g., catheter or stone).

Surgical interventions

- If obstruction cannot be quickly relieved or if anatomic abnormalities are uncovered, then urological consultation is strongly advised.
- Intermittent catheterization is preferable to an indwelling catheter whenever possible. The use of sterile vs. non-sterile technique with intermittent catheterization makes no difference in UTI rates.
- Pts with condom catheters have fewer UTIs than those pts with indwelling catheters (0.08 vs. 0.21 UTIs per pt/mo). Candidates for condom catheters must be alert and have intact skin.

Prevention of cUTI

- Meatal cleaning, antibiotics in the foley bag and systemic antibiotics are ineffective for preventing catheter associated UTIs.
- Effective measures include: aseptic insertion, maintaining a closed system, avoiding obstruction or backflow, and removing the catheter as soon as possible.
- Either a computer-driven or pre-printed prompt system to regularly assess the need for urinary catheters may reduce catheter use in the hospital.
- Bladder scanning whenever bladder distension is suspected may help avoid unnecessary catheter insertions.

FOLLOW UP

- Urological consultation is advised if obstruction cannot be quickly relieved or if anatomic abnormalities are uncovered.
- Infectious diseases consultation is advised if unusual pathogens are identified or if the pt fails to respond to therapy.

OTHER INFORMATION

- Culture and sensitivity are mandatory. The wide array of pathogens and increasing abx resistance often make empiric treatment inaccurate.
- Renally secreted agents are always preferable when treating UTIs.

- Asymptomatic bacteriuria, candiduria or pyuria does not need to be treated, except in pregnancy, children, renal transplant pts, and neutropenia. Remember to treat the pt and not the culture result.
- Follow up cultures are not required if the pt is clinically improving.
- Antibiotic prophylaxis for most pts with risk factors for recurrent, complicated UTI is not recommended. The risk of resistance outweighs the slight reduction in infection rate. Renal transplant pts in the post-op period are an exception and may benefit from prophylaxis.

BASIS FOR RECOMMENDATIONS

Naber KG, Bergman B, Bishop MC, et al. EAU guidelines for the management of urinary and male genital tract infections. Urinary Tract Infection (UTI) Working Group of the Health Care Office (HCO) of the European Association of Urology (EAU). *Eur Urol,* 2001; Vol. 40; pp. 576–88.
Comments: European guidelines for the diagnosis and treatment of uncomplicated and complicated UTIs.

Lundstrom T, Sobel J. Nosocomial candiduria: a review. *Clin Infect Dis,* 2001; Vol. 32; pp. 1602–7.
Comments: An excellent review of the issues surrounding candiduria.

Stamm WE, Hooton TM. Management of urinary tract infections in adults. *N Engl J Med,* 1993; Vol. 329; pp. 1328–34.
Comments: Review of uncomplicated and complicated UTIs.

URINARY TRACT INFECTION, RECURRENT (WOMEN)

Noreen A. Hynes, MD, MPH

PATHOGENS

- *Escherichia coli*
- *Staphylococcus saprophyticus*
- Other Enterobacteriaceae
- Enterococcus spp.

CLINICAL

- Two or more symptomatic UTIs (dysuria, frequency, urgency, hematuria, and suprapubic discomfort not associated with voiding) within a 12-mo period following clinical resolution of each previous UTI after treatment with antimicrobial agents.
- The majority of cases are among women have no anatomical or physiological abnormality related to the urinary tract, therefore investigation for urinary tract abnormalities is unlikely to be of benefit; subgroups that would benefit from investigation are not clearly defined.
- **Reinfection**: a type of recurrent UTI caused by a different pathogen strain at any time or the original infecting strain >13 days after Rx of the original UTI.
- **Relapse**: a type of recurrent UTI caused by the same species as that causing the original UTI within 2 wks after Rx.
- **Premenopausal women:** risks include history of first episode of acute cystitis before the age of 15 yrs, a mother with a history of UTIs, frequent sexual intercourse, new sex partner within the past yr, nonsecretor of ABH blood group antigens, P1 genetic phenotype, and short distance between the urethra and anus.
- **Postmenopausal women:** risks are associated the presence of incontinence, a cystocele or post-void residual (nl PVR # 50–100 ml) (Obst Gyn 2007;110:827); other risk factors include a history of a premenopausal UTI and being a nonsecretor of ABH blood group antigens and with local tissue changes due to decreased local estrogen (elevated vaginal pH and the absence of vaginal lactobacilli may play a role).
- No association between pre- and post-coital voiding patterns, douching, use of hot tubs, frequent use of pantyhose or tights, or BMI and recurrent UTI.
- Pregnant women have an increased risk of recurrent UTI from 6–24 wks gestation due to changes in the uro-genital tract (see UTI in Pregnancy module, p. 88).

DIAGNOSIS

- Point of care confirmation of diagnosis: 1) dipstick positive leukocyte esterase test or positive nitrite (75% sensitive, 82% specific); or 2) >100 CFU/mL on midstream clean-catch urine culture or 3) >9 WBCs/HPF.
- Culture and sensitivity only if UTI recurs within 7 days of completion of therapy for initial UTI or second UTI.

- Diagnostic imaging and other testing for urinary tract abnormalities is usually not indicated. Isolation of *Proteus* sp requires an evaluation for renal stones beginning with a CT or renal ultrasound.

TREATMENT

Continuous Prophylaxis

- TMP-SMZ 1/2 SS tab (40 mg/200 mg) PO qhs or TMP 100 mg PO qhs, if *E. coli* resistance locally to these agents <20% × 6–12 mos.
- Nitrofurantoin 100 mg PO qhs × 6–12 mos.
- Ciprofloxacin 125 mg PO qhs × 6–12 mos.
- Norfloxacin 200 mg PO qhs × 6–12 mos.
- Cefaclor 250 mg PO qhs × 6–12 mos.
- See UTI in pregnant women for regimens in pregnancy.
- Long-term antibiotic prophylaxis (>12 mos). Has not been adequately evaluated in randomized controlled clinical trials and may be of benefit although is likely to have a significant side effect profile and effect on antibiotic resistance.

Postcoital Regimens (within 2 hrs of coitus)

- TMP-SMZ 1/2 single strength tab (40 mg/200 mg) PO postcoitally × 1 (if TMP-SMZ-resistant *E. coli* prevalence locally <20%).
- Ofloxacin 100 mg PO or norfloxacin 200 mg PO or ciprofloxacin 125 mg PO—postcoitally × 1.
- Nitrofurantoin 50–100 mg PO postcoitally × 1.
- See UTI in pregnant women for regimens in pregnancy.

Self-Treatment (at onset of symptoms)

- TMP-SMZ 1/2 SS tab (40 mg/200 mg) PO qhs × 3 days (if TMP-SMZ-*resistant E. coli* prevalence locally <20%).
- See Urinary tract infections in pregnant women for regimens in pregnancy.
- Nitrofurantoin 100 mg PO once daily × 3 days.
- Norfloxacin 200 mg PO once daily × 3 days.
- Ciprofloxacin 125 mg PO once daily × 3 days.

Other Prevention Modalities

- **Cranberry juice and cranberry-containing products for prophylaxis**. There is some evidence from 2 RCTs that cranberry juice (using "fresh" juice) may decrease the number of UTIs over a 12-mo period in child-bearing aged women. Data for children or elderly men and women not clear. The optimal dose is also uncertain.
- **Methenamine hippurate**: insufficient data to support recommendation for use for continuous prophylaxis.
- **Voiding after intercourse**: no data to support the recommendation.
- *Lactobacillus* **species vaginal suppositories**: use of probiotic *Lactobacillus* spp. is only beginning to be studied but may have a role in the future; small clinical trials with too few subjects upon which to base recommendations.
- **Topical vaginal estrogen in postmenopausal women**: use is controversial. May wish to consider in women with >2 recurrent UTI/yr where >20% of local *E. coli* isolates are resistant to both trimethoprim-sulfamethoxazole and fluoroquinolones.
- Heat-killed uropathogen vaginal suppository vaccines: Phase II clinical trials have been conducted and show some promise especially in preventing recurrent UTI associated with uropathogenic *E. coli*.

OTHER INFORMATION

- No published national guidelines; recommendations based on Clinical Evidence 2000;3:961–8, literature review, and author's opinion.
- 80–90% of recurrent UTIs are reinfections; one-third with original strain; recurrent acute uncomplicated cystitis occurs in 12–27% with previous UTI; ratio of recurrent cystitis to recurrent pyelo = 18:1.
- Women >54 yrs old are more likely to have a recurrence after an initial UTI than younger women.
- <5% of women with recurrent UTI have an underlying anatomical or functional abnormality as the cause; in absence of abnormalities associations include maternal hx of UTI, blood-group secretor status.

BASIS FOR RECOMMENDATIONS

Hooton TM. Recurrent urinary tract infection in women. *Int J Antimicrob Agents,* 2001; Vol. 17; pp. 259–68.

Comments: An excellent synthesis of all existing information regarding recurrent urinary tract infections in healthy women.

Melekos MD, Asbach HW, Gerharz E, et al. Post-intercourse versus daily ciprofloxacin prophylaxis for recurrent urinary tract infections in premenopausal women. *J Urol,* 1997; Vol. 157; pp. 935–9.

Comments: Non-randomized, non-blinded study of 70 pts who received prophylaxis as single dose post intercourse vs group of 65 receiving daily dose of ciprofloxacin 125 mg PO. Regimens followed for 12 mos. Long term post-coital prophylaxis was equally effective to daily prophylaxis. The former approach uses approximately 1/3 the amount of drug, hence making it a less expensive option.

Brumfitt W, and Hamilton-Miller JM. A comparative trial of low dose cefaclor and macrocrystalline nitrofurantoin in the prevention of recurrent urinary tract infection. *Infection,* 1995; Vol. 23; pp. 98–102.

Comments: Randomized, non-blinded study of 128 women, age 18–90 yrs with hx of at least 4 episodes of UTI w/ sx in preceding 12 mos. One group received 250 mg cefaclor hs, the other 50 mg macrocrystalline nitrofurantoin hs. Prophylaxis was for 12 mos. There was no difference in clinical efficacy (80%) in the 2 groups and in both there was a 5-fold reduction in recurrences. Nitrofurantoin had a higher side effect profile than cefaclor.

URINARY TRACT INFECTIONS IN PREGNANCY

Noreen A. Hynes, MD, MPH

PATHOGENS

- *Escherichia coli*: 80–85% of isolates
- *Staphylococcus saprophyticus: 3–8%*
- Group B beta-hemolytic *Streptococcus* (GBS): 1–2%
- Other *Enterobacteriaceae*
- *Enterococcus* spp.
- Other organisms less common and include: other Enterobacteriaceae, *P. aeruginosa,* group D streptococci, enterococci, and rarely *H.influenzae,* M.tuberculosis, anaerobes, salmonella, shigella, adenovirus type 11, ureaplasma, and mycoplasma spp. Chlamydia trachomatis can cause urethritis with dysuria and pyuria but is not associated with cystitis or acute pyelonephritis.

CLINICAL

- **Asymptomatic bacteriuria (ASB)**: occurs in 2.5–11% (vs 3–8% in non-pregnant women). Risk increases with age, multiparity, sexual activity, low SES (5-fold), sickle cell trait (2-fold), gestational diabetes, previous hx of UTI, urinary tract abnormalities. Adverse outcomes of untreated ASB: premature or low-birth weight infant, early pregnancy loss, pyelonephritis during pregnancy (20–30-fold) compared with women without bacteriuria, hypertension. Rx decreases risk of pyelonephritis to 1–4% and improves fetal outcomes. Screening urine cx at end of 1st trimester recommended based on clinical outcomes and cost effectiveness. Rx all that meet lab definition.
- **Acute bacterial cystitis (ABC)**: urgency, frequency, suprapubic discomfort, no fever, no flank pain.
- **Acute bacterial pyelonephritis (ABP)**: fever, flank pain, with or without signs/sx of lower tract UTI. Nausea/vomiting may be present. Pathognomonic = tenderness to palpation/percussion over CVA. This is one of the most severe complications of pregnancy; occurs in 1–2% of pregnant women; majority in 2nd, 3rd trimester: 1st trimester (2% of all cases), 2nd trimester (52% of all cases), 3rd trimester (46% of all cases). Hospitalize for initial treatment period.
- Prevalence in USA of UTI (ASB, ABC or ABP) during pregnancy is 28.7% in whites and Asians, 30.1% in blacks, and 41.1% in Hispanics.

MORE CLINICAL

Physiological factor predisposing to UTI in pregnancy

- Weight of enlarging uterus impinging on bladder with resulting urinary stasis.
- Ureteral smooth muscle relaxation secondary to increased progesterone effect contributing to urinary stasis.
- Aminoaciduria. The fractional excretion of alanine, glycine, histidine, serine, and threonine is increased. Other amino acids (leucine, lysine, phenylalanine, cysteine, taurine, and

tyrosine are elevated in 1st half of pregnancy only). Increase concentration postulated to increase adherence of *E. coli* to the urothelium.

- Glucosuria. Glucose excretion increases 100 × compared to non-pregnant state due to impaired resorption of glucose. Glucose in static urine promotes growth of microorganisms.

Hydroureter of pregnancy

- A physiological change of pregnancy.
- Extends to level of pelvic brim.
- Dilatation begins by the 7th wk of pregnancy and progresses until term.
- Both mechanical and hormonal changes contribute.
- Right ureter is more affected than the left.
- Post-partum ureters return to normal in most pts by 2 mos.

Bladder location: In 3rd trimester bladder changes to become an abdominal rather than pelvic organ and has decreased tone secondary to hormonal changes.

Group B beta hemolytic Streptococcus (GBS)

- Intrapartum transmission can cause neonatal pneumonia, meningitis, sepsis, and death.
- GBS asymptomatic bacteriuria is treated if found at end of 1st trimester screening.
- GBS causing symptomatic UTI is treated if it occurs.
- Additional screening: universal vaginal and rectal screening of all women at 35–37 wks gestation with rx of positives.

DIAGNOSIS

- **Asymptomatic bacteriuria**: screen for asymptomatic bacteriuria with urine culture in pregnant women at 12–16 wks gestation or at the first prenatal visit, if later (Grade A recommendation).
- **Asymptomatic bacteriuria**: ≥100,000 cfu/mL of urine with same organism identified in a pregnant woman on 2 consecutive midstream clean-catch urine cx samples with no clinical signs or symptoms of a UTI. Leucocyte esterase and nitrate tests are not useful for dx in asymptomatic pts as it is not specific for asx bacteriuria.
- **Acute bacterial cystitis**: ≥100,000 cfu/mL on midstream clean-catch urine culture or ≥100 cfu/mL of urine from a bladder catheterization specimen (avoid cath unless no other option as this may increase risk of infection).
- **Acute bacterial pyelonephritis**: ≥100,000 cfu/mL on midstream clean-catch urine culture or ≥100 cfu/mL of urine from a bladder catheterization specimen (avoid cath unless no other option as this may increase risk of infection). Blood cx does not add anything to the routine management.
- **Routine imaging of urinary tract**: no role in dx. Consultation with a specialist recommended if you suspect structural abnormalities.

TREATMENT

Empiric Therapy for Asymptomatic Bacteriuria and Cystitis (Pregnancy)

- Nitrofurantoin 100 mg PO four times a day × 7 days.
- Cephalexin 200–500 mg PO four times a day × 3–7 days.
- Cefuroxime axetil 250 mg PO twice daily × 3–7 days.
- Adjust as necessary when culture results return.

Empiric Therapy for Acute Pyelonephritis (Pregnancy)

- Single dose IV in emergency department then home with oral may be an option for clinically stable and treatment adherent pts.
- Cefazolin 1 g IV q8h until afebrile × 48 hrs, then change to PO to complete 14 days.
- Ceftriaxone 1 g IV or IM q24h until afebrile × 48 hrs, then change to PO to complete 14 days.
- Mezlocillin 1–3 g IV q6h until afebrile × 48 hrs, then change to PO to complete 14 days.
- Piperacillin 4 g IV q8h until afebrile 48 hrs, then change to PO to complete 14 days.
- Adjust as necessary upon return of culture results.

FOLLOW UP

Post treatment

- Test of cure 1 wk after completion of rx.
- Periodic screening throughout pregnancy following treatment for ASB, ABC or ABP.
- After pyelonephritis, some experts recommend daily suppressive therapy with nitrofurantoin until delivery.

Culture negative at end of first trimester

- No recommendation for or against subsequent screening due to absence of data. A single urine culture costs approximately $40.

OTHER INFORMATION

- Contraindicated abx in treating UTI during pregnancy: tetracyclines, trimethoprim, sulfa-containing agents. Can cause congenital cardiac and cleft defects.

BASIS FOR RECOMMENDATIONS

U.S. Preventive Services Task Force. Screening for asymptomatic bacteriuria in adults: U.S. Preventive Services Task Force reaffirmation recommendation statement. *Ann Intern Med*, 2008; Vol. 149; pp. 43–7.

Comments: This is a reaffirmation statement of the 2004 U.S. Preventive Services Task Force recommendation statement for asymptomatic bacteriuria in adults. The one Grade A recommendation is to screen for asymptomatic bacteriuria with urine culture in pregnant women at 12 to 16 wks gestation or at the first prenatal visit, if later. These guidelines do **not** recommend screening asymptomatic men or nonpregnant women.

Nicolle LE, Bradley S, Colgan R, et al. Infectious Diseases Society of America guidelines for the diagnosis and treatment of asymptomatic bacteriuria in adults. *Clin Infect Dis*, 2005; Vol. 40; pp. 643–54.

Comments: Infectious Disease Society of America guideline for the definition and management of asymptomatic bacteriuria (ASB) of adults. ASB in women is as 2 consecutive voided urine specimens with isolation of the same bacterial strain in quantitative counts $>10^5$ cfu/mL in an asymptomatic woman or 1 catheterized urine specimen with 1 bacterial species isolated in a quantitative count $>10^2$ cfu/mL. Guideline recommendations for pregnant women include: (1) pregnant women should be screened for bacteriuria by urine culture at least once in early pregnancy, and they should be treated if the results are positive, (2) the duration of antimicrobial therapy should be 3–7 days, (3) periodic screening for recurrent bacteriuria should be undertaken following therapy, and 4) no recommendation is made for or against repeated screening of culture-negative women in later pregnancy.

Warren JW, Abrutyn E, Hebel JR, et al. Guidelines for antimicrobial treatment of uncomplicated acute bacterial cystitis and acute pyelonephritis in women. Infectious Diseases Society of America (IDSA). *Clin Infect Dis*, 1999; Vol. 29; pp. 745–58.

Comments: Infectious Disease Society of America guideline for the treatment of uncomplicated bacterial cystitis and acute pyelonephritis in women.

DIAGNOSIS

APPENDICITIS see p. 194 in Pathogens Section

DIARRHEA, COMMUNITY-ACQUIRED, ACUTE

John G. Bartlett, MD

PATHOGENS
- Norovirus
- *Campylobacter jejuni*
- *Salmonella* species
- *Shigella* species
- Enteroaggregative *E. coli* (EAEC)
- Enterohemorrhagic *Escherichia coli* (EHEC)
- *Giardia lamblia*
- Other causes of acute community-acquired diarrheal disease: **Bacteria**: *Yersinia enterocolitica*, Vibrio species, and possibly *Plesiomonas shigelloides*. **Viruses**: rotavirus, norovirus (formerly Norwalk agent) enteric adenovirus, calicivirus, astrovirus, small round virus, coronavirus. **Parasites**: *Strongyloides stercoralis*. Non-infectious causes: adverse drug reactions, irritable bowel syndrome, inflammatory bowel disease (ulcerative colitis or Crohn's disease), radiation or ischemic bowel disease, partial bowel obstruction, endocrine disorders among others.

CLINICAL
- Hx (symptoms): severity, bloody?, duration, fever, tenesmus, symptomatic dehydration.
- Hx (epidemiology): outbreak?, travel, antibiotic exposure, underlying diseases.
- Traveler's diarrhea (developing countries): enterotoxigenic *E. coli* (dx and rx empirically w/ fluoroquinolone) main cause, others include Norovirus, *Salmonella*, *Shigella*, *Giardia*, *C. jejuni*.
- Bloody stool: *E. coli* 0157 (avoid abx), *E. histolytica*, inflammatory bowel disease.
- Antibiotic exposure: especially broad spectrum beta-lactams, fluoroquinolones or clindamycin. *C. difficile* (20%), antibiotic-induced carbohydrate malabsorption in others. Community-acquired *C. difficile* now described without known antibiotic exposure or hospitalization.
- Critical Historical Data: (1) severity of symptoms: blood, fever, dehydration, vomiting; (2) place: recent travel to developing countries, *E. coli*, *Salmonella*, *Shigella*, Plesiomonas, Norwalk agent; (3) antibiotic-associated: carbohydrate malabsorption 75%, *C. difficile* 20%, *Klebsiella oxytoca*, *S. aureus*, *C. perfringens*; (4) Parasites: Giardia, *E. histolytica*, Strongyloides: (5) Most common bacteria: *Salmonella*, *C. jejuni*, *Shigella*; (6) Bloody: *E. histolytica*, *E. coli* 0157; (7) Outbreak: Norovirus, *Salmonella*; (8) Viral: Norovirus, adenovirus, astrovirus, coronovirus, calicivirus; (9) Foodborne outbreaks: *Salmonella*, *C. jejuni*.

DIAGNOSIS
- Fecal leukocytes: suggestive of *C. jejuni*, *C. difficile*, *Salmonella*, *Shigella*.
- Lab: stool culture for *Salmonella*, *Shigella*, *C. jejuni* +/- *E. coli* 0157:H7, *Yersinia*, vibrio (seasonal).
- Lab (if abx exposure): *C. difficile* most use stool toxin assay either cytotoxin (toxin B) or EIA (toxin A or A and B) or PCR (toxigenic strains *of C. difficile*).
- Lab (parasite): standard O and P for *E. histolytica*. Commonly special AFB stain/trichrome stains ordered for detection of, *isospora*, *cyclospora*. Giardia antigen (EIA).

TREATMENT
Sequential Evaluation
- Assessment: dehydration, duration, evidence of inflammation (fever, blood, tenesmus).
- Symptomatic rx: hydration + loperamide (initial 4 mg PO, then 2 mg q each loose stool [16 mg/day max]).
- Management by setting: travel, outbreak, nosocomial, abx exposure.

- Stool study: travel-related, *E. coli*. Outbreak—*Salmonella*, norovirus. Abx hx?—*C. difficile*. Bloody—*E. coli* 0157:H7, *E. histolytica*.
- Empiric abx (if indicated usually for severe infections): ciprofloxacin 500 mg twice daily PO × 3 days. If travel related: cipro/levo 1–3 days, if sx >7 days—use metronidazole 500 mg three times a day PO × 7–10 days.
- Reportable infections: *Salmonella*, *Shigella*, *E. coli* 0157:H7, *cyclospora*, *giardia*.

Pathogen Specific Therapy (IDSA CID 2001;32:331)

- **Shigella**: ciprofloxacin 500 mg PO twice daily × 3 days or levofloxacin 500 mg PO once daily × 3 days. Treat for 7–10 days if immunocompromised.
- **Salmonella** (abx treatment if severe, >50 yrs, valve disease, severe atherosclerosis, cancer, AIDS, uremia): ciprofloxacin 500 mg PO twice daily × 5–7 days, TMP-SMX DS twice daily PO × 5–7 days, ceftriaxone 2 g IM/IV × 5–7 days. Treat for 14 days if immunocompromised (or if relapsing disease).
- **C. jejuni**: erythromycin 500 mg PO twice daily × 5 days (quinolone resistance high).
- **E. coli, enterohemorrhagic (Shiga toxin—bloody diarrhea)**: no antibiotic, as abx rx may increase toxin release.
- **C. difficile**: stop implicated drug + metronidazole 250 mg PO every other day × 10 days or oral vancomycin 125 mg PO every other day × 10 days.
- **Giardia:** metronidazole 250–750 mg three times a day PO × 7–10 days or tinidazole 2 g PO × 1 dose.
- **Cyclospora:** TMP-SMX 1DS PO twice daily × 7–10 days. If immunocompromised: TMP-SMZ 1DS every other day. × 10 days, followed by TMP-SMZ thrice weekly.
- **E. histolytica**: metronidazole 750 mg three times a day PO × 5–10 days + paromomycin 500 mg three times a day PO × 7 days. Alternative treatment: tinidazole 2 g PO every day × 3 days followed by paromomycin, iodoquinol, or diloxanide furoate.
- **Isospora:** TMP-SMX 1DS twice daily PO × 7–10 days. If immunocompromised: TMP-SMZ 1DS every other day × 10 days, followed by TMP-SMZ thrice weekly.
- **Aeromonas and Plesiomonas (severe or prolonged):** cipro 500 mg PO twice daily × 3 days or TMP-SMX 1DS PO twice daily × 3 days or ofloxacin 300 mg PO twice daily × 3 days.

Non-Specific Therapy

- Rehydration: mild diarrhea take clear juices and soups with small frequent feedings.
- Moderate-severe: use oral rehydration solution (ORS) such as Ceralyte, Pedialyte, or other w/ Na/K and glucose (50–100 ml/kg/q3–4 hrs). Unable to drink, use NG tube or IV D5W + ¼ NS + 20 mEq/L KCl.
- Severe: IV Ringers lactate (preferred) or NS 20 mL/kg until improved perfusion, then 100 ml/kg ORS PO in 4 hr or D5W/ ½ NS IV.
- Food should match stool: watery—soups, broth, yogurt, soft drinks, Jello +/– saltines; some formed—rice, bread, broiled fish, chicken, baked potato.
- Avoid milk, milk products, caffeine, fried foods, spicy foods.
- Antimotility agents: avoid w/ *E. coli* 0157 (bloody diarrhea) and *C. difficile*.
- Consider antimotility agents after r/o *E.coli* 0157 and *C.difficile*: loperamide (OTC) 4 mg, then 2 mg q loose stool (16 mg/day max).

Follow Up

- Outbreak: if *Salmonella* or Norovirus suspected, notify health dept.
- Reportable: Cholera, *Salmonella*, *Shigella*, *E. coli* 0157, *Giardia*.

Other Information

- Highest priorities: rehydration, treat shigellosis (fluoroquinolone), avoid antibiotics with bloody diarrhea (*E. coli* 0157).
- Inflammatory diarrhea (fecal WBC, tenesmus, fever): think Salmonella, Shigella, *C. jejuni*, *C. difficile*, Yersinia. Obtain stool culture if bloody or severe.
- Most common = norovirus, occurs both sporadic and epidemic (hospitals, nursing homes, cruise ships, events), waterborne.
- Foodborne outbreaks: *Salmonella*, *E. coli* 0157, norovirus, Yersinia, Vibrio (seafood), *C. jejuni* (poultry).

DIAGNOSIS

BASIS FOR RECOMMENDATIONS

Thielman NM, Guerrant RL. Clinical practice. Acute infectious diarrhea. *N Engl J Med*, 2004; Vol. 350; pp. 38–47.

Comments: Clinical review basis; (1) Assessment: dehydration, duration, evidence of inflammation (blood, fever, tenesmus); (2) Symptom Rx: hydration, loperamide; (3) Management by setting: outbreak, travel, abx, clinical features; (4) Stool analysis: travelers—*Salmonella, Shigella, C. jejuni, E. coli* 0157, *C. dif*; Nosocomial: *C. difficile*; Bloody: *E. coli* 0157; Persistent: Giardia, *Cyclospora*, Isospora; (5) Antibiotic Rx based on sx and agent; (6) Report to health department.

Guerrant RL, Van Gilder T, Steiner TS, et al. Practice guidelines for the management of infectious diarrhea. *Clin Infect Dis*, 2001; Vol. 32; pp. 331–51.

Comments: These guidelines are the basis of the recommendations for the module. The highest priorities (1) treating shigellosis, traveler's diarrhea and *C. jejuni*; (2) evaluating the diarrhea (stool character, fever, blood, tenesmus), outbreak, antibiotic exposure, travel hx, exposure to seafood and raw milk; and (3) avoidance of abx when Shiga toxin producing strains of *E. coli* (e.g., O157:H7) are suspected.

DIARRHEA, COMMUNITY-ACQUIRED, PERSISTENT/CHRONIC

Christopher F. Carpenter, MD and Aditi Swami, MD

PATHOGENS
- *Giardia lamblia*
- *Entamoeba his*tolytica
- *Clostridium difficile*
- *Campylobacter jejuni*
- *Salmonella* species
- *Shigella* species
- Enterohemorrhagic *Escherichia coli* (EHEC)
- Other pathogenic *Escherichia coli*
- Other infectious causes

MORE PATHOGENS

*Enterotoxigenic, Enteropathogenic, Enteroinvasive, and Enteroaggregative; Enterohemorrhagic *E. coli* (EHEC) also known as Shiga toxin-producing *E. coli* (STEC).

**Other infectious causes include: *Aeromonas* species, *Plesiomonas species*, *Cryptosporidium parvum, Microsporidia, Yersinia* species, *Vibrio* species, *Clostridium perfringens*, Rotavirus, Norovirus/Calicivirus, Enteric adenovirus, Astrovirus, small round viruses, Coronavirus, Herpes simplex virus, and Cytomegalovirus, *Cyclospora cayetanensis, Isospora belli*, and *Strongyloides stercoralis.*

CLINICAL
- Persistent diarrhea is defined as diarrheal disease lasting longer than 1–2 wks but less than 4 wks; diarrhea lasting longer than 4 wks is considered chronic diarrhea.
- Most infectious causes of acute diarrhea generally resolve within 2 wks of onset; on the other hand, most of these infectious causes can also cause persistent or chronic diarrhea.
- Definitions of diarrhea in the United States or Western Europe, where low residual diets are the norm, may include: stools weighing >200 g, >3 stools/day, and decreased fecal consistency.
- Non-infectious causes of diarrhea are increasingly common as the duration of diarrhea increases.
- Irritable bowel syndrome (IBS—see Diagnosis section below) should be considered in pts with persistent or chronic complaints and associated abdominal pain.

DIAGNOSIS
- Initial evaluation: fecal leukocytes or stool lactoferrin, occult blood test, stool culture, *C. difficile* toxin assay, O and P (including trichrome stain), giardia antigen, rotavirus EIA, viral cultures. Assays for norovirus not yet for routine use. For chronic diarrhea, also consider stool pH, wt. (g/day), 72 hr fecal fat (on 75–100 g/day fat).
- 2nd tier eval: trial lactose-free diet, CBC w/ diff., ESR/CRP, metabolic panel, TSH, T4, gastrin, radiographs (AXR, Abd. CT, UGI w/ SBFT, contrast enema), sigmoid/colon endoscopy w/ biopsies
- 3rd tier eval: VIP, substance P, calcitonin, histamine (high output and hypokalemia); urine 5-HIA acids (flushing); alkalinization assays, phenolphthalein, and anthraquinone (?laxative

abuse); fecal electrolytes/osmolality; urine studies w/ thin-layer chromatography for bisacodyl; enteroclysis, bile acid or other breath tests for bacterial overgrowth.

- Concern for organic (vs. functional) diarrhea: higher output (>400 g/day in western countries), shorter duration (<3 mos), nocturnal, continual, sudden onset, wt. loss >5 kg, potentially elevated ESR/CRPP, anemia, low albumin.

- **Non-infectious causes of persistent and chronic diarrhea:** include inflammatory bowel disease (ulcerative colitis, Crohn's disease, collagenous colitis, microscopic/lymphocytic colitis), steatorrhea, carbohydrate malabsorption, adverse drug reactions, food additives, previous gastrointestinal or gall bladder surgery, adrenal insufficiency, thyroid disease, diabetes, laxative abuse, ischemic bowel disease, radiation enteritis or colitis, and idiopathic (functional, e.g., irritable bowel syndrome) diarrhea.

- Other less common non-infectious causes include factitious diarrhea, hormone-producing tumors, infiltrative disorders, epidemic chronic diarrhea (e.g., Brainerd diarrhea and milk, untreated water-associated diarrhea), chronic idiopathic diarrhea, fecal incontinence, Celiac disease, and food allergy.

- **Irritable bowel syndrome:** IBS = abd, pain, and abnormal bowel habits (constipation, diarrhea, or both) w/o source.

TREATMENT

Symptomatic Medications and Measures:

- Fluid replacement is an important component of treatment, especially in pts with significant dehydration where it is often the most important component.

- Oral replacement with oral rehydration solutions (ORS); commercially available packets include Cera Lyte generic ORS, the WHO ORS, Rehydralyte, Pedialyte, Resol, and Rice-Lyte.

- IV replacement with 0.9% NS with 20 mEq KCL or with Lactated Ringers solution should be used in pts with moderate to severe diarrhea or in pts not tolerating oral replacement.

- Antimotility agents, such as loperamide 4 mg PO, then 2 mg PO past each loose stool to a maximum of 16 mg/day are of benefit; avoid with *C. difficile* diarrhea, enterohemorrhagic *E. coli* diarrhea.

- Diphenoxylate with atropine and tincture of opium offer no major advantage over loperamide; all of these agents should be avoided in pts with dysentery and/or EHEC infection (may result in HUS) as well as *C. difficile* diarrhea.

- Other recommendations: lactose-free (e.g., milk, cheese) diet, caffeine avoidance, Metamucil, bismuth subsalicylate, Kaolin-containing agents, and probiotics.

- Gatorade, fruit juices, and soft drinks are hyperosmolar and deficient in electrolytes and thus are sub-optimal replacements for pts with significant dehydration.

- These drinks may be sufficient in otherwise healthy pts who are mildly ill; additional electrolytes from soups or saltine crackers will be supplemental.

Empiric Therapy:

- In cases where an initial evaluation has been unrevealing, and further studies are more invasive and place the pt at risk, consideration of an empiric trial is reasonable.

- Use metronidazole for suspected protozoal diarrhea or a fluoroquinolone for suspected bacterial diarrhea as empiric therapy with the potential risks and benefits explained to the pt.

- Metronidazole 250–500 mg PO three times a day for 10 days.

- Ciprofloxacin 500 mg PO twice daily for 3–5 days, Norfloxacin. 400 mg PO twice daily for 3–5 days, or Ofloxacin 300 mg PO twice daily for 3–5 days are reasonable empiric choices.

- If pt has history of recent antibiotic therapy, would consider empiric *C. difficile* treatment (while awaiting stool toxin assays): for mild to moderate diarrhea—metronidazole 500 mg PO three times a day for 10 days, and for severe diarrhea—vancomycin 125 mg PO q6h for 10–14 days.

- Trimethoprim-sulfamethoxazole may be considered for empiric treatment of pts at high risk for Cyclospora infections.

Pathogen Specific Therapy:

- Specific therapy for the 3 most common causes of infectious persistent or chronic diarrhea (giardia, amebiasis, and *C. difficile*) is generally indicated.

- First-line therapy for all 3 includes metronidazole; amebiasis requires the addition of an agent active against cysts (paromomycin or iodoquinol or diloxanide furoate).

- *Specific treatment is indicated for bacterial enteritis caused by *Shigella* sp. and possibly *C. jejuni*; isolated *Salmonella* sp. intestinal disease should not be treated with antibiotics due to possibly prolonging carrier state.
- *EHEC treatment is controversial and we recommend holding treatment due to concern that certain antibiotics have been demonstrated to induce toxin synthesis and release. Furthermore, both trimethoprim-sulfamethoxazole and fluoroquinolones may promote hemolytic uremic syndrome.
- *Fluoroquinolone-resistant strains of *C. jejuni* have been identified in many parts of the world, hence macrolides are preferred such as azithromycin.
- A hypervirulent strain of *C. difficile* (BI/NAP1, toxinotype III) resulting in increased morbidity and mortality, has emerged in North America and Europe; virulence factors of the epidemic strain include increased toxin production, the presence of binary toxin, quinolone resistance, and increased sporulation capacity. Its role as a cause of chronic diarrhea is unknown. Description of "community-acquired" *C. difficile* without known exposure to antibiotics described.

OTHER INFORMATION

- Chronic diarrhea is generally caused by non-infectious etiologies, whereas acute diarrhea is mostly due to self-limited infections.
- Depending on the definition used, chronic diarrhea occurs in 3–18% of Americans; irritable bowel syndrome with abdominal pain makes up a majority of pts in the studies with higher estimates. There is a growing literature of irritable bowel syndrome occuring following enteric infections, especially traveler's diarrhea.
- With an extensive workup including hospital evaluation when required, only approximately 10% of pts with chronic diarrhea remain undiagnosed.
- Immunocompromised pts (e.g., HIV-infected pts) with persistent/chronic diarrhea: consider *Giardia*, *Cryptosporidium*, *Cyclospora*, *Isospora belli*, *Microsporidia*, and *M. avium* complex.

BASIS FOR RECOMMENDATIONS

Sellin JH. A practical approach to treating pts with chronic diarrhea. *Rev Gastroenterol Disord*, 2007; Vol. 7 Suppl 3; pp. S19–26.
Comments: Guideline for management of chronic diarrhea

Guerrant RL, Van Gilder T, Steiner TS, et al. Practice guidelines for the management of infectious diarrhea. *Clin Infect Dis*, 2001; Vol. 32; pp. 331–51.
Comments: Guidelines for treatment of community-acquired, traveler's, nosocomial, and persistent diarrhea developed on behalf of the Infectious Diseases Society of America.

DIARRHEA, TRAVELER'S

Lisa Spacek, MD, PhD

PATHOGENS

- Enterotoxigenic *Escherichia coli*
- Enteroaggregative *Escherichia coli*
- *Salmonella* species
- *Shigella* species
- *Campylobacter jejuni*
- *Aeromonas* species
- *Plesiomonas* species
- *Vibrio parahaemolyticus*
- Rotavirus
- Noroviruses
- *Giardia lamblia*
- *Cyclospora cayetanensis*
- *Cryptosporidium parvum*
- *Entamoeba histolytica*

CLINICAL
- Definition: sudden onset watery diarrhea, 3 or more loose stools in 24 hrs with one enteric symptom: nausea, vomiting, abdominal cramps, fever, fecal urgency. Tenesmus and bloody stools suggest dysentery.
- Hx: onset 5–15 days after arrival at destination, illness often self-limited; duration 1–5 days.
- Host factors increasing risk: immunosuppression, hypochlorhydria, inflammatory bowel disease, diabetes mellitus, AIDS.
- Disease etiology diverse. Bacterial enteric pathogens most commonly isolated. Viral outbreaks sporadic (e.g., cruise ship-associated). Parasitic pathogens rare and associated with longer duration of symptoms.
- Fever, anorexia, malaise and abd tenderness +/− nausea and vomiting.
- Usually mild illness with brief duration, infrequent stools, and minimal symptoms.
- Severe illness/dysentery associated with fever, frequent small bowel movements with blood and mucus.

DIAGNOSIS
- Presence of fecal leukocytes suggests inflammation (non-viral).
- Stool culture: looking for *E. coli*, *Shigella*, *Salmonella*, *Campylobacter*, *Aeromonas*, *Plesiomonas*; Shiga toxin assay.
- Giardia Ag ELISA. Stool for O and P.

TREATMENT
Non-specific and Empiric Therapy
- Treatment based on symptom severity includes rehydration, antimotility agent loperamide, and antibiotics. May reduce duration of diarrhea (CID 2006;43:1499).
- Mild illness, 1–2 stools/24 hrs, minimal symptoms: loperamide 4 mg PO loading dose, then 2 mg PO after each loose stool (max 16 mg/24 hrs) or bismuth subsalicylate two 262 mg tabs chewed four times per day or 30 ml PO q1h (max 8 doses/24 hrs).
- Moderate illness, >2 stools/24 hrs, watery diarrhea: fluoroquinolone, single dose of once daily fluoroquinolone may be adequate plus loperamide; for dysentery, complete 3 days course of abx.
- Severe illness/dysentery, >6 stools/24 hrs, fever, bloody stools: fluoroquinolone therapy to complete 3-day course.
- Fluoroquinolone: ciprofloxacin (500 mg PO twice daily or 750 mg PO single dose), levofloxacin (500 mg PO q24h).
- Rifaximin, a nonabsorbable antibiotic FDA approved for noninvasive *E. coli,* 200 mg PO three times daily × 3 days, equivalent to ciprofloxacin for noninvasive pathogens (*AJTMH* 2006;74:1060), not recommended for systemic infections or diarrhea complicated by fever, bloody stool or persistent symptoms >24–48 hrs.
- Bismuth preparations contain salicylate, two tabs four times a day comparable to 3–4 adult aspirins, avoid additional salicylates, do not use bismuth subsalicylate with oral anticoagulants, may cause blackening of tongue and stool.
- Avoid bismuth subsalicylate (BSS) when using a tetracycline, combination will decrease tetracycline absorption. Avoid BSS in travelers with renal insufficiency. Cipro absorption not affected by bismuth [L Rambout et al, AAC 1994].
- Prevention: handwashing before eating, water purification, avoid raw fruits and vegetables unless peeled, choose steaming hot foods.
- Azithromycin (1 g single dose or 500 mg once daily × 3 days) in regions with fluoroquinolone-resistant *Campylobacter species*, Thailand and southeast Asia.

Pathogen specific therapy
- *C. jejuni:* azithromycin 500 mg PO once daily × 3 days or ciprofloxacin 500 mg PO twice daily (consider regional resistance to fluoroquinolones in SE Asia, India, Latin America) or erythromycin stearate 500 mg PO q6h × 5 days (erythro resistance rarely reported).
- Cryptosporidium: nitazoxanide 500 mg PO twice daily × 3 days. If AIDS: HAART and nitazoxanide 500 mg PO twice daily × 14 days.
- Cyclospora: TMP-SMZ 1DS PO twice daily × 7–10 days.

- *E. histolytica:* metronidazole 750 mg PO q8h × 10 days or tinidazole 2 g PO once daily × 3 days, followed by luminal agent, paromomycin 500 mg q8h PO × 7 days (*NEJM* 2003;348:1565).
- Enterotoxigenic *E. coli:* ciprofloxacin 750 mg single dose PO or 500 mg PO twice daily × 3 days (for severe disease), rifamixin 200 mg PO q8h × 3 days (for non-invasive disease).
- Enterohemorrhagic *E. coli* (Shiga-toxin producing *E. coli* -STEC): if suspect/bloody diarrhea, **avoid** antibiotics and antimotility agents, reserve antibiotics for severe illness.
- Giardia: tinidazole 2 g PO × 1 dose or nitazoxanide 500 mg PO twice daily × 3 days.
- *Salmonella*, non-typhi, treat if severe illness, pt <1 yr or >50 yrs, prostheses, vascular grafts, valvular heart disease, severe atherosclerosis, ca, uremia: ciprofloxacin 500 mg PO twice daily × 5–7 days or azithromycin 1 g PO once daily then 500 mg PO q24 × 6 days.
- *Shigella:* ciprofloxacin 500 mg PO twice daily × 3 days or TMP-SMZ 1DS PO twice daily × 3 days or azithromycin 500 mg PO × 1 day then 250 mg PO once daily × 4 days.
- *Vibrio cholerae:* azithromycin 1 g PO × 1 dose or doxycycline 300 mg PO × 1 dose or tetracycline 500 mg PO q6h × 3 days or TMP-SMZ 1DS PO twice daily × 3 days or ciprofloxacin 500 mg × 1 dose. Primary treatment is rehydration.
- *Vibrio parahaemolyticus*: Antibiotics do not shorten illness. Rehydration. Fluoroquinolones for severe disease.

OTHER INFORMATION

- Prevent and treat dehydration, reduce symptoms and duration of illness with empiric self-therapy. Prompt self-treatment can reduce duration to 1 day or less (Emerg Med Clin N Am 2008;26:499).
- Dysentery or inflammatory diarrhea likely bacterial, consider stool culture, treat with antibiotics. **Avoid** antibiotics in proven or suspected Enterohemorrhagic *E. coli* (STEC) to avoid toxin production.
- Persistent diarrhea >2 wks likely parasitic infection. Check giardia ELISA, serial stool exams for ova and parasites, *C. difficile* toxin assay.
- Self-reported lower incidence (29 versus 60 cases/100 persons-mos) of travelers' diarrhea in long-term/military travelers (>1 mo) compared to short-term business/leisure travelers attributable to limited exposure to contaminated food and water (*Am J Trop Med Hyg* 2006;74:891).
- Vaccination of travellers for enterotoxigenic *E. coli* reduced rate of more severe episodes of TD but did not reduce overall rate of diarrhea (Vaccine 2007;25:4392). Inactivated, oral Vibrio cholerae whole cell/B subunit vaccine (Dukoral, SBL Vaccine) against heat-labile ETEC estimated to benefit <7% of travelers (*Lancet Infect Dis* 2006;361).

BASIS FOR RECOMMENDATIONS

Hill DR, Ericsson CD, Pearson RD, et al. The practice of travel medicine: guidelines by the Infectious Diseases Society of America. *Clin Infect Dis,* 2006; Vol. 43; pp. 1499–539.
Comments: IDSA travel medicine guidelines.

Guerrant RL, Van Gilder T, Steiner TS, et al. Practice guidelines for the management of infectious diarrhea. *Clin Infect Dis,* 2001; Vol. 32; pp. 331–51.
Comments: Complete reference for recommended therapy. Guidelines provide basis for treatment of specific pathogens listed in this module.

DIVERTICULITIS

Christopher F. Carpenter, MD and Aditi Swami, MD

PATHOGENS

- As a rule, infections are polymicrobial with a predominance of anaerobes and Gram-negative bacilli
- Anaerobes, including Bacteroides species
- Gram-negative bacilli, including Enterobacteriaceae
- Enterococcus (pathogenic role of enterococci remain controversial)

CLINICAL

- Diverticulosis increases with age: 50% of people >60 yrs old have diverticulosis, and 10–25% of those with diverticulosis develop diverticulitis.

- Although diverticulosis is unusual in younger adults (<40 yrs old), incidence is increasing and often it is associated with more severe complications in this age group (with increased need for surgery).
- In westernized societies, a low-fiber diet is believed to be the primary contributing factor to diverticulosis and diverticulitis.
- Primary symptoms include LLQ pain that can be intermittent or constant, fever, and altered bowel habits (either diarrhea or constipation).
- Complicated diverticulitis involves abscess, free perforation, fistula, or obstruction.
- Differential includes IBD, ischemic colitis, appendicitis, infectious colitis, PID, pyelonephritis, colon cancer.

DIAGNOSIS

- PE: fever, LLQ tenderness that may localize, +/− rebound and guarding; mass may be palpable, may also have abdominal distention or urinary symptoms.
- Lab: leukocytosis w/ left shift frequent.
- Dx: often clinical (like appendicitis); CT used in pts with atypical presentations or more severe/complicated illness (unresponsive to abx or concern of abscess/rupture).
- CT criteria include: presence of sigmoid diverticula, pericolonic fat inflammation (streaking), colonic wall thickening, pericolic or distant abscesses, and extraluminal air.
- CT sensitivity 90–95% but specificity 72%.
- Ultrasound, barium enema, and endoscopy may have a limited role in select pts.

TREATMENT

Inpatient treatment

- IV antibiotics, bowel rest, +/− TPN and NG tube.
- Ampicillin-sulbactam 3.0 g IV q6h or ticarcillin-clavulanate 3.1 g IV q6h (for community-acquire/mild-moderate disease) or piperacillin-tazobactam 3.375 g IV q6h or 4.5 g IV q8h (nosocomial, severe).
- Third or 4th generation cephalosporin **or** fluoroquinolone **or** aztreonam, **plus** metronidazole (moxifloxacin has an FDA indication as monotherapy for intra-abdominal infection but *B. fragilis* coverage inadequate).
- Cefoxitin 1–2 g IV q6h (mild to moderate disease).
- Ampicillin 2 g IV q6h **plus** gentamicin 1.7 mg/kg IV q8h **plus** either metronidazole 1.0 g IV loading dose then 0.5 g IV q6h.
- Ertapenem 1 g IV q24h (for pts with a high risk of resistant pathogens, consider imipenem-cilastatin 500 mg IV q6h, meropenem 1 g IV q8h, or doripenem 500 mg IV q8h).
- Tigecycline 100 mg loading dose then 50 mg IV q12h (mild to moderate disease).
- Duration (average) 5–10+ days, usually may d/c abx with clinical improvement: benign exam, afebrile, resolution of leukocytosis, return of bowel function. Option to convert to oral therapy (below) to complete course.

Outpatient treatment

- Oral antibiotics (see below), clear liquids, low-fiber diet, most improve within 2–3 days.
- Amoxicillin-clavulanic acid 500 mg PO three times a day or 875 mg PO twice daily.
- Ciprofloxacin 500 mg PO twice daily or levofloxacin 500 mg PO every day **plus** metronidazole 500 mg PO q6h.
- Moxifloxacin 400 mg PO q24h (+/− metronidazole 500 mg PO q6h).
- Trimethoprim-sulfamethoxazole DS twice daily PO **plus** metronidazole 500 mg PO q6h.
- Duration (average) 5–10+ days, usually may d/c abx with clinical improvement: benign exam, afebrile, resolution of leukocytosis, return of bowel function.

Surgical Treatment

- If abscess present, percutaneous drainage may offer temporizing intervention for localized perforation w/o generalized peritonitis or severe illness; resection performed later.
- Resection +/− diversion may be required for perforation with generalized peritonitis and/or pneumoperitoneum.
- Recurrence after 1st attack 20–30%; after 2nd 30–50%. Resection is thus recommended for consideration on a case-by-case basis after 2nd/3rd attack.
- Perforation rates in immunosuppressed and post-operative pts higher.
- Laparoscopic sigmoidectomy viable approach for delayed resection in selected pts in the hands of an experienced surgeon.

DIAGNOSIS

- Pts with recurrent complicated attacks, fistula or abscess development, younger age, or immunocompromise may require surgical intervention.
- Consider pts acceptable for outpatient management: mild illness, tolerating oral intake, supportive social situation, and no significant comorbidity or other risk factors for complications.

OTHER INFORMATION
- High fiber diets (fruits, vegetables, etc.) may reduce the risk of developing diverticular disease.
- Diverticulosis alone without signs or symptoms of diverticulitis does not warrant the use of antibiotics.
- Pts w/ severe disease who cannot tolerate oral intake or have risk factors for complicated course (immunosuppression, elderly, significant comorbid illness) should be hospitalized.
- Diverticulosis and diverticulitis do not increase the patient's risk for polyps and colorectal neoplasia.

BASIS FOR RECOMMENDATIONS

Rafferty J, Shellito P, Hyman NH, et al. Practice parameters for sigmoid diverticulitis. *Dis Colon Rectum,* 2006; Vol. 49; pp. 939–44.
Comments: Update of guidelines from the American Society of Colon and Rectal Surgeons (ASCRS).

Solomkin JS, Mazuski JE, Baron EJ, et al. Guidelines for the selection of anti-infective agents for complicated intra-abdominal infections. *Clin Infect Dis,* 2003; Vol. 37; pp. 997–1005.
Comments: Consensus evidence-based guidelines from IDSA, SIS, ASM, and SIDP.

H. PYLORI–RELATED PEPTIC ULCER DISEASE

Paul G. Auwaerter, MD

PATHOGENS
- *Helicobacter pylori*
- *H. pylori* intrinsically resistant to sulfonamides, trimethoprim and vancomycin.
- Metronidazole resistance estimated 22–39%.
- Clarithromycin resistance ~11–12%, in some studies up to 24%.
- Amoxicillin or tetracycline resistance is rare.

CLINICAL
- *H. pylori* colonization increases risk of peptic ulcer disease (PUD), noncardia gastric adenocarcinoma and gastric lymphoma.
- Abx treatment may significantly impact PUD and MALT (strongest treatment indications).
- Persistent dyspepsia (in those not receiving NSAIDs) and positive *H. pylori* serology in those <45 yrs old recommended in those without weight loss, bleeding, anemia or dysphagia—antibiotic treatment is recommended as initial therapy as risk of gastric cancer is low. Benefit of eradication appears to occur in a subset of pts with functional dyspepsia.
- Whether to test and treat for *H. pylori* in pts with dyspepsia, GERD, pts taking NSAIDs, iron deficiency anemia or at risk for gastric cancer remains controversial.
- Three drug therapy is recommended norm. Quadruple or sequential drug therapy often employed for treatment failures.

DIAGNOSIS
- Definite indications to diagnose (and treat): *H. pylori*–associated PUD, history of PUD not previously treated for *H. pylori*, gastric MALT lymphoma, post-endoscopic treatment of early gastric carcinoma.
- Direct histologic demonstration of the organism on endoscopic biopsy specimens (>95% sensitive and specific).
- Positive urease test on endoscopic biopsy specimens (>95% sensitive, but reduced sensitivity post-treatment).
- Positive results from labeled urea breath test (rapid, inexpensive and >95% sensitive and specific, but reduced sensitivity post-treatment [90%]). This technology is becoming more widely available.

- Positive IgG serum antibody (~85% sensitive, 79% specific) **but** cannot distinguish active from remote infection. Of no utility post-treatment. Treatment decision based upon positive serology discouraged.
- Culture of *H. pylori* is actually the least sensitive diagnostic test (70–80% sensitive, difficult to perform).
- Stool antigen test >90% sensitivity, specificity and non-invasive.
- If low pretest probability—use urea breath test or fecal antigen test (superior to predicative value of antibody test). What this means for clinicians is that antibody testing fine for high prevalence populations (urban areas, immigrant populations), but for most of U.S., prevalence rate is <20%, then antibody testing helpful if negative, but positive result "no better than a coin toss in predicting active infection."

TREATMENT
First-Line Regimens
- Optimal treatment regimen unclear despite many trials performed to date.
- Standard first line (recommended): proton pump inhibitor (PPI) + clarithromycin 500 mg twice daily + amoxicillin 1 g twice daily [Available as Prevpac using PPI lansoprazole]. Eradication 70–85%. Duration 10–14 days*.
- If penicillin allergy: PPI + clarithromycin 500 mg twice daily + metronidazole 500 mg twice daily. Duration 10–14 days. Eradication rate probably less than 70–85%.
- **Sequential therapy** (may be helpful to improve eradication rates, especially if clarithromycin resistance exists): PPI + amoxicillin 1000 mg twice daily × 5 days then PPI + clarithromycin 500 mg twice daily + tinidazole 500 mg twice daily × 5 days. Efficacy >90% in published studies. Whether this approach should replace standard regimens are under study.
- **Quadruple therapy:** bismuth subsalicylate 525 mg PO four times a day + tetracycline 500 mg four times a day + metronidazole 250–500 mg four times a day + ranitidine 150 mg twice daily or PPI. Duration = 10–14 days*. Eradication rate 75–90%. May use with PCN allergy.
- Alternative: ranitidine bismuth citrate 400 mg twice daily + clarithromycin 500 mg twice daily + amoxicillin 1 g twice daily. Duration = 7–10 days.
- Metronidazole containing regimens may have reduced efficacy due to common resistance.
- Specific diagnosis and tests of cure are not necessary in pts who only have duodenal ulcers.
- PPIs: omeprazole 20 mg PO twice daily × 10 days, esomeprazole 40 mg PO once daily × 10 days, lansoprazole 30 mg PO twice daily × 10 days, pantoprazole 40 mg PO once daily × 10 days, rabeprazole 20 mg PO twice daily × 7 days.
- * denotes FDA approved regimens.

Salvage Regimens
- Often used for treatment failures following three drug regimen.
- Avoid antibiotics previously prescribed, if possible. Use alternative three drug, or four drug regimen as above.
- PPI + bismuth subsalicylate 525 mg four times a day + tetracycline 500 mg twice daily + metronidazole 500 mg twice daily. Duration 7–14 days. Eradication rate ~68%. Inexpensive but high pill burden and increased side effects.
- PPI + amoxicillin 1000 mg twice daily + levofloxacin 500 mg twice daily × 10 days. Eradication rate = 87%. Regimen not yet studied in U.S., but widely chosen for salvage.
- Alt: PPI + moxifloxacin 400 mg once daily + rifabutin 300 mg once daily × 7 days (eradication rate 78–83% with clarithromycin or metronidazole resistant organisms) or PPI + rifabutin 300 mg once daily + amoxicillin 1000 mg twice daily (87% eradication rate).
- PPIs: omeprazole 20 mg PO twice daily × 10 days, esomeprazole 40 mg PO once daily × 10 days, lansoprazole 30 mg PO twice daily × 10 days, pantoprazole 40 mg PO once daily × 10 days, rabeprazole 20 mg PO twice daily × 7 days.

Two drug regimens (FDA approved)
- Dual therapy well-studied, but lower eradication rates (60–85%) make them no longer recommended. Potential use for the pts intolerant of clarithromycin or metronidazole.
- PPI + either clarithromycin 500 mg three times a day or amoxicillin 1 g twice daily for 2 wks then PPI for 2 more wks (PPI = omeprazole 40 mg every day or lansoprazole 30 mg three times a day).

- Ranitidine bismuth citrate (RBC) 400 mg twice daily + clarithromycin 500 mg three times a day or twice daily for 2 wks then RBC for 2 more wks.

FOLLOW UP

- Treatment failure: 5–>12% pts fail initial eradication attempts. Among first line therapy, increasing failure rates (15–30%) ascribed to increasing clarithromycin resistance.
- Note: eradication rates lower in 7 days regimens compared to 14 days courses.
- Confirmation of eradication recommended by stool antigen or breath test especially in pt with *H. pylori*–associated ulcer, continued dyspepsia, MALT lymphoma or resected gastric CA.

OTHER INFORMATION

- Multiple regimens exist. Main treatment indication is PUD. Clarithromycin resistance has been increasing.
- *H. pylori* does not appear to cause GERD or most routine non-ulcerative dyspepsia. Treatment in these conditions (without ulcers) is controversial but advocated by some, mainly because a subset of dyspepsia pts do seem to benefit.
- Note that *H. pylori* infection is common in the population and of uncertain significance. No evidence supports routine screening and treatment in order to reduce the risks of gastric cancer.
- Testing and treatment also recommended for those with atrophic gastritis and 1st degree relatives of pts with gastric cancer.

BASIS FOR RECOMMENDATIONS

Chey WD, Wong BC. Practice Parameters Committee of the American College of Gastroenterology. American College of Gastroenterology guideline on the management of *Helicobacter pylori* infection. *Am J Gastroenterol*, 2007; Vol. 102; pp. 1808–25.
Comments: Basis for diagnosis and treatment recommendations in this module. Some recommendations (e.g., PPI + amoxicillin + levofloxacin) not yet validated within the U.S.

PANCREATITIS AND PANCREATIC ABSCESS

Robin McKenzie, MD

PATHOGENS

- The most common causes of pancreatitis are noninfectious (see below). Infectious causes include the following pathogens:
- Viruses: mumps, coxsackie virus, CMV, varicella-zoster, HSV, HIV, hepatitis B
- Bacteria: mycoplasma, mycobacteria, *Legionella*, Leptospira, *salmonella*
- Fungi: cryptococcus (HIV), PCP, *aspergillus*
- Parasites: toxoplasma, *cryptosporidia*, ascaris
- Infected phlegmon (necrosis) and pancreatic abscess: usually caused by bowel flora and polymicrobial (Gram-negative, Gram-positive, and anaerobic organisms). Resistant bacterial and fungal infection may occur, especially if pts have received prior antibiotics.

CLINICAL

- Most common known causes of pancreatitis are alcohol and gallstones. Many cases idiopathic.
- Medications causing pancreatitis include HIV medications (ddI and d4T with lactic acidosis and hepatic steatosis, 3TC in children, IV/aerosolized pentamidine, TMP-SMX), INH, rifampin, erythromycin, and other medications, e.g., valproic acid.
- Other causes include hypertriglyceridemia (fasting TG >1000, may be associated with protease inhibitors), post-ERCP, acute HIV infection, AIDS with OIs (CMV, toxoplasmosis, MAC, PCP, cryptosporidiosis), pancreatic or periampullary cancer, vasculitis (polyarteritis nodosa, SLE), alpha-1-antitrypsin deficiency and other genetic disorders. Many cases remain idiopathic.
- Typical history (acute pancreatitis): acute onset of constant, upper abdominal pain that may radiate to back with nausea +/– vomiting. Presentation varies from no symptoms to shock/coma.
- Exam may be notable for fever, tachycardia, epigastric tenderness. Hemorrhagic discoloration of flanks (Grey-Turner's sign) or periumbilical area (Cullen's sign) in ~1% cases.

DIAGNOSIS

DIAGNOSIS

- Amylase: usually >3× normal in acute pancreatitis but may be normal. Increased amylase also caused by renal insufficiency, intestinal or fallopian tube disease, macroamylasemia, acidosis, various medications, HIV infection.
- Lipase: usually >3× normal, more specific than amylase. Mild increases also occur with renal insufficiency, bowel disease, DKA, macrolipasemia, medications, and HIV. Lipase remains elevated longer than amylase.
- ALT >3× ULN in a nonalcoholic pt strongly suggests gallstone pancreatitis, but a lower value does not exclude the diagnosis.
- Contrast-enhanced CT useful to R/O other diagnoses and stage severity of pancreatitis. Not indicated for mild disease unless dx uncertain. Necrosis (lack of enhancement) best identified several days after presentation. The percent of glandular necrosis correlates with mortality rate. MRI more sensitive for mild pancreatitis and more specific for categorizing fluid collections as necrosis, abscess, hemorrhage or pseudocyst, but less clinical correlation available with MRI.
- If cause not obvious (medications, EtOH) consider U/S, MRCP, CT or endoscopic U/S to detect gallstones or biliary tract disease. ERCP and sphincterotomy may be indicated to remove impacted gallstones and obtain fluid for Gram-stain and cx if infection present (e.g., bacterial cholangitis or OI suspected for HIV+ pt with low CD4).
- CT- or U/S-guided FNA or placement of drainage catheter indicated if infected necrosis suspected or abscess seen on imaging.

TREATMENT

Initial therapy

- Stop any suspected causative medications (e.g., ddI).
- Give IV fluids (avoid hemoconcentration).
- Control pain (often requires narcotics).

Antibiotics

- Infection of pancreatic necrosis probably caused by translocation of gut flora. Infection rate proportional to extent of necrosis.
- No prophylactic abx for mild pancreatitis: may cause superinfection with resistant bacteria and Candida.
- For acute, severe pancreatitis (>30% necrosis by CT), previous studies supported use of imipenem 500 mg IV q6h as prophylaxis. More recent trials do not support this recommendation. Prophylactic ABX for necrotizing pancreatitis are not recommended. Instead, if infection suspected, obtain aspirate for Gram-stain and culture, begin empiric antibiotics, and continue ABX only if culture is positive.
- Infected necrosis usually presents in 2nd or 3rd wk. Both sterile and infected necrosis may cause abdominal pain, fever, leukocytosis. CT- or US-guided aspiration needed for culture dx.
- Choice of abx for infected necrosis ideally based on cx results. GI flora (aerobes and anaerobes) often present. Abx with good penetration: carbapenems (imipenem, meropenem, doripenem, or ertapenem), fluoroquinolones (ciprofloxacin, levofloxacin, moxifloxacin), ceftazidime, cefepime, metronidazole, clindamycin, fluconazole.
- For empiric Rx consider carbapenem (doripenem 500 mg IV q8h, imipenem 500 mg IV q8h, or meropenem 1 g IV q8h) alone or fluoroquinolone (ciprofloxacin 400 mg IV q8h, levofloxacin 500 mg IV q24h, moxifloxacin 400 mg IV q24h) + metronidazole 500 mg IV q6–8h.

Nutritional support

- Mild pancreatitis: start clear liquids early and advance diet as tolerated.
- Severe pancreatitis: begin enteral nutrition as soon as possible. NJ feeding usually used, but NG as safe in a recent small study (Eatock).
- Give parenteral nutrition only if adequate enteral feeding not tolerated.

FOLLOW UP

Stage severity

- Calculate APACHE II score on admission: ≥8 in HIV-negative pt and ≥9–14 in HIV+ pt predicts severe course.
- Ranson criteria (table below in 'more' section) less predictive in HIV+ pts: >3 in HIV-negative pt and ≥4 in HIV+ pt suggests severe course.

- Obtain contrast-enhanced CT unless pancreatitis is mild. Necrosis best detected 2–3 days after admission. Necrosis >30% predicts mortality >20%.
- Measure CRP: >21 mg/dL on day 2–4 and >12 end of first wk predict severe pancreatitis.
- Early deaths (first 2 wks) primarily due to multisystem organ failure.

Diagnosis and treatment of complications (including infected phlegmon/abscess)

- Later deaths due to local and systemic infection.
- Infected necrosis must be diagnosed (CT-guided aspirate) and drained (percutaneously or surgically). If blood cxs negative and no evidence of sepsis, drainage may be delayed to allow organization of necrotic area.
- Early ERCP indicated for severe gallstone pancreatitis. Cholecystectomy usually performed before discharge in mild cases or within a few mos in complicated cases.

MORE FOLLOW UP

Ranson criteria:

On admission	Within 48 hrs
Age >55 yr	Hct decrease >10%
WBC >16,000/mm³	BUN increase >5 mg/dL
LDH >350 IU/L	Ca <8 mg/dL)
AST >250 IU/L	PaO_2 < 60 mm Hg
Glucose >200 mg/dL	Base deficit >4 mEq/L
	Fluid sequestration >6 L

BASIS FOR RECOMMENDATIONS

Bai Y, Gao J, Zou DW, et al. Prophylactic antibiotics cannot reduce infected pancreatic necrosis and mortality in acute necrotizing pancreatitis: evidence from a meta-analysis of randomized controlled trials. *Am J Gastroenterol,* 2008; Vol. 103; pp. 104–10.

Comments: This meta-analysis of 7 trials involving 467 pts showed no significant difference in rates of infected pancreatic necrosis or mortality among pts who received prophylactic antibiotics vs. controls who did not.

Dellinger EP, Tellado JM, Soto NE, et al. Early antibiotic treatment for severe acute necrotizing pancreatitis: a randomized, double-blind, placebo-controlled study. *Ann Surg,* 2007; Vol. 245; pp. 674–83.

Comments: This is the second randomized, double-blind, placebo-controlled trial of prophylactic antibiotics for severe acute pancreatitis. In this trial 50 pts received meropenem, and 50 received placebo. As in the previous blinded, placebo-controlled study, there was no difference in the rate of infection or death.

Whitcomb DC. Clinical practice. Acute pancreatitis. *N Engl J Med,* 2006; Vol. 354; pp. 2142–50.

Comments: ERCP with endoscopic sphincterotomy performed by an experienced endoscopist recommended for gallstone pancreatitis with bile-duct obstruction.

Isenmann R, Rünzi M, Kron M, et al. Prophylactic antibiotic treatment in pts with predicted severe acute pancreatitis: a placebo-controlled, double-blind trial. *Gastroenterology,* 2004; Vol. 126; pp. 997–1004.

Comments: First placebo-controlled, double-blind trial of prophylactic antibiotics for severe acute pancreatitis. Pts with necrosis on CT scan or CRP >15 mg/dL randomized to receive ciprofloxacin and metronidazole (N = 58) or placebo (N = 56). No difference in rate of infected necrosis or mortality.

BACTERIAL VAGINOSIS

Noreen A. Hynes, MD, MPH

PATHOGENS

- Disruption of normal vaginal flora ecology with alteration in the relative concentrations of various microorganisms including a depletion of lactobacilli and a proliferation of anaerobic bacteria such as *Gardnerella vaginalis*, *Mobiluncus* species, *Mycoplasma hominis*, *Prevotella* species, and *Atopobium vaginae*.
- A dense biofilm is present in which *G. vaginalis* predominates over other species.

CLINICAL

- 50% of women are asymptomatic; BV is less likely to be seen in sexually inexperienced women. Prevalence higher at earlier stages of menstrual cycle.
- **Sx:** offensive, fishy smelling vaginal discharge without associated soreness, itching, or irritation.
- **Signs:** thin, white, homogeneous discharge coating the walls of the vagina and the vestibule.
- **Risk factors for BV acquisition:** cigarette smoking, receptive anal intercourse before vaginal intercourse, vaginal intercourse, sex with an uncircumcised male partner, detection of HSV-2 serum antibodies prior to the diagnosis of BV, lack of H_2O_2-producing lactobacilli.
- Lab dx required! BV is NOT an infection; it is a disruption of the normal vaginal ecology that results in signs and symptoms.
- BV is a clinical syndrome resulting form replacement of normal peroxide-producing *Lactobacillus* sp in the vagina with high concentrations of anaerobic bacterial (e.g., *Mobiluncus* sp and *Prevotella* sp), *G. vaginalis*, and *Mycoplasma hominis*. BV is the most common cause of vaginal discharge or malodor. The cause of this microbial alteration is not known. Women who have never been sexually active are rarely affected. Treatment of the male partner has never been shown to be effective in preventing relapse.
- BV associated with increased risk of adverse obstetrical and gynecological clinical outcomes: (1) preterm delivery, (2) upper genital tract infections, (3) pelvic inflammatory disease.
- Also increases risk of acquiring HIV infection.
- Treatment is suboptimal with cure rates of only 60–80% and high recurrence/reinfection rates.

DIAGNOSIS

- Gold standard = Gram-stain to determine relative concentration of the various bacterial morphologic forms. This is not commonly used.
- Amsel criteria (need 3 of 4): (1) thin, white, homogeneous discharge; (2) clue cells on microscopy; (3) pH of vaginal fluids >4.5, (4) release of fishy odor on adding 10% KOH (+ whiff test).
- Nugent criteria (on Gram-stain): normally lactobacillus predominates. With BV predominantly *Gardnerella* and/or *Mobiluncus* morphotypes are seen with few or absent Lactobacilli. Training is required to properly interpret slides.
- Card test for detection of elevated pH and trimethylamine (QuickVue Advance Quidel, San Diego, CA) may have some utility.
- Card test for prolineaminopeptidase (Pip Activity TestCard, Quidel, San Diego, CA) may have some utility.
- A DNA probe-based test for high concentrations of *Gardnerella vaginalis* may have some utility in diagnosis. Cervical Pap smear of limited utility.
- Cultures for *Gardnerella vaginalis* NOT recommended. It is not specific as *G. vaginalis* can be recovered from almost all women with BV and 58% without BV.

TREATMENT

Nonpregnant women (HIV negative or positive)

- **Recommended:** metronidazole (MTZ) 500 mg PO twice daily × 7 days.
- Metronidazole gel 0.75%, one full applicator (5 g) intravaginally twice daily × 5 days.

- Clindamycin cream 2%, one full applicator (5 g) intravaginally qhs × 7 days.
- Note: single 2 g dose of metronidazole no longer recommended due to low efficacy.
- **Alternatives:** clindamycin 300 mg PO twice daily × 7 days.
- Clindamycin ovules 100 mg intravaginally qhs × 3 days.
- Benefits of treatment in the non-pregnant woman: relief of vaginal sx and signs, reduction of risks for infectious complications after abortion or hysterectomy, possible reduction of HIV acquisition if exposed, possible reduction of PID.

Pregnancy w/ sx or no sx but H/O previous pre-mature birth
- Optimal treatment regimen is unclear.
- **Recommended:** metronidazole 500 mg PO twice daily × 7 days.
- Metronidazole 250 mg PO three times a day × 7 days.
- Clindamycin 300 mg PO twice daily × 7 days.
- Benefits treating asymptomatic high-risk pregnant woman: conflicting evidence exists for asx women at low risk for pre-term delivery as some studies indicate decreased risk of pre-term deliver while others show no reduction. These findings have led some experts to recommend screening and treatment of asymptomatic high-risk women. Screening and treatment, if given, should be conducted at the first prenatal visit.

Allergy/intolerance to metronidazole
- Preferred: clindamycin cream 2%, 1 full applicator (5 g) intravaginally qhs × 7 days [do not use in pregnancy].
- Systemic intolerance to metronidazole (not *a bona fide* allergy): metronidazole gel 0.75%, 1 full applicator (5 g) intravaginally daily × 5 days.

FOLLOW UP
- In non-pregnant women: no follow-up if symptoms resolve. Instruct to return if symptoms recur; may wish to use a different regimen from that used originally in recurrences.
- Women with multiple recurrences should be referred to an infectious disease specialist. Long-term treatment may be needed in such cases.
- Pregnant women: follow-up evaluation 1-mo after completion of treatment.
- BV may be more persistent in HIV-infected women and may recur and require longer treatment.

OTHER INFORMATION
- Treat ALL pregnant women w/ sx. BV is associated w/ adverse outcomes (PROM, postpartum endometritis, chorioamnionitis, preterm birth, post-cesarean wound infection). Consider treatment of asx pregnant women w/ history of previous preterm birth.
- Associated risks for developing BV: douching, IUDs, multiple or new sex partners. Vinegar and water douches do not treat BV!
- A true STD only in women-who-have-sex-with-women; partners require treatment. Sexually associated in all other women; partners do not need treatment.
- BV is the most prevalent cause of vaginal sx among childbearing aged women; may be seen in up to 50% of women seen in public STD clinics. Self-dx of vaginitis is usually incorrect.
- Use of probiotics in prevention or treatment (and reduction of recurrent) BV is conflicting, and therefore use cannot be recommended at this time.

BASIS FOR RECOMMENDATIONS

Centers for Disease Control and Prevention, Workowski KA, and Berman SM. Sexually transmitted diseases treatment guidelines, 2006. *MMWR Recomm Rep*, 2006; Vol. 55; pp. 1–94.

Comments: The CDC treatment guidelines provide clinicians with a readily available reference for STD treatments recommended by a panel of national and international experts in STD diagnosis, treatment, prevention, and control. These guidelines available electronically from: http://www.cdc.gov/std/treatment/

CERVICITIS

Noreen A. Hynes, MD, MPH

PATHOGENS
- **Majority of cervicitis cases:** no organism identified
- *Chlamydia trachomatis* (CT)
- *Neisseria gonorrhoeae* (NG)

- *Trichomonas vaginalis* (TV)
- Herpes Simplex Virus (HSV)
- *Mycoplasma genitalium* (a suspect but unproven cause)

CLINICAL

- Frequently asymptomatic, but some women have abnormal vaginal discharge or intermenstrual vaginal bleeding.
- Cervicitis may be a sign of upper genital tract infection (endometritis), therefore, must assess for clinical findings of pelvic inflammatory disease.
- Frequent douching may cause cervicitis, so all pts should be asked about douching; this is a diagnosis of exclusion before testing for infectious agents.
- **Major signs:** purulent or mucopurulent endocervical exudate visible in the endocervical canal or on an endocervical swab (mucopurulent cervicitis) and friability, bleeding after gentle passage of swab though cervical os.
- Hypertrophic cervicitis: an intensely erythematous, raised, irregular area radiating outward from the cervical os that bleeds easily with contact (common in chlamydial cervicitis).
- Nabothian cysts, benign pearly white/yellow, nonfriable entities w/ clear mucous within may be seen in the transition zone of cervix and do not require Rx.
- Leukorrhea: >10 neutrophils per oil-immersion field on Gram-stained slide of cervical secretions collected after the endocervix has been cleaned off is has been associated with chlamydia (CT) and gonorrhea (GC) but has low predictive value.
- Gram-negative intracellular diplococci on Gram-stain is specific for gonococcal cervical infection but very insensitive (seen in on 50% of women with GC cervicitis).
- Routine confirmatory laboratory tests from collected cervical specimens should be performed for GC, CT, trichomonas vaginalis (TV) and vaginal sample to test for bacterial vaginosis (BV). Cervicitis is a major risk factor for both HIV acquisition and transmission, therefore test for HIV.

DIAGNOSIS

- The preferred screening test for CT and GC is a nucleic acid amplification test (NAAT). It can be performed on either endocervical or urine samples. If unavailable, followed by a non-NAAT such as nucleic acid hybridization test (such as GenProbe), EIA, or DFA.
- Culture is the gold standard but is expensive, difficult to preform, and less sensitive than a NAAT.
- Screening tests provide a presumptive diagnosis. In places with prevalence <2% of CT, a second NAAT test would be needed to confirm the first screening test.
- Test for TV by culture or antigen-based testing (saline wet preparation is insensitive).
- Test for bacterial vaginosis (BV) and treat if present.
- Routine testing for HSV in this setting is not recommended.
- No commercial tests are available for *Mycoplasma genitalium.*

TREATMENT

Presumptive Treatment Based on Risk Profiles Before Test Results

- **Presumptive treatment indications:** (1) ≤25 yrs, (2) new sexual partner in the last 90 days, (3) multiple sexual partners, (4) unprotected sex, (5) if follow-up cannot be ensured, (6) if a non-NAAT diagnostic test is used.
- **Presumptive treatment coverage:** CT and GC if the prevalence of GC in the pt population targeted (young age or facility prevalence) is >5%.
- **Presumptive Treatment Regimen:** azithromycin 1 g PO once OR doxycycline 100 mg PO bid/ × 7 days (adolescents and adults), azithromycin 1 g PO once OR amoxicillin 500 mg PO tid × 7 days (in pregnancy). Consider concurrent Rx for GC if prevalence of GC is high in the pt population under assessment (e.g., detention center, female prisoners <25 yrs, STD clinic in high prevalence area).
- GC treatment: See *Neisseria gonorrhoeae* on p. 301. *N. gonorrhoeae* resistance rates to fluoroquinolone antibiotics have increased to >25% in some U.S. cities and are no longer recommended for use in treatment of gonococcal infections at any site.
- Treat most recent sex partners, even if last partner >60 days before diagnosis.

Recurrent and Persistent Cervicitis

- **Persistent cervicitis:** reevaluate for possible reexposure to an STD and reassess for BV. Assess if all partners treated. Management of persistent cervicitis of unknown etiology is undefined.
- If high-risk profile for re-exposure, treat for GC and CT at time of presentation and prior to return of laboratory results. Otherwise, test for CT, GC, TV, BV and await results and treat accordingly.
- If cervix appears to have a necrotic area: test for syphilis by dark field microscopy or collect slide sample and submit slide to state lab for direct fluorescent treponemal antibody test.
- No validated, approved lab test for *M. genitalium.*
- Women with persistent symptoms that are clearly due to cervicitis despite treatment: cervical Pap test indicated along with referral to a gynecologist.

Gram-stain consistent with Gonorrhea (intracellular Gram-negative diplococci)

- Presumptively treat for GC as well as CT (this is the standard of care; see *Neisseria gonorrheae* in Pathogens section, p. 301, for recommended Rx).
- Uncomplicated GC cervicitis: a single dose of ceftriaxone (125 mg IM), cefixime (400 mg PO), AND treatment for CT with either azithromycin 1 g PO one time OR doxycycline 100 mg PO bid × 7 days. If the woman is pregnant, doxycycline is contraindicated and either azithromycin (as noted) or amoxicillin 500 mg PO tid × 7 days can be used. *N. gonorrhoeae* resistance rates to fluoroquinolone antibiotics have increased to >25% in some U.S. cities and are no longer recommended for use in treatment of gonococcal infections.

Cervicitis in HIV-infected Women

- Provide the same treatment as HIV negative women with cervicitis.

FOLLOW UP

- Females <20 yrs should be strongly encouraged to return for rescreening in 3–6 mos after a CT or GC dx.
- CT: for non-pregnant women, with non-persistent cervicitis, if treated with azithromycin, doxycycline, erythromycin, ofloxacin, or levofloxacin, a test-of-cure is NOT recommended.
- CT in pregnancy: Repeat testing (preferably with a NAAT) 3 wks after completion of Rx is recommended to ensure therapeutic cure. Do not retest sooner as false positive rates are high before 3 wks.
- GC: for non-pregnant women, with non-persistent cervicitis, if treated with cefatriaxone, cefixime, ciprofloxacin, ofloxacin, or levofloxacin a test-of-cure is NOT recommended.
- Persistent GC: will require antimicrobial sensitivity, therefore a sample of endocervical secretions for culture, with a request for sensitivity testing, rather than other testing modality should be sent to the laboratory.
- Recurrent infection with CT or GC over a 90–120 day period: consider advising pt to be retested 3 mos after treatment due to elevated risk for pelvic inflammatory disease.
- TV: no follow-up needed for women who become asymptomatic with treatment.

OTHER INFORMATION

- Risk Profile: Treatment decisions must consider prevalence of pathogens in the community and the risk profile of the pt examined including age, number of sexual partners, previous history of an STD, recent history of an STD or STD syndrome in any sexual partner, number of sex partners of patient's sex partners.

BASIS FOR RECOMMENDATIONS

Centers for Disease Control and Prevention (CDC). Update to CDC's sexually transmitted diseases treatment guidelines, 2006: fluoroquinolones no longer recommended for treatment of gonococcal infections. *MMWR Morb Mortal Wkly Rep*, 2007; Vol. 56; pp. 332–6.

Comments: Fluoroquinolones (FQ) have been used in the U.S. for the treatment of gonorrhea since 1993. Since 2000, FQ resistance among *Neisseria gonorrhoeae* isolates reported by the Centers for Disease Control and Prevention (CDC)-sponsored sentinel surveillance system, the Gonococcal Isolate Surveillance System (GISP) has been steadily increasing. Data available from the GISP for 2005 and preliminary data from 2006 demonstrate FQ resistant gonorrhea continues to increase among heterosexuals as well as men who have sex with men. Rates among heterosexual men are now as high as 26.6% in some cities. Therefore, on 13 April 2007, the CDC revised its *2006 Sexually Transmitted Diseases Treatment Guidelines* and no longer recommend the use of any FQ for the treatment of proven or suspect gonorrhea at any site of infection.

Centers for Disease Control and Prevention, Workowski KA, Berman SM. Sexually transmitted diseases treatment guidelines, 2006. *MMWR Recomm Rep*, 2006; Vol. 55; pp. 1–94.

Comments: These STD guidelines were developed by CDC in consultation with a large group of national STD experts. These new guidelines update those published in 2002 and include an expanded diagnostic evaluation for cervicitis as discussed in this module include cervicitis caused by *Trichomonas vaginalis*. This is the first time that tinidazole is listed among the recommended treatment options for *T. vaginalis*.

MASTITIS

Paul G. Auwaerter, MD

PATHOGENS

- Noninfectious
- *Staphylococcus aureus*
- Group A beta hemolytic strep
- Peptostreptococcus
- Prevotella species

CLINICAL

- Breast infection ranging from erythematous nodule to abscess formation.
- Bacterial mastitis usually with unilateral wedge-shaped induration, erythema, warmth, elicited pain, and fever.
- Common affliction (2–33%) of nursing mothers, usually 1st 3 mos, peak = 2 to 3 wks postpartum.
- Lactation mastitis may or may not be infectious as acute inflammation of breast tissue. Sx may include malaise, fever, unilateral redness, and tenderness of breast tissue.

DIAGNOSIS

- Mastitis usually clinical diagnosis, but breast milk cx may discriminate infectious vs. noninfectious—but normal milk may have >1000 colonies/cc organisms skin flora.
- DDX: breast engorgement/milk stasis that is often bilateral and lacking fever/erythema. Breast CA must be considered in unilateral findings, esp. nonlactating women. TB mastitis: consider in endemic area.

TREATMENT

Nursing Mothers

- Supportive: analgesics (ibuprofen preferred as not transferred to milk) and hot compresses. Also change breastfeeding patterns, ensure drainage of breast milk by regular emptying.
- To facilitate let down, initiate nursing w/ uninfected breast first.
- No consensus on when nursing should be discontinued during active infection, most favor continued nursing as it may aid response.
- If bacterial process, usually staphylococcal origin. Use beta-lactamase stable penicillin (since breastfeeding). Dicloxacillin 500 mg PO four times a day or cephalexin 500 mg PO four times a day 10–14 days.
- If abscess formation occurs, I and D, stop nursing, consider IV abx: nafcillin or oxacillin 2.0 g IV q4h or cefazolin 1.0 g q8h IV. Clindamycin 600 mg q8 or vancomycin 1 g q12h IV alternative if PCN allergic or concern for MRSA.
- With abscess, use breast pump to empty q2h or when engorged. May resume feeding when abscess, erythema resolved.
- Full antibiotic course should be taken even if symptoms resolve within 24–48 hrs.
- True fungal mastitis rare but can occur. Yeast often cultured from sore/cracked nipples but of unclear significance.

Recurrent Mastitis

- Cause may be inadequate Rx or breast abscess. Assess for breast abscess by USG before assuming due to resistant bacteria and changing abx.
- USG may be unhelpful as features of breast abscess nonspecific, and focal tenderness alone may be indicative of need for drainage.

Nonpuerperal mastitis or abscess

- Often bilateral black/green nipple discharge. Duct ectasia, aging breast w/ varicoceles may be cause. Bxp may show plasma cell mastitis w/ necrosis and inflammation, may also r/o CA.

- May be self-limited. Some authorities believe antibiotics unhelpful, and frequent I and D offers only temporary relief. Definitive treatment with complete excision of involved duct system.
- Subareolar location may include anaerobes, otherwise likely staphylococcal.
- Frank abscess require drainage.
- If abx employed, clindamycin 600 mg IVq8 or 300 mg PO q6h, or amox/clav 500 mg PO three times a day.

OTHER INFORMATION

- For primary care practitioner, safest to assume all mastitis in nonlactating pt is inflammatory carcinoma until proven otherwise.
- Decreased lactation mastitis seen over past few yrs often ascribed to increased breastfeeding rather than infant formula practices.
- Milk stasis major risk factor for mastitis: e.g., changing or skipped feedings, poor positioning, switching breasts prior to complete drainage, maternal or infant illness, abundant milk supply.
- Antibiotics may control bacterial infection if present, but w/ lactation mastitis they do not correct underlying cause. MUST promote milk drainage.

BASIS FOR RECOMMENDATIONS

Barbosa-Cesnik C, Schwartz K, Foxman B. Lactation mastitis. *JAMA*, 2003; Vol. 289; pp. 1609–12.

Comments: Review article highlights many of the controversial issues regarding diagnosis and management. The authors suggest there is strong evidence to continue with breastfeeding and also push for culturing milk to sort out if significant bacterial infection is present.

PELVIC INFLAMMATORY DISEASE (PID)

Noreen A. Hynes, MD, MPH

PATHOGENS

- *Chlamydia trachomatis*
- *Neisseria gonorrhoeae*
- *Trichomonas vaginalis*
- Anaerobes (vaginal flora)
- Enteric Gram-negative rods (vaginal flora)
- *Mycoplasma genitalium* (vaginal flora)
- *Gardnerella vaginalis* (vaginal flora)
- *Haemophilus influenzae* (vaginal flora)
- *Mycoplasma hominis* (vaginal flora)
- *Ureaplasma urealyticum* (vaginal flora)
- *Streptococcus agalactiae* (vaginal flora)
- Other less common or rare organisms: *Treponema pallidum*, *Mycobacterium tuberculosis*, *Actinomyces israeli*.

MORE PATHOGENS

Herpes simplex virus, type 2: virus has been isolated from the endometrium and fallopian tubes of women with acute PID, but its role pathogenesis remains unproven although evidence is beginning to suggest that HSV-2 alone may cause endometritis. It's role in salpingitis and tubal scarring remains to be defined. The viral role in facilitating the movement of lower tract bacteria to the upper tract has been suggested but has yet to be systematically studied.

CLINICAL

- Two-thirds of cases are considered to be due to sexually transmitted infections (most often chlamydia or gonorrhea but mixed flora common); one-third (particularly in older women) are commonly polymicrobial and with a higher risk of tubo-ovarian abscess. Risk factors to assess on history and physical examination include young age, douching, bacterial vaginosis, gynecologic surgery, smoking, HIV infection.
- This is a spectrum of inflammatory disorders of the upper female genital tract that is hard to diagnosis and can include: endometritis, salpingitis, tubo-ovarian abscess, and pelvic peritonitis. Clinical dx is imprecise but is best due to lack of reliable, readily available laboratory dx tools. Delays in dx and rx probably contributes to sequelae including scarring of

the fallopian tubes with subsequent ectopic pregnancy, chronic pelvic pain, infertility. Some cases are asymptomatic and others thought to be very mild but still with adverse outcomes.

- **Clinical dx (minimum criteria to initiate empiric treatment):** 1 or more of the following—cervical motion tenderness on bimanual pelvic examination or uterine tenderness or adnexal tenderness. Symptomatic PID has a positive predictive value for salpingitis of 65% to 90% compared with laparoscopic diagnosis. No single sign or symptom is both sensitive and specific enough for making the PID clinical dx. Symptomatic women may present with a chief complaint of lower abdominal pain, abnormal vaginal discharge, abnormal uterine bleeding, dyspareunia, menometrorrhagia, pain at the time of menses, nausea, vomiting, fever.

- **Other clinical criteria to enhance specificity of dx:** majority of cases—abnormal cervical or vaginal mucopurulent discharge or abundant WBC on saline wet prep of vaginal secretions (if neither found, consider seeking other causes than PID as cause of pelvic pain); other clinical criteria include oral temp >38.3°C (>101°F), elevated erythrocyte sedimentation rate, elevated C-reactive protein, laboratory documentation of cervical infection with *N. gonorrhoeae* or *C. trachomatis*.

- **Fitz-Hugh-Curtis syndrome:** also known as perihepatitis, can be an extrapelvic manifestation of PID secondary to inflammation of the liver capsule and diaphragm Acutely presents with severe right upper quadrant pain (RUQ) over the gall bladder area, with or without pain referral to the right shoulder, pleuritic pain that increases with movement or Valsalva maneuver. Other features including fever and night sweats may also be noted. If untreated chronic RUQ pain may ensue. Can occur with or without the minimum criteria for PID diagnosis. Between 10–30% of women with PID develop this syndrome, incidence highest in areas where there is high prevalence of gonorrhea. Periappendicitis can also be seen.

- **Indications for hospitalization:** unable to exclude a surgical emergency, severe illness (nausea/vomiting/high fever), tubo-ovarian abscess present, HIV-infected with low CD4 count, other cause of immunodeficiency, lack of response after 72 hrs of outpatient treatment, pregnant women (could see PID in 1st trimester) because of high risk of maternal mortality, fetal wastage, preterm delivery. Some experts recommend hospitalization of nulligravida teens to insure adherence with treatment regimen.

- **DDx:** ectopic pregnancy, acute appendicitis, and functional pain.

- Empiric PID therapy is unlikely to impair dx or management of other cause of lower pelvic pain.

MORE CLINICAL

- **Frequency of PID:** In the USA, disease afflicts more than 1 million women/yr.
- **Annual costs:** approx. $4.2 billion.
- **Location of care:** >90% now managed as outpatients; approx 250,000 hospitalizations/yr.
- **Frequency of complications:** a. *Ectopic pregnancy:* 12–15% in women who have had at least 1 episode of PID. b. *Tubal infertility:* 12–50% increasing risk with the number of episodes of PID. c. *Chronic pelvic pain:* may be as high as 18% after first clinical episode of PID.

DIAGNOSIS

- This is a clinical dx as outlined above. Other modalities that increase specificity of the diagnosis are NOT recommended as part of routine diagnosis. Additional studies (see following) may have a role in some cases.
- Laparoscopy to diagnosis salpingitis or tubo-ovarian abscess and to collect samples for a more complete bacterial diagnosis.
- Endometrial biopsy to search for histopathological evidence of endometritis (will not be seen on laparoscopy).
- Transvaginal sonography or MRI looking for thickened, fluid-filled fallopian tubes with or without free pelvic fluid or tubo-ovarian abscess.
- Doppler studies looking for tubal hyperemia or other evidence of pelvic infection.

TREATMENT
Oral/Outpatient Treatment of Mild to Moderately Severe Acute PID

- Ceftriaxone 250 mg IM × 1 PLUS doxycycline 100 mg PO twice daily × 14 days with or without metronidazole 500 mg PO twice daily × 14 days.
- Cefoxitin 2 g IM PLUS probenecid 1 g PO × 1 PLUS doxycycline 100 mg PO twice daily × 14 days with or without metronidazole 500 mg PO twice daily × 14 days.

- Other parenteral 3rd generation cephalosporin PLUS doxycycline 100 mg PO twice daily × 14 days with or without metronidazole 500 mg PO twice daily × 14 days.

Inpatient/Parenteral Regimens for PID

- Cefotetan 2 g IV q12h (no longer available in U.S.) or cefoxitin 2 g IV q6h PLUS doxycycline 100 mg IV or PO q12h for at least 24 hrs after clinical improvement, then outpatient regimen to complete 14 days.
- Clindamycin 900 mg IV q8h plus gentamicin loading dose IV/IM (2 mg/kg), then 1.5 mg/kg q8h or 5 mg/kg once daily for at least 24 hrs after clinical improvement, then change to outpatient regimen to complete 14 days.
- Alternative parenteral regimen: ampicillin/sulbactam 3 g IV q6h PLUS doxycycline 100 mg IV or PO q12h for at least 24 hrs after clinical improvement; then change to outpatient regimen to complete 14 days.

Alternative Oral Regimens if Parenteral Therapy Not Feasible

- If community prevalence and risk of gonococcal infection is low (<5%): Levofloxacin 500 mg PO once daily or ofloxacin 400 mg PO q12h with or without metronidazole 500 mg IV q8h, for at least 24 hrs after clinical improvement, then change to outpatient regimen to complete 14 days. Tests for gonorrhea must be performed prior to instituting treatment and the pt managed as follows if the test is positive for *N. gonorrhoeae*: (1) if a non-culture test is used and is positive, a parenteral cephalosporin regimen is recommended; (2) if culture for gonorrhea is positive, treatment should be based upon results of antimicrobial susceptibility. If the the isolate is fluoroquinolone resistant or resistance cannot be assessed, parenteral cephalosporin therapy is recommended.

Penicillin or Cephalosporin Allergic Patients

- Pts with a history of cephalosporin or penicillin allergy should be referred to a specialist for evaluation and possible desensitization prior to treatment with either a penicillin or cephalosporin.
- In areas where <5% of all gonococcal isolates identified by culture and sensitivity testing in the past 6 mos have been found to be fluoroquinolone resistant providers may consider use of levofloxacin as outlined above under "Alternative Oral Regimens if Parenteral Therapy Not Feasible".
- Spectinomycin efficacy in the treatment of pelvic inflammatory disease is too low and should not be used for treatment.

BASIS FOR RECOMMENDATIONS

Centers for Disease Control and Prevention (CDC). Update to CDC's sexually transmitted diseases treatment guidelines, 2006: fluoroquinolones no longer recommended for treatment of gonococcal infections. *MMWR Morb Mortal Wkly Rep*, 2007; Vol. 56; pp. 332–6.

Comments: Fluoroquinolones (FQ) have been used in the U.S. for the treatment of gonorrhea since 1993. Since 2000, FQ resistance among *Neisseria gonorrhoeae* isolates reported by the Centers for Disease Control and Prevention (CDC)-sponsored sentinel surveillance system, the Gonococcal Isolate Surveillance System (GISP) has been steadily increasing. Data available from the GISP for 2005 and preliminary data from 2006 demonstrate FQ resistant gonorrhea continues to increase among heterosexuals as well as men who have sex with men. Rates among heterosexual men are now as high as 26.6% in some cities. Therefore, on 13 April 2006, the CDC revised its *2006 Sexually Transmitted Diseases Treatment Guidelines* and no longer recommend the use of any FQ for the treatment of proven or suspect gonorrhea at any site of infection.

Centers for Disease Control and Prevention, Workowski KA, Berman SM. Sexually transmitted diseases treatment guidelines, 2006. *MMWR Recomm Rep*, 2006; Vol. 55; pp. 1–94.

Comments: The CDC treatment guidelines provide clinicians with a readily available reference for STD treatments recommended by a panel of national and international experts in STD diagnosis, treatment, prevention and control. These guidelines available electronically from: http://www.cdc.gov/

Korn AP, Landers DV. Gynecologic disease in women infected with human immunodeficiency virus type 1. *J Acquir Immune Defic Syndr Hum Retrovirol*, 1995; Vol. 9; pp. 361–70.

Comments: Good overview of gyn disease encountered in HIV-infected women and altered natural histories and refractoriness to standard therapies. Supports need for inpatient treatment initially for PID if HIV-infected woman is AIDS-defined.

Kahn JG, Walker CK, Washington AE, et al. Diagnosing pelvic inflammatory disease. A comprehensive analysis and considerations for developing a new model. *JAMA*, 1991; Vol. 266; pp. 2594–604.

Comments: No statistically significant predictor of PID found when reviewing studies from 1969 through 1990. No single or combined diagnostic indicators found to reliably predict PID. Therefore, high index of suspicion needed even when symptoms subtle to ensure earliest possible treatment.

VAGINAL DISCHARGE

Noreen A. Hynes, MD, MPH

PATHOGENS
- *Trichomonas vaginalis* (vaginitis and ectocervicitis)
- *Candida albicans* (vaginitis)
- *Gardnerella vaginalis* (bacterial vaginosis)
- *Mycoplasma hominis* (bacterial vaginosis)
- *Mobiluncus* species (bacterial vaginosis)
- *Peptostreptococci* (bacterial vaginosis)
- *Bacteroides species* (bacterial vaginosis)
- *Neisseria gonorrhoeae* (endocervicitis)
- *Chlamydia trachomatis* (endocervicitis)
- Herpes simplex virus (endocervicitis and ectocervicitis)
- *Mycoplasma genitalium* (endocervicitis, possible urethritis)

CLINICAL
- The complaint of vaginal discharge and visual inspection of the discharge is non-specific and **cannot** be relied upon to differentiate etiologies. More than 1 pathogen/process may be present. Additional testing is required!
- History: ask about the presence and characteristics of vaginal discharge: odor, external dysuria, pruritis, vaginal soreness or irritation, dyspareunia.
- Physical examination: (1) inspect external genitalia and palpate inguinal lymph nodes, (2) characterize discharge in terms of color, consistency, volume, (3) speculum examination to evaluate vaginal mucosa for erythema and presence of discharge on vaginal walls, evaluation of cervix for discharge, erythema, petechiae, edema, ulceration, and collect samples for testing pH of vaginal fluid and for microscopy (saline and KOH mounts).
- **Trichomoniasis:** pruritis—occasional complaint. Discharge—profuse, yellow-green to grey, homogeneous, with or without a mild fishy odor. Vulvovaginal area—usually erythematous. Cervix—ectocervical erythema, colpitis macularis ("strawberry cervix") caused by punctate hemorrhages is pathognomonic but infrequently seen.
- **Bacterial vaginosis:** pruritis—occasional complaint. Discharge—homogeneous, white to grey, with fishy odor coating the vaginal walls. Vulvovaginal area—minimal or no erythema. Cervix—normal.
- **Uncomplicated vulvovaginal candidiasis (VVC):** non-immunocompromised woman and sporadic or infrequent episodes and has mild to moderate clinical findings that is likely to be due to *C. albicans.* Pruritis—very common and may be severe. Discharge—scant to moderate, white, clumped or curd-like, adhering to vaginal walls, with little or no odor. Vulvovaginal area—erythematous often with mucosal swelling. Cervix—infrequent ectocervical erythema.
- **Complicated vulvovaginal candidiasis (VVC):** immunocompromised woman (uncontrolled diabetes, debilitation, immunosuppression, or pregnant) or with risk of non-albicans candidiasis or with recurrent VVC (>3 episodes of symptomatic VVC/yr) or severe VVC (severe pruritis, widespread vulvar erythema with mucosal swelling, excoriations and fissures large amount of white and clumped or curd-like discharge adhering to vaginal walls often with associated ectocervical erythema).
- **Gonorrhea, chlamydia and HSV:** pruritis—rare. Discharge—yellowish, if present, homogeneous, with little or no odor. Vulvovaginal area—no erythema. Cervix—mucopurulent drainage from the os commonly seen.
- **Mycoplasma genitalium:** cervicitis and mucopurulent cervicitis; possible urethritis. Discharge may be seen; dysuria not uncommon; not associated with pruritis.

DIAGNOSIS

- The 3 most common causes of vaginal discharge in women are trichomoniasis, bacterial vaginosis, and vulvovaginal candidiasis.
- **Trichomoniasis:** point of care diagnosis includes clinical exam findings and pH of discharge >4.5 (sensitivity = 56%, specificity = 50%); wet mount—motile trichomonads (60–70% sensitive compared with culture) and increased PMNs (ratio of PMNs to vaginal epithelial cells >1:1 but can also be seen in gonorrhea, chlamydia, and HSV discharge). 10% KOH slide yields positive "whiff" test (increase in foul fishy odor upon the addition of 10% KOH to vaginal discharge sample) in some cases. Other non-microscopy based FDA-cleared point of care diagnostics are >83% sensitive and >97% specific and include: OSOM Trichomonas Rapid Test (Genezyme Diagnostics, Cambridge, MA) which takes 10 minutes (83% sensitivity, 98.8% specificity). Culture using Diamond's media and commercially available culture based tests such as the InPouch system are 90–95% sensitive and >95% specific.
- **Bacterial vaginosis (BV):** point of care clinical diagnosis includes 3 of 4 criteria (Amsel Criteria—sensitivity = 92%, specificity = 77%) being present (1) homogeneous discharge adherent to vaginal wall, (2) pH of discharge >4.5 (sensitivity = 97%, specificity = 64%); (3) wet mount—clue cells (exfoliated vaginal squamous epithelial cells covered with bacteria so that the cell appears granular and obscuring the cell boarders) and few PMNs, and (4) 10% KOH slide—positive "whiff" test. When a microscope is not available at the point of care, card tests for elevated pH and amines are available (sensitivity 89–91%, specificity >95% if pH >4.7). A DNA probe test for high concentration of *G. vaginalis* (Affirm VP III, Becton Dickinson), may be of use. Culture for *G. vaginalis* or other organisms associated with BV is not recommended due to very low specificity. The Nugent Criteria is the diagnostic gold standard and is a scoring system based on Gram-stain of vaginal discharge. See Bacterial Vaginosis module on p. 104 for more information.
- **Uncomplicated vulvovaginal candidiasis (VVC):** point of care clinical diagnosis includes clinical exam findings and pH of discharge 4.0–4.5 (normal); wet mount—budding yeast, pseudohyphae (40%–60% sensitive), and few PMNs; 10% KOH slide—negative "whiff" test and clearer view of yeast (increases sensitivity to 60%–75%). Positive test findings must be interpreted in light of clinical signs and symptoms as 10%–20% of asymptomatic women vaginal colonization with *Candida species.*
- **Recurrent vulvovaginitis candidiasis (complicated VVC):** vaginal culture required as *C. glabrata* do not form pseudohyphae and are hard to identify with microscopy; nonalbicans species found in 10%–20% of pts.
- **Gonorrhea:** Gram-stain of cervical discharge with >30 PMNs per high-power field and intracellular Gram-negative diplococci is 50%–60% sensitive; culture on selective media has a sensitivity of 86%–96%; DNA probe has almost equivalent sensitivity to culture; nucleic acid amplifications tests (NAATs) are 95%–98% sensitive.
- **Chlamydia:** tissue culture has a sensitivity of 70%–80% and a specificity of 100% but is not widely available; enzyme immunoassay sensitivity is 73%–95% sensitive for cervical specimens; direct fluorescent anti body test is 50% to 81% sensitive; DNA probe is slightly more sensitive than culture; nucleic acid amplification tests (NAATs) are 85%–95% sensitive and 99% specific.
- **Herpes simplex virus:** Tzanck smear of a cervical ulcer (diagnostic feature is multinucleated giant cells) has a sensitivity of 50%; culture sensitivity is 100% if cervical vesicles are sampled but as low as 33% in late stage ulcers. Type-specific HSV serology is only of use if seroconversion can be demonstrated.
- *Mycoplasma genitalium*: transcription mediated assay and polymerase chain reaction are both research assays only and not FDA cleared. Culture is the standard method but growth is slow and may takes wks before it can be read as positive.

TREATMENT

Pathogen/Clinical Syndrome Specific Treatment in Non-Pregnant Women

- *Trichomonas vaginalis*: metronidazole or tinidazole 2 g PO × 1. Alternative treatment: metronidazole 500 mg PO twice daily × 7 days.
- **Bacterial vaginosis:** metronidazole 500 mg PO twice daily × 7 days; metronidazole gel 0.75%, 1 full applicator (5 g) intravaginally, once daily × 5 days; clindamycin cream, 2%, 1 full

applicator (5 g) intravaginally qhs × 7 days. Alternative treatments include: clindamycin 300 mg PO twice daily × 7 days; clindamycin ovules 100 g intravaginally qhs × 3 days.

- **Uncomplicated vulvovaginal candidiasis (VVC):** intravaginal agents: 6 agents and 14 regimens (see pathogen specific therapy below for partial listing), 4 of which are OTC given × 1, 3 or 7 days depending upon dose. Oral agent: fluconazole 150 mg PO × 1 dose.
- **Recurrent vulvovaginal candidiasis (complicated VVC):** remission therapy to include either (1) intravaginal agent: any of the same agents used for uncomplicated VVC but for 7–14 days or (2) oral agent: fluconazole 100 mg, 150 mg, or 200 mg PO every 3rd day for a total of 3 doses (day 1, 4, and 7). Maintenance therapy to follow: fluconazole 100 mg, 150 mg or 200 mg PO every wk × 6 mo. Alternative maintenance therapy: topical clotrimazole 200 mg (2 tablets) intravaginally twice weekly; clotrimazole 500 mg (5 tablets) intravaginally every wk; or other topical treatments intermittently.
- **Severe vulvovaginal candidiasis (complicated VVC):** intravaginal agent—any of the same agents used for uncomplicated VVC but for 7–14 days or oral agent—fluconazole 150 mg PO every 3 days for a total of 2 doses (day 1 and day 4).
- **Nonalbicans vulvovaginal candidiasis (complicated VVC):** Optimal rx is unknown. Refer to a specialist to assist with treatment.
- **Vulvovaginal candidiasis in HIV infected women (complicated VVC):** Treat as for uncomplicated VVC or with a regimen for recurrent or severe VVC as indicated by history and physical findings.
- *Neisseria gonorrhoeae:* ceftriaxone 125 mg IM × 1 or cefixime 400 mg PO × 1. *N. gonorrhoeae* resistance rates to fluoroquinolone antibiotics have increased to >25% in some U.S. cities and are no longer recommended for use in treatment of gonococcal infections at any site. Spectinomycin is no longer available in the U.S. for women allergic to cephalosporins. Manage cephalosporin allergic women in consultation with an expert.
- **Chlamydia trachomatis:** azithromycin 1 g PO × 1 or doxycycline 100 mg PO twice daily × 7 days. Alternatives: erythromycin base 500 mg PO q6h 7 days or erythromycin ethylsuccinate 800 mg q6h × 7 days or ofloxacin 300 mg PO twice daily × 7 days or levofloxacin 500 mg PO daily × 7 days.
- **Herpes simplex virus:** use a 7–10 days regimen of acyclovir 400 mg PO three times a day or acyclovir 200 mg PO 5 times per day or famciclovir 250 mg PO q8h or valacyclovir 1 g PO twice daily.
- **Mycoplasma genitalium:** azithromycin 1 g PO × 1 or doxycycline 100 mg PO twice daily × 7 days.

Pathogen or Clinical Syndrome Specific Treatment in Pregnancy

- *Trichomonas vaginalis:* infection (definitely) and treatment (possibly) associated with perinatal morbidity, therefore risks and benefits need to be discussed. Consider deferring treatment until >37 wks gestation. Metronidazole 2 g PO × 1 may be used. If post-partum and breastfeeding, do not breastfeed for 12–24 hrs following treatment.
- **Bacterial vaginosis:** metronidazole 500 mg PO twice daily × 7 days or metronidazole 250 mg PO q8h × 7 days or clindamycin 300 mg PO twice daily × 7 days.
- **Vulvovaginal candidiasis:** only topical azole therapies should be used × 7 days.
- *Neisseria gonorrhoeae:* ceftriaxone 125 mg IM × 1 or cefixime 400 mg PO × 1. Spectinomycin is no longer available in the U.S. for women allergic to cephalosporins. Manage cephalosporin allergic women in consultation with an expert.
- *Chlamydia trachomatis:* azithromycin 1 g PO × 1 or amoxicillin 500 mg PO q8h × 7 days.
- **Herpes simplex virus (severe or first episode only):** acyclovir 400 mg PO q8h × 7–10 days or acyclovir 200 mg PO 5 times per day × 7–10 days.

OTHER INFORMATION

- Directly observed, single dose therapy is preferred whenever possible to insure treatment and to decrease ongoing transmission.
- BV and candidiasis are considered sexually associated rather than sexually transmitted diseases. However, in women who have sex with women BV has been shown to be sexually transmitted.

DIAGNOSIS

- Initial Rx: use best available evidence provided by point-of-care tests AND a risk assessment of the cause for discharge in each pt. NO one agent is available to treat all of the likely causes.
- Other non-infectious causes of vaginal discharge must also be considered including desquamative inflammatory vaginitis, retained foreign body (e.g. tampon), allergic vaginitis, and invasive carcinoma of the cervix.
- The majority of male partners of women with *T. vaginalis* have asymptomatic infection and need to be examined and offered treatment. Reinfection by untreated asymptomatic partners could lead to a misdiagnosis of possible drug-resistant infection.

BASIS FOR RECOMMENDATIONS

Centers for Disease Control and Prevention (CDC). Update to CDC's sexually transmitted diseases treatment guidelines, 2006: fluoroquinolones no longer recommended for treatment of gonococcal infections. *MMWR Morb Mortal Wkly Rep*, 2007; Vol. 56; pp. 332–6.

Comments: Fluoroquinolones (FQ) have been used in the U.S. for the treatment of gonorrhea since 1993. Since 2000, FQ resistance among *Neisseria gonorrhoeae* isolates reported by the Centers for Disease Control and Prevention (CDC)-sponsored sentinel surveillance system, the Gonococcal Isolate Surveillance System (GISP) has been steadily increasing. Data available from the GISP for 2005 and preliminary data from 2006 demonstrate FQ resistant gonorrhea continues to increase among heterosexuals as well as men who have sex with men. Rates among heterosexual men are now as high as 26.6% in some cities. Therefore, on 13 April 2006, the CDC revised its *2006 Sexually Transmitted Diseases Guidelines* and no longer recommends the use of any FQ for the treatment of proven or suspect gonorrhea at any site of infection.

Centers for Disease Control and Prevention, Workowski KA, Berman SM. Sexually transmitted diseases treatment guidelines, 2006. *MMWR Recomm Rep*, 2006; Vol. 55; pp. 1–94.

Comments: These STD guidelines were developed by CDC after consultation with a group of professionals knowledgeable in the field of STDs. The information in this report updates the Sexually Transmitted Diseases Treatment Guidelines, 2002. Included in these updated guidelines are an expanded diagnostic evaluation for cervicitis and trichomoniasis; new antimicrobial recommendations for trichomoniasis; discussion of the role of *Mycoplasma genitalium* and trichomoniasis in urethritis/cervicitis and treatment-related implications; and increasing prevalence of quinolone-resistant *Neisseria gonorrhoeae* in MSM.

HEENT

CERVICAL FASCIAL (PERIMANDIBULAR) SPACE INFECTIONS

John G. Bartlett, MD

PATHOGENS
- *Bacteroides species*
- *Prevotella* spp.
- *Fusobacterium nucleatum*
- *Peptostreptococcus*
- *Streptococcus species* including *S. milleri*
- *Fusobacterium necrophorum*
- *S. aureus* including MRSA
- Potential complications: septic phlebitis

CLINICAL
- Definition: infection involving the spaces created by facial insertions along the mandible.
- Presentation: tender swelling along mandible (usually with local and systemic signs of infection). Differential dx: parotitis, lymph node infection, actinomycosis.
- Major spaces involved: submandibular and parapharyngeal.
- Serious space infections: (1) Submandibular spaces (Ludwig's angina), (2) Retropharyngeal space (behind esophagus) and (3) Lateral pharyngeal space—jugular venom septic phlebitis (Lemierre's syndrome).
- Signs include tender swelling along the mandible—differential dx includes parotitis, actinomycosis, peritonsillar abscess or lymphadenitis.
- Cause: dental source most common; other—foreign body, tonsillitis or pharyngitis, malignancy, surgery.

DIAGNOSIS
- CT scan defines space infections with great clarity.
- Needle aspiration for bacteriology ± cytology.

TREATMENT
Life-threatening space infections
- Lemierre's Syndrome: most respond to antibiotic treatment and do not require anticoagulation, vein ligation or surgical drainage.
- Ludwig's angina: secure airway (intubation or tracheostomy) antibiotics +/− surgical drainage.
- Retropharyngeal abscess: secure airway (tracheostomy prn) + antibiotics. Surgery if unresponsive to antibiotics.

Antibiotics
- Principles: (1) Anatomic definition—obtain CT scan, (2) Drainage—ENT/oral surgery, (3) Airway protection, (4) abx should be directed against anaerobes and streptococci.
- **Preferred:** clindamycin 300 mg PO four times a day or 600 mg IV q8h.
- **Alternatives:** ampicillin-sulbactam (Unasyn) 3 g IV q6h or amoxicillin-clavulanate (Augmentin) 875 mg PO twice daily.
- **Alternatives:** Metronidazole (Flagyl) 500 mg PO twice daily-four times a day (+ penicillin or amoxicillin).
- Imipenem (Primaxin) 0.5–1 g IV q6h (or meropenem or ertapenem).
- Piperacillin-tazobactam (Zosyn) 3.375 g IV q6h or any beta-lactam/beta-lactamase inhibitor combination.
- *S. aureus*: oxacillin/nafcillin 1–2 g IV q6h if MSSA, vancomycin 15 mg/kg IV q12h if MRSA.

Miscellaneous
- Drainage: critical component of treatment. Usually surgical drainage, sometimes needle aspiration is adequate.
- Dental care: dental infections are usually the underlying cause—a tooth that needs extraction or a complication of a dental procedure.
- Lemierre's syndrome—role of surgery and anticoagulants is unclear.

DIAGNOSIS

BASIS FOR RECOMMENDATIONS

Vieira F, Allen SM, Stocks RM, et al. Deep neck infection. *Otolaryngol Clin North Am*, 2008; Vol. 41; pp. 459–83, vii.

Comments: Deep neck infections: Complications include airway obstruction, jugular vein thrombosis, descending mediastinitis, ARDS, sepsis and DIC Primary sources—dental, salivary gland, foreign body, tonsil infection, malignancy. Bacteriology—mixed flora with anaerobes.

DENTAL INFECTIONS

Spyridon Marinopoulos, MD

PATHOGENS

- *Streptococcus mutans*
- pigmented Bacteroides (Porphyromonas and Prevotella)
- *Streptococcus milleri*
- *Actinomyces viscosus*
- Peptostreptococcus

CLINICAL

- **Dental caries:** no sx. Chalky white lesion turns golden-brown then dark/black with central cavitation. Pain suggests progression to pulp infection (pulpitis).
- **Pulpitis:** sharp-to-dull throbbing pain, tooth specific or generalized, may refer to ear/temple/neck/opposite jaw (rare). May be early/reversible or progress to late/irreversible stage with necrosis.
- Early: sensitive to temperature change, sweet stimuli, worse w/ reclining, spontaneously better in secs. Late: pain severe, persistent, often poorly localized, worse with any stimulus including air.
- PE: grossly decayed tooth. If not obvious, localize by percussing with or asking pt to bite on tongue blade. Exquisite pain suggests progression to periapical abscess.
- **Periapical abscess:** exquisite tooth pain w/ touch/chewing. Loss of temp sensitivity. Fever, LN, tooth mobility (tooth feels higher/longer) +/– soft tissue edema.

TREATMENT

Miscellaneous

- Warm saline rinses.
- NSAIDs +/– weak opioid analgesics for pain control.
- Early/reversible pulpitis: removing carious lesion and filling of cavities with inert material may be sufficient to arrest disease.
- Late/irreversible pulpitis requires endodontic therapy (root canal treatment) or extraction of involved tooth.
- Note: persistent root canal infection is associated w/ *Candida albicans*. Eradicate w/ calcium hydroxide/camphorated paramonochlorophenol/glycerin or 0.12% chlorhexidine digluconate/zinc oxide.
- Periapical abscess requires I&D + endodontic therapy (root canal treatment) or extraction of diseased tooth. Abx are adjunctive only.
- Prevention is essential and involves meticulous dental care and frequent dental visits to eliminate dental caries.

Antibiotics

- Abx commonly used for the rx of periapical abscess, but generally not needed in healthy pts w/ pulpitis alone. Use if systemic sxs/signs of infection. Treat for 3 days, then reassess. Occasionally treatment needed for 7 days.
- Penicillin VK 500 mg PO q6h × 7 days. Switch/broaden coverage if no better after 48 hrs.
- Cephalexin 500 mg PO q6h × 7 days. Switch/broaden coverage if no better after 48 hrs.
- Clindamycin 300 mg PO q6h × 7 days in pen-allergic pts or if pen/ceph ineffective. First-line in more severe cases, if anaerobes predominant (after day 3) or beta-lactamase resistance a concern.
- Penicillin VK 500 mg PO q6h + metronidazole (Flagyl) 500 mg PO q6h × 7 days excellent for broader Gram-positive and anaerobic coverage when pen alone ineffective.
- Augmentin 500 mg PO q8h × 7 days if pen/ceph ineffective. First-line in more severe cases, if anaerobes predominant (after day 3) or beta-lactamase resistance a concern.

- Moxifloxacin 400 mg PO q24h × 7 days covers Strep and anaerobes and is an excellent alternative in more severe cases and if pen allergy.
- Limited use: erythromycin 500 mg PO q6h × 7 days alternative to penicillin but less active against anaerobes and certain mouth flora and there is emerging resistance. Clindamycin preferred.
- Azithromycin 500 mg PO × 1 then 250 mg PO daily × 4 days (Z-pak) or clarithromycin (Biaxin) 500 mg PO q12h × 7 days more expensive alternatives to erythromycin w/ similar concerns re resistance.
- Non-preferred: doxycycline 200 mg PO × 1 then 100 mg PO daily × 7 days or tetracycline 250 mg PO q6h × 7 days in pen-allergic pts. Very limited use as many streptococci and anaerobes resistant. Clindamycin preferred.

OTHER INFORMATION

- The etiology of dental infections is dental caries, which can be prevented by meticulous dental hygiene and frequent dental visits.
- Treatment of infection must always involve treatment of the offending tooth +/– abscess drainage if necessary. Abx may be used for periapical abscess but not needed in healthy pts with pulpitis alone.
- Potential complications include sinusitis, cavernous sinus thrombosis, Ludwig's angina, retro/parapharyngeal abscess, osteomyelitis, endocarditis, brain abscess, necrotizing fasciitis.
- Infection may spread into fascial planes and extend into face/neck soft tissues if bacteria aggressive or host compromised. Dysphagia/drooling suggest retro/parapharyngeal infection, a medical emergency.
- Refer to dentist ASAP if (1) severe, acute pain unrelieved with analgesics or removal of thermal stimuli; (2) trauma; (3) new or enlarging orofacial swelling; (4) uncontrolled bleeding; (5) fever.

BASIS FOR RECOMMENDATIONS
Author opinion.

EPIGLOTTITIS

John G. Bartlett, MD

PATHOGENS

- *Haemophilus influenzae,* less commonly other pathogens implicated: *S. pneumoniae,* other Streptococcus species.
- Respiratory tract viruses.
- Immunocompromised hosts (only): *Candida albicans,* Kaposi's sarcoma, Gram-negative bacilli, *Aspergillus.*

CLINICAL

- Sore throat with odynophagia and fever, +/– drooling, stridor dyspnea, hoarseness.
- Has become a rare condition in children since *H. influenza* type b vaccination.
- Direct visualization shows cherry red epiglottis with tongue blade exam, or by direct or indirect laryngoscopy (caution: don't attempt this exam unless there's setup for airway control).
- Leukocytosis with shift—prognostic.
- Lab: X-ray of lateral neck shows enlarged epiglottis, but not sensitive or specific. CT scan may help.
- Chest XR shows accompanying pneumonia in up to 25%.

DIAGNOSIS

- Clinical diagnosis although lateral neck soft tissue X-ray or neck CT or flexible laryngoscopy may help.
- Diagnosis requires visualization of epiglottis with tongue blade, laryngoscope, or lateral neck XR—don't manipulate airway or send for XR without being prepared for emergent intubation.

TREATMENT
Antibiotic
- Principles: maintain airway + empiric abx targeting.
- Preferred abx: cefotaxime 2–3 g IV q6–8h × 7–10 days or ceftriaxone 1–2 g IV q24h × 7–10 days.
- Cefuroxime 0.75–1.5 g IV q6–8h × 7–10 days.
- Ampicillin-sulbactam (Unasyn) 1.5–3 g IV q6h × 7–10 days.
- Ticarcillin-clavulanate (Timentin) 3.1 g IV q4–6h × 7–10 days.
- Piperacillin-tazobactam (Zosyn) 3.375 g IV q4–6h × 7–10 days.
- Levofloxacin (Levaquin) 500 mg IV qday × 7–10 days.
- Moxifloxacin (Avelox) 400 mg IV qday × 7–10 days.

Maintain airway
- Manage in ICU, maintaining airway is most critical.
- Indications for intubation or tracheostomy: dyspnea, stridor and/or drooling.
- Laryngoscopy showing narrowed airway correlates with need for artificial airway.

Anti-inflammatory and miscellaneous agents
- Prednisone (or other steroid) is often given although utility is not known and dose is arbitrary (usually 40–60 mg).
- Hydration, oxygen, analgesics.

OTHER INFORMATION
- Major decision is managing airway—tracheostomy or intubate or observation in ICU—adults usually observed.
- *H. influenzae* is the major identifiable treatable pathogen; many cases in adults are culture negative and are thought to be viral.

BASIS FOR RECOMMENDATIONS
Mayo-Smith MF, Spinale JW, Donskey CJ, et al. Acute epiglottitis. An 18-yr experience in Rhode Island. *Chest*, 1995; Vol. 108; pp. 1640–7.
Comments: Indications for artificial airway: dyspnea, strider, drooling, rapid progression, or significant swelling. Mortality in this series was 3% in adults.

GINGIVITIS/PERIODONTITIS

Spyridon Marinopoulos, MD

PATHOGENS
- *Prevotella gingivalis* and *P. intermedia*
- *Actinobacillus actinomycetemcomitans*
- *Treponema denticola*
- *Bacteroides forsythus*
- *Capnocytophaga* sp.
- *Peptostreptococcus micros*
- Spirochetes
- Gram-negative anaerobes

CLINICAL
- **Gingivitis:** gums bleed with minor injury/spontaneously +/– edema/erythema. HIV gingivitis (linear gingival erythema): brightly inflamed band of marginal gingiva +/– bleeding/pain/ rapid destruction.
- Acute necrotizing ulcerative gingivitis (NUG) or trench mouth: fetid breath, blunting of interdental papillae and ulcerative necrotic gingival sloughing +/– fever/regional LN. Noma (ref module) precursor.
- **Periodontitis:** inflamed gingiva w/ loss of supportive connective tissues. No sx. PE: bone craters w/ increased gingival pocket (probing) depth and tooth mobility. XR may show bone loss.
- Necrotizing ulcerative periodontitis (NUP): rapidly progressive painful gingival tissue and alveolar bone destruction w/ eventual necrosis, progresses from NUG. Impaired host. If HIV, CD4 usually <200.
- Periodontal abscess: acute, tender, purulent inflammation in gingival wall of periodontal pocket + fluctuance +/– sinus tract +/– regional LN +/– tender/sensitive adjacent teeth + fever if severe.

- Predisposing factors to poor gingival and periodontal health include pregnancy (hormonal shifts), smoking, diabetes, HIV, leukemia, Down syndrome, other immune/leukocyte disorders (Job's syndrome, leukocyte adhesion deficiencies, Chediak-Higashi syndrome, Papillon-Lefevre syndrome, chronic granulomatous disease), exogenous immunosuppression (chemotherapy), head and neck radiation, medications causing gingival hyperplasia (nifedipine/other Ca blockers, dilantin, cyclosporin) or Xerostomia etc.

DIAGNOSIS
- Clinical diagnoses, see above.

TREATMENT
Miscellaneous/Topical Antibacterial
- Gingivitis/periodontitis: plaque removal w/ scaling and root planing (SRP) q3–6 mo can rx most pts w/ no need for abx. Prevention involves meticulous hygiene w/ brushing, flossing and regular dental visit.
- Initiate rx w/ scaling and root planing (SRP)+ home hygiene. Consider antibacterial mouthwash (see below) if pts unwilling/unable to comply w/ home hygiene measures. Assess for response 1–3 mo post rx.
- Exceptions: (1) fulminant types (2) disease caused *by A. Actinomycetemcomitans* (Aa)—including juvenile and some adult—not responsive to SRP alone and requires post-SRP adjunctive systemic abx.
- Chlorhexidine (PerioGard) 0.12% oral rinse 15cc twice daily between dental visits reduces bacterial flora/prevents plaque advancement. May cause tooth staining and promote bacterial resistance w/ prolonged use.
- Refractory +/– recurrent periodontitis: obtain culture prior to initiation of treatment. If sites of disease few, treat w/ SRP + local-delivery abx. If extensive disease, treat SRP + systemic abx (see below).
- Local delivery adjunct to SRP (applied once): minocycline 1 mg microsphere (Arestin)/tetracycline 12.7 mg fiber (Actisite)/doxycycline 10% gel (Atridox)/chlorhexidine 2.5 mg chip (PerioChip).
- Other therapies: (submicrobial dose) doxycycline hyclate (Periostat) 20 mg PO q12h × 90 days (up to 9 mo) reduces periodontitis by inhibiting collagenase. Effect small but significant. Useful as adjunct to SRP.
- Periodontal abscess: NSAIDs +/– weak narcotic opioids for pain control. I&D is primary treatment w/ abx supportive if systemic sx (fever, LN, etc.). Refer to dentist within 24 hrs.

Systemic antibiotics
- Comment: although scaling and root planing (SRP) alone is effective in most pts w/ periodontal disease, strong evidence exists for use of abx as adjunct to SRP in severe/refractory/aggressive cases.
- Juvenile periodontitis: tetracycline 250 mg PO q6h or doxy/minocycline 200 mg PO × 1 then 100 mg PO twice daily × 14 days. If no success/aggressive disease: amoxicillin 500 mg + metronidazole 250 mg PO q8 × 7 days.
- Refractory +/– recurrent periodontitis: culture prior to initiation of treatment. If sites of disease few, Rx SRP + local-delivery abx (see above). If extensive disease, Rx SRP + systemic abx (below).
- If c+s unavailable and no prior abx hx: tetracycline 250 mg PO q6h or doxy/minocycline 200 mg PO × 1 then 100 mg PO twice daily × 14 days. Alt: amox/clav 250–500 mg PO q8h × 10 days. PCN allergy: clindamycin 150–300 mg PO q6h × 7–10 days.
- More aggressive disease: amox 500 mg + metronidazole 250 mg PO q8h × 7 days. PCN allergy: clindamycin 150–300 mg PO q6h × 10 days very effective. Alternative: metronidazole 500 mg + cipro 500 mg PO q12h × 7 days.
- ANUG (Trench Mouth) /NUP/HIV-NUG/HIV-NUP: metronidazole 250 mg + amox/clav 250 mg PO q8h × 7 days (+ nystatin rinses 5 ml four times a day or fluconazole 200 mg PO once daily × 7–14 days if HIV+ especially given candida overgrowth w/ abx use).
- Pen allergy: metronidazole 500 mg PO + ciprofloxacin 500 mg PO q12h × 7 days (+ nystatin rinses 5 ml four times a day or fluconazole 200 mg PO once daily × 7–14 days if HIV+ esp given candida overgrowth w/ abx use).

- Periodontal abscess: abx controversial. Use if severe/systemic sx always in conjunction w/ I&D. Cover anaerobes. Traditionally treat 7 days, but also acceptable 3 days then reassess if further therapy required.
- Augmentin 500 mg PO q8h or (PCN allergy) metronidazole 500 mg PO q8h. Rx failure: when possible, obtain c+s and tailor abx accordingly. Rx failure empiric rx: clindamycin 300 mg PO q6h.

OTHER INFORMATION

- Gingivitis and periodontitis are preventable; meticulous oral hygiene and regular dental visits are key. Rx consists of scaling and root planing +/− adjunctive abx.
- Use abx adjunctively in fulminant/aggressive/recurrent disease. Prefer topical if few teeth involved, but systemic justified in more diffuse/severe disease. C+s may aid appropriate abx selection.
- Gingivitis/periodontitis may represent initial presentation of systemic illness: DM, HIV, leukemia, other immune. Also consider meds causing gingival hyperplasia: dilantin, nifedipine, cyclosporin, etc.
- HIV-positive pts present with fulminant disease. Unique bacterial flora includes Gram-negative anaerobes, enterobacteriaceae and fungi. Must cover Candida. Refer urgently.
- Potential complications include tooth loss, sinusitis, cavernous sinus thrombosis, Ludwig's angina, retro/parapharyngeal abscess, osteomyelitis, endocarditis, brain abscess. CAD and CVA risk association also reported.

BASIS FOR RECOMMENDATIONS

Author opinion.

HORDEOLUM (STYE)/CHALAZION

Spyridon Marinopoulos, MD

PATHOGENS

- Hordeolum: *S. aureus*
- Chalazion: non-ID causes

CLINICAL

- **Hordeolum (stye):** infection of Zeiss/Moll tear glands in eyelid margin (external) or meibomian gland in tarsal plate (internal hordeolum). Acute inflammation of eyelid with abscess formation.
- Clinical: tender swelling of eyelid and erythema. Abscess points internally or externally. Self-limited, spontaneously drains in 5–7 days, but may progress to cellulitis or chalazion especially if internal.
- Ddx: eyelid tumor, blepharitis, conjunctivitis, periorbital cellulitis.
- **Chalazion:** granuloma develops as foreign body reaction to lipid produced by meibomian gland. May arise from internal hordeolum or with sebum plugging tear gland opening and causing obstruction.
- Clinical: painless, rubbery, palpable nodule at margin of lid or higher. If large, may cause visual disturbance by pressing on and deforming the cornea.
- Predisposing factors: hordeolum—staph blepharitis; chalazion—seborrheic blepharitis and rosacea.

DIAGNOSIS

- Clinical diagnosis most commonly (see above).
- Occasionally may require culture (hordeolum) or biopsy (chalazion) to rule-out malignancy.

TREATMENT

General Measures

- **Hordeolum (Stye):** most will drain spontaneously within 3–4 days following pointing, especially if external. Internal may persist and progress to chalazion.
- Warm compresses 4–5 ×/day × 10–15 min per session essential to help open pore and promote drainage. Scrubbing eye with neutral soap (Dove, Ivory or baby shampoo) may hasten recovery.

- If external, relief of pain and resolution are hastened if pointing lesion is pricked with fine sterile needle. Apply antibiotic ointment post procedure. Do not attempt for internal hordeolum.
- Refer to ophthalmology for I&D if no improvement by day 3 of conservative therapy +/− antibiotics.
- **Chalazion:** may resolve spontaneously if duct of gland opens. Warm compresses 4–5 ×/day × 10–15 min per session × 1 mo will help soften plug. ~50% will resolve. If no resolution, refer to ophthalmology.
- Ophthalmologists may treat by incision and curettage, intralesional steroid injection or both.
- Intralesional steroid injection with 0.05–0.3 mL of 5 mg/dL triamcinolone effective, but may depigment overlying skin in darkly pigmented individuals. Expect resolution in 1–2 wks.
- Steroid injection good for children, pts allergic to local anesthesia and lesions close to lacrimal drainage system. Also no eye patching required, less in-office time/cost and can treat multiple lesions in same visit.
- Outpatient incision and curettage preferred for hard lesions of >6 mos duration, for possibly infected chalazia, when skin depigmentation is a concern, and is the only recourse if steroid injection is ineffective.
- Combined incision, curettage and intralesional corticosteroid injection may be more effective for pts with large, recurrent and multiple chalazia.

Antibiotics

- Hordeolum (Stye): generally systemic abx unnecessary unless there is associated periorbital cellulitis (rare). However, oral abx may be indicated in moderate to severe cases of internal hordeola.
- Hordeolum (external): erythromycin ophthalmic ointment (E-mycin, Eryc) 0.5-inch into conjunctival sac twice daily four times a day × 7 days or sulfacetamide 10% ophthalmic oint 0.5-in ribbon twice daily four times a day × 7 days.
- Hordeolum (internal, mild cases): erythromycin ophthalmic oint (E-mycin, Eryc) 0.5-inch into conjunctival sac twice daily four times a day × 7 days or sulfacetamide 10% ophthalmic oint 0.5-in ribbon twice daily four times a day × 7 days.
- Hordeolum (internal, moderate or severe cases): dicloxacillin 500 mg PO q6h × 7 days or cephalexin 500 mg PO q6h × 7 days.
- Alternatives (pen or ceph allergy): clindamycin 300 mg PO q6h × 7 days or clarithromycin 500 mg PO q12h × 7 days or azithromycin 500 mg PO once then 250 mg PO daily × 5 days (Z-PAK).
- **Chalazion:** not an infectious disease as lesion generally is sterile. However, chronic oral tetracycline or doxycycline may treat recurrent chalazia via effect on fatty acid production by tear glands.

Treatment Regimen Details

Conservative treatment of chalazia

- Method by Perry and Serniuk (80% of chalazia resolved by 4 wks).

Eyelid hygiene

- Prepare saline solution using $\frac{1}{2}$ tsp table salt in 1qt warm H20.
- Soak sterile cotton ball with soln and place on eye with lid closed until cool.
- Continue × 10 min replacing cotton balls as soon as they cool.

Eyelash cleansing

- Clean eyelashes twice daily by brushing gently with cotton tipped applicator soaked in above solution.

Other Information

- Hordeolum (stye): warm compresses primary rx with topical abx secondary and oral abx only in moderate to severe cases if hordeolum internal. Refer if no improvement by day 3 of rx.
- Preauricular lymph node involvement and fever are not consistent with diagnosis and may suggest a more serious infection (e.g., periorbital cellulitis) requiring aggressive systemic therapy.
- Chalazion: refer for incision and curettage or intralesional steroids if compresses not effective. R/O sebaceous cell, basal cell or meibomian gland CA if persistent or recurrent. There are a few reported cases of distant malignancies (mesothelioma, renal cell CA) or vasculitis (Wegners) presenting as chalazion.

BASIS FOR RECOMMENDATIONS
Lederman C, Miller M. Hordeola and chalazia. *Pediatr Rev*, 1999; Vol. 20; pp. 283–4.
Comments: A concise review article on the pathophysiology and management of hordeola and chalazia.
Author opinion.

LARYNGITIS

John G. Bartlett, MD

PATHOGENS
- Parainfluenza virus
- Influenza
- Coronavirus
- Rhinovirus
- Adenovirus
- Herpes simplex virus
- Metapneumovirus

MORE PATHOGENS

Viral	Non-viral	Rare
Parainfluenza virus	C. pneumoniae	Coccidioides immitis
Influenza virus	C. diphtheriae	C. neoformans
Coronavirus (Non-SARS)	M. pneumoniae	M. tuberculosis
Respiratory syncytial virus	Group A streptococci	Blastomyces dermatitidis
Rhinovirus	H. influenzae	H. capsulatum
Adenovirus	M. catarrhalis	Paracoccidioidomycosis
Herpes Simplex	S. pneumoniae	Leishmaniasis

CLINICAL
- Hoarseness or harsh voice with deep pitch +/– episodic aphonia.
- Usually accompanied by symptoms of an URTI.
- Most common non-ID cause: GERD.

DIAGNOSIS
- Usually a clinical diagnosis.
- Laryngoscopy may demonstrate hyperemic vocal cords and (for enigmatic cases) provide ability to obtain tissue for histopathology and culture.

TREATMENT
Treatment for Viral URTI
- Nasal decongestants: pseudoephedrine 120 mg bid. Also others e.g., Actifed, Cardec or sprays—Afrin, Dristan, Neo-Synephrine.
- Antihistamines: 1st generation drugs, e.g., Benadryl, Atarax, etc.
- Ipratropium (Atrovent): 2 sprays each nostril 3–4 ×/day.
- If allergic rhinitis suspected: loratadine (Claritin) 10 mg/day and nasal steroids.
- NSAIDS: naproxen (Aleve) not ibuprofen.

Other Treatments
- Principles: treatment = voice rest. Common causes: viral URTI and GERD. If conditions persists, need to r/o rare disorders such as TB, malignancy.
- Humidity may improve speech and throat pain.
- Antimicrobials are not useful. Exceptions: HSV, TB, Candida, *M. catarrhalis.*
- Prednisone: 60–80 mg/day with rapid taper (may be tried for opera singers and others who urgently need their voice).

- Treat common cold if appropriate—see above.
- Non-ID causes: GERD (trial PPI × 1–2 mos), allergy, tumors, anabolic steroids.

FOLLOW UP
- Lack of resolution should prompt otolaryngology consultation to rule out polyps, malignancy (especially in smokers), rare ID causes (e.g., TB).

OTHER INFORMATION
- Antibiotic trials have not shown benefit despite possible role for treatable pathogens such as *H. influenzae* or *S. pneumoniae*.
- Symptomatic treatment is voice rest and humidification. Pts who need their voice—consider prednisone 60–80 mg/days w/ rapid taper.
- Most common non-ID cause: GERD—Rx w/antacids. Rare cause is tuberculosis—laryngeal TB is the most contagious form of TB.
- Prolonged laryngitis requires referral to ENT to see if vocal cord structural abnormality exists.

BASIS FOR RECOMMENDATIONS
Snow V, Mottur-Pilson C, Gonzales R, et al. Principles of appropriate antibiotic use for treatment of nonspecific upper respiratory tract infections in adults. *Ann Intern Med*, 2001; Vol. 134; pp. 487–9.
Comments: These are the guidelines from ACP/ASIM on management of URIs which includes laryngitis. Main Rx is symptomatic; antibiotics are discouraged.

MASTOIDITIS

Daniel J. Lee, MD and Ophir Handzel, MD

PATHOGENS
- *S. pneumoniae*
- *Haemophilus influenzae*

CLINICAL
- Sx may include: mastoid tenderness with erythema, fluctuance, increased projection of outer ear accompanied by otalgia with aural fullness/decreased hearing, middle ear pus/fluid/bubbles, fever.
- Main indications for abxs: pain, erythema, fever. Abx-steroid ear drops not indicated unless TM perforation present with otorrhea. Otherwise, TM erythema/middle ear fluid not treated with drops.
- Complications: spontaneous TM perforation, coalescent mastoiditis (mastoid abscess dx'ed by CT), bacterial labyrinthitis (constant vertigo and hearing loss), neck abscess, meningitis, facial nerve palsy, sigmoid sinus thrombosis, epidural abscess.
- Myringotomy in clinic setting for adult pts will aid in obtaining cultures, guiding abx therapy, and improve pain. Topical antibiotic drops can then be used with oral/IV abxs.

DIAGNOSIS
- AOM on otoscopy (or imaging showing coalescent mastoiditis) with local inflammatory signs over the mastoid.
- Culture not routine (and not obtainable) until spontaneous TM rupture, myringotomy, or mastoidectomy performed. Cultures may be helpful in chronic mastoiditis with infection, failure to multiple therapies or immunocompromised pt.
- High Resolution temporal bone CT scan (≤1mm cuts, axial and coronal) can demonstrate destruction of mastoid bone septation (coalescence) diagnostic for acute mastoiditis, as well as identify other underlying problems (e.g., cholesteatoma) or the presence of a mastoid cortex subperiosteal abscess.
- MRI + contrast is helpful to rule out or better define intracranial complications (such as associated brain abscess), when indicated.
- Fluid in mastoid air cells seen on CT/MRI is insufficient to make the diagnostic of mastoiditis as acute otitis media is often associated with fluid in mastoid due to the continuation of the air cell system between these two compartments.

TREATMENT

Uncomplicated Acute Mastoiditis

- PO abx, close followup indicated for healthy pt with otitis media and mild mastoid tenderness, erythema. Obtain temporal bone CT to r/o abscess (if so identified, then requires IV abx/tympanostomy/mastoidectomy).
- Amoxicillin-clavulanate 875 mg PO twice daily × 14 days.
- Cefuroxime axetil 500 mg PO twice daily × 14 days.
- Alt: clindamycin 300 mg PO three times a day × 14 days.

Chronic, recurrent or complicated mastoiditis

- IV abx, temporal bone CT, otology consultation for tympanostomy +/− mastoidectomy indicated for severe pain, recurrent infection, proptotic ear, complications (meningitis or immunocompromised).
- Duration of IV abx based on clinical improvement, and timing of tympanostomy/mastoidectomy.
- Following surgery, PO abx typically given for 3–4 wks with selection guided by surgical cultures.
- **Empiric options:** clindamycin 600 mg IV q8h + Cefuroxime 0.75–1.5 g IV q6–8h.
- Vancomycin 15 mg/kg IV q12h + ceftriaxone 1–2 g IV q24h.
- Moxifloxacin 400 mg IV/PO q24h.
- Ampicillin/sulbactam 1.5–3 g IV q6h.
- Consider tubercular mastoiditis in pt with risk factors and refractory disease.

FOLLOW UP

- Prompt referral to otologist/otolaryngologist important-for tympanostomy +/− mastoidectomy as complications are common in undertreated cases.

OTHER INFORMATION

- Acute mastoiditis almost always accompanied by acute/chronic otitis media. Mastoiditis without otitis media ("masked mastoiditis") is more common after previous abx rx.
- Fluid in mastoid air cells with mild post-auricular erythema/tenderness may be managed with oral abx and close followup—Keep a low threshold for IV abx/tympanostomy for increasing pain/fever/swelling.
- Pathogens responsible for mastoiditis may be changing due to the influence of vaccinations (e.g., pneumococcal conjugate vaccine); strains are potentially more virulent and drug resistant.

BASIS FOR RECOMMENDATIONS

Gate G, ed. *Current Therapy in Otolaryngology-Head and Neck Surgery*, 6th ed, 1998.

Comments: Recommendations used to form the basis of recommendations in this novel. MRSA is not yet been identified as a common problem with acute mastoiditis.

OTITIS EXTERNA

Daniel J. Lee, MD and Ophir Handzel, MD

PATHOGENS

- *Pseudomonas aeruginosa*
- *Staphylococcus aureus*
- Corynebacterium spp.
- Aspergillus
- Candida

CLINICAL

- A painful and/or itchy ear, otorrhea, hx of local trauma (e.g., Q-tips), eczema, or water exposure ("swimmer's ear").
- Exam: diffuse ear canal erythema and/or edema, periauricular adenopathy.
- R/O furuncle/abscess if findings localized.
- If pinna nontender consider middle ear pathology.
- Ddx: otitis media with tympanic membrane rupture, herpes zoster oticus, polychondritis, cellulitis, eczema, bullous or granular external otitis.
- **Complications (common):** conductive hearing loss, narrowing of external auditory canal. **Rare:** malignant otitis externa (MOE +/− cranial nerve involvement) seen in diabetics,

immunocompromised states, also facial nerve paralysis w/ progression to involve CN IX, X, XI and XII +/– skull osteomyelitis.

- Indications usually for topical abx.

DIAGNOSIS

- Based on physical examination findings and compatible hx.
- Obtain cultures in recalcitrant, chronic or recurrent infections.
- Indication for biopsy: chronic infections resistant to aggressive topical/oral therapy, presence of granulation tissue (r/o aggressive fungal infxn/malignancy).
- Indications for labs: r/o immunocompromised state (diabetes, HIV, etc.) or autoimmune disease (e.g., Wegner's). Temporal bone CT only to assess for malignant otitis externa (MOE), not for routine infections.

TREATMENT

General principles

- Typical indications for topical therapy: otalgia, swelling, and otorrhea.
- Add oral antibiotics for recurrent infections or those resistant to local rx, severe sx's, extension beyond the external auditory canal, poorly controlled diabetics, immunocompromised pts.
- Treatment should include analgesia, if needed.

Uncomplicated bacterial infection-primary therapy

- Neomycin+polymyxin + hydrocortisone (Cortisporin Otic): 4 drops three times a day × 7–10 days (prescribe suspension not solution that burns).
- Ciprofloxacin + steroid (Cipro HC): 3–4 drops three times a day × 7–10 days.
- Alt: Ofloxacin (Floxin): 10 drops once daily or twice daily × 7–10 days (often used by PCPs in the setting of TM perforation or tympanostomy tube, but most otolaryngologists will use Cortisporin suspension or Cipro HC).
- Tobramycin (Tobradex ophth): 3–4 drops three times a day × 7 days (use only if TM intact).
- Gentamicin (Garamycin ophth): 3–4 drops three times a day × 7 days (use only if TM intact).
- Acetic acid+propylene glycol+hydrocortisone 1% (VoSol HC): 4–6 drops three times a day × 10 days.
- Ciprofloxacin 0.3%/dexamethasone 0.1% (Cipro/dex): 4 drops twice daily × 7–10 days.

Uncomplicated fungal infection: primary therapy

- Debridement and dry ear hygiene crucial in otomycosis.
- Acetic acid + propylene glycol + hydrocortisone 1% (VoSol HC) 4–6 drops three times a day × 10 days.
- Acetic acid (Domeboro Otic) 4–6 drops four times a day × 10 days.
- Clotrimazole (Lotrimin solution) 3–4 drops twice daily × 7 days.

Severe/recurrent bacterial infection

- Aggressive aural toilet by an otologist/otolaryngologist essential for severe infxn, placement of ear wick for stenotic external canal to facilitate topical therapy.
- Surgery not indicated for recurrent or chronic infection—controversial for malignant otitis externa.
- Add oral drug therapy to topical treatment: ciprofloxacin 500 mg PO twice daily × 10–14 days.
- Ofloxacin 400 mg PO twice daily × 10–14 days.
- In poorly responsive severe otitis externa, consider parenteral antipseudomonal therapy; use cx + sensitivities to guide selection.

FOLLOW UP

- Referral to otolaryngologist or otologist essential in severe otitis externa.
- Outpatient debridement using binocular otomicroscopy essential.

OTHER INFORMATION

- Pathophysiology: maceration of external canal skin (mechanical/chemical damage), allergy, diabetes, resulting in atrophy of sebaceous and cerumen glands, increase in canal pH.
- Stenotic canals impairing administration of drops require temporary wick placement. Strict dry ear precautions while showering/bathing (use cotton ball/Vaseline/hair dryer).
- Diabetics: strict glucose control essential.

BASIS FOR RECOMMENDATIONS

Rosenfeld RM, Singer M, Wasserman JM, et al. Systematic review of topical antimicrobial therapy for acute otitis externa. *Otolaryngol Head Neck Surg*, 2006; Vol. 134; pp. S24–48.

DIAGNOSIS

Comments: This is a meta-analysis of the clinical literature and reviews topical therapy for acute otitis externa. A total of 18 studies were reviewed, showing that topical therapy alone (antimicrobial, antimicrobial+steroid, or quinolone preparation) is highly effective for acute otitis externa with cure rates of 65 to 80% within 10 days of therapy.

Rosenfeld RM, Brown L, Cannon CR, et al. Clinical practice guideline: acute otitis externa. *Otolaryngol Head Neck Surg*, 2006; Vol. 134; pp. S4–23.

Comments: These are clinical practice guidelines from the AAO-HNSF. They formulate recommendations for the diagnosis and treatment of acute otitis externa in pts older than 2 yrs based on the evidence available in the literature. Although pathogens such as fungi and viruses are discussed as well, emphasis is on bacterial infections. It is intended to be used by those treating pts in the primary care setting as well as specialists.

OTITIS MEDIA

Daniel J. Lee, MD and Ophir Handzel, MD, LLB

PATHOGENS
- *S. pneumoniae*
- *Haemophilus influenzae*

CLINICAL
- Onset of sx is usually acute, typical sx: otalgia, aural fullness, decreased hearing +/– fever.
- Exam (otoscopy): erythema, TM bulging, or fluid/pus behind TM, reduced TM mobility on insufflation (TM color, bulging and mobility). Weber test: 512 Hz tuning fork—lateralizes to involved ear. Take note if facial n. function is abnormal.
- Main indications oral abx's: pain, TM erythema, fever. Presence of middle ear fluid alone— not strict indication for abx. Abx-steroid ear drops for purulent otorrhea.
- Cultures not routine (and not obtainable) until spontaneous TM rupture or myringotomy performed—cultures may be helpful in chronic draining infection resistant to multiple therapies.
- Imaging: fine-cut temporal bone CT indicated for chronic infection, concern for middle ear mass, retraction pocket, cholesteatoma, or if febrile +/– mastoid erythema, otalgia and OM.
- Obtain hearing test, if a question of non-conductive hearing loss arises.
- Complications: common—conductive hearing loss, mastoiditis, TM perforation; rare— labyrinthitis/vertigo, facial palsy, meningitis, Gradenigo's syndrome (abducens palsy/ retroorbital pain/OM).

DIAGNOSIS
- Most cases diagnosed clinically based upon symptoms and exam findings above.

TREATMENT
Uncomplicated acute otitis media (non-immunocompromised adults)
- Amoxicillin 500 mg PO three times a day × 7–10 days.
- Cefuroxime (Ceftin) 500 mg PO twice daily × 7–14 days.
- Ceftriaxone 1 g IM (Rocephin) every other day × 3 doses.
- Cefpodoxime 200 mg PO twice daily × 7–10 days.
- Alt (beta-lactam allergy or fails initial rx): cefdinir 300 mg PO twice daily/600 mg PO once daily, clindamycin 300 mg PO 3–4 times a day, +levofloxacin (Levaquin) 500 mg PO every day, moxifloxacin (Avelox) 400 mg PO every day—all × 7–10 days.
- Amoxicillin/clavulanate use as primary therapy for immunocompromised or diabetic pt.

Uncomplicated acute otitis media (immunocompromised adults) or recurrent/chronic otitis media
- Amoxicillin/clavulanate (Augmentin) 875 mg PO twice daily (or 500 mg PO three times a day) × 10–14 days.
- Amoxicillin / clavulanate use as primary therapy for immunocompromised or diabetic pt.
- Cefpodoxime 200 mg PO twice daily × 7–10 days.
- Alt: cefdinir 300 mg PO twice daily/600 mg PO once daily × 7–10 days or clindamycin 300 mg three times a day × 7–10 days (PCN allergy).
- Referral to specialist to r/o chronic otomastoiditis or cholesteatoma in setting of chronic OM.

Adjunctive therapy for otitis media
- Address risk factors for eustachian tube dysfunction: smoking/allergies/sinusitis/GERD.
- Nasal decongestants: pseudoephedrine 120 mg + topical vasoconstrictors—oxymetazoline nasal sprays 2 puffs three times a day × 3–4 days only (may use OTC preparations such as

Afrin, Neosynephrine, Dristan). Although they may provide relief from congestive symptoms, decongestants alone do not improve the healing of AOM nor help prevent complications.

- For pts with suspected RT allergy consider the use of antihistamines such as loratadine (Claritin) 10 mg PO every day or fexofenadine (Allegra) 60 mg PO twice daily.
- Analgesia: NSAIDs—ibuprofen (Motrin) 400 mg PO three times a day × 5 days, celecoxib (Celebrex) 200 mg PO once daily × 5 days. Acetaminophen (Tylenol) can also be used. Local analgesics (e.g., Auralgan) may provide an additional benefit when TM intact.
- For persistent infection, intractable pain, or complications listed above, referral to specialist essential. Most adults tolerate myringotomy +/− tympanostomy tube placement in clinic setting.
- Severe vertigo/facial palsy/mastoid abscess/meningitis requires tympanostomy and ventilation tube placement, hospital admission, temporal bone CT, cultures/LP, intravenous antibiotics, possible surgical drainage.

FOLLOW UP
- Local and systemic symptoms should improve or resolve in 24–72 hrs. Consider pathogenic role of drug resistant *H. influenza* or *S. pneumoniae*, or unusual pathogens in non-responders.
- Chronic effusion following antibiotic therapy w/o otalgia does not warrant abx's. Pt with muffled hearing and fluid (clear or amber) but no otalgia managed with decongestants/nasal steroids/referral.

OTHER INFORMATION
- Much of the evidence available in the literature concerns the pediatric age group; may not be directly applicable to adults. In contrast to the pediatric population, observation is not a recommended treatment choice for adults with AOM, as course may not be as benign in non-pediatric populations.
- Anti-pneumococcal vaccinations may change the profile of pathogenic bacteria by increasing prevalence of less-common pathogens (e.g., *S. aureus* [MRSA]) and strains of pneumococcus not included in the vaccines.
- Topical steroid/antibiotic ear drops not helpful in acute OM unless tympanic perforation present with otorrhea.
- Otorrhea and tenderness of pinna is otitis externa, not OM, which can be managed with topicals alone; oral abx not useful unless pt diabetic, immunocompromised.
- "Muffled hearing" should not be treated w/antibiotics/decongestants unless obvious otitis media present and tuning forks testing is compatible with conductive hearing loss, as it may represent sudden neural hearing loss rather than AOM; neural hearing loss is considered an otologic emergency requiring high dose steroids and referral to an otologist.

BASIS FOR RECOMMENDATIONS

Pichichero ME, Brixner DI. A review of recommended antibiotic therapies with impact on outcomes in acute otitis media and acute bacterial sinusitis. *Am J Manag Care*, 2006; Vol. 12; pp. S292–302.

Comments: This is a nice meta-analysis reviewing recent studies on antibiotic therapy for acute otitis media. Amoxicillin and amoxicillin/clavulanate are considered first line therapies for AOM, followed by 2nd and 3rd generation cephalosporins such as cefdinir, cefpodoxime, ceftriaxone, and cefuroxime. Cefdinir in several studies has been shown to be an effective agent in pts with AOM and penicillin allergies.

American Academy of Pediatrics Subcommittee on Management of Acute Otitis Media. Diagnosis and management of acute otitis media. *Pediatrics*, 2004; Vol. 113; pp. 1451–65.

Comments: Practice guidelines for the diagnosis and treatment of pediatric acute otitis media from the subcommittee on the management of AOM, American Academy of Pediatrics. The guidelines include a comprehensive description of the symptoms and signs of AOM, applicable to a large extent to the adult population but most recommendations within are directed toward pediatric populations.

PAROTITIS

John G. Bartlett, MD

PATHOGENS
- Mumps
- *Staphyloccocus aureus*
- Anaerobes

DIAGNOSIS

Clinical

- Hx for bacterial parotitis: severe pain, tenderness, erythematous swelling—pre-auricular to angle of jaw.
- Predisposing factors: elderly, dehydration, anticholinergic drugs, Sjögren's syndrome, duct stones or duct atresia, diabetes, immunosuppression, HIV/AIDS [DILS-diffuse infiltrative lymphocytic syndrome].
- PE: fever, toxicity, tender swelling along the mandible with purulent drainage from parotid duct.
- Suppurative (bacterial) usually unilateral (as opposed to bilateral viral) + predisposing cause. Pain is intense and aggressive, analgesic therapy is needed.
- Lab: blood cx +/− cx and Gram-stain of drainage (Stenson's duct) or aspirate.
- Anatomic studies for stone: CT, ultrasound or sialography.
- Ddx enlarged parotid: mumps, sarcoid, Sjogrens, tumor (CA, benign, lymphoma), TB, HIV (especially immune reconstitution post-ART).
- Ddx for tender submandibular swelling: cervical adenitis, perimandibular space infections and actinomycosis.
- Mumps: acute parotid swelling not otherwise explained—usually in previously vaccinated young adults.

Diagnosis

- Evaluate by CT/US and aspirate/bxp.
- Mumps: show seroconversion or positive mumps IgM, or virus recovered from parotid duct by viral culture or RT-PCR.
- Suspect mumps: if fever, malaise, earache along with bilateral tender swelling of parotid gland.

Treatment

Antibiotics (bacterial parotitis)

- Principles: cause—stone in duct, dehydration or viral. Empiric abx for *S. aureus* if bacterial (often unilateral, while viral = bilateral); surgical drainage usually unnecessary. Must rule out non-infectious causes of parotid swelling.
- MRSA: vancomycin 15 mg/kg IV q12h or linezolid 600 mg PO/IV q12h.
- Anaerobes or *S. aureus* (if sensitive): clindamycin 600 mg IV q8h.

Surgery

- May probe duct or get CT, US or sialogram to detect stone.
- Acute suppurative parotitis rarely requires surgery for drainage and decompression.
- Sialoscopic probing often needed if duct stricture exists.
- Main concern with surgery: facial nerve palsy.

Non-bacterial causes

- Diagnosis with enigmatic parotid enlargement: fine needle aspiration (FNA) to detect neoplasm.
- Mumps: Warm compresses, analgesics. Supportive care only for mumps parotitis.

General Measures

- Prevention: increase oral fluid intake, chew hard candy especially citrus to promote salivary flow.
- Artificial saliva: expensive and doesn't last.
- Oral pilocarpine 5–10 mg PO three times daily may help stimulate saliva production.
- Prevention of episodes: discontinue predisposing medications, e.g., anticholinergics such as tricyclics, diphenhydramine (Benadryl), etc.

Chronic or Recurrent

- Prevention: discontinue predisposing medications, e.g., anticholinergics such as tricyclics, diphenhydramine (Benadryl), etc.
- Usually due to duct obstruction or reduced saliva production (xerostomia).
- Consult otolaryngology. Need sialogram +/− siladenoscopy.
- Other options to consider: surgery to ligate duct, ductoplasty, parotidectomy.

Follow Up

- Prevention: prior mumps immunization does not guarantee prevention of mumps in adolescents or adults due to waning immunity.

OTHER INFORMATION
- *S. aureus* the major cause of suppurative parotitis—usually unilateral and causes severe toxicity. Empiric therapy should cover *S. aureus* (MRSA).

BASIS FOR RECOMMENDATIONS
Author opinion.
Comments: No guidelines exist regarding therapy for salivary gland infections.

PHARYNGITIS, ACUTE

John G. Bartlett, MD

PATHOGENS
- *Streptococcus pyogenes* (Group A Streptococcus)
- *Neisseria gonorrhoeae* (rare)
- *Arcanobacterium haemolyticum* (can mimic *S. pyogenes*, most often in college-aged students, also accompanied by diffuse macular rash)
- *Corynebacterium diphtheria* (rare)
- Coronavirus
- Parainfluenza virus
- Rhinovirus
- Respiratory Syncytial virus
- Epstein-Barr Virus
- Herpes Simplex virus
- HIV (acute infection)

CLINICAL
- Pharyngeal pain +/− dysphagia, URI symptoms, cough (if present suggests viral not bacterial cause), fever, and other constitutional sx.
- PE: red throat +/− purulent exudate (exudative tonsillitis).
- Ddx of sore throat: epiglottitis, peritonsillar abscess, retropharyngeal abscess, thyroiditis, oropharyngeal or laryngeal tumor.

DIAGNOSIS
- Strep pharyngitis: microbial detection w/ positive rapid antigen test (75–90% sensitivity) or throat cx (slow but accurate).
- Clinical Strep diagnosis (often called Centor criteria), need 3 of 4: fever, tonsillar exudate, no cough and tender cervical lymphadenopathy.
- GC: culture throat, note special request for micro lab.
- Influenza: rapid test or clinical (epidemic + typical sx of fever and cough, etc.)
- Acute HIV: plasma HIV RNA + risk.
- EBV: monospot or EBV-specific serologies + atypical lymphs on differential.

TREATMENT
Streptococcal pharyngitis
- Principles: 90% cases (in adults) are viral; therefore give pencillin or erythromycin only if: (1) (+) strep Ag or (2) (+) throat culture. Centor clinical criteria is poorly predicative.
- Lab tests GAS: rapid antigen tests (80–90% sensitive and available in minutes) or throat culture (90% sensitive, but culture delays treatment 24–48 hrs).
- Preferred: penicillin VK 250 mg PO four times a day or 500–1000 mg PO twice daily × 10 days or penicillin benzathine 1.2 mil units IM × 1.
- Pen allergy: erythromycin estolate 500 mg PO twice daily or three times a day × 10 days, or azithromycin (Z-pack) PO or clarithromycin (Biaxin) 1 g × R PO or 500 mg PO twice daily × 5 days.
- Cefpodoxime (Vantin) 200 mg twice daily PO × 5 days.
- Cefadroxil 500 mg twice daily PO × 5 days.
- Loracarbef (Lorabid) 200 mg twice daily × 5 days.

Gonococcal pharyngitis
- Preferred: ceftriaxone 125 mg IM × 1 dose + doxycycline 100 mg PO twice daily × 7 days (for risk of concomitant chlamydia).

- Azithromycin (Zithromax) 2 g PO × 1 dose.
- Ciprofloxacin no longer preferred due to concern for resistance. See *Neisseria gonorrhea* module for additional details (p. 301).

Miscellaneous agents

- *N. gonorrhoeae*: request culture and treat for gonococci + Chlamydia-ceftriaxone + doxycycline.
- *Arcanobacterium haemolyticum:* weakly acid fast bacteria, a Gram-positive bacillus that causes pharyngitis in healthy young adults often with an associated rash. Sensitive to beta-lactams, macrolides and clindamycin.
- Influenza (efficacy only if treatment started within 48h sx onset): zanamivir (Relenza) 10 mg twice daily inhaled, oseltamivir (Tamiflu) 75 mg PO twice daily either combined empirically with amantadine or rimantidine if circulating strains of influenza with neuraminidase inhibitor resistance. Each × 5 days.
- Acute HIV: See HIV/AIDS, Acute Retroviral Syndrome (p. 138).
- HSV: acyclovir 400 mg PO three times daily × 5–10 days, valacyclovir (Valtrex) 1 g PO twice daily × 5–10 days, famciclovir (Famvir) 250 mg PO twice daily × 5–10 days.
- Diphtheria (C. diphtheriae): erythromycin 500 mg PO four times daily × 14 days, TMP-SMX 1 DS PO twice daily × 14 days.

FOLLOW UP

- No test-of-cure required.

OTHER INFORMATION

- Recent meta-analysis shows cephalosporins superior to penicillin (CID 2004;38:1526) but experts still like penicillin best.
- Some experts treat strep based on Centor clinical criteria (ACP) but others treat only with lab-proven strep (IDSA).
- Dx: (Centor criteria) hx of fever, exudative tonsillitis, no cough, tender cervical LN. Some recommend empiric Rx when 3 of 4 are present but others think strep Ag detection helps prevent abx abuse.
- Reasons to treat: prevent rheumatic fever (rare) and peritonsillar abscess (rare), reduce spread (usually non-contagious in 48 hrs), relieve suffering (modest benefit).
- Greatest concern about spread is with pediatric pts.

BASIS FOR RECOMMENDATIONS

Bisno AL, Gerber MA, Gwaltney JM, et al. Practice guidelines for the diagnosis and management of group A streptococcal pharyngitis. Infectious Diseases Society of America. *Clin Infect Dis*, 2002; Vol. 35; pp. 113–25.

Comments: Guidelines for managing pharyngitis in adults from IDSA. The main difference w/ the ACP/CDC guidelines is that the IDSA guidelines accept only group A strep as the cause only if it is detected by culture of a rapid antigen test. The concern with the more liberal ACP/CDC guidelines which accept clinical criteria that appear to overtreat about 50% of cases. Bisno et al. argue that overtreating is unnecessary and undertreating is not terrible since rheumatic fever has nearly disappeared (1) the clinical response is modest or nil, (2) adults do not pose a public health problem, (3) quincy has become rare.

Snow V, Mottur-Pilson C, Cooper RJ, et al. Principles of appropriate antibiotic use for acute pharyngitis in adults. *Ann Intern Med*, 2001; Vol. 134; pp. 506–8.

Comments: Guidelines from 2 panels: one representing the CDC and the other representing ACP/ASIM. Guidelines were nearly identical. Both endorse use of the Centor clinical criteria, the use of strep antigens assays for a bacteriological dx, treatment only for those with 3–4 Centor criteria or a positive strep antigen assay and use if penicillin as the drug of choice.

SINUSITIS, ACUTE

John G. Bartlett, MD

PATHOGENS

- Rhinovirus and other viruses
- *S. pneumoniae*
- *Haemophilus influenzae*
- Less common pathogens include *M. catarrhalis, S. aureus* and anaerobes

- Main causes: viral URI, allergy, anatomical defect, smoking, dental infection, swimming.
- Classification: acute: <4 wks, subacute: 4–12 wks, chronic >12 wks.
- Bacterial infection rare w/ less than 7 days sx.
- Viral infections and allergies are much more common causes of sinus congestion than acute bacterial sinusitis (ABS).
- Symptoms include nasal obstruction, face pressure or pain, rhinorrhea, reduced sense of smell.
- Purulent nasal drainage +/– maxillary or frontal pain/tenderness or decreased transillumination.
- Physical examination usually not helpful.
- Complications: orbital infection, meningitis, brain abscess or cavernous sinus thrombosis— all very rare.

DIAGNOSIS
- Only 0.2–10% clinical sinusitis cases are bacterial—on average, likely 2% of all cases.
- Recommended tests with routine case: <u>nothing</u>—no culture, no CT scan and no x-ray.
- Cultures are not useful unless taken directly from sinuses. Valid microbiology studies require sinus puncture or endoscopy and are rarely done, for uncomplicated ABS.

TREATMENT
Antibiotics
- Principles: most sinusitis is viral or allergic; usual indication for abx are symptoms >7 days.
- Indications for abx: nasal purulence + symptoms that are severe or persists >10 days or worse at 7 days.
- Nearly all antibiotic treatment is empiric.
- Preferred abx: amoxicillin 0.5–1.5 g PO three times a day × 10–14 days; amoxicillin/clavulanate 875/125 mg PO twice daily, or cefpodoxime 200–400 mg twice daily × 10–14 days.
- Alt: azithromycin 2 g × 1 dose or 500 mg PO once daily × 3 days; clarithromycin 500 mg PO twice daily × 14 days, doxycycline 100 mg PO twice daily or TMP-SMX DS twice daily PO × 10–14 days.
- Severe, non-responsive or hx of recent antibiotic use: fluoroquinolone (levofloxacin 500 mg PO daily or moxifloxacin 400 mg PO daily) or amoxicillin/clavulanate 875/125 PO twice daily × 5–14 days).
- Abx cost (above regimens AWP): amoxicillin $9–20, doxycycline $9, amoxicillin/clavulanate $55, TMP-SMX $3–12, azithromycin $45, cefprozil $21, other cephalosporins $100–170, ciprofloxacin $24, other FQs $91–100.

Adjunctive
- Systemic decongestants: pseudoephedrine 120 mg + sedating antihistamine PO twice daily × 1–2 wks (OTC preps as Actifed, Advil, Allerest, Contac, Dristan, etc), ASA, acetaminophen or ibuprofen.
- Topical nasal sprays: oxymetazoline nasal spray 2 sprays twice daily × 5 days (OTC preps available as Afrin, Dristan, Vicks, Sinex nasal sprays)—avoid use >5 days.
- Allergic rhinitis: loratadine (Claritin) 10 mg PO once daily and flunisolide spray (Flonase) 2 sprays each nostril/days.
- Not proven effective: vitamin C, inhaled steam, zinc.

Complicated Sinusitis
- Consider if periorbital edema, erythema, face pain +/– mental status change.
- Obtain CT imaging and otolaryngology consultation.
- Use ceftriaxone, ciprofloxacin, levofloxacin, moxifloxacin, amoxicillin/clavulanate.
- Endoscopy +/– drainage by an otolaryngologist.

TREATMENT REGIMEN DETAILS
Preferred antibiotics (Otolaryngology—Head and Neck Surgery, 2004; 130:1)
- Usual: amoxicillin (1.5–4.5 g/days), amox-clavulanate, cefpodoxime, cefdinir, cefuroxime.
- Beta-lactam allergy:
- fluoroquinolone Recent antibiotic exposure: fluoroquinolone, amox-clavulanate, clindamycin + cefixime. No improvement 72 hrs: fluoroquinolone, amoxicillin 3–4.5 g/days, clindamycin + cefixime, amoxicillin-clavulanate.
- Complications: Orbital cellulitis, frontal bone osteomyelitis, extradural or subdural empyema.

FOLLOW UP
- Unresponsive to abx at 72 hrs—image and change abx to fluoroquinolone or amoxicillin-clavulanate.

OTHER INFORMATION
- Most colds are complicated by viral sinusitis and do not respond to abx.
- Dx is clinical—usually avoid routine x-ray, CT scan or culture.
- If abx treatment initiated—amoxicillin is usual first choice, but may need higher doses (e.g., 3 g/day).

BASIS FOR RECOMMENDATIONS

Piccirillo JF. Clinical practice. Acute bacterial sinusitis. *N Engl J Med*, 2004; Vol. 351; pp. 902–10.

Comments: Frequency of bacterial infections in all cases of rhinosinusitis 0.5–2%; in cases seen in general medical clinic 50%, in ENT referral up to 80%. Symptomatic therapy: little evidence it works. Antibiotic selection: no evidence newer drugs work better than amoxicillin, TMP-SMX, doxycycline. Indications for abx: symptoms that persist 10 days or get worse at 7 days. Allergic rhinitis: loratadine or other antihistamines work; nasal steroids probably work.

Snow V, Mottur-Pilson C, Hickner JM, et al. Principles of appropriate antibiotic use for acute sinusitis in adults. *Ann Intern Med*, 2001; Vol. 134; pp. 495–7.

Comments: GUIDELINES from 2 panels; one representing the CDC and the other representing ACP/ASIM. Guidelines were nearly identical. The recommendations included: No routine cultures or imaging, abx treatment only for those with severe symptoms or sx lasting >7 days and preferential use of amoxicillin as the drug of choice.

Hickner JM, Bartlett JG, Besser RE, et al. Principles of appropriate antibiotic use for acute rhinosinusitis in adults: background. *Ann Intern Med*, 2001; Vol. 134; pp. 498–505.

Comments: GUIDELINES from 2 panels; one representing the CDC and the other representing ACP/ASIM. Guidelines were nearly identical. The major difference is that the CDC guideline fails to define an antibiotic. Instead it says that abx should be given to cover *S. pneumoniae* and *H. influenzae*.

SINUSITIS (OR RHINOSINUSITIS): SUBACUTE/CHRONIC

Raj Sindwani, MD, FACS, FRCSC and Ralph Metson, MD

PATHOGENS
- Bacteriology of chronic sinusitis less well defined than acute sinusitis [*Streptococcus pneumoniae, Haemophilus influenzae, Moraxella catarrhalis*] although flares of chronic sinusitis may be cause be the usual acute pathogens just noted.
- Polymicrobial flora typically, increased Gram-negative organisms and possibly anaerobes.
- *Pseudomonas aeruginosa, Staphylococcus aureus* more common in nosocomial and immunocompromised infections.
- Controversy exists over role of fungi in chronic sinusitis. Suggestion that fungal elements may be inciting an eosinophil-mediated immune response in sinonasal mucosa.

CLINICAL
- Sinusitis definitions: inflamed sinonasal mucosa. Acute bacterial sinusitis (ABS): symptoms lasting for up to 4 wks. Subacute sinusitis: lasting between 4 and 12 wks. Chronic sinusitis (CRS): sx longer than 12 wks.
- Pathophysiology: obstruction of ventilation and drainage of ostiomeatal complex and sinus outflow tract causing retained secretions and subsequent infection. Chronic sinusitis is considered an inflammatory condition.
- Sx: facial pain or headache, nasal blockage, nasal discharge, postnasal drip, hyposmia, fatigue, inflamed mucosa, purulent secretions. Transillumination not helpful. Endoscopy helpful but not required.
- Tests: initial—no x-rays or CT scans. Culture—not needed and difficult to access. Other tests only for consideration of alternative diagnoses: allergy, cystic fibrosis, Wegener's.
- Imaging: CT sinuses obtained only after maximal medical therapy trial has failed for chronic sinusitis or to rule out complications in acute sinusitis. CT best modality, necessary for preoperative work-up. Plain x-ray insufficient bony detail of osteomeatal complex.
- Indications for ENT referral: recurrent or chronic infection not responsive to medical management, suspected anatomic abnormality (e.g., deviated nasal septum or polyps), concern over underlying disease (e.g., sinonasal malignancy, granulomatous diseases) or complications of sinusitis.

DIAGNOSIS
- Acute sinusitis is a clinical diagnosis, no imaging necessary.

- In chronic sinusitis, post therapy noncontrast CT scan often helpful in planning management strategy (role of surgery, etc.), but unnecessary for true diagnosis. Contrast CT may be useful if concerned for osteomyelitis or spread of infection beyond sinuses.
- Chronic sinusitis: other options include nasal endoscopy, nasal/sinus cultures, allergy testing.

TREATMENT
Adjuvant pharmacotherapy

- Intranasal steroid sprays: fluticasone (Flonase), mometasone (Nasonex), triamcinolone (Nasacort)—2 sprays each nostril/days for prolonged period.
- Systemic decongestant: pseudoephedrine 120 mg + sedating antihistamine PO twice daily (OTC preparations—Actifed, Contac, Dristan).
- Topical decongestant spray: oxymetazoline nasal spray 2 sprays twice daily × 4 days only (OTC preparations—Afrin, Dristan, Vicks, Sinex nasal sprays).
- Antihistamine (systemic or topical): loratadine (Claritin) 10 mg PO qday or fexofenadine (Allegra) 60 mg PO twice daily or 180 mg PO qday; astelin—only topical antihistamine available.
- Pain relief: ASA, acetaminophen, ibuprofen, naproxen or other NSAID.
- Others: nasal saline irrigation especially helpful for chronic management, inhaled steam.
- Immunotherapy: specific allergy treatment, if appropriate.
- Systemic steroids: acute or chronic use in selected pts—allergies, polyps, asthma.
- Leukotriene antagonists: used in some severe pts, particularly those with comorbid asthma—uncertain benefit at present.

Antibiotics

- Principles: prolonged antibiotic therapy for 3–6 wks with appropriately selected agent (similar to those used for acute infections). Some controversy exists as to efficacy of this approach.
- **Preferred**: amoxicillin/clavulanate (Augmentin) 875 mg PO q8h × 3–6 wks.
- **Alternatives:** clindamycin (Cleocin) 300 mg PO q8h × 3–6 wks.
- Cefuroxime axetil (Ceftin) 500 mg PO twice daily × 3–6 wks.
- Cefprozil (Cefzil) 500 mg PO twice daily × 3–6 wks.
- Clarithromycin (Biaxin) 500 mg PO twice daily × 3–6 wks.
- Levofloxacin (Levaquin) 500 mg PO qday × 3–6 wks.
- Moxifloxacin (Avelox) 400 mg PO qday × 3–6 wks.
- Use of antifungal agents for chronic sinusitis unproven and not currently recommended.

Surgery

- Goal of "functional endoscopic sinus surgery" (FESS) to restore physiologic ventilation and drainage of sinuses.
- Indications: recurrent/chronic infection not responsive to medical therapy with demonstrated abnormalities on endoscopy and/or CT scan, and orbital or intracranial complications of sinusitis.
- Risks of sinus surgery: bleeding, infection, orbital injury, intracranial injury or CSF leak, and risks of general anesthesia—major complications are rare.
- Surgery plays important role in management of chronic sinusitis, ongoing medical therapy often still required.
- Endoscopic sinus surgery is outpatient surgery that is very well tolerated by pts.
- Computer-aided sinus surgery using surgical navigation systems may improve efficacy and safety of procedures, and is considered state-of-the-art.
- Outcomes studies using validated scientific instruments have demonstrated beneficial effects of sinus surgery on disease-specific symptoms and general quality of life scores.
- Balloon sinus dilation: new (yet unproven) tool used for ESS. Special balloon catheters used to dilate sinus openings in place of traditional surgical instruments. Balloon dilatation applicable only to sphenoid, frontal and maxillary (complicated) sinuses. The ethmoid sinuses are not addressed, which is major short-coming leaving most procedures performed as "hybrids" (part of surgery done with and part without balloon dilation). Increased costs and lack of results are other major issues. Little to no outcomes data presently available.

OTHER INFORMATION

- Mainstay of medical therapy is prolonged course of antibiotics. Duration required uncertain, most recommend 3–6 wks.

- Most common adjuvant therapy: intranasal steroid spray and saline irrigation.
- Important to address predisposing factors: allergies, nasal foreign body (NG tube, packing), anatomic abnormalities (septal deviation), illnesses (asthma, cystic fibrosis).
- Chronic sinusitis often requires surgical intervention.

BASIS FOR RECOMMENDATIONS

Dubin MG, Liu C, Lin SY, et al. American Rhinologic Society member survey on "maximal medical therapy" for chronic rhinosinusitis. *Am J Rhinol*, 2007; Vol. 21; pp. 483–8.

Comments: American Rhinologic Society (ARS) survey (43% response rate) finding that most consider maximal medical therapy for CRS to be nasal steroid spray and prolonged antibiotics (median 3.1–4.0 wks). In the hands of these experts, "rarely or never used" treatments included: oral or topical antifungals, nebulized medications, or IV antibiotics.

Meltzer EO, Hamilos DL, Hadley JA, et al. Rhinosinusitis: establishing definitions for clinical research and pt care. *J Allergy Clin Immunol*, 2004; Vol. 114; pp. 155–212.

Comments: Overview of disease and diagnostic/therapeutic recommendations.

DIAGNOSIS

HIV/AIDS

CRYPTOCOCCAL MENINGITIS

John G. Bartlett, MD

PATHOGENS

- *Cryptococcus neoformans*
- Four serotypes (A to D) described based upon the capsule components. Three varieties described as causing human disease *C. neoformans v. neoformans* (most common), *v. gattii*, and *v. grubii* (recently established).
- *C. gattii*, unlike *C. neoformans*, is mostly seen in healthy hosts.

CLINICAL

- Principles: most common cause of meningitis in AIDS pts (CD4 <100). Increased rates also seen with iatrogenic immunosuppression (steroids), organ transplantation, cancer chemotherapy, lymphoma, idiopathic CD4 lymphopenia, anti-TNF inhibitor therapy, diabetes.
- About 10–20% are afflicted pts are normal hosts (but often elderly) and they have better prognosis.
- Hx: headache and fever +/– visual changes, cranial nerve deficits, meningismus, seizures. Symptoms may be minimal and subacute or even chronic (e.g., fever or headache only).
- PE: fever, meningeal signs uncommon, vesicular skin lesions may be present in disseminated cases.

DIAGNOSIS

- Dx: positive fungal culture or cryptococcal Ag (CrAg) in CSF. Supportive if blood culture or serum CrAg positive.
- If focal neurological findings exist or obtundation, obtain CT imaging before LP.
- Lab: CSF cryptococcal Ag positive >95% (serum ~100%), India ink positive stain in CSF ~75%, CSF fungal culture >95%.
- Typical CSF profile: protein 30–150 mg/dl, monos 0–100. Opening pressure >200 mm H_2O in 75%.

TREATMENT

Antifungal therapy

- **Preferred (induction phase):** amphotericin B 0.7 mg/kg/day IV + flucytosine 25 mg/kg q6h PO × >14 days, then fluconazole 400 mg PO once daily × 8 wks, then fluconazole 200 mg PO once daily until CD4 >200 × 6 mos on HAART.
- Renal insufficiency: liposomal amB 4–6 mg/kg/day IV + flucytosine (above dose) × >14 days (induction phase).
- Intolerance or failure: fluconazole 800–1200 mg/day /PO flucytosine 100 mg/kg/day PO × 6 wks then fluconazole 200 mg PO once daily (reserve for mild cases). Monitor flucytosine levels.
- Maintenance regimen: fluconazole 200 mg/day PO (preferred). Fluconazole intolerance: itraconazole 200 mg PO twice-daily.
- Maintenance duration: forever, unless CD4 >200 × 6 mos, or treat for 12 mos and remains asymptomatic.
- 5FC use: monitor especially if renal insufficiency exists. Peak (2 hrs post dose) should be <75 μg/mL.

Management of increased intracranial pressure

- If opening pressure (OP) >250 mm H_2O: CSF drainage until <200 mm H_2O or >50% reduction. Repeat daily until OP stable.
- If elevated pressure persists despite daily lumbar drainage: consider lumbar drain or VP shunt.

FOLLOW UP

- No LP necessary at end of acute treatment phase unless new or persisting sx.
- Serum cryptococcal antigen is not helpful in follow-up and CSF cryptococcal Ag is not routinely followed.

DIAGNOSIS

- Treatment failure: fluconazole resistance rare, susceptibility tests—not recommended. Check OP as often an explanation for ongoing symptoms and continue recommended treatment.

OTHER INFORMATION
- Perform LP whenever cryptococcus is found at any site, or if serum antigen positive.
- Always measure opening pressure.
- Serum cryptococcal Ag assay sensitivity 95%. Not useful to follow response or helping ascertain if relapse has occurred.
- Lumbar puncture drainage (often repeated) to control intracranial pressure is critical.
- Primary prophylaxis not recommended.

BASIS FOR RECOMMENDATIONS
Dismukes WE. Antifungal therapy: lessons learned over the past 27 yrs. *Clin Infect Dis*, 2006; Vol. 42; pp. 1289–96.
Comments: Review of multiple NIH-sponsored trials in AIDS pts: (1) Ampho B + 5FC beat Ampho B alone; (2) Ampho B beat fluconazole; (3) for maintenance fluconazole beat itraconazole; and (4) maintenance fluconazole can be safely discontinued with immune reconstitution.

Masur H, Benson C, Holmes. Guidelines for Prevention and Treatment of Opportunistic Infections in HIV-Infected Adults and Adolescents (http://AIDSinfo.nih.gov).
Comments: Source document for recommendations given here–June, 2008 edition.

PNEUMOCYSTIS JIROVECII (PNEUMOCYTIS CARINII)

John G. Bartlett, MD

PATHOGENS
- *Pneumocystis jirovecii* (formerly *P. carinii*)
- Note: historically *P. jiroveci* when renamed in 1999/2002 as believed to be a protozoan, but once clearly a fungal species, it is now properly termed *P. jirovecii* according to the International Code of Botanical Nomenclature.

CLINICAL
- Clinical: cough (no sputum), fever and dyspnea evolving over 2–4 wks (AIDS), over 5–14 days (non-AIDS). Formerly *P. carinii* (PCP).
- Always found in a compromised host: AIDS, organ transplant, cancer chemotherapy, chronic steroids, severe malnutrition.
- Studies: CXR w/ bilateral interstitial infiltrates, hypoxemia or oxygen desaturation w/ exercise. Elevated LDH, CD4 count <250/mm³ (AIDS).
- Up to 20% of AIDS pts with PCP will have a negative chest x-ray, but CT scan will have positive findings.

DIAGNOSIS
- Definitive dx: demonstration of *P. jirovecii* cysts on induced sputum or bronchoscopy specimen.

TREATMENT
Antibiotics
- Principles: 1. Host: CD4 <250 or other compromise. 2. DX: induced sputum +/or bronchoscopic lavage. 3. Treatment: multiple options +/− prednisone. Expect slow response.
- **Preferred:** TMP-SMX 5 mg/kg q8h (dose based upon trimethoprim component) PO or IV × 21 days.
- **Alternatives:** dapsone 100 mg/day PO + trimethoprim 5 mg/kg q8h PO × 21 days.
- Clindamycin 1.8–2.4 g/day IV or 300–450 mg PO q6h + primaquine 15–30 mg base/day PO × 21 days.
- Atovaquone 750 mg (5 ml) PO w/ food twice daily × 21 days.
- Pentamidine IV 3–4 mg/kg/day × 21 days.

Prednisone
- Indications for prednisone: p_aO2 ≤70 mm/Hg or A-a gradient >35 mm Hg.
- Steroid regimen: prednisone 40 mg PO twice daily × 5 days, then 40 mg PO every day × 5 days, then 20 mg PO every day × completion of antibiotic therapy.

Failure to Respond/Adverse Drug Reactions

- Drug failure: consideration if failure to improve, or progression at 5 days or later; (not before 5 days).
- Oral regimens: TMP-SMX, dapsone + TMP, clindamycin-primaquine all considered equally effective for mild/moderate disease.
- IV regimens: TMP-SMX and pentamidine considered equally effective. Pentamine IV: concern for serious side effects.
- Switch therapy: usually works w/change for drug toxicity, often fails if prompted by "failure" of initial Rx.
- Clindamycin + primaquine: may be optimal oral regimen for switch therapy due to treatment failure (Arch Int Med 2001;161:1529).

OTHER INFORMATION

- PCP is always fatal if untreated. Hospitalized pts w/ PCP have 15–20% mortality despite recommended treatment.
- Rate of reactions to TMP-SMX in AIDS pts is 30–40%, especially fever, pruritis, rash, GI intolerance. Less common: hepatitis, neutropenia
- Evolving developments: PCR for detection, possible TMP-SMX resistance, *P. jiroveci* carriage in healthy hosts and possible role in chronic lung disease.
- Trimetrexate no longer manufactured for U.S. market (2006).

BASIS FOR RECOMMENDATIONS

Benson CA, Kaplan JE, Masur H, et al. Treating opportunistic infections among HIV-exposed and infected children: recommendations from CDC, the National Institutes of Health, and the Infectious Diseases Society of America. *MMWR Recomm Rep,* 2004; Vol. 53; pp. 1–112.

Comments: Basis for recommendations made in this module.

RETROVIRAL SYNDROME, ACUTE

John G. Bartlett, MD

PATHOGENS

- Human immunodeficiency virus

CLINICAL

- Definition: HIV infection prior to seroconversion.
- Consider when typical (mononucleosis-like) symptoms occur, sometimes as enigmatic fever occur in a pt at risk or "Monospot negative mononucleosis syndrome."
- Signs and symptoms of acute retroviral syndrome (symptomatic disease): fever (96%), lymphadenopathy (74%), pharyngitis (70%, not exudative), rash (70%, maculopapular face, trunk, extremities, mucosal ulceration), myalgia/arthralgia (54%), diarrhea (32%), headache (32%), nausea +/− vomiting (27%), hepatosplenomegaly (14%), neurologic sx (12%). Oral or genital ulceration may be noted.
- Asymptomatic or trivial illness in 20–50%.
- Lab: Rapid test showing Ag positive, Ab negative or HIV viral load >10,000 c/mL and serology negative or indeterminant;seroconversion must follow and typically occurs 4–2 wks post-transmission).
- Other labs: frequent lymphopenia and transaminase elevations.

DIAGNOSIS

- Diagnosis: plasma HIV RNA by PCR testing, considered positive >10,000 copies/ml. Note: false-positives noted with viral load <10,000 at low levels in 3–5% of population.
- Confirm seroconversion with conventional HIV serology.

TREATMENT

Treatment

- Benefit of early treatment is unclear. Refer to trial if possible. If Rx treating (preferred): 2 NRTIs + boosted PIs (ATV, DRV) or EFV + 2 NRTIs. PI-based HAART preferred if baseline resistance tests not available.
- Possible benefit of HAART: reduce symptoms and prevent transmission. Theoretical: Reduce HIV set point, limit viral heterogenicity, and preserve HIV immune response.

- Disadvantages to HAART: drug toxicity, cost, need for lifetime of treatment and possible viral resistance.
- HAART = 2 NRTIs (usually ABC/3TC or TDF/FTC) plus boosted PI or NNRTI (click on drug specific comments to find individual dosing and other information).
- Duration of HAART: appropriate duration is unknown, but may be a lifetime.
- Resistance (genotype) testing: indicated for immediate use (if treated) or future use.

Treatment: Counseling and Baseline Tests

- Prevention: acute retroviral syndrome associated with the highest VL in blood and genital secretions. WARN pt of transmission risks.
- Adherence: critical for viral suppression and prevention of resistance emergence.
- Counsel re: risks of drugs including lipodystrophy, intolerance, resistance and cost.
- Standard baseline tests: obtain CD4, HIV PCR, HIV genotypic resistance test, CBC, chemistry panel, toxoplasma serology, VDRL, Hepatitis BsAg and Hepatitis C serology, PPD, lipid profile and FBS.
- Acute infection—virus tropism to GALT (GI track) with depletion of 50% of CD4 cells— massive CD4 loss in 3 wks.

OTHER INFORMATION

- Guidelines for antiretroviral agents in adults and adolescents from the DHHS (11/08 http://www.aidsinfo.nih.gov/) and IAS-USA At least half of pts are asymptomatic seroconversions.
- Benefit of early treatment is unproven, but this may be the optimal time to start Rx
- IAS-USA and DHHS guidelines recommend baseline HIV resistance testing to show transmitted resistance and help regimen selection now or later; this is advocated (but do not delay initial treatment for these results).
- Resistance test results and knowledge of antiretroviral use in source pt may help initial decision.
- Acute infection—virus tropism to GALT (GI tract) with depletion of 50% of CD4 cells— massive loss in 1st 3 wks.

BASIS FOR RECOMMENDATIONS

Hammer SM, Eron JJ, Reiss P, et al. Antiretroviral treatment of adult HIV infection: 2008 recommendations of the International AIDS Society-USA panel. *JAMA,* 2008; Vol. 300; pp. 555–70.

Comments: Guidelines from IAS-USA: No clear recommendation for ART for acute HIV.

Neurologic

ASEPTIC MENINGITIS

Michael Melia, MD and Paul G. Auwaerter, MD

PATHOGENS

- **Viral:** enteroviruses (including Coxsackie, echo), HSV (primarily Type 2), arboviruses (West Nile virus, others), LCMV, mumps, influenza, parainfluenza, measles, EBV, CMV, VZV, HHV-6, parvovirus B19, acute HIV infection.
- **Bacterial:** *Borrelia burgdorferi, rickettsial* spp., leptospira spp., syphilis, *Brucella* spp., *Mycoplasma pneumoniae*, parameningeal infection (e.g., bacterial sinusitis or otitis), meningitis as a consequence of endocarditis.
- **Fungal:** cryptococcus, coccidioides, candida, histoplasma, blastomycosis.
- **Parasitic:** *Toxoplasma gondii* (more commonly encephalitic), Amoeba spp.
- **Recurrent:** often due to HSV (formerly called Mollaret's meningitis)
- **Non-infectious causes:** carcinomatous (primary or metastatic, lymphoma or leukemia), drug-induced (e.g., TMP-SMX, INH, ibuprofen, allopurinol), CNS vasculitis, CNS sarcoidosis, Bechet's syndrome, vaccines, benign lymphocytic meningitis, intravenous immunoglobulin, Vogt-Koyanagi-Harada syndrome, SLE.

CLINICAL

- Annually 36,000 hospitalizations. Most common cause is viral w/ enteroviruses leading cause (55–90%), seen mostly in summer and fall.
- Enteroviruses [more than 60 serotypes, including Polioviruses, Coxsackieviruses (23 Type A, 6 Type B strains), Echoviruses (28 strains), and newer numbered enteroviruses] are picornaviruses, 2nd most common viral infection in humans after rhinovirus. Infants infected>children>adults. Highly contagious, by fecal-oral spread (children) or respiratory (adult). Incubation 7–10 days. Only 1/1000 infected develops meningitis.
- Clinical: varies with pathogen and host age and immune status, but typically fever, headache (often more prominent than in bacterial meningitis), photophobia, nausea/vomiting, rash (depending on etiology), diarrhea, flu-like illness, meningeal signs, and lethargy without obtundation.
- Review history of travel and exposures: rodents (LCMV, leptospirosis), ticks (Lyme, rickettsial), TB, sexual activity (HSV, HIV, syphilis), endemic/epidemic (West Nile virus), IDU (HIV, endocarditis).
- Other etiologies: drug-induced meningitis (NSAIDs, co-trimoxazole), parameningeal foci (epidural abscess, epidermoid cyst), and malignancy (lymphoma, carcinoma).
- Physical Examination: meningismus, cranial nerve palsies, rash (depending on cause), acute flaccid paralysis (WNV, polio), genital herpes ($>\frac{1}{3}$ of primary genital HSV-2 infections in women are accompanied by meningitis; 11% in men).
- Lab: CSF with 10–<1,000 WBC typical, mostly monos, (but PMNs may be seen early in course), elevated protein, glucose nl, neg culture and Gram-stain.

DIAGNOSIS

- CT or MRI should not show any acute brain pathology.
- Craniocervical and sinus imaging (MRI or CT) should be considered to rule out parameningeal focus.
- Dx studies should include: CSF-WBC, protein, glucose, VDRL, crypt Ag, standard cultures including C&S, fungal, AFB; PCRs for Enterovirus, HSV, VZV; Lyme serology (if in endemic region), RPR. Other tests per suspicions.
- Enterovirus CSF PCR superior to viral culture.
- Consider WNV serology/PCR or other arbovirus serologies (e.g., Western Equine encephalitis, Eastern Equine encephalitis, St. Louis Encephalitis, etc.).
- Appropriate studies depend on exposures/risks: HIV (viral load qualitative), Lyme serology, RPR/CSF VDRL.
- Suspect w/ CSF WBC <500/ml, monos, protein <80. Enteroviral PCR helpful, can shorten abx administration, speed hospital discharge.

DIAGNOSIS

TREATMENT

Viral meningitides

- Supportive care for most (hydration, electrolyte repletion, pain management). Observe for SIADH. Seizures rare. Progressive downhill course argues against most viral meningitides (may be meningoencephalitis).
- Enteroviral meningitis: pleconaril appeared promising but drug was not FDA approved and no longer available for compassionate use.
- Agammaglobulinemic pts with chronic enteroviral meningitis (rare): IVIG administer 350–>400 mg/kg IV q3wks to maintain serum IgG >500–800 mg/dL +/– initial intrathecal therapy.
- HSV-2 meningitis: treat for neurologic sx such as urinary retention or weakness: acyclovir 10 mg/kg IV q8h × 10–14 days, can likely switch to valacyclovir 1 g PO three times a day w/ improvement (experience limited)
- Recurrent HSV-2 meningitis (formerly called Mollaret's meningitis): prevent with acyclovir 400 mg twice daily/three times a day PO, famciclovir 250 mg PO twice daily, or valacyclovir 500 mg PO once daily.
- VZV meningitis: treat if compromised hosts and severe infection: acyclovir 10 mg/kg IV q8h × 10–14 days.
- Acute HIV infection: consider HAART (See Acute Retroviral Syndrome p. 138)

Bacterial/Fungal/Mycobacterial Meningitis

- Refer to specific pathogen or diagnosis module.

OTHER INFORMATION

- Confusion may arise with partially treated meningitis: may rx empirically for bacterial meningitis or preferably repeat LP in 12 hrs off therapy.

BASIS FOR RECOMMENDATIONS

Rotbart HA. *Infections of the central nervous system* (2nd ed), Scheld M, Whitley R, Durack D (Eds), Raven, New York. 1997; Vol. 23.

Comments: Comprehensive review of evaluation and management of the pt with aseptic meningitis.

BACTERIAL MENINGITIS, ACUTE COMMUNITY-ACQUIRED

Paul G. Auwaerter, MD

PATHOGENS

- *S. pneumoniae*
- *N. meningitidis*
- *Listeria monocytogenes*
- *Haemophilus influenzae*
- *Streptococcus agalactiae (Group B)*
- *Enterococcus*
- *Streptococcus pneumoniae* and *Neisseria meningitidis* are responsible for 80 percent of all cases
- The overall species-specific infection rates (from 1995 U.S. data from CDC): Streptococcus pneumoniae 47%, Neisseria meningitidis 25%, Group B streptococcus 12%, Listeria monocytogenes 8%, and Haemophilus influenzae 7%, with an overall incidence of 2.4 cases per 100,000 population (inclusive of neonates, children, and adults).
- Note the incidence of Haemophilus influenzae type b meningitis in children has been dramatically reduced with the introduction of the vaccine in 1986; most cases of *H. influenzae* meningitis are secondary to non serotype b organisms or serotype b infections in non-vaccinated children and adults.
- Rates of community-acquired infection with specific pathogens strongly influenced by age.
- Children and young adults 2–29 yrs: *N. meningitidis* 60%, *S. pneumoniae* 27%, group B streptococcus 5%, *H. influenzae* 5%, *L. monocytogenes* 2%.
- Adults 30–59 yrs: *S. pneumoniae* 61%, *N. meningitidis* 18%, *H. influenzae* 12%, *L. monocytogenes* 2%.
- Adults >60: *S. pneumoniae* 61%, *N. meningitidis* 18%, *H. influenzae* 12%, *L. monocytogenes* 6%, Group B streptococcus 3%.

CLINICAL

- Clinical sx: neck stiffness, headache, and altered mental status usually present, fever common but may be absent especially in elderly. Also rash or myalgia complaints.
- Signs: Kernig's/Brudzinski's sign (present ≤ 5%), nuchal rigidity (30%), jolt accentuation of headache, cranial nerve palsies or other focal neurologic findings, rash (petechial, purpura fulminans), seizures.
- Brudzinski's sign—pt supine, flex the neck; flexion of the hips and knees is positive Brudzinski's sign. Kernig's sign—pt's leg flexed at knee and hip, straighten knee; discomfort behind the knee with full extension is a positive Kernig's sign.
- Classic triad (fever, neck stiffness, and altered mental status) found in only 44 percent, but almost all present with at least two out of four symptoms—headache, fever, neck stiffness, and altered mental status (as defined by a score below 14 on the Glasgow Coma Scale).
- Usual sequence for severely ill pts with suspected meningitis: stat empiric antibiotics —>CT if needed —>LP.

MORE CLINICAL

CSF normal values

OP = 5–15 mm Hg or 65–195 mm H_2O

WBC = <5–10 monos, no polys

protein = 15–45 mg/dL, may be higher in elderly

glucose = 40–80 mg/dL; CSF/blood ratio >0.6 (with abruptly high serum glucose, usual ratio is 0.3)

DIAGNOSIS

- LP: perform promptly in all pts. Consider CT first if focal neuro findings, papilledema, or severely depressed sensorium or defer if bleeding risks high (coagulopathy, thrombocytopenia)—to avoid brain herniation or bleeding risks.
- CSF: typical results OP >30 cm (nl <17 cm), WBC >500 cells/ml with >80% neutrophils, glucose <40 mg/dL (or <2/3 plasma), and protein >200 mg/dL.
- CSF: predictors of pyogenic meningitis: WBC >2000 or PMNs >1200; glucose <34, protein >220 (JAMA 1989; 262:2700).
- Gram-stain and sensitivities of blood and CSF cultures direct later decisions.
- Other adjunctive laboratory studies: blood and CSF cultures, antigen detection (rarely helpful for adults except partially treated meningitis), CSF PCR (viral causes, e.g., enterovirus, HSV).

TREATMENT

Empiric Treatment: Children and Adults

- Age 2–50 yrs likely etiologies = S. pneumoniae and *N. meningitidis*: vancomycin 15 mg/kg IV q8–12h (maintain serum trough concentrations of 15–20 μg/mL) plus either ceftriaxone 2 g IV q12h or cefotaxime 2 g IV 4–6 hrs.
- Age >50 likely etiologies = S. pneumoniae, L. monocytogenes, and GNB: ampicillin 2 g IV q4h + vancomycin 15 mg/kg IV q8–12h (maintain serum trough concentrations of 15–20 μg/mL) plus either cefotaxime 2 g IV q4–6 hrs or ceftriaxone 2 g IV q 24 or q12h (4 g/day max).
- Pen/ceph allergy: chloramphenicol 1 g IV q6h + vancomycin +/– rifampin 300 mg PO or IV twice-daily.
- Dexamethasone (10 mg IV q6h × 4 days) recommended 15–20 min. prior/along side first abx infusion for suspected pneumococcal meningitis. Some would give to all cases of bacterial meningitis (controversial). Continue for 4 days but discontinue if not bacterial meningitis (some would d/c if not pneumococcal meningitis). Most benefit seen with pneumococcal meningitis.
- Pen/ceph allergy: chloramphenicol 1 g IV q6h + vancomycin +/– rifampin

Pathogen–Specific Treatment

- S. pneumoniae (pcn sens—MIC <0.1 μg/ml): pcn G, cefotaxime, ceftriaxone, chloramphenicol. Rx >10 days.
- S. pneumoniae (pcn MIC >1.0 μg/ml): vancomycin +/– rifampin.
- *N. meningitidis*: penicillin, cefotaxime, ceftriaxone; treat for 7 days minimum.
- H. influenzae: cefotaxime, ceftriaxone, chloramphenicol; Rx 10 days min.
- Listeria: ampicillin +/– gentamicin, (2nd line alt. TMP-SMX). Rx 14–21 days.

DIAGNOSIS

- Enterobacteriaceae (*E. coli*, etc.): cefotaxime, ceftriaxone, meropenem, aztreonam, any +/– aminoglycoside, Rx at least 21 days.
- *P. aeruginosa*: ceftazidime, cefepime, piperacillin, aztreonam, meropenem + aminoglycoside IV (consider intrathecal only in refractory cases).

Prevention

- Conjugated pneumococcal vaccine offers reduction in invasive pneumococcal infections such as meningitis in children, and perhaps indirectly in adults.
- Antibiotic prophylaxis not required for pneumococcal meningitis, but recommended for *N. meningitidis* and *H. influenzae*. ONLY FOR CLOSE CONTACTS (individuals who frequently sleep and eat in the same dwelling with an index case, e.g., family, day care contacts, boyfriend/girlfriend).
- *N. meningitidis*: prophylaxis for household, daycare and intimate contacts and HCWs with secretion contact (intubation etc.): cipro 500 mg PO × 1 or rifampin 600 mg q12h × 4 doses. *H. influenzae* prophylaxis (rifampin 20 mg/kg—up to max of 600 mg/day–qdx4)—considered in unvaccinated household contacts <4 yrs old; unvaccinated day care contacts <2 yrs old, multiple cases should prompt prophylaxis for all children and personnel.

TREATMENT REGIMEN DETAILS

Recommendations based on Gram-stain characteristics or positive culture

Gram-positive diplococci: usually *S. pneumoniae*—vancomycin plus either ceftriaxone or cefotaxime.

Large Gram-negative diplococci: usually *N. meningitidis*—penicillin G, ceftriaxone, cefotaxime Gram-positive bacilli or coccobacilli: usually *L. monocytogenes* (don't dismiss as diphtheroid)— ampicillin +/– aminoglycoside.

Gram-negative bacilli: usually *H. influenzae* (may appear as coccobacilli),—cefotaxime or ceftriaxone OR Enterobacteriaceae or *P. aeruginosa*—cefotaxime or ceftriaxone or ceftazidime +/– aminoglycoside.

Other drug dosing: ceftazidime 50–100 mg/kg up to 2 g IV q8h, gentamicin or tobramycin 5 mg/kg IV once-daily, penicillin G 4 million units IV q4h, piperacillin 3–4 g IV q4h, nafcillin/oxacillin 1.5–2 g IV q4h, aztreonam 1.5–2.0 g IV q6h TMP-SMX 4–5 mg/kg/day IV q6h, rifampin 600 mg.

Intrathecal doses (consider with clinical failure >48–72h abx): gentamicin 4–8 mg q24h, tobramycin 4–8 mg q24h, amikacin 5–7.5 mg q24h, vancomycin 5–20 mg q24h (note: only use preservative free abx preparations)

FOLLOW UP

- Repeat LP if no clinical response after 48 hrs of appropriate antimicrobial therapy. This may be especially important if drug-resistant pneumococcal meningitis documented and pt receiving dexamethasone and vancomycin. Gram-stain of CSF should be negative after 24 hrs of appropriate antimicrobial therapy.

OTHER INFORMATION

- Since dexamethasone now considered standard for pneumococcal meningitis, most pts will receive at least one dose of dexamethasone empirically if antibiotics expeditiously administered before return of any diagnostic studies (Gram-stain, CSF antigen studies). Empiric choices may be narrowed by Gram-stain and culture and sensitivity results.
- Must give abx rapidly—main issue is sequence of CT, LP and Abx. Most cases: LP >Abx. If papilledema, non-cranial focal neurologic or severe CNS suppression: Abx >CT >LP. Delay in antibiotic administration contributes to increased morbidity and mortality.
- Role of corticosteroids in low income countries appear less helpful in lessening morbidity or mortality.

BASIS FOR RECOMMENDATIONS

van de Beek D, de Gans J, Tunkel AR, et al. Community-acquired bacterial meningitis in adults. *N Engl J Med*, 2006; Vol. 354; pp. 44–53.

Comments: Review article discusses management, including ICU care for the typically very ill meningitis pts.

Tunkel AR, Hartman BJ, Kaplan SL, et al. Practice guidelines for the management of bacterial meningitis. *Clin Infect Dis*, 2004; Vol. 39; pp. 1267–84.

Comments: Most recent Guideline statement that serves as a basis for this module's recommendations.

BRAIN ABSCESS

Paul G. Auwaerter, MD

PATHOGENS

- In 80–90% of abscesses, multiple organisms are found.
- Streptococci most common single organisms identified (30–50%), but anaerobic or other aerobic organisms can predominate.
- Gram-negatives are more common in infants.
- Fungal causes include *candida* spp., *aspergillus*, *zygomycetes*.
- Most series of pyogenic abscess ~25% unknown source (cryptogenic).
- **Source or host specifics:** <u>paranasal sinusitis:</u> microaerophilic (*S. intermedius* group) and anaerobic strep, *Haemophilus* species, Bacteroides spp., *Fusobacterium* spp., *Prevotella* sp. <u>Otogenic infection:</u> aerobic and anaerobic streptococci, Enterobacteriaceae, *Pseudomonas aeruginosa*, *Prevotella* spp., *B. fragilis*. <u>Odontogenic infection:</u> *S. viridans* and anaerobic streptococci, Bacteroides spp., *Fusobacterium* spp., *Prevotella* spp., *Actinomyces* spp. Endocarditis: *Staphylococcus aureus*, *S. viridans*, Enterococcus. Lung abscess: microaerophilic and anaerobic streptococci, *Actinomyces* species, *Fusobacterium* species, *Nocardia* species, *Prevotella*. <u>Penetrating trauma:</u> *Staphylococcus aureus*, aerobic streptococci, Clostridium species, Enterobacteriaceae. <u>Postoperative:</u> *Staphylococcus epidermidis*, *S. aureus*, Enterobacteriaceae, *Pseudomonas aeruginosa*. <u>Right to left shunt (congenital heart disease):</u> microaerophilic and aerobic strep. <u>Compromised host (AIDS, cancer chemotherapy, chronic steroids, lymphoma):</u> toxoplasmosis, nocardia, EBV lymphoma, TB, fungal. <u>Immigrant:</u> cysticercosis, echinococcus, TB (tuberculoma).

CLINICAL

- Symptoms of mass lesion: headache, nausea and vomiting, seizures, mental status changes, fever (50% only). Focal neurologic signs.
- CT or MRI: hypodense lesion(s) with diffuse (cerebritis) or peripheral/ring (abscess) enhancement +/− surrounding edema. Often occur at grey/white matter junction. Confusion w/ neoplasia not uncommon.
- Ddx includes tumor, rarely hemorrhage. Though bacterial etiology most common, if AIDS or immune-suppressed or immigrant need to also consider TB, fungi, parasitic causes (see complete pathogens list).
- Complications include rupture (ventriculitis/meningitis), coma, neurologic sequelae (25–45%), death.

DIAGNOSIS

- Dx: gold standard is aspiration/surgery with examination of contents and Gram-stain and cultures.
- Send specimens for: (1) Gram-stain, aerobic and anaerobic culture; (2) AFB stains, mycobacterial cx; (3) KOH smear, fungal culture; (4) Stain for toxoplasma; and (5) histopathological examination.
- Putative dx with compatible clinical picture/imaging +/− positive blood cx or known source.
- Lumbar puncture contraindicated, yields little specific data.
- HIV testing should be performed, as a positive result will change the differential diagnosis.

TREATMENT

Empiric antimicrobial therapy

- May be based on predisposing condition. Efforts should be made to aspirate or drain to help guide therapy. Exceptions: multiple abscesses, difficult locations, (+) blood culture, poor surgical risk.
- Unknown: cefotaxime 2 g IV q4–6h or ceftriaxone 2 g IV q12h + metronidazole 500 mg IV q6h.
- Odontogenic infection: penicillin G 4 MU IV q4h + metronidazole 500 mg IV q6h.
- Sinusitis: cefotaxime 2 g IV q4–6h or ceftriaxone 2 g IV q12h + metronidazole 500 mg IV q6h.
- Otitis/mastoiditis: cefotaxime 2 g IV q4–6h or ceftriaxone 2 g IV q12h or cefepime 2 g IV q8h + metronidazole 500 mg IV q6h.
- Endocarditis: vancomycin 15 mg/kg IV q8–12h or nafcillin/oxacillin 2 g IV q4h + gentamicin 1 mg/kg IV q8h.
- Lung abscess/empyema: penicillin G 4 MU IV q4h + metronidazole 500 mg IV q6h.

- Trauma/post-neurosurgical: vancomycin 1 g IV q8–12h + ceftazidime 2 g IV q8h or cefepime 2 g IV q8h.
- *Nocardia* suspected: add trimethoprim/sulfamethoxazole 5–6 mg/kg IV q6–8h.
- Duration of therapy unclear. Common course is 4–8 wks, longer times especially if not drained. Treat until sufficient response by neuroimaging (note time to mean resolution 4 mos, but may take up to a yr or more by MRI enhancement changes).

Pathogen-directed therapy (may combine)
- Streptococci (PCN sensitive): penicillin G 4 MU q4h or ampicillin 2 g IV q4h.
- *S. aureus* (MSSA): nafcillin or oxacillin 2 g IV q4h.
- MRSA: vancomycin 15 mg/kg IV q8–12h (dose by level, trough suggested 20 mg/dL for CNS penetration).
- Strep, GNB, *H.influenzae*: cefotaxime 2 g IV q4–6h or ceftriaxone 2 g IV q12h or cefepime 2 g IV q12h.
- Anaerobes: metronidazole 500 mg IV every 6 hrs and clindamycin 600–1200 mg IV q6–8h.
- GNB, anaerobes: meropenem 2 g IV q8h.
- *H. influenzae*, GNB, strep: ciprofloxacin 400 mg IV q8h or levofloxacin 750 mg IV q24h.
- GNB: aztreonam 2 g IV q6–8h.
- *Nocardia*: trimethoprim/sulfamethoxazole 10–20 mg/kg IV divided every 6–8 hrs (highest dosage for nocardiosis). See Nocardia module (p. 305) for other alternatives.
- Cysticercosis: albendazole 400 mg PO twice daily 8–30 days or praziquantel 15 mg/kg three times a day PO × 15 days.

Adjunctive and Surgical Therapy
- Surgical options: generally either stereotactic aspiration of abscess by burr hole placement OR surgical drainage by craniotomy.
- Dexamethasone (10 mg IV load, then 4 mg q6h) may be needed if there is significant mass effect (increased ICP) and/or neurological decline.
- Concern for elevated intracranial pressure may require additional neurosurgical consideration for ventriculostomy or shunt placement.
- Sz risk is 35–80%. Phenytoin or other anticonvulsant may be required to prevent seizures.
- Lesions <2.5–3.0 cm may respond to medical therapy alone.
- No clear data exist showing superiority of aspiration vs. excision.

FOLLOW UP
- Duration of therapy unclear. Common course is 4–8 wks, longer times especially if not drained.
- Treat until sufficient response by neuroimaging (note time to mean resolution 4 mos, but may take up to a yr or more by MRI enhancement changes).
- Recurrence ~8%.

OTHER INFORMATION
- Pts with cerebritis small abscess (<3 cm), multiple abscesses often treated empirically.
- Indications for surgery for dx/drainage: large abscess, abscess refractory to empiric therapy, immunocompromised host.
- Coma at presentation bodes for poor outcome regardless of treatment.

MORE INFORMATION
Unusual pathogens should be suspected in pts from Latin America (cysticercosis—check serology) or in compromised hosts with AIDS, chronic steroids, cancer chemotherapy, etc.—(toxoplasmosis, nocardia, TB, crypto, etc.—See AIDS).

BASIS FOR RECOMMENDATIONS
Wispelwey B, Dacey RG, Scheld WM. Brain abscess. In: Scheld WM, Whitley RJ, Durack DT, eds. *Infections of the Central Nervous System.* 2nd ed. Philadelphia: Lippincott-Raven, 1997; pp. 463–493.
Comments: Comprehensive review of the subject. There has been little new data to change antimicrobial practice since this publication.

Author opinion.

Comments: Little prospective data is available, so recommendations based on small series, case reports and expert opinion.

ENCEPHALITIS

Paul G. Auwaerter, MD

PATHOGENS

- **Viruses:** Herpes Simplex Virus (most common sporadic form in U.S.)
- CMV, VZV and EBV
- Common arboviruses causing encephalitis in the U.S. are: St. Louis encephalitis virus, Eastern Equine encephalitis virus, Western Equine encephalitis virus, Venezuelan Equine encephalitis virus La Crosse, Colorado tick fever.
- West Nile Virus
- Enterovirus (more commonly causes meningitis), polio virus
- Japanese encephalitis virus: seen in SE Asia, Japan, Korea, N' Australia
- Murray Valley encephalitis virus: Australia
- Powassan virus (tick-borne): New England, Canada, Asia
- Rabies
- Tick-borne encephalitis virus: central Europe through Eurasia
- Adenovirus
- Hendra virus, Nipah virus: Australia, SE Asia
- Other less common viral etiologies include: mumps, measles, rubella (these can also cause post-infectious CNS disease), influenza, rabies, human herpesvirus-6, EBV. CMV, VZV possible especially in immune suppressed. B virus (post-monkey bite). Acute HIV infection may occasionally present with encephalitis.
- **Bacteria:** *A naplasma phagocytophilum:* vector same as Lyme disease, *Ixodes scapularis*
- Bartonella species: *B. bacilliformis*, *B. henselae*
- *Borrelia burgdorferi*
- *Coxiella burnetti* (Q fever)
- *Ehrlichia chaffeensis:* transmitted by the Lone Star tick
- *Listeria monocytogenes*
- *Mycobacterium tuberculosis*
- *Mycoplasma pneumoniae:* more common in children, controversial cause
- *Rickettsia rickettsii* (RMSF): Dog tick, most common vector
- *T. pallidum* (syphilis)
- *Tropheryma whipplei*
- **Parasites:** Amoebic encephalitis is most commonly caused by *Naegleria fowleri* or Acanthamoeba species.
- *Baylisascaris procyonis*
- Gnathostomiasis
- *Plasmodium falciparum*
- *Taenia solium*
- *Toxoplasma gondii*
- Trypanosomiasis (*T. brucei rhodesiense, T. brucei gambiense*)
- **Fungi:** Coccidioides species
- *Cryptococcus neoformans*
- *Histoplasma capsulatum*

CLINICAL

- Fever, cognitive deficits, focal neurologic signs (often rapidly progressive), and/or seizures of preceded by non-specific/flu-like prodrome. Review travel, sexual contact, tick/insect hx.
- Obtain hx looking for epidemiological include: geography, exposure to vectors, time of yr, travel hx, animal contact, recent vaccines, occupational exposure (esp lab workers).
- PE: meningeal signs (meningoencephalitis); abnormal mental status with ataxia, hemi-paresis, aphasia, cranial nerve involvement and psychosis possible.
- Ddx: among most common—arboviruses (summer-fall), HSV (most common sporadic cause), enterovirus (summer-fall), toxic/metabolic explanations, CNS vasculitis, paraneoplastic syndromes, post-infectious or post-immunization encephalitis/ encephalomyelitis (e.g., ADEM).

DIAGNOSIS

Possible etiologic agents of encephalitis based on epidemiology and risk factors. CID 2008;47:303

Epidemiology or Risk Factor	Possible Infectious Agent(s)
Agammaglobulinemia	Enteroviruses, Mycoplasma pneumoniae
Age	
Neonates	Herpes simplex virus type 2, cytomegalovirus, rubella virus, Listeria monocytogenes, Treponema pallidum, Toxoplasma gondii
Infants and children	Eastern equine encephalitis virus, Japanese encephalitis virus, Murray Valley encephalitis virus (rapid in infants), influenza virus, La Crosse virus
Elderly persons	Eastern equine encephalitis virus, St. Louis encephalitis virus, West Nile virus, sporadic CJD, L. monocytogenes
Animal contact	
Bats	West Nile virus, Eastern equine encephalitis virus, Western equine encephalitis virus, Venezuelan equine encephalitis virus, St. Louis encephalitis virus, Murray Valley encephalitis virus, Japanese encephalitis virus, Cryptococcus neoformans (bird droppings)
Cats	Rabies virus, Coxiella burnetii, Bartonella henselae, T. gondii
Dogs	Rabies virus
Horses	Eastern equine encephalitis virus, Western equine encephalitis virus, Venezuelan equine encephalitis virus, Hendra virus b
Old World primates	B virus
Rodents	Eastern equine encephalitis virus (South America), Venezuelan equine encephalitis virus, tick-borne encephalitis virus, Powassan virus (woodchucks), La Crosse virus (chipmunks and squirrels), Bartonella quintanab
Sheep and goats	C. burnetii
Skunks	Rabies virus
Swine	Japanese encephalitis virus, Nipah virus
White-tailed deer	Borrelia burgdorferi
Immunocompromised persons	Varicella zoster virus, cytomegalovirus, human herpesvirus 6, West Nile virus, HIV, JC virus, L. monocytogenes, Mycobacterium tuberculosis, C. neoformans, Coccidioides species, Histoplasma capsulatum, T. gondii

Ingestion items	
Raw or partially cooked meat	*T. gondii*
Raw meat, fish, or reptiles	Gnanthostoma species
Unpasteurized milk	Tick-borne encephalitis virus, *L. monocytogenes*, *C. burnetii*
Insect contact	
Mosquitoes	Eastern equine encephalitis virus, Western equine encephalitis virus, Venezuelan equine encephalitis virus, St. Louis encephalitis virus, Murray Valley encephalitis virus, Japanese encephalitis virus, West Nile virus, La Crosse virus, Plasmodium falciparum
Sandflies	*Bartonella bacilliformis*
Ticks	Tick-borne encephalitis virus, Powassan virus, *Rickettsia rickettsii*, *Ehrlichia chaffeensis*, Anaplasma phagocytophilum, *C. burnetii* (rare), *B. burgdorferi*
Tsetse flies	*Trypanosoma brucei gambiense*, *Trypanosoma brucei rhodesiense*
Occupation	
Exposure to animals	Rabies virus, *C. burnetii*, Bartonella species
Exposure to horses	Hendra virus
Exposure to Old World primates	B virus
Physicians and health care workers	Varicella zoster virus, HIV, influenza virus, measles virus, *M. tuberculosis*
Veterinarians	Rabies virus, Bartonella species, *C. burnetii*
Person-to-person transmission	Herpes simplex virus (neonatal), varicella zoster virus, Venezuelan equine encephalitis virus (rare), poliovirus, nonpolio enteroviruses, measles virus, Nipah virus, mumps virus, rubella virus, Epstein-Barr virus, human herpesvirus 6, B virus, West Nile virus (transfusion, transplantation, breast feeding), HIV, rabies virus (transplantation), influenza virus, *M. pneumoniae*, *M. tuberculosis*, *T. pallidum*
Recent vaccination	Acute disseminated encephalomyelitis
Recreational activities	
Camping/hunting	All agents transmitted by mosquitoes and ticks (see above)
Sexual contact	HIV, *T. pallidum*
Spelunking	Rabies virus, *H. capsulatum*
Swimming	Enteroviruses, *Naegleria fowleri*

Season	
Late summer/early fall	All agents transmitted by mosquitoes and ticks (see above), enteroviruses
Winter	Influenza virus
Transfusion and transplantation	Cytomegalovirus, Epstein-Barr virus, West Nile virus, HIV, tick-borne encephalitis virus, rabies virus, iatrogenic CJD, *T. pallidum*, A. phagocytophilum, *R. rickettsii*, *C. neoformans*, Coccidioides species, *H. capsulatum*, *T. gondii*
Travel	
Africa	Rabies virus, West Nile virus, *P. falciparum*, *T. brucei gambiense*, *T. brucei rhodesiense*
Australia	Murray Valley encephalitis virus, Japanese encephalitis virus, Hendra virus
Central America	Rabies virus, Eastern equine encephalitis virus, Western equine encephalitis virus, Venezuelan equine encephalitis virus, St. Louis encephalitis virus, *R. rickettsii*, *P. falciparum*, *Taenia solium*
Europe	West Nile virus, tick-borne encephalitis virus, *A. phagocytophilum*, *B. burgdorferi*
India, Nepal	Rabies virus, Japanese encephalitis virus, *P. falciparum*
Middle East	West Nile virus, *P. falciparum*
Russia	Tick-borne encephalitis virus
South America	Rabies virus, Eastern equine encephalitis virus, Western equine encephalitis virus, Venezuelan equine encephalitis virus, St. Louis encephalitis virus, *R. rickettsii*, *B. bacilliformis* (Andes mountains), *P. falciparum*, *T. solium*
Southeast Asia, China, Pacific Rim	Japanese encephalitis virus, tick-borne encephalitis virus, Nipah virus, *P. falciparum*, Gnanthostoma species, *T. solium*
Unvaccinated status	Varicella zoster virus, Japanese encephalitis virus, poliovirus, measles virus, mumps virus, rubella virus

Possible etiologic agents of encephalitis based on clinical findings CID 2008;47:303

Clinical Presentation	Possible Infectious Agent
General findings	
Hepatitis	*Coxiella burnetii*
Lymphadenopathy	HIV, Epstein-Barr virus, cytomegalovirus, measles virus, rubella virus, West Nile virus, Treponema pallidum, Bartonella henselae and other Bartonella species, Mycobacterium tuberculosis, Toxoplasma gondii, Trypanosoma brucei gambiense

Parotitis	Mumps virus
Rash	Varicella zoster virus, B virus, human herpesvirus 6, West Nile virus, rubella virus, some enteroviruses, HIV, Rickettsia rickettsii, Mycoplasma pneumoniae, *Borrelia burgdorferi*, *T. pallidum*, *Ehrlichia chaffeensis*, Anaplasma phagocytophilum
Respiratory tract findings	Venezuelan equine encephalitis virus, Nipah virus, Hendra virus, influenza virus, adenovirus, M. pneumoniae, C. burnetii, M. tuberculosis, *Histoplasma capsulatum*
Retinitis	Cytomegalovirus, West Nile virus, *B. henselae*, *T. pallidum*
Urinary symptoms	St. Louis encephalitis virus (early)
Neurologic findings	
Cerebellar ataxia	Varicella zoster virus (children), Epstein-Barr virus, mumps virus, St. Louis encephalitis virus, *Tropheryma whipplei*, *T. brucei gambiense*
Cranial nerve abnormalities	Herpes simplex virus, Epstein-Barr virus, *Listeria monocytogenes*, *M. tuberculosis*, *T. pallidum*, *B. burgdorferi*, *T. whipplei*, Cryptococcus neoformans, Coccidioides species, *H. capsulatum*
Dementia	HIV, human transmissible spongiform encephalopathies (sCJD and vCJD), measles virus (SSPE), *T. pallidum*, *T. whipplei*
Myorhythmia	*T. whipplei* (oculomasticatory)
Parkinsonism (bradykinesia, masked facies, cogwheel rigidity, postural instability)	Japanese encephalitis virus, St. Louis encephalitis virus, West Nile virus, Nipah virus, *T. gondii*, *T. brucei gambiense*
Poliomyelitis-like flaccid paralysis	Japanese encephalitis virus, West Nile virus, tick-borne encephalitis virus; enteroviruses (enterovirus-71, coxsackieviruses), poliovirus
Rhombencephalitis	Herpes simplex virus, West Nile virus, enterovirus 71, *L. monocytogenes*

DIAGNOSIS

- MRI normal in many cases early on. May show temporal lobe changes (in HSV) or more diffuse involvement.
- EEG abnl in many cases HSV encephalitis with characteristic temporal lobe spikes. Should be performed in all pts to rule out non-convulsive seizure activity.
- Lab: obtain CSF if safe to do so, usually w/ mononuclear cells and increased protein; CSF PCR, CSF culture (viral cx of limited value), or serology (based on suspected agents: IgM, acute/convalescent IgG or CSF).
- HSV PCR should be performed on all pts with encephalitis. If negative, repeat within 3–7 days in pts with compatible findings if not other diagnosis secured.
- Note: negative PCR test is not absolute evidence that the certain infection is not extant.
- Consider brain biopsy in pts with continued deterioration despite acyclovir.
- Many cases without known etiology despite extensive testing.

DIAGNOSIS

MORE DIAGNOSIS

Special Diagnostic testing considerations: adapted from CID 2008;47:303.

Viruses: CSF PCRs for HSV, VZV, EBV, Enterovirus, West Nile virus (WNV), also CMV, JC, HHV-6 in immunocompromised pts. DFA or PCR of respiratory secretions for respiratory viruses. Viral cx (respiratory, nasopharynx, stool). Serology for EBV, HIV. Acute/convalescent serology for St. Louis encephalitis virus (SLEV), Eastern equine encephalitis virus (EEEV), Venezuelan equine encephalitis virus (VEEV), LaCrosse virus, WNV. CSF IgM: WNV, SLEV, VZV.

Bacteria: blood and CSF cxs. Acute/convalescent serology *Mycoplasma pneumoniae*. Respiratory PCR for *M. pneumoniae*.

Rickettsieae/Ehrlichiae: PCR blood for *Ehrlichia chaffeensis, Anaplasma phagocytophilum*. Acute/convalescent serology for *R. rickettsii, E. chaffeensis, A. phagocytophilum*. DFA and/or PCR skin rash for *R. rickettsii*. Blood smear exam for morulae.

Spirochetes: Serum RPR/FTA, CSF VDRL, FTA-ABS. EIA with reflex to Western blot for *Borrelia burgdorferi*.

Mycobacteria: CXR. CSF AFB culture/smear, PCR. Culture tissue/respiratory secretions/PCR of any non-CNS involved organ.

Fungal: Blood, CSF cx. Serum and CSF cryptococcal Ag. Urine/CSF Histoplasma Ag.

Protozoa: cytopathologic examination, *Toxoplasma gondii* IgG.

TREATMENT

General recommendations and empiric therapy

- Important to consider treatable causes and use empiric therapy. Therefore, acyclovir 10 mg/kg q8h should be used in all pts with suspected encephalitis. Doxycycline (200 mg load then 100 mg q12h) should be also considered in anyone with potential tick exposure that may transmit Rocky Mt Spotted fever, other rickettsial infection including ehrlichia.
- Supportive care is all that can be done for most pts.
- Many cases of encephalitis without an identifiable cause or due to a virus without known therapy.

Viral encephalitis—Treatable causes

- HSV: acyclovir 10 mg/kg IV q8h × 14–21 days. In neonates: 20 mg/kg IV q8h × 21 days. If good response not seen, f/u LP and treat until HSV PCR negative.
- VZV: acyclovir 10–15 mg/kg IV q8h × 10–14 days. Alt: ganciclovir.
- CMV: ganciclovir 5 mg/kg IV q12h × 14–21 days; then 5 mg/kg IV every day for maintenance. Some combine ganciclovir w/ foscarnet 90 mg/kg IV q12h w/ 90–120 mg/kg IV every day for maintenance, especially with HIV CMV CNS infection. Reduce immune suppression, if possible. Consider HAART in HIV pts. Note: cidofovir penetrates into CSF poorly, not recommended.
- B virus: ganciclovir 5 mg/kg IV twice daily or acyclovir 15 mg/kg IV q8h × >14 days or until all CNS sx resolve, then acyclovir 800 mg PO 5 times daily or valacyclovir 1 g PO three times a day indefinitely. See B virus module for details.
- HHV-6: case reports suggest ganciclovir or foscarnet may help. Follow CMV recommendations.

Nonviral encephalitis

- Listeria: Ampicillin 2 mg IV q4h + gentamicin 5 mg/kg/day IV divided q8h × 3–6 wks.
- Listeria (alternative): TMP/SMX 15 mg/kg/day IV divided q6h × 3–6 wks.
- Toxoplasmosis: Pyrimethamine 100–200 mg PO once (loading dose), then 50–100 mg PO every day + sulfadiazine 4–8 g PO every day + folinic acid 10 mg PO every day × minimum 6 wks.
- Toxoplasmosis: Pyrimethamine 100–200 mg PO once (loading dose), then 50–100 mg PO every day + clindamycin 900 mg IV q6h + folinic acid 10 mg PO every day × minimum 6 wks.

Prevention

- Tick-borne encephalitis virus: flavivirus infection seen in Western Europe through Eurasia. Serology to diagnose. No effective treatment known. Immunization thought to be >95% effective.
- Japanese encephalitis virus: vaccine available, recommended for people living in rural, rice-growing parts of Asia or who are traveling to such regions with extended stay and for laboratory workers at risk for exposure.

Postinfectious/postvaccination related

- Acute disseminated encephalomyelitis: neurology consultation, high-dose corticosteroids recommended. Plasma exchange or IV IgG could be considered.

FOLLOW UP

- Relapse rate of HSV encephalitis may be 5% or more. Negative HSV PCR in CSF portends for better outcome, less relapse—especially in neonates.

OTHER INFORMATION

- HSV is critical to treat rapidly; clues-fever, sz, MS/personality change, focal neuro deficits, temporal lobe involvement on MRI. Always start empiric acyclovir while awaiting test results.
- HSV clues (cont'd)-CSF showing RBCs and elevated protein (HSV meningitis); no HSV skin lesions seen in the majority.
- Suspected or proven HSV: acyclovir IV; if dx studies neg—may need brain bx

BASIS FOR RECOMMENDATIONS

Tunkel AR, Glaser CA, Bloch KC, et al. The management of encephalitis: clinical practice guidelines by the Infectious Diseases Society of America. *Clin Infect Dis*, 2008; Vol. 47; pp. 303–27.
Comments: First comprehensive guideline ever published for encephalitis.

Ziai WC, Lewin JJ. Advances in the management of central nervous system infections in the ICU. *Crit Care Clin*, 2006; Vol. 22; pp. 661–94; abstract viii–ix.
Comments: Includes strategies in critically ill pts that may require ICU monitoring.

EPIDURAL ABSCESS

Eric Nuermberger, MD

PATHOGENS

- *S. aureus*
- Enterobacteriaceae
- Streptococcal species
- *Pseudomonas aeruginosa*
- Mycobacterium tuberculosis
- After spinal procedure: *S. aureus*, coagulase-negative staphylococci, Gram-negative bacilli (including *Pseudomonas*), *Aspergillus* (after steroid injections)
- Immunocompromised host (AIDS, steroids, transplants): *Candida species, Aspergillus* species, *Cryptococcus neoformans, Nocardia asteroides, Mycobacterium tuberculosis and* other *mycobacteria*
- Foreign-born: *M. tuberculosis*

CLINICAL

- Sx: fever (60–80%), focal vertebral pain, tenderness to percussion, radicular pain, or paresthesias along involved nerve roots.
- Evidence of spinal cord compression: motor weakness, bowel or bladder dysfunction, sensory changes, paralysis (possibly depressed respiratory fxn if cervical cord involved).
- Obtain blood culture, CT-guided aspiration of abscess, or operative Gram-stain and culture (preferably before abx).

DIAGNOSIS

- Dx: radiographic evidence (usually MRI) of inflammation in the epidural space (frequently accompanied by diskitis or vertebral osteomyelitis).

TREATMENT
Antimicrobial therapy

- Antimicrobial therapy alone may be attempted in the absence of neurologic deficit with close monitoring if the infectious etiology is known (e.g., + blood culture).
- Initial empiric therapy may be guided by concomitant or recent infection elsewhere (e.g., bacteremia/line sepsis, skin/soft tissue infection/decubitus, dental infection, UTI).
- Minimal empiric therapy must cover *S. aureus* (including MRSA based on local epidemiology and pt risk factors).
- Expand coverage for aerobic Gram-negative bacilli in pts with recent spinal surgery or intravenous drug use.
- Empiric therapy should be modified by culture results.

- Duration of therapy typically 2–4 wks IV, then orally to complete 6–8 wks or until CRP normal.
- No clear role for follow-up imaging unless symptoms fail to resolve, new symptoms arise or CRP remains elevated.

Drug regimens (for suspected pathogens)
- Use culture and susceptibility data to guide final choices.
- Staph (MSSA)/Strep: nafcillin or oxacillin 2 g IV q4h or cefazolin 2 g IV q8h.
- Clindamycin 600 mg IV q6h.
- MRSA, coagulase-negative staphylococci: vancomycin 25–30 mg/kg IV × 1, then 15–20 mg/kg IV q8–12h (dose by levels, trough 15–20 goal).
- Strep/enterococci: penicillin 3–4 MU IV q4h or ampicillin 2 g IV q4h.
- Enterobacteriaceae: ceftriaxone 1–2 g IV q12h or cefotaxime 2 g IV q6–8h.
- Gram-negatives: ceftazidime 2 g IV q8h or cefepime 2 g IV q12h.
- Ciprofloxacin 400 mg IV q12h or levofloxacin 750 mg IV once daily or moxifloxacin 400 mg IV once daily (early conversion to oral possible).
- Anaerobes: metronidazole 500 mg IV q6h (early conversion to oral possible).
- Staph/Gram-negatives/anaerobes: ampicillin/sulbactam 3 g IV q6h or ticarcillin/clavulanate 3.1 g IV q4h or piperacillin/tazobactam 3.375 g IV q4–6h.
- Staph/Gram-negatives/anaerobes: imipenem 500–1000 mg IV q6h or meropenem 1–2 g IV q8h.

Drainage
- Urgent surgical or percutaneous drainage together with IV antibiotics remains the treatment of choice.
- The surgical standard is decompressive laminectomy with complete debridement.
- Drainage must be performed emergently for eligible pts with acute neurological (especially motor) deficit.
- CT-guided aspiration and/or drainage has been used successfully in absence of neurologic deficits.

OTHER INFORMATION
- Infecting organism should always be sought! Abscess cultures positive in up to 90%. Blood cultures in 60–70%. Culture for anaerobes, mycobacteria, and fungi when suspected.
- Drainage must be performed emergently for eligible pts with neurologic deficit, as improvement is strongly related to the rapidity of surgical intervention.
- Likelihood of neurologic recovery very low if surgery delayed >24–36 hrs after onset of paralysis.
- Antibiotic therapy alone may be considered if the pt is not a surgical candidate, has no neurologic deficit, and/or has interval improvement in pain, neurologic status, fever, leukocytosis.
- Paralysis of more than 2–3 days duration may be another indication for nonsurgical management.

MORE INFORMATION
Progression to paralysis may occur over hrs. All pts must be monitored closely for new or worsening neurologic deficit indicating need for further drainage.

BASIS FOR RECOMMENDATIONS
Darouiche RO. Spinal epidural abscess. *N Engl J Med*, 2006; Vol. 355; pp. 2012–20.

Comments: Current review by an authority in the field. Maintains surgical drainage with antibiotics as treatment of choice. Most poor outcomes associated with delays in diagnosis and suboptimal management. Table 1 describes common pitfalls in diagnosis and treatment.

PRION DISEASES

Khalil G. Ghanem, MD

PATHOGENS
- Prions

CLINICAL
- **Classification:** (1) familial [fatal familial insomnia (FFI) and Gerstmann-Straussler Scheinker disease (GSS)], (2) sporadic (85% of cases) [Creutzfeldt-Jakob disease (sCJD), (3) acquired from suspected agent [variant-CJD (vCJD)], (4) iatrogenic CJD (iCJD) [kuru]. All forms universally fatal.

- **sCJD:** rapidly progressive dementia with 2 or more findings: (startle) myoclonus, cortical blindness, pyramidal signs, cerebellar signs, extrapyramidal signs, or mutism.
- Typical age 45–75 yrs; CT/MRI normal or with atrophy. EEG: pseudoperiodic complexes are diagnostic; CSF profile bland but protein 14-3-3 usually +; brain biopsy if dx unclear.
- **vCJD:** depression, anxiety, withdrawal, peripheral sensory symptoms; then ataxia, chorea, athetosis; then dementia. Onset in young (20's) adults; incubation ~10 yrs;
- EEG: pseudoperiodic complexes are diagnostic; CSF profile bland but protein 14-3-3 usually +; brain biopsy if dx unclear.
- **iCJD:** progressive cerebellar syndrome and behavioral disturbances, or like sCJD. Can be young; incubation variable depending on source of exposure ranging from 6 mos–19 yrs.
- **Familial:** highly variable clinical syndromes; consider in all presenile dementias and ataxias irrespective of familial history; PrP analysis reveals diagnostic codon 129 mutations.
- Animal TSE: scrapie (sheep and goat), bovine spongiform encephalopathy (BSE—cattle), chronic wasting disease (deer and elk), transmissible mink encephalopathy (mink); found in zoo animals and domestic cats.

DIAGNOSIS

- EEG may show pseudoperiodic complexes, considered diagnostic.
- CT or MRI may be normal or display atrophy.
- CSF with normal CSF glucose/protein and without pleocytosis, but protein 14-3-3 usually positive for sCJD or vCJD.
- Brain biopsy definitive.

TREATMENT

Prevention

- Universal system of precautions currently in place is adequate for dealing w/ pts: gloves in handling bodily fluids, masks, eyewear, and gowns for extensive blood or fluid exposures.
- Sterilization controversial: suggested methods include steam autoclaving at 132°C × 1 hr; immersion in 1 N NaOH × 1 hr; concentrated (>3 M) guanidine thiocyanate.
- Others have suggested 4.5 hrs of steam autoclaving at 121°C and 15 lbs atmospheric pressure.
- Banning feeding of ruminant proteins to ruminants yielded control of the BSE epidemic.
- The American Red Cross and FDA have restrictions on importing European blood products and on accepting European and UK donations because of possible transmission of vCJD via blood transfusion.

Treatment

- Treatment with agents such as idoxuridine, acyclovir, amphotericin, and interferon have been unsuccessful.
- There are no FDA licensed treatments for any of the human TSE.
- There have been case reports of stabilization w/ various agents including amantadine and vidarabine, but no trials have been performed.
- Several new investigational agents are being evaluated.

FOLLOW UP

- Negative CSF 14-3-3 should not rule-out CJD in pts with compatible clinical syndrome.

OTHER INFORMATION

- Prions not thought to contain DNA/RNA. May cause disease in both humans and animals; resistant to radiation, heat, nucleases, and alcohols. Annual rate of sCJD is 1.5 per million/yr.
- Epidemiological studies suggest that the number of new cases should remain relatively low in view of the recent decline in the number of cases.
- Negative CSF 14-3-3 should not rule-out CJD in pts with compatible clinical syndrome.
- Transmission of TSE: ingestion of contaminated foods, iatrogenic (equipment/organs contaminated with neural tissue from infected source: dura mater grafts and human growth hormone most common sources), genetic (familial variants). No documented transmission w/ blood transfusions to date, although theoretical risk w/ vCJD.

MORE INFORMATION

BSE epidemic in U.K. (late 80s–early 90s) a result of rendering process used (1970s–1980s) that did not inactivate BSE agent, transferring it from bovine to bovine (practice of feeding cattle the waste of other cattle); thought to have resulted in the human cases of vCJD seen in Britain, France, and Germany (late 90s–00s) via ingestion of contaminated meat. Exact number of cases of vCJD in Europe (especially U.K.), although limited, may still increase as exact duration of incubation period unknown. Epidemiological studies suggest that the number of new cases should remain relatively low in view of the significant decline in the number of cases.

Basis for Recommendations

Aguzzi A. Prion diseases of humans and farm animals: epidemiology, genetics, and pathogenesis. *J Neurochem*, 2006; Vol. 97; pp. 1726–39.

Comments: Extensive review article that summarizes the current state of knowledge on the epidemiology and pathogenesis of prion diseases.

CNS SHUNT INFECTIONS

Paul G. Auwaerter, MD

Pathogens

- *Coagulase-negative staphylococci*
- *S. aureus*
- *Streptococcal species*
- *Gram-negative bacteria*
- Propionibacterium species
- *Candida species*
- Vast majority CSF shunt infections caused by normal skin commensals. Coagulase-negative staphylococci 40–45%, *S. aureus* 25%. *P. acnes* uncommon (usually less than 8% most series), diphtheroids (rare). Pts with CSF shunts have an increased risk of meningitis caused by traditional pathogens (*S. pneumoniae, N. meningitidis, H. influenzae*), often treatable without shunt revision.

Clinical

- Fever (variable 14–92%), shunt malfunction causing raised intracranial pressure (headache, nausea or vomiting, altered mental status). Traditional meningeal symptoms less common.
- PE: erythema and tenderness of skin over tubing.
- **Proximal shunt involvement:** meningitis or ventriculitis (30%), shunt malfunction. Non-communication between ventricle and meninges (i.e., reason for shunt such as aqueductal stenosis) may mean meningeal signs will not develop.
- **Distal shunt involvement:** ventriculoperitoneal (VP) shunts: abdominal pain, focal or generalized peritonitis, intraabdominal abscess, perforated viscus.
- Ventriculoatrial shunts: sepsis, positive blood cultures, right-sided endocarditis, shunt nephritis, hepatosplenomegaly.

Diagnosis

- Shunt tap revealing CSF leukocytosis (cells >10/mm³, may see eosinophilia) +/− elevated protein. CSF may be near normal.
- Positive CSF Gram-stain or culture.
- If normal CSF formula and recovery of organism that may be a contaminant, repeat tap and culture. Recovery of organism ×2 very suggestive of infection.
- VP shunt: ultrasound or CT imaging may reveal free flowing or loculated fluid collection(s) or abscess(es).
- VA shunt: obtain blood culture ×2.
- Note: CSF and blood cultures should be ordered for anaerobic growth and extended culture (7–10 days) to enhance recovery of *Propionibacterium acnes*.

Treatment

General Considerations: shunt revision

- Complete removal favored over partial shunt removal with temporary external ventricular drain usually recommended. Partial revisions usually with high failure rates (up to 80%).
- Approaches: (1) Two stage: removal of entire shunt, placement of CSF external drain (if needed), replacement of shunt when CSF sterile [typically 48–72 hrs minimum]. (2) One stage: removal of entire shunt with immediate replacement of shunt followed by antibiotics. (3) Conservative management: antibiotics alone without shunt removal, generally only considered for clinically stable pts with low-virulence pathogens such as coagulase-negative Staphylococci, *P. acnes*.

- Efficacy: (1) Two stage: 88% cure, (2) One stage: 64%, (3) Conservative management: 34%.
- If possible, monitor CSF for up to 3 days off antibiotics before placement of permanent shunt to document CSF sterility.
- Timing/need for new shunt or continued external drainage based on neurosurgical considerations.
- Antibiotic treatment for 3–14 days (exact duration not well studied).
- IV antibiotics may be continued for an additional 7–14 days from shunt revision.

Parenteral therapy (empiric)
- Vancomycin 15 mg/kg IV 12 hrs (strive for trough level ~20 µg/mL) + ceftazidime 2 g IV q8h.
- Vancomycin 15 mg/kg IV q12h + cefepime 2 g IV q12h.
- For PCN allergic, consider ciprofloxacin 400 mg IV q8h to replace cephalosporin choice.

Parenteral therapy (organism known)
- Use antimicrobial sensitivities to guide therapy.
- Coagulase-negative staphylococci or *S. aureus* (MRSA): vancomycin 15 mg/kg IV q12h +/– rifampin 600 mg IV or PO q24h.
- *S. aureus* (MSSA): nafcillin or oxacillin 2 g IV q4h +/– rifampin 600 mg IV or PO q24h.
- *S. aureus*: TMP/SMX 4–5 mg/kg/day (of trimethoprim component) q8h.
- GNB: ceftriaxone 2 g IV q12h or cefepime 2 g IV q12h or meropenem 2 g IV q8h or aztreonam 2 g IV q6h. Choose on sensitivities. Intrathecal aminoglycosides rarely required for shunt-related infections.
- *P. acnes*, Streptococci: penicillin G 4 MU or ampicillin 2 g IV q4h +/– gentamicin 1–1.7 mg/kg q8h (add gentamicin for Group B streptococcal and enterococcal infections).
- Fungi: Amphotericin B 0.6–1.0 mg/kg IV q24h or liposomal AmB 5 mg/kg/day (exact recommendation based on recovered organism).

Intrathecal antibiotics
- Consider if intravenous antibiotic therapy and shunt removal have failed to clear infection within 48–72 hrs or clinical condition worsening.
- Vancomycin 5–20 mg daily.
- Aminoglycosides: gentamicin 4–8 mg, tobramycin 4–8 mg or amikacin 15–50 mg. Preservative free preparations should be used, as preservative is associated with an increased risk of seizures.
- Colistin 10 mg
- Amphotericin B 0.1–0.5 mg
- Do not give β-lactams by intrathecal route due to increased seizure risk.
- Use troughs to guide intraventricular dosing. Some use the inhibitory quotient = CSF trough/MIC. If >10–20 × this should be sufficient to achieve sterilization.

FOLLOW UP
- Failure to improve: remove temporary drain, change abx or increase dose, add rifampin (for GPC) or give intraventricular abx.

OTHER INFORMATION
- Obtain CSF (aspirate directly from shunt or reservoir), blood (VA shunt), peritoneal fluid (VP shunt), distal shunt tip (roll on plate do not put in broth).
- Antibiotics should be selected for bactericidal activity and ability to penetrate the CSF space to exceed the MIC of the infecting organism.
- Parenteral abx therapy and complete replacement of shunt is successful in >~88% of cases versus 36% for abx alone or partial revision of shunt.
- CSF cultures are generally negative within 2 days of removal/externalization and appropriate abx therapy.

BASIS FOR RECOMMENDATIONS

Tunkel AR. Cerebrospinal fluid shunt infections. *Principles and Practice of Infectious Diseases*, 6th ed, 2005; pp.

Comments: Little good prospective data exists to back recommendations, so much is based on single center experience and expert opinion.

Tunkel AR, Hartman BJ, Kaplan SL, et al. Practice guidelines for the management of bacterial meningitis. *Clin Infect Dis*, 2004; Vol. 39; pp. 1267–84.

Comments: Guidelines for meningitis, mainly addressing community-acquired and nosocomial varieties.

BRONCHIECTASIS

Paul G. Auwaerter, MD

PATHOGENS

- *S. pneumoniae*
- *Haemophilus influenzae*
- *Moraxella catarrhalis*
- *Pseudomonas aeruginosa*
- Mycobacterium avium complex
- Other mycobacteria (atypical)
- *Aspergillus fumigatus*

MORE PATHOGENS

- *A. fumigatus* can lead to allergic bronchopulmonary aspergillosis (ABPA) in pts with asthma and cystic fibrosis. It can also colonize the airways of pts with chronic lung diseases. Similarly, MAI cultures may represent colonization or a true pathogen.

CLINICAL

- Definition: pathologic, irreversible dilation of one or more proximal, medium-sized bronchi due to destruction of the bronchial walls.
- Consequence of pulmonary infections (esp. bacterial pneumonia (untreated), TB, endemic fungi) or host disorders; e.g., cystic fibrosis, other structural lung dz, immune disorder/ Kartagener's.
- Study of 150 adults in UK found 53% idiopathic, 29% post-infectious, 8% immune defect related, 7% allergic bronchopulmonary aspergillosis, 4% aspiration, 3% Young's syndrome, 3% cystic fibrosis, 3% rheumatoid arthritis, 1.5% ciliary dysfunction, <1% miscellaneous.
- Sx: chronic cough, purulent sputum, hemoptysis, fever, weight loss. PE: fetid breath, clubbing, basilar crackles, rhonchi.
- CXR: tram tracks, toothpaste shadows, clustered cysts (may be normal in 84% of pts w/ bronchiectasis seen on CT).
- High Resolution CT: gold standard to secure dx of bronchiectasis; dilation of bronchi >1.5 times as wide as nearby vessel, bronchial wall thickening, lack of normal tapering, cysts.
- Diagnosis of flare (four of the following): change in sputum, increased dyspnea, increased cough, fever, increased wheezing, fatigue, decreased PFT's, new infiltrate, change in lung exam.
- In highly immunized societies, host defect explanations as cause for bronchiectasis are now much more common, then historically when mostly all due to post-infectious sequelae—and therefore should be explored.

MORE CLINICAL

- Clinical presentation of bronchiectasis difficult to distinguish from chronic bronchitis. Epidemiology depends on the population. Prior to widespread immunizations and antibiotic rx, majority of cases were post-infectious. Now most cases due to systemic diseases including congenital abnormal, immunodeficiencies, sequelae of toxic inhalations, rheumatic dz, and others (complete ddx outlined in Barker article).
- Classification system using terms cylindrical, saccular or cystic bronchiectasis has no clinical or therapeutic application.

TREATMENT

Outpatient (bacterial bronchiectasis flare)

- Some suggest inhaled fluticasone 500 µg twice daily along with physical therapy and exercise therapy first before considering prolonged use of antibiotics with good lung penetration (e.g., macrolides such as clarithromycin).
- Preferred: oral fluoroquinolone but use sputum cultures to guide therapy.
- Ciprofloxacin 750 mg PO twice daily or levofloxacin 500–750 mg PO q24h.

- Moxifloxacin 400 mg PO q24h, if chosen drug provides little coverage for *P. aeruginosa*.
- All abx recommendations are for 10–14 days for initial treatment of an acute flare. Some may treat 3–6 wks for recurrences.
- Treatment of bacterial bronchiectasis flare may often yield excellent results even in pts known MAI positive. Bacterial cultures of sputum may help guide therapy.
- Treatment of experienced CF pts can be challenging with highly resistant organisms.

Hospitalized patient

- Recommendations for ill pts requiring hospitalization or pts failing oral therapy.
- IV antipseudomonal beta-lactam (consider change to oral abx once improved). Use sputum culture sensitivities to guide therapy.
- Piperacillin 3.0–4.0 g IV q4–6 hrs.
- Ticarcillin 3.0 g IV q4–6 hrs.
- Cefepime 1–2 g IV q12 hrs.
- Ceftazidime 1–2 g IV q8–12 hrs.
- All abx recommendations are for 10–14 days. Some may treat 3–12 wks for recurrences.

Pathogen specific

- *P. aeruginosa*: ciprofloxacin oral or IV, antipseudomonal penicillin IV(piperacillin, ticarcillin), 3rd or 4th gen cephalosporin IV (ceftazidime, cefepime), TOBI (300 mg inhaled twice daily × 28 days).
- *H. influenzae*: amox/clav, 2nd or 3rd gen cephalosporin, TMP-SMX, fluoroquinolone.
- *M. catarrhalis*: amox/clav, 2nd or 3rd generation cephalosporin, TMP-SMX, fluoroquinolone.
- MAI: clarithromycin 500 mg PO twice daily, ethambutol 15–25 mg/kg/day PO once daily, rifampin 600 mg PO once daily (rifabutin 300 mg PO once daily) × 12–18 mos.
- Allergic bronchopulmonary aspergillosis: corticosteroids plus itraconazole.

Prophylactic strategies

- Consideration for pts who relapse soon after therapy. Three basic strategies described although little good data to guide preference:
- **Prolonged antibiotics:** at least 4-wk course.
- **Aerosolized antibiotics:** most commonly used on alternating mos.
- **Pulsed IV antibiotics:** e.g., 2–3 wks parenteral abx, separated by 4–8 wks without abx.
- Metaanalyses of prolonged oral antibiotics showed benefit in terms of decreased sputum production and purulence but no impact upon lung function, mortality, or rate of exacerbations.
- **Inhaled antibiotics:** gentamicin 40 mg inhaled twice daily or tobramycin (TOBI) 300 mg twice daily × 4 wks are common regimens. Others have used ceftazidime 1 g inhaled daily or tobramycin 100 mg inhaled twice daily for longer periods such as 1 yr.

Non-antimicrobial therapy

- Mucolytics: studies in bronchiectasis have been mixed or need further study. Oral bromhexine 30 mg three times daily, rDNase I 2.5 mg once or twice daily, inhaled mannitol 300–400 mg daily.
- Anti-inflammatories: may work much as in asthma, e.g., fluticasone 500 µg twice daily. Studies have suggested decreased sputum production but no overall benefit to better lung function or decreased rates of flares. Leukotriene inhibitors, such as Singulair, have not been studied in this population.
- Bronchodilators: good studies don't exist, but used by some for symptomatic improvement.
- Respiratory therapy: chest physiotherapy often employed, but unclear impact based on available studies.
- Surgery: historically of great value when no antibiotics existed. Now considered occasionally in well-localized disease, or if process has advanced to life-threatening.

OTHER INFORMATION

- Acute exacerbations (4 of the following): change in sputum, increased dyspnea, increased cough, fever, increased wheezing, fatigue, decreased PFTs, new infiltrate, change in PE.
- Recombinant human DNAase 2.5 mg twice daily may be especially beneficial in tx of pts with CF.
- Mucolytic therapy never proven beneficial and not commonly recommended.

BASIS FOR RECOMMENDATIONS

ten Hacken NH, Wijkstra PJ, Kerstjens HA. Treatment of bronchiectasis in adults. *BMJ*, 2007; Vol. 335; pp. 1089–93.

Comments: Helpful review of both antibiotic and non-antibiotic strategies.

Rosen MJ. Chronic cough due to bronchiectasis: ACCP evidence-based clinical practice guidelines. *Chest*, 2006; Vol. 129; pp. 122S–131S.

Comments: Document reviews background and basis for recommendations in this module.

BRONCHITIS, ACUTE UNCOMPLICATED

John G. Bartlett, MD

DIAGNOSIS

PATHOGENS

- Viruses: rhinovirus, parainfluenza virus, coronavirus, RSV, metapneumovirus
- Influenza: the only routinely treatable virus
- *Chlamydophila pneumoniae*
- *Mycoplasma pneumoniae*
- Pertussis (*Bordetella pertussis*)
- Other offenders: allergens, smoking, toxic fumes

CLINICAL

- Hx: acute upper respiratory tract infection, cough is the predominant complaint.
- PE: fever is most common with influenza or parainfluenza infection. Lung exam may reveal rhonchi or wheezing, but no crackles or evidence of lung consolidation.
- Differential dx of cough: subclinical asthma, postnasal drip and allergies, pertussis, CHF, GERD, neoplasm, ACE inhibitor reaction.

DIAGNOSIS

- Clinical diagnosis based on compatible symptoms and lack of concerning findings on exam (r/o pneumonia).
- Indications for chest X-ray: abnormal vital signs (P > 100, T $> 38°C$, RR > 20) or rales or cough >3 wks.

TREATMENT

Treatment: etiology-based

- Principles: dx = URI + cough. Clinician should rule-out asthma, GERD, cancer or postnasal drip. CXR if abnormal vital signs to R/O pneumonia. No treatment (no antibiotics) unless concern for pertussis.
- Indications for antimicrobials: suspected pertussis or influenza. If influenza suspect, agents consider anti-influenza agents if sxs <48 hrs.
- Influenza (see Influenza module): consider anti-flu drug(s) if onset of symptoms <48 hrs. In 2009–2010 season, pandemic H1N1 influenza A is excepted to be the predominant circulating species, and only oseltamivir or zanamivir is recommended. See CDC website for most up to date recommendations: Updated Interim Recommendations for the Use of Antiviral Medications in the Treatment and Prevention of Influenza for the 2009–2010 Season. In hospitalized pts, drugs may benefit even if given beyond 48 hrs of symptom onset.
- Exceptions to antibiotic (NICE in UK) recommends: antibiotics if severe-associated disease, immunosuppressed pts or age >65 plus diabetes, heart failure or hospitalization within the past yr.
- Cough medications: contain codeine or dextromethorphan.
- Common cold: dexbrompheniramine + sedating antihistamine (Actifed, Contac, Dimetapp, etc.), naproxen 500 mg three times a day PO $\times$ 5 days and/or Atrovent nasal spray.
- Allergic rhinitis: for example, loratadine 10 mg PO once daily.
- Sinusitis: above +/– antibiotic if severe symptoms or >7 days of sx. (Efficacy is unclear).
- AECB: (see "Bronchitis, Acute Exacerbation of Chronic").
- Cough or bronchospasm (infectious-induced): albuterol by inhaler, 2 inhalations q4–6h. May be more effective in those with demonstrable reductions in peak flow capacity.
- If cough lasts >3 wks: should r/o asthma, GERD, pertussis, cancer.

Suspected or confirmed pertussis

- Antibiotics should not be used for bronchitis except for suspected or confirmed pertussis.
- Most adults with pertussis lack typical sx due to partial immunity. Major clues: severe coughing paroxysms >3 wks, whoop, or post-tussive emesis.
- Preferred tests: nasopharyngeal swab for PCR and/or culture (not sensitive).

- Pertussis: erythromycin 500 mg PO four times a day × 14 days or azithromycin (Zpak 500 mg, then 250 mg PO once daily × 4 days). Most use azithromycin due to erythromycin side effects.
- Alternatives: TMP-SMX 1 DS twice daily PO × 14 days or clarithromycin 500 PO twice daily × 14 days.

FOLLOW UP
- Pt acceptance of non-antibiotic treatment is better if it is called "a chest cold" rather than "bronchitis."
- If abnormal vital signs (T > 38°C, P > 100, RR > 20) and not obviously influenza—get chest XR to exclude pneumonia.
- However, non-use of antibiotics is less clear than often stated based on review by NICE (as summarized above).

OTHER INFORMATION
- Multiple well-controlled studies show antibiotics are not justified, but given in up to 70% of pts regardless.
- Academicians keep saying antibiotics don't work, but Cochrane library says they do based on careful data analysis. The best explanation is mild benefit which doesn't justify to cost or risk.
- Review by NICE recommends antibiotics for those with co-morbidities and advanced age.
- Abx indications: severe exacerbations of chronic bronchitis, some vulnerable hosts, some influenza cases, or pertussis.

BASIS FOR RECOMMENDATIONS

Snow V, Mottur-Pilson C, Gonzales R, et al. Principles of appropriate antibiotic use for treatment of acute bronchitis in adults. *Ann Intern Med*, 2001; Vol. 134; pp. 518–20.
Comments: See reference: Gonzales R, Bartlett JG, Besser RE, et al. *Ann Intern Med*, 2001;134:521. Recommendations are nearly identical.

Gonzales R, Bartlett JG, Besser RE, et al. Principles of appropriate antibiotic use for treatment of uncomplicated acute bronchitis: background. *Ann Intern Med*, 2001; Vol. 134; pp. 521–9.
Comments: Guidelines from 2 Panels: one representing the CDC and the other representing ACP/ASIM. Guidelines were nearly identical. They say: (1) X-ray to r/o pneumonia if VS are abnormal (HR >100/ml), RR >24/min, temp >38°C) or if chest exam is abnormal; (2) suspect cough variant asthma with cough worse at night, with exercise, or with cold; (3) non-viral microbial pathogens are *C. pneumoniae, M. pneumonia*, and *B. pertussis*; only pertussis requires treatment w/abx; (4) most with URI are due to flu, paraflu 3, RSV, coronavirus, rhinovirus or adenovirus; (5) 8/8 clinical trials show no benefit with abx.

Irwin RS, Madison JM. The diagnosis and treatment of cough. *N Engl J Med*, 2000; Vol. 343; pp. 1715–21.
Comments: The authors provide the "Primary Care" Guidelines For Acute Cough. Management is based on chronicity and cause. Acute bronchitis is treated as viral infection + managing associated conditions—viral URI, sinusitis, allergic rhinitis, exacerbation chronic bronchitis, or pertussis. Chronic cough (>3 wks) is classified as asthma, GERD, or postnasal drip syndrome.

CHRONIC BRONCHITIS, ACUTE EXACERBATIONS

John G. Bartlett, MD

PATHOGENS
- *Haemophilus influenzae* (most important)
- *Streptococcus pneumoniae*
- *Moraxella catarrhalis*
- Viruses: influenza, rhinovirus, parainfluenza, RSV
- Other offenders: allergens, smoking, toxic fumes, etc.

CLINICAL
- Principles: about half of AECB are caused by bacterial infection.
- Increased sputum production, increased cough, increased dyspnea note significant AECB flare.
- PE: increased respirations, wheezing, rhonchi, cyanosis +/– fever.

DIAGNOSIS
- Definition: increased over baseline in cough, sputum and sputum purulence in pt with chronic bronchitis (chronic bronchitis defined as cough + sputum × 3 yrs).
- Obtain chest X-ray to R/O pneumonia, CHF, effusion, mass lesion or pneumothorax.

- Lab: sputum Gram-stain and culture, not advocated routinely.
- Arterial blood gases or pulse oximetry if pt seriously ill. Spirometry—probably not useful.
- Severity: judge by pulse oximetry, blood gases, FEV-1.

TREATMENT

Antibacterials

- Supportive care includes bronchodilators (albuterol, ipratropium bromide), corticosteroids, oxygen (see below).
- Abx indications: severe acute exacerbations with increased cough, sputum volume and sputum purulence.
- **Preferred (ACP):** amoxicillin 500–875 mg PO three times a day or doxycycline 100 mg PO twice daily × 10–14 days.
- **Alternatives:** amoxicillin/clavulanate (Augmentin) 875 mg PO twice daily × 10–14 days.
- Azithromycin 500 mg, then 250 mg PO once daily × 4 days, or clarithromycin 500 mg PO twice daily or 1 g (Biaxin XR) PO once daily × 10–14 days.
- Cefuroxime axetil (Ceftin) 500 mg PO twice daily; cefprozil (Cefzil) 500 mg PO twice daily; cefpodoxime (Vantin) 200–400 mg PO twice daily or cefdinir (Omnicef) 600 mg PO once daily. All 10–14 days.
- **Severe or recent abx:** moxifloxacin (Avelox) × 5 days or levofloxacin (Levaquin) 500 (or 750 mg) mg PO once daily × 7 days.
- **Influenza (efficacy in ambulatory pts seen if used within 48 hrs):** oseltamivir (Tamiflu) 75 mg twice daily × 5 days; avoid zanamivir due to possible exacerbation of wheezing from inhalant powder. Unclear if oseltamivir-resistant virus will circulate in 2009–2010 season as in past, expect predominant species to be oseltamivir-susceptible pandemic H1N1 influenza A virus; however, check CDC website for latest recommendations: Updated Interim Recommendations for the Use of Antiviral Medications in the Treatment and Prevention of Influenza for the 2009–2010 Season.

Supportive Care (most important)

- Prednisone: If FEV, <50% predicted: prednisone 30–40 mg/days PO × 7–10 days or nebulized budesonide.
- Inhaled bronchodilators: albuterol 2.5 mg nebs four times a day (may titrate up to q30 min) or 2 puffs four times a day by metered inhaler +/– spacer when stable and/or ipratropium (Atrovent) 0.25–0.5 mg inhaled q6h–8h.
- Hospitalized pts: methylprednisolone 125 mg IV q6h × 3 days, then PO prednisone 60 mg/days × 4–7 days, 40 mg/days × 8–11 days, 20 mg/days × 12–15 days.
- Hospitalized pts: O_2 2–4 L by nasal cannula; to keep pulse oximeter >91%; if need increase or pCO_2 > 45 use Venturi mask. Risk with higher O_2 administration is respiratory failure, so close monitoring recommended if pt is known CO_2 retainer.
- Aminophylline/theophylline: potentially serious side effects and not effective; avoid or use with caution + measure levels at 8–12 hrs.
- Inhaled metered dose steroids: not generally indicated for acute therapy.
- Non-invasive positive-pressure ventilation; requires trained physician.
- Not effective: chest PT, methylxanthine bronchodilators (e.g., theophylline), mucolytic agents.
- Opportune time for smoking cessation counselling.

OTHER INFORMATION

- Common non-bacterial causes of AECB: viral infections, allergens, pollution.
- Must r/o pneumonia (x-ray), subclinical asthma (PFTs), and respiratory failure (ABG).
- Abx in 3 categories: cheap, old, and proven (amox, doxy,); better activity vs *S. pneumo* and *H. flu* (oral cephs, amox-clav); drugs w/ clout but concern re: abuse (levofloxacin, moxifloxacin).
- Main issues: role of *H. influenzae* and role of newer drugs to reduce hospitalizations and to delay next exacerbation?

BASIS FOR RECOMMENDATIONS

Global strategy for the diagnosis management and prevention of COPD. Global Initiative for Chronic Obstructive Lung Disease (GOLD). 2007 (accessed 7/1/08).

Comments: Initiative from NIH and WHO to guide management: Indication for Abx: (1) 3 symptoms (increased dyspnea, increased sputum purulence, increased volume and (2) require mechanical ventilation. Diagnostic evaluation: (1) bronchodilator reversibility test, chest x-ray, and arterial blood gas and (2) sputum culture.

Stoller JK. Clinical practice. Acute exacerbations of chronic obstructive pulmonary disease. *N Engl J Med,* 2002; Vol. 346; pp. 988–94.

Comments: Review of guidelines: *Brit Thor Soc 1997: Tetracycline, amoxicillin; *Am College Chest Phys 2001: Amox, tetra, TMP-SMX; *European Resp Society 1995: Amox or tetra; *ATS: Doxy or amoxicillin.

EMPYEMA

John G. Bartlett, MD

PATHOGENS

- *S. pneumoniae*
- Anaerobes
- *Streptococcus aginosus*
- *S. aureus,* including community-acquired MRSA

CLINICAL

- Empyemas are rare. Pleural effusions occur in 30–40% of pneumonias, while empyemas in only 0.5–2%.
- Major cause in CAP is anaerobic bacteria. Major nosocomial cause (usually after chest surgery) is *S. aureus.* Major new cause is community-acquired MRSA.
- Symptoms of pneumonia + pleurisy.
- Fulminant course in healthy host: usually MRSA, especially if following influenza as a bacterial superinfection.
- Exam consistent with signs of effusion (dullness, decreased fremitus, decreased/absent breath sounds).

DIAGNOSIS

- Chest XR (or ultrasound or CT scan) shows effusion, but empyema dx requires pleural fluid analysis showing pus and positive Gram-stain or positive culture for likely pathogen, or effusion with pH <7.0.
- Perform thoracentesis, if free-flowing fluid >10 mm on lateral decubitus x-ray.
- Pleural fluid tests: Gram-stain, culture, pH, WBC, LDH, AFB stain/cx, glucose, cytology.
- Gram-stain—important clues for bacteriology and abx selection on day 1. Polymicrobial flora often indicates anaerobes. "Putrid" empyema always means anaerobes. GPC in clusters— *S. aureus.* GPC in chains—*S. pneumonia* or *S. milleri.*

TREATMENT

Antibiotics: anaerobes +/- aerobes

- Principles: dx by pleural fluid with pus or pH <7.0 or positive culture for pathogen/Gram-stain. Rx: drainage + abx. Recovery: often slow.
- Community-acquired and fulminant course—suspect MRSA, especially if young previously healthy person, with influenza or necrotizing pneumonia.
- Standard empiric rx: (covers most anaerobes, MSSA, GPC, and GNB; not MRSA): imipenem 0.5–1 g IV q6h (or meropenem or doripenem) or piperacillin-tazobactam 3.375 g–4.5 g q6h IV.
- Abx AnO$_2$ (putrid pus or mixed bacterial Gram-stain)[preferred]: clindamycin 600 mg IV q8h, then 300 mg PO q6–8h or beta-lactams/BLI: ampicillin/sulbactam (Unasyn) 1.5–3.0 g IV q6h (or piperacillin/tazobactam or ticarcillin/clavulanate) then amoxicillin/clavulanate (Augmentin) 875 PO twice daily.
- Anti-anaerobe and GNB coverage: imipenem 0.5–1.0 g IV q6h, meropenem 1 g q8h, doripenem 500 mg IV q8h, or ertapenem 1 g IV q24h.
- *S. pneumoniae/S. aginosus* complex: cefotaxime 1 g IV q8h or ceftriaxone 1 g IV every day then amoxicillin 500–750 mg PO four times a day.
- *S. pneumoniae/S. aginosus* (alt rx/penicillin resistant): moxifloxacin 400 mg PO IV/day or levofloxacin 750 mg PO IV/day.
- *S. aureus* (MSSA): oxacillin or nafcillin 2 g IV q4–6h IV, then cephalexin (Keflex) 500 mg PO four times a day.
- *S. aureus* (MRSA or pen allergy): vancomycin 15 mg/kg q12h (1 g q12h) or linezolid 600 mg IV/PO twice daily.

- MRSA (alt): use sensitivities to guide choice, consider clindamycin for CA MRSA.
- GNB: cefotaxime/ceftriaxone/fluoroquinolones, adjust abx based on sensitivities.

Pleural drainage

- Principles: (1) pleural fluid → drain, (2) empyema → chest tube, (3) incomplete drainage → fibrinolytics and/or thoracotomy, (4) loculated effusion → thoracotomy or video-assisted thoracic surgery (VATS).
- CT evidence of pleural peel—usually requires decortication.
- Fibrinolytics (not generally recommended): streptokinase (250,000 IU/day), urokinase (100,000 IU/day) or streptokinase plus streptodornase (Varidase).
- Loculated effusions: tube + thrombolytics. If drainage incomplete: thoracotomy.
- pH 7.0–7.2 or LDH >1000: consider chest tube if loculated or large effusion.
- pH <7.0 or glucose <40 or pus: chest tube.
- pH >7.2, glucose >40, LDH <1000: (repeat) thoracentesis.
- Streptokinase: if chest tube placed, consider instillation of 250,000 units twice daily × 3 days.

Follow Up

- THE critical facet is adequate drainage with thoracentesis +/− tube placement, thoracotomy tube (open or closed) or decortication.
- Delay in surgical drainage is the major cause of long LOS.

Basis for Recommendations

Mandell LA, Wunderink RG, Anzueto A, et al. Infectious Diseases Society of America/ American Thoracic Society consensus guidelines on the management of community-acquired pneumonia in adults. *Clin Infect Dis,* 2007; Vol. 44 Suppl 2; pp. S27–72.

Comments: Guidelines include discussion of complicated pneumonia and pleural effusions.

Light RW. Management of parapneumonic effusions. *Chest,* 1991; Vol. 100; pp. 892–3.

Comments: The author reviews his MANAGEMENT GUIDELINES for empyema based on pleural fluid analysis: (1) pH <7.0 or glucose <40 mg/dL—chest tube; (2) pH 7.0–7.2 or LDH >1,000 IU/L—consider chest tube if effusion is loculated or large; (3) pH >7.2 and glucose >40 mg/dL and LDH <1,000 IU/L—no chest tube; repeat thoracentesis if pt does not respond or effusion increases.

INFLUENZA

John G. Bartlett, MD

Pathogens

- Influenza A (H1N1 and H3N2, seasonal)
- Influenza B (seasonal)
- Influenza (Novel H1N1, swine influenza 2009)

Clinical

- Typical uncomplicated influenza sx w/ abrupt onset fever, myalgia, headache, malaise, dry cough, sore throat, and rhinitis. Children have more otitis media, nausea/vomiting.
- Common complications: bacterial sinusitis, otitis, exacerbation of chronic bronchitis, pneumonia, asthma, cardiac decompensations, diabetic, or other chronic disease worsening.
- Spread: respiratory droplets within 6 feet of infected person; less common is hand contact.
- Prevention: >6 feet from case, other basics include cover sneezes, hand hygiene, and stay home; masks—surgical or N95 mask.
- Adults infectious from day one prior sx until day 7 in adults, day 10 in children. Viral shedding may be prolonged for wks or mos in immunosuppressed pts. Highest viral load in first 48 hrs.
- Children can routinely shed >10 days.
- Most vulnerable (seasonal flu): infants (<2 yrs), elderly, hospitalized, compromised host, pregnancy, and co-morbidities—especially pre-existing heart and lung disease.
- Bacterial superinfections (pneumonia): *S. pneumoniae* (most common), *S. aureus* (most serious).
- Pandemic H1N1: (1) different from seasonal flu in age distribution (most <65 yrs) and (2) most vulnerable to serious complications: pregnancy, babies <6 mo, persons 6 mos–25 yrs, <65 yrs with co-morbidities (chronic diseases, asthma, diabetes, immunodeficiency) and obesity. Note: 20–30% of hospitalizations and deaths are in pts with no

co-morbidities; about 20% have bacterial superinfections and the rest have ARDS secondary to influenza.

DIAGNOSIS

- Gold standard: RT-PCR superior to viral culture (which is only 70% sensitive) > rapid tests (40%–60% sensitive).
- Physician clinical dx influenza (epidemic, fever + typical sx) is as sensitive as rapid DFA test (~70% sensitivity) but less specific. Fever $\geq 100°F$ especially important sign in clinical dx.
- Major competing diagnoses: parainfluenza, RSV, adenovirus, metapneumovirus, rhinovirus, coronavirus.

TREATMENT

Influenza Treatment

- Consider treat in persons with symptoms <48 hrs and persons who are likely to have a serious outcome even if >48 hrs (high risk of serious infection or hospitalized pts).
- See CDC recommendations for 2009 flu season: "Updated Interim Recommendations for the Use of Antiviral Medications in the Treatment and Prevention of Influenza for the 2009–2010 Season" (www.cdc.gov). Prior 2008–09 season recommendations were based on early dominance of (seasonal) H1N1 and astonishing oseltamivir resistance rates in H1N1 (98%).
- Treatment options (2009): as of Oct 2009 circulating strains almost entirely novel H1N1 influenza A, so use oseltamivir or zanamivir (chronic lung disease and asthma are contraindications).
- Dosing, base on knowledge of susceptability of circulating strains: oseltamivir 75 mg PO twice daily × 5 days; zanamivir 10 mg (2 puffs) twice daily × 5 days. Use amantadine 100 mg twice daily or 200 mg daily × 5 days and rimantidine <65 yrs 100 mg PO twice daily × 5 days, if >65 yrs 100 mg PO twice daily × 5 days.

Influenza Prophylaxis

- Preferred (by everybody): all school-aged children, all children 6 mos–59 mos, persons ≥ 50, pts with chronic diseases/immunosuppression and for healthcare workers, women who will become pregnant during influenza season, all residents of long-term care facilities, healthy household contacts (including children) who could transmit infection to people at risk, especially if infant <6 mos of age in house. Need 2 wks for response.
- Immunization: (1) trivalent inactivated vaccine (TIV) given yearly, reformulated annually, (2) live-attenuated vaccine (LAIV) given intranasally (only age 4–49 yrs). See "Influenza Prophylaxis" module for details including pandemic influenza recommendations.
- Tiered priority (seasonal influenza, if vaccine in short supply): persons >65 yrs or <23 mos, chronic illness, pregnancy or health care workers.
- Immediate protection: give antivirals (70–80% effective) + vaccine (2 wks required for antibody response).
- ACIP 2008 changes and updated recommendations: a) emphasis of giving 2 doses of vaccine to all children ages 6 mos–8 yrs, b) if children 6 mos–8 yrs receive only one dose in their first yr of immunization, they should receive two the following yr, c) all children ages 6 mos—18 yrs should be immunized, d) all adults >50 yrs, e) adults 18–50 yrs with comorbidities, f) recommendation that health-care administrators consider HCW immunization part of their pt safety initiatives.
- Chemoprophylaxis 2009 flu season: oseltamivir 75 mg PO once daily or zanamivir 2 puffs daily for H1N1 (swine) strain.
- Antiviral prophylaxis given for at least 7 days following close contact or up to 6 wks during community outbreak.

Symptomatic treatment

- Naprosyn 500 mg PO three times a day, ASA (don't use for children <12 yrs because of risk of Reyes syndrome), etc.
- Cough: medications w/ codeine or dextromethorphan.
- Sedating antihistamine preparations: e.g., Actifed, Contact, Dimetapp, etc.
- Atrovent nasal spray.
- Albuterol nasal spray 2 whiffs q4–6h prn.

- Bacterial pneumonia: (1) Major pathogens are *S. pneumoniae,* Group A strep and *S. aureus;* (2) Two patterns—<u>concurrent infection</u> (influenza culture positive) or <u>influenza resolving and bacterial superinfection</u> at 5–10 days (influenza culture negative, serology positive.
- MRSA is a major concern, and can have rapid onset morbidity/mortality. Clues: young adult, seriously ill, hemorrhagic or necrotizing pneumonia, leukopenia or erythroderma. Treat with vancomycin (15 mg/kg q12h, goal trough level 15–20 mcg/mL) or linezolid 600 mg IV q12h (linezolid often preferred due to better lung penetration).

OTHER INFORMATION

- Avian influenza A (H5N1, see "Influenza, avian" module) in Asia—highly lethal and no current human vaccine. Annual cases have decreased after 2004, due to control in poultry but still shows high lethality and epidemiologic center has shifted to Egypt.
- Seasonal influenza is major cause of serious disease in persons >65 yrs, nursing home residents and persons w/ chronic dz—lung, heart, liver/renal failure, diabetes, etc. Associated with high rates of cardiovascular deaths.
- Oseltamivir anti-influenza drugs reduce duration sx by average 1–2 days if started <48 hrs of onset of sx; benefit is greater if started early (at 12 hrs after onset of illness) and if sx severe. Now advocated for hospitalized pts regardless of duration symptoms.
- CDC weekly flu updates: T: 888–232–3228, fax: 888–232–3299 (doc. #361100), or http://www.cdc.gov/flu/weekly

MORE INFORMATION

Lab tests: Most cost $30–60, use nasopharyngeal or throat swab, and are best <72 hrs after symptom onset.

Test method: RT-PCR is now the gold standard. Novel H1N1 strain not well detected by rapid diagnostic tests or DFA; RT-PCR preferred

Test	Time to report	Sensitivity
PCR, RT-PCR	2 hrs.	Very high—gold standard
DFA	2–4 hrs.	
Culture	2–10 days	Moderately high
Serology	days-wks	Not useful

Clinical features usually adequate if influenza is circulating in the community.

BASIS FOR RECOMMENDATIONS

Fiore AE, Shay DK, Broder K, et al. Prevention and control of seasonal influenza with vaccines: recommendations of the Advisory Committee on Immunization Practices (ACIP), 2009. *MMWR Recomm Rep,* 2009; Vol. 58; pp. 1–52.

LUNG ABSCESS

John G. Bartlett, MD

PATHOGENS

- *S. aureus* including MRSA
- Anaerobes
- Aerobic and microaerophilic strep including *S. anginosus* complex
- Gram-negative bacteria, especially *Klebsiella*
- Legionella
- Nocardia
- Actinomyces
- Group A streptococci
- *H. influenzae* (type b)
- Mycobacteria: *M. tuberculosis,* MAI, *M. kans*asii
- Fungi: aspergillus, cryptococcus, coccidioides, histoplasmosis, blastomycosis

CLINICAL

- Clinical: cough, fever, sputum that is often putrid, +/– weight loss. Chronic course often with night sweats, predisposition to aspiration and/or pleurisy.

- PE: fever and signs of pneumonia +/– pleural effusion +/– terrible gingivitis.
- MRSA—rare, but serious and becoming more common. Suspect with recent or concurrent influenza illness or evidence of necrotizing pneumonia and shock in young adults or adolescents.
- Rupture into pleural space may result in thoracic empyema.

DIAGNOSIS

- CXR or CT scan showing parenchymal infiltrate with cavity.
- CT scan provides best anatomical definition—recommended when x-rays are equivocal, cases of uncertain cause, and cases that do not respond to antibiotics.
- Sputum bacteriology: useless with anaerobes except for putrid smell. *S. aureus* should be seen (Gram-stain) and grown easily in presentations of CAP.
- Leukocytosis and anemia common with chronic abscess; leukopenia common with MRSA.
- Differential diagnosis of air-fluid level cavity on CXR: TB, MAC, empyema, malignancy, cyst, fungi, nocardia.
- Bronchoscopy, once routine in all lung abscess pts, now reserved for cases with atypical presentation or cases that do not respond to treatment.

TREATMENT

Antibiotic therapy

- Principles: diagnosis by CXR/CT shows cavity. Main cause = anaerobes. Need to rule-out TB, Ca, etc. Usual treatment: clindamycin (especially if putrid). Bronchoscopy if atypical presentation or failure to respond.
- **Preferred:** clindamycin 600 mg IV q8h, then clindamycin 300 mg PO four times a day × 3 mos or until CXR shows small stable lesion or is clear.
- Ampicillin + sulbactam (Unasyn) 1.5–3 g IV q6h, then amoxicillin-clavulanate (Augmentin) 875 mg PO twice daily or clindamycin 300 mg PO four times a day as above.
- **Alternatives:** piperacillin-tazobactam (Zosyn) 3.375 g IV q6h, then amoxicillin-clavulanate (Augmentin) 875 mg PO twice daily or clindamycin 300 mg PO four times a day.
- Imipenem (Primaxin) 0.5–1 g IV q6–8h or meropenem or doripenem, then clindamycin 300 mg PO four times a day or amoxicillin-clavulanate (Augmentin) 875 mg PO twice daily.
- MRSA: linezolid 600 mg IV q12h or vancomycin 15 mg/kg IV q12h.
- Most "non-specific" lung abscesses are treated empirically with clindamycin and respond, but may require 3 mos. or longer course.
- Most pts are treated with IV antibiotics until clinical improvement, then receive oral antibiotics × 2–3 mos or until a f/u CXR is clear or shows a small, stable residual lesion.

Antibiotics-Special hosts, settings

- Compromised host, e.g., AIDS: consider TB, *P. aeruginosa*, *nocardia*, *cryptococcus*, *aspergillus*, PCP, *Rhodococcus equi*, MAC, *M. kansasii*, lymphoma.
- Nosocomial: *S. aureus*, GNB, especially *Klebsiella*.
- Post-influenza: *S.aureus* including community-onset MRSA.
- Nursing home: anaerobes, GNB, *S. aureus*.
- Injection drug user: aspiration w/ anaerobes and streptococci, or septic emboli due to tricuspid endocarditis usually due to *S. aureus* or *Streptococcus viridans*.
- Fulminant illness: *S. aureus*, *Klebsiella* species.

Drainage and Surgery

- Most pts have already drained abscess spontaneously via bronchus and need only abx.
- Bronchoscopic drainage or physical therapy—not generally useful.
- Percutaneous transthoracic drainage—indicated in refractory lung abscess cases.
- Postural drainage—often done but probably plays no role in treatment and may be dangerous.
- Resectional surgery—usually a lobectomy or pneumonectomy, if necessary.
- Resection indications (rare): failure to respond to abx treatment usually due to abscess cavity >6 cm diameter, complicated/serious associated diseases, or GNB.

FOLLOW UP

- Abx treat duration—until CXR clear or small stable residual scar (arbitrary).

OTHER INFORMATION

- Most common cause is anaerobic infection due to aspiration.
- Must R/O mycobacteria (esp. TB), fungi (endemic fungi such as histoplasmosis, coccidioidomycosis, blastomycosis, cryptococcosis), cancer, infected cysts, and CA-MRSA.

DIAGNOSIS

- Clues to anaerobes: putrid discharge, chronic course, predisposition to aspiration (decreased consciousness, dysphagia, or gingivitis).
- Community-acquired pneumonia + abscess often occurs post-influenza—concern for *S. aureus*, must treat rapidly usually with vancomycin or linezolid.
- The epidemic MRSA (USA 300 and 400 strains) usually cause rapid septic course in pts with influenza who have pulmonary necrosis and shock.

BASIS FOR RECOMMENDATIONS

Mandell LA, Wunderink RG, Anzueto A, et al. Infectious Diseases Society of America/ American Thoracic Society consensus guidelines on the management of community-acquired pneumonia in adults. *Clin Infect Dis*, 2007; Vol. 44 Suppl 2; pp. S27–72.

Comments: Guideline recommendations for treatment of CAP infections.

Bartlett JG. Anaerobic bacterial infections of the lung and pleural space. *Clin Infect Dis*, 1993; Vol. 16 Suppl 4; pp. S248–55.

Comments: Review of pulmonary infections with high yield of anaerobes—lung abscess, aspiration pneumonia and empyema. Major pathogens are *Peptostreptococcus*, Prevotella, Fusobacteria, and Bacteroides. Clindamycin is the only drug that is extensively tested and proven to be superior to penicillin.

PNEUMONIA, ASPIRATION

John G. Bartlett, MD

PATHOGENS

- Anaerobes
- *Staphylococcus aureus*
- Streptococcus species
- Gram-negative bacilli

CLINICAL

- Three forms based on aspiration: bacterial (infection), acid (chemical pneumonia) or water/ vegetal (obstruction).
- Infection: pts usually aspiration prone (dysphagia, decreased consciousness), fever, cough, infiltrate (comprise ~10% of community-acquired pneumonia).
- Acid-related pneumonia: sudden dyspnea +/– cyanosis, fever, wheezing, often ARDS-like picture.
- Obstruction: vegetal (peas and beans, etc.), water (drowning).
- Lab: chest X-ray—if no infiltrate = no significant disease.

DIAGNOSIS

- Clinical diagnosis mostly.
- Sputum Gram-stain and culture may be supportive of bacterial explantation.

TREATMENT

Infection

- Principles: suspect if aspiration prone pt + infiltrate + cough/fever.
- Pathogens: <u>community-acquired</u>—anaerobes and streptococci; <u>healthcare-associated</u>—GNB, *S. aureus* +/– anaerobes.
- Anaerobic aspiration pneumonia (preferred): clindamycin 600 mg IV q8h or 300 mg PO four times a day (+/– fluoroquinolone) × 10 days.
- Alt: amoxicillin-clavulanate (Augmentin) 875 mg PO twice daily × 10 days, or ampicillin-sulbactam (Unasyn) 1.5–3 g IV q6h or piperacillin-tazobactam (Zosyn) 3.375 g IV q6h, or imipenem link (Primaxin) 0.5–1 g IV q6h. All × 10 days.
- Community-acquired pneumonia with questionable aspiration: use fluoroquinolone + clindamycin or beta-lactam/beta-lactamase inhibitor (IDSA guidelines).
- Nosocomial case: see "Pneumonia, Hospital-Acquired" module—for anaerobes use imipenem, piperacillin-tazobactam (Zosyn), or clindamycin + GNB coverage +/– vancomycin 15 mg/kg q12h.

Chemical/Acid

- Principles: fulminant onset w/ dyspnea, decreased O_2, infiltrate +/– wheezing. Suction pt + supportive care.
- Suction: to remove particles, fluid, etc.
- Support: IV fluids, ventilatory support (ARDS).

- Controversial: positive pressure ventilation, colloids, corticosteroids, and antibiotics.
- Steroids: not useful in 2 controlled trials.
- ABX: unnecessary, but usually given.

Obstruction/Prevention

- Obstruction with foreign body: consider bronchoscopy.
- Obstruction at laryngeal level: Heimlich maneuver.
- Obstruction with fluids: tracheal suction.
- Prevention: maintain upright or semi-upright position (documented benefit).
- Controversial for prevention: tracheostomy, nasogastric or PEG tubes, gastric pH increase.
- Prevention with endotracheal tube: continuous aspiration of subglottic secretions = possible benefit.
- Prevention with gastric paresis: postpyloric feeding tube.
- Nutrition: feeding/gastric tubes may be necessary but don't lower aspiration risk.

Follow Up

- Infection: 10% of community acquired pneumonia, usual pathogens: anaerobes and streptococci. Treat w/ clindamycin or beta-lactam/beta-lactamase inhibitor.
- Anaerobic Treatment: clindamycin, imipenem, piperacillin-tazobactam, ampicillin-sulbactam. Possibly effective: moxifloxacin, macrolides.

Other Information

- Nosocomial cases: bacteriology and Rx different—GNB + *S. aureus* +/– anaerobes.
- Chemical pneumonitis: 3 outcomes—rapid recovery, ARDS, or superinfection.

Basis for Recommendations

Mandell LA, Wunderink RG, Anzueto A, et al. Infectious Diseases Society of America/American Thoracic Society consensus guidelines on the management of community-acquired pneumonia in adults. *Clin Infect Dis,* 2007; Vol. 44 Suppl 2; pp. S27–72.

Comments: Guidelines states "Anaerobic coverage is clearly indicated only in the classic aspiration pleuropulmonary syndrome in pts with a history of loss of consciousness as a result of alcohol/drug overdose or after seizures in pts with concomitant gingival disease or esophageal motility disorders."

Marik PE. Aspiration pneumonitis and aspiration pneumonia. *N Engl J Med,* 2001; Vol. 344; pp. 665–71.

Comments: Review of the topic with division of syndromes into chemical pneumonia due to acid aspiration (aspiration pneumonitis) and bacterial infection (aspiration pneumonia). For the former, the review shows no treatment with established benefit.

PNEUMONIA, COMMUNITY-ACQUIRED

John G. Bartlett, MD

Pathogens

- *Streptococcus pneumoniae*
- *Haemophilus influenzae*
- *Moraxella catarrhalis*
- *Chlamydophila pneumoniae*
- Legionella species
- *Mycoplasma pneumoniae*
- viruses: influenza, RSV, parainfluenza, adenovirus 14

Clinical

- Hx: cough, fever, and sputum production, dyspnea +/– GI symptoms, or pleurisy.
- PE: fever, tachypnea, rales, or evidence of consolidation.
- Site of care—use judgment + PSI or CURB –65 (1 pt for decreased consciousness, increased BUN, respiratory rate >30/min and BP <90 systolic plus age >65 yrs): score 0–1 = outpt treatment.

Diagnosis

- Chest XR nearly always shows an infiltrate. PCP is a major exception.
- Preferred diagnostic test for major pathogens. *S. pneumoniae*: blood culture, sputum Gram-stain and culture, urine antigen assay.
- Legionella: urine antigen assay and culture on selective media (BCYE). *C. pneumoniae*: no test is FDA cleared. *M. pneumoniae*: IgM in pediatric populations only.

- *S. aureus, Moraxella catarrhalis, H. influenzae,* other GNB: blood culture, sputum Gram-stain and culture.

TREATMENT
Outpatient (Empiric)
- **Outpatient and uncomplicated:** doxycycline or macrolide.
- Doxycycline 100 mg twice daily PO × 7–10 days.
- Azithromycin 500 mg PO every day × 3 days (Tri-pak)or 2 g PO × 1 dose (Zmax).
- Clarithromycin 1 g (XR) PO every day or 500 mg twice daily PO × 7 days.
- **Outpatient and comorbidity (COPD, diabetes, CHF, etc) and/or recent abx:** above drugs or use fluoroquinolone.
- Fluoroquinolones: levofloxacin 750 mg daily PO × 5 days or moxifloxacin 400 mg daily PO × 7 days or gemifloxacin 320 mg PO × 7 days.

Hospitalized patient (Empiric, non-ICU)
- **Preferred (IDSA guidelines, non-ICU)** either 1. fluoroquinolone (alone) or 2. [ceftriaxone or cefotaxime] **and** [erythromycin, azithromycin or clarithromycin] as dosed below.
- Levofloxacin (Levaquin) 750 mg IV/PO q24h or moxifloxacin (Avelox) 400 mg PO/IV q24h × 7–10 days.
- Ceftriaxone (Rocephin) 1 g IV q24h or cefotaxime 1 g IV q8h, each combined with a macrolide.
- Azithromycin 500 mg IV/PO every day × 3 days usually with ceftriaxone or cefotaxime.
- **Aspiration pneumonia:** clindamycin 600 mg IV q8h + fluoroquinolone. Other choices include Augmentin (oral) or Zosyn, Unasyn or Timentin (parenteral).
- **Influenza +/– bacterial superinfection** (*S. pneumoniae > S. aureus*): ceftriaxone or cefotaxime +/– oseltamivir 75 mg twice daily × 5 days. Consider MRSA, add vancomycin 15 mg/kg IV q12h or linezolid 600 mg IV/PO q12h.
- If structural disease of lung exists, consider covering for *P. aeruginosa.*

Hospitalized patient (Empiric, ICU)
- **Inpatients, ICU treatment:** cefotaxime 1 g IV q8h, ceftriaxone 1 g IV q24h or ampicillin-sulbactam 3 g IV q6h PLUS either azithromycin 500 mg IV q24h or moxifloxacin 400 mg IV q24 or levofloxacin 750 mg IV q24h.
- If penicillin allergy: use respiratory fluoroquinolone (moxifloxacin or levofloxacin as above) and aztreonam 2 g IV q6–8h.
- **Pseudomonas aeruginosa:** if considered one of 3 options—(1) add an antipneumococcal, antipseudomonal beta-lactam (piperacillin/tazobactam 4.5 g IV q6h or 3.375 q4h, cefepime 1–2 g IV q8h, imipenem 1 g q6–8h, or meropenem 2 g IV q8h) plus either ciprofloxacin 400 mg IV q8h or levofloxacin 750 mg IV q24h.
- (2) any of the above beta-lactam plus an aminoglycoside (gentamicin, tobramycin or amikacin) and azithromycin or (3) any of the above beta-lactams plus an aminoglycoside (gentamicin, tobramycin or amikacin) and an antipneumococcal fluoroquinolone (levofloxacin or moxifloxacin). For penicillin-allergic pts, substitute aztreonam for above b-lactam.
- **MRSA:** if concerned, add vancomycin 15 mg/kg IV q12h or linezolid 600 mg IV/PO q12h.

Pathogen Specific
- *S. pneumoniae* (pen-sens): amoxicillin, ceftriaxone, cefotaxime, cefpodoxime, cefprozil, or macrolide—until afebrile 3 days.
- *S. pneumoniae* (pen-resistant): levofloxacin, moxifloxacin, vancomycin, linezolid, telithromycin.
- MRSA: linezolid 600 mg IV/PO q12h.
- MSSA: oxacillin or nafcillin 3 g IV q6h or cefazolin 1 g IV q6h.
- Mycoplasma or chlamydia: macrolide or doxycycline × 7 days.
- Legionella: azithromycin × 3–5 days or fluoroquinolone × 7 days.
- *H. influenzae*: doxycycline, 2nd or 3rd gen. cephalosporin or fluoroquinolone × 1–2 wks.
- Influenza: zanamivir or oseltamivir × 5 days. Initiate even if beyond 48 hrs onset if pt with severe illness or hospitalized. See CDC website for latest recommendations, especially if oseltamivir-resistant virus is circulating: Updated Interim Recommendations for the Use

of Antiviral Medications in the Treatment and Prevention of Influenza for the 2009–2010 Season.

- Anaerobes: clindamycin or amoxicillin-clavulanate (Augmentin) or ampicillin-sulbactam (Unasyn) or piperacillin-tazobactam (Zosyn).

FOLLOW UP

Major debate: roles of Mycoplasma and Chlamydia, and need for fluoroquinolones. See http://www.journals.uchicago.edu/doi/pdf/10.1086/511159 for IDSA Guidelines on CAP.

- IV->PO switch: clinically improving, $pO_2 > 92$, T $< 38°C$, p < 100, RR < 24, able to take pills, GI tract works.

OTHER INFORMATION

- Pts with cough and abnormal vital signs should have a chest x-ray. If negative—no abx; if infiltrate—use abx.
- Medicare "rules" for hospitalized pts: administer abx within 6 hrs, abx per IDSA/ATS guidelines, smoking cessation, pneumovax + influenza vaccines.

BASIS FOR RECOMMENDATIONS

Mandell LA, Wunderink RG, Anzueto A, et al. Infectious Diseases Society of America/American Thoracic Society consensus guidelines on the management of community-acquired pneumonia in adults. *Clin Infect Dis,* 2007; Vol. 44 Suppl 2; pp. S27–72.

Comments: IDSA/ATS Guidelines for CAP: (1) Outpatients: doxycycline or macrolide; (2) Hospitalized pts: respiratory fluoroquinolone or ceftriaxone + macrolide and (3) ICU: (FQ or macrolide) + beta-lactam.

PNEUMONIA, HOSPITAL-ACQUIRED

John G. Bartlett, MD

PATHOGENS

- *S. aureus:* MRSA > MSSA
- Gram-negative bacilli: *Klebsiella*, Enterobacter, *E. coli*, *Pseudomonas aeruginosa*, *S. maltophilia*, Acinetobacter spp.
- Most recent dreaded: KPC (carbapenemase) producing Klebsiella—hard to detect and hard to treat.
- *Legionella* spp.
- Anaerobes (aspiration)
- Viruses: influenza, RSV, parainfluenza

CLINICAL

- Pneumonia symptoms (fever, purulent respiratory secretions +/− dyspnea) + pulmonary infiltrate on CXR or CT, acquired >48–72 hrs after hospitalization. Leukocytosis may be noted.
- Lab: culture of blood, sputum, endotracheal aspirate, and/or bronchoscopic specimen.
- Preferred micro study is bronchoscopy with quantitative culture or ET tube aspirate.
- Most common agents: Gram-negative bacilli and *S. aureus* (MRSA).
- Organisms to ignore: *Staphylococcus epidermidis*, *Enterococcus* spp., all Gram-positive rods other than *Nocardia* and *B. anthracis*, *Candida* species.
- Biggest problems to treat: *P. aeruginosa*, Acinetobacter spp.

DIAGNOSIS

- Preferred micro study by some experts is bronchoscopic lavage with quantitative culture—but need is controversial.
- Obtain expectorated sputum and blood for cultures. If concern exists, also need viral studies (Influenza, RSV, etc.)
- *Legionella*: urinary antigen, sputum PCR or sputum culture (requires BCYE media).

TREATMENT

Antibiotics—empiric

- Empiric abx based on risk of multiply-resistant (MDR) pathogens. Knowledge of local antibiogram helpful.
- Risk of multiple-drug resistant (MDR) pathogen: hospitalization > 4 days, admitted from chronic care facility, abx received within past 90 days, immunosuppression, high rates of abx resistance in region or facility.

- **Low risk of MDR:** ceftriaxone 2 g/day IV, levofloxacin 750 mg, ciprofloxacin 400 mg q8h IV or moxifloxacin 400 mg q24h IV, ampicillin-sulbactam 2 g IV q6h or ertapenem 1 g IV q24h.
- **High risk of MDR:** empiric treatment should cover *P. aeruginosa*, other GNB (e.g., ESBLs, *Klebsiella, Acinetobacter*, etc.), *S. aureus* (MRSA) using (1) beta-lactam and (2) fluoroquinolone or aminoglycoside and (3) vancomycin or linezolid. High concern for ESBL should prompt use of carbapenem.
- Antipseudomonal beta-lactams (IV, chose one): cefepime 1–2 g q8–12h or ceftazidime 2 g q8h or imipenem 0.5–1.0 g q6h or meropenem 1 g q8h or piperacillin-tazobactam 4.5 g q6h **Plus** one of the following: a) levofloxacin 750 mg IV q24h or ciprofloxacin 400 mg IV q8h or b) gentamicin 7 mg/kg/day, tobramycin 7 mg/kg/day or amikacin 20 mg/kg/day IV (goal is trough levels: gentamicin/tobramycin < 1 µg/ml, amikacin < 4–5 µg/ml) **Plus** MRSA coverage: a) vancomycin 15 mg/kg IV q12h (trough > 15 µg/mL) or linezolid 600 mg IV q12h.
- Follow-up at 48–72h (clinically improved): pretreatment culture(s) negative, consider stopping abx. If culture positive, de-escalate regiment to specific pathogen, treat for 7–8 days.
- Follow-up at 48–72h (clinically unimproved): if culture negative, look for alternative causes. If cx positive, adjust abx accordingly.

Pathogen specific

- *Pseudomonas aeruginosa*: use sensitivity tests to guide choice, e.g., ceftazidime, ciprofloxacin, cefepime, aztreonam, imipenem, meropenem, piperacillin +/– aminoglycoside (tobramycin or amikacin) × 8 days. Some treat longer (10–14 days) for Pseudomonas pneumonitis as opposed to other specific pulmonary pathogens.
- Coliforms: *in vitro* tests needed.
- Anaerobes (aerobic GNB usually more important in mixed infections): ampicillin/sulbactam, ticarcillin/clavulanate, piperacillin/tazobactam, clindamycin, imipenem, ertapenem.
- *S. aureus*: (MSSA)–oxacillin or nafcillin. (MRSA)—or penicillin allergy: vancomycin or linezolid.
- *Legionella*: levofloxacin 750 mg IV q24h, moxifloxacin 400 mg IV q24 × 7–10 days or azithromycin 500 mg IV q24h × 5 days.
- Duration: generally 7–8 days of therapy judged sufficient, although some consider *P. aeruginosa* to be an exception.

Prevention

- Prevention recommendations based on 2003 meta-analysis (Ann Int Med 2003;138:494).
- Semi-recumbent position, if possible.
- Sucralfate instead of H_2 blocker or proton pump inhibitor in order to preserve gastric acidity.
- Subglottic aspiration, use if available.
- Decontamination of gut, works but not recommended.
- Infection control by institutional guidelines.

OTHER INFORMATION

- Frequency of nosocomial pneumonia is 0.5% of all hospitalized pts, 15–20% of ICU pts and 20–60% of ventilated pts.
- Usual dx criteria are fever, infiltrate and purulent respiratory secretions. Many pts w/ these findings have other conditions—pulmonary infarcts, CHF, atelectasis, etc.
- Major pathogens are GNB (50–70%), *S. aureus* (15–30%), *Legionella* (4%), or viral (10–20%).
- Role of bronchoscopy (protected brush catheter or BAL) for bacterial studies is controversial—some love it, some hate it. If used, the methodology must be precise for specimen collection and micro.

BASIS FOR RECOMMENDATIONS

No authors listed. Guidelines for the management of adults with hospital-acquired, ventilator-associated, and healthcare-associated pneumonia. *Am J Respir Crit Care Med*, 2005; Vol. 171; pp. 388–416.
Comments: Guidelines that serve as basis for recommendations.

Collard HR, Saint S, Matthay MA. Prevention of ventilator-associated pneumonia: an evidence-based systematic review. *Ann Intern Med*, 2003; Vol. 138; pp. 494–501.
Comments: (1) semi-recumbent position-consider if tolerated; need more studies; (2) Sucralfate vs H_2 antagonists to prevent ulcer; 4/7 meta-analysis showed benefit other show trend; consider if low risk for GI bleed; (3) Selective abx decontamination- 7 metaanalyses w/ >40 publications-all show reduced pneumonia rates but not recommended due to concern for abx abuse; (4) Subglottic aspiration-1/3 studies showed benefit; consider; (5) Oscillating bed-5/6 studies showed benefit; consider in surg pts and neuro pts; (6) Less frequent circuitry-4/4 studies showed no benefit; (7) Enteral feeding-4 studies showed no difference.

DIAGNOSIS

TUBERCULOSIS, ACTIVE

Timothy Sterling, MD

PATHOGENS
- *Mycobacterium tuberculosis*
- *Mycobacterium bovis*

CLINICAL
- Hx: pulmonary TB = cough >2 wks, fever, night sweats, weight loss, hemoptysis, SOB, chest pain.
- Disseminated TB = fevers, weight loss, organ involvement. Also see TB meningitis module for CNS disease.
- CXR: upper lobe infiltrate classic (may be cavitary); atypical presentations especially in children or if HIV+; adenopathy.
- Sputum AFB smear—50% sensitive.
- AFB culture—80% sensitive.
- PCR: best for sputum with positive AFB smear, expensive.
- Tuberculin skin test and IFN-gamma release assays cannot distinguish active disease from latent infection.

DIAGNOSIS
- Culture is the gold-standard; it also allows for determining drug susceptibility.
- PCR (nucleic acid amplification) tests can be performed directly on clinical specimens in untreated pts. Sensitive in smear + pulmonary pts. Less sensitive in smear-negative and extrapulmonary specimens.
- AFB smear provides indication of infectiousness, i.e., AFB smear-positive more infectious than smear-negative.
- IFN-gamma release assays (QuantiFERON-Gold, T.SPOT.TB) have been approved by the FDA for diagnosis of TB infection and disease, but they cannot distinguish between infection and disease.

TREATMENT
Adults
- Typically four drugs used for 8 wks, then using susceptibilities 2 or 3 drugs (usually INH + RIF) are used for balance of duration.
- **Initial therapy:** INH 5 mg/kg (300 mg max) + RIF 10 mg/kg (600 mg max) + PZA 15–30 mg/kg (2 g max) + EMB 15–25 mg/kg (1.6 g max) + vit B6 50 mg—all PO and dosed once daily.
- Can use rifabutin in place of rifampin in persons on HIV-1 protease inhibitors, NNRTI, methadone. Dose adjustments necessary, TB always treated first unless pt already on HAART.
- Check drug susceptibilities when available. Treat with at least 2 drugs to which M. tb is susceptible.
- Treatment duration determined by site of disease, response to therapy.
- Usual duration 6 mos, but 9 mos if cavitary disease and cx (+) after 2 mos.
- For meningitis treatment, see Meningitis, TB.
- Bone/joint TB: longer duration typical, usually 9–12 mos.
- Refer to health department so pt. can receive directly-observed therapy (DOT).
- Dosing less frequently than daily is possible, but must be done via DOT.

Children
- **Initial therapy:** INH 10–15 mg/kg (300 mg max) + RIF 10–20 mg/kg (600 mg max) + PZA 15–30 mg/kg (2 g max) + EMB 15–20 mg/kg (1g max)–all PO and dosed once daily.
- After first 2 mos of treatment can decrease to INH + RIF if drug-susceptible (or presumed source case has drug-susceptible TB if culture and susceptibilities are unknown for the child).
- Use EMB only if can monitor visual acuity (e.g., usually age >8 yrs).
- Can use rifabutin in place of rifampin in persons on HIV protease inhibitors, NNRTI. Dose adjustments necessary.
- Check drug susceptibilities; treat with at least 2 drugs to which M. tb is susceptible.
- Rx duration determined by site of disease, response to therapy.
- Refer to health department so pt. can receive directly observed therapy (DOT).
- Dosing less frequently than daily is possible, but must be done via DOT.

Infection Control

- TB isolation: cough >2 wks + abnormal CXR.
- Can discontinue if 3 sputums (expectorated or induced) are AFB smear-negative. Three expectorated can be within 24 hrs if one specimen is from early AM.
- If AFB smear-positive or on TB treatment, can discontinue infection control after 2 wks of treatment, clinical improvement, and AFB smear-negative. Special concern if pt will be transferred to high-risk setting (e.g., nursing home, homeless shelter, contact with immunocompromised persons).

Follow Up

- Refer all cases to local health dept for treatment and contact investigation.
- Directly-observed therapy (DOT) preferred for both adults and children.
- If adverse drug reactions prompt change in 4 or later 2 drug therapy, this is best done is close consultation with a health expert in TB or infectious diseases.

Other Information

- Guidelines based on ATS/CDC Guidelines. Am J Respir Crit Care Med 2003;167:603-62. This includes a new recommendation to extend treatment to 9 mos if cavitary disease plus cx + after 2 mos.
- TB Rx in HIV-infected pt: concern re: drug interactions, immune reconstitution inflammatory syndrome (IRIS), drug toxicity.

Basis for Recommendations

Kaplan JE, Benson C, Holmes KK, et al. Guidelines for Prevention and Treatment of Opportunistic Infections in HIV-Infected Adults and Adolescents. *MMWR*, 2009; Vol. 58; pp. 1–198.
Comments: Additional updates on concomitant TB/HIV treatment.

Blumberg HM, Burman WJ, Chaisson RE, et al. American Thoracic Society/Centers for Disease Control and Prevention/Infectious Diseases Society of America: treatment of tuberculosis. *Am J Respir Crit Care Med*, 2003; Vol. 167; pp. 603–62.
Comments: These guidelines include new recommendation to extend treatment to 9 mos if cavitary disease plus cx + after 2 mos of Rx. Also new: INH+RPT once/wk may be given in continuation phase if noncavitary disease, sputum smear-neg after 2 mos, and pt HIV-negative.

TUBERCULOSIS, LATENT

Timothy Sterling, MD

Pathogens

- *Mycobacterium tuberculosis*

Clinical

- Evidence of latent infection (and indication to treat) based on mm induration on tuberculin skin test (TST), TB risk.
- Unless risk factors present, routine TST not advocated.
- **5mm:** HIV+, close contact of TB case, fibrosis on CXR, or immunosuppressed (e.g., prednisone >15 mg/day for >1 mo).
- **10 mm:** recent immigrant, injection drug user, resident/employee of prison, jail, nursing home, hospital, shelter, diabetes, renal failure, leukemia/lymphoma, weight loss, gastrectomy; child <4 yrs.
- Recent converter: >10 mm increase in induration within 2 yrs of last negative PPD.
- If meet above high-risk criteria, treat regardless of age.
- **15mm:** all others.
- Interferon gamma release assays (QuantiFERON TB-Gold, T.SPOT.TB) may also be used. Like the TST, they do not distinguish between active TB and latent infection.

Diagnosis

- The tuberculin skin test (TST) has been used for >100 yrs. Low sensitivity in immunocompromised persons. Low specificity due to false-positive tests from BCG and environmental mycobacteria.
- Obtain CXR if skin test +. Obtain sputum AFB if CXR abnormal and/or symptomatic. Must rule out active TB before starting treatment for latent infection.

- Interferon-gamma release assays like QuantiFERON TB-Gold and T.SPOT.TB are more specific than the TST, particularly in persons with prior BCG vaccination, but may also have decreased sensitivity in immunocompromised pts. CDC has guidelines for the use of these assays.
- Both QuantiFERON TB-Gold and T.SPOT.TB are FDA-approved.

TREATMENT

HIV-seronegative Adults
- **Preferred:** isoniazid 5 mg/kg (300 mg max) PO every day × 9 mos. Pyridoxine (vit B6) 50 mg PO every day may decrease neuropathy risk.
- **Alt:** rifampin 10 mg/kg (600 mg max) PO every day × 4 mos. [be wary of interactions with rifampin: antiretrovirals, methadone, oral contraceptives, anticoagulants, steroids, etc.].
- Monitoring for toxicity: INH—baseline LFTs in pts at increased risk of hepatotoxicity (HIV+, hx of liver disease, EtOH, pregnant or <3 mos post-partum).
- RIF/PZA (2 mos) not recommended by CDC due to hepatotoxicity.

HIV-seropositive Adults
- Isoniazid 5 mg/kg (300 mg max) PO every day × 9 mos. Pyridoxine (vit B6) 50 mg PO every day may decrease neuropathy risk.

Children <18 yrs
- Isoniazid 10–20 mg/kg (300 mg max) every day × 9 mos. Pyridoxine (vit B6) generally unnecessary.

FOLLOW UP
- For pts receiving INH, follow for signs and symptoms of hepatotoxicity such as loss of appetite, nausea, abdominal pain, etc. Routine LFT testing is unnecessary if clinically well.

OTHER INFORMATION
- Must exclude active TB before treatment of latent infection (TLI).
- If HIV+, eligible for TLI if close contact of TB case even if skin-test negative, or prior TLI.

BASIS FOR RECOMMENDATIONS

Blumberg HM, Leonard MK, Jasmer RM. Update on the treatment of tuberculosis and latent tuberculosis infection. *JAMA*, 2005; Vol. 293; pp. 2776–84.

Comments: Update on the treatment of latent infection.

UPPER RESPIRATORY INFECTIONS

John G. Bartlett, MD

PATHOGENS
- *Rhinovirus*
- *Influenza virus*
- *Coronavirus*
- *Respiratory syncytial virus* (RSV)
- *Parainfluenza virus*
- *Metapneumovirus*
- *Adenovirus*

CLINICAL
- Acute infection, usually of viral origin, involving the upper airways and often sinuses, pharynx, larynx, or bronchi, i.e., sinusitis, laryngitis, pharyngitis and bronchitis.
- PE: depends on area of involvement, e.g., red throat, nasal pus (yellow or green), etc.

DIAGNOSIS
- Dx: clinical syndrome with nasal secretion +/− nasal obstruction. No cultures needed. Note: allergies often mimic URTIs.
- Often accompanied by pharyngitis and/or acute cough.
- Differential diagnosis: most often, allergic rhinitis (pollutants).
- Need to R/O pneumonia, epiglottitis, cervical deep space infection, thrush (HIV).
- Pathogen detection: New PCR-based method to detect 12 viral pathogens in respiratory secretions (FDA cleared).

TREATMENT
Common cold

- Principles: viral infection—symptomatic treatment +/− antiinfluenza agent. For allergy—topical steroids, and non-sedating antihistamines (loratadine, etc).
- Preferred (Irwin NEJM 2000; 343:1715): nasal decongestants, sedating antihistamines, anticholinergic and antiinflammatory agents (see below).
- Decongestants: pseudoephedrine and sedating antihistamine such as dexbrompheniramine, brompheniramine chlorpheniramine, diphenhydramine carbinoxamine—OTC as Actifed, Atrofed, Cardec, etc.
- Anticholinergic: ipratropium bromide nasal spray (Atrovent 0.6%) 2 sprays each nostril 3–4 ×/day.
- Oral decongestant: pseudoephedrine, 120 mg PO twice daily (available OTC).
- Nasal sprays: oxymetazoline nasal solutions (0.05%)—Afrin, Allerest, Dristan, Neo-Synephrine, 2–3 gtts/nostril twice daily. Otrivin, Vicks vapor inhaler, etc: 2–6 sprays/nostril no more than q2–10h.
- Anti-inflammatory agents: ASA, acetaminophen, naproxen (Aleve)(not ibuprofen).
- Antihistamines—sedating 1st generation: preferred—diphenhydramine (Benadryl), hydroxyzine (Atarax).
- Heated humidified air.

Allergic basis

- Nasal steroids such as fluticasone (Flonase), flunisolide (Nasalide), beclomethasone (Beconase), triamcinolone (Nasacort), budesonide (Rhinocort)—all 2 sprays twice daily.
- Antihistamine—2nd generation nonsedating such as fexofenadine (Allegra) 60 mg PO twice daily or loratadine (Claritin) 10 mg PO once daily.
- Avoid allergen exposure.

Controversial/prevention

- Zinc gluconate lozenges 13–23 mg Zn, 1q2h while awake: conflicting data.
- Vitamin C: probably no benefit.
- Humidified hot air.
- Prevention: avoid hand contact and aerosol; flu vaccine or anti-influenza agents; fresh air circulation in office (*rhinovirus*).
- Avoid active and passive smoking.
- Gargling water ≥3 ×/day.
- "10 foot rule": Pts with URIs need to be ≥10 feet from others in waiting rooms, etc.

OTHER INFORMATION

- Viral URIs are a major cause of sinusitis, otitis, bronchitis, laryngitis, exacerbations of bronchitis and asthma.
- URI does not benefit from antibiotics, but is a major cause of antibiotic abuse.

BASIS FOR RECOMMENDATIONS

Snow V, Mottur-Pilson C, Gonzales R, et al. Principles of appropriate antibiotic use for treatment of nonspecific upper respiratory tract infections in adults. *Ann Intern Med*, 2001; Vol. 134; pp. 487–9.

Comments: The authors emphasize the frequent abuse of antibiotics in this condition. Review of controlled trial data does not support it.

Irwin RS, Madison JM. The diagnosis and treatment of cough. *N Engl J Med*, 2000; Vol. 343; pp. 1715–21.

Comments: The authors Recommend the Following Treatment for The Common Cold: dexbrompheniramine 6 mg + pseudoephedrine 120 mg* twice daily × 1 wk; or naproxen 500 mg three times a day × 5 days or ipratropium (0.06%) nasal spray, 2 spays/nostril 3–4 ×/days × 4 days. Importance of 1st vs 2nd generates antihistamine stressed. (*if not hypotensive)

Sepsis—Syndromes

SEPSIS—UNKNOWN SOURCE

John G. Bartlett, MD

PATHOGENS

- *E. coli*
- Other Enterobacteriaceae—*Klebsiella, Enterobacter*, etc.
- Non-fermenters: Pseudomonas, *Serratia*
- *Staphylococcus aureus*
- Toxin mediated: Staphylococcal or streptococcal toxic shock, *C. difficile, C. sordellii*
- *S. pneumoniae, N. meningitis*
- *Candida* species
- Other causes (less common): *Salmonella enteritidis, S. typhi, Plasmodium falciparum, Listeria monocytogenes.*

CLINICAL

- Classic signs sepsis: fever, chills and hypotension.
- Systemic inflammatory response syndrome (SIRS): 2 or more of the following: fever (T>38°C) or hypothermia (T<36°C), tachycardia (HR>90), tachypnea (RR>20), leukocytosis (WBC>12,000 or differential w/ >10% bands).
- Systemic inflammatory response syndrome (SIRS): sepsis + non-infectious processes, e.g., burns, pancreatitis.
- Sepsis: SIRS + infection (e.g., positive blood culture).
- Sepsis syndrome: infection + temperature >38.3°C or <35.6°C + pulse >90 + RR >20 + either—altered mental status, p_aO_2 <75, increased lactate or oliguria.
- Severe sepsis: sepsis + organ failure, decreased perfusion (lactic acidosis, oliguria, altered mental status) **or** low BP.
- Septic shock: hypotension despite fluids + lactic acidosis, oliguria, altered mental status.
- **Special populations:** Neonatal (< 1 wk): Group B streptococci, *E. coli*. HIV with CD4 < 50–100: MAC, CMV, TB, line sepsis, ABC hypersensitivity, Cryptococcus. Injection drug users: *S. aureus*, esp. MRSA. Splenectomized pts: *Streptococcus pneumoniae, Haemophilus influenzae, Neisseria meningitidis, Capnocytophaga canimorsus*. Neutropenic: GNB, Aspergillus. Traveler: malaria, salmonellosis. Healthy young adult: toxic shock syndromes (*S. aureus* or group A strep), *N. meningitidis,* Rocky Mt Spotted fever, bioterrorism (anthrax, plague, etc.), hantavirus.
- Diagnostic clues: Ecthyma gangrenosum—*Pseudomonas aeruginosa;* petechiae or purpura—*Neisseria meningitidis* or Rickettsial infection.

DIAGNOSIS

- Clinical definitions as above.
- Blood cultures typically positive but may not be so in toxic shock syndromes, RMSF, malaria, etc.
- Obtain blood cultures × 2 (1 via each access device) + urine cx + other suspect sources.

TREATMENT

Antibiotic selection (all parenteral)

- Empiric: piperacillin-tazobactam 3.375–4.5 g IV q6h + vancomycin 15 mg/kg q12h +/− tobramycin 5–7 mg/kg/day—starting within 1 hr of pt presentation.
- Alt: aminoglycoside, e.g., gentamicin or tobramycin 5 mg/kg/day or amikacin 15 mg/kg/day all IV.
- Alt: beta-lactam (IV, choose one): cefotaxime 2 g q6h, ceftriaxone 1 g q12h, cefepime 2 g q12h, ceftazidime 2 g q8h, imipenem 0.5–1 g q6h, meropenem 1 g q8h or piperacillin-tazobactam 3.375 g q6h.
- Vancomycin should be dosed 15 mg/kg q12h if normal renal function with trough goal of 10–15 mcg/mL.
- Neutropenia: ceftazidime, imipenem or cefepime +/− aminoglycoside.
- Intra-abdominal sepsis: ticarcillin-clavulanate, piperacillin-tazobactam, imipenem, meropenem, doripenem; all +/− aminoglycoside.

- Fast administration of correct antibiotics probably yields more survival advantage than fluids, pressor agents or steroid administration.
- Refine antibiotics when culture results available.

Tissue perfusion maneuvers

- Resuscitation: rapid IV fluids, then packed RBC to Hct >30% and/or dobutamine <20 µg/kg/min.
- Resuscitation goals: CVP 8–12 mm Hg, mean arterial pressure >65, urine output >0.5 ml/kg/hr; venous O_2 sat >70%.
- Fluids: colloids and crystalloids are both equally effective.
- Vasopressors: norepinephrine (usual adult: 0.1 mg/kg/min then 0.05 mcg/kg/min) or dopamine (2–25 µg/kg/min) to keep BP >65 systolic.
- Inotropic agent: dobutamine to increase cardiac output.
- Glycemic control: blood glucose <150 mg/dL.
- Control Source of infection if so identified (e.g., interventional radiology drainage, surgery).
- Blood: transfuse if Hgb <7 g/dL, target goal Hgb >7–9 g/dL.
- Activated protein C (drotrecogin): APACHE >25, septic shock, >1 organ dysfunction and no bleeding risks. Dose 24 mcg/kg/hr continuous IV infusion × 96 hrs.
- Hypoxemia: PEEP (concern for barotrauma).
- No longer advocated (2008): corticosteroids or intensive insulin therapy.

OTHER INFORMATION

- Septic shock (persistent hypotension): blood cx positive in 50%, mortality is 30%–50%.
- Sepsis mortality increased by: wrong abx, increased age, nosocomial origin, resp > abd > urinary infections, underlying disease, complications (decreased BP, decreased temp, anuria), shock.
- Complications: bleeding, leukopenia, thrombocytopenia, acidosis, oliguria, jaundice, DIC, CHF, ARDS.

BASIS FOR RECOMMENDATIONS

Dellinger RP, Carlet JM, Masur H, et al. Surviving Sepsis Campaign guidelines for management of severe sepsis and septic shock. *Crit Care Med*, 2004; Vol. 32; pp. 858–73.
Comments: The basis for management of septic shock recommended here in this module.
The Medical Letter. Treatment guidelines for the Medical Letter: choice of antibacterial drugs. *Med Letter*, 2004; Vol. 2; p. 13.
Comments: Basis for antibiotic selection for sepsis without a known source in these recommendations.

STAPHYLOCOCCAL TOXIC SHOCK SYNDROME

Joel Blankson, MD, PhD

PATHOGENS

- Methicillin Sensitive *Staphylococcus aureus* (MSSA)
- Methicillin Resistant *Staphylococcus aureus* (MRSA)
- Toxin occurs in ~1% of *S. aureus* strains.

CLINICAL

- CDC TSS dx based upon 5 clinical criteria.
- **Fever:** T > 38.9°C. **Hypotension:** SBP <90 in adults or < 5th percentile for children <16 yrs, includes orthostatic hypotension (pts commonly faint or are dizzy upon standing).
- **Rash:** diffuse macular erythroderma often sunburn-like. Later, **d esquamation** of palms and soles usually involved, typically 1–2 wks after onset of illness.
- **Multisystem involvement (3 or > of following)** a) GI: vomiting, diarrhea at onset, b) musculoskeletal: CPK > 2X nl or severe myalgia c) Renal: BUN/creatinine > 2X nl or sterile pyuria.
- d) Hepatic: bilirubin, AST or ALT > 2X nl, e) Hematologic: plts < 100 000/mm³, f) CNS: altered mental status without focal neurologic signs. g) mucous membranes: red eyes, mouth and vagina.
- Negative Cx for other explanation e.g., blood, throat, or CSF cultures (Cx can be positive for *S. aureus*). There should not be an increase in titer to Rocky Mountain spotted fever, leptospira, rubeola antibodies.

DIAGNOSIS

- Tampon use has been a historical risk factor, but is now less common due to a change in manufacture.

DIAGNOSIS
- Based upon clinical symptoms and microbiology listed above.
- Serology for TSS toxin is usually negative.

TREATMENT
Clindamycin 900 mg IV q8hrs + oxacillin 2 g IV q 4 hrs for methicillin sensitive *S. aureus* (MSSA).
- Clindamycin 900 mg IV q8hrs + vancomycin 1 g IV q12 hrs for methicillin resistant *S. aureus* (MRSA). Some favor linezolid instead of vancomycin or clindamycin if MRSA is a concern, mainly due to protein synthesis inhibition.
- Consider IVIG: 2 g/kg IV X 1, repeat in 48 hrs if pt remains unstable.
- Supportive care and ICU monitoring.

OTHER INFORMATION
- *S. aureus* produces the enterotoxins, TSST-1, SEB, and SEC. These toxins are superantigens capable of activating up to 25% of T cells.
- Therapy guided at stopping toxin production. Clindamycin inhibits protein synthesis and is the drug of choice if susceptible.
- Most pts with Staph TSS have been shown to lack antibodies to the toxin, and pooled IVIG contains these antibodies to this common antigen.
- No controlled studies exist for IVIG therapy in *S. aureus* TSS, but a small study showed a decrease in mortality in Streptococcal TSS.
- A mortality rate of 3–5% is generally quoted for *S. aureus* TSS.

BASIS FOR RECOMMENDATIONS
Russell NE, Pachorek RE. Clindamycin in the treatment of streptococcal and staphylococcal toxic shock syndromes. *Ann Pharmacother*, 2001; Vol. 34; pp. 936–9.
Comments: This review article summarizes the experimental data on the efficacy of clindamycin in the treatment of staphylococcal and streptococcal toxic shock syndromes.

STREPTOCOCCAL TOXIC SHOCK SYNDROME

Joel Blankson, MD, PhD

PATHOGENS
- *Streptococcus pyogenes* (Group A)

CLINICAL
- Severe multiorgan system illness with abrupt onset that requires the following findings:
- Clinical signs of severe disease **A. Hypotension:** SBP <90 or <5th percentile in children AND **B. Multisystem involvement:** 2 or more of the following systems:
- **1. Renal:** creatinine > 2X baseline **2. Hematologic:** P \ plts < 100, 000/mm³ or diss. intravascular coagulopathy **3. Hepatic:** bilirubin, AST/ALT >2x nl. **4. Pulmonary:** ARDS **5. Derm:** generalized erythematous rash that may later desquamate. Soft tissue necrosis, including necrotizing fasciitis, myositis, or gangrene.
- Ddx includes: *S. aureus* (toxic shock syndrome), RMSF, *Leptospira interrogans, Neisseria meningitidis, Streptococcus pneumoniae.*
- Recent studies have reported a >40% case fatality rate.

DIAGNOSIS
- Isolation of *S. pyogenes* [Group A Streptococci] A. from a normally sterile site (e.g. blood, CSF) B. from a non sterile site (e.g. throat, superficial skin lesion).
- Clinical sx as described above.

TREATMENT
- Surgical debridement essential for GAS associated necrotizing fasciitis or myositis.
- Clindamycin 900 mg IV q8hrs + PCN G 4 million units IV q4hrs for GAS.
- Consider IVIG: the studied dose in RCT is 1 g/kg (day 1) and 0.5 g/kg (days 2 and 3).
- Supportive cares and ICU monitoring.

DIAGNOSIS

OTHER INFORMATION

- *S. pyogenes* produces exotoxins SPEA, SPEB, and SPEC. These toxins are superantigens capable of activating up to 25% of T cells. Therapy guided at stopping toxin production.
- Clindamycin inhibits toxin synthesis and is the drug of choice.
- A small comparative observational study showed a decrease in mortality in Streptococcal TSS associated with IVIG tx.
- A follow up double blind, placebo controlled study found decreased mortality (but did not reach statistical significance) in Streptococcal TSS associated with IVIG tx.
- Early surgical intervention is crucial for fasciitis or myonecrosis. Suspect when pain is out of proportion to exam.

BASIS FOR RECOMMENDATIONS

Russell NE, Pachorek RE. Clindamycin in the treatment of streptococcal and staphylococcal toxic shock syndromes. *Ann Pharmacother*, 2001; Vol. 34; pp. 936–9.

Comments: This review article summarizes the experimental data on the efficacy of clindamycin in the treatment of staphylococcal and streptococcal toxic shock syndromes.

VASCULAR CATHETER–ASSOCIATED INFECTION

John G. Bartlett, MD

PATHOGENS

- Coagulase-negative staphylococcus (37%)
- *Staphylococcus aureus* (13%)
- Enterococcus (13%)
- Gram-negative bacilli (14%)
- Candida species (8%)
- Origins of most pathogens: skin, contamination of catheter hub, contaminated infusion solution, or hematogenous seeding.

CLINICAL

- Bacteremia: fever + no alternate source + same pathogen peripheral blood and significant growth from catheter tip.
- Catheter colonization: significant growth from catheter tip only (>15 colonies) with negative peripheral blood cultures.
- **Phlebitis:** suspect if hot, red, and tender at catheter exit site. **Tunnel infection:** hot, red and tender if >2 cm from skin exit site.
- Sites of infection: 1. blood = bacteremia, 2. catheter insertion site: phlebitis (may be due to chemical or infection), 3. pocket, and 4. complicated: sepsis, phlebitis, and/or associated abscess.

DIAGNOSIS

- Obtain two sets of blood cultures, at least one peripheral.
- Central venous catheters: may roll tip, if >15 colonies, suggests line colonized/source.
- If negative blood cultures, and catheter tip culture negative, seek other source or consider mycobacterial infection.

TREATMENT

Removable central venous catheters (CVCs)

- DX: obtain 2 blood cultures (at least 1 peripheral blood cx, PBC): d/c CVC, culture catheter tip, insert new line.
- Empiric abx: if seriously ill—low BP, organ failure.
- PBC negative and CVC >15 colony forming units (CFU): monitor for infection and blood cultures if known heart valve disease, neutropenia, *Candida* or *S. aureus*.
- PBC positive + CVC positive due to coagulase-negative staphylococci: d/c CVC + treat with abx 7 days OR keep CVC + use IV abx IV + abx lock solution × 10–14 days.
- PBC and CVC both positive due *to S. aureus* : d/c CVC + obtain TTE/TEE. If echocardiography without vegetation treat with appropriate abx 14 days. If vegetation found treat for endocarditis.
- PBC and CVC both positive with complication (endocarditis, osteomyelitis, septic phlebitis): d/c CVC + abx 4–6 wks for identified pathogen.
- PBC and CVC both positive due to GNB or *Candida*: d/c CVC + use appropriate abx × 14 days.

Tunneled CVCs

- Tunnel or mediport infection w/ abscess (negative blood cxs): d/c line + abx × 10–14 days.
- Complication (e.g., septic phlebitis, endocarditis, osteomyelitis): d/c line + appropriate abx 4–6 wks.
- Coagulase negative staphylococci: keep line + use appropriate abx and abx lock treatment × 10–14 days.
- *S. aureus*: if TEE is negative for vegetation (no endocarditis), d/c line + abx 14 days.
- GNB: d/c line + use appropriate abx 10–14 days OR keep line if pt stable + treat with abx IV + abx lock therapy × 14 days.
- *Candida albicans* or other Candida species: d/c line + appropriate antifungal × 14 days from last positive blood cx. Consider echocardiogram, ophthalmological exam to rule out endocarditis or endophthalmitis.

Miscellaneous information

- Once permanent line removed: consider replacement only after bacteremia/fungemia clears.
- Empiric abx: goal to cover MRSA and resistant Gram-negative pathogens. Examples, vancomycin + ceftazidime or cefepime.
- CVC culture: roll tip on agar plate. If >15 CFU or sonicated tip >10^2 CFU = infection.
- Hemodialysis catheters: colonization occurs in 10–55%, if bacteremia occurs complications such as endocarditis, osteomyelitis, septic phlebitis not uncommon.
- Septic thrombophlebitis: d/c line, surgical consultation for potential vein ligation/removal, abx × 4–6 wks.
- Indications for 6 wks of IV therapy with *S. aureus* line sepsis for presumed endocarditis: (1) persistent fever × >72 hrs; (2) prosthetic valve; or (3) positive blood culture at 72 hrs.

Antibiotic lock solutions

- Rationale is that local antibiotic concentrations are 40–120 × greater than peak blood concentrations.
- Consider abx lock therapy only in uncomplicated infections, typically non-tunneled coagulase negative staphylococcal infections or uncomplicated tunneled cath/port infections with CoNS, *S. aureus,* or Gram-negative bacilli.
- Don't use if complicated infection, candidal infections.
- Always use in combination with systemic antibiotics.
- 1–5 mg/ml of abx + heparin 50–100 u **or** saline to fill lumen of catheter (typically 2–5 ml).
- Dwell time of solution in catheter should be at least 12 hrs.
- Vancomycin (1–5 mg/ml), gentamicin (1–2 mg/ml) and amikacin (1–2 mg/ml) typically used. Others: cefazolin (5 mg/ml), ceftazidime (0.5 mg/ml), ciprofloxacin (1–2 mg/ml). Most solutions stable for 72 hrs at 37°C.
- Ethanol lock a recent proposal to salvage long-term catheters. Typically regimen is to place solution in for 12–24 hrs/day × 5 days. Solution is 25–50% ethyl alcohol or medical-grade ethanol to fill lumen(s).

Prevention

- CVC are 5–10 × more likely to be the source of line sepsis than peripheral line.
- CVC or PICC line insertion: use maximal barrier precautions.
- Catheters impregnated with antimicrobials or antiseptics can decrease risk in first 14 days.
- Antibiotic lock (flushing and filling catheter w/ abx solution): may reduce incidence of bacteremia but risks propagating resistance.
- Routine replacement of non-clinically infected CVCs and peripheral lines is not necessary.

OTHER INFORMATION

- Main dx issue: matching blood culture and catheter tip cultures.
- Main rx issues: (1) line removal: peripheral-D/C line; CVC-line salvage option best with coagulase-negative Staphylococci; (2) duration abx treatment—usually 7–14 days.
- Feared complications: *S. aureus*—endocarditis, septic phlebitis and osteomyelitis; *Candida*—endophthalmitis; GNB—septic shock.
- Infection within 7 days of catheter insertion, pathogens most likely from skin. If >7 days after insertion, likely due to hub contamination.

BASIS FOR RECOMMENDATIONS

O'Grady N, et al. Guidelines for Prevention of Intravascular Cathether-Related Infections. *Clin Infect Dis*, 2002; Vol. 35; pp. 1281–307.

Comments: IDSA Guidelines for Prevention of IV Cathether-Associated Infections.

Mermel LA, Farr BM, Sherertz RJ, et al. Guidelines for the management of intravascular catheter-related infections. *Clin Infect Dis*, 2001; Vol. 32; pp. 1249–72.

Comments: This document is basis for recommendations given here. Guidelines are given for all types of lines-peripheral, CVC, CVC w/ tunneled procedure, pockets for IV devices hemodialysis cath. They provide a review of 514 episodes of septicemia in association with tunneled cath which showed successful cath salvage in 342(67%). The greatest success was w/ *S. epidermidis* infections. A review of 3 observational studies showed cath removal is associated w/ a more rapid response when *S. AUREUS* is involved. A review of 40 cases of bacteremia managed with lock therapy permitted line salvage in all cases.

DIAGNOSIS

Soft Tissue

BITE WOUNDS

John G. Bartlett, MD

PATHOGENS
- *Pasteurella multocida* (cats and dogs)
- *Capnocytophaga canimorsus* (dogs)
- *Eikenella corrodens* (humans)
- *Streptococcus* spp. (all bites), especially *S. anginosus*
- *Staphylococcus aureus* (all bites)
- *Staphylococcus intermedius* (dogs)
- Anaerobes (all bites), especially *Prevotella* spp.

CLINICAL
- Module recommendations includes bites of humans, cats, dogs, bats (not insects).
- Bite-related infections may cause cellulitis, abscesses, purulent tenosynovitis, septic arthritis and osteomyelitis (especially puncture injuries).
- Human bite wounds or closed fist injuries may be minimized or falsely reported by pt, so press for accurate history. Consider any injury over the MCPs as potential for infection.

DIAGNOSIS
- Wound <8 hrs old: crush or puncture wound, scratches (too early for infection).
- Wound >8 hrs old: examine for signs of infection such as fever, cellulitis, purulent drainage, abscess.
- Gram-stain and culture for aerobes/anaerobes important (swab or tissue).
- Radiographs to assess for osteomyelitis.

TREATMENT
General care
- Principles: (1) clean and debride, (2) Abx (severe early or late and infected) usually amoxicillin/clavulanate (875 mg PO twice daily), (3) tetanus toxoid, (4) animal bite—consider rabies (rare except w/ bat exposure in U.S.).
- Clean wound: copious soap and water, alcohol, povidone-iodine; puncture wound—use high pressure irrigation w/20 ml syringe with #18 needle.
- Debride necrotic tissue; immobilize and elevate extremity.
- Wound closure: usually not sutured except early uninfected wound and facial wounds; use adhesive strips to approximate edges.
- Tetanus vaccine hx: if <u>≤3 doses or unknown</u> and minor wound—use tetanus toxoid (Td) series 0.5 ml at 0, 1–2 mos and 6–12 mos. Severe injury: Td series + tetanus immune globulin.

Antibiotic prophylaxis and treatment
- **Prophylaxis indications:** severe injury <8 hrs, crush injury; bone or joint penetration, wound of face, hand, or genitals; immunosuppressed host.
- Preferred prophylaxis: amoxicillin/clavulanate (Augmentin) 875/125 mg PO twice daily × 7 days.
- Alternative: moxifloxacin (Avelox) 400 mg PO once daily × 7 days.
- Alternatives: amoxicillin, doxycycline, cefuroxime (active vs. most oral flora of man and animals).
- **Treatment of infection** (established infection, hospitalized pts, preferred): ampicillin-sulbactam (Unasyn) 1–2 g IV q6h or ticarcillin-clavulanate (Timentin) 3–6 g IV q4–6h.
- Alternatives: cefoxitin 1–2 g IV q6h or moxifloxacin 400 mg IV q24h.
- Outpatient treatment (preferred): amoxicillin/clavulanate (Augmentin) either 875/125 mg PO twice daily or 2000 (XR)/125 mg twice daily.
- Alt: moxifloxacin 400 mg PO once daily, azithromycin 500 mg PO, then 250 mg once daily.

Rabies Prophylaxis
- (1) Wash wound with soap; (2) capture animal (if possible without injury), (3) report to public health department.
- Do not keep or handle bats and get them out of enclosures.

- Presumed exposure: dog or cat with suspected rabies; presumed risk with bite from raccoon, skunk, bat, fox.
- Reality issue: 1990–2003 record with 30 human cases in U.S., 28 had no prior hx of bite and most were bat associated.
- Rabies prophylaxis (see Rabies module, p. 437): (1) wound cleansing ASAP—alcohol or iodine; (2) vaccine × 5 IM doses; (3) RIG-expensive, scarce and only for severe bites.
- Vaccine: Imovax (800-822-2463) or RabAvert (PCEC) 1 ml day 0, 3, 7, 14, and 28 (800-244-7668) Rabipur (outside U.S.) 1 ml IM days 0, 3, 7, 14, and 28.
- RIG (800-822-2463) 20 IU/ kg—1/2 IM and 1/2 into wound.
- No human-human transmission except cases with organ transplant (2004).

FOLLOW UP
- All bite wounds managed as an outpatient should have follow-up within 1–2 days of initial diagnosis and treatment, especially to see if infection prevented/arrested and/or surgical attention required.

OTHER INFORMATION
- Bacteriology: oral flora of donor and or skin flora of recipient (*S. aureus*).
- Oral flora: dogs—*P. multocida, C. canimorsus,* anaerobes; cats—*P. multocida, anaerobes,* humans—Streptococci, Eikenella, anaerobes.
- Rabies prophylaxis—worry about bats, raccoons and skunks; dogs in developing countries; only 2 non-bat animal bites associated rabies cases in U.S. 1990–2003.
- Most wounds are left open with approximation of edges using adhesive strips; suture only clean wounds and face wounds (cosmetic issue).

BASIS FOR RECOMMENDATIONS
Rupprecht CE, Gibbons RV. Clinical practice. Prophylaxis against rabies. *N Engl J Med*, 2004; Vol. 351; pp. 2626–35.
Comments: Source of recommendations given here.

Talan DA, Citron DM, Abrahamian FM, et al. Bacteriologic analysis of infected dog and cat bites. Emergency Medicine Animal Bite Infection Study Group. *N Engl J Med*, 1999; Vol. 340; pp. 85–92.
Comments: Multicenter study of the bacteriology of dog and cat bites seen in emergency rooms. The major isolates were *S. aureus, Pasteurella multocida,* and anaerobes.

CELLULITIS/ERYSIPELAS see p. 33 in Dermatologic Section

GAS GANGRENE

John G. Bartlett, MD

PATHOGENS
- *Clostridium perfringens*
- *Clostridium novyi*
- *Clostridium septicum*
- *Clostridium histolyticum*
- *Clostridium sordellii* (toxic shock after childbirth and with contaminated heroin injections)

CLINICAL
- Severe pain within 24 hrs, then rapid progression w/ fever, shock, hemolysis, renal failure. Wound shows tense edema that changes color: white to bronze to dark with blebs.
- Other processes often accompanying include hemolytic anemia, leukocytosis, and renal failure. Clinical course rapid.
- Ddx: streptococcal (Group A strep) myonecrosis, necrotizing fasciitis, *Vibrio vulnificus,* *Aeromonas* spp.

DIAGNOSIS
- Aspirates of bullae or muscle show "box-car" Gram-positive bacilli on Gram-stain.
- Cx of blood, muscle or bullae yield *Clostridia* spp., usually *C. perfringens.*
- X-rays shows gas in tissue.
- CT scan w/ evidence of myonecrosis.
- Note: less than 1% of cultures blood and infected tissues yielding *Clostridia* spp. represent gas gangrene—most isolates represent contaminants and some are mixed infections. Must correlate cx with clinical scenario.

DIAGNOSIS

TREATMENT

Antibiotics

- Principles: rare but critical to dx early. Dx based on hx of injury/surgery + severe pain + soft tissue changes + CT/MRI. Need surgeon + abx ASAP.
- Preferred: clindamycin 600–900 mg IV q6h + penicillin 2–4 million units IV q4h × 10–28 days (covers clostridia + streptococci and the 5% of clostridia that are clindamycin-resistant.
- Alt: clindamycin 600–900 mg IV q6h + cefotaxime 2–4 g IV q8h or imipenem 0.5–1 g IV q8h × 10–28 days (or meropenem, doripenem or ertapenem: covers clostridia, strep species, potential mixed infection w/ GNB).
- PCN allergy: clindamycin or chloramphenicol 1 g IV q6h.
- Most active *in vitro*: pen G, ampicillin, metronidazole, piperacillin, chloramphenicol, cefotaxime, imipenem. Clindamycin often used to reduce toxin production.
- Clostridia antitoxin: no longer available.
- Drugs that inhibit toxin at subinhibitory concentrations: clindamycin, metronidazole, tetracycline, chloramphenicol, and linezolid.
- Experimental gas gangrene response better to clindamycin, tetracycline, or chloramphenicol than penicillin or hyperbaric O_2.

Surgery

- Mutilating surgery or amputations often required.
- May need re-op daily to debride necrotic tissue.
- Uterine gas gangrene: total hysterectomy.
- Typhlitis (cecal inflammation with *C. tertium*): usually medical management, while *C. septicum*—may require laparotomy with resection.

Hyperbaric oxygen

- Role of hyperbaric O_2 debated.
- Advantages: often demarcates viable tissue to facilitate surgery, surgeons at O_2 chambers often have extensive experience.
- Disadvantages: pt transportation may delay critical surgery, unconvincing clinical response data.

OTHER INFORMATION

- Skin lesions with bullae ddx: necrotizing fasciitis, necrotizing synergistic cellulitis, Aeromonas infections, *Vibrio vulnificus*.
- Other serious soft tissue infections: necrotizing fasciitis (mixed coliforms + anaerobes or strep), myonecrosis (strep or clostridial), Aeromonas (fresh/brackish water exposure), Vibrio spp. (sea/oyster).
- Need surgical consultation immediately.

BASIS FOR RECOMMENDATIONS

Stevens DL, Bisno AL, Chambers HF, et al. Practice guidelines for the diagnosis and management of skin and soft-tissue infections. *Clin Infect Dis*, 2005; Vol. 41; pp. 1373–406.

Comments: Guidelines for treating gas gangrene are to use clindamycin + penicillin. Role of hyperbaric oxygen is unclear.

NECROTIZING FASCIITIS

John G. Bartlett, MD

PATHOGENS

- Mixed aerobic-anaerobic bacteria
- Group A streptococcus (GAS), *S. pyogenes*
- *Clostridium perfringens*
- Community-acquired MRSA
- *Vibrio vulnificus*

CLINICAL

- Infection extending along fascial plane—usually an extremity, perianal area, genitals (Fournier's).
- Clinical: severe pain, severe systemic toxicity, process with rapid spread, fever, skin necrosis with bullae, tense edema, and/or black-blue discoloration.

- Some pts have preceding injury or surgery; some do not.
- Differential diagnosis: 1. Cellulitis: treated with antibiotics and NO surgery (big difference), 2. Gas gangrene, 3. Vibrio vulnificus, 4. Soft tissue infection, 5. Myositis.
- Pus with anaerobic infection is "dishwater gray," has a characteristic putrid smell, and Gram-stain/culture of pus shows mixed flora.
- 3 major bacterial patterns: Group A streptococci, mixed anaerobes + coliforms, or MRSA (USA 300). Distinguish by GS and cx of exudate, bullae, aspirate, or blood.
- Mixed anaerobic infections are most common form—also requires rapid surgery.
- Host specific etiologies: a) diabetes, steroids: mucormycosis, b) burns, neutropenia: Pseudomonas gangrenous cellulitis, c) Exposure to aquacultured fish: *Streptococcus iniae*, d) Exposure to fresh/brackish waters: *Aeromonas* spp. and *Vibrio vulnificus*, e) Systemic infection: *N. meningitidis, Ps. aeruginosa.*

DIAGNOSIS
- Lab: CT scan or MRI showing fascial plane infection.
- Some pts should not be delayed by imaging studies, but rather have rapid surgical consultation and proceed to OR.

TREATMENT

Antibiotic treatment
- Principles: diagnosis by CT/MRI or surgery. Surgery urgent. Abx vs. strep (clindamycin) or anaerobes + coliforms (e.g., intra-abdominal sepsis regimens) and MRSA (vancomycin, clindamycin, or linezolid).
- Empiric regimen: Linezolid 600 mg IV q12h + either meropenem 1 g IV q8h or piperacillin/tazobactam 3.375 g IV q6h.
- Mixed infection with coliforms + anaerobes (preferred): cefotaxime 2–4 g IV q8h + either clindamycin 600 mg IV q8h or metronidazole 500 mg IV/PO q6h.
- Alternative: ampicillin/sulbactam (Unasyn) 1.5–3 g IV q6h or piperacillin/tazobactam (Zosyn) or ticarcillin/clavulanate (Timentin) or imipenem (Primaxin).
- Group A strep: clindamycin 600 mg IV q8h + penicillin 2–4 million units IV q4h.
- Community acquired MRSA: linezolid 600 mg IV q12h or vancomycin 1 g IV q12h.
- Modify antibiotic regimen when the pathogen is defined: (1) strep: give clindamycin + penicillin, (2) mixed anaerobes + coliforms: use regimen for intra-abdominal sepsis.

Surgery
- Incision + debridement mandatory.
- May require daily re-debridements.

Other treatment
- Supportive care: hydration, treatment of renal failure, wound care.
- Hyperbaric O_2: merit is debated. Problem is transfer of seriously ill pt and uncertain benefit.
- Hyperbaric O_2 (cont'd): possible benefit = surgeons affiliated. w/ facilities often expert regarding management of serious soft tissue infections, especially the need for extensive surgery and reoperation.
- Toxic-shock (streptococcal): IVIG (>2 batches: some use 50 g/dose, others 0.4 g/kg q6h IV).
- Infection control: Group A strep *and S. aureus* (MRSA), use contact precautions.
- Infection control: some consider Gr A strep transferable to family members, household contacts and healthcare workers, but risk is small.

FOLLOW UP
- Causes for alarm with soft tissue infection: (1) severe pain, (2) systemic toxicity, (3) bullae, (4) cutaneous necrosis, (5) gas in tissue, (6) tense edema.

OTHER INFORMATION
- Immediate Rx: (1) initiate abx vs. strep (clind +/– pen) and anaerobes/coliforms (regimens for intra-abd sepsis) and MRSA (clind+/–linezolid/vancomycin). (2) need surgeon ASAP. (3) if time available, obtain CT can or MRI to define extent of problem.
- Two major complications with Gr A streptococcal necrotizing fasciitis: rapid extension with necrosis and toxic shock syndrome.

BASIS FOR RECOMMENDATIONS
Stevens DL, Bisno AL, Chambers HF, et al. Practice guidelines for the diagnosis and management of skin and soft-tissue infections. *Clin Infect Dis*, 2005; Vol. 41; pp. 1373–406.
Comments: IDSA guidelines include those for necrotizing skin, skin structure and deeper infections.

Author opinion.
Comments: Additional information beyond existing guidelines.

PYOMYOSITIS

John G. Bartlett, MD

PATHOGENS

- *Staphylococcus aureus*—including MRSA
- Gram-negative bacilli (infrequent)
- Mixed infections with anaerobes
- Streptococci including *S. pneumoniae*
- Immunocompromised hosts (especially AIDS): aspergillus, mycobacteria (TB, MAI), salmonella, other Gram-negative bacilli

CLINICAL

- Presentation with painful, tender, localized swelling over muscle + fever. Larger muscle involved, typically (iliopsoas, quadriceps).
- Risk factors: HIV, IDU, penetrating trauma, tropical exposure ("tropical pyomyositis"), diabetes, steroids, cirrhosis.
- May be single or multiple sites and may result from trauma or occur spontaneously.
- Most common sites are large leg muscles, (quadriceps, gluteus, and psoas).
- Differential dx: necrotizing fasciitis, gas gangrene, cellulitis, carbuncle, streptococcal myositis, phlebitis.

DIAGNOSIS

- CT scan or MRI demonstrates muscle abscess.
- Aspiration of abscess (by surgery or CT/US guided) yields pus, usually yielding *S. aureus.*
- Bacteremia may accompany.

TREATMENT

Treatment based on Gram-stain/culture of aspirate

- *S. aureus* sensitivity to methicillin will dictate use of alternatives to beta-lactams, usually vancomycin but sometimes clindamycin, TMP-SMX, linezolid. Determine by *in vitro* testing. Unusual organisms guided by culture and susceptibility testing.
- Preferred: *S. aureus* (MSSA), use nafcillin/oxacillin 2 g IV q6h or cefazolin 500–1000 mg IV q8h × 14–28 days.
- *S. aureus* (MSSA and pen allergy): clindamycin, TMP-SMX, vancomycin.
- *S. aureus* (MRSA): vancomycin 15 mgkg IV q12h or linezolid 600 mg q12h PO/IV × 14–28 days.
- Staph, Strep, or anaerobes: clindamycin 600 mg IV q8h × 14–28 days.
- Anaerobes: ampicillin-sulbactam (Unasyn) 1.5–3 g IV q6h or clindamycin or piperacillin-tazobactam or ticarcillin-clavulanate or imipenem.

Surgery

- Open drainage or CT/US-guided aspirate with drainage.
- Complicated cases may require fasciotomies and debridement.
- Some respond to empiric antibiotic treatment vs. *S. aureus* without drainage.

OTHER INFORMATION

- *S. aureus* is most common pathogen.
- Predisposing conditions: HIV, IDU, penetrating trauma, tropical exposure ("tropical pyomyositis"), diabetes, steroids, cirrhosis.

BASIS FOR RECOMMENDATIONS

Harbarth SJ, Lew DP. Pyomyositis as a nontropical disease. *Current Clinical Topics in Infect Dis. Remington J, Swartz MN (Eds), Blackwell Science Publ*, 1997; pp. 37–50.
Comments: Emphasizes DIFFERENCES IN NON-TROPICAL CASES including associated conditions in about 50–60% including diabetes, cirrhosis, steroids, Felty syndrome, leukemia, sickle cell disease, HIV.

Author opinion.
Comments: No guidelines exist regarding therapy of pyomyositis.

GENITAL ULCER ADENOPATHY SYNDROME/GENITAL ULCER DISEASE (GUD)

Noreen A. Hynes, MD, MPH

PATHOGENS

- Herpes simplex virus
- *Treponema pallidum* (primary syphilis or chancre)
- *Haemophilus ducreyi* (chancroid)
- *Chlamydia trachomatis* L1, L2 and L3 serovars causing lymphogranuloma venereum (LGV)
- *Klebsiella granulomatis* (formerly *Calymmatobacterium granulomatis*) causing granuloma inguinale (donovanosis)
- Rarer infectious causes of genital ulcer adenopathy syndrome include: *Phthirus pubis-Sarcoptes scabei* pyoderma, *Trichomonas vaginalis, Entamoeba histolytica.*
- Non-infectious causes include: trauma, fixed drug eruption, Reiter's syndrome, Behcets syndrome.

CLINICAL

- Genital ulcers enhance the acquisition and transmission of HIV therefore offer HIV counseling and testing to all pts with genital ulcer disease (GUD).
- **Laboratory diagnosis is key:** accuracy of clinical diagnosis is inadequate and coinfection with >1 pathogen occurs in 5% to 10% of all cases. The diagnostic accuracy of clinical diagnosis is highest for chancroid (80%) and least for the other causes of GUD: genital HSV (22%), primary syphilis (55%) and LGV (27%).
- **Ulcer and adenopathy location**: men—ulcers may be found on the prepuce (uncircumcised), coronal sulcus (circumcised), near the frenulum, or on the penile shaft; women—ulcers may occur on the labia, on the vaginal walls, on the cervix, on the inner thigh or the fourchette; look for rectal or perianal area ulcers in those who engage in anal receptive intercourse; lymph nodes draining the inguinal regions are primarily affected in GUD; femoral lymph nodes are less frequently affected.
- **Herpes simplex virus (type 1 or type 2):** begins usually as multiple grouped superficial vesicles seen 2–7 days after sexual contact with an infected person, that quickly become superficial painful superficial ulcers without induration and with a red, smooth base; bilateral tender inguinal adenopathy is common along with constitutional symptoms. This classic pattern is most likely to be seen in primary clinical episodes of HSV. Pain and lymphadenopathy are less common in recurrent disease. Subtle immunological abnormalities in antibody-dependent cytotoxicity and in the complement system may account for the recurrent disease phenotype.
- **Primary syphilis (chancre):** painless, well-defined single–multiple ulcer(s) seen 2–4 wks after sexual contact; ulcer base is usually red, smooth, and shiny with firm, indurated edges (the consistency of an Oxford shirt collar buttonhole); unilateral or bilateral painless lymphadenopathy without suppuration or associated constitutional symptoms. This classic pattern is only seen in about 50% of cases.
- **Chancroid:** also called "soft chancre"; painful, single or multiple (1–3), deep and defined or irregular ulcers seen 3–7 days after sexual contact with an infected person; ulcer has a yellow-gray rough base, with soft induration; unilateral or bilateral tender inguinal adenopathy is seen and may suppurate. Constitutional symptoms are rare. Up to 10% of persons with chancroid may be co-infected with syphilis.
- **Lymphogranuloma venereum (LGV):** variably painful, usually single ulcer that is transient and often missed leading to diagnosis at a later stage of infection; the initiating lesion varies from papule, pustule, vesicle to ulcer occuring 10–14 days after sexual contact with an infected person. This initial lesion precedes unilateral or bilateral variably tender lymphadenopathy by 7 to 30 days. In men, the "groove sign" or enlargement of the lymph nodes above and below the inguinal ligament, may be seen (but can also be seen in

chancroid). Inguinal buboes may become fluctuant and rupture. Women may have pelvic pain or symptoms of proctitis due to lymphatic spread to the rectal mucosa region. Increasingly reported among men who have sex with men in North America and Europe; may also present with proctitis.

- **Granuloma inguinale (donovanosis):** painless, single or multiple ulcer(s) presenting 1–4 wks after sexual contact with an infected person; the firmly indurated ulcer can have either well-defined or irregular borders and may appear hypertrophic or verrucous with a red, beefy and rough base that is usually friable; not associated with true lymphadenopathy—instead there is subcutaneous spread of granulomata (hence the name granuloma inguinale) which leads to pseudobubo formation; constitutional symptoms are rare. Healing usually proceeds inward from the ulcer margins. Relapse can occur 6–18 mos after apparently effective rx.

DIAGNOSIS

- **GUD diagnostic workup:** test for syphilis (darkfield microscopy, if available, and serology) and **HSV** (culture), Test for chancroid (culture), LGV (cell culture) and granuloma inguinale (tissue smear or biopsy) if the sexual history identifies epidemiological characteristics that increase risk (such as sexual contact in an endemic area).
- **Primary (and secondary) syphilis definitive diagnosis**: visualization of the spirochete by either positive darkfield microscopy or direct immunofluorescent (IF) staining of a sample collected from the base of the ulcer, from a mucous patch on the genitalia (not from mouth or rectum), or aspirated from enlarged, painless lymph node. Serological screening tests (e.g., RPR/VDRL) are variably positive at this stage.
- **Primary (and secondary) syphilis presumptive diagnosis:** 2 types of serological tests are needed for diagnosis—nontreponemal tests (such as the RPR and VDRL) and treponemal tests (such as the fluorescent treponemal antibody absorbed [FTA-ABS] and the *T. pallidum* particle agglutination [TP-PA]). The non-treponemal test, usually correlates with disease activity and is applied first and if positive the treponemal test is performed on the specimen. These tests may be negative in early primary syphilis when only the definitive diagnostic tests are positive—RPR is 80% sensitive in primary syphilis; the FTA-ABS is 86%–100% sensitive for primary syphilis. The treponemal tests tend to remain positive for life whereas the RPR undergoes seroreversion, therefore, the treponemal test cannot be applied solely in active early infection.
- **Genital herpes:** Cell culture is preferred test but sensitivity and specificity is dependent upon stage of the lesion: 95% sensitivity for vesicular stage; 50% in the ulcer stage; sensitivity is lower for recurrent lesions and declines rapidly as lesions begin to heal; PCR for HSV DNA is more sensitive but are not FDA cleared for use on genital specimens; use of Tzanck preparation smears are insensitive (67% in the vesicular stage; 50% in ulcer stage); type-specific serologic tests based upon the HSV-specific glycoprotein G2 (HSV-2) and glycoprotein G1 (HSV-1) may have a role in certain settings such as recurrent genital symptoms or atypical symptoms with negative culture, clinical diagnosis of HSV without laboratory confirmation, and a partner with laboratory-confirmed genital HSV. In general, serological tests do not have a role in the laboratory confirmation of an initial suspect case of genital HSV.
- **Chancroid:** Definitive diagnosis is by culture to identify *H. ducreyi*. The test is only 75% sensitive compared with PCR from genital swabs but PCR is a research tool only.
- **LGV:** Culture is the definitive diagnostic tool but the recovery rate is only 50%; serologic testing by complement fixation (CF) or microimmunofluorescence (MIF) cannot distinguish among other *Chlamydia* species. Positive titers >1:256 by CF or >1:128 with MIF strongly suggest LGV although invasive *C. trachomatis* serovars D-K can also give high titers.
- **Granuloma inguinale (Donovanosis):** Giemsa or Wright stain of crushed tissue smears or biopsy specimen looking for Donovan bodies (bacillary organisms within histiocytes). Donovan bodies found in only 60%–80% of cases using smear or biopsy.

TREATMENT
Genital Herpes Regimens
- 1st clinical episode: acyclovir 400 mg PO q8h × 7–10 days or acyclovir 200 PO 5 × days × 7–10 days or famciclovir 250 mg PO q8h × 7–10 days or valacyclovir 1 g PO twice daily × 7–10 days.

- Episodic Rx of recurrent HSV: Use 5 days (5–10 days in HIV +): acyclovir 400 mg PO q8h; acyclovir 800 mg PO twice daily famciclovir 125 mg PO twice daily or valacyclovir 1 g PO twice daily. Other regimens: acyclovir 800 mg PO q8h × 2 days; famciclovir 1 g PO twice daily × 1 days; valacyclovir 500 mg twice daily PO × 3 days.
- Suppressive daily therapy for recurrent disease (without HIV): acyclovir 400 mg PO twice daily; famciclovir 250 PO twice daily; valacyclovir 500 mg PO once daily; valacyclovir 1.0 g PO once daily.
- Suppressive daily therapy for recurrent disease (HIV infected): acyclovir 400–800 mg PO q8–12h; famciclovir 500 PO twice daily; valacyclovir 500 mg PO once daily (DO NOT USE 1 G twice daily dosing).
- Acyclovir resistant HSV (other oral RX don't work): foscarnet 40 mg/kg IV q8h until clinical resolution; cidofovir gel 1% to lesions once daily × 5 days may work (requires pharmacy compounding).
- Severe disease or complications requiring hospitalization: acyclovir 5–10 mg/kg IV q8h × 2–7 days or until clinical improvement. Change to PO to complete 10 days.

Primary Syphilis Regimens
- Benzathine penicillin G (BPG) 2.4 million units IM × 1.
- Penicillin allergy (not for use in pregnancy): doxycycline 100 mg PO twice daily × 14 days; or tetracycline 500 mg PO q6h × 14 days; or in persons with non-IgE-mediated penicillin allergy-ceftriaxone 1 g IV or IM once daily × 8–10 days. Azithromycin is no longer recommended due to treatment failures.
- HIV-infected: benzathine penicillin G 2.4 million units IM × 1 (some recommend qwk × 3). In penicillin allergic persons with HIV infection BPG after desensitization is preferred, but if can't be done, use regimens above for those with penicillin allergy although data on efficacy in HIV-infected persons has not been studied.
- Pregnant woman: Must ALWAYS be treated with penicillin; desensitize if penicillin-allergic. Tetracycline and doxycycline are contraindicated in pregnancy; erythromycin should not be used because it does not reliably cure the infected fetus; data are insufficient on the use of ceftriaxone for the treatment of maternal syphilis or the prevention of congenital syphilis and therefore, should not be used.

Chancroid Regimens
- Azithromycin 1 g orally × 1
- Ceftriaxone 250 mg IM × 1
- Ciprofloxacin 500 mg PO twice daily × 3 days (contraindicated in pregnant and lactating women)
- Erythromycin base 500 mg PO q6h × 7 days

Lymphogranuloma venereum (LGV) Regimens
- Doxycycline 100 mg PO twice daily × 21 days.
- Pregnant women: Erythromycin base 500 mg PO q6h × 21 days.
- Azithromycin (unproven regimen but some STD specialists believe it is effective): 1 g PO qwk × 3 wk.
- HIV infected persons: Give the same regimens as for HIV uninfected persons but may need to give for longer if resolution of symptoms is delayed.

Granuloma Inguinale (Donovanosis) Regimens
- Doxycycline 100 mg PO twice daily for at least 3 wks and until all lesions have completely healed. This is the preferred regimen. Some STD specialists recommend adding gentamicin 1 mg/kg IV q8h if there is no subjective improvement in symptoms at 72 hrs.
- Alternative regimens (all for at least 3 wks and until all lesions have completely healed): azithromycin 1 g PO qwk; or ciprofloxacin 750 mg twice daily; or erythromycin base 500 mg PO q6h; or trimethoprim-sulfamethoxazole 1 double strength (160 mg/800 mg) tab PO twice daily.
- Pregnant and lactating women: erythromycin 500 mg PO q6h for at least 3 wks and until all lesions have completely healed. Consider the addition of a parenteral aminoglycoside such as gentamicin 1 mg/kg IV q8h at the outset of treatment. Doxycycline and ciprofloxacin are contraindicated in pregnant women; ciprofloxacin should be avoided in lactating women.

FOLLOW UP

- **Genital HSV:** sex partners should be offered evaluation and counseling. Symptomatic sex partners should be evaluated and treated in the same way as pts with genital lesions. Asymptomatic sex partners of symptomatic persons should be interviewed regarding a history of symptomatic genital lesions and offered type-specific serologic testing for HSV infection.
- **Primary syphilis:** persistent signs or sx or recurrence of signs or sx or if the pt has a sustained (i.e., ≥6 mo after rx) four-fold increase in nontreponemal titer compared with baseline titer at the time of treatment a treatment failure is likely to have occurred or the pt has been reinfected. Evaluate for HIV and perform lumbar puncture with CSF analysis (reinfection cannot be reliably differentiated from treatment failure) as a treatment failure may signal the presence of unrecognized CNS infection. If CSF is negative, retreat with benzathine penicillin G 2.4 million units weekly × 3 wks. Sex partners in the 90 days prior to diagnosis should be treated presumptively for incubating syphilis; sex partners exposed >90 days prior to diagnosis in the pt need to be evaluated for syphilis.
- **Chancroid:** Reexamine in 3–7 days after starting rx; success if pt complains of decrease in sx at 72 hrs and ulcers improve objectively within 7 days of starting rx. If no clinical improvement reconsider if dx is correct; if there is coinfection with another STD or HIV, if non-adherent to regimen prescribed, if *H. ducreyi* strain is resistant to selected antibiotic. Time to complete healing depends on size of initial ulcer; uncircumcised men heal more slowly. If drainage of suppurating lymph nodes needed, incision and drainage is preferred to needle aspiration as is less likely to require repeat drainage. Treat all sex partners regardless of the presence or absence of signs or symptoms if they had sexual contact with the pt during the 10 days preceding patient's onset of symptoms and thereafter.
- **Lymphogranuloma venereum (LGV):** follow-up until signs and symptoms have completely resolved; persons who have had sexual contact with the pt within the 60 days before onset of the patient's sx should be examined, tested for urethral, cervical, or rectal chlamydia infection, and treated with a standard chlamydia regimen (azithromycin 1 g PO once or doxycycline 100 mg PO twice daily × 7 days.
- **Granuloma inguinale (donovanosis):** follow-up until all signs and symptoms have resolved; sexual contacts in the 60 days before the onset of symptoms in the pt should be examined and offered rx.

OTHER INFORMATION

- No single agent affords reliable therapy for all causes of genital ulcer adenopathy syndrome.
- All genital ulcer diseases facilitate the acquisition and transmission of HIV infection.
- HSV is the most common cause of GUD in U.S. Recurrent painful ulcers preceded by vesicles is usually HSV.
- In an area with a high incidence or increasing incidence of syphilis, all pts presenting with genital ulcers with or without adenopathy should be treated for syphilis at the time of presentation.

BASIS FOR RECOMMENDATIONS

Centers for Disease Control and Prevention, Workowski KA, Berman SM. Sexually transmitted diseases treatment guidelines, 2006. *MMWR Recomm Rep*, 2006; Vol. 55; pp. 1–94.

Comments: The CDC treatment guidelines provide clinicians with a readily available reference for STD treatments recommended by a panel of national and international experts in STD diagnosis, treatment, prevention, and control. These guidelines available electronically from cdc: www.cdc.gov.

HAEMOPHILUS DUCREYI (CHANCROID) see p. 269 in Pathogens Section

HERPES SIMPLEX VIRUS see p. 416 in Pathogens Section

HUMAN PAPILLOMAVIRUS (HPV) see p. 423 in Pathogens Section

NEISSERIA GONORRHOEAE see p. 301 in Pathogens Section

PROCTITIS (SEXUALLY TRANSMITTED)

Noreen A. Hynes, MD, MPH

DIAGNOSIS

PATHOGENS

- *Neisseria gonorrhoeae*
- *Chlamydia trachomatis*
- *Herpes Simplex Virus*
- *Treponema pallidum*
- *Chlamydia trachomatis*, Lymphogranuloma venereum (LGV) serovars
- Men who have sex with men (MSM) enteric pathogens: may include Salmonella spp, Shigella spp, *Entamoeba histolytica,* and *Giardia lamblia* may be sexually transmitted. In the right setting these should be considered and appropriate testing carried out.
- Severely immunocompromised pts: CMV proctocolitis may be seen but is considered to be a reactivation of a previously acquired infection.

CLINICAL

- Proctitis increases risk of HIV acquisition by up to 9-fold in receptive anal intercourse.
- Proctitis represents inflammation of the rectal mucosa, i.e., above the pectinate line (also called the anorectal line or dentate line) to 15 cm on sigmoidoscopy. Proctocolitis is inflammation extending from >15 cm above the anorectal line into the sigmoid colon. Infections of the anal canal, lined with squamous epithelium (from the anal verge or introitus to the pectinate line) are often considered within the definition of proctitis although technically separate.
- **History:** it is important to ask about anal receptive intercourse in all pts presenting with anal discharge, tenesmus, anorectal pain or found to signs and symptoms consistent with vaginitis, cervicitis or urethritis. Up to 10% of American women surveyed engage in anal receptive intercourse on a regular basis.
- **General signs and symptoms:** tenesmus (painful spasm of the anal sphincter accompanied by an urgent desire to evacuate bowel with involuntary straining, resulting in little or no stool) with or without constipation is the most frequent symptom), anorectal pain, mucopurulent discharge with or without hematochezia. Proctocolitis presents with proctitis, diarrhea, bloating, and abdominal pain.
- Site specific clinical manifestations: anal canal—very painful due to abundant sensory nerve endings (HSV and syphilis). Rectum—if concomitant anal infection absent, infection likely to be painless. Chlamydial and gonococcal proctitis usually asymptomatic.
- **Gonococcal proctitis:** when symptomatic may present with pruritis ani, mucopurulent discharge, pain and tenesmus with or without constipation. If untreated, rectal abscess can result. Visualization may not be possible due to pain but rectal swab for culture should be collected. If proctoscopy possible, spectrum from normal mucosa to visible pus with contact bleeding may be seen.
- **Chlamydia (non LGV) proctitis:** when symptomatic, may be indistinguishable from milder forms of symptomatic gonococcal proctitis with pruritis ani, mucoid rather than mucopurulent discharge, and peri-anal pain. If visualization possible, proctoscopy findings range from normal mucosa to erythema with or without edema and possible contact bleeding. Consider LGV in symptomatic MSM.
- **LGV proctitis:** in industrialized countries is seen almost exclusively in MSM (outbreaks reported in several European countries); painless shallow pustule or ulcer usually not noted at the site of inoculation (primary stage). Anogenital syndrome is one of 2 common second stage manifestations occurring 3–6 mos after the first stage. Constitutional symptoms of fever, myalgia, arthralgias, anorexia, general malaise often noted. Symptoms of proctitis or proctocolitis may be seen with severe pain, anal discharge that may be bloody or mucopurulent or mixed, tenesmus, constipation. Untreated LGV proctitis/proctocolitis may lead to tissue destruction with fistula or stricture formation. It is critically important to distinguish this from Crohn's disease to avoid inappropriate and potentially damaging intervention.
- **Herpes proctitis:** usually proctitis is an extension from perianal and anal infection; grouped vesicles that become very painful shallow ulcers; associated with moderate to severe pain on

attempted defecation tenesmus, bloody or mucopurulent discharge. HSV-2 accounts for 85% of cases; HSV-1 for 15%; immunocompromised pts may have severe HSV proctitis; urinary retention with rectal pain and constipation suggests HSV infection in pts diagnosed with proctitis.

- **Syphilitic proctitis:** primary syphilis (chancre) confined to the perianal and anal areas and does not cause proctitis. A painless ulcer with a clean base and indurated edges with the consistency of an oxford shirt collar buttonhole may be noted; secondary syphilis, if it causes proctitis is usually as an extension from the anal area and usually occurs after resolution of the chancre. Perianal condylomata lata may be seen with rectal mucosal patches (oval-to-crescentic erosions or shallow ulcers of about 1 cm diameter), covered by a grey mucoid exudate and with an erythematous border; patches may coalesce or there may be *de novo* serpiginous lesions, sometimes termed snail track ulcers); generalized skin rash with or without involvement of the palms and soles. Fever, lymphadenopathy are commonly seen.

DIAGNOSIS

- **General diagnosis:** light microscopy—>4 PMNs/high power field on Gram-stain of anorectal secretions; collect specimens for syphilis dark field microscopy (if available), Gram-stain and cultures (gonorrhea, chlamydia, herpes) and syphilis serology; cultures for gonorrhea should also be obtained from urethra, pharynx, and cervix (in women). In MSM pts, consider stool cx for enteric pathogens, stool O and P for parasites.

- **Gonococcal proctitis:** culture only for diagnosis; nucleic acid amplification tests (NAAT) have been cleared by FDA for testing of genital specimens (cervical and male urethral swabs and urine), but the performance of NAATs has not been adequately evaluated for use in rectal or oropharyngeal gonorrhea [a CDC-sponsored trial to examine the use of NAAT for gonorrhea at these anatomic sites is being conducted at the University of Alabama and results are anticipated within 2009.

- **Chlamydia (non-LGV) proctitis:** culture for diagnosis; nucleic acid amplification tests (NAAT) have been cleared by FDA for testing of genital specimens (cervical and male urethral swabs and urine), but the performance of NAATs has not been adequately evaluated for use in rectal or oropharyngeal chlamydia.

- **LGV proctitis:** culture of specimen collected from involved area of rectal mucosa; there are no data on efficacy of NAAT for rectal specimens; if inguinal lymph adenopathy or bubo noted, aspiration specimen may be tested for *C. trachomatis* by culture, direct immunofluorescence or nucleic acid detection. Genotyping needs to be requested to distinguish LGV from non-LGV chlamydia. Complement fixation serology (titer >1:64) can support but not prove the diagnosis. Do NOT wait for laboratory confirmation to treat if this dx is suspected.

- **Herpes proctitis:** herpes virus culture or polymerase chain reaction.

- **Syphilitic proctitis:** dark field microscopy of sample collected from a mucus patch (if available) to demonstrate spirochetes; syphilis serology (rapid plasmin reagin [RPR] tests combined with a confirmatory test such as the fluorescent treponemal antibody absorbed [FTA-Abs] is 100% sensitive for diagnosing secondary syphilis).

- If proctocolitis indicated by symptoms or findings on sigmoidoscopy, then cultures for *Campylobacter* sp, salmonella, shigella and stool O and P exam for *E. histolytica* and *Giardia lamblia* are indicated. These pathogens are traditionally not considered to be sexually transmitted but may be in MSM and others engaging in receptive anal intercourse.

TREATMENT

Initial Empiric Therapy (Presumed Gonorrhea or Chlamydia)

- Ceftriaxone 125 mg IM once plus doxycycline PO twice daily × 7 days.
- Cefixime 400 mg PO × 1 plus doxycycline PO twice daily × 7 days.
- Ciprofloxacin 500 mg PO × 1 (do not use in MSM) plus doxycycline PO twice daily × 7 days.
- Ofloxacin 400 mg PO × 1 (do not use in MSM) plus doxycycline PO twice daily × 7 days.
- Levofloxacin 250 mg PO × 1 (do not use in MSM) plus doxycycline PO twice daily × 7 days.

HSV proctitis, first clinical episode

- Acyclovir 400 mg 5 × per days × 10 days.
- Valacyclovir 1 g PO twice daily × 7–10 days.
- Famciclovir 250 mg PO three times a day × 7–10 days.

HSV proctitis suppression after 4 bouts/yr
- **No HIV infection:** acyclovir 400 mg PO twice daily or famciclovir 250 mg PO twice daily or valacyclovir 1 g PO once daily.
- **HSV proctitis in AIDS:** acyclovir 5–10 mg/kg IV q8h until clinical resolution, then acyclovir 400–800 mg PO twice daily-three times a day or famciclovir 500 mg PO twice daily or valacyclovir 500 mg PO twice daily.

Syphilitic Proctitis
- Benzathine penicillin G 2.4 g IM × 1.
- Penicillin allergic (non-pregnant woman): doxycycline 100 mg PO twice daily × 14 days.

Lymphogranuloma venereum (LGV) proctitis
- Doxycycline 100 mg PO twice daily × 21 days.

FOLLOW UP
- All pts with symptomatic proctitis should have follow-up within 72 hrs to assess symptom resolution; pts with LGV should be followed up every wk thereafter to assess response to rx and to determine if longer treatment is needed.
- Partners of pts should be examined and treated based upon the diagnoses determined by laboratory testing.
- Pts with laboratory-confirmed LGV should have a test of cure 4–5 wks after completion of therapy.

BASIS FOR RECOMMENDATIONS

Centers for Disease Control and Prevention, Workowski KA, Berman SM. Sexually transmitted diseases treatment guidelines, 2006. *MMWR Recomm Rep*, 2006; Vol. 55; pp. 1–94,

Comments: The CDC treatment guidelines provide clinicians with a readily available reference for STD treatments recommended by a panel of national and international experts in STD diagnosis, treatment, prevention, and control. These guidelines available electronically from: http://www.cdc.gov/

TREPONEMA PALLIDUM (SYPHILIS) see p. 338 in Pathogens Section

Surgical Infections

APPENDICITIS

Christopher F. Carpenter, MD and Aditi Swami, MD

PATHOGENS
- Polymicrobial process, as a rule
- Enterobacteriaceae
- Anaerobes
- Enterococcus

CLINICAL
- The diagnosis of appendicitis in young men is usually straight forward; differential diagnosis is much broader in premenopausal women and older adults.
- 5–10% lifetime risk, higher in males, peak age 15–25 but affects all age groups.
- More than 250,000 appendectomies are performed in the U.S. each yr; approximately 15–20% have normal appendix (relatively higher in premenopausal women, young children, and the elderly).
- Mortality 1/600 (higher in the elderly); diagnostic accuracy varies by gender, male 78–92%, female 58–95%.
- Differential diagnoses include gynecologic causes (PID, ruptured ovarian cyst, ectopic pregnancy, etc.), gastroenteritis, UTI, Crohns disease, renal colic, abdominal pain of unknown origin, and ileocecitis or mesenteric adenitis (e.g., Yersiniae).

DIAGNOSIS
- Despite advances in imaging and laboratory studies in recent yrs, pt history and physical exam (often serial exams) remain the cornerstone of diagnosis.
- Hx/PE: abdominal pain and tenderness progressing to rigidity, with migration of pain from the periumbilical region to the right lower quadrant. McBurney's point tenderness (located approximately one third of the distance from the anterior superior iliac spine to the umbilicus).
- Rovsing's sign: referral of pain to the RLQ with palpation of the LLQ. Psoas sign: pain with active extension of the right hip. Obturator sign: pain with internal rotation of the right hip.
- Lab: leukocytosis with left shift non-specific and may be absent; evaluate other potential causes (UA, beta-HCG, etc.).
- Ultrasound and CT are useful adjuncts to clinical impression. CT appears to be more accurate and more likely to provide alternative diagnoses. Imaging is most beneficial in equivocal cases.
- Observation or laparoscopy may also be of benefit in equivocal cases.

TREATMENT
General Points
- Surgical removal of appendix is definitive treatment.
- The differentiation between simple appendicitis and gangrenous appendicitis/perforated appendicitis with peritonitis should determine the length of antibiotic administration.
- Simple appendicitis requires ONLY preoperative antibiotic prophylaxis.
- Gangrenous appendicitis and perforated appendicitis with peritonitis require a therapeutic abx course; 3 to 5 days is likely sufficient but longer courses may be indicated in complicated cases.

Surgery
- Prompt surgical intervention in acute appendicitis (either with our without rupture and secondary peritonitis) is mainstay of treatment.
- A normal appendix seen in 15–20% of cases; rates higher in young children, premenopausal women, and elderly.
- Perforation rates remain approximately 20%, higher in young (40–57%) and elderly (55–70%).
- No consensus on optimal approach: open vs. laparoscopic appendectomy.

Single agent prophylaxis or treatment
- Ticarcillin-clavulanate 3.1 g IV q6h
- Ampicillin-sulbactam 3.0 g IV q6h
- Piperacillin-tazobactam 3.375 g IV q6h or 4.5 g IV q8h
- Tigecycline 100 mg IV × 1 then 50 mg IV q12h
- Ertapenem 1000 mg IV q day
- Doripenem 500 mg IVq8h
- Use of piperacillin-tazobactam or doripenem is likely more appropriate for severe cases of intra-abdominal infection, or pts with recent antibiotic exposure.

Combination prophylaxis or treatment
- Combination of metronidazole (0.5 g IV q6–8h, load with 15 mg/kg if life threatening) with one of the following:
- Cefazolin 1–2 g IV q8h
- Ceftriaxone 2.0 g IV q24h
- Cefotaxime 2.0 g IV q6–8h
- Cefepime 2.0 g IV q12h
- Ciprofloxacin 400 mg IV q12h
- Levofloxacin 500 mg IV q24h
- Aztreonam 1 g IV q8hr—2 g IV q6h
- Gentamicin or tobramycin 2.0 mg/kg loading dose then 1.7 mg/kg q8h IV; once-a-day (5–6 mg/kg/day) dosing may be considered.

FOLLOW UP
- Generally low complication rate.

OTHER INFORMATION
- Laparoscopy helpful with diagnostic accuracy, especially in women ages 16–39.
- Studies of non-operative management have not demonstrated comparable outcomes with surgery.
- The Appendicitis Inflammatory Response (AIR) score is a recently developed clinical diagnostic tool.

BASIS FOR RECOMMENDATIONS
Solomkin JS, Mazuski JE, Baron EJ, et al. Guidelines for the selection of anti-infective agents for complicated intra-abdominal infections. *Clin Infect Dis*, 2003; Vol. 37; pp. 997–1005.
Comments: Consensus guidelines from IDSA, SIS, ASM, and SIDP for treatment of IAI. Due for publication of an update in 2010.

CHOLANGITIS

Christopher F. Carpenter, MD and Aditi Swami, MD

PATHOGENS
- Frequently polymicrobial
- *E. coli*
- Klebsiella species
- Enterobacter species
- Enterococcus (unclear relevance)
- Anaerobes (unclear relevance)
- Pathogenic role of enterococci and anaerobes not well defined and empirical coverage for these organisms is not usually required.
- Resistant pathogens may be encountered in pts with health care-associated infections and empirical coverage should be adjusted accordingly

CLINICAL
- Infectious cholangitis results from bacterial infection in the setting of an obstructed biliary tree.

- Sources of obstruction: gallstones (50%), strictures, biliary or pancreatic malignancy, sclerosing cholangitis, iatrogenic (occluded stent or drain), parasitic (rare in developed world).
- Obstruction alone is not sufficient to cause cholangitis.
- Mirrizi syndrome is the common hepatic duct obstruction caused by extrinsic compression from an impacted stone in the cystic duct.
- Charcot's triad of intermittent chills/fever, jaundice, and RUQ pain present in 50–70%.
- Reynold's pentad includes Charcot's triad along with altered mental status and hypotension and is associated with increased morbidity and mortality.
- Iatrogenic causes of cholangitis include ERCP, percutaneous transhepatic cholangiography, and biliary stents.
- Primary sclerosing cholangitis (PSC) is non-infectious.

DIAGNOSIS

- Diagnosis often made clinically, but requires imaging confirmation.
- Hx: Charcot's triad of intermittent chills/fever, jaundice, RUQ pain. RUQ pain less likely in pts w/ biliary stent or endoprosthesis—though fever and jaundice remain common.
- Pts may present early in the course of infection with only fever.
- PE: RUQ tenderness present in two-thirds, but peritoneal signs less common.
- Labs: leukocytosis, hyperbilirubinemia (90%), elevated alkaline phosphatase/GGT, AST, ALT; blood cultures often positive.
- Evaluate source of jaundice. US if gallstones suspected, CT scan if malignancy suspected.
- A normal US does not rule out cholangitis.
- Cholangiography needed to define etiology; treat underlying cause WHEN STABLE. Pts w/ fever, RUQ pain, jaundice, confusion, and hypotension require rapid evaluation and treatment.
- MRCP increasingly utilized in suspected malignancy and diagnosis of duct stones (US less sensitive).
- ERCP should not be utilized solely for diagnosis if less risky studies are available; it is best utilized when likelihood of intervention is high, e.g., high likelihood of common bile duct stone in acute cholangitis.

TREATMENT

Treatment of acute cholangitis (Severe/health-care associated)

- Piperacillin-tazobactam 3.375 g IV q6h or 4.5 g IV q8h
- Cephalosporins (ceftriaxone 1–2 g IV qday or cefepime 1–2 g IV q8h); consider additional coverage for anaerobes (metronidazole 500 mg IV q6–8h) and enterococci, clinical relevance of ceftriaxone association with biliary sludge unclear
- Ticarcillin-clavulanate 3.1 g IV q6h
- Tigecycline 100 mg IV times one dose then 50 mg IV qday
- Imipenem 0.5 g IV q6h if at high risk of resistant pathogens
- Meropenem 1.0 g IV q8h if at high risk of resistant pathogens
- Doripenem 500 mg IV q8h if at high risk of resistant pathogens
- Pts unresponsive to antibiotics may require drainage (T-tube), or surgery (gallstones)

Treatment of acute cholangitis (mild-moderate disease/not health-care associated)

- Ampicillin-sulbactam 3.0 g IV q6h.
- Ertapenem 1 g IV qday.
- Fluoroquinolones (ciprofloxacin 400 mg IV q12h, levofloxacin 500 mg IV qday, or moxifloxacin 400 mg IV/PO qday), consider additional coverage for anaerobes with ciprofloxacin and levofloxacin (metronidazole 500 mg IV q6–8h).
- Cefoxitin 1–2 g IV q6h (if available).
- Ampicillin 2 g IV q6h plus gentamicin 1.7 mg/kg IV q8h, consider additional coverage for anaerobes (metronidazole 500 mg IV q6–8h).

TREATMENT REGIMEN DETAILS

- Use of ursodeoxycholic acid and/or antibiotics for the **prevention** of biliary stent occlusion or infection **not routinely recommended.**

FOLLOW UP
- If severe, treat for 7–10 days; modify antibiotic choice for local pathogens and resistance patterns.

OTHER INFORMATION
- Antibiotics are indicated in all pts with acute cholangitis. Bactibilia alone is not cholangitis, and obstruction does not always imply infection.
- Pts who present seriously ill and who are not responding to antimicrobial and supportive therapy will require emergent drainage.
- Gallstones account for more than 50% of cases. Can occur post-cholecystectomy.
- Occlusion of the bile duct from stricture (benign or malignant), bile stents, or parasites account for most non-gallstone causes.

BASIS FOR RECOMMENDATIONS
Solomkin JS, Mazuski JE, Baron EJ, et al. Guidelines for the selection of anti-infective agents for complicated intra-abdominal infections. *Clin Infect Dis*, 2003; Vol. 37; pp. 997–1005.
Comments: Consensus evidence-based guidelines from IDSA, SIS, ASM, and SIDP.

Mazuski JE, Sawyer RG, Nathens AB, et al. The Surgical Infection Society guidelines on antimicrobial therapy for intra-abdominal infections: evidence for the recommendations. *Surg Infect (Larchmt)*, 2002; Vol. 3; pp. 175–233.
Comments: Current evidenced based recommendations from the Surgical Infection Society.

CHOLECYSTITIS

Christopher F. Carpenter, MD and Aditi Swami, MD

PATHOGENS
- Usually inflammatory and noninfectious
- If infectious, frequently polymicrobial
- *E. coli*
- *Klebsiella species*
- *Enterobacter species*
- *Enterococcus*
- *Escherichia coli* and *Klebsiella species* are the most common Enterobacteriaceae; less common spp. include Enterobacter and Proteus
- Pathogenicity unclear for organisms cultured in bile/gall bladder unless also recovered in blood
- Anaerobes are less significant unless bile duct to bowel anastomosis or fistula present; if so, the most common organisms include *Clostridium species* and *Bacteroides species*
- Pathogenic role of enterococci and anaerobes are otherwise not well defined and empirical coverage not usually required

CLINICAL
- Gallstones occurs in approximately 3–20% of the population worldwide, with more than 80 percent being asymptomatic.
- Acute cholecystitis develops in 1–3% of those with symptomatic gallstones, accounting for 3 to 9% of hospital admissions for acute abdominal pain.
- No single history, exam, or laboratory finding is sufficient for diagnosis; combination of findings and clinical gestalt more likely to lead to diagnosis with imaging study to confirm.
- Most often caused by gallstones (>90%); acalculous cholecystitis (i.e., cholecystitis without gallstones) occurs typically in otherwise critically ill pts.
- Acute cholecystitis is usually noninfectious.

DIAGNOSIS
- Hx: nausea/vomiting and RUQ pain (often following fatty meal) with fever. Predisposition: female sex, multiparity, obesity, recent pregnancy, sickle cell.
- Lab: elevated WBC, variable elevation of alkaline phosphatase, bilirubin, and transaminases; increased amylase may occasionally occur.
- US for gallstones, may see edema/pericholecystic fluid, or probe causes RUQ tenderness; color-flow doppler shows hyperemia. Hepatobiliary scans (e.g., Tech-HIDA) is > expensive but, slightly

more sensitive (US sensitivity >92–95%, HIDA >97%.). CT with little role except to exclude other diagnoses.
- Rebound and guarding are less commonly found and indicate peritonitis.
- Hyperbilirubinemia may suggest CBD stones or Mirrizzi's syndrome (obstruction by a stone impacted in Hartman's pouch).
- Diaphragmatic irritation may lead to right shoulder pain.
- Majority of pts have gallbladder-associated symptoms prior to the development of acute cholecystitis.
- Murphy's sign (inspiratory arrest during deep palpation over the gallbladder) not highly sensitive but quite specific.
- Jaundice, hypoactive bowel sounds, and a palpable mass may also be present.
- Technetium-HIDA is less specific in acalculous cholecystitis and ultrasonography plays a larger role in diagnosis as does percutaneous cholecystostomy.

TREATMENT
Antibiotic Treatment of acute cholecystitis
- Acute cholecystitis is usually only an inflammatory process w/ o infection; however, most pts are covered with antibiotics. If infected, most are polymicrobial.
- Uncomplicated cholecystitis: treat with operation and antibiotics for 24–48 hrs, if operation delayed treat for 3–5 days. Persistent fever/SIRS or illness indicates complication.
- Choice of antibiotic depends on whether community-acquired without comorbidities or prior abx [consider amp/sulbactam, ticar/clav, ertapenem, cefoxitin, moxifloxacin] or pt abx-experienced, recent GI surgeries or comorbidities [pip/tazo, meropenem, imipenem, FQ/metronidazole, cephalosporin/metronidazole].
- **Mild-moderate:** ampicillin-sulbactam 3.0 g IV q6h.
- Ticarcillin-clavulanate 3.1 g IV q6h.
- Ertapenem 1 g IV qday.
- Fluoroquinolone (ciprofloxacin 400 mg IV q12h, levofloxacin 500 mg IV every day, or moxifloxacin 400 mg IV every day).
- ceftriaxone 1–2 g IV every day or cefepime 1–2 g IV q12h; clinical relevance of ceftriaxone association with biliary sludge unclear.
- Cefoxitin 1–2 g IV q6h (if available).
- Tigecycline 100 mg IV times one dose then 50 mg IV q12h.
- **Severe/nosocomial/prior antibiotics:** Piperacillin-tazobactam 3.375 g IV q6h or 4.5 g IV q8h, meropenem 1 g IV q8h or imipenem 0.5 g IV q6h. Doripenem 500 mg IV q8h.

Surgical Treatment
- Laparoscopic cholecystectomy preferred if possible; early cholecystectomy (soon after admission) should be considered in the majority of cases; some surgeons still advocate delayed surgery.
- Laparoscopic cholecystectomy in the extremely elderly is safe and well tolerated, but may be associated with a higher conversion rate, increased morbidity, and a longer hospital stay.
- Open cholecystectomy if technically needed.
- Percutaneous drainage or cholecystostomy if unable to tolerate above.
- Early/emergent intervention is indicated in acalculous cholecystitis due to risk of gangrene and/or perforation: either percutaneous drainage via cholecystostomy, or CCY.

Prophylaxis for cholecystectomy
- Indicated for all cholecystectomy operations in pts with acute cholecystitis.
- Prophylaxis for routine cholecystectomy also indicated in high-risk pts (age >70, nonfunctioning gallbladder, obstructive jaundice, or common duct stones).
- Also advocated by many clinicians for endoscopic retrograde cholangiopancreatography.
- Cefazolin + metronidazole or cefotetan 1–2 g IV within 60 minutes prior to surgical incision.
- Antibiotics not needed beyond the operating room time unless suspicion of infection (implies treatment and not prophylaxis).

FOLLOW UP
- Early symptoms related to inflammation.
- Late signs, symptoms and complications likely infectious.

- Duration of antibiotics: if early surgery, would discontinue antibiotics 24 hrs post-op; if surgery delayed, would consider treatment for 3–5 days maximum. Continued SIRS/sepsis suggests complication and further workup indicated.

OTHER INFORMATION

- Pts with acute cholecystitis require hospitalization, and the definitive treatment is cholecystectomy.
- Over 90% of pts have calculus cholecystitis. Acalculous cholecystitis has different epidemiology (less predominant in females and often associated with other acute events, e.g., trauma).
- Chronic cholecystitis is **not** an indication for antibiotic treatment. Should elective cholecystectomy be performed, preoperative prophylaxis should only be considered in high-risk pts.

BASIS FOR RECOMMENDATIONS

National Surgery Infection Prevention Project. Antimicrobial prophylaxis for surgery: an advisory statement from the National Surgical Infection Prevention Project. *Clin Infect Dis*, 2004; Vol. 38; pp. 1706–15.
Comments: Summary of national recommendations for select cardiac, vascular, orthopedic (arthroplasty), gynecologic (hysterectomy), and colorectal surgeries.

Solomkin JS, Mazuski JE, Baron EJ, et al. Guidelines for the selection of anti-infective agents for complicated intra-abdominal infections. *Clin Infect Dis*, 2003; Vol. 37; pp. 997–1005.
Comments: Consensus evidence-based guidelines from IDSA, SIS, ASM, and SIDP.

DIVERTICULITIS see p. 97 in GI Section

HEPATIC ABSCESS

Christopher F. Carpenter, MD and Aditi Swami, MD

PATHOGENS

- Gram-positive cocci: *Streptococcal* spp. (especially *S. intermedius* group), enterococci, and *S. aureus.*
- Anaerobes: *Bacteroides* species, *Fusobacterium* sp, *Actinomyces* sp, *Clostridium* sp, etc.
- Enterobacteriaceae (*E. coli*, *Klebsiella* spp., etc.) and other GNR.
- *Yersinia enterocolitica*: rare cause of liver abscess, consider underlying hemochromatosis.
- *Candida species.*
- *Entamoeba histolytica*: liver abscesses may complicate up to 10% of the cases of amebic colitis.
- *Echinococcus granulosus*: most common cause of hydatid cysts.

CLINICAL

- Generally occurs in middle-aged adults (40's and 50's).
- Signs and symptoms include fever +/– RUQ pain, tenderness w/ hepatomegaly. Some may only have fever (60%) associated with chills and malaise, and presentation may be subacute or chronic including weight loss, anorexia, and occasionally mental status changes.
- Rarely, pts can present with sepsis and peritoneal signs from intraperitoneal rupture of the abscess.
- Diaphragmatic irritation may refer pain to the right shoulder +/or cough or pleural rub.
- Approximately 50% of pts have a solitary abscess.
- Majority of abscesses involve in the right hepatic lobe (~75%), less commonly left (20%) or caudate (5%) lobes.
- Classified by presumed origin. Up to 50% from biliary tract (cholangitis); rest from hepatic artery (bacteremia), portal vein (abdominal source, e.g., diverticulitis), contiguous focus (local abscess or cholecystitis) or penetrating trauma. Many are of cryptogenic origin.
- Underlying disease typically is the primary determinant of outcome.
- Entamoeba histolytica causes amoebic liver abscess, with spread to the liver via the portal system during colitis and usually manifesting as right lobe solitary lesions; it is rare in the Untied States, occuring almost exclusively in immigrants and travelers, and men are at higher risk for invasive disease.

- Echinococcal, or hydatid, cysts, are most commonly caused by *Echinococcus granulosus* and usually acquired from canines; rarely seen in the United States, and usually asymptomatic until symptoms develop due to size of enlarging cyst or leakage/rupture.

DIAGNOSIS

- For pyogenic liver abscess(es), positive blood cultures up to 50%, with alkaline phosphatase and WBC counts frequently elevated. Hyperbilirubinemia with or without jaundice occurs in <50% of pts.
- Although dx may be suggested on plain films (e.g., gas within the abscess), CT, US, and MRI are the imaging modalities of choice in suspected liver abscess or FUO (fever of unknown origin).
- CT or US-guided percutaneous or surgical drainage should be considered in all cases of hepatic abscess for diagnostic confirmation and culture.
- Positive amebic or echinococcal serology helps differentiate parasitic liver abscess from pyogenic, especially in nonendemic areas. It cannot distinguish between active and prior infection.
- Uncomplicated small abscesses due to *Entamoeba histolytica* in endemic areas may not require aspiration; consider empirical rx.

TREATMENT

Drainage and General Management

- Abscess drainage is the optimal therapy for pyogenic liver abscesses.
- Aspirate should be sent for Gram-stain and aerobic/anaerobic culture; evaluation for fungal and mycobacterial pathogens and *E. histolytica* should be considered based on epidemiologic factors.
- CT or US-guided percutaneous needle aspiration +/- catheter drainage initial method of choice with success in up to 90% of cases; if drainage inadequate, surgical drainage may be required.
- Percutaneous aspiration without catheter placement has recently been found to have similar success rates as catheter placement, with repeat aspiration required in approximately 50%.
- Complications of percutaneous drainage include perforation of adjacent abdominal organs, pneumothorax, hemorrhage and leakage of abscess contents in peritoneum.
- General recommendations are for at least one wk of drainage with CT follow-up.
- Surgical drainage may be primary treatment in setting of: complex abscess, multiple abscesses, percutaneously unreachable abscess, or additional surgical problem is present; drainage may be done laparoscopically.
- Hepatotomy generally successful approach, but improvements in percutaneous techniques make it secondary management in most cases.
- Medical management should be considered in pts with high risk for drainage or with small/multiple abscesses not amenable to drainage.

Antibiotic treatment

- Empiric coverage should include Enterobacteriaceae, enterococci, anaerobes, and in certain situations staphylococci and streptococci. In stable pt may defer abx until post-aspiration/drainage.
- In pts who have received adequate drainage, duration of treatment depends on resolution of fever and leukocytosis (often 14–42 days total).
- Longer courses (up to several mos) may be required in the pt who is inadequately drained or treated solely medically.
- Follow-up imaging studies should be performed to determine resolution, utilizing CT and/or US.
- Consider empiric antifungal rx in immunosuppressed pts at risk for chronic disseminated candidiasis (CDC, a.k.a. hepatosplenic candidiasis, also see *C. albicans* module).
- Culture results may help narrow coverage, but for pyogenic abscess do not discontinue anaerobic coverage given difficulty culturing these organisms.
- Empiric Rx: ampicillin 2.0 g IV q6h plus gentamicin 1.7 g IV q8h plus metronidazole 0.5 g IV q8h until diagnostic cultures have returned to refine regimen.
- Alt: cefotaxime 2.0 g IV q8h or ceftriaxone 2.0 g IV q24h plus metronidazole 0.5 g IV q8h.

- B-lactam/B-lactamase inhibitors (e.g., piperacillin-tazobactam) are reasonable alternatives; metronidazole should be included if amebic abscess is in the differential.
- Fluoroquinolone (ciprofloxacin, levofloxacin, or moxifloxacin) plus metronidazole also an alternative; often used as an oral regimen for prolonged therapy.

Amebic hepatic abscess

- Metronidazole (750 mg PO three times a day × 7–10 days) as a tissue agent, followed by a luminal agent to eliminate residual colonic colonization, usually paromomycin 500 mg three times a day PO × 7 days.
- Alternatives tissue agents (in place of metronidazole): tinidazole 800 mg three times a day or 2 g daily × 3–5 days.
- Alternative luminal agents (in place of paromomycin): iodoquinol (650 mg three times a day × 20 days) or diloxanide furoate (500 mg three times a day × 10 days).
- Percutaneous aspiration has no clear role in therapy, but consider for diagnosis if uncertain (serology pending) or no response to appropriate therapy.
- Predictors of need for aspiration include age >55 yrs, abscesses >5 cms, involvement of both lobes of liver and failure of medical therapy after 7 days.

Hydatid (Echinococcal) cyst

- Most commonly *E. granulosus*. Serology usually helpful in most cases.
- In pts with rupture of the cyst in the biliary tree, transient but markedly elevated levels of alkaline phosphatase and bilirubin may occur. Hyperamylasemia and eosinophilia occur in up to 60%.
- Surgical resection standard intervention.
- In pts with uncomplicated cysts, PAIR (Percutaneous puncture with CT or US guidance, followed by aspiration, Injection of a protoscolicidal agent such as hypertonic saline or ethanal, and finally re-aspiration 15 minutes later) is becoming more accepted treatment of choice due to high success rates with low morbidity.
- Open or percutaneous (PAIR) procedures should be combined with albendazole treatment.

OTHER INFORMATION

- Frequently polymicrobial; single/multiple lesions occur in approximately a 1:1 ratio, with the majority in the right lobe (especially when solitary); cryptogenic abscesses are generally solitary.
- Untreated, the mortality rate associated with pyogenic hepatic abscess approaches 100%, with treatment in some series it is below 15%; the latter mortality is dependent upon underlying disease.
- Recurrence is more frequent after simple percutaneous aspiration without placement of a temporary drain, or in pts in whom drains are removed too early.
- Abscesses are frequently associated with chronic medical conditions (e.g., diabetes mellitus) hematologic disease (e.g., leukemia), and chronic granulomatous disease (*Staphylococcus aureus*).
- Chronic disseminated candidiasis (CDC, a.k.a. hepatosplenic candidiasis) occurs in immunosuppressed pts, e.g., bone marrow transplant recipients.

BASIS FOR RECOMMENDATIONS

Solomkin JS, Mazuski JE, Baron EJ, et al. Guidelines for the selection of anti-infective agents for complicated intra-abdominal infections. *Clin Infect Dis*, 2003; Vol. 37; pp. 997–1005.
Comments: Consensus, evidence-based general guidelines from IDSA, SIS, ASM, and SIDP.

INTRA-ABDOMINAL ABSCESS

Christopher F. Carpenter, MD and Aditi Swami, MD

PATHOGENS

- If identified, location of source of infection (e.g., site of perforation—stomach, duodenum, jejunum, ileum, appendix, or colon) defines likely flora
- Health-care associated flora more likely when infections are complications of prior intraabdominal operations or procedures
- Anaerobes including *Bacteroides* spp., *Fusobacterium* spp., *Clostridium* spp., *Actinomyces* spp., etc.

DIAGNOSIS

- Enterobacteriaceae
- Other Gram-negative bacilli
- Enterococci
- Candida species
- Occasionally, Gram-positives including *Staphylococcus aureus*

CLINICAL
- Broad range of presenting complaints: pts may only present with malaise/anorexia or weight loss; others present acutely ill in septic shock with an acute abdomen.
- Non visceral abscesses develop after gastrointestinal perforation from local disease (diverticulitis, etc.), trauma, or surgical intervention; Subsequent secondary peritonitis then becomes walled off by inflammatory adhesions, loops of intestine, mesentery or omentum, and other abdominal viscera; intra–abdominal abscess also may develop after primary peritonitis (spontaneous bacterial peritonitis).
- Sx: fever, pain, nausea, vomiting, anorexia.
- PE: local tenderness, possibly a palpable mass; postoperative assessment for abscess confounded by analgesics and incisional pain, with over half presenting within 10 days of initial operation.
- Lab: elevated WBC, direct aspiration yielding positive Gram-stain/culture, blood cultures positive ~25% depending on site.

DIAGNOSIS
- CT most helpful. US and MRI used occasionally. MRI not used for drainage guidance.
- CT or US-guided percutaneous or surgical drainage should be considered in all cases for diagnostic confirmation, microbiologic evaluation, and therapy.
- Indium and Gallium scanning rarely required for this diagnosis with the advent of these imaging newer modalities.

TREATMENT
Primary therapy: abscess drainage
- CT or US-guided percutaneous needle aspiration with subsequent catheter drainage is considered by many as the first line of therapy; if drainage is inadequate surgery may be required.
- Surgery used primarily after percutaneous therapy has failed, when it has stabilized condition for primary surgical therapy, or when concurrent surgical source control needed.
- Infected pancreatic necrosis not well suited to percutaneous therapy because of cellular debris.
- If an enteric abscess unrelated to a surgical procedure is encountered, must consider the possibility of an underlying necrotic cancer.

Adjunctive antibiotic treatment
- Empiric coverage (i.e., when the microbiologic source of infection is unknown) should include coverage of Enterobacteriaceae, enterococci, and anaerobes.
- After adequate drainage, at least 5–10 days of antibiotic coverage is indicated, with duration in part based on resolution of fever and leukocytosis, severity of infection, and clinical response. Duration of therapy has not been subjected to rigorous study. If the underlying surgical problem has been controlled (source) short course of antibiotics maybe appropriate.
- Empiric coverage may be broadened or cautiously narrowed on the basis of the abscess and blood cultures results.
- **Mild-moderate infections:** ticarcillin-clavulanate 3.1 g IV q6h or ampicillin-sulbactam 3.0 g IV q6h or ertapenem 1 g IV q24h.
- Alternative combination therapy for mild-moderate infections: ciprofloxacin 400 mg IV q12h or levofloxacin 500 mg IV once daily plus metronidazole 500 mg IV q6–8h; moxifloxacin 400 mg IV once daily +/– metronidazole. Cefazolin 1–2 g IV q8h + metronidazole.
- **Severe and/or nosocomial infections:** piperacillin-tazobactam 3.375 g IV q6h or 4.5 g IV q8h, imipenem 0.5 g IV q6h or meropenem 1.0 g IV q8h, ciprofloxacin 400 mg IV q12h or levofloxacin 500 mg IV once daily plus metronidazole 500 mg IV q6–8h; moxifloxacin 400 mg IV once daily + metronidazole, doripenem 500 mg IV q8h.

- Alternatives for severe and/or nosocomial infections: cefotaxime 2 g IV q8h or ceftriaxone 2 g IV once daily or cefepime 2 g IV q8h plus metronidazole 500 mg IV q6–8h. Aztreonam 1–2 g IV q8h + metronidazole.

FOLLOW UP

- On-demand re-laparotomy rather than a planned re-laparotomy may be associated with better results in selected cases.
- Source control is essential. The open abdomen approach is occasionally necessary to control the source of infection.
- If no clinical response within 3–5 days of antibiotic therapy and drainage, consider re-imaging to look for undrained collections, other processes.
- Follow up CT scan/US and/or sinograms needed to show resolution of source and abscess.
- Useful clinical parameters to follow include imaging studies, temperature, white blood cell count, and possibly serum C-reactive protein.

OTHER INFORMATION

- Multiple factors, including severity of illness, bacteremia, multiple abscesses, and location of abscess are predictive of mortality (even with treatment mortality may still approach 30% depending on the population).
- Percutaneous drainage should be utilized IF possible and surgical source is controlled.
- Rate of recovery of yeast from intraoperative specimens of a perforated viscus was >30% and was associated with death and complications. Consider anti-fungal treatment if recovery of yeast from cultures and pt not clinically improving, or repeated recovery of yeast from cultures.
- Non-visceral intra-abdominal abscesses should be considered polymicrobial in nearly all cases.
- Local susceptibility patterns (e.g., for *Pseudomonas*, etc.) should be considered in the decision for empiric coverage for hospital-acquired infections.

BASIS FOR RECOMMENDATIONS

Solomkin JS, Mazuski JE, Baron EJ, et al. Guidelines for the selection of anti-infective agents for complicated intra-abdominal infections. *Clin Infect Dis*, 2003; Vol. 37; pp. 997–1005.

Comments: IDSA, SIS, ASM, and SIDP consensus guidelines.

PERITONITIS, SPONTANEOUS BACTERIAL AND SECONDARY

Christopher F. Carpenter, MD and Aditi Swami, MD

PATHOGENS

- *Escherichia coli*
- *Klebsiella species*
- Enterobacter species
- Other Enterobacteriaceae
- *Streptococcus pneumoniae*
- Streptococci and enterococci
- Polymicrobial (secondary peritonitis)
- Anaerobes (secondary peritonitis)

CLINICAL

- Pts with ascites, fever (may be low-grade or absent) and/or abdominal pain should be evaluated for spontaneous bacterial peritonitis (SBP, also known as primary peritonitis) or other forms of peritonitis.
- Other signs/symptoms (e.g., encephalopathy) may be the only clues of SBP. The abdomen in SBP often has mild diffuse discomfort but rarely is it consistent with classic findings of secondary peritonitis.
- SBP should be suspected in all pts with ascites and clinical decompensation.
- The possibility of SBP should be considered in (1) all cirrhotic pts on admission to hospital; (2) all pts with ascites who develop hepatic encephalopathy, renal impairment, or altered GI motility; and (3) all pts with ascites suffering from a GI bleed (empirical treatment/prophylaxis may be indicated).
- Secondary peritonitis = peritonitis with a surgically amenable source (e.g., appendicitis, diverticulitis; routinely polymicrobial).

DIAGNOSIS

- Tertiary peritonitis = relatively new term referring to persistence of peritonitis/abscess following apparent adequate treatment of primary or secondary peritonitis.

DIAGNOSIS

- SBP clinical findings: fever (70%), ascites (may be small amount), abdominal pain/tenderness (50%); many will have no classic findings to suggest infection.
- SBP diagnostic criteria: ascites with >250 PMN cells/ml with positive cultures and no surgically amenable intraabdominal source of infection.
- SBP variant forms: culture-negative neutrophilic (PMN >250) ascites (CNNA—up to 40%) and monomicrobial non-neutrophilic (PMN <250) bacterascites (MNB).
- Secondary peritonitis clinical findings: more commonly with peritoneal findings of an acute abdomen—rebound tenderness and guarding, sepsis, and radiographic findings defining the source and revealing free air and potentially early abscess development.
- Differentiation of SBP from secondary peritonitis (if surgical source not identified): secondary peritonitis results in much higher WBC count (often >10,000), with polymicrobial culture results.
- Culture of ascitic fluid in a blood culture bottle may result in a higher culture yield for SBP (from 50% conventional to approximately 80%).

TREATMENT

SBP Treatment

- Cefotaxime 2 g IV q8h or ceftriaxone 1 g IV once daily.
- Recent single center report of effectiveness of cefotaxime + albumin in reducing mortality and irreversible renal impairment.
- Ciprofloxacin 400 mg IV q12h or levofloxacin 500 mg IV once daily or moxifloxacin 400 mg IV once daily.
- Ofloxacin has been reported effective as an oral alternative at 400 mg PO twice daily.
- Ticarcillin-clavulanate 3.1 g IV q6h or piperacillin-tazobactam 3.375 g IV q6h or 4.5 g IV q8h or ampicillin-sulbactam 3.0 g IV q6h.
- Ertapenem 1.0 g IV once daily; for pts with resistant pathogens: imipenem 500 mg IV q6h, meropenem 1.0 g IV q8h, or doripenem 500 mg IV q8h.
- Cefepime 1–2 g IV q8h for pts with resistant pathogens.
- Use ascitic culture results to refine antibiotic choice (if necessary).
- Repeated paracentesis may be considered; PMN's <250 with negative culture support an abbreviated course (<5 days).
- Duration of 5–7 days likely adequate; traditional 10–14 days is longer than needed unless complicated pts or positive blood cultures.
- Culture-negative neutrophilic ascites (CNNA) has clinical, prognostic, and therapeutic characteristics similar to spontaneous bacterial peritonitis (SBP) and should be treated in a similar fashion. Pts with monomicrobial non-neutrophilic bacterascites (MNB) typically respond similar to CNNA and SBP if the pt is symptomatic; asymptomatic pts usually do not need antibiotics and observation is appropriate, but consideration of TB should be entertained.

SBP prophylaxis

- Prophylaxis recommended **after** first episode of SBP (secondary prophylaxis); benefits for other indications, e.g., after variceal bleeding or in pts with low ascitic fluid protein, etc. (primary prophylaxis) controversial, especially with concerns of resistance promotion.
- Trimethoprim-sulfamethoxazole 1 DS PO once daily.
- Norfloxacin 400 mg PO once daily.
- Ciprofloxacin 750 mg PO once weekly

Secondary Peritonitis Treatment

- Supportive therapy.
- Operative management is indicated to eliminate the source of contamination, reduce the bacterial load, and prevent recurrence.
- Empiric antimicrobial coverage should include coverage of Gram-negative aerobes, Gram-positive cocci, and anaerobes.

- Upper tract source (e.g., perforated ulcer) usually predominantly Gram-positive infections; lower tract (distal small bowel or colon) generally results in anaerobic and Gram-negative aerobes.
- Duration can generally be limited to 5 to 7 days, longer if leukocytosis/left shift and fever are slow to resolve or source control inadequate.
- Ticarcillin-clavulanate 3.1 g IV q6h or piperacillin-tazobactam 3.375 g IV q6h or 4.5 g IV q8h or ampicillin-sulbactam 3.0 g IV q6h.
- Metronidazole **plus** 3rd/4th generation cephalosporin **or** fluoroquinolone **or** aztreonam.
- Ertapenem 1.0 g IV once daily; for pts with resistant pathogens: imipenem 500 mg IV q6h or meropenem 1.0 g IV q8h or doripenem 500 mg IV q8h.

Catheter-associated Peritonitis

- Treat CAPD-associated peritonitis empirically with vancomycin plus Gram-negative coverage, pending cultures.
- Catheter may need removal (especially for yeast, *S. aureus*, *Pseudomonas aeruginosa*, and *Stenotrophomonas maltophilia*).

OTHER INFORMATION

- Pts with cirrhosis and ascites have a 1 yr risk of SBP as high as 29%.
- Peritonitis associated with chronic ambulatory peritoneal dialysis (CAPD). Requires coverage of *Staphylococcus aureus*, coagulase-negative staphylococci, Enterobacteriaceae, *Pseudomonas aeruginosa*, and *Candida* spp.
- Several other potential causes of peritonitis: tuberculosis, chemical peritonitis, malignant ascites with carcinomatosis, familial Mediterranean fever (FMF), or systemic lupus erythematosis (SLE), etc.

BASIS FOR RECOMMENDATIONS

Piraino B, Bailie GR, Bernardini J, et al. Peritoneal dialysis-related infections recommendations: 2005 update. *Perit Dial Int*, 2005; Vol. 25; pp. 107–31.

Comments: International guideline update for peritoneal dialysis-related infections.

Solomkin JS, Mazuski JE, Baron EJ, et al. Guidelines for the selection of anti-infective agents for complicated intra-abdominal infections. *Clin Infect Dis*, 2003; Vol. 37; pp. 997–1005.

Comments: Consensus evidence-based guidelines from IDSA, SIS, ASM, and SIDP.

SPLENIC ABSCESS

Christopher F. Carpenter, MD and Aditi Swami, MD

PATHOGENS

- Gram-negative bacilli, *especially E. coli* and *Salmonella* spp.
- *Staphylococcus aureus.*
- *Streptococci* and *enterococci.*
- Anaerobes.
- *Candida* spp.
- Mycobacteria.
- Rarely, *Brucella* spp. may cause splenic abscesses.
- Polymicrobial in up to 25% including anaerobes.
- As the most common cause of splenic abscess is bacteremia from a distant site (e.g., endocarditis, UTI, pancreatitis, GI tract, etc.), the likely pathogens are determined by the original focus as well as other underlying risk factor(s).
- Neutropenia and chronic corticosteroid use predispose to candida splenic abscesses.
- Chronic disseminated candidiasis (formerly hepatosplenic candidiasis) often include frank candidal splenic abscesses.

CLINICAL

- Hematogenous spread is most common cause (septicemia, endocarditis, IDU, etc.); other risk groups include immunosuppressed individuals (e.g., HIV, steroid use, chemotherapy, underlying illness, etc.), trauma, contiguous spread, etc.
- More common in men, with an age range from 6 mos to over 90 yrs.
- Other high risk groups include pts with hemoglobinopathies (e.g., sickle cell disease), diabetes mellitus; up to 20% may not have an identifiable predisposing underlying disease.

DIAGNOSIS

- Generalized abdominal (15–70%) or LUQ (40–50%) pain, fever (85–95%), and LUQ tenderness (40–60%), usually subacute (2–4 wks or longer); splenomegaly in 30–50%.
- Diaphragmatic irritation may result in referred left shoulder pain, +/– a pleuritic component. Also may have anorexia and malaise.
- Localizing signs of splenic abscess may be overshadowed by underlying illness/risk factor such as endocarditis, pancreatitis, neutropenia, and injection drug use.
- Lab: leukocytosis w/ left shift common (60–80%). Blood cxs may be positive in 20–83% of pts w/ multiple splenic abscess but only 14% w/ solitary abscess.
- Multiple abscesses the norm in pts with hematogenous origin; were more likely of GNR origin and have a higher mortality rate.

DIAGNOSIS

- Clinical diagnosis is inherently difficult.
- Plain radiographs may reveal abnormalities, e.g., an effusion or infiltrate, but are non-specific, and radionuclide scans are of little utility.
- Need CT or MRI as imaging procedures of choice; ultrasound reasonable alternative.
- CT findings suggesting infection: (1) gas, (2) progressive increase in size, (3) subcapsular extension with free adjacent fluid.
- With consistent imaging findings, diagnosis may be further confirmed with positive blood cultures.
- Biopsy/aspiration may be required establish or exclude infection.

TREATMENT

Drainage

- Due to relative rarity of splenic abscesses, most information garnered from small case series.
- Optimal management includes drainage if feasible. Small or multiple abscesses may respond to abx alone, especially if pathogen known.
- CT or US-guided percutaneous needle aspiration (potentially with drain placement for larger abscesses) is considered initial drainage method of choice; if drainage inadequate, may require surgical drainage.
- Splenectomy or splenotomy are the standard surgical approaches for pts w/ unresolving abscesses or after failure despite percutaneous drainage + abx.
- Splenectomy performed only if splenotomy unfeasible.
- EUS-guided drainage also being evaluated as therapeutic option; experience extremely limited.
- Due to risk of post splenectomy sepsis, early immunization against encapsulated organisms with pneumococcal, *Haemophilus influenzae* type b, and meningococcal vaccines should be pursued if splenectomy is under consideration (ideal timing at least 2 wks prior to splenectomy).

Antibiotic treatment considerations

- Empiric coverage directed toward *S. aureus, Strep* spp., Gram-negative rods and anaerobes, e.g., ampicillin-sulbactam, piperacillin-tazobactam, ceftriaxone + metronidazole; consider vancomycin if suspect MRSA.
- If source of splenic abscess known (e.g., a pt with a contiguous intraabdominal infection), empiric coverage should be directed appropriately.
- Empiric coverage should be narrowed to pathogen-specific coverage once blood and/or abscess culture results available.
- Follow-up imaging studies guide duration; antibiotics may be discontinued once resolution of the abscess is documented (if splenectomy not performed) granted no other foci of infection persist.
- In pts w/ adequate drainage or resection, duration of 10–14 days abx may be adequate.
- Longer courses (up to 6 wks) may be required in pts w/ inadequate drainage or treated medically (e.g., pt with endocarditis or chronic disseminated candidiasis).
- Empiric antifungal treatment should be considered in immunosuppressed pts at risk for chronic disseminated candidiasis (see *Candida* module).
- Useful clinical parameters to follow include imaging studies, temperature, white blood cell count, and potentially serum C-reactive protein.

OTHER INFORMATION

- Over half are solitary lesions, more commonly with associated endocarditis (60–85%); less common in immunosuppressed pts.
- Other organs w/ abscesses in approximately one-fourth of pts, more commonly in pts with multiple splenic abscesses (40–50%). Most common other organ: liver.
- Chronic disseminated candidiasis (CDC, a.k.a. hepatosplenic candidiasis) occurs in pts with prolonged profound immunosuppression, e.g., stem cell transplant recipients.
- CDC manifests as multiple small abscesses in the spleen, liver, kidneys, and other solid organs. Typically pts become febrile and their lesions become visible once neutropenia resolves.
- Untreated, the mortality rate associated with splenic abscess is near 100%; with drainage and adjunctive antibiotics, it drops to below 15%.

BASIS FOR RECOMMENDATIONS

Ng KK, Lee TY, Wan YL, et al. Splenic abscess: diagnosis and management. *Hepatogastroenterology*, 2002; Vol. 49; pp. 567–71.

Comments: Case series and review of diagnosis and management.

SURGICAL PROPHYLAXIS

Paul G. Auwaerter, MD

PATHOGENS

- Coagulase negative staphylococci (especially cardiac surgery and hardware associated surgeries)
- *Staphylococcus aureus*
- Streptococcal species
- Enterobacteriaceae (GI)
- Anaerobes (GI)

CLINICAL

- Surgical prophylaxis refers to the administration of antibiotics in pts with no signs of infection to reduce the risk of post-operative wound infections.
- Antibiotics should be given prior to procedures where the risk of contamination is high (e.g., gastrointestinal surgery) or the consequences of infection would be very serious (e.g., cardiac surgery).
- Antibiotics should cover the predominant flora of the operative site. Staphylococci and streptococci for most cases. Anaerobes and enterobacteriaceae for GI cases.
- Effectiveness of antibiotics most dependent upon having tissue levels of the antibiotic at time of initial skin incision. In prolonged surgery, antibiotics may need to be redosed; however, there has been no convincing data to document efficacy for post-operative administration of antibiotics for prophylactic measures.
- Most guidelines give option to substitute vancomycin for cefazolin in hospitals with "high" rates of MRSA, but this is no well defined.
- Please see table (p. 209) for complete recommendations.

TREATMENT

General Considerations

- For procedures not listed below and for important dosing information, see treatment table (pp. 210–211). For redosing, see Follow-Up section. Cefotetan is now available again in U.S.
- In general, clean cases (most plastic surgery and dermatologic surgery) do not require pre-operative prophylaxis.
- Efficacy based upon having antibiotics in skin and soft tissue at time of first surgical incision.
- All antibiotic administration <u>must be completed at the time of surgical incision</u> and no more than <u>1 hr prior</u> (except higher doses of vancomycin infused in prior 2 hrs).
- **Antibiotic administration specifics:** β-lactams (cefazolin, other cephalosporins and ampicillin/sulbactam): may be given IV or IV push over 3–5 minutes, all reach adequate skin levels within minutes—hence can be given just prior to surgery. Also, cefuroxime may be substituted for cefazolin in all indications.

- Vancomycin: infuse over 1 hr (2 hrs for higher doses), entire dose must be administered prior to skin incision. Vancomycin (wt based dosing recommendations): <70 kg—1 g, 71–99 kg—1.25 g, >100 kg—1.5 g; all IV q12h.
- Clindamycin: infuse over 10–20 m.
- Ciprofloxacin: infuse over 1h, entire dose must be administered prior to skin incision.
- If pt already receiving antibiotics: vancomycin—redose if 8 hrs elapsed from last dose, if <8 hrs give ½ dose. For other antibiotics, hold usual dose until 1hr prior to incision.
- Any aminoglycoside may be substituted for Gram-negative coverage.

General surgery
- Cefotetan again available, but alternatives include cefoxitin 1 g IV, or cefazolin 2 g IV + metronidazole 500 mg IV or ampicillin/sulbactam 3 g IV. Ertapenem 1 g compared favorably to cefotetan in one study and FDA approved, but many reluctant to use a carbapenem due to resistance, expense concerns. Also, data suggest mechanical bowel cleansing regimens may be unnecessary for bowel surgery.
- Appendectomy (uncomplicated, if complicated or perforated treat as peritonitis): cefotetan 2 g IV. PCN allergy: clindamycin 600 mg IV plus gentamicin 5 mg/kg.
- Cholecystectomy open or laparoscopic prophylaxis, gastrectomy, hepatectomy: cefotetan 2 g IV. PCN allergy: clindamycin 600 mg IV +/– gentamicin 5 mg/kg.
- Colon surgery/whipple procedure: neomycin and erythromycin (or metronidazole), 1 g each PO at 1, 2, and 11 pm day before surgery. IV: cefotetan 2 g or cefoxitin 2 g or ampicillin/sulbactam 3 g IV pre-op. [Some combine PO and IV]. PCN allergy: clindamycin 600 mg IV + gentamicin 5 mg/kg IV pre-op.
- Inguinal hernia repair: uncomplicated, prophylaxis not recommended. Complicated, recurrent or emergent: cefotetan 2 g IV or cefoxitin 2 g or ampicillin/sulbactam 3 g IV; PCN allergy: clindamycin 600 mg IV +/– gentamicin 5 mg/kg.
- PEG: cefazolin 2 g IV or cefotetan 2 g IV. PCN allergy: clindamycin 600 mg IV +/– gentamicin 5 mg/kg.
- Penetrating abdominal trauma: cefotetan 2 g IV. PCN allergy: clindamycin 600 mg IV + gentamicin 5 mg/kg IV.
- Mastectomy: no abx recommended. Mastectomy with LN dissection: cefazolin 2 g IV, PCN allergy: clindamycin 600 mg IV+ gentamicin.
- Small bowel or colon surgery: cefotetan 2 g IV. PCN allergy: clindamycin 600 mg IV +/– gentamicin 5 mg/kg.
- Whipple procedure or pancreatectomy: cefotetan 2 g IV. PCN allergy: clindamycin 600 mg IV +/– gentamicin 5 mg/kg.

Gynecologic surgery
- Cesarean section: cefazolin 2 g IV after cord clamping, if β-lactam allergy use clindamycin 600 mg IV.
- Hysterectomy (abdominal or vaginal): uncomplicated—cefazolin 2 g. Complicated: cefotetan 2 g IV. PCN allergy: clindamycin 600 mg IV + gentamicin.
- Repair of cystocele or rectocele: cefazolin 2 g. PCN allergy: clindamycin 600 mg IV.
- Dilation and curettage: uncomplicated, no prophylaxis needed. Complicated: cefazolin 2 g IV. PCN allergy: clindamycin 600 mg IV.

Orthopedic surgery
- Joint replacement: cefazolin 2 g IV. PCN allergy: vancomycin IV. Infuse before inflation of tourniquet.
- Open reduction of fracture: cefazolin 2 g IV pre-op, continue 24 hrs for closed hip fractures (open fractures should be treated as infected, use cefazolin 2 g IV q8h × 10 days). PCN allergy: vancomycin IV pre-op and then dosed for duration as cefazolin.
- Lower limb amputation: cefotetan 2 g IV. PCN allergy: gentamicin 5 mg/kg IV + clindamycin 600 mg IV.
- Laminectomy: cefazolin 2 g IV. PCN allergy: clindamycin 600 mg IV.
- Spinal fusion: cefazolin 2 g IV. PCN allergy: clindamycin 600 mg IV or vancomycin IV.
- Arthroscopic surgery: no data support prophylaxis.

Cardiac or vascular surgery
- Uncomplicated median sternotomy/uncomplicated heart transplant: cefazolin 2 g IV. PCN allergic: vancomycin IV.

- Heart transplant w/ previous VAD, MRSA colonization/infection: cefazolin 2 g IV plus vancomycin IV. PCN allergy: vancomycin IV.
- May continue dosing for 24 hrs after surgery, median sternotomy only. For open chest, continued prophylaxtic antibiotics until 24 hrs post closure (48 hrs for VAD).
- Pacemaker/AICD placement: cefazolin 2 g IV. PCN allergy: clindamycin 600 mg IV.
- LVAD/BIVAD placement: vancomycin IV plus ciprofloxacin 400 mg IV plus fluconazole 400 mg IV.
- Carotid surgery prophylaxis unnecessary unless considered high risk.

FOLLOW UP
- Further antibiotics are unnecessary following most surgical procedures, except as noted.
- Abx must be redosed during lengthy procedures, depending on drug used and its pharmacodynamics. Optimal redosing time of all agents is not known but general guidelines are given.
- **Redosing schedule:** ampicillin/sulbactam 3 g IV q2h (note T½ is 1.0–1.2 hrs).
- Cefazolin 2 g IV q4h (q2h for cardiac surgery); cefazolin also should be re-dosed q 1500 ml blood loss.
- Cefuroxime 1.5 g IV q3–4h. Cefoxitin 1–2 g IV q3–4h.
- Clindamycin 600 mg IV q8h
- Ciprofloxacin 400 mg IV q8h
- Gentamicin 5 mg/kg IV dose generally does not require redosing. If using gentamicin 2 mg/kg dose, then redose q8h.
- Metronidazole 500 mg IV q8h
- Vancomycin (wt based): <70 kg—1g, 71–99 kg—1.25 g, >100 kg—1.5 g; all IV q12h.

OTHER INFORMATION
- Some studies indicate antibiotics should be given no more than 2 hrs prior to case, but newer data suggest 1 hr or less for optimal efficacy.
- Single dose of antibiotic (with intraoperative redosing if needed) appear to be equivalent to pre and post-procedure antibiotic administration, therefore post-procedure antibiotics are not recommended.
- Hot topic: recommendations regarding vancomycin use in era of increasing MRSA and CA-MRSA.

MORE INFORMATION
Peri-operative Antibiotic Prophylaxis
To Prevent Surgical Site Infection
Note: **Never** "split" doses: give the full dose at one time!
Dosing Antibiotics should **not** be given more than 1 hr prior to incision (2 hrs for vancomycin).
Redosing suggestions listed immediately below each drug name in *italics*.

Weight (kg)	Cefa-zolin Q2–4h (Cardiac Q2h)	Cefo-tetan Q8h	Vanco-mycin Q12h	Clin-damycin Q8h	Metron-idazole Q8h	Gen-tamicin redos-ing not needed	Ampicil-lin/Sul-bactam Q2h
<70 kg	2 g	2 g	1 g	600 mg	500 mg	5 mg/kg	3 g
71–99	2 g	2 g	1.25 gs	600 mg	500 mg	5 mg/kg	3 g
>100	2 g	2 g	1.5 gs	600 mg	500 mg	5 mg/kg	3 g
Admin-istration	IV Push	IV Push	1–2 hrs infusion	10–20 minute infusion	1 hr infusion	30 minute infusion	IV Push

Also Re-Dose for Every 1500 CC Of Blood Loss Or Hemodilution.
Note on endocarditis prophylaxis: Pts receiving pre-op antibiotics to prevent an SSI generally do **not** need additional antibiotics for endocarditis prophylaxis.
Pts with orthopedic hardware also do not appear to need additional prophylaxis beyond what is recommended for the case.

Procedure	Prophylaxis Recommendations	PCN Allergy Alternate Prophylaxis
Transplant Surgery		
Renal transplant/adult live liver donor	Cefotetan 2 g IV	Clindamycin 600 mg IV plus Ciprofloxacin 400 mg
Liver transplant	Cefotetan 2 g IV	Clindamycin 600 mg IV
Pancreas or pancreas/kidney transplant	Cefotetan 2 g IV	Clindamycin 600 mg IV plus Ciprofloxacin 400 mg I
Plastic Surgery		
Tissue expander insertion/all flaps	Cefazolin 2 g IV	Clindamycin 600 mg IV
Rhinoplasty	No prophylaxis or cefazolin 2 g IV	No prophylaxis or Clindamycin 600 mg IV
Thoracic Surgery		
All cases except esophageal	Cefazolin 2 g IV	Clindamycin 600 mg IV
Esophageal cases	Cefotetan 2 g IV	Clindamycin 600 mg IV
Lung transplant	Piperacillin-tazobactam 4.5 g IV	Vancomycin IV plus ciprofloxacin 400 mg IV. If cystic fibrosis pt, use pre-transplant sputum cultures to guide recommendations.
Urologic Surgery		
Transrectal prostate biopsy	Cefotetan 2 g IV	Ciprofloxacin 500 mg PO/IV
Transurethral surgery (TURP, TURBT, ureteroscopy, cystouretoscopy)	Cefazolin 2 g IV	Gentamicin 5 mg/kg/day
Radical, retropublic prostatectomy OR nephrectomy	Cefazolin 2 g IV	Clindamycin 600 mg IV pre-op
Prostatectomy (TURP or peritoneal)	If sterile urine: ciprofloxacin 500 mg PO or 400 mg IV pre-op only if high-risk procedure. No data to support prophylaxis if pre-procedure urine cultures are sterile and procedure is low risk.	

Procedure	Prophylaxis Recommendations	PCN Allergy Alternate Prophylaxis
Penile or other prosthesis	Cefazolin 2 g IV or vancomycin IV +/− gentamicin 5 mg/kg IV.	Clindamycin 600 mg IV or vancomycin IV either +/− gentamicin 5 mg/kg IV.
Radical cystectomy, cystoprostatectomy OR anterior exoneration	Cefotetan 2 g IV	Clindamycin 600 mg IV plus gentamicin 5 mg/kg IV
Lithrotripsy	Cefazolin 2 g IV	Gentamicin 5 mg/kg IV
Head and Neck Surgery		
Major procedure with incision of oral, sinus or pharyngeal mucosa, major neck dissection, or parotid surgery	Cefotetan 2 g IV	Clindamycin 600 mg IV
Tonsillectomy	Clindamycin 600 mg IV	
Thyroid/parathyroid surgery	Prophylaxis not recommended.	
Vascular surgery		
All cases (except carotid surgery, unnecessary)	Cefazolin 2 g IV	Vancomycin IV
Neurosurgery		
Craniotomy, spinal fusion, laminectomy, shunt placement	Cefazolin 2 g IV	Clindamycin 600 mg IV or vancomycin IV
Interventional Radiology		
Biliary/GI Procedure (including chemo/radio- ablation, splenic embolization)	Cefotetan 2 g IV	Gentamicin 5 mg/kg IV plus metronidazole 500 g IV
Urologic Procedure	Cefazolin 2 g IV	Gentamicin 5 mg/kg IV
Implantable Venous Access Port (e.g., Mediport)	Cefazolin 2 g IV	Clindamycin 600 g IV
Tunneled Catheters	No prophylaxis recommended	
Lymphangiogram, vascular malformation ablation, fibroid treatment	Cefazolin 2 g IV	Clindamycin 600 mg IV

There are no recommendations for antibiotics for these pts in cases where they are not indicated for SSI prevention.

BASIS FOR RECOMMENDATIONS

Cosgrove S, Avdic E. Johns Hopkins Antibiotic guidelines: treatment recommendations for inpatients. *The Johns Hopkins Antibiotic Management Program*, 2008–2009.

Comments: Guideline strategies used at Johns Hopkins Hospital, written and directed by Sara Cosgrove and Edina Avdic. Modules recommendations reflect these recommendations with similar options to reflect formulary differences at other institutions.

Antimicrobial prophylaxis for surgery. *Treat Guidel Med Lett*, 2006; Vol. 4; pp. 83–8.
Comments: Another guideline, from a recognized authority that offers similar suggestions and a more thorough discussion of indications and rationale.

SURGICAL SITE INFECTIONS (SSI)

Christopher F. Carpenter, MD and Aditi Swami, MD

PATHOGENS
- Staphylococcus aureus (often MRSA)
- Coagulase-negative staphylococci
- Gram-negative bacilli
- *Enterococcus*
- *Streptococcus* spp.
- Anaerobes (depending on site)
- Candida species may be isolated in culture; treatment is controversial

CLINICAL
- SSI Rate: overall estimates range up to 5%, accounting for up to one-fourth of all nosocomial infections.
- Appropriate antibiotic prophylaxis and other perioperative care interventions could reduce the rate of SSI by over 50%.
- In general, SSI risk factors include pre-existing medical illnesses, e.g., diabetes; prolonged operations (site specific), and contaminated or dirty wounds.
- Traditional wound classification system (clean, clean-contaminated, contaminated, and dirty-infected) alone does not adequately predict infection risk.
- To quantify risk factors, NNIS system assigns one point for ASA score of 3 or more on a 5 point scale, operation lasting longer than 75th percentile of the average duration for that procedure, and a contaminated or dirty procedure.
- SSI Risks using this system: 0 risk factors—1.5%, 1 risk factor—2.9%, 2 risk factors—6.8%, and 3 risk factors—13%, with all surgeries combined risk of 2.8%.
- Most postoperative SSIs occur a median of 12 days (3–28 days, 25–75%) after surgery; more rapid presentations suggest toxin producing pathogens, e.g., Clostridium spp., *Streptococcus pyogenes*.
- Estimated costs range from $400 for superficial SSI to >$30,000 for severe organ/space SSIs.

DIAGNOSIS
- Surgical site infection (SSI) = wound infection; types include superficial (skin and subcutaneous tissue), deep incisional (fascia and muscle), or organ/space infection.
- PE: erythema, tenderness, drainage, fluctuance, +/− fever.
- Cellulitis: infection of the skin with erythema without drainage or fluctuance.
- Abscess: localized collections of purulent material within tissue.
- Necrotizing soft tissue infection (rare postoperatively: *Streptococcus pyogenes* or Clostridium perfringens): rapidly spreading and invasive infection resulting in necrosis (of fascia −> necrotizing fasciitis, of muscle −> myonecrosis). Process may start as early as 24 hrs after surgery, considerably earlier than pedestrian SSIs.

TREATMENT
Surgical site infections or dirty wound coverage
- For dirty wounds, antimicrobial coverage should be considered treatment, not prophylaxis.
- The length of treatment for dirty wounds is controversial; durations as short as 24 hrs have been recommended; treatment duration for infected wounds is dependent upon severity, surgical debridement (if needed) and clinical response.
- Coverage for SSI and dirty wounds should include Gram-positive organisms, and in special circumstances Gram-negative and anaerobic organisms (e.g., perforated viscus).
- For general wound infections, cefazolin 1–2 g IV q8h is often adequate. Vancomycin, linezolid, tigecycline, or daptomycin may be required in pts with or at risk for resistant Gram-positive pathogen infections (e.g., MRSA) or with serious beta-lactam allergies.

DIAGNOSIS

- Coverage for wounds infections with increased risk of Gram-negative or anaerobic infection: beta-lactam beta-lactamase inhibitor combination (e.g., piperacillin-tazobactam), cefotetan or cefoxitin, cefazolin + metronidazole, or clindamycin + gentamicin.
- The presence of prosthetic material (e.g., mesh) markedly increases the risk of treatment failure and often successful treatment requires removal.
- Tetanus immunization booster should be addressed with all wounds.

Clean-contaminated wound prophylaxis
- Antimicrobial prophylaxis indicated. See Surgical Prophylaxis module (p. 207).
- Cefazolin 1–2 g IV sufficient for majority of surgeries.
- Vancomycin 15 mg/kg IV in pts with serious beta-lactam allergies or at high risk for methicillin-resistant *Staphylococcus aureus* infection.
- Cefoxitin or cefotetan 1–2 g IV, cefazolin 1–2 g + metronidazole 500 mg, ertapenem 1000 mg, or a beta-lactam/beta-lactamase inhibitor combination (e.g., ampicillin-sulbactam) should be considered in pts at high risk for anaerobic SSI, e.g., colorectal operations.
- Mechanical bowel preparation and oral antibiotics often considered in colorectal operations, e.g., neomycin plus erythromycin base, 1 g each, at 1, 2, and 11 pm the day prior to an 8 am surgery; though unclear if any additional benefit of oral antibiotics when IV antibiotic prophylaxis also used.

Clean-wound prophylaxis
- In general, antimicrobial prophylaxis is not routinely recommended in clean wound operations. See Surgical Prophylaxis module (p. 207) for more details.
- Exceptions include operations where infection outcome could be catastrophic, such as craniotomy or cardiac surgery, or with implantation of prosthetic devices.
- Cefazolin 1–2 g IV within 60 minutes prior to surgical incision is the primary recommendation for most procedures.
- Vancomycin 15 mg/kg IV in pts with serious beta-lactam allergies or at high risk for methicillin-resistant *Staphylococcus aureus* infection.
- Intranasal mupirocin may reduce *Staphylococcus aureus* infections in colonized pts.
- Decontamination of nasopharynx and oropharynx with <u>Chlorhexidine gluconate</u> may be helpful in the prevention of cardiac surgery infections and nasal carriage of <u>*Staphylococcus aureus*</u>.
- Full body wash with Chlorhexidine gluconate solution or prep controversial.

OTHER INFORMATION
- Primary treatment is to open/drain the wound. Antibiotics not indicated unless cellulitis is present or fascia involved.
- Optimal prevention involves appropriate choice of antibiotic (usually cefazolin), timing (within 60 minutes of incision), and duration (<24 hrs). SSI surveillance decrease rates of infection.
- Rapidly developing wounds on postoperative day 1 or 2, either with or without systemic toxicity, should raise suspicion of infection with *Clostridium species* or *Streptococcus pyogenes*.
- Hair removal should be performed using clippers and not razor blades because the latter is associated with an increase in SSIs.
- Temperature control, glucose control, wound space oxygenation, and smoking cessation all potentially decrease SSI.

BASIS FOR RECOMMENDATIONS

Bratzler DW, Houck PM, Surgical Infection Prevention Guideline Writers Workgroup. Antimicrobial prophylaxis for surgery: an advisory statement from the National Surgical Infection Prevention Project. *Am J Surg*, 2005; Vol. 189; pp. 395–404.

Comments: Summary of national recommendations for select cardiac, vascular, orthopedic (arthroplasty), gynecologic (hysterectomy), and colorectal surgeries in surgical journal.

Bratzler DW, Houck PM, Surgical Infection Prevention Guidelines Writers Workgroup, et al. Antimicrobial prophylaxis for surgery: an advisory statement from the National Surgical Infection Prevention Project. *Clin Infect Dis*, 2004; Vol. 38; pp. 1706–15.

Comments: Summary of national recommendations for select cardiac, vascular, orthopedic (arthroplasty), gynecologic (hysterectomy), and colorectal surgeries in ID journal.

VASCULAR GRAFT INFECTIONS

Christopher F. Carpenter, MD and Aditi Swami, MD

PATHOGENS

- *Staphylococcus aureus*
- Coagulase negative staphylococci
- Gram-negative bacteria, e.g., *Escherichia coli*
- Streptococci and enterococci
- Anaerobes rarely associated, more frequent with aortic grafts.

CLINICAL

- Rates of prosthetic vascular graft infection (PVGI) range between 1 and 6%, including between 0.5 and 5% for aortic graft infections (likely closer to 1%) and ranging up to 12% for peripheral lower extremity grafts; rates for infection of endovascular grafts appear much lower.
- Mortality rates are high, especially for aortic graft infections, with marked morbidity (limb loss, etc. in up to 50%) even with aggressive interventions.
- Risk factors for infection include groin incision, wound infection, and wound complication; other risk factors may include immunosuppressive therapy, diabetes mellitus, cancer, and immunologic disorders.
- Approximately 35% of infections are caused by staphylococci, with *S. aureus* more likely early and coagulase-negative staphylococci more likely late, and approximately 25% of infections are polymicrobial.
- For hemodialysis vascular access infections: central venous catheters (CVC) and arteriovenous grafts (AVG) have an increased infection and mortality risk when compared to arteriovenous fistula (AVF).
- With hemodialysis vascular access infections, silent infection is common and positive indium scan may indicate infection, EVEN in the absence of clinical signs of graft infection; clotted grafts may have occult infection as well. Staphylococcal pathogens most common, with Gram-negative rods occuring in approximately 20%. Resection and prolonged antibiotics mandatory, especially with *Staphylococcus aureus*. Initial access goal should be to preserve native fistula, and avoid using CVC or AVG unless absolutely required.

DIAGNOSIS

- Draining sinus or an inflammatory pulsatile mass at the graft site strongly suggests infection, as does local cellulitis that is poorly responsive to antibiotics or that rapidly recurs.
- CT and MRI findings that suggest vascular graft infection include peri-graft fluid, ectopic air, abnormal tissue planes or soft tissue swelling, and pseudoaneurysm formation, especially when multiple.
- Nonspecific findings include fever, leukocytosis with left shift, and elevated inflammation markers (ESR, CRP); absence of other signs of graft infection should prompt a thorough workup for other causes.
- Blood cultures (2) are mandatory but may not reflect non-luminal infection of grafts.
- Gastrointestinal bleeding in pts with intra-abdominal grafts is suggestive of enteric erosion and vascular graft infection, especially when other signs or symptoms of infection are present. Specifically, endoscopic evidence of bleeding in the third or fourth portion of the duodenum is strongly suggestive of enteric erosion from an abdominal aortic graft.
- Occasionally, exploratory surgery is required to confirm the diagnosis of graft infection; a poorly incorporated/adherent graft to peri-graft tissue is the most suggestive intraoperative finding.
- In most pts pseudoaneurysm and/or graft occlusion are not by themselves indicative of vascular graft infection; however, aortic graft thrombosis may be associated with infection in up to 25% of pts.
- Evidence of septic emboli or hypertrophic osteoarthropathy are rare but when present strongly suggest vascular graft infection.

TREATMENT
Preoperative Antimicrobial Prophylaxis

- Cefazolin 2 g IV administered within 60 minutes before skin incision.

- Vancomycin 15 mg/kg IV administered within 60 minutes before skin incision (only pts with significant penicillin or cephalosporin allergy or at high risk of MRSA infection); consider enteric GNR coverage, especially for procedures involving the groin.
- Duration of prophylaxis of 24–48 hrs likely more than adequate and longer duration not recommended.

Primary Surgical Therapy

- Optimal treatment involves explantation of the graft, extensive debridement of infected and necrotic tissue, reperfusion of the peri-graft and distal tissue, and appropriate antimicrobial coverage for an appropriate duration.
- Surgery is the gold standard for treating vascular graft infections.
- Staged: extra-anatomic bypass followed in a few days by graft removal.
- Sequential: extra-anatomic bypass followed immediately by graft removal.
- Simultaneous: graft excision either before or after in line graft replacement using new prosthetic graft, autogenous graft, or homograft.
- Partial: sub-total graft resection, usually reserved for situations where only well-defined short segments of graft are infected.
- Non-surgical: no resection of the infected graft (only pts with superficial wound infection); requires prolonged antibiotic course. Exceptions: bleeding or occlusion, sepsis, or Dacron graft.
- Antibiotic coverage should be guided by culture of blood, local fluid collection(s), and graft material, when available.

Empiric Adjunctive Antibiotic Therapy

- Cefazolin 1–2 g IV q8h, nafcillin or oxacillin 1–2 g IV q4h unless at risk for MRSA.
- Vancomycin 15 mg/kg IV q12h.
- Would consider enteric GNR coverage depending on location of surgery.
- Duration is dependent on the type of surgery performed and the extent of the infection; 7–10 days after complete resection is a reasonable starting point in uncomplicated pts.
- Empirical coverage for MRSA or MRSE should be considered in all pts, especially in those with chronic kidney disease and/or frequent hospitalizations and in areas with high rates of nosocomial- and/or community-associated MRSA.
- Consider anaerobic coverage (e.g., metronidazole) for abdominal aortic graft infections.

OTHER INFORMATION

- Between 1 and 5% of pts develop vascular graft infection; the rate primarily depends on graft site and pt population.
- The infection rate is highest for infrainguinal grafts at 2–5%; for aortofemoral grafts the rate is 1–2%, and for aortic grafts approximately 1%.
- Polymicrobial infections are not infrequent and should be considered when deciding upon empiric coverage or narrowing coverage.
- Staphylococcus species and Enterobacteriaceae account for the majority of infections and in general, empiric coverage should be directed to cover these pathogens.
- Vacuum assisted closure (VAC) treated synthetic vascular graft infections in the groin appear to be at greater risk of developing infection-related complications.

MORE INFORMATION

- Empiric coverage of Pseudomonas aeruginosa and Enterococcus species is not generally recommended.

BASIS FOR RECOMMENDATIONS

Perera GB, Fujitani RM, Kubaska SM. Aortic graft infection: update on management and treatment options. *Vasc Endovascular Surg*, 2006; Vol. 40; pp. 1–10.
Comments: Nice recent review of controversies in management of aortic graft infections.

Antimicrobial prophylaxis for surgery. *Treat Guidel Med Lett*, 2006; Vol. 4; pp. 83–8.
Comments: Concise review of antimicrobial prophylaxis in surgery.Barie PS. Often, antibiotics are continued even after the surgery is complete. This article examines several studies that have looked at the optimal number of doses that should be given as surgical prophylaxis. The conclusion is that continuing antibiotics after surgery is not better than single doses, given before the incision and re-dosed for long cases and blood loss. Modern surgical antibiotic prophylaxis and therapy-- less is more. *Surg Infect (Larchmt)*, 2000; Vol. 1 pp. 23–9

FEVER IN THE RETURNED TRAVELER see p. 455 in Management Section

---

MALARIA see p. 387 in Pathogens Section

RESPIRATORY TRACT INFECTIONS: IN THE RETURNED TRAVELER see p. 462 in Management Section

---

TRYPANSOMIASIS

Paul G. Auwaerter, MD and Joseph Vinetz, MD

MICROBIOLOGY

- Protozoan hemoflagellates agents of human African Sleeping Sickness.
- Trypanosoma brucei complex of which two subspecies exist: *T. b. gambiense* causes West African sleeping sickness, *T. b. rhodesiense* causes East African sleeping sickness.
- Zoonotic disease of cattle, transmitted by painful bite of TseTse (not preventable with DEET) in rural African locales.

CLINICAL RELEVANCE

- Humans are the epidemiological reservoir of transmission for *T. brucei gambiense*, which accounts for vast majority (>99%) of cases. Game animals are reservoirs for *T. b. rhodesiense*.
- Ongoing epidemic in Africa from coast to coast. *T. brucei gambiense* widely found in West and Central Africa; *T. b. rhodesiense* in small areas of East/Southeast Africa.
- Stages described: (1) ulcerated chancre at site of bite, (2) systemic symptoms develop following venous/lymphatic spread including fever, lymphadenopathy and pruritus, (3) meningoencephalitic symptoms reflect CNS invasion with symptoms including somnolence, headaches, behavioral disturbances that ultimately progress to coma.
- Stage I: trypanosome negative or CSF wbc < 10 cells/mm^3. Stage II: trypanosome positive or CSF wbc >10cells/mm^3.
- Course of illness: *T. b. rhodesiense* presents more quickly and progresses faster than *T. b. gambiense*.
- Rare cause of illness in returned traveler.
- Dx: demonstration of parasites. Motile trypanosomes seen in serous fluid expressed from chancres, aspirates of lymph nodes, wet prep of blood, bone marrow, CSF (in late stages). Trypanosomes can be seen in Giemsa stained thick blood smears; parasites cycle so repeated blood smears may be necessary. Concentration techniques may facilitate identification (e.g., centrifugation, in blood examine the buffy coat).
- In sleeping sickness, parasites can be seen in CSF. Parasitemia is higher with Rhodesian form and parasites easier to demonstrate in blood.
- Xenodiagnosis by inoculation of pt fluid into rats or mice offers good sensitivity, but only available in certain research labs and helpful only with *T. b. rhodesiense* infection.
- Serological diagnosis: CATT (Card agglutination test for trypanosomes, Institute of Tropical Medicine, Lab. of Serology, Nationalestraat 155, B-2000 Antwerp, Belgium); seek advice from Centers for Disease Control in U.S., as serology testing considered of limited help given variable sensitivity and specificity. In addition, *T. b. rhodesiense* seroconversion only occurs well after initial symptom onset.

SITES OF INFECTION
- Cutaneous: inoculation chancre at site of TseTse fly bite.
- Lymph: 1–2 cm, soft, painless numerous and mobile cervical lymph nodes (Winterbottom's sign); cervical in Gambian form; submandibular, axillary, inguinal in Rhodesian form.
- Systemic: Gambian form: intermittent fever, headache, myalgia for mos to yrs; Rhodesian form: more acute presentation.
- CNS: progressive somnolence, occasional meningitis and focal neurologic forms that progresses to loss of consciousness and coma.

TREATMENT
General principles
- Determine geographic origin of infection, and whether CNS involved. Both determine which drugs to use.
- Ulcerated skin lesions in a person from an endemic area should suggest the possibility of human African trypanosomiasis (HAT).
- Determine whether a pt has early vs. late stage disease by lumbar puncture. Presence of >20 WBCs/uL of CSF indicates late disease.

T. brucei gambiense
- **Early, hemolymphatic stage** (preferred): pentamidine isethionate IM4 mg/kg up to 300 mg/day × 7 days.
- Alternative: suramin, use 100–200 mg test dose IV then 1 g IV on days 1, 3, 7, 14, and 21.
- **Late stage with CNS involvement**: eflornithine 100 mg/kg IV q6h × 14 days or melarsoprol 2.2 mg/kg/day IV × 10 days (see subheading below on drug use).
- Combination [NECT] regimen: eflornithine 400 mg/kg IV q12h dosing × 7 days plus nifurtimox 15 mg/kg PO q8h × 10 days.
- Combination regimen: low dose melarsoprol 1.2 mg/kg/day and nifurtimox 7.5 mg/kg PO twice daily × 10 days was more effective than melarsoprol alone.
- Note: One study found fewer side effects with eflornithine than melarsoprol, NECT regimen perhaps favored when drug can be administered. Also, eflornithine not considered active against T. b. rhodesiense; obtain drug from CDC or WHO.
- Relapses: post-pentamidine, use melarsoprol or eflornithine as above; post-eflornithine—use melarsoprol as above.
- Melarsoprol-resistant parasites described, and increasingly reported.

T. brucei rhodesiense
- Early stage: suramin use 100–200 mg test dose IV then 1 g IV on days 1, 3, 7, 14, and 21.
- Late stage: melarsoprol 2.0–3.6 mg/kd × 3 days, after day 7 use 3.6 mg/kg/day × 3 days, then repeat regimen again after 7 days.
- Relapses: post-suramin, use melarsoprol as above; post-melarsoprol—use second course of melarsoprol, 3 × 4 daily injections, all doses at 3.6 mg/kg (up to 180 mg).

Melarsoprol-induced encephalopathy
- Arsenical drug, may cause encephalopathy. Steroids may prevent development of encephalopathy.
- Prevention: prednisolone 1 mg/kg up to 40 mg/day started 1–2 days before first dose of melarsoprol, continued to last dose, tapered over 3 days.
- Treatment: anti-convulsants, IV steroids, epinephrine.
- Pretreatment for Tbg: 1–2 doses of 4 mg/kg pentamidine 24–72 hrs before 1st injection of melarsoprol.
- Pretreatment for Tgr: 2–3 doses of suramin (5, 10, 20 mg/kg) IV over 3–5 days before 1st injection of melarsoprol.
- Reduced with newly reported regimen for T. brucei gambiense.

FOLLOW UP
- In T. b. gambiense infection, expect up to 20% of pts may not respond (melarsoprol was study drug, Lancet 1999;353:1113).

OTHER INFORMATION
- Gambian sleeping sickness surging dramatically in Central Africa.
- Manufacture of eflornithine in U.S. now primarily for restoring baldness with side benefit of providing treatment for orphan disease.

BASIS FOR RECOMMENDATIONS

[No authors listed]. *The Medical Letter*, 2007; Vol. 5; pp. e1–e14.

Comments: Guidelines used in this module, although combination therapies such as lower dose melarsoprol/nifurtimox and nifurtimox/eflornithine deserve strong consideration for Stage II HAT therapy of *T. b. gambiense*.

Pépin J, Milord F. The treatment of human African trypanosomiasis. *Adv Parasitol*, 1994; Vol. 33; pp. 1–47.

Comments: Drug treatment of the human African trypanosomiasis is toxic, and often fails in advanced cases.

TRYPANOSOMA CRUZI

Joseph Vinetz, MD and Paul G. Auwaerter, MD

MICROBIOLOGY

- Protozoan parasite causes S. American trypanosomiasis (Chagas' Disease).
- Transmitted in rural Latin America by bite of "kissing bug" of the species *Rhodnius* or triatomine bug.
- Also present in zoonotic reservoirs/insect vectors in southern U.S. but transmission to humans rare.

CLINICAL RELEVANCE

- Capable of causing an incurable chronic infection of the heart, esophagus, and colon. Most infected are asymptomatic.
- Suspect acute infection w/ hx suggestive of exposure (immigration, travel, lab accident); usually non-specific systemic sxs, occasionally severe myocarditis.
- Immigrants can be chronic carriers hence no longer solely a rural Latin American disease, estimated ~100,000 chronic carriers in U.S.
- Chronic *T. cruzi* carriers have potential to transmit parasite through blood supply (7 cases reported in past 20 yrs).
- Can be opportunistic CNS disease in AIDS
- Death usually a consequence of cardiac arrhythmias or heart failure.
- Acute dx immunocompetent: parasites seen on wet preps or Giemsa-stain of blood or buffy coat, acute serology of limited utility.
- Acute dx immunocompromised: bxp for parasites in bone marrow, LN, epimyocardium, skin, CSF, pericardial fluid. Specialized labs—blood cx, PCR, or xeno-dx (lab bugs feed on suspected cases).
- Chronic dx: serologic detection *T. cruzi*-specific IgG. Parasites difficult or impossible to find. PCR, blood cx, xenodiagnosis in specialized labs.
- FDA has approved a new serological test for screening for Chagas carriers; blood supply now starting to be screened.

SITES OF INFECTION

- **Acute disease:** (1) chagoma: red, indurated lesion at site of inoculation; (2) Romana's Sign in conjunctiva; (3) systemic: fever, malaise, face/leg edema, general lymphadenopathy, hepatosplenomegaly.
- Cardiac: severe myocarditis in acute Chagas' disease,
- **Intermediate stage** Chagas' Disease is characterized by resolution of acute illness after 4–8 wks without treatment, then lack of symptoms, subpatent parasitemia, easily detectable antibodies.
- **Chronic disease** involves heart and GI systems. Involvement of CNS only in immunocompromised host.
- Cardiac: occurs in 10–30% of chronic infection resulting in biventricular dilation, mural thrombi, left ventricular apical aneurysm, CHF, syncope, arrhythmia, thromboembolism, death.
- GI: megadisease of esophagus, colon; manifestations—dysphagia, constipation, abdominal pain.
- CNS: disease reactivation described in AIDS, including meningoencephalitis and brain abscess-like lesion.

TREATMENT

Acute Chagas' Disease

- Benznidazole: 5 mg/kg/day PO for 60 days. Not available in United States.
- Benznidazole available from the Centers for Disease Control Drug Service (404) 639-3670 under an Investigational New Drug protocol.
- Nifurtimox: <u>adults</u>, 8–10 mg/kg/day, <u>children</u> 1–10 yrs, 15–20 mg/kg/day, <u>adolescents</u>, 12.5 to 15 mg/kg/day; doses divided 4 × /day for 90–120 days. Available from CDC Drug Service (404) 639-3670.

Intermediate Stage Chagas' Disease

- Controversial; unknown whether treatment forestalls chronic complications; substantial toxicity.

Chronic Chagas' Disease

- Pharmacologic treatment is not indicated.
- Cardiac: symptomatic; pacemakers, drug treatment for CHF, cardiac transplantation.
- Megaesophagus: treat as for idiopathic achalasia, i.e., balloon dilation of lower esophageal sphincter, botulinum toxin, or surgery.
- Megacolon/colonic dysfunction: symptomatic; high fiber diet, manual disimpaction, surgical intervention for toxin megacolon, volvulus, or decompression.
- Some consider treatment in pts pending organ transplantation, immunocompromise or advanced HIV infection (using acute Chagas' recommendations).

BASIS FOR RECOMMENDATIONS

Bern C, Montgomery SP, Herwaldt BL, et al. Evaluation and treatment of chagas disease in the United States: a systematic review. *JAMA,* 2007; Vol. 298; pp. 2171–81.

Comments: Comprehensive review highlights the many knowledge gaps. Immunocompromised/pending organ transplant or HIV-infected pts should be treated according to these authors although there is slender evidence.

Villar JC, Marin-Neto JA, Ebrahim S, et al. Trypanocidal drugs for chronic asymptomatic *Trypanosoma cruzi* infection. *Cochrane Database Syst Rev,* 2002; Vol. CD003463.

Comments: This analytical review found that there was promising but inconclusive evidence for the use of anti-*T. cruzi* drugs in the treatment of chronic asymptomatic infection. Demonstration of the presence of the organism in blood likely indicates a higher likelihood of some response to therapy, at least in terms of preventing further end-organ damage.

TAENIA SOLIUM/CYSTICERCOSIS see p. 391 in Pathogens Section

SECTION 2
PATHOGENS

Bacteria

ACINETOBACTER BAUMANNII

John G. Bartlett, MD

MICROBIOLOGY

- Aerobic Gram-neg coccobacilli or rods, often mistaken for Neisseria or Moraxella on Gram-stain.
- Common in environment (water, soil) and hospital (catheters, lotions, ventilation equipment).
- Grows on standard agar media.
- *A. baumannii* is the major species of Acinetobacter. Others occasional human pathogens include *A. calcoaceticus, A. lwoffi, A. junii, A. johnsonii,* and *A. baylyi.*
- *A. baumannii* is low grade pathogen affecting compromised hosts (immunosuppression, post-surgical, ventilator-associated pneumonia, burn wounds, ICU pts, device-associated infections, and malnutrition).

CLINICAL

- Emerging as important global, pan-resistant GNB nosocomial pathogen.
- Clearly pathogenic when recovered from blood and normally sterile body sites.
- May cause nosocomial epidemics from contaminated common sources, e.g., ventilation equipment, catheters, etc.
- Diagnosis by standard aerobic bacterial culture.
- Lab isolations often meaningless (representing colonization) unless from (1) normally sterile site, (2) found as a dominant pathogen, (3) outbreak and/or (4) good clinical correlation.

SITES OF INFECTION

- Usually a cause of nosocomial infections
- Pneumonia: nosocomial, especially ventilator-associated
- Septicemia: often catheter-associated, or consequence of HAP or VAP
- Wounds: burns, war wounds acquired in Iraq, natural disasters—hurricanes/earthquakes
- Rare: meningitis (post-neurosurgical), liver abscess, endocarditis, urinary tract infections, brain abscess
- Community-acquired: reports from Iraqi war theater, one major report from New Zealand

TREATMENT

Antibiotic

- Antibiotic selection guided by *in vitro* sensitivity tests—most active: imipenem, ampicillin/sulbactam, cefepime, colistin, tigecycline, and amikacin.
- Imipenem (Primaxin): 0.5–1 g IV q6h (Preferred—Med Letter 2004;2:21).
- Ampicillin/sulbactam (Unasyn): 3 g q4h (sulbactam is the active component).
- Tigecycline (Tygacil): 100 mg IV, then 50 mg IV q12h.
- Ceftriaxone: 1–2 g IV every day or cefotaxime 2–3 g IV q6–8h.
- Ciprofloxacin (Cipro): 400 mg IV q8–12h or 750 mg PO twice daily (or levofloxacin, or moxifloxacin).
- Cefepime (Maxipime): 1–2 g IV q8h.
- TMP-SMX: 15–20 mg (TMP)/kg/day IV divided 3 or 4 doses/day or 2 DS PO twice daily.
- Amikacin: 7.5 mg/kg q12h IV or 15 mg/kg/day IV.
- Pan-resistant isolates: colistin 5 mg/kg/day IV divided q12h +/– imipenem or ampicillin/sulbactam.
- Colistin 2.5 mg/kg IV q12h.

Outbreaks

- Notify infection control.
- Emphasize barrier precautions and hand washing.
- Identify common source—water, ventilators, catheters, endoscopes, feeding tubes, etc.

Other Information

- Acinetobacter has become major nosocomial pathogen, especially as a multiply resistant GNB in ICU.

- Major culture sources: blood, respiratory secretions, and urine.
- Nosocomial pathogen that colonizes skin, dry surfaces and water, including hand lotion, ventilation equipment, and catheters.
- Important pathogen in war (Iraq) and disasters (tsunami).

BASIS FOR RECOMMENDATIONS

Murray CK, Hospenthal DR. Treatment of multidrug resistant Acinetobacter. *Curr Opin Infect Dis*, 2005; Vol. 18; pp. 502–6.

Comments: Drugs that are usually active include imipenem, amikacin, ampicillin-sulbactam, colistin, rifampin and tigecycline.

ACTINOMYCES

John G. Bartlett, MD

MICROBIOLOGY
- Thin, branching Gram-positive bacillus.
- Microaerophilic, grow best anaerobically. **Very** fastidious.
- Agents: *A. israelii, A. gerencseriae, A. naeslundii, A. odontolyticus, A. viscosus, A. meyer,* and *Propionibacterium propionicum.*
- Normal flora of mouth, gut, genital tract.
- Diagnosis is often made by histopathology—not by culture, even when suspected.

CLINICAL
- Nearly always part of a mixed infection—especially w/ *Actinobacillus actinomycetemcomitans, Eikenella corrodens, Bacteroides* spp, *Streptococcus* spp.
- Characteristic chronic lesion: dense fibrosis ("woody"), draining fistulae, "sulfur granules," infection may advance through tissue planes with no respect for anatomical boundaries.
- Diagnosis: characteristic Gram-stain (filamentous rods) in tissue or sulfur granule with radiating Gram-positive bacilli seen on histopathology or by culture.
- Recovery important only if from normally uncontaminated sources, e.g., cleanly obtained tissue, needle aspirates, **or** examination of sulfur granules, etc.
- Main differential is nocardia. Looks similarly on Gram-stain, but nocardia is weakly AFB and is usually disease of an immunocompromised host.

SITES OF INFECTION
- Oral cervico-facial ("lumpy jaw")
- Pelvic infection (IUD-associated)
- Thoracic: pneumonia, mass lesion (may be confused with malignancy)
- Intra-abdominal: abscess or mass lesion
- Musculoskeletal
- Osteonecrosis of jaw: post-chemotherapy
- Cardiac: endocarditis (The "A" of HACEK, *Actinobacillus actinomycetemcomitans* [*Aggregatibacter actinomycetemcomitans*])
- CNS: meningitis, encephalitis, brain abscess
- Disseminated (rare)

TREATMENT
Antibiotics
- Preferred: penicillin G 18–24 mil units IV/day × 2–6 wks, then amoxicillin 500–750 mg PO three times a day/four times a day × 6–12 mos; oral therapy alone may be adequate.
- Alt: doxycycline 100 mg twice daily IV × 2–6 wks, then 100 mg PO twice daily × 6–12 mos; erythromycin 500 mg PO four times a day × 6–12 mos.
- Clindamycin 600 mg IV q8h × 2–6 wks, then 300 mg PO four times a day × 6–12 mos.
- Other agents (limited data): clarithromycin, azithromycin, imipenem, cefotaxime/ceftriaxone.
- Not active: metronidazole, TMP-SMX, ceftazidime, aminoglycosides, oxacillin, fluoroquinolones.

Miscellaneous
- Surgery usually reserved for suspected neoplasm, to establish diagnosis, lesion in vital area (epidural, CNS, etc.) or unresponsiveness to abx.

PATHOGENS

- Surgical procedures: debulking, excision of fistula tracts, abscess drainage.

FOLLOW UP

- Use of high dose and long duration of antibiotics justified by tradition and perceived need for penetration into dense fibrotic tissue.

OTHER INFORMATION

- Disease is "**Actinomycosis**" caused by one of 6 actinomyces agents, most commonly *A. israelii.*
- **Suspect**: characteristic lesion (hard, chronic inflammatory mass (+/– sinus tracts) passing through tissue planes) and micro (Gram-stain ID culture often negative).
- A newly recognized entity is associated with osteonecrosis of the mandible.
- Most abx are active except metronidazole.

Comparison with Nocardia
Agents
Actinomyces: Agents of actinomycosis
Nocardia: *N. asteroides*
Gram-stain
Actino: Filamentous, GPB
Nocardia: Filamentous GPB
Modified AFB
Actino: Negative
Nocardia: Positive (weakly)
Source
Actino: Mouth flora
Nocardia: Soil
Host
Actino; Previously healthy, poor dentition
Nocardia: Decreased cell mediated immunity
Clinical features
Actino: Indurated, fistula
Nocardia: Indurated with sulphur granules
Course
Actino: Indolent
Nocardia: Indolent
Rx
Actino: Penicillin G, ampicillin/amoxicillin, antipseudomonal PCNs, most cephalosporins, macrolides, tetracycline, imipenem, clindamycin
Nocardia: TMP-SMX, imipenem, amikacin, linezolid

BASIS FOR RECOMMENDATIONS

Author opinion.

Comments: No professional society guideline statements exist for the treatment of actinomycoses. Long duration of antibiotic therapy guided by case series reports and expert opinion.

AEROMONAS

Paul G. Auwaerter, MD

MICROBIOLOGY
- Gram-negative bacillus, facultative anaerobe. Oxidase positive, lactose-fermenting, motile.
- Found in warmer climes, primarily fresh or brackish water.
- *A. hydrophila* is the most common and important human pathogen, also *A. caviae* and *A. veronii* biovar sobria.

CLINICAL
- Pathogen that can cause severe skin/soft tissue infection and sepsis, often in the immunocompromised, typically after tissue injury exposed to fresh water.
- Risk factors for severe infection: immunocompromise, diabetes, hepatobiliary disease (cirrhosis).
- Cellulitis can be severe and spread rapidly, often within hrs following exposure. Infection into deeper tissues may cause necrotizing fasciitis or myonecrosis.
- Ddx (skin/soft tissue necrotizing infections): two groups—monomicrobial (group A Strep, *S. aureus*, *Vibrio vulnificus*, microaerophilic Strep species such as *Peptostreptococcus*) and polymicrobial (such as necrotizing cellulitis or necrotizing fasciitis). Also: catfish spine envenomation or other aquatic animal-related bites/stings.
- Dx: culture of infected tissue, abscess, blood or other fluid.
- Role in gastroenteritis remains controversial; studies equivocal in demonstrating role (similar to *Plesiomonas*). Usually causes sporadic rather than outbreak illness.
- Diarrhea usually watery, often self-limiting. May have positive stool lactoferrin or fecal leukocytes. Usually a mild-moderate diarrhea, but can be severe enough to cause hospitalization.
- Dx (GI illness): some labs do not routinely culture, others do.

SITES OF INFECTION
- GI: gastroenteritis/dysentery (children may be severe, adults less so or chronic). Peritonitis (rare).
- Skin/soft tissue infection: cellulitis (may be fulminant with necrotizing features). Often polymicrobial, combined with *S. aureus* or enteric flora.
- Sepsis: bacteremia often associated with malignancy, hepatobiliary disease such as cirrhosis; less commonly with diabetes.
- Bone: osteomyelitis, septic arthritis.
- CNS: meningitis (rare).
- Cardiac: endocarditis (rare).

TREATMENT
General measures
- Diarrheal illness usually self-limiting and only requires supportive care.
- Most pts with soft-tissue infection do not present with diarrhea.
- Soft tissue infection: early fasciotomy may be required. Obtain early surgical consultation with any suspected infection.

Antibiotic treatment
- Usually active: aminoglycosides (gentamicin, amikacin > tobramycin), fluoroquinolones, carbapenems, aztreonam, third-generation cephalosporins.
- Usually not active: penicillin, ampicillin, cefazolin, ticarcillin, streptomycin. *Aeromonas* spp. are frequent ß-lactamase producers.
- Variable resistance: piperacillin, amoxicillin/clavulanate, ticarcillin/clavulanate, TMP-SMX, tetracycline, chloramphenicol.
- Use culture susceptibility data to guide final selection. There have been no trials examining antibiotic selection or duration.
- **Diarrheal illness** (consider if not self-limiting, or if severe): ciprofloxacin 500 mg PO twice daily. Alt: TMP-SMX 1 DS PO twice daily (note: high resistance to sulfa agents described in Taiwan and Spain).
- Empiric antibiotics for severe skin and skin structure infections should include coverage for Streptococcal and Staphylococcal (including MRSA) species.

PATHOGENS

- **Skin/soft tissue infection (mild):** ciprofloxacin 500 mg PO twice daily or levofloxacin 500 mg once daily.
- **Skin/soft tissue infection (severe) or sepsis:** ciprofloxacin 400 mg IV q8h or levofloxacin 750 mg IV q24 (plus for suspicion of water-based injury, empiric coverage for *Vibrio* [doxycycline 100 mg twice daily, although FQ may also cover] plus vancomycin 15 mg/ kg IV q12h +/– clindamycin or linezolid for inhibition of Gram-positive toxin production). Alternatives to fluoroquinolones for Aeromonas coverage include carbapenems (ertapenem, doripenem, imipenem or meropenem), ceftriaxone, cefepime and aztreonam.

Prevention

- Water-related injuries should be cleaned thoroughly. Some use fluoroquinolones as a prophylactic measure, although there is no data to support this approach. Development of infection after water exposure should prompt culturing for *Aeromonas* and *Vibrio* species with appropriate antibiotic coverage.
- Risk of infection with use of medicinal leeches.
- Frequent recommendations include using a cephalosporin (e.g., cefuroxime, ceftriaxone or cefixime) or a fluoroquinolone (e.g., ciprofloxacin or levofloxacin) during treatment with medicinal leeches. *Aeromonas* isolates from leeches have been described as uniformly susceptible to fluoroquinolones.
- Duration of antibiotic use is 3–5 days; some recommend continuing until wound or eschar resolves.
- External decontamination of the leeches with chlorhexidine is insufficient.

FOLLOW UP

- When bacteremia accompanies severe soft tissue infections, mortality rates in published series have ranged between 25–70%.

OTHER INFORMATION

- Rapidly evolving cellulitis after fresh or brackish water injury/exposure should prompt concern for *Aeromonas, Erysipelothrix* or *Vibrio* spp. infection.
- Odd pearl: medicinal use of leeches has been implicated in transmission of *Aeromonas* causing infection.
- Evidence cited for *Aeromonas* as a diarrheal pathogen includes a) recovered more frequently in pts with diarrhea than asx pts; b) lack of other pathogen identified in pts with diarrhea; c) presence of enterotoxins expressed; including demonstration of diarrhea in animal model; and d) improvement of diarrhea with antibiotics.

BASIS FOR RECOMMENDATIONS

Stevens DL, Bisno AL, Chambers HF, et al. Practice guidelines for the diagnosis and management of skin and soft-tissue infections. *Clin Infect Dis*, 2005; Vol. 41; pp. 1373–406.

Comments: General measures for managing necrotizing soft tissue infections, although there are no specific recommendations for *Aeromonas*.

Author opinion.

Comments: No guidelines or clinical trials exist to determine the best therapy for GI or non-GI *Aeromonas* infections. Recommendations based upon reports of *in vitro* susceptability profiles.

BACILLUS SPECIES

Paul G. Auwaerter, MD

MICROBIOLOGY

- Facultative anaerobe or aerobic spore-forming usually Gram + rods. See Anthrax module, p. 2.
- Ubiquitous in decayed organic matter and soil. Some species are part of normal flora.
- Potential human pathogens include *B. cereus, B. subtilis, B. megaterium, B. circulans, B. sphaericus*.

CLINICAL

- *B. cereus* capable of producing enterotoxins causing emesis and diarrhea. Presentation mimics *C. perfringens* food poisoning.
- Actual infection rare, most isolates considered culture contaminates. Standard culture methods for tissue, fluids, or blood.

- Risk factors for actual infection: IDU, sickle cell, intravascular catheters, cancer, AIDS, immune suppression, neutropenia.
- Diagnosis of foodborne outbreak: confirmation of *B. cereus* requires either (1) isolation of strains of the same serotype from the suspect food and feces or vomitus of the pt, (2) isolation of large numbers of a *B. cereus* serotype known to cause foodborne illness from the suspect food or from the feces or vomitus of the pt, or (3) isolation of *B. cereus* from suspect foods and determining their enterotoxigenicity by serological (diarrheal toxin) or biological (diarrheal and emetic) tests. The rapid onset time to symptoms in the emetic form of disease, coupled with some food evidence, is often sufficient to diagnose this type of food poisoning (source FDA: http://vm.cfsan.fda.gov/~mow/chap12.html).

SITES OF INFECTION

- Food poisoning: *B. cereus* w/ 2 forms. Emetic: 1–6 hrs after ingestion contaminated usually starchy food, e.g., fried rice. Diarrheal: 10–12 hrs after eating e.g. tainted meats, milk, vegetables, etc. w/ watery diarrhea, tenesmus lasting <2–10 days.
- Bacteremia: uncommon, may complicate mixed infections including surgical wounds or infected necrotic tumors. Source of pseudobacteremia: contaminated blood cx, gloves, syringes, etc. Often transient bacteremia of no significance in IDU population.
- Meningitis, brain abscess: uncommon presentations, may complicate otitis, mastoiditis, neurosurgical procedures, and shunts.
- Ocular: primary pathogen of post-traumatic endophthalmitis, risk factor also IV drug use. May also cause keratitis, orbital abscess, conjunctivitis, dacryocystitis.
- Endocarditis: rare complication in IVDU population. TV endocarditis mostly indolent in nature.
- Soft tissue: rare reports of fasciitis.
- Pneumonia: rare pathogen of compromised host. May mimic *B. anthracis*-type presentation.

TREATMENT

Serious Bacillus Infections

- First consider if isolate a contaminate or part of significant infection. Repeatedly positive cultures should give weight to a truly pathogenic role.
- Most species sensitive to penicillins, cephalosporins, FQ, and AG. Exception: *B. cereus* often resistant to beta-lactams. Antibiotic sensitivities extremely variable for Bacillus spp.
- *B. cereus* most common isolate in significant infections. Vancomycin 15 mg/kg IV q12h drug of choice based on *in vitro* case reports. Often resistant to beta-lactam antibiotics.
- Alt: clindamycin (600 mg IV q8h) reported w/ successful outcomes.

B. cereus Food Poisoning

- Self-limited, no antibiotics necessary.
- Supportive therapy, hydration, and anti-emetics.
- **Prevention:** fried/boiled rice should be maintained >60°C or rapidly cooled <8°C to avoid room temperature germination of spores and toxin.

Endophthalmitis

- Rapid, massive destruction of vitreous/retina in IDU's or posttraumatic w/ ring abscess within 48 hrs ~pathognomic *B. cereus* panophthalmitis.
- Early ophthalmological consultation, culture ocular fluids. Early vitrectomy and intravitreal abx advocated.
- Intravitreal clindamycin 450 μg and gentamicin 400 μg. Some advocate intravitreal dexamethasone. Prognosis for sight retention poor.
- Intravitreal abx combined with systemic antibiotics (see choices under Serious Bacillus Infections).

Endocarditis

- Well-described but rare complication seen in IDUs. Most blood cx's in IDU positive for bacillus are contaminates or represent transient bacteremia.
- Evidence of valvular involvement should be sought by echocardiography to prove endocarditis. Tricuspid valve involvement most common. Course indolent.
- Successful treatment reported with either vancomycin (15 mg/kg IV q12h) or clindamycin (600 mg IV q8h).

PATHOGENS

OTHER INFORMATION
- Blood culture isolates are mostly contaminates until proven otherwise, especially in IDU population.
- Ocular infections devastating and require quick intervention.
- Gram-stain similarity may stoke concern in pneumonia, meningitis, and soft-tissue presentations until culture results rule-out *B. anthracis*.

BASIS FOR RECOMMENDATIONS

Fekete, T. Bacillus Species and Related Genera Other than *Bacillus anthracis*. Mandell, Bennett, and Dolin: Principles and Practice of Infectious Diseases, 6th ed., 2005 Churchill Livingstone, Chap 206.

Comments: No guideline statements exist for systemic infections with *B. cereus* and related species.

Author opinion.

Comments: Latest recommendations for safe food preparation and handling. www.cfsan.fda.gov/list.html.

BACTEROIDES FRAGILIS

John G. Bartlett, MD

MICROBIOLOGY
- Small, pleomorphic Gram-negative anaerobic bacillus.
- Easily grown relative to other anaerobes.
- Colonizes virtually all human colons.

CLINICAL
- Abscessogenic—causes abscesses at nearly all anatomical sites, especially below the diaphragm.
- Most common agent of anaerobic bacteremia.
- Usually part of polymicrobial infection from a colonic source.
- Most common pathogen in intra-abdominal sepsis except biliary infections and spontaneous bacterial peritonitis.
- Infrequently found above diaphragm except for otogenic brain abscess.
- Detection: rarely cultured unless anaerobic cultures ordered. Suspect with mixed flora on Gram-stain, intraabdominal/pelvic infection, putrid pus.
- Culture (anaerobically) only uncontaminated specimens: blood, peritoneal specimens, etc.

SITES OF INFECTION
- Intra-abdominal: peritonitis, abscess, appendicitis, diverticulitis, post-op wound infection, liver abscess, cholangitis.
- Gynecologic infections: PID, tubo-ovarian abscess, post gynecologic surgery wound infection, endometritis, pelvic cellulitis, pelvic abscess.
- Soft tissue: necrotizing fasciitis, diabetic foot infections, decubitus ulcers.
- Bacteremia.
- Abscesses: otogenic brain abscess, intra-abdominal abscess, pelvic abscess, soft tissue abscess (below diaphragm), perirectal abscess.
- Gut: enterotoxin producing strains may cause secretory diarrhea.

TREATMENT
Empiric antibiotics, mixed infection
- Recommendations assume polymicrobial infection and empiric treatment of *B. fragilis*.
- Monotherapy: imipenem (Primaxin) or other carbapenem (ertapenem, meropenem, doripenem) 0.5–1.0 g IV q6h, piperacillin-tazobactam (Zosyn) 3.375 g IV q6h, ampicillin-sulbactam (Unasyn) 1–2 g IV q6h, tigecycline (Tygacil) 100 mg IV, then 50 mg IV q12h.
- Combination therapy: metronidazole 0.75–1.0 g IV q12h + cefotaxime 1.5–2 g IV q6h, aztreonam 1–2 g IV q8h or ceftriaxone 1 g IV q12h.

Surgery
- Drain abscesses; exceptions: most tubo-ovarian abscess, some (small or multiple) brain and liver abscesses respond to abx alone.
- Source control: repair anastomotic leaks, perforations.
- Surgery for appendicitis, etc.

OTHER INFORMATION
- Abx for intra-abdominal sepsis: treat *B. fragilis* and *E. coli*; this covers everything common and important in most cases.
- *B. fragilis* is the most common cause of anaerobic bacteremia—"sepsis for surgeons."
- *B. fragilis* is often suspected (intra-abd or pelvic sepsis), sometimes seen (Gram-stain w/ mixed flora), occasionally smelled (putrid) and rarely cultured.
- Abx always active against *B. fragilis*: metronidazole, imipenem (Primaxin), piperacillin/ tazobactam (Zosyn). Resistance increasing: clindamycin, cefoxitin, cefotetan and moxifloxacin—none of these drugs are advocated for use in serious anaerobic infections.

BASIS FOR RECOMMENDATIONS
Solomkin JS, Mazuski JE, Baron EJ, et al. Guidelines for the selection of anti-infective agents for complicated intra-abdominal infections. *Clin Infect Dis,* 2010 (in press).

Comments: Recommendations assume major pathogens are *B. fragilis* and *E. coli.* Mild-moderate: Amp-sulbactam (Unasyn) ticar-clavulanate (Timentin) or ertapenem. Severe: Pip-tazo or imipenem/meropenem. Combination therapy: Metro + cefazolin, fluoroquinolone, 3rd generation cephalosporin or aztreonam. **Note:** Clindamycin and cefoxitin are no longer recommended as 1st line drugs for IAS due to increased resistance by *B. fragilis.*

BACTEROIDES SPECIES

Joseph Vinetz, MD

PATHOGENS

MICROBIOLOGY
- Pleomorphic, Gram-negative, anaerobic bacilli, easily cultivated.
- Clinically important spp.: *B. fragilis, B. thetaiotaomicron, B. vulgatus, B. distasonis, B. ovatus, B. uniformis, B. caccae.*

CLINICAL
- See separate *B. fragilis* (previous module) for information on that species.
- Normal component of intestinal, oral, vaginal flora.
- Most significant in polymicrobial infections, abscesses.
- Virtually all members of genus sensitive to metronidazole, carbapenem, beta-lactam/beta-lactamase inhibitor combinations, so speciation not usually important.
- Culture only uncontaminated specimens: blood, peritoneal, pleural empyema, or other abscess aspirates.
- Recent emergence of multiply-drug resistant *B. fragilis.*

SITES OF INFECTION
- Intra-abdominal: abscess (often polymicrobial) associated with ruptured viscus, intestinal surgery (especially *B. fragilis*); liver abscess (especially with abnormal anatomy or stone); infected pancreatic pseudocyst.
- CNS: brain abscess often in association with other bacteria, and as consequence of chronic sinusitis, chronic otitis media; subdural empyema; epidural abscess.
- Oral cavity, upper respiratory tract: tooth abscess, periodontitis, peritonsillar abscess (in association with other bacteria), sinusitis (chronic), parotiditis (unusual).
- Lung: aspiration pneumonia or necrotizing pneumonia, lung abscess, empyema.
- GU: Bartholin's cyst abscess, PID, tuboovarian abscess, endometritis, chorioamnionitis, post-ob/gyn surgical wound infections.
- Bloodstream: common isolate, often indicates a primary source (intra-abdominal in one-half to two-thirds of cases).
- Skin/soft tissue: human/animal bites, post-surgical, necrotizing fasciitis; decubitus and diabetic ulcers.
- Bone: osteomyelitis especially polymicrobial in association with decubitus ulcer, other local contamination.

TREATMENT
Antimicrobial agents
- Recommendations assume polymicrobial infection and empiric treatment of *Bacteroides* species including *B. fragilis.*
- Monotherapy: piperacillin/tazobactam (Zosyn) 3 g IV q6h, ampicillin/sulbactam 1–2 g q6h, imipenem 500 mg IV q6h, meropenem 1 g IV q8h or doripenem 500 mg IV q8h.

- Community-acquired, moderately severe: ampicillin/sulbactam (as above), moxifloxacin 400 mg IV/PO q24h or ticarcillin/clavulanate 3 g IV q6h.
- Nosocomial or severe: piperacillin/tazobactam or carbapenem (as above) +/– aminoglycoside.
- Alternative combination therapy: metronidazole 0.75–1.0 g IV q12h + gentamicin or tobramycin 5 mg/kg/day IV or cefotaxime 1.5–2 g IV 6h or ceftriaxone IV 1 g q12h or ciprofloxacin 400 mg IV q8h.

Adjunctive therapy

- Surgical or percutaneous catheter drainage of abscess.
- Exception: most tubo-ovarian abscesses, some brain (multiple or ≤2 cm) and liver abscesses respond to abx alone.
- Hyperbaric oxygen not demonstrated to be useful in clinical trials, and is of only theoretical benefit.

Surgical Prophylaxis

- Many (e.g., The Medical Letter) recommend cefazolin + metronidazole or ampicillin/sulbactam as surgical prophylaxis when anaerobic bacteria leakage likely.

OTHER INFORMATION

- Abx for intra-abdominal sepsis—treat *B. fragilis* and *E. coli*; this covers everything common and important.
- *B. fragilis* most common species causing anaerobic bacteremia.
- *Prevotella melaninogenicus* common species in lung abscess, oto/odontogenic infection.
- Abxs active against 99% Bacteroides spp: metronidazole, imipenem, piperacillin/tazobactam; no longer considered to be reliable for significant infections—clindamycin, cefoxitin, cefotetan due to increasing resistance.

BASIS FOR RECOMMENDATIONS

See *B. fragilis* references on p. 229.

BARTONELLA SPECIES

John G. Bartlett, MD

MICROBIOLOGY

- Small fastidious intracellular pleomorphic Gram-negative bacilli.
- Bartonella has 19 known species, 6 cause human disease: *B. henselae*, *B. bacilliformis*, *B. quintana*, *B. vinsonii*, *B. elizabethae* and *B. koehlerae*.
- Best seen with Warthin-Starry silver stain or a Brown–Hopps tissue Gram-stain.
- Major reservoir of *B. henselae* is cats—50% of cats are seropositive and transmit by saliva contact or scratching ("cat scratch fever").

CLINICAL

- Epidemiology: cats (kittens > cats, owners w/ CSD), lice (homeless w/ fever) and AIDS pts (bacillary angiomatosis, peliosis hepatis).
- *B. henselae* (cat source): Cat scratch disease [typically a pustule forms at scratch site after 3–12 days perhaps surrounded by additional pustules then within 1–3 wks a finding of regional LN proximal to initial lesion which is what usually prompts MD visit. LN often fluctuant], hepatosplenomegaly most commonly. Less common, bacillary angiomatosis (AIDS), peliosis hepatis.
- *B. quintana* (louse-born): urban trench fever, a cause of FUO (fever of unknown origin) in homeless.
- Miscellaneous syndromes: FUO (fever of unknown origin), hepatosplenomegaly, culture negative endocarditis, ocular infections especially uveitis, neurologic syndromes.
- Dx: Warthin-Starry stain tissue and/or serology (IFA >1:256 w/ acute infection, >1:800 correlates with chronic infection (sensitivity specification variable). Other: hard to culture (takes 2–6 wks and low yield); PCR—probably best, but difficult and experimental; skin test—useless and risky.

SITES OF INFECTION

- Skin nodule +/– regional adenopathy, fever: Cat Scratch disease (CSD).
- Conjunctivitis + preauricular node: Parinaud oculoglandular syndrome.
- Ocular: neuroretinitis.

- Liver +/– spleen: peliosis hepatitis.
- CNS: encephalitis, myelitis, aseptic meningitis.
- Skin nodules: bacillary angiomatosis (seen in AIDS pts, often resemble KS lesions).
- Endocarditis: culture negative.
- FUO (fever of unknown origin) with bacteremia: especially seen in homeless and alcoholics.

TREATMENT
Treatment

- Cat scratch disease: no abx; if extensive adenopathy, azithromycin 500 mg × 1 dose.
- Retinitis: doxycycline 100 mg twice daily + rifampin 300 mg twice daily all PO × 4–6 wks.
- Bacillary angiomatosis: erythromycin 500 mg PO four times a day or doxycycline 100 mg PO twice daily × >3 mos.
- Peliosis hepatitis: erythromycin 500 mg PO four times a day or doxycycline 100 mg PO twice daily × 4 mos.
- Oroya fever: ciprofloxacin 500 mg PO twice daily × 10 days.
- Endocarditis: gentamicin 3 mg/kg/day divided q8h IV × 14 days + ceftriaxone 2 g/day IV × 6 wks +/– doxycycline 100 mg PO twice daily × 6 wks.

OTHER INFORMATION

- Most common: (1) Cat scratch disease = cat injury—nodule + node, (2) bacillary angiomatosis seen w/ AIDS—skin nodules appear like KS lesions.
- Most serious infections: endocarditis (mortality 25%), CNS (encephalopathy), neuroretinitis.
- Bartonella spp. have been observed in ticks, significance regarding human disease is unclear.

BASIS FOR RECOMMENDATIONS

Rolain JM, Brouqui P, Koehler JE, et al. Recommendations for treatment of human infections caused by Bartonella species. *Antimicrob Agents Chemother*, 2004; Vol. 48; pp. 1921–33.

Comments: Review by major authority. Diseases and species in the genera. *B bacilliformis*-Oroya fever; *B henselae*-CSD, bacillary angiomatosis, bacteremia, neuroretinitis, endocarditis, peliosis hepatitis; *B quintana*: bacteremia, trench fever, endocarditis; *B elizabethae*: endocarditis. Treatment recommendations, these are the source for the recommendations in this module.

BORDETELLA SPECIES

Paul G. Auwaerter, MD

MICROBIOLOGY

- Bordetella are small aerobic Gram-negative coccobacilli. *B. pertussis* is most common etiology of whooping cough and exclusively a human pathogen. *B. parapertussis* leads to less severe but similar symptoms. Fastidious, needs special media (such as charcoal blood agar with cephalexin, Regan Lowe or Bordet-Gengou media) for isolation.
- *B. bronchiseptica* (kennel cough), *B. holmesii* rarely been implicated to cause human respiratory disease.
- *B. trematum* is rarely found in wounds and ear infections.
- *B. hinzii*, *B. homesii* uncommon cause of sepsis in immunocompromised hosts.
- *B. avium* is a pathogen identified only in birds.

CLINICAL

- Typical pertussis infection lasts several wks and consists of 3 stages. **Catarrhal stage:** rhinorrhea, mild fever, coryza and mild cough (1–2 wks, infants may have apnea/respiratory distress) followed by **paroxysmal stage** with increased cough with spells of repetitive usually dry cough, followed by sudden inspiratory effort (whoop) and post-tussive emesis (2–6 wks). **Convalescent stage:** decreasing frequency and severity of coughing episodes (≥2 wks).
- Clinical incubation 5–21 days (7 day average). Consider pts infectious from catarrhal prodrome stage until 3 wks after symptom onset.
- Clinical manifestations vary. Highest mortality in infancy, often under-recognized in adolescents and adults who may have prominent hacking cough but lack characteristic whoop. Prior immunization can lead to atypical presentations.
- In adults, *B. pertussis* most commonly presents as a chronic dry cough that is misdiagnosed as bronchitis (estimated that 13–20% of adults with prolonged cough). Average duration of cough approximately 50 days.

PATHOGENS

- Adult incidence is estimated to be 1–2 cases/1000 adults per yr, highest in adolescents and adult healthcare workers, but this may change with Tdap.
- Suspect pertussis in pts with 2 wks of cough and evidence of (a) coughing paroxysms, (b) inspiratory "whoop," (c) post-tussive emesis.
- 20% of people with acute pertussis may develop radiographic infiltrates.
- Gold standard for dx of pertussis is culture of nasopharyngeal secretions. Nasal aspirates have greater yield than swabs (use Dacron). Cultures should be plated on Bordet-Gengou medium for 7 days.
- Due to the low sensitivity of culture (only 1–3% positive in pts with 3 wks of cough), diagnosis often clinical. PCR-based assays have been developed for respiratory secretions that are increasingly available clinically, and may be the most sensitive test (reportedly 73–100%). There is little standardization with available PCR-based tests. Either culture or PCR recommended and of highest yield if performed within 3 wks of cough onset, or 4 wks from onset of symptoms.
- Standardized serological assays are specific but sensitivity ranges 20–90% compared to culture/PCR. They are usually for research epidemiology. Pertussis toxin (PT) IgG or IgA ideally performed in acute (<2 wks of illness onset) and convalescent (4 wks after symptom onset) serum may support diagnosis. This is often more helpful in adults and adolescents who have lower rates of culture and PCR positivity. Some studies have found that a single high titer is indicative of recent infection (e.g. >100 U/ml anti-PT IgG).

MORE CLINICAL

CDC Definitions for pertussis (2005)

- **Clinical case:** cough ≥2 wks with one of the following: paroxysms of cough, inspiratory "whoop," or post-tussive emesis without other cause.

Laboratory criteria for diagnosis

- Isolation of *B. pertussis* from clinical specimen **or**
- PCR positive for *B. pertussis*

Case classification

- **Probable:** meets clinical case definition, not laboratory confirmed or epidemiologically linked to laboratory confirmed case.
- **Confirmed:** acute cough of any duration that is lab confirmed by culture or case meets clinical case criteria and is confirmed by PCR or epidemiologically linked to confirmed case.

SITES OF INFECTION

- Respiratory disease: laryngobronchitis, pneumonia (less common) usually *B. pertussis*. *B. parapertussis* less common cause of whooping cough.
- Complications: urinary incontinence, post-tussive vomiting, hearing loss, development of hernias, pneumothorax, aspiration, rib fractures, carotid artery dissection, death (rare in adults).

TREATMENT

B. pertussis* and *B. parapertussis

- Empiric treatment recommended if strongly suspecting diagnosis, consider infection control/isolation of pt and treatment of vulnerable contacts.
- Antibiotic treatment unlikely to shorten duration of illness if started more than one wk after symptom onset, but mainly benefits by shortening infectious period and therefore decreasing transmission.
- *In vitro*, most strains are sensitive to both macrolides and fluoroquinolones, but resistant to beta-lactams.
- Rarely, strains of *B. pertussis* resistant to erythromycin have been identified.
- Macrolides are the first line of therapy. Most experience has been with erythromycin, but trials have found azithromycin and clarithromycin to be equally effective and better tolerated.
- **Preferred (adults/adolescents):** azithromycin 500 mg PO × 1 dose then 250 mg PO daily for days 2–5 or clarithromycin 500 mg twice daily × 7 days.
- **Alt (adults/adolescents):** trimethoprim-sulfamethoxazole DS twice daily PO × 14 days is a second-line treatment option for pts who are intolerant of macrolides. Erythromycin 250 mg

PO four times daily × 14 days used less commonly now due to worse side effect profile and longer duration compared to azithromycin and clarithromycin.

- Infection in infants under age 6 mos, may require hospitalization due to complications of hypoxemia, apnea, poor feeding.
- **<1 mo:** azithromycin recommended, 10 mg/kg daily × 5 days (erythromycin, clarithromycin and TMP-SMX not recommended)
- **1–5 mos:** azithromycin recommended, 10 mg/kg daily × 5 days, or clarithromycin 15 mg/kg twice daily × 7 days or erythromycin 10 mg/kg PO four times daily × 14 days, TMP-SMX contraindicated.
- **>6 mos-children:** azithromycin recommended, 10 mg/kg (500 mg max) daily × 5 days, or clarithromycin 15 mg/kg (1 g daily max) twice daily × 7 days or erythromycin 10 mg/kg PO (2 g daily max) four times daily × 14 days, TMP-SMX 4 mg/40 mg per kg twice daily × 14 days.
- TMP-SMX should only be used in pts ≥2 mos of age who are allergic or intolerant of macrolides or who have a macrolide-resistant strain.
- Although fluoroquinolones have excellent *in vitro* sensitivity profiles, clinical experience for *B. pertussis* is limited.

Antibiotic Prophylaxis
- Since transmitted through person-person aerosolized droplets, and highly contagious (80% attack rate), secondary prophylaxis recommended.
- Administer antibiotic prophylaxis if within 3 wks of exposure to index pt (note: incubation period is 5–21 days with 7–10 days average).
- Use drugs with same duration as in treatment section.

Immunization Adolescents and Adults
- New recommendations to immunize adolescents and adults are efforts to decrease the reservoir and transmission of pertussis in these populations and to infants.
- Whole-cell vaccines are inexpensive and effective therefore are still used by many countries, although acellular vaccines are used by most developed countries due to lower adverse events than whole-cell vaccines. For adolescents and adults, given as Tdap (tetanus-diphtheria-acellular pertussis) vaccine.
- **Tdap recommendations:** 1. A single dose of Tdap should replace the next dose of Td for adults aged 19 to 64 yrs as part of the every-10-yr Td boosting schedule.
- Most common side effect from acellular vaccine is large (often painless) local reactions at vaccine site in ~1–2%, highest in those who received acellular booster after the initial series.
- A single dose of Tdap should be administered to adults who have close contact with infants less than 6 mos of age. The optimal interval between Tdap and the last Td is 2 yrs or greater, but shorter intervals are acceptable.
- Women of childbearing age should receive Tdap before conception or immediately postpartum prior to hospital discharge/birthing center, if they have not previously received Tdap or last immunization >2 yrs. Tdap is not approved for use during pregnancy, and usually Td is recommended if needed (or plan to have Tdap immediately post-partum).
- All adolescents aged 11 to 12 should receive a single dose of Tdap.
- Adolescents aged 13 to 18 should receive Tdap if they received the last Td more than 5 yrs previously, or in less than 2 yrs for special circumstances such as close contact with an infant or in an outbreak.
- Contraindications Tdap: history of anaphylactic reaction to a Tdap vaccine component, or a history of encephalopathy within 7 days of receiving a pertussis vaccine that cannot be attributed to another cause. Precautions include Guillain-Barré syndrome less than 6 wks after a previous dose of tetanus toxoid, moderate or severe acute illness (with or without fever), unstable neurologic condition, or a history of an Arthus hypersensitivity reaction after a dose of tetanus or diphtheria toxoid.

FOLLOW UP
- Eradication of *B. pertussis* especially important in high-risk pts: infants, healthcare workers, pregnant women in third trimester.

OTHER INFORMATION
- Increasing recognition of cases and modern diagnostics such as PCR, (25,827 in 2004 (2004 rate: 8.5 cases per 100,000 population) and likely many more not diagnosed.

PATHOGENS

- The classic lymphocytosis associated with acute *B. pertussis* is more common in children than adults.
- Increasing incidence in adults may be due to waning immunity.
- Most mortality occurs from infection within first 6 mos of life including complications of pneumonia, seizures, encephalopathy, and complications of severe coughing (cerebral hypoxia, pulmonary hypertension).
- Adults and adolescents are a primary source of transmission to >60% of infants hospitalized with pertussis.

BASIS FOR RECOMMENDATIONS

Murphy TV, Slade BA, Broder KR, et al. Prevention of pertussis, tetanus, and diphtheria among pregnant and postpartum women and their infants recommendations of the Advisory Committee on Immunization Practices (ACIP). *MMWR Recomm Rep,* 2008; Vol. 57; pp. 1–51.

Comments: Document deals with use of Tdap in pregnancy and post-partum. The following is directly pasted from the abstract: (1) receive Tdap in the immediate postpartum period before discharge from hospital or birthing center, (2) may receive Tdap at an interval as short as 2 yrs since the most recent Td vaccine, (3) receive Td during pregnancy for tetanus and diphtheria protection when indicated, or (4) defer the Td vaccine indicated during pregnancy to substitute Tdap vaccine in the immediate postpartum period if the woman is likely to have sufficient protection against tetanus and diphtheria. Although pregnancy is not a contraindication for receiving Tdap vaccine, health-care providers should weigh the theoretical risks and benefits before choosing to administer Tdap vaccine to a pregnant woman. This report (1) describes the clinical features of pertussis, tetanus, and diphtheria among pregnant and postpartum women and their infants, (2) reviews available evidence of pertussis vaccination during pregnancy as a strategy to prevent infant pertussis, (3) summarizes Tdap vaccination policy in the United States, and (4) presents recommendations for use of Td and Tdap vaccines among pregnant and postpartum women.

Tiwari T, Murphy TV, Moran J, et al. Recommended antimicrobial agents for the treatment and postexposure prophylaxis of pertussis: 2005 CDC Guidelines. *MMWR Recomm Rep,* 2005; Vol. 54; pp. 1–16.

Comments: Basis for drug recommendations for treatment and prophylaxis used in this module.

BORRELIA SPECIES

Paul G. Auwaerter, MD

MICROBIOLOGY

- **Epidemic relapsing fever [RF]**, person-person transmission of Borrelial species (like typhus) by human body louse *(Pediculus humanus).*
- Worldwide infection (ex. S' Pacific), spirochete, helical 5–40 μm long with 3–10 spirals.
- **Sporadic endemic relapsing fever** is tick-borne (Ornithodoros soft ticks), reservoirs include rodents and small animals.
- *B. recurrentis* only causes epidemic louse-borne RF [LBRF], but >15 Borrelia spp. cause endemic tick-borne RF [TBRF].
- In North America, essentially all cases have been associated w/ 2 spp. of ticks: *O. hermsii* and *O. turicatae*. The 3 main agents of TBRF in U.S. are *B. hermsii*, *B. parkeri*, and *B. turicatae*. Microscopic inspection cannot distinguish bacterial spp. *B. hermsii* can be identified by monoclonal antibody, and most Borrelia spp. can be sorted by PCR analysis using genome species-specific markers though neither of these are routinely available in most commercial laboratories. *Borrelia duttonii*, transmitted by the *Ornithodoros moubata* tick vectors is a cause of TBRF in Tanzania, and other parts of Africa. It tends to be more severe than usual TBRF.

CLINICAL

- RF tends to cause high fever, chills, headache, myalgia and nausea that recur every wk or ten days for several mos. Recurrences tend to be less severe. See sites of infection (below) for more info.
- Epidemic LBRF occurs usually in poor socioeconomic settings, war, famine. LBRF occurs endemically in parts Central/East Africa, Peru, and Bolivia.
- Tick-borne RF (most often acquired in warm climates, w/ 2,000–7000 ft. elevation preferred by Ornithodoros soft ticks. In U.S., mostly in Cascades, Sierra Nevada, Rockies and limestone caverns of Texas.

- Many cases of tick-borne RF in the United States have been associated with travel to Lake Coeur D'Alene (Idaho), Packer Lake, Big Bear Lake, and Lake Tahoe (California and Nevada). Outbreaks have been described in Spokane County, Washington; Estes Park, Colorado; and the North Rim of the Grand Canyon.
- Ddx: includes Colorado tick fever, yellow and dengue fever, African hemorrhagic fevers, leptospirosis, LCMV, malaria, bartonella, enterovirus, rat bite fever.
- Dx: obtain Wright- or Giemsa-stained blood smear during fever showing spirochetemia. This is considered diagnostic of relapsing fever. 4 × serologic rise (reference labs only). Culture and PCR methods available only at certain reference labs.
- Mortality greater in untreated LBRF than TBRF. Even w/ rx, LBRF has 5% mortality compared to only rare deaths due to TBRF.
- TBRF and LBRF tend to have similar clinical characteristics; however, LBRF tends to be more severe. LBRF cases typically have more liver/CNS bleeding complications and extensive petechiae.

SITES OF INFECTION

- General: fever—initially lasts 3–6 days, may be associated w/ shock (especially LBRF). After remittance, fever may return in 7–10 days, usually less severe. Louse-borne single relapse; tick-borne multiple.
- General: fevers associated with headache, myalgia/arthralgia. Relapse episodes tend to be shorter, ~2–3 days.
- Heme: DIC, thrombocytopenia.
- GI: abd pain, n/v, diarrhea, jaundice (10%); hepatosplenomegaly (LBRF>>TBRF), splenic rupture (rare).
- Cutaneous: rash (25%), may turn petechial. Eschar at tick bite site rare.
- CNS: altered mental status/photophobia (common); cranial nerve palsy, other focal neurologic deficits or frank meningitis (rare).
- Pulmonary: dry cough, ARDS described (in recent TBRF series from Lake Tahoe region, 16% with hypoxia, 5% with ARDS).
- Cardiac: myocarditis
- Ocular: uveitis

TREATMENT

Tick-Borne Relapsing Fever

- Majority of TBRF cases likely self-limited, without requiring abx rx.
- Preferred: doxycycline 100 mg PO twice daily × 5–10 days.
- Alt: erythromycin 500 mg PO four times a day 5–10 days.
- If meningitis/encephalitis present, use ceftriaxone 2 g IV q12h × 14 days.
- Untreated TBRF infection mortality ~5%.
- Jarisch-Herxheimer reaction (severe rigor, fever, low BP) may occur post-abx. More commonly seen in LBRF.
- Jarisch-Herxheimer reaction may be life-threatening. 2 hr post-initial abx observation period recommended.

Louse-Borne Relapsing Fever

- Preferred: single dose tetracycline 500 mg PO.
- Alt: erythromycin 500 mg PO × 1.
- Single dose therapy effective with few cases of relapse.
- Untreated louse-borne infection mortality ~40%.
- Jarisch-Herxheimer rxn (severe rigor, fever, low BP) may occur post-abx
- Jarisch-Herxheimer reaction may be life-threatening. 2 hr post-initial abx observation period recommended.

Prevention

- Avoid rodent and tick-infested dwellings and infested natural sites, such as animal burrows or caves. Many cases in U.S. acquired by sleeping in tick-infested cabins.
- Education especially important for visitors to mountain resort areas.
- Rodent proof dwellings.

PATHOGENS

- Avoid arthropod vectors; DEET sprays of uncertain help; for TBRF tick inspection generally not helpful since soft ticks are nocturnal biters, leaving host by morning.
- De-lousing, good personal hygiene or insect sprays in dwellings may help control epidemic LBRF.
- Doxycycline 200 mg on day 1 then 100 mg daily days 2–5 shown to provide post-exposure prevention of tick-borne relapsing fever in the Israeli army study performed in an area of high endemicity and suspected tick exposure.

OTHER INFORMATION
- In U.S., TBRF occurs generally only west of Mississippi. Suspect if febrile illness with rural, mountainous exposure esp. sleeping in primitive cabins, or if there is rodent exposure. Bite often inapparent, lasting for less than 30 minutes (when host asleep)—hence pts unaware of tick bite.
- Epidemic LBRF clinically similar and confused with epidemic typhus (*Rickettsia prowazekii*) as both spread by body louse.
- Relapsing nature has been attributed to antigenic variation in spirochetes.
- High-level spirochetemia characteristic of RF w/ >10,000 organisms/hpf; however, during afebrile/asx stages they're undetectable.
- Recent MMWR report suggestive that pulmonary complications of TBRF including ARDS may be more common than previously reported.

BASIS FOR RECOMMENDATIONS
Dworkin MS, Schwan TG, Anderson DE. Tick-borne relapsing fever in North America. *Med Clin North Am*, 2002; Vol. 86; pp. 417–33, viii–ix.
Comments: Nicely comprehensive recent review of RF that emphasizes most cases have been acquired from exposure to rustic tick-infested cabins and caves.

BRUCELLA SPECIES

Joseph Vinetz, MD

MICROBIOLOGY
- Aerobic, Gram-negative coccobacilli causing brucellosis.
- Zoonotic disease, most important species: *B. abortus* (cattle), *B. melitensis* (goat).

CLINICAL
- Major endemic regions: Mediterranean (Spain, Portugal, Italy, Greece); Middle East; Latin America (Peru, Mexico, Argentina); not infrequently seen in Texas, Arizona and California among Mexican immigrants.
- In developed countries, rare; may be in immigrants who ingest raw goat milk/cheese; abattoir workers/vets; potential from bison in Yellowstone and other areas.
- Presentation varies: (1) Acute febrile disease is systemic, non-focal; (2) Relapsing/"undulant form" (Malta fever) arthritis, hepatic; (3) chronic may be cyclic or localized.
- Laboratory data: low or nl hemoglobin; WBC <4000/ul in 20%, lymphocytosis in 50%; AST/ALT/alkaline phosphatase often elevated.
- Dx: blood culture (15–30% of cases positive). Isolated organism differentiates acute from chronic infections.
- Lab cultures common cause of infection of laboratory workers through aerosolization, thus cultures should be done in a laminar flow hood; potentially weaponizable as BT agent (category B BT agent). Notify lab if considering diagnosis.
- Serological diagnosis: agglutination titer >1:160 considered diagnostic; titers can be lower. 2-mercaptoethanol treatment of serum destroys IgM. If agglutination titer decline post-2Me, acute infection dx'd.
- Dx of relapsing infection: rising agglutination titers. Culture of blood lower yield, may require bone marrow culture.
- Dx of chronic focal or systemic disease: requires high index of suspicion. Serology may be negative, may require bone marrow culture.

SITES OF INFECTION

- Systemic: fever, generalized myalgia/arthralgia, chills, night sweats, anorexia, lethargy.
- Bone/joint: arthritis, often severe and disabling; involvement of back, hips, spondylitis, sacroilitis psoas abscess, etc.
- GU: epididymo-orchitis.
- Renal: pyelonephritis, glomerulonephritis.
- Neuro: cerebral (papilledema, cranial neuritis, meningoencephalitis, brain abscess); spinal (polio-like, cord compression (abscess), cauda equina syndrome, myelopathy, transverse myelitis); peripheral.
- Musculoskeletal: sacroiliitis, can clinically mimic acute pyogenic spondylodiskitis.
- Psychiatric: depression, chronic fatigue, especially during chronic brucellosis and during convalescence.

TREATMENT

First Line Combination Therapy
- Doxycycline 100 mg PO/IV twice daily × 45 days **plus** streptomycin 1 g/IM/day for first 14 days or gentamicin for first 7 days; total duration of therapy 6 wks or longer.

Second Line Combination Therapy
- Doxycycline 100 mg twice daily **plus** rifampin 600–900 mg/day × 6 wks.
- Ciprofloxacin 500 mg/twice daily **plus** rifampin 600 mg/day × 30 days.
- Ciprofloxacin + doxycycline 30-day regimen suggested to be equivalent to doxycycline + rifampin 45-day regimen in open, randomized trial of 40 pts.

Third Line Combination Therapy
- Trimethoprim-sulfamethoxazole 160/800 mg three times a day **plus** gentamicin (240 mg IM/day or 5 mg/kg IM/day for pts <50 kg) for first 5 days.

Treatment of Children
- 7 yrs or older: same as adults.
- 6 yrs or younger: rifampin 10 mg/kg/day × 4 wk **plus** streptomycin 30 mg/kg/day IM (max: 1 g) (14 days) or gentamicin 2.5 mg/kg every day (7 days) IM **or plus** TMP-SMZ (5 mg/kg TMP component) × 4 wk.

Pregnancy
- Rifampin 900 mg q24 **or** rifampin 600 mg q24 **plus** streptomycin or gentamicin as above.

MORE TREATMENT

- A recent randomized non-blinded clinical trial suggested that adding amikacin (7.5 mg/kg IM bid) to doxycycline/rifampin led to more rapid resolution of signs and symptoms of infection but was insufficiently powered to detect a difference in relapse rates.

OTHER INFORMATION

- Serological diagnosis may miss *B. canis* infections (which is nonetheless rare in humans).
- Neuropsychiatric illness, particularly depression, has been noted after microbiological cure even w/ declining antibody titers. Retreatment without active infection not effective in reducing psych sxs.

BASIS FOR RECOMMENDATIONS

Solera J, Espinosa A, Martínez-Alfaro E, et al. Treatment of human brucellosis with doxycycline and gentamicin. *Antimicrob Agents Chemother,* 1997; Vol. 41; pp. 80–4.

Comments: This article discusses efficacy and response rates of this gentamicin-containing regimen that is an alternative to a streptomycin-containing regimen. Of importance, there is further evidence that prolonging the doxy regiment to 45 days reduces the relapse rate.

BURKHOLDERIA CEPACIA COMPLEX

John G. Bartlett, MD

MICROBIOLOGY

- Now called *B. cepacia* complex (Bcc) with 3 species: *B. cepacia, B. cenocepacia,* and *B. multivorans.* Nonfermenting aerobic Gram-negative rod.
- Easily grown on standard media.

- Ubiquitous: water, soil, plants.
- Waterborne, nosocomial, opportunistic pathogen.
- Formerly known as *Pseudomonas cepacia*.

CLINICAL
- Predisposing conditions: cystic fibrosis, chronic lung disease, chronic granulomatous disease, sickle cell disease, burn pts, oncology pts.
- Common cause of outbreaks due to contaminated substances.
- Diagnose by standard culture. If from non-sterile source, must from distinguish colonization clinically.

SITES OF INFECTION
- Pneumonia
- Bacteremia +/– shock and DIC
- Cystic fibrosis: range from colonization to pneumonia, including necrotizing pneumonia
- Bronchiectasis
- Post-lung transplant pneumonia
- Ecthyma gangrenosum
- Burn wound sepsis
- Endophthalmitis
- Endocarditis (rare), especially heroin addicts

TREATMENT
- Sensitivities must guide therapy. Most active drugs are minocycline, doripenem, meropenem and ceftazidime.
- Preferred (if sensitive): ceftazidime 2 g IV q8h, imipenem 1 g IV q6h, meropenem 1–2 g IV q8h or minocycline 100 mg IV/PO twice daily.

OTHER INFORMATION
- Abx recommendations based upon Medical Letter (Med Letter 2004;2:21) and CF Referral Center (http://synergy.columbia.edu).
- Opportunistic pathogen, especially in cystic fibrosis, CGD and sickle cell disease.
- Cystic fibrosis: usually colonizes, may cause pneumonia or fulminant infection (sepsis).
- Resistant to abxs commonly used empirically for sepsis. Usually resistant to cefepime.

BASIS FOR RECOMMENDATIONS
Choice of antibacterial drugs. *Treat Guidel Med Lett*, 2004; Vol. 2; pp. 13–26.
Comments: Recommendations are used for this module.

BURKHOLDERIA MALLEI

John G. Bartlett, MD

MICROBIOLOGY
- Aerobic small slender Gram-negative rod causes disease known as glanders in animals (esp. horses) and rarely humans.
- Hard to see on Gram-stain. Grows slowly, best with glycerol. If suspected, warn lab since it can pose a lab hazard.
- May be erroneously identified as *Pseudomonas* sp. by standard microbiologic testing.

CLINICAL
- Primarily an infection of horses in Asia, Africa, and S. America, rarely acquired from soil. Most human cases described in SE Asia a result of animal transmission.
- One reported case in U.S. from 1947–2003 which was lab acquired.
- Major concern is bioterrorism—using antibiotic resistant strain for aerosol. If organism isolated, suspect bioterrorism and notify public health offices.
- Acute glanders may produce a localized infection with ulceration following inoculation in the skin often associated with lymphadenopathy. Lung infections may present as pneumonia, lung abscesses and pleural effusion. Acute bloodstream infections can be rapidly fatal.
- The chronic form of glanders often produces multiple abscesses within liver, spleen, or extremities.
- Diagnosis is usually by culture of blood, pus, or affected tissue or respiratory secretions. PCR test may be available. Serology is not available.

SITES OF INFECTION
- Subcutaneous nodule/skin ulcer +/– adenopathy
- Oral ulcer
- Pulmonary—acute or chronic
- Disseminated—liver and spleen abscesses
- Adenopathy
- Ocular

TREATMENT
Treatment
- If organism isolated suspect bioterrorism—quarantine pt and give antibiotics (refined by *in vitro* susceptibilities).
- TMP-SMX 5 mg/kg (TMP component) IV or PO q8h or imipenem 0.5–1 g q4–6h IV (max 4 g/day).
- Other possible options: gentamicin, doxycycline, ciprofloxacin, ceftazidime, piperacillin.
Treatment–Miscellaneous
- Multiple cases (consider bioterrorism): need *in vitro* tests to define proper antibiotic.
- Pts should be isolated—*B. mallei* spread by aerosol.
- Prophylaxis for exposed persons—no guidelines—consider using doxycycline or ciprofloxacin.
- Contact state/local bioterrorism authorities—see http://www.bt.cdc.gov/emcontact/#State.

OTHER INFORMATION
- Only one U.S. case since 1947, occuring in bioterrorism lab worker.
- Major concern—bioterrorism using antibiotic resistant strain with aerosol delivery.
- Range of disease: 1) skin +/– lymph only, 2) lung-acute/chronic or 3) disseminated liver/spleen/lung abscesses.
- One U.S. case in past 50 yrs—means there is nearly no experience with antibiotics except in animals and *in vitro*.

BASIS FOR RECOMMENDATIONS
Author opinion.

Comments: No formal guidelines exist for treatment.

CAMPYLOBACTER AND RELATED SPECIES

Paul G. Auwaerter, MD

MICROBIOLOGY
- Gram-negative bacteria with curved bacillary appearance on Gram-stain. Oxidase positive.
- *C. jejuni* (see *C. jejuni* [p. 240] module for information specific to this species) most common member.
- Other members include *C. coli, C. fetus, C. lari* described in this module.
- Worldwide zoonosis, with *C. fetus* causing abortion in cattle and sheep.
- Helicobacter spp. closely related (e.g., *H. pylori* formerly *C. pylori*) *H. cinaedi, H. fennelliae, H. pullorum, H. westmeadii, H. canadensis* described as causing human illness such as enteritis and sepsis, often in immunocompromised.

CLINICAL
- Non-jejuni spp. tend to cause extra-intestinal illness. *C. fetus* subsp. *fetus* most human common pathogen of this type. Infections acquired from ingesting infected animal excreta contaminating meat.
- Typical extra-intestinal Campylobacter infection affects debilitated hosts. Can infect normal hosts, but less common.
- Homosexual men appear at increased risk probably due to sexual practices.
- Dx: blood culture isolate may take 4–14 days to grow. If attempting to culture *C. fetus* or other species from feces [rarely achieved], alert micro lab for 37°C requirements and media without cephalosporins.

PATHOGENS

SITES OF INFECTION
- Bacteremia: may be prolonged, w/ relapsing fever. Source inapparent.
- Endovascular: may cause endocarditis, mycotic acronyms especially abdominal aorta. Predilection to cause septic thrombophlebitis.
- GI: diarrheal disease can occur with "atypical campylobacter" (non-*C. jejuni* spp.), but generally less severe and self-limited.
- Meningoencephalitis: rare, seen in neonates and adults.
- Cellulitis: described especially in immune suppressed with Helicobacter spp.

TREATMENT
Gastrointestinal
- Uncommon, usually self-limited in normal hosts [non-*C. jejuni* infections].
- Supportive care, rehydration (oral or IV).
- Antibiotics rarely needed in normal hosts, but in very ill or if sx persist >7 days may choose from agents listed below.
- Erythromycin 250 mg PO 4 times a day × 7 days or clarithromycin 500 mg PO twice daily or azithromycin 500 mg PO once daily [would **not** use for severe or systemic illness because of resistance concerns].
- Ciprofloxacin 500 mg twice daily PO an alternative and may be preferred due to increasing resistance reports in non-*C. jejuni* spp.

Extra-intestinal infections
- If possible susceptibility tests should guide choices due to increasing resistance. Agents listed generally sensitive except as noted.
- Campylobacter and Helicobacter spp. usually resistant to penicillins and cephalosporins; exceptions amoxicillin, ampicillin and ticarcillin/clavulanate (but not sulbactam or tazobactam).
- Serious infections: gentamicin 5 mg/kg/day IV or imipenem 1 mg IV q6h or ceftriaxone 2 g IV q12h.
- Endovascular infections prefer aminoglycoside (4–6 wk) perhaps combined with carbapenem. CNS prefer ceftriaxone or chloramphenicol (2–3 wk).
- Atypical campylobacter or *H. cinaedi* infections acquired in developing countries often resistant to erythromycin, tetracycline.

OTHER INFORMATION
- *C. fetus* and related infections may be fatal in cirrhotics, diabetics or severely compromised pts.
- Survival in the very ill probably dependent on the timeliness of initiating proper antibiotic.
- Systemic campylobacter infections deserve parenteral therapy. Erythromycin **not** always effective and should be avoided.

BASIS FOR RECOMMENDATIONS
Guerrant RL, Van Gilder T, Steiner TS, et al. Practice guidelines for the management of infectious diarrhea. *Clin Infect Dis*, 2001; Vol. 32; pp. 331–51.
Comments: Guidelines for the management of Campylobacter-related diarrhea are included here.

Author opinion.
Comments: No guidelines exist for non-gastrointestinal infections.

CAMPYLOBACTER JEJUNI

Paul G. Auwaerter, MD

MICROBIOLOGY
- Spiral-shaped bacteria well adapted to birds (carriage is asymptomatic). Raw chicken in U.S. frequently contaminated with organism.
- Major cause of diarrhea (either #1 or #2 cause in U.S. trading with Salmonella). *C. jejuni* causes 99% of Campylobacter infections. For non-*C. jejuni* infections, see "Campylobacter and related species" (previous module).
- Often food-borne cause of human diarrhea. Cases occur summer > winter.

CLINICAL

- Typical diarrhea, abdominal cramping and fever arise 2–5 days after exposure. Typically acquired from raw meat or contaminated cutting-boards used to prepare food. Person-person spread rare. Large outbreaks most often from unpasteurized milk or contaminated water.
- Campylobacter enteritis: ~8% w/ visible blood in stool, ~52% occult blood +, 59% w/ fever and 45% had abdominal tenderness.
- Rare cause of bacteremia (especially in immune compromised), meningitis and endocarditis.
- Guillain-Barre syndrome is preceded by Campylobacter infection in 20–50% of cases.
- Dx: stool cx (special media and 42°C required to grow Campylobacter; lab notification may be required when considering this organism).

SITES OF INFECTION

- GI: diarrhea, colitis, acute abdominal pain, pseudo-appendicitis.
- Systemic (rare): bloodstream infection, meningitis, focal abscesses.
- Musculoskeletal: occasional cause of post-infectious arthropathy or *erythema nodosum*.
- Neurologic: Guillain-Barré syndrome (post-infectious).

TREATMENT

Gastroenteritis

- Rehydration essential. Most pts do not require antibiotics and sx last <1 wk. Exceptions: high fevers, bloody stools, prolonged illness (sx >1 wk), pregnancy, HIV and other immunosuppressed states.
- Estimated rates of FQ resistance ~10% but may raise to 55% if associated with foreign travel to SE Asia. Pts with FQ-resistant Campylobacter may have more severe or prolonged infection.
- **Preferred:** erythromycin stearate 500 mg PO q12h × 5 days. Azithromycin is probable alternative but not as well studied.
- **Alt:** ciprofloxacin 500 mg PO q12h × 5 days (wary of resistance, especially if acquired SE Asia).
- *Campylobacter* species also are generally susceptible to aminoglycosides, chloramphenicol, clindamycin and carbapenems as considerations if parenteral therapy required.
- Extraintestinal infections should be treated longer (e.g., 2–4 wks).

Prevention

- Poultry stocks nearly universally contaminated with *Campylobacter* spp.
- Handwashing, thorough cooking of food (internal temperature of 170–180°C) especially poultry.
- Use of poorly cleaned cutting boards, food preparation utensils that cross-contaminate other foods are common ways of causing infection.
- Avoid unpasteurized milk.

OTHER INFORMATION

- Most infections self-limited, not requiring abx. In U.S., the most common cause of bloody diarrhea is not Campylobacter *but* E. coli O157:H7 infection.
- Fluoroquinolone resistance increasingly common (animal husbandry use of FQ driving resistance), so erythromycin preferred drug that most clinicians prescribed azithromycin.
- Increasing quinolone resistance noted to *C. jejuni* especially in overseas travelers.
- Certain clones of Campylobacters appear to be associated with Guillain-Barre syndrome (LPS-019+), but are typically no longer present enterically at neurological presentation.
- Campylobacter is quite sensitive to complement-mediated effects, therefore, is uncommonly found in the bloodstream.

BASIS FOR RECOMMENDATIONS

Guerrant RL, Van Gilder T, Steiner TS, et al. Practice guidelines for the management of infectious diarrhea. *Clin Infect Dis,* 2001; Vol. 32; pp. 331–51.

Comments: A review by an expert panel. For diarrhea caused by *Campylobacter jejuni,* erythromycin is recommended as treatment of choice. Data indicates that for pts with Campylobacter gastroenteritis, 8% had visible blood in stool, 52% had occult blood +, 59% had fever and 45% had abdominal tenderness.

PATHOGENS

CAPNOCYTOPHAGA CANIMORSUS

Paul G. Auwaerter, MD

MICROBIOLOGY

- *C. canimorsus* (previously known as DF-2, dysgonic fermenter) and *C. cynodegmi* (previously known as DF-2 like organism) are facultatively anaerobic Gram-negative rod, part of normal oral flora of dogs and cats.
- Other *Capnocytophaga* species may be part of normal human oral flora or dental plaque.
- Organism has a long, fusiform appearance on Gram-stain, making it distinctive enough to consider morphologic identification pending cx results.
- Organisms considered fastidious by micro lab.
- Most strains are resistant to polymyxin, fusidic acid, fosfomycin and trimethoprim. Variably active: erythromycin, quinolones, metronidazole, vancomycin, aminoglycosides.

CLINICAL

- May cause fulminant sepsis following dog > cat bites, particularly in asplenic pts, alcoholics or immune suppressed.
- Many pts have hx of dog/cat bite or scratch.
- Infection may be mild to severe, including shock, DIC, acral gangrene, disseminated purpura, renal failure, meningitis and pulmonary infiltrates.

SITES OF INFECTION

- Soft tissue (dog > cat bites): cellulitis
- Bacteremia/sepsis: risk of severe infection increased in asplenics, alcoholics
- CNS: meningitis
- Cardiac: endocarditis (rare)

TREATMENT

Severe Cellulitis/Sepsis or Endocarditis

- Preferred: beta-lactam/beta-lactamase inhibitor (e.g., ampicillin/sulbactam 3 g IV q6h), penicillin G 2–4 million units q4h IV (if non-beta-lactamase producing).
- Alt: ceftriaxone 1–2 q IV q24h, or meropenem 1 g IV q8h.
- Clindamycin 600 mg IV q8h may be combined with above agents especially in pts with complicated infections or immunocompromise.
- Note that resistance to aztreonam described, and variable susceptibility reported to TMP-SMX and aminoglycosides.
- For endocarditis, alternatives to penicillins not well established, duration: 6 wks. For non-endocarditis infections, duration not well established, but most authorities recommend at least 14–21 days of therapy.

Mild Cellulitis/Dog or Cat Bites

- Preferred: amoxicillin/clavulanate 500 mg PO 3 times a day or 875 mg PO twice daily, or amoxicillin 500 mg PO 3 times a day. Since pathogen of bites usually not known, empiric amoxicillin/clavulanate usually selected.
- Alt: clindamycin 300 mg PO 4 times a day, doxycycline 100 mg PO twice daily or clarithromycin 500 mg PO twice daily or moxifloxacin 400 mg PO once daily.

Meningitis or brain abscess

- Use ceftriaxone 2 g IV q12h + ampicillin 2 g IV q4h, combination antibiotic coverage favored by some in serious infections, but can likely simplify to single agent with clinical improvement based upon susceptibility testing in pts with meningitis.
- Imipenem/cilastin 1000 mg q6–8h + clindamycin 600 mg IV q8h (if beta-lactamase producing or polymicrobial brain abscess).

Prevention

- Although no firm data supports this recommendation, many clinicians do give prophylaxis for dog/cat bites in asplenic pts with amoxicillin/clavulanate for 7–10 days.

OTHER INFORMATION

- Consider *C. canimorsus* in all dog bite infections, or any fulminant infection in asplenics.
- Cx results or *in vitro* susceptibilities may be delayed due to slow growth of organism in the lab.

- All asplenic pts after a dog bite should be considered to undergo antibiotic prophylaxis, e.g., amoxicillin/clavulanate.
- Other Capnocytophaga spp. include *C. ochracea* that is a colonizer of normal human oral flora. The bacteria may be associated with periodontal disease, and bacteremia/sepsis has been described in cancer/neutropenic pts.
- *C. sputigena*, *C. gingivalis* found in dental plaques.

MORE INFORMATION

- The above organisms have variable susceptability to beta-lactams and metronidazole, while generally sensitive to clindamycin, macrolides, fluoroquinolones and carbapenems. *C. cynodegmi* is a closely related organism to *C. canimorsus*, and is associated with dog bites. Antibiotic susceptibilities are likely similar.

BASIS FOR RECOMMENDATIONS

Jolivet-Gougeon A, Sixou JL, Tamanai-Shacoori Z, et al. Antimicrobial treatment of Capnocytophaga infections. *Int J Antimicrob Agents*, 2007; Vol. 29; pp. 367–73.

Comments: Thorough review emphasizes that *Capnocytophaga* spp. are commensal species of the oral flora/dental plaque rather than truly implicated as causes of periodontal disease in humans. Article also gives table with recommendations for less common infections. Authors favor combination therapy for serious infections in immunocompromised hosts especially if using linezolid or clindamycin.

Goldstein EJ. Current concepts on animal bites: bacteriology and therapy. *Curr Clin Top Infect Dis*, 1999; Vol. 19; pp. 99–111.

Comments: Lovely review by one of the most knowledgeable clinicians in this arena.

CHLAMYDIA TRACHOMATIS

Noreen A. Hynes, MD, MPH

MICROBIOLOGY

- 3 subsets: (1) D-K biovars—genital tract chlamydia—worldwide STD causing cervicitis, urethritis, PID, epididymitis, (2) L-serovars causing lymphogranuloma venereum (LGV), (3) A-C biovars causing trachoma.

CLINICAL

- The STD forms (biovars D-K and L-serovars) enhance the acquisition and transmission of HIV.
- **Genital tract chlamydia D-K biovars:** up to 70% infections in women are asymptomatic; up to 40% of men are asymptomatic.
- D-K biovars: Can cause mucopurulent cervicitis (MPC), dysuria-pyuria syndrome, PID, and perihepatitis in women. 70% of perihepatitis due to CT. Can cause adverse outcome in newborn.
- D-K biovars: Leading cause of PID, believed to cause "silent salpingitis" therefore must screen for CT. Thought to be leading cause of infertility in women.
- Genital tract chlamydia, particularly those caused by serotype G and LGV L2 strain appear to be linked to cancer. Serotype G and infection over time with multiple serotypes linked to cervical squamous cell carcinoma.
- **D-K biovars screening tests:** nucleic acid amplification tests (NAAT) are more sensitive than non-nucleic acid amplification tests (hybridization tests such as GenProbe, EIA, or DFA)—although all are adequate for screening. In locations where prevalence is >2%, some experts believe NAATs can be considered confirmatory. Otherwise, when positive, provide only a presumptive diagnosis; culture, that is less sensitive than a NAAT is the gold standard for diagnosis. NAATs are most sensitive when used on endocervical and intraurethral samples with slightly less sensitivity in urine. NAATs cannot be used on rectal or pharyngeal samples—culture or DFA should be requested for such samples, are more sensitive (85%) than most previous tests but have less specificity; if CT prevalence is <2% in an area, another type of NAAT should be used to confirm a positive result. The specificity of the screening tests are variable. Point of care rapid tests are not recommended for routine screening.

PATHOGENS

- **LGV L serovars:** cause STD lymphogranuloma venereum (LGV) associated w/ genital ulcer-adenopathy syndrome and proctocolitis. Seen mostly in the developing world and in the developed world among men who have sex with men.
- **Trachoma A-C biovars:** cause of hyperendemic blinding trachoma, usually among children in the developing world.

Environmental contamination may lead to false positive results using nucleic acid amplification tests. Disinfection with dilute bleach solution of surfaces following a pt visit can help to decrease contamination risk.

SITES OF INFECTION

- Genito-urinary tract: urethritis, cervicitis, PID, epididymitis, prostatitis (rare).
- Rectum: proctitis
- Colon: colitis and proctocolitis.
- Eye: conjunctivitis, trachoma

TREATMENT

CT cervicitis/urethritis (D-K biovars)

- Recommended regimen: azithromycin 1 g PO × 1 (preferred if adherence is an anticipated problem). Consider concurrent Rx for gonococcal infection if prevalence of gonorrhea is high in pt population where infection was likely acquired.
- Recommended regimen: doxycycline 100 mg PO twice daily × 7 days. Consider concurrent Rx for gonococcal infection if prevalence of gonorrhea is high in pt population where infection was likely acquired.
- Alternative regimen (2nd line): erythromycin base 500 mg PO four times a day × 7 days.
- Alternative regimen (2nd line): erythromycin ethylsuccinate 800 mg PO four times a day × 7 days.
- Alternative regimen (2nd line): ofloxacin 300 mg PO twice daily × 7 days. Not for use in HI, CA, MA, NY City, Pacific Basin, where rates of fluoroquinolone-resistant gonorrhea is high unless gonorrhea ruled out.
- Alternative regimen (2nd line): levofloxacin 500 mg PO every day × 7 days. Not for use in HI, CA, MA, NY City, Pacific Basin, where rates of fluoroquinolone-resistant GC is high unless gonorrhea ruled out.

CT cervicitis in pregnant women (D-K biovars)

- Recommended regimen: azithromycin 1 g PO × 1 (test of cure required 3 wks after end of treatment preferably using a nucleic acid amplification test—NAAT)
- Recommended regimen: amoxicillin 500 mg PO three times a day × 7 days (test of cure required 3 wks after preferably using a nucleic acid amplification test—NAAT)
- Alternative regimen (2nd line): erythromycin base 500 mg PO four times a day × 7 days (test of cure required 3 wks after preferably using a nucleic acid amplification test—NAAT)
- Alternative regimen (2nd line): erythromycin base 250 mg PO four times a day × 14 days (Test of cure required 3 wks after preferably using a nucleic acid amplification test—NAAT)
- Alternative regimen (2nd line): erythromycin ethylsuccinate 800 mg four times a day × 7 days (Test of cure required 3 wks after preferably using a nucleic acid amplification test—NAAT)
- Alternative regimen (2nd line): erythromycin ethylsuccinate 400 mg four times a day × 14 days (Test of cure required 3 wks after preferably using a nucleic acid amplification test—NAAT)

Other GU-related infections

- Epididymitis: ceftriaxone 250 mg IM × 1 + doxycyline 100 mg PO twice daily × 10 days. Alt: ofloxacin 300 mg PO twice daily or levofloxacin 500 mg once daily, either × 10 days. See "Epididymitis" module, p. 75.
- Pelvic inflammatory diseases: **Oral** (recommended): levofloxacin 500 mg PO every day × 14 days or ofloxacin 400 mg PO twice daily × 14 days with or without metronidazole 500 mg PO twice daily × 14 days. Alternative: ceftriaxone 250 mg IM × 1 or cefoxitin 2 g IM × 1 with probenecid 1 g PO concurrently × 1 **plus** doxycycline 100 mg PO twice daily × 14 days with or without metronidazole 500 mg PO twice daily × 14 days. **Parenteral** (preferred): cefotetan 2 g IV q12h or cefoxitin 2 g IV q6h **plus** doxycycline 100 mg PO or IV q12h for at least 24 hrs, then change to PO regimen (above) to complete 14 days of Rx. Also see "Pelvic Inflammatory Disease" module, p. 109.

- Proctitis/proctocolitis: (D-K biovars): ceftriaxone 125 mg IM × 1 **plus** doxycycline 100 mg PO twice daily × 7 days. Also see notes in separate "Proctitis/Proctocolitis" module for proper management.
- Lymphogranuloma venereum (recommended regimen): doxycycline 100 mg PO twice daily × 21 days. Alternative regimen: erythromycin base 500 mg PO four times a day × 21 days.

HIV-infected persons (D-K biovars)
- Treat same as HIV-uninfected persons.

Ocular Infections
- Acute inclusion conjunctivitis: same as non-LGV chlamydia genital tract infection outlined above.
- Trachoma: azithromycin 1 g PO × 1 dose.

OTHER INFORMATION
- When rectal involvement suspected, culture or DFA only (inhibitors obscure other tests). In cases of severe proctitis always consider LGV. Requires longer therapy.
- Retest all women with genital tract CT 3 mos after treatment due to high reinfection rate (this is **not** a test of cure!); providers should retest all women treated for chlamydia whenever they next seek medical care for any reason within the 3–12 mos following initial Dx, regardless of whether or not the pt believes her sex partners have all been treated.
- Test of cure not needed if **recommended** (as opposed to alternative) regimens used (**Except** in pregnant women—test of cure needed in all pregnant women regardless of regimen due to the possible sequelae in the mother and neonate if infection persists).
- Counsel pts to refrain from sexual activity for sexually transmitted CT infections for 7 days after completion of RX. **Treat all partners!**

MORE INFORMATION
- Controversy re: existence of doxycycline resistant CT exists and its clinical relevance.
- Nucleic acid based tests if repeated less than 3 wks after RX may yield false positive results.
- In adults, acute inclusion conjunctivitis, usually unilateral usually results from autoinoculation with infected genital secretions; about 10% of teens with keratoconjunctivitis will have CT infection. Scarring does not occur as with trachoma.

BASIS FOR RECOMMENDATIONS

American Academy of Pediatrics. 2006 Red Book: Report of the Committee on Infectious Diseases. *AAP, Elk Grove Village, IL*, 2006.

Comments: This is the pediatric "bible" for infectious disease treatment in the pediatric age-group. The AAP specifically recommends screening sexually active adolescents and other women aged 20–24, especially if at risk and that sex partners should be treated. Previously infected adolescents are a high priority for repeat testing for C trachomatis, usually 3 to 6 mos after initial infection and should be rescreened. Among pregnant women, then recommend screening and treatment of sex partners. Retesting for infection using nucleic acid amplification test should occur no sooner than 4 wks (this differs from CDC STD guidelines) after completing regimens with erythromycin or amoxicillin.

Centers for Disease Control and Prevention, Workowski KA, Berman SM. Sexually transmitted diseases treatment guidelines, 2006. *MMWR Recomm Rep*, 2006; Vol. 55; pp. 1–94.

Comments: The 2006 CDC treatment guidelines provide clinicians with a readily available reference for STD treatments recommended by a panel of national and international experts in STD diagnosis, treatment, prevention and control. Noteworthy new updates to the Guidelines include newly available evidence: (1) The latest information on the presentation, appropriate screening, and treatment of STDs among men who have sex with men; (2) New evidence on the benefits of rescreening for chlamydia and gonorrhea; (3) Recommendations for partner-delivered therapy for gonorrhea and chlamydia, if other strategies for reaching partners are not likely to succeed; (4) New medications and treatment regimens to treat chlamydia and trichomoniasis and decrease herpes simplex virus 2 (HSV2) transmission; and (5) information on the new HPV vaccine. These guidelines available electronically at: http://www.cdc.gov/std/treatment/

Peterman TA, Tian LH, Metcalf CA, et al. High incidence of new sexually transmitted infections in the yr following a sexually transmitted infection: a case for rescreening. *Ann Intern Med*, 2006; Vol. 145; pp. 564–72.

Comments: This critically important study focuses on the expanded need for rescreening CT infected persons at periodic intervals. This is the report of a secondary analysis using data collected during the multicenter randomized, controlled trial of HIV prevention counseling with a rapid HIV test or a standard HIV test (RESPECT-2). The trial was conducted in from Feb 1999 to Dec 2000; for this analysis there were 2419 eligible (51% women; 49% men) persons with evaluable data from 3 public STD clinics in Denver, CO; Long Beach, CA; and Newark, NJ. Participants were tested for *C. trachomatis, N. gonorrhoeae*, and *T. vaginalis* infections at time of study entry, at each quarterly follow-up visit, and at other visits not related to the study that occurred during the 12-mo follow-up period. 25.8% of women vs 14.7% of men had 1 or more new infections; 11.9% women vs 9.4% men acquired *C. trachomatis*; 6.3% of women vs 7.1% of men acquired *N. gonorrhoeae,*

PATHOGENS

and 12.8% of women had *T. vaginalis*—men were not assessed for this infection. If infected at baseline, the risk for infection was high at 3 and 6 mos (16.3 per 100 three-mo intervals) and remained high at 9 and 12 mos (12.0 per 100 three-mo intervals). 66.2% of participants reported no symptoms. The implication of this analysis is that Rx of a new STD case is unlikely to eliminate a reservoir of infection in the community. Behavioral change is critical to prevent reinfection.

CHLAMYDOPHILA PNEUMONIAE

John G. Bartlett, MD

MICROBIOLOGY
- Obligate intracellular bacteria. Grows like a virus (requires cell culture systems) but is a bacterium with RNA and DNA.
- As intracellular parasite, requires host cell for ATP/GTP.
- Elementary body is metabolically inactive form, has rigid cell wall that permits survival outside cell. Inside cell is seen as inclusion body.
- Incubation period: average 21 days.

CLINICAL
- Major cause of respiratory infections (causes % of): pharyngitis 1%, sinusitis 5%, bronchitis 5–10%, community-acquired pneumonia 5–15%.
- May cause atypical pneumonia, manifests as URI (rhinitis, laryngitis) + cough + patchy infiltrate, slow onset and prolonged sx with cough >2 wks; reinfection is less severe.
- Asymptomatic carriage in pharynx reported, but uncommon.
- Dx: most common is MIF serology—technically hard and poor interobserver correlation. This is the most common method used in studies but validity is questionable and FDA has not cleared it. Serology not currently recommended for clinical diagnosis.
- Culture with tissue culture best (but research labs only), PCR (experimental but looks promising).
- Other associated syndromes: exacerbations asthma, otitis media, endocarditis, erythema nodosum, Guillain-Barre syndrome, encephalitis (all rare).

SITES OF INFECTION
- Upper respiratory tract: pharyngitis, sinusitis, laryngitis, bronchitis
- Lung: pneumonia
- CNS: association with Guillain-Barre syndrome
- Cutaneous: cases seen as causing erythema nodosum
- Asthma: exacerbations of asthma (children and adults)
- Ear: otitis media
- Cardiac: endocarditis (rare)
- Role in cardiovascular disease is doubtful.

TREATMENT
Pneumonia
- Macrolides: erythromycin 250–500 mg PO four times a day × 10–14 days, clarithromycin 500 mg twice daily × PO 10–14 days (or Biaxin XL 1 g PO daily) or azithromycin (Zithromax) 250–500 mg PO once daily × 10 days.
- Doxycycline: 100 mg twice daily PO × 10–14 days.
- Fluoroquinolones: levofloxacin (Levaquin) PO/IV 750 mg q24h, moxifloxacin (Avelox) PO/IV 400 mg q24, all × 10–14 days.
- Other agents also *active in vitro:* tetracycline, doxycycline. Not active: any beta-lactam, trimethoprim/sulfamethoxazole or other sulfas.

URTIs
- Pharyngitis: treat Group A streptococci only, no antibiotic required for *C. pneumoniae* pharyngitis.
- Bronchitis: no antibiotic required.
- Sinusitis: treat if symptoms remain beyond 7–10 days.

OTHER INFORMATION
- Common cause (5–15%) of URIs, bronchitis and pneumonia, but abx indicated only for pneumonia.

- Seroprevalence is 50% by 20 yrs, 75% by 60 yrs.
- Clinician rarely knows *C. pneumoniae* as proven cause of any given pneumonia, therefore must treat empirically.
- Role in coronary artery disease—supported by serologic studies, antigen in plaque 40–100%, mouse and rabbit models but abx trials are not supportive of role.

BASIS FOR RECOMMENDATIONS

Mandell LA, Wunderink RG, Anzueto A, et al. Infectious Diseases Society of America/American Thoracic Society consensus guidelines on the management of community-acquired pneumonia in adults. *Clin Infect Dis,* 2007; Vol. 44 Suppl 2; pp. S27–72.

Comments: Recommendations of ATS/IDSA for management of community-acquired pneumonia. All empiric regimens including an agent that targets *C. pneumoniae*—macrolide, tetracycline or fluoroquinolone.

Gonzales R, Bartlett JG, Besser RE, et al. Principles of appropriate antibiotic use for treatment of acute respiratory tract infections in adults: background, specific aims, and methods. *Ann Intern Med,* 2001; Vol. 134; pp. 479–86.

Comments: Rationale why even if *C. pneumoniae* URTIs could be easily diagnosed, treatment is usually not required.

CHLAMYDOPHILA PSITTACI

Joseph Vinetz, MD and Paul G. Auwaerter, MD

PATHOGENS

MICROBIOLOGY

- Old taxonomy: *Chlamydia psittaci*
- May appear Gram-negative, spherical, (0.4–0.6 microns in diameter). Intracellular bacteria.
- Agent of endemic avian chlamydiosis and epizootic outbreaks in mammals.
- Typical epidemiology: birds excrete infectious organisms in discharge from eyes, beaks, excrement.

CLINICAL

- Systemic infection transmitted by respiratory route, most commonly associated in humans with atypical pneumonia.
- Approximately 80 U.S. cases reported annually, probably under-recognized and under-reported. Rare (<1%) cause of community acquired pneumonia. Hx of bird exposure (particularly a pet) key to dx.
- Usual incubation period: 5–21 days.
- Humans acquire after contact w/ sick or asymptomatic bird; contacts may be close (kissing parrot), casual (pigeon exposure in park, pet store), lawn mower aerosolization of dead wild birds.
- Presentations: non-specific (fever and malaise), typhoidal (fever, bradycardia, splenomegaly) and atypical pneumonia. Headache an often prominent feature. Fatality rate as high as 20% if untreated.
- Radiologic manifestations: no pathognomonic pattern. CXR can include nodular densities, interstitial densities, segmental and lobar consolidation and pleural effusion.
- Ddx: *Coxiella burnetii, Mycoplasma pneumoniae, Chlamydia pneumoniae,* Legionella species and respiratory viruses such as influenza.
- Dx: cx possible, rarely done (requires cell cx, agent is biohazard risk, so notify micro lab). Serology: microimmunofluorescence assay, IgM >1:16 or seroconversion (MIF or complement fixation) w/ 4 × rise titer over 4–6 wks.
- Single high titer IgG (>1:32) supports presumptive diagnosis. Serology does not differentiate from other chlamydial infections, particularly *Chlamydophila pneumoniae.*

MORE CLINICAL

Case definition:

Confirmed case of psittacosis: compatible clinical illness with laboratory confirmation by one of three methods: a) positive culture of respiratory secretions; b) 4-fold rise in antibody titer against *C. psittaci* (to a reciprocal titer of 32 between paired acute- and convalescent-phase serum specimens collected at least 2 wks apart) as demonstrated by complement fixation (CF) or microimmunofluorescence (MIF); or c) IgM detected against *C. psittaci* by MIF (to a reciprocal titer of 16). Probable case of psittacosis: compatible clinical illness and a) the pt is epidemiologically linked to a confirmed human case of psittacosis or b) a single antibody titer of 32, demonstrated by CF or MIF, is present in at least one serum specimen obtained after onset of symptoms. Most diagnoses are established by using serologic methods in which paired sera are tested for chlamydial antibodies by CF test. However, because chlamydial CF antibody is not species-specific, high CF titers also can result from *C. pneumoniae* and *C. trachomatis* infections.

Information about laboratory testing is available from most state public health laboratories. Few commercial laboratories have the capability to differentiate Chlamydia species. The following laboratories accept human specimens to confirm *C. psittaci*:

Focus Diagnostics, Cypress, CA (800) 445–4032: immunofluorescence, PCR, culture. Lab Corp, Burlington, NC (800) 334–5161: Culture, polyclonal antibody determination. Specialty Labs, Santa Monica, CA (800) 421–4449; microimmunofluorescence.

SITES OF INFECTION

- Pulmonary: dyspnea, cough, no sputum, rales on auscultation, CXR findings often more dramatic than abnormalities appreciated on exam. Pleural rub (less common). Occasional progression to ARDS.
- Systemic: fever, malaise, myalgia, chills (may be predominant presentation), severe headache plus atypical pneumonia suggestive of *C. psittaci* infection.
- Cardiac: relative bradycardia in presence of fever, pericarditis, myocarditis, dilated cardiomyopathy, culture-negative endocarditis.
- Liver: hepatitis including jaundice.
- Heme: Coombs-positive hemolytic anemia, hemophagocytic syndrome with pancytopenia, cold agglutinins, DIC.
- CNS: stroke due to emboli of endocarditis, cranial neuropathy including VIII nerve-related hearing loss, ataxia, transverse myelitis, meningitis, encephalitis.
- Dermatologic: pink, blanching maculopapular rash (Horder's spots). This rash is rarely seen.

TREATMENT

Doxycycline
- Preferred: 100 mg twice daily (IV until PO can be tolerated) for 10 to 21 days.
- Duration of therapy unclear, controversial whether prolonged course prevents relapse.

Tetracycline
- Tetracycline 500 mg PO four times a day × 10–21 days.
- Less convenient dosing than doxycycline.

Azithromycin
- Azithromycin 250 mg to 500 mg PO daily × 7 days.
- Dosing based *on in vitro* and animal model data, no human clinical data available.

Erythromycin
- Erythromycin 500 mg IV or PO q6h.
- Clearly inferior to tetracyclines, inferior to azithromycin in animal models. Good clinical data unavailable.

OTHER INFORMATION

- Can present from mild to fulminant illness. Often systemic manifestations predominate early in infection. Chest x-ray manifestations may be more dramatic than expected on the basis of H and P.
- Typical presentation: abrupt onset of fever, chills, headache (often severe), malaise, and myalgia. A nonproductive cough is often accompanied by dyspnea and chest tightness.
- Other features: pulse-temperature dissociation, enlarged spleen and rash (Horder's spots) suggest psittacosis in pts with community-acquired pneumonia.
- Auscultatory findings can underestimate the extent of pulmonary involvement; radiographic findings include lobar or interstitial infiltrates.

BASIS FOR RECOMMENDATIONS

Mandell LA, Wunderink RG, Anzueto A, et al. Infectious Diseases Society of America/American Thoracic Society consensus guidelines on the management of community-acquired pneumonia in adults. *Clin Infect Dis*, 2007; Vol. 44 Suppl 2; pp. S27–72.

Comments: Guidelines for community-acquired pneumonia, with coverage of atypical agents recommended and covering *C. psittaci* empirically in such cases.

Cunha BA. The atypical pneumonias: clinical diagnosis and importance. *Clin Microbiol Infect*, 2006; Vol. 12 Suppl 3; pp. 12–24.

Comments: A very useful recent review of the differential diagnosis and diagnostic approaches of atypical pneumonia, including psittacosis.

CITROBACTER SPECIES

Paul G. Auwaerter, MD

MICROBIOLOGY

- Enteric Gram-negative bacilli. Normal part of gut flora.
- May be mistakenly identified as Salmonella; colonies on plates resemble *E. coli*.
- Species associated w/ infection most commonly *C. freundii*, *C. amalonaticus*, and *C. koseri* (previously known as *C. diversus*).

CLINICAL

- Mostly a nosocomial pathogen found in compromised hosts, pts aged >60 yrs, and neonates.
- Commonly causes UTIs, pneumonia, line infections.
- Beta-lactamases frequently expressed. Nosocomial isolates may be highly resistant to multiple abx.

SITES OF INFECTION

- GU: UTI
- CNS: meningitis, brain abscess (mostly *C. koseri* in newborns)
- Pulmonary: nosocomial pneumonia (must distinguish from colonization)
- Bacteremia: frequently part of polymicrobial infection
- Endocarditis: rare reports
- Soft tissue: associated with superficial and deep infections, post-op wound infections
- GI: intraabdominal infection, usually part of polymicrobial flora

TREATMENT

General principles

- UTI's may be treated by monotherapy, hopefully an oral fluoroquinolone or TMP-SMX.
- More serious infections empirically should be treated at least initially with either cefepime or carbapenem if Citrobacter suspected.
- Aminoglycosides generally have activity and may be selected in combination, especially if ESBL suspected and using cephalosporin-based beta-lactam.
- For meningitis (adult recommendations only given in this guide), would employ third/fourth generation cephalosporin or meropenem.
- Susceptibility results should guide therapy; potential for multiple drug resistance, including ESBL.

Citrobacter koseri

- Preferred: ceftriaxone 1–2 g IV q12–24, cefotaxime 1–2 g IV q6h or cefepime 1–2 IV q8h.
- Alt: ciprofloxacin 400 mg IV q12h (or 500 mg PO q12h for UTI), imipenem 1 g IV q6h, doripenem 500 mg IV q8h, meropenem 1–2 g IV q8h, aztreonam 1–2 g IV q6h, or TMP-SMX 5 mg/kg q6h IV (or DS PO twice daily for UTI).
- Usually ampicillin resistant, but may be sensitive to first generation cephalosporins.

Citrobacter freundii

- More antibiotic resistance generally identified with this species.
- Preferred: meropenem 1–2 g IV q8h or imipenem 1 g IV q6h or doripenem 500 mg IV q8h, cefepime 1–2 g IV q8h, ciprofloxacin 400 mg IV q12h (or 500 mg PO twice daily for UTI), or aminoglycoside (e.g., gentamicin 5 mg/kg/day).
- Alt: piperacillin/tazobactam 3.375 mg q6h IV, aztreonam 1–2 g IV q6h or TMP-SMX 5 mg/kg q6h IV (or DS PO twice daily for UTI).
- Usually carbenicillin sensitive, cephalothin resistant.

OTHER INFORMATION

- Usually a nosocomial pathogen. Has been described as cause of outbreaks in healthcare facilities.
- Bacteremia often polymicrobial in ~50% of pts.
- Brain abscesses are rarely a complication of meningitis, with the exception of *C. koseri* infections in neonates with rates of ~70%.

BASIS FOR RECOMMENDATIONS

Author opinion.

Comments: No specific guidelines exist for therapy of Citrobacter infection; however, based on infection may wish to see modules on UTI, complicated intra-abdominal infection, hospital acquired pneumonia, catheter infections, etc.

PATHOGENS

CLOSTRIDIUM BOTULINUM

John G. Bartlett, MD

MICROBIOLOGY
- Gram-positive spore-forming, anaerobic rod.
- Found worldwide.
- Produces neurotoxin.

CLINICAL
- Forms: foodborne (outbreaks), infant ("floppy baby"), wound (IDU), inhalation (bioterrorism), iatrogenic (cosmetic treatment), unclassified.
- U.S.: 100 cases/yr (infant 71, foodborne 24, wound 3). Types A and B most common, E in Alaska.
- Clinical: (1) 4-Ds (diplopia, dysarthria, dysphoria, dysphagia), (2) afebrile, (3) alert, (4) descending flaccid paralysis, (5) normal CSF and MRI, EEG = fasciculations.
- Suspect in settings of cranial nerve palsy, descending symmetrical paralysis while maintaining alertness, afebrile.
- Wound botulism causes regional (limb) paralysis. In U.S. seen mainly in IDU skin poppers with black tar heroin with small abscess at injection site.
- Ddx: myasthenia, Eaton-Lambert, tick paralysis, Guillain-Barré, magnesium intoxication, CVA, paralytic shellfish toxins, nerve gas, CO or organophosphates poisoning.
- Dx: toxin in sera, stool, food; cx—wound, stool.
- Foodborne: take 3 day food history. Most are 2–3 days cases following ingestion of home canned food.
- Lethal dose (70 kg man): 0.15 µg IV, 0.9 µg inhalation, 70 µg PO.

SITES OF INFECTION
- Neurologic system (toxin only)
- Wound infection/colonization
- GI: infant botulism, mostly age <1 yr, colonization gut yields *in vivo* toxin.

TREATMENT
Notifications and Antitoxin/General Therapy
- Suspected botulism (see Botulism module): immediate clinical consult and give antitoxin.
- CDC hotline 770-488-7100; antitoxin and toxin assay: call State Health Dept or CDC.
- Public health emergency (report immediately), contact state health department or CDC 770-488-7100.
- Concern of bioterrorism?: 404-639-2206 (day)/ 404-639-2880.
- Tests: obtain botulin toxin assay of stool, vomit, blood.
- Immediate rx (CDC): trivalent antitoxin (A 7,500 IU, B 5,000 IU, and E 5,000 IU) 1 vial diluted 1:10, IV infusion over 30 min. preferably <24h post symptoms onset.
- Antitoxin, equine: hypersensitivity reactions in 9%, anaphylaxis in 2%.
- Mechanical ventilation required in 20–40% adults and may continue for 3–6 mos.
- Miscellaneous support: IV hydration, tube feedings, abx for ID complications.

Prevention and Epidemiology
- Destroy spores w/ heat 120°C × 30 min (pressure cooker).
- Prevent germination: lower pH, refrigerate, freeze, dry, add salt, sugar, or Na nitrate.
- Inactivate toxin: heat to 85°C × 5 min.
- Water-chlorine + hypochlorite (bleach) = sporicidal.

OTHER INFORMATION
- Recommendations from CDC [see http://www.cdc.gov/ncidod/dbmd/diseaseinfo/files/botulism.pdf] and CID 2005;41:1167.
- Consult state health department or CDC immediately.
- Sequence w/ all forms: toxin absorbed → blood → nerve endings → cranial nerves → descending flaccid paralysis.
- Major risk: respiratory failure, may require ventilatory support × 3–6 mos.
- Rx antitoxin ASAP if suspected. Get from State Health Dept or CDC. Use 1 vial IV.

BASIS FOR RECOMMENDATIONS
Sobel J. Botulism. *Clin Infect Dis*, 2005; Vol. 41; pp. 1167–73.

Comments: Review of topic with clinician physicians' protocol for first response: notify health department and give antitoxin.

CLOSTRIDIUM DIFFICILE

John G. Bartlett, MD

MICROBIOLOGY

- Spore-forming anaerobe.
- Produces toxins A and B—both cause colitis in humans.
- Epidemiology: colon colonization 3% in healthy adults, but 20–40% for hospitalized pts.

CLINICAL

- **Risk for disease**: hospitalized or chronic care facility, elderly age and antibiotic exposure.
- **Antibiotic risk** (rank order), **High**: clindamycin, 3rd generation cephalosporins, fluoroquinolones; **Medium**: penicillins and cephalosporins (1st, 2nd, 4th gen), carbapenems, macrolides TMP/SMX; **Low**: metronidazole, tetracyclines, vancomycin, aminoglycosides; No risk: sulfa, nitrofurantoin, linezolid.
- **Clinical presentations**: diarrhea and cramps +/– fever, may be acute or chronic.
- **Complications**: ileus and toxic megacolon, hypoalbuminemia, shock, renal failure, leukemoid reaction.
- **Diagnosis**: toxin assay—95% of U.S. labs use EIA which has false negatives rate of ~30%. Other tests: cytotoxin (preferred, but expensive and delayed results .48 hrs) or detection of bacterium by culture or "common antigen"—false positives in hospitalized pts. PCR for toxin B gene is sensitive, but expensive and technically demanding.

SITES OF INFECTION

- Colon: colitis/pseudomembranous colitis, toxic megacolon
- Enteritis: only 7 cases reported with small bowel involvement only
- Extra colonic infection: rare and usually not important
- Reactive arthritis (post diarrheal): rare and not HLA-B27 linked

TREATMENT

Antibiotics

- Principles: positive toxin assay, d/c implicated abx, avoid narcotics, infection control (contact isolation) +/– metronidazole or vancomycin (oral).
- Toxin assay negative and high clinical probability: repeat test + treat empirically but only if seriously ill.
- Metronidazole 250 mg PO four times a day or 500 mg PO three times a day × 10 days ($12.00/10 days).
- Vancomycin 125 mg PO four times a day × 10 days (as IV form or puvule, $708.00 AWP), use for moderate–severely ill pts.
- Seriously ill or using metronidazole with delayed response: vancomycin 125–500 mg PO four times a day. (standard is 125 mg four times a day using pulvules (expensive) or IV vancomycin solution given PO (hospital frequently use this strategy to reduce cost).
- Response: average time to formed stools: 5–7 days.

Special Considerations

- If need systemic abx for ongoing infection (other than *C. difficile*): use oral vancomycin or metronidazole + agent unlikely to cause *C. difficile* if possible: IV vancomycin, macrolide, sulfa, doxycycline, aminoglycoside, or narrow spectrum beta-lactam.
- Supportive care: IV hydration or oral fluids.
- Avoid antiperistaltics (Lomotil, loperamide, opiates).
- Clues to severe disease: ileus, WBC >20,000, sepsis, renal failure, PMC by endoscopy, anasarca.
- Ileus or vomiting: IV metronidazole 500 mg q8h +/– vancomycin PO (500 mg 4 × a day) by NG tube and/or retention enema.
- Surgery: total colectomy if severely ill and unresponsive to PO vancomycin +/– IV metronidazole, especially if toxic megacolon.
- Follow infection control procedures (see below).

Multiple relapses

- Metronidazole 250 mg PO four times a day (first episode only) or vancomycin 125 mg PO four times a day × 10 days, then one of the following:
- Vancomycin 125 mg PO every other day (pulse dosing) × 6 wks or longer.

PATHOGENS

- Vancomycin taper/pulse: 125 mg PO four times a day × 10 days, then 125 mg twice daily × 2 wks, then 125 mg/day × 2 wks then 125 every other day × 6 wks or longer.
- Cholestyramine 4 g PO three times a day × 4–6 wks (do not co-administer with PO vanco).
- *Saccharomyces boulardii* 500 mg PO four times a day from day 6 of vancomycin × 4–6 wks.
- Alt: IVIG 400 mg/kg IV q3 wks (experimental).
- Alt: stool from healthy donor via enema or NG tube (works well but liability concerns).

Infection Control

- Single room with toilet or cohort cases.
- Wash hands w/ soap and water (epidemics).
- Vinyl gloves and gowns.
- No rectal thermometers.
- Clean room w/ 10% household bleach.
- Epidemics (hospitals and nursing homes): control abx use, especially clindamycin, broad-spectrum cephalosporins, and FQs.

FOLLOW UP

General

- Relapse after initial therapy occurs in up to 25% of pts.
- See treatment section, "multiple relapses."
- No need for test of cure, or documentation of *C. difficile* clearance.

OTHER INFORMATION

- Guidelines: metronidazole PO preferred—IDSA (CID 2001;32:331); SHEA (Inf Con Hosp Ep 1995;16:459) CDC (MMWR 1995;44:RR-12).
- *C. difficile* causes 20% of antibiotic-associated diarrheas and >95% of pseudomembranous colitis.
- Clinical clues: hx of prior abx + diarrhea, colitis (cramps, fever), elevated WBC, hypoalbuminemia.
- Response to treatment is rapid: if diarrhea persists >5–7 days, question dx or consider concurrent IBD, lactose deficiency, medication effect, etc. Relapses (3–21 days) post metronidazole or vancomycin in up to 25%.
- Prevention: control abx use, especially clindamycin as prophylaxis. Vancomycin/metronidazole to carriers increases risk.

DETAILED INFORMATION

other

- NAP1 strain (also called BI, NAP1 and ribotype 027): new epidemic strain recognized in Quebec in 2002, now global.
- Causes more disease, more serious disease, disease that is more refractory to treatment and more likely to relapse.
- Highly resistant to fluoroquinolones (more common) and more toxin A and B production (more serious disease).
- Clinician will usually not know if pt has this strain since only rare labs culture stool for *C. difficile*, but knowing this does not change therapy or infection control practice.

BASIS FOR RECOMMENDATIONS

Dubberke ER, Gerding DN, Classen D, et al. Strategies to prevent clostridium difficile infections in acute care hospitals. *Infect Control Hosp Epidemiol*, 2008; Vol. 29; Suppl 1 pp. S81–92.

Comments: Review of infection control principles emphasizing barrier precautions need for single rooms or cohorting, soap and water for hand hygiene, room cleaning with 1:16 household bleach and antibiotic stewardship.

Guerrant RL, Van Gilder T, Steiner TS, et al. Practice guidelines for the management of infectious diarrhea. *Clin Infect Dis*, 2001; Vol. 32; pp. 331–51.

Comments: IDSA guidelines which include: 3 day rule—with nosocomial diarrhea, test only for *C. dif* because no other enteric pathogen is likely; Rx—Metronidazole 250 mg four times a day or 500 mg three times a day × 10 days; Test—EIA for *C. dif* toxin.

CLOSTRIDIUM SPECIES

John G. Bartlett, MD

MICROBIOLOGY

- Obligate anaerobic Gram-positive bacillus, belonging to the Firmicutes. Individual cells are rod-shaped.
- Capable of endospore formation.
- Clostridia: normal colonic flora including *C. perfringens* in 50% and *C. difficile* in 3%.
- Members causing human disease include *C. perfringens, C. sordelli. C. septicum, C. tertium.*
- See separate modules for *C. tetani, C. botulinum,* and *C. difficile.*

CLINICAL

- Most disease toxin mediated: gas gangrene (alpha toxin) w/ myonecrosis and sepsis. Tetanus (*C. tetani*, tetanus toxin) w/ neurotoxin. Botulism (*C. botulinum*, botulinum toxin) w/ paralysis. Colitis (*C. difficile* toxin A and B) with colitis (*C. perfringens* (enterotoxin)) with diarrhea or *C. sordellii* (lethal toxin) with therapeutic abortion.
- Soft tissue disease often with gas formation: crepitant cellulitis, gas forming cellulitis, emphysematous cholecystitis.
- Bacteremia: significant if occuring in the setting of gas gangrene or neutropenic typhlitis.
- Dx: need for anaerobic culture of blood, tissue, other body fluid.
- If part of mixed flora: common with infections from normal gut or genital flora where Clostridia are part of mixed flora and pathogenic role is questionable.

SITES OF INFECTION

- GI tract: food poisoning, botulism, enteritis necroticans, typhlitis, antibiotic-associated diarrhea, and colitis.
- Bacteremia: usually a contaminant except if specifically occuring within the setting of gas gangrene or typhlitis.
- Soft tissue infection: gas gangrene, crepitant cellulitis, or necrotizing fasciitis.
- Intra-abdominal sepsis: peritonitis and intra-abdominal abscess (polymicrobial), emphysematous cholecystitis.
- Separate sections on tetanus, botulism and *C. difficile* infections.
- Uterine infection: *C. sordelli.*

TREATMENT

Soft tissue infections

- **Gas gangrene:** aggressive surgery and penicillin 20 MU/ IV per 24 hrs and clindamycin 600 mg IV q8h or metronidazole 500 mg IV q6h.
- Hyperbaric oxygen: controversial and less important than immediate surgery.
- **Crepitant cellulitis/necrotizing fasciitis:** debridement and penicillin 20 MU/day IV, clindamycin 600 mg IV q8h, metronidazole 500 g IV or PO q6h or imipenem 1 g IV q6h.

Toxin-mediated

- **Neutropenic enterocolitis:** clindamycin or metronidazole or imipenem.
- Surgery: most *C. sordellii* require surgery while most *C. tertium* do not.
- ***Clostridium perfringens* type A food poisoning:** supportive care, diarrhea usually resolves <24 hr.
- ***C. sordellii:*** IV support, clindamycin.
- Botulism (see separate module): trivalent antitoxin (A/B and E) available from CDC: 404-639-3670.
- Tetanus (see separate module): tetanus toxoid and human TIG 500 IU IM and metronidazole 500 mg IV q6h and benzodiazepines.
- *C. difficile* colitis: d/c implicated abx and use metronidazole 250 mg PO q6h or vancomycin 125 mg PO four times a day × 7–10 days (see module *C. difficile*).

Miscellaneous infections

- **Emphysematous cholecystitis:** urgent cholecystectomy, ticarcillin-clavulanate, piperacillin-tazobactam, imipenem.
- **Bacteremia:** usually a contaminant unless accompanies gas gangrene or necrotizing enterocolitis.

PATHOGENS

- **Mixed infection:** cover mixed anaerobic infection with imipenem, beta-lactam/beta-lactamase inhibitor or combination metronidazole/clindamycin and a cephalosporin.
- **Septic abortion due to** *C. sordellii*: associated with therapeutic abortion, septic shock and WBC .30,000/mL.

OTHER INFORMATION

- Most pathology is toxin-mediated with toxins that have great clout: gas gangrene, botulism, tetanus, *C. difficile*, typhlitis
- Surgery critical with gas gangrene; also often important for cholecystitis, crepitant cellulitis, typhlitis.
- Most blood culture isolates are not clinically important unless there is evidence of neutropenic enterocolitis or gas gangrene.
- Clostridial disease is usually a clinical dx sometimes supported by Gram-stain (distinctive GPB), culture of blood/soft tissue or toxin assay (*C. difficile*).
- ABX active vs. most clostridia species: PCN, ampicillin, chloramphenicol, cefotaxime, piperacillin. Less active: cefoxitin, clindamycin, metronidazole, ceftazidime. If mixed infection suspected—need to broaden coverage.

BASIS FOR RECOMMENDATIONS

Stevens DL, Bisno AL, Chambers HF, et al. Practice guidelines for the diagnosis and management of skin and soft-tissue infections. *Clin Infect Dis*, 2005; Vol. 41; pp. 1373–406.

Comments: Guidelines include recommendations for necrotizing fasciitis and clostridial infections.

Author opinion

Comments: No guidelines exist for clostridial bacteremia or other non-soft tissue infections.

CLOSTRIDIUM TETANI (TETANUS)

Paul G. Auwaerter, MD

MICROBIOLOGY

- Gram-positive bacillus, obligate anaerobe.
- Spore wide spread in soil and animal feces.
- Rod-shaped appearance on Gram-stain often likened to drumsticks or tennis rackets.
- Toxin, tetanospasmin, causes tetanus: unopposed muscle spasm, contraction due to interference of toxin with neurotransmitters (including GABA and glycine).

CLINICAL

- Although tetanus is rare in the developed world, it is still an important cause of death worldwide and has a high case fatality rate. The highest incidence of tetanus infections are found in Africa and Southeast Asia, while there are only between 50 and 70 cases in the United States each yr. Worldwide, neonatal tetanus most common presentation from infected umbilical stump.
- Classic triad of rigidity, muscle spasm, and autonomic dysfunction.
- Trismus or lock jaw is the presenting complaint in 75% of cases due to masseter spasm, if extends to facial muscles causes classic "risus sardonicus" (painfully grinning face).
- **Generalized tetanus:** most commonly, muscles of head and neck affected first with caudal spread to entire body.
- Waves of opisthotonos (back arches with head and ankles moving toward another), highly characteristic and due to spasms of back musculature.
- **Localized tetanus:** spasm, restricted to a limited part of body due to lower toxin loads. Associated with a lower mortality.
- **Cephalic tetanus:** usually localized cranial nerve dysfunction and follows head trauma or a middle ear infection. Associated with a high mortality.
- Incubation period from the injury to first sx averages 7–10 days (range 1–60 days).
- Autonomic nervous system involvement can include labile blood pressure, arrhythmias, diaphoresis, urinary retention, and temperature dysregulation.
- The diagnosis is usually made clinically based on history and physical findings. *C. tetani* is very infrequently recovered from wounds (requires anaerobic culture).

SITES OF INFECTION

- Commonest worldwide: infantile tetanus due to umbilical stump infection (secondary to poor birth delivery hygiene).
- Usually follows recognized injury contaminated with soil, manure, or rusted metal.
- Also can complicate burns, ulcers, gangrene, necrotic snake bites, middle ear infections, septic abortions, intramuscular injections, and surgery.
- Increasing incidence in some areas associated with high prevalence of injection drug use.

TREATMENT

Neutralization of unbound toxin

- Human tetanus immune globulin 3000–6000 units IM for active tetanus.
- Tetanus toxoid should be administered at a separate site if vaccination status is unknown or if greater than 5 yrs since last booster.
- Tetanus prophylaxis (500 U IM) should be given for contaminated wounds if <3 Td doses or unknown vaccination status

Removal of infection source

- Debridement of wounds should be considered when appropriate.
- Metronidazole has replaced penicillin as the antibiotic of choice due to a better safety profile and improved outcomes.
- Recommend: metronidazole 7.5 mg/kg q6hrs given IV or PO (not to exceed 4 g/day).
- Alternative: penicillin can be given in doses of 10–20 million units/day IV.
- Other alternatives: erythromycin, tetracycline, chloramphenicol, and clindamycin.

Control of rigidity and spasms

- Sedation with benzodiazepines mainstay of treatment.
- Some recommend magnesium infusions to control spasms as it is non-sedating.
- When sedation alone is inadequate, neuromuscular blocking agents may be used in conjunction with mechanical ventilation.

Control of autonomic dysfunction

- Most importantly, aggressive fluid resuscitation of up to 8 L per day in some pts may be required.
- Alpha and beta adrenergic blockers have been used with variable results and should be used only with caution.

Supportive measures

- Intubation and mechanical ventilation are often necessary.
- Since mechanical ventilation is usually required for several wks, early tracheotomy often performed.
- Early enteral nutritional support important.
- Use of life support measures in intensive care units has decreased mortality from nearly 50% to approximately 10%.

Prevention

- Readily preventable with proper immunization.
- See tetanus vaccine module (p. 747) for details.
- Forms: single tetanus toxoid (TT), diphtheria toxoid (dT or DT), combinations with diphtheria and pertussis (DTwP, DTap, dTaP, or DtaP). Generally administer as combination for protection against tetanus (meaning with diphtheria or acellular pertussis toxoids). Tdap now recommended as one time immunization during ages 12–65. Over age 65, use Td.
- Recovery from clinical tetanus does not provide protective immunity, therefore immunization still recommended.

OTHER INFORMATION

- Decreased prevalence in developed countries is due to successful implementation of vaccination programs.

BASIS FOR RECOMMENDATIONS

Cook TM, Protheroe RT, Handel JM. Tetanus: a review of the literature. *Br J Anaesth*, 2001; Vol. 87; pp. 477–87.
Comments: Review of the supportive management that is the basis for recommendations here.

PATHOGENS

CORYNEBACTERIUM DIPHTHERIAE

Paul G. Auwaerter, MD

MICROBIOLOGY

- Pleiomorphic Gram + bacillus (club-shaped), facultative anaerobe. Humans are only known hosts.
- Diphtheria caused by exotoxin-producing strains.
- Virulent *C. diphtheria* strains carry a bacteriophage with the diphtheria toxin gene. Without of the bacteriophage, the microbe is unable to cause serious disease.

CLINICAL

- Capable causing tonsillitis/pharyngitis, cervical LN/swelling, palatal paralysis, and T<103°F.
- Classic gray-white membrane covering posterior pharynx. Toxigenic strains capable of causing carditis and neuritis.
- Now rare, diphtheria often confused with severe strep throat, Vincent's angina or glandular fevers.
- Emerging **non-toxigenic** strains cause endocarditis, arthritis and recurrent sore throat.
- Dx: throat or nasopharyngeal swab. Transport rapidly and alert micro lab for special media. Rapid dx possible if lab has IFA staining of a 4-hr culture.

SITES OF INFECTION

- Pharyngeal: malaise, fever, sore throat with gray-white membrane covering tonsils, palate, uvula and posterior pharynx.
- Laryngeal/bronchial: spread of membrane can cause dyspnea and cyanosis on basis of obstruction.
- Cardiac: toxin-related ~1–2 wks after illness w/ 1st deg. block, AV dissociation, arrhythmias, myocarditis. Some cardiac effects seen 10–25% pts. Myocarditis/advanced blocks = 60–90% mortality.
- Neurologic: toxin-related paralysis of pharyngeal muscles, with possible CN palsies, and subsequent motor neuropathy of limbs.
- Cutaneous: chronic, nonhealing wound w/ grayish membrane. Seen mostly in tropics. In U.S., homeless, alcoholics, native Americans. Most strains non-toxigenic, role in pathogenesis of ulcer often unclear.

TREATMENT

Prevention

- Primary series age >7 yrs (Td, toxoids now generally Tdap): two doses IM 4 wks apart, 3rd dose 6–12 mos later.
- Booster: Tdap or Td (if >65 yrs) every 10 yrs.
- Pts with clinical diphtheria should still receive toxoid immunization during convalescent phase, since infection may not be immunogenic.
- For infected pts, maintain strict isolation procedures: contact and respiratory.

Diphtheria treatment

- Equine hyperimmune antiserum reduces mortality by neutralizing toxin prior to cellular entry. Critical to administer ASAP w/ presumptive Dx.
- Hypersensitivity to horse proteins determined by 1:100 dilution antitoxin scratched or pricked into skin. If neg. proceed w/ 0.02 ml of 1:1000 dilution. Have epinephrine available if necessary.
- Reaction requires desensitization protocol.
- **Antitoxin:** 20,000–40,000 U pharyngeal disease <48 hrs; 40–60,000 U nasopharyngeal; 80–120,000 U for extensive disease, brawny neck or sx >72 hrs. Give IV (severe disease) or IM.
- **Antibiotics:** Procaine PCN G (<20 lbs: 300,000 U; >20 lbs: 600,000 U) IM q12h until pt can swallow then PCN Vk 125–250 mg PO four times a day or erythromycin 125–500 mg PO four times a day for 14 days total. Parenteral erythromycin (20–25 mg/kg IV q6h max 4 g/day) can be substituted in the β-lactam allergic pt.
- Clindamycin (600 mg IV q8h) probably an acceptable alternative.
- Antibiotics may decrease toxin production.
- Serum sickness occurrence 10%.
- Antitoxin available from CDC (770-488-7100).
- Consider early tracheostomy or intubation if laryngeal involvement exists. Supportive care should also include telemetry to monitor for cardiac complications.

C. diphtheriae carrier
- Erythromycin preferred (250–500 mg PO four times a day).
- If compliance uncertain, administer benzathine PCN G 600,000–1,200,000 units IM × 1.

Endocarditis treatment
- Selection based on case report usage, so not well studied.
- Penicillin G or ampicillin IV × 4–6 wks.
- Often combined with an aminoglycoside.

Follow Up
- Culture nasopharynx 2 wks after illness to ensure eradication.

Other Information
- Administer antitoxin ASAP with presumptive dx. **Don't** wait for confirmation.
- Most deaths in first 3–4 days from asphyxiation or myocarditis.
- Public health threat. Must identify contacts and carriers to limit spread. Humans only known reservoir.
- Immunized pts may acquire disease.

Basis for Recommendations

Broder KR, Cortese MM, Iskander JK, et al. Preventing tetanus, diphtheria, and pertussis among adolescents: use of tetanus toxoid, reduced diphtheria toxoid and acellular pertussis vaccines recommendations of the Advisory Committee on Immunization Practices (ACIP). *MMWR Recomm Rep,* 2006; Vol. 55; pp. 1–34.
Comments: New guidelines for immunization incorporating the acellular pertussis component into tetanus and diphtheria vaccines.

MacGregor RR. Corynebacterium diphtheriae. *Principles and Practice of Infectious Diseases, 6th ed,* 2005; Vol. Chap 202; pp. 2457–2465.
Comments: Chapter outlines antibiotic treatment recommendations for clinical infection and carrier state eradication.

COXIELLA BURNETII

John G. Bartlett, MD

Microbiology
- Small, obligate intracellular Gram-negative bacillus.
- Excreted from feces, urine, and milk of infected animals.
- Organisms are hardy.
- Can survive in environment as resistant to heat, desiccation, and often disinfectants.

Clinical
- **Epidemiology:** global zoonosis, rare in the U.S.
- **Primary reservoirs:** cattle, sheep, and goats most commonly implicated. Less common: cats, dogs, arthropods.
- **Acquisition:** mammals (usually asymptomatic) shed *C. burnetii* in stool, urine, milk, birth products. Highest bacterial loads seen in placenta. Acquired by inhalation, often from dust contaminated by infected feces or birth material. Tick-borne and human-human transmission rarely described.
- **Occupational risk:** farmers, vets, abattoir workers, lab workers.
- **Diagnosis:** serology (IFA) (1) acute disease (pneumonia) show seroconversion or anti-phase II Ab, (2) chronic anti-phase I Ab. PCR (blood, heart valve) is 60% sensitive and 100% specific. Immunohistochemistry, PCR or cell culture techniques can also be used.
- **Reportable infection** in U.S.; bioterrorism category B agent.
- Other abnormalities: thrombocytopenia, valvular vegetations.

Sites of Infection
- Asymptomatic (60%)
- **Acute:** Flu-like illness, pneumonia (typical or atypical presentations or FUO w/ "incidental" pneumonia), or hepatitis
- **Chronic:** endocarditis (90% pts have prosthetic valve or other pre-existing cardiac abnormality, other groups at risk include those with immunosuppression, e.g., transplant pts, active malignancy)

PATHOGENS

- **Chronic, other:** pneumonia (FUO w/ "incidental" pneumonia), hepatitis, rare-pericarditis, myocarditis, aseptic meningitis, osteomyelitis, chronic fatigue
- **Risks for chronic infection:** prosthetic valve and immunosuppression
- Many cause chronic (post-infectious) fatigue syndrome and travel related FUO (fever of unknown origin) (rare).

TREATMENT
Antibiotic regimens
- **Active *in vitro*:** tetracyclines, macrolides, TMP-SMX, rifampin, fluoroquinolones.
- Inactive: β-lactams, aminoglycosides.
- Acute pneumonia (ATS/IDSA guidelines, CID 2007;44:S27): doxycycline 100 mg PO or IV twice daily × 14–21 days. Alternative: macrolide ± rifampin or fluoroquinolone (levofloxacin or moxifloxacin).
- Hepatitis: doxycycline 100 mg PO twice daily × 2 wks (duration arbitrary).
- Endocarditis (Karakousis, et al, JCM 2006;44:2283): doxycycline 100 mg PO or IV twice daily + chloroquine 200 mg PO three times a day × ≥18 mos (indefinitely or until phase I IgG <1:200, Raoult CID 2001;33:312). Some recommend treating ≥3 yrs (Levy AAC 1991;35:533).

OTHER INFORMATION
- Occupational disease from cattle, goat, sheep; also parturient cats.
- Dx is serology w/ evidence of seroconversion (pneumonia) or high titers (endocarditis).
- Main forms: "atypical pneumonia" (multilobar consolidation), nonspecific fever, and endocarditis.
- Chronic endocarditis usually is prosthetic valve endocarditis. Chronic infection often w/ "autoimmune" phenomenon, e.g., rash, (+) rheumatoid factor, Coombs' test (+).

BASIS FOR RECOMMENDATIONS
Mandell LA, Wunderink RG, Anzueto A, et al. Infectious Diseases Society of America/American Thoracic Society consensus guidelines on the management of community-acquired pneumonia in adults. *Clin Infect Dis*, 2007; Vol. 44 Suppl 2; pp. S27–72.
Comments: Used for Q fever pneumonia recommendations.

Karakousis PC, Trucksis M, Dumler JS. Chronic Q fever in the United States. *J Clin Microbiol*, 2006; Vol. 44; pp. 2283–7.
Comments: Review of 7 U.S. cases of prosthetic valve endocarditis with farm exposure (5), male sex (7), phase I IgG elevated (7), aortic valve involvement (7) and treatment with valve replacement (4).

Fenollar F, Fournier PE, Carrieri MP, et al. Risks factors and prevention of Q fever endocarditis. *Clin Infect Dis*, 2001; Vol. 33; pp. 312–6.
Comments: The authors review 102 cases of Q fever endocarditis in France. Of these 95 (93%) had predisposing valve disease. The abx regimen advocated with doxycycline + chloroquine for 12 mo w/ follow-up serology q3 mos for the next 2 yrs. The risk of Q fever endocarditis in those with acute Q fever + a predisposing valve lesion was 39%.

Marrie T. Coxiella burnetii. *Chapter 177 IN: Principles and Practice of Infectious Disease, 5th Ed, Mandell G, Bennett J, Dolin R, Churchill Livingstone, 2000*, p. 2043.
Comments: The author, noted for his experience with Q fever pneumonia, summarizes the various forms of Coxiella burnetii infection. The pneumonia has 3 forms—"typical," atypical pneumonia, fulminant pneumonia, or FUO (fever of unknown origin) with pneumonia as an incidental finding. The dx is serology and the treatment is doxycycline.

EHRLICHIA SPECIES

Paul G. Auwaerter, MD

MICROBIOLOGY
- Cause of tick-borne infection in humans.
- **Human Monocytic Ehrlichiosis (HME):** due to *Ehrlichia chaffeensis*, transmitted by *Amblyomma americanum* (Lone Star tick) and possibly other tick vectors such as *Dermacentor variabilis* (American dog tick).
- **Human Granulocytic Anaplasmosis (HGA):** formerly known as Human Granulocytic Ehrlichiosis (HGE). Organism is now known as *Anaplasma phagocytophilum* transmitted by *Ixodes scapularis* (deer tick) and on the West Coast, the western blacklegged tick (Ixodes pacificus)—same as Lyme disease (*Borrelia burgdorferi*).
- *E. ewingii*: canine pathogen that rarely infects humans, infection now termed "human ewingii ehrlichiosis."

CLINICAL

- **HME:** Seen mostly in areas from NJ to Ill to Tx.
- Suspected exposure endemic area spring-fall. Abrupt febrile, flu-like illness, HA, N/V, abdominal pain. Abnl LFT's, leukopenia, decreased plts. common. ~30% have maculopapular rash +/– petechiae.
- Children: HME presentation differs with rash in 67%, more frequent cytopenias, more neuro sxs.
- **HGA:** Seen in same areas as Lyme disease: NE, MidAtlantic, Upper Midwest. Also Europe.
- Sx similar to HME but less rash (10%). Can see leukopenia and thrombocytopenia, but neutropenia distinguishes from HME. Generally milder illness than HME. Coinfection w/ Lyme or Babesia possible.
- Elderly/immunosuppressed/asplenics at risk for severe disease (HME>HGA)—multiorgan failure including. ARDS, renal failure, CNS abnormalities, coagulopathies.
- Dx HME or HGA: confirmed case as a) 4x rise IFA titer from acute to convalescent or >1:256 or b) PCR detection or c) visible morulae and IFA >64. Probable case if single titer 1:64–128.
- Serological testing yields 90–95% sensitivity if performed with acute/convalescent serology after 3–4 wks. Sensitivity of PCR is 60–90% prior to antibiotics for acute infection. Blood smear is only 2–38% for HME and 25–75% for HGA.

SITES OF INFECTION

- Systemic: fever, headache, nausea, rigor, myalgia, nausea, vomiting, abdominal pain w/ average ~7 days post tick-bite.
- Monocytes or lymphocytes: HME—few pts (~7%) w/ morulae (mulberry-like clusters) in monos or lymphs.
- Granulocytes: HGA—morulae much more common in HGE (20–80%) than in HME.
- Liver: liver function test abnormalities common, jaundice less so.
- Heme: thrombocytopenia, leukopenia, anemia.

TREATMENT

HME or HGA: Adults

- Do not wait for confirmatory dx, treat w/ clinical suspicion. Delayed treatment may increase mortality, normally ~3%, especially in immunosuppressed.
- Doxycycline 100 mg PO/IV twice daily standard as ddx often includes RMSF and tx empirical. Duration uncertain, but at least >3 days after last fever [min. 5–7 days]. Often quick clinical response <48 hr except ICU pts.
- In toxic pts, some use 200 mg loading dose of doxycycline.
- Duration of treatment is 10 days. Should also be sufficient for early Lyme disease treatment.
- Pregnancy or doxycycline intolerance: rifampin 600 mg PO/IV daily × 7–10 days for HGA. Choices for HME unclear but may respond to rifampin or chloramphenicol 500 mg four times a day. Note: rifampin is not effective therapy for Lyme disease.
- *In vitro* resistance to chloramphenicol, macrolides, PCNs and AG's, and clinical data scanty so routine use cannot be strongly recommended. Quinolones have activity, but limited clinical data.
- Treatment is not recommended for asymptomatic pts who are merely seropositive or who are seropositive with vague, subjective and chronic complaints.

HME or HGA: Children

- Doxycycline 2 mg/kg IV/PO q12h (max 200 mg/day).
- Children <8 yrs without Lyme disease, treat for 4–5 days (or 3 days after resolution of fever) to minimize chances of drug toxicity.
- Children ≥8 yrs may receive full 10-day treatment.
- Children treated for less than 10 days should be closely monitored to ensure resolution of infection.
- If co-infected with Lyme disease, at the conclusion of doxycycline then give amoxicillin 50 mg/kg in 3 divided doses (max 500 mg/dose) or cefuroxime 30 mg/kg in 2 divided doses (max 500 mg/dose) × 14 days.

FOLLOW UP

- Persistence of fever >48 hrs after start of doxycycline should prompt reconsideration of diagnosis and/or consideration of rare babesia co-infection.

PATHOGENS

259

OTHER INFORMATION

- Summertime fever, headache especially in association with liver function test abnormalities and thrombocytopenia should prompt consideration of tick-borne illness: HME, HGA, Rocky Mountain Spotted Fever, babesiosis > Lyme disease—all based on locale and exposure risk.
- Spectrum of illness may range from subclinical to moderate to severe. About 40% HME pts require hospitalization. Abnl LFT's with leukopenia or thrombocytopenia clinical tip-off in pt w/ tick exposure.
- No randomized clinical trials exist to define optimal antibiotic choice or treatment. Chronic infection has not been described.
- Immune compromised pts at risk of severe illness, and common lab abnormalities in ICU may not trigger consideration of infection.
- *Ehrlichia ewingii* (agent of canine ehrlichiosis) has been described in humans. Seen mostly in immunocompromised pts from Missouri, Oklahoma, and Tennessee. Treatment is doxycycline 100 mg PO twice daily 7–14 days.

BASIS FOR RECOMMENDATIONS

Wormser GP, Dattwyler RJ, Shapiro ED, et al. The clinical assessment, treatment, and prevention of lyme disease, human granulocytic anaplasmosis, and babesiosis: clinical practice guidelines by the Infectious Diseases Society of America. *Clin Infect Dis*, 2006; Vol. 43; pp. 1089–134.
Comments: Recommendations for HGA presented in these IDSA recommendations.

Chapman AS, Bakken JS, Folk SM, et al. Diagnosis and management of tickborne rickettsial diseases: Rocky Mountain spotted fever, ehrlichioses, and anaplasmosis—United States: a practical guide for physicians and other health-care and public health professionals. *MMWR Recomm Rep*, 2006; Vol. 55; pp. 1–27.
Comments: Document is directed to help clinicians consider tick-borne infections in their ddx, add empiric doxycycline while ordering diagnostic studies that if positive should be reported to local health departments.

Olano JP, Walker DH. Human ehrlichioses. *Med Clin North Am*, 2002; Vol. 86; pp. 375–92.
Comments: Review article by leading Ehrlichial investigator that serves as basis for HME recommendations.

EIKENELLA CORRODENS

Paul G. Auwaerter, MD and Joseph Vinetz, MD

MICROBIOLOGY

- Facultatively anaerobic, fastidious, Gram-negative coccobacillary organism.
- Pits agar on culture plates (only ~50% of such colonies produce this pitting). Grows best if enhanced by 3–10% CO_2.
- Often found as a component of mixed infections.
- Member of HACEK group of endocarditis-associated bacteria (*Haemophilus* spp., *Actinobacillus*, *Cardiobacterium*, *Eikenella*, *Kingella*).

CLINICAL

- Component of normal human periodontal flora.
- Common component of soft tissue infections related to human bites, especially clenched fist injuries, rarely from cat/dog bites.
- Course of infection typically indolent (>1 wk from injury to clinical manifestations of infection).
- Also cause of head and neck infections, respiratory tract infections such as aspiration pneumonia/lung abscess.
- Definite evidence of *Eikenella corrodens* diagnosed by culture. May also be seen as component of polymicrobial process.

SITES OF INFECTION

- Human bite wounds: clenched fist injury most common, also affects nail biters (rare).
- Head and neck: periodontitis, floor of mouth infections, internal jugular septic thrombophlebitis.
- Heart: endocarditis, particularly after IV drug abuse.
- Lung: lung abscess, aspiration pneumonia, septic emboli from head and neck, infective thrombophlebitis.
- GI: intraabdominal abscess.

- Gyn: occasionally associated with IUD, orogenital trauma.
- GU: genital ulcer (rare), urinary tract infection(rare).

TREATMENT

Human bite/soft tissue infections

- Often present within polymicrobial infection.
- Surgical drainage of any abscess, critical for optimal management.
- Severe infection/parenteral therapy: ampicillin/sulbactam 1.5–3 g IV q6h. Other beta-lactam/ beta-lactamase inhibitors (BL/BLI) also effective.
- Oral regimen: amoxicillin/clavulanate 250–500 mg PO three times a day or 875/125 mg PO twice daily.
- Third generation cephalosporins in standard doses as effective as BL/BLIs but ceftriaxone better for continued once daily outpt management.
- Additional therapy against frequently polymicrobial infections may need to be added, e.g., metronidazole.
- Alternatives (beta-lactam allergy): doxycycline 100 mg IV/PO twice daily, moxifloxacin 400 mg once IV/PO daily or levofloxacin 500 mg IV/PO once daily, although less clinical experience, isolates are usually sensitive.
- No role for clindamycin, metronidazole unless added for polymicrobial therapy.
- Aminoglycosides: no role, no synergy even in endocarditis.

Head and neck infections

- Same as for human bite.

Endocarditis

- Preferred: third generation cephalosporins (ceftriaxone 1 g IV q12h, cefotaxime 1–2 g IV q8h or cefepime 1–2 g IV q8h).
- Insufficient clinical data for definitive recommendations.
- PCN, ampicillin useful, but recent emergence of beta lactamase-producing isolates makes these second tier drugs. Few laboratories do sensitivity testing; prudent to avoid these agents unless *in vitro* susceptibility data obtained.
- Aminoglycosides: no role, no synergy even in endocarditis.

Other sites of infection

- As for human bite.
- In case of pulmonary empyema, drainage necessary.

OTHER INFORMATION

- Surgical drainage of collections essential.
- Consider polymicrobial infection especially in skin and soft tissue/HEENT/lung infection so that antibiotic selection also covers *Strep species*, *S. aureus*, and anaerobes.
- Can be isolated in pure culture or in polymicrobial culture.

BASIS FOR RECOMMENDATIONS

Choice of antibacterial drugs. *Treat Guidel Med Lett,* 2007; Vol. 5; pp. 33–50.
Comments: For non-endocarditis recommendations.

Baddour LM, Wilson WR, Bayer AS, et al. Infective endocarditis: diagnosis, antimicrobial therapy, and management of complications: a statement for healthcare professionals from the Committee on Rheumatic Fever, Endocarditis, and Kawasaki Disease, Council on Cardiovascular Disease in the Young, and the Councils on Clinical Cardiology, Stroke, and Cardiovascular Surgery and Anesthesia, American Heart Association: endorsed by the Infectious Diseases Society of America. *Circulation,* 2005; Vol. 111; pp. e394–434.
Comments: Basis for endocarditis recommendations.

ENTEROBACTER SPECIES

Lisa A. Spacek, MD, PhD and Joseph Vinetz, MD

MICROBIOLOGY

- Gram-negative, aerobic, motile bacilli of *Enterobacteriaceae* family.
- Major pathogenic spp., *E. cloacae* (most common), *E. aerogenes, E. gergoviae,* and *Pantoea agglomerans. E. sakazakii* now classified as *Cronobacter.*

PATHOGENS

261

- Drug resistance is due to expression of chromosomal AmpC beta-lactamases that are constitutive and inducible, as well as plasmid-encoded extended-spectrum beta-lactamases (ESBLs).
- Presence of beta-lactams is required for activation of inducible beta-lactamases, which may not be detected on initial testing.

CLINICAL

- Common cause of nosocomial infections including ventilator-associated pneumonia, burn and surgical wound infections, catheter or device-related infections, and post-neurosurgical meningitis.
- *E. sakazakii*, now *Cronobacter*, is an opportunistic pathogen that causes meningitis, necrotizing enterocolitis and septicemia in low-birth weight infants and neonates; known as a contaminant in non-sterile powdered infant formulas.
- Resistant to ampicillin, first-generation cephalosporins, and macrolides. Beta-lactamases produced during treatment with beta-lactams, occurs more commonly at infection sites with limited antibiotic penetration, e.g., pneumonia and osteomyelitis.

SITES OF INFECTION

- UTI: catheter, instrumentation-associated.
- Pulmonary: pneumonia, predominantly nosocomial, ventilator-associated.
- Soft tissue: wound infection, burns, surgical sites. May lead to sepsis and/or be part of polymicrobial infection in dirty sites such as decubitus ulcer.
- Bacteremia: catheter, device-associated.
- CNS: meningitis, mostly nosocomial, related to neurosurgery.
- Neonatal: necrotizing enterocolitis, sepsis, and meningitis. *E. cloacae* and *Cronobacter* in NICU outbreaks.

TREATMENT
Serious infections

- For suspected infections, double empiric coverage with synergistic antibiotics recommended until susceptibilities known to avoid emergence of resistance during treatment of severe infections: piperacillin-tazobactam 3.375–4.5 g IV q6h **plus** aminoglycoside (gentamicin, tobramycin or amikacin) or fluoroquinolone, e.g., ciprofloxacin 400 mg IV q8–12 hrs.
- For coverage of ESBLs, imipenem 500 mg IV q6h **or** meropenem 500–1000 mg IV q8h **or** doripenem 500 mg IV q8h.
- Cefepime 2 g IV q8h, drug resistance while on therapy may develop.

UTI without systemic signs

- Remove bladder catheter; straight catheterize pt until pyuria clears.
- Single agent such as fluoroquinolone appropriate (ciprofloxacin 250 mg PO twice daily) or agent based upon susceptibility profile.

OTHER INFORMATION

- Remove infected hardware if possible (bladder catheter, endotracheal tube, peripheral IV or central line, peritoneal dialysis catheter, etc.).
- Consider *Enterobacter* spp. as similar to *P. aeruginosa* because both can develop resistance to antibiotics during the course of therapy, necessitating double antibiotic coverage for serious infections.

BASIS FOR RECOMMENDATIONS

Jacoby GA. AmpC beta-lactamases. *Clin Microbiol Rev*, 2009; Vol. 22; pp. 161–82.

Comments: This review of AmpC beta-lactamases details constitutive, inducible and plasmid-transmitted antibiotic resistance in *Enterobacteriaceae* as well as detection and treatment.

Paterson DL, Bonomo RA. Extended-spectrum beta-lactamases: a clinical update. *Clin Microbiol Rev*, 2005; Vol. 18; pp. 657–86.

Comments: Extended-spectrum beta-lactamases (ESBLs) are a rapidly evolving group of beta-lactamases which share the ability to hydrolyze third-generation cephalosporins and aztreonam yet are inhibited by clavulanic acid. Carbapenems are the treatment of choice for serious infections due to ESBL-producing organisms, yet carbapenem-resistant isolates have recently been reported.

ENTEROCOCCUS

Lisa A. Spacek, MD, PhD and Joseph Vinetz, MD

MICROBIOLOGY

- Enterococci are facultatively anaerobic, Gram-positive cocci that grow in short chains under extreme conditions, i.e., 6.5% NaCl, pH 9.6, temp range from 10–45°C, and in the presence of bile salts. Can be found in soil, water, food, and are significant component of normal colonic flora. Also, in oropharyngeal and vaginal secretions.
- Relatively low virulence; adheres to extracellular matrix proteins, adheres to urinary tract epithelia, and produces biofilms. Enterococci can be multidrug resistant and difficult to eradicate.
- Intrinsically resistant to beta-lactams due to inner cell wall penicillin-binding proteins. High level beta-lactam resistance is increasing in *E. faecium*, but uncommon in *E. faecalis*. Resistant to TMP-SMX, as organism uses exogenous folate to overcome anti-folate synthesis mechanism.
- Relatively impermeable to aminoglycosides, adequate drug concentrations may be achieved with addition of a cell-wall agent and result in bactericidal effect at ribosomal target. Ribosomal mutation and decreased aminoglycoside transport may confer high-level resistance. Some may remain susceptible to streptomycin.
- Vancomycin resistant enterococci (VRE): *E. faecium (60%)* >> *E. faecalis* (2%) reported in nationwide surveillance study (SCOPE). Plasmid-mediated VanA and VanB phenotypes confer high-level vancomycin resistance. Other types are variably resistant.

CLINICAL

- Cause of UTIs, most often catheter or instrumentation-associated, bacteremia due to enterococcal UTI occurs infrequently.
- Cause of bacteremia and meningitis (nosocomial bacteremia not routinely associated with endocarditis); meningitis in setting of head trauma, s/p neurosurgery or CNS anatomic defects; peritonitis; and a component of mixed aerobic/anaerobic flora in intra-abdominal, pelvic, wound, decubitus ulcers and diabetic foot infections.
- Risk factors: prolonged hospitalization, hemodialysis, ICU stays and broad spectrum abx therapy, esp. anaerobic abx.
- Association of VRE with high morbidity and mortality most significant in debilitated hosts. Independent association of VRE bacteremia and mortality is inconsistent, may also serve as a marker of severe illness.
- Nonantimicrobial treatments include: catheter removal, percutaneous or surgical drainage, incision and drainage, and debridement.
- Use contact isolation to prevent nosocomial spread on hands of caregivers. Wash hands, leave stethoscope and BP cuff in room.
- No reliable means to terminate VRE colonization.

SITES OF INFECTION

- Cardiac: endocarditis
- Bacteremia: central venous catheter-associated
- GI/GU: UTI, complication of intestinal, pelvis or biliary tract surgery, cholangitis
- CNS: meningitis, in setting of neurosurgery, abnl CNS anatomy, and head trauma

TREATMENT

Endocarditis

- Test for susceptibility to penicillin and vancomycin and high-level resistance to gentamicin and streptomycin. Combination therapy with cell wall-active agents PLUS aminoglycosides is standard of care for infections requiring bactericidal activity, e.g., endocarditis, meningitis, and enterococcemia in neutropenic host.
- Ampicillin 2 g IV q4h **or**-penicillin G 18–24 million U/24h IV continuously or divided q4h **plus** gentamicin 1 mg/kg IV q8h. Treat 4–6 wks for native valve and at least 6 wks for prosthetic valve. Maintain penicillin, ampicillin, and vancomycin trough levels above MIC.
- To avoid nephrotoxic and ototoxic effects, shorter course of aminoglycosides (median, 14 days) to treat susceptible enterococci accepted in Sweden with 81% cure rate. Longer course of

synergistic regimen preferred for prosthetic valves, large vegetations, or in setting of decreased sensitivity to antibiotics.

- If pt allergic to penicillin, vancomycin 15 mg/kg IV q12h recommended (target trough between 15–20 mcg/mL). Consider penicillin desensitization for serious infections.
- If penicillin resistance due to beta-lactamase, use ampicillin-sulbactam **plus** gentamicin **or** vancomycin **plus** gentamicin. If due to intrinsic penicillin resistance, use vancomycin **plus** gentamicin. If high-level gentamicin resistance encountered, test streptomycin. Streptomycin 7.5 mg/kg q12h IV/IM. Trough concentration <10 µg/ml.
- For multi-drug resistant *E. faecalis*, use imipenem/cilastin **plus** ampicillin **or** ceftriaxone **plus** ampicillin. Synergy may be achieved with beta-lactam combinations due to different penicillin-binding protein targets.
- For multi-drug resistant *E. faecium* use linezolid or quinupristin-dalfopristin. Treat for at least 8 wks.
- In setting of multidrug resistance or inability to achieve synergistic bactericidal effect, treatment success limited to <50% with antimicrobials alone, consider valve replacement.
- Daptomycin is generally not recommended for enterococcal endocarditis.

Bacteremia, catheter-related infections

- If ampicillin/penicillin susceptible, ampicillin 2 g IV q4–6h **or** ampicillin **plus** gentamicin 1 mg/kg q8h.
- Ampicillin resistant and vancomycin susceptible or penicillin allergy, vancomycin 15 mg/kg IV q12h (target trough 15–20 mcg/mL) **plus** gentamicin 1 mg/kg q8h **or** linezolid 600 mg q12h **or** daptomycin 6 mg/kg per day.
- If ampicillin and vancomycin resistant, linezolid 600 mg q12h **or** daptomycin 6 mg/kg IV per day **or** quinupristin-dalfopristin 7.5 mg/kg IV q8h.
- Quinupristin-dalfopristin is **not** effective against *E. faecalis*.
- Remove catheter and replace at new site if needed.

UTI, intra-abdominal, and wound infections

- Penicillin or ampicillin are preferred agents, vancomycin in setting of penicillin allergy or high-level penicillin resistance.
- Uncomplicated urinary tract infections with susceptible strains: amoxicillin 875 mg PO twice daily × 7–10 days; if penicillin allergy, nitrofurantoin 50–100 mg PO four times a day × 7–10 days.

Treatment of VRE

- Linezolid 600 mg IV q12h. Bacteriostatic, resistance may emerge during therapy. Major risk, myelosuppression, esp. thrombocytopenia after 2 wks of therapy. Due to excellent CSF penetration, may be used to treat VRE meningitis.
- Quinupristin/dalfopristin (*E. faecium* only) 7.5 mg/kg IV q8h. Bacteriostatic, resistance may emerge during therapy. Adverse reaction, phlebitis (administer via central venous catheter) arthralgia/myalgia.
- Daptomycin 6 mg/kg per day. Bactericidal, approved for right-sided *S. aureus* endocarditis, however, daptomycin-resistance has emerged during treatment of VRE infection. Some use higher dose of daptomycin 8–10 mg/kg.
- Tigecycline 100 mg IV loading dose, then 50 mg IV q12h. Approved for complicated skin-skin structure and intra-abdominal infection.
- For VRE UTI, fosfomycin 3 g PO × 1 dose.
- In non-invasive infections, nonantimicrobial interventions including catheter or foreign body removal, drainage of closed space infection, and wound debridement, may offer adequate treatment.

BASIS FOR RECOMMENDATIONS

Mermel LA, Allon M, Bouza E, et al. Clinical practice guidelines for the diagnosis and management of intravascular catheter-related infection: 2009 update by the Infectious Diseases Society of America. *Clin Infect Dis,* 2009; Vol. 49; pp. 1–45. **Comments:** 2009 updated guidelines for treatment of intravascular catheter-related infections. For details regarding *E. faecalis* and *E. faecium*, see www.hopkins-abxguide.org

Segreti JA, Crank CW, Finney MS. Daptomycin for the treatment of Gram-positive bacteremia and infective endocarditis: a retrospective case series of 31 pts. *Pharmacotherapy,* 2006; Vol. 26; pp. 347–52.

Comments: In this small retrospective case series of 31 pts, 6 of 11 pts with VRE bacteremia and/or infective endocarditis who were treated with daptomycin died. Recommendation to avoid daptomycin for treatment of VRE endocarditis, despite bactericidal activity.

Baddour LM, Wilson WR, Bayer AS, et al. Infective endocarditis: diagnosis, antimicrobial therapy, and management of complications: a statement for healthcare professionals from the Committee on Rheumatic Fever, Endocarditis, and Kawasaki Disease, Council on Cardiovascular Disease in the Young, and the Councils on Clinical Cardiology, Stroke, and Cardiovascular Surgery and Anesthesia, American Heart Association: endorsed by the Infectious Diseases Society of America. *Circulation,* 2005; Vol. 111; pp. e394–434.

Comments: Guidelines and recommendations for the management of enterococcal endocarditis, among many other recommendations. Endorsed by the Infectious Disease Society of America.

Stevens DL, Bisno AL, Chambers HF, et al. Practice guidelines for the diagnosis and management of skin and soft-tissue infections. *Clin Infect Dis,* 2005; Vol. 41; pp. 1373–406.

Comments: Guidelines and recommendations for the management of skin and soft tissue infections, including in compromised hosts, due to enterococci, among other pathogens. Published as Guidelines from the Infectious Disease Society of America.

ERYSIPELOTHRIX RHUSIOPATHIAE

Paul G. Auwaerter, MD and Joseph Vinetz, MD

MICROBIOLOGY

- Aerobic, thin, pleomorphic Gram-positive rod.
- Zoonotic infection that more commonly infects turkeys, pigs, and other animals than humans.
- *E. rhusiopathiae* is only genus within species.

CLINICAL

- Cause of erysipeloid.
- Zoonosis, major reservoir domestic swine, but also from wide variety of animals.
- Major animal reservoirs: pigs, sheep, fish, shellfish, domestic fowl.
- Major syndromes: mild skin form as known as erysipeloid (most common); diffuse cutaneous form (rare); sepsis/endocarditis (rare).
- Intrinsically resistant to vancomycin, which commonly might be used empirically unless the organism is properly identified and distinguished from diphtheroids (*Corynebacterium* spp.) and Lactobacillus.
- Dx: erysipeloid—cx of skin bx. Lab can confuse with diphtheroids, coryneforms, but *E. rhusiopathiae* distinguished by H_2S production and unlike most cellulitis syndromes is frequently associated with positive blood cxs.

SITES OF INFECTION

- Skin: erysipeloid (cellulitis, "Rosenbach's Rouget") purplish-red, spreading patch, raised border, central clearing, starts at site of inoculation. Can have bullous forms with dissemination.
- Cardiovascular: endocarditis occurs on normal valves (50%), usually aortic. Large, shaggy, ulcerated vegetations typical, often occurs in context of sepsis.
- Lymph: ~10% of cellulitis cases have associated lymphangitis or regional lymphadenopathy.
- General: sepsis (rare, most common in immunocompromised hosts); metastatic skin lesions (rare).

TREATMENT

Localized infection

- Penicillin: single dose of benzathine PCN 1.2 million U, or PCN VK 250 mg PO four times a day × 5–7 days or daily procaine PCN 600,000–1.2 million U IM per day for 5–7 days.
- Erythromycin 250 mg PO four times a day × 5–7 days.
- Doxycycline 100 mg PO twice daily × 5–7 days.

Disseminated skin infection

- As for localized infection.
- Assess for endocarditis.

Sepsis/Endocarditis

- Penicillin 2.4 million U IV/day in 4 divided doses × 4–6 wks +/− streptomycin 1 g IV/day or gentamicin 1 mg/kg IV q8hr for first wk.

- Evidence for aminoglycoside need is limited.
- Valve replacement may be necessary.

OTHER INFORMATION
- Prevention: education of occupational risk groups. Use gloves. Vaccination of susceptible herds (not possible for aquatic sources).
- Organism always resistant to vancomycin.

BASIS FOR RECOMMENDATIONS

Reboli AC, Farrar WE. Erysipelothrix rhusiopathiae. *Principles and Practice of Infectious Diseases, 6th ed, Chap 207*, 2005.

Comments: Given rarity, there are no prospective data upon which to base recommendations. MIC/MBC *in vitro* data have tended to guide recommendations.

ESCHERICHIA COLI

Paul G. Auwaerter, MD

MICROBIOLOGY
- Gram-negative rod, *Enterobacteriaceae* w/ human strains as (1) commensal bowel flora, (2) intestinal pathogenic (enteric/diarrheogenic), (3) extraintestinal pathogenic.
- Predominant facultative anaerobe of normal human colonic flora.
- *E. coli* easy to grow from sterile specimens. Stool cx: only if chronic diarrhea (need reference lab to ID) or suspect O157:H7 (cx all bloody diarrhea) use sorbitol-MacConkey agar or perform Shiga EIA.
- ~ 90% strains lactose fermenter; some *diarrheogenic E. coli* strains, including many of the EIEC strains, typically lactose negative. Indole test 99% (+).

CLINICAL
- Most common cause of UTI, neonatal meningitis, traveler's diarrhea. Seen often w/ intra-abdominal infections. Not an uncommon cause of nosocomial pneumonia, line-infections, post-operative wound infections.
- *E. coli* O157:H7 spectrum—10% nonbloody diarrhea; 90% hemorrhagic colitis, 10% (pts <10 yrs) hemolytic-uremic syndrome [HUS]; <5% w/ intestinal and extraintestinal complications.
- **Enterotoxigenic *E. coli* (ETEC):** major cause of traveler's diarrhea.
- **Enteroadherent *E. coli* (EAEC):** cause of travel-related diarrhea.
- **Enteroinvasive *E. coli* (EIEC):** bloody diarrhea, presentations similar to Shigella often with abdominal pain. Fecal leukocytes often present.
- **Entero-pathogenic *E. coli* (EPEC):** watery diarrhea of infants. Role of antibiotic therapy unclear.
- **Enteroaggregative *E. coli* (EAEC):** food-borne, enteric pathogen. May be persistent, especially children in less-developed countries. Cipro and rifampin shown to decrease illness duration.
- **Shiga toxin-producing *E. coli* (STEC):** serotype O157:H7 best known cause although non-O157 may predominate in some geographic regions; zoonotic, food or waterborne enteric illness; occurs in epidemics; cause of hemolytic uremic syndrome (HUS), the leading cause of acute renal failure in children. Diarrhea may be bloody. Leading causes include undercooked meats (ground beef), vegetables, fruits, prepared foods, or contaminated water. Non-O157 strains identified by stool or supernatant testing by EIA for shiga toxin.
- Non-O157 STEC diarrhea may not be bloody, more frequent in some geographic areas. It may be missed by culture as many are sorbitol positive.

SITES OF INFECTION
- GU: acute cystitis, pyelonephritis, renal abscess, prostatitis, PID
- GI: traveler's diarrhea (enterotoxigenic > enteroinvasive > enteroadherent strains); intra-abdominal abscess, peritonitis (secondary and SBP)
- Lung: nosocomial pneumonia
- Bloodstream: bacteremia/sepsis secondary to UTI, GI/biliary tract, venous catheters

- Skin/soft tissues: cellulitis—often in diabetics, debilitated w/ decubiti or ulcers; myositis/fasciitis, post-operative wound infections
- CNS: neonatal meningitis, occasional adult nosocomial or geriatric meningitis, brain abscess

TREATMENT

Uncomplicated UTI

- See Bacterial Cystitis, Bacterial Prostatitis and Bacterial Pyelonephritis Modules in the Diagnoses section for additional information.
- Preferred agents (IDSA/AUA Guidelines): TMP-SMX DS or fluoroquinolones.
- Preferred: TMP-SMX DS PO twice daily × 3-day (short course) if local resistance is known to be <10–20%.
- Alt: ciprofloxacin 250 mg PO twice daily (or 500 mg XR once daily) × 3 days; levofloxacin 250 mg PO once daily × 3 days.
- Nitrofurantoin 100 mg PO four times daily or nitrofurantoin macrocrystals (Macrobid) 100 mg PO twice daily × 7 days.
- Fosfomycin 3 g sachet PO × 1 dose.
- For older pts, those with comorbidities (e.g., diabetes mellitus) use 7–10 days course.

Bacteremia/Pneumonia/Pyelonephritis/Other

- Sensitivity data once known should guide abx selection.
- *E. coli* extended-spectrum beta-lactamase (ESBL) strains increasingly common, consider in nosocomial situations, severe infections requiring ICU care—consider initial carbapenem +/– aminoglycoside use. FQ-resistance rising, so should not rely upon in empirically serious infections.
- Ceftriaxone 1–2 g IV q24h or other third or fourth generation cephalosporin.
- Ciprofloxacin 400 mg IV q12h or 500 mg PO q12h, levofloxacin 500 mg PO/IV q24h, moxifloxacin 400 mg IV/PO q24h (do not use moxifloxacin for UTI due to low urinary concentrations).
- Ampicillin (if sensitive) 2 g IV q6h.
- TMP-SMX (if sensitive) 5–10 mg/kg/day divided q6–8h IV.
- Alt: imipenem, meropenem, ertapenem, doripenem; ceftazidime, cefepime; cefazolin or cefuroxime (if sensitive); aztreonam; ticarcillin, piperacillin; piperacillin-tazobactam; aminoglycosides; tigecycline (intra-abd or skin/soft tissue).
- Ampicillin-sulbactam 3 g IV q6h (rates of resistance may be as high as 50–60% in hospitalized pts) +/– gentamicin 1.5 mg/kg/q8h or 5–7 mg/kg/day IV.
- Gentamicin 5 mg/kg/day or tobramycin 5 mg/kg/day IV (monotherapy generally not recommended for bacteremia/pneumonia).
- Duration: 7–14 days therapy course.

Hemolytic-Uremic Syndrome E. coli O157:H7

- HUS defined by triad of hemolytic anemia, thrombocytopenia, and renal failure. Seizures may be common.
- No antibiotics should be used if suspected/documented. Studies suggest increased HUS toxicity in children if abx used.
- No anti-motility agents.
- Notify public health authorities promptly.

Gastroenteritis (non-O157:H7)

- See Traveler's Diarrhea module.
- If treatment required (severe sx): ciprofloxacin 500 mg PO twice daily; ofloxacin 300 mg PO twice daily; norfloxacin 400 mg PO twice daily; TMP-SMX DS PO twice daily; rifamixin 200 mg three times a day—all drugs given for 3 days, except bloody diarrhea × 5 days.
- Do not use rifamixin 200 mg PO three times a day if invasive disease suspected as it is not absorbed from lumen, so no systemic levels of drug.
- Laboratory confirmation of *E. coli*-induced diarrhea usually unavailable. Most treatment is empiric.
- Dx of ETEC or EAEC requires EIA, DNA probe testing. Many strains resistant to TMP-SMX and doxycycline.
- Alt: bismuth subsalicylate 1048 mg PO four times a day × 5 days; enteroinvasive (EIEC) ampicillin 500 mg PO or 1 g IV four times a day × 5 days; Enteropathogenic (EPEC) neomycin 50 mg/kg/divided q8h or furazolidone 100 mg PO four times a day either × 3–5 days.

PATHOGENS

FOLLOW UP

- Follow-up urine or blood cultures not routinely necessary to document clearance of infection if pt responding to agent deemed susceptible.

OTHER INFORMATION

- Increasingly, *E.coli is* resistant to ampicillin (~30–45%) and ciprofloxacin (~15%).
- Urine culture is not needed for management of a routine uncomplicated UTI.
- Diagnosis of UTI should be accompanied by an abnormal urine analysis (abnl dip: leukocyte esterase +, nitrites +, or abnl microanalysis).
- If hemolytic-uremic syndrome suspected, abx should not be given; stool should be cultured on sorbitol-MacConkey agar (notify microbiology) or perform EIA for shiga toxins.

BASIS FOR RECOMMENDATIONS

Guerrant RL, Van Gilder T, Steiner TS, et al. Practice guidelines for the management of infectious diarrhea. *Clin Infect Dis,* 2001; Vol. 32; pp. 331–51.

Comments: A review by an expert panel. For diarrhea caused by *E. coli,* the panel recommends oral TMP-SMX or an oral quinolone for enteropathogenic and enteroinvasive strains. For *E.coli* O157-H7 both anti-motility and antibiotic agents should be avoided.

Warren JW, Abrutyn E, Hebel JR, et al. Guidelines for antimicrobial treatment of uncomplicated acute bacterial cystitis and acute pyelonephritis in women. Infectious Diseases Society of America (IDSA). *Clin Infect Dis,* 1999; Vol. 29; pp. 745–58.

Comments: A review by an expert panel. On the basis of available data the panel recommended 3 day courses of therapy for uncomplicated cystitis with either TMP-SMX or a quinolone. Beta lactam drugs are less effective and should be second line choices. Acute pyelonephritis should be managed with a quinolone or TMP-SMX for 14 days in the non-pregnant female with normal anatomy of the GU tract. If the infection is due to a Gram + pathogen then ampicillin-sulbactam +/– an aminoglycoside should be used. No guideline update scheduled although catheter-associated UTI guideline due in 2010.

FRANCISELLA TULARENSIS

John G. Bartlett, MD

MICROBIOLOGY

- Small, pleomorphic, aerobic Gram-negative bacillus.
- Culture: poor or no growth on standard media. Requires addition of cysteine, e.g., thioglycolate or Legionella media.
- Considered a laboratory hazard. Notify lab if considering diagnosis when submitting specimens.

CLINICAL

- Epidemiology: acquired from tick exposure or contact with rabbits (skinning or aerosolized carcass, e.g., cutting hay, lawn, etc.) or bioterrorism.
- Tularemia endemic SE/Western U.S. and New England islands. Most cases are ulceroglandular, <200 cases/yr.
- Bioterrorism: pneumonia + pleuritis + hilar adenopathy. In this differential dx: anthrax, plague.
- Six clinical forms (see below)—all have incubation period 3–5 days (range 1–21 days), often with abrupt onset of fever.
- Pneumonia presentation: sudden fever, prostration, dry cough. CXR: infiltrates + hilar adenopathy.
- Pathophysiology: (1) bite/abrasion → nodule/ulcer → node → sepsis, or, (2) inhalation → pneumonia/pharyngitis → sepsis.
- Diagnosis: DFA stain, PCR, serology +/– standard cultures, BUT hard to grow and lab hazard (notify micro lab if suspecting). Culture and identification requires >1 wk. If suspecting this dx, obtain blood and sputum cxs.
- Confirmed case: compatible case + positive PCR, positive culture or 4× rise in serology.
- Pneumonia: case fatality with treatment <2%, without treatment 7%.

SITES OF INFECTION

- Ulceroglandular: skin ulcer + adenopathy
- Glandular: adenopathy only
- Oculoglandular: conjunctivitis + preauricular nodes

- Oropharyngeal: pharyngitis
- Pneumonia: acquired by inhalation
- Septicemia: bacteremia

TREATMENT

Treatment

- Indications: tularemia or fever or flu-like illness within 14 days of presumed exposure.
- Preferred: streptomycin 1 g IM twice daily or gentamicin 5 mg/kg/day IV × 10 days.
- Alt (efficacy unproven): doxycycline 100 mg IV twice daily or chloramphenicol 1 g IV q6h or ciprofloxacin 400 mg IV twice daily. Rx until stable then PO for 14–21 days (total).
- Pregnancy: gentamicin 5 mg/kg/day IV × 10 days. Alt: use ciprofloxacin.

Post Exposure Prophylaxis

- Preferred: doxycycline 100 mg PO twice daily or ciprofloxacin 500 mg PO twice daily × 14 days.

Disease Control/Bioterrorism Considerations

- Notify Infection Control (or other facility contact) and local public health dept if bioterrorism suspected.
- Pathogen not spread by person-to-person transmission. No isolation necessary.
- Alert micro lab—need biological safety level 2.
- Surface decontamination: 10% bleach and soapy water.
- Clothing: clean w/ soapy water.

OTHER INFORMATION

- Pneumonic form—must consider bioterrorism. Outbreak in Martha's Vineyard (early 2000s) due to lawn mowing and bush cutting that aerosolized bacteria from infected animals.
- Epidemic pneumonia ddx: Legionella, influenza, histoplasmosis, anthrax, Q fever, plague.

BASIS FOR RECOMMENDATIONS

Dennis DT, Inglesby TV, Henderson DA, et al. Tularemia as a biological weapon: medical and public health management. *JAMA,* 2001; Vol. 285; pp. 2763–73

Comments: Differential dx: anthrax, plague, Q fever or tularemia. Micro dx could require >1 wk. Dominant form: pneumonic, but would expect some cases of ocular, pharyngeal, glandular, ulceroglandular. Abx resistance reported with doxycycline, chloro, and streptomycin. Dx by cx (requires >1 wk). DFA, PCR, etc. available in special labs.

Cross JT., Penn RL. Francisella tularensis (Tularemia). *Chapter 216 in Principles and Practice Infectious Diseases, 5th Ed.* Mandell G, Bennett J, Dolin R, Eds. Churchill Livingston, 2000; pp. 2393.

Comments: Pathogen: pleomorphic gram-negative coccobacillus. Infectious dose: 10–50 organisms via skin or lungs. Clinical features: 6 classic forms. Abrupt onset: fever, chills, malaise +/– cough, abd pain, diarrhea. Fever lasts over 32 days w/o Rx. Forms: ulceroglandular, glandular, oculoglandular, pharyngeal, typhoidal, pneumonic.

HAEMOPHILUS DUCREYI (CHANCROID)

Noreen A. Hynes, MD, MPH

MICROBIOLOGY

- Fastidious, facultative anaerobic Gram-negative coccobacillus.
- Requires hemin (X factor) for growth but no requirement for NAD (V factor); 3 types of nutritionally enriched media needed for growth.
- Specific molecular techniques used to identify likely geographic origin of strains.
- Organism found within the granulocytic infiltrate of the ulcer and colocalized with neutrophils and fibrin at the ulcerative stage of disease.

CLINICAL

- Uncommon in U.S. When occurs in U.S., usually in discrete outbreaks but can be endemic in some areas. Decreasing in endemic regions of the developing world for unclear reasons.
- Painful genital ulcer disease with adenopathy.
- Painful inguinal adenitis (buboes) occur in up to 40%, may suppurate. Autoinoculation of non-genital sites such as eyes and fingers occasionally seen.
- Trauma/abrasion needed for introduction of infection. Painful ulcer + regional painful LN in $\frac{1}{3}$ of pts. Painful ulcer + suppuration = high probably of chancroid.

- Chancroid ulcer classically ragged w/ undermined edges, sharply demarcated, no induration; purulent, dirty grey base. Ulcer w/ friable base; bleeds if scraped. Men >1 ulcer in ~50%. Many women asx.
- Up to 10% co-infected with syphilis therefore **must** Rx for **both.**
- Communicable until the ulcer heals. Heals with or without Rx but Rx speeds healing. Increases risk of HIV acquisition and transmission.
- **Definitive diagnosis**: (1) Requires identification of *H. ducreyi* on special culture media that are not widely available. (2) Even with special media, sensitivity is only about 80%, using more than 1 of the 3 media that will support growth may increase recover of the organism. (3) There is no nationally-available FDA-approved PCR test for *H. ducreyi* but some commercial labs may have developed their own PCR test.
- **Probable diagnosis**: (1) Criteria can be used for clinical and surveillance purposes. (2) Probable case defined if the following criteria are met: a. pt has 1 or more painful genital ulcers. b. pt has no evidence of *T. pallidum* infection on darkfield microscopy of ulcer exudate or by a serologic test for syphilis performed at least 7 days after onset of ulcers. c. the clinical presentation, appearance of ulcers and, if present, regional lymphadenopathy, are typical for chancroid. d. a test for HSV performed on the ulcer exudate is negative. (3) Painful ulcer + tender LN seen in $\frac{1}{3}$ of pts; when suppurative LN also seen these signs almost pathognomonic.

Sites of Infection
- Genitalia: genital ulcer(s)
- Inguinal lymph nodes: following small, missed genital ulcer or with genital ulcer
- Conjunctivae: autoinoculation from genitalia source
- Fingers: can follow autoinoculation or foreplay

Treatment
Recommended regimens
- Azithromycin 1 g PO × 1.
- Ceftriaxone 250 mg IM × 1.
- Ciprofloxacin 500 mg PO twice daily × 3 days.
- Erythromycin base 500 mg PO four times a day × 7 days.

Regimens in pregnancy
- Ceftriaxone 250 mg IM × 1.
- Erythromycin base 500 mg PO four times a day × 7 days.
- Azithromycin: safety and efficacy in pregnancy and lactation not firmly established.

Treatment in HIV infection or uncircumcised men
- Some experts recommend the 7-day erythromycin course due to slow healing in these groups of pts.
- Efficacy of azithromycin and ceftriaxone unknown in this group. Use only if follow-up is ensured.

Management of fluctuant buboes
- Incision and drainage is probably preferred treatment in those not adequately responding to antibiotics alone.
- Bubo aspiration is simpler and safer than I and D, but reaspiration often needed; sinus tracts may form.

Other management considerations
- Follow-up: exam all pts 3–7 days after initiation of Rx. If no clinical improvement: (1) reassess dx, (2) consider coinfection w/ another STD or HIV, (3) consider noncompliance, (4) antibiotic-resistance.
- Sex partners: all sex partners during the 10 days prior to sx to the present should be examined and treated regardless of symptoms.
- Candidates for longer Rx and close follow-up: HIV-infected persons; uncircumcised men.
- All pts should be offered HIV testing at the time of chancroid diagnosis; retest all pts for syphilis and HIV 3 mos after chancroid dx is made if initial tests negative.

Follow Up
- Time to complete healing is dependent upon the size of the ulcer.
- Large ulcers usually require >2 wks.

- Fluctuant lymphadenopathy takes longer to resolve than ulcers.
- Healing of ulcer in uncircumcised men and HIV-infected persons may take longer than in circumcised men and HIV uninfected persons, respectively.

OTHER INFORMATION
- Uncircumcised men may be at higher risk; take longer to cure.
- No immunity develops after single infection.
- More commonly diagnosed in men, especially if partners include commercial sex workers.
- Incubation is 3–5 days, may be as long as 14 days.

BASIS FOR RECOMMENDATIONS
Centers for Disease Control and Prevention, Workowski KA, Berman SM. Sexually transmitted diseases treatment guidelines, 2006. *MMWR Recomm Rep,* 2006; Vol. 55; pp. 1–94.

Comments: The CDC treatment guidelines provide clinicians with a readily available reference for STD treatments recommended by a panel of national and international experts in STD diagnosis, treatment, prevention, and control. These guidelines available electronically from: http://www.cdc.gov/

Mayaud P and McCormick D. 2001 National guideline for the management of chancroid. *Clinical Effectiveness Group (Assn of GUM and MSSVD) (www.mssvd.org.uk).* 2001.

Comments: This is the UK's guideline for chancroid. It provides an excellent synthesis of our current understanding of this STD with a comprehensive supporting bibliography. All UK guidelines include auditable outcome measures that may be of use to STD clinic directors and HMOs in the U.S.

HAEMOPHILUS INFLUENZAE

Paul G. Auwaerter, MD

MICROBIOLOGY
- Small aerobic Gram-negative coccobacilli found mainly in the respiratory tract.
- Six types generally recognized (Types a–f).
- Encapsulated, type B strain (with capsular antiphagocytosis and anticomplement virulence factors) accounts for most invasive and bacteremic pneumonia.
- Non-typeable strains less invasive and cause more otitis media, epiglottitis, acute exacerbations of chronic bronchitis (AECB), sinusitis, and nonbacteremic pneumonia. Biofilm formation may play role in upper respiratory tract infections.
- Fastidious organism; factors X (hemin) and V (nicotinamide-adenine-dinucleotide) required for growth on chocolate agar.

CLINICAL
- Major cause of bacterial otitis media, sinusitis, conjunctivitis, and community-acquired pneumonia.
- Infant Hib vaccination has made childhood meningitis, epiglottitis, bacteremia, and septic arthritis very uncommon in the U.S.
- Sensitivity of Gram-stain and cx probably ~50% for pneumonia. Confusion may arise due to oropharyngeal and tracheal colonization which is higher especially in smokers.
- Polysaccharide capsular antigen studies sometimes helpful in establishing rapid diagnosis in meningitis. Positive in 80–90% of *H. influenzae* meningitis.
- Up to 50% of strains worldwide produce beta-lactamase, meaning ampicillin or amoxicillin should only be used for significant infections if susceptibility is known.

SITES OF INFECTION
- Lung: acute exacerbations of chronic bronchitis (AECB), community acquired pneumonia
- HEENT: epiglottis, sinusitis, otitis media, periorbital cellulitis
- Bloodstream: bacteremia, rarely endocarditis
- CNS: meningitis (incidence markedly reduced with use of Hib vaccine, rare in adults)
- Musculoskeletal: septic arthritis (often weight-bearing joints), osteomyelitis
- Eye: conjunctivitis (subtype aegyptius (*H. influenzae* biotype 3): aka Brazilian purpuric fever)

TREATMENT
Non-threatening infections: Adults
- Examples: otitis media, acute exacerbation of chronic bronchitis (AECB), sinusitis.
- Amoxicillin-clavulanate 500 mg PO three times a day or 875 mg PO twice daily.

PATHOGENS

- Amoxicillin 500 mg PO three times a day. Expect resistance (25–50%), but use if sensitive or empirically treating certain infections (e.g., sinusitis or otitis media).
- TMP-SMX DS tabs 1 tab PO twice daily (some resistance ~7–10%).
- Cefuroxime 250–500 mg PO twice daily.
- Moxifloxacin 400 mg PO once daily, levofloxacin 500 mg PO daily.
- Azithromycin 500 mg PO × 1 then 250 mg daily × 4 days; clarithromycin 500 mg twice daily or XL 2 tabs 500 mg daily. Macrolides have inferior *iv vitro* susceptibility profiles compared to beta-lactam/beta-lactamase inhibitors and quinolones. Clinical significance usually uncertain.
- Treatment duration: otitis (10–14 days), AECB (5 days [quinolone]–14 days), sinusitis (10–14 days).

Meningitis
- Dexamethasone (0.15 mg/kg) 15–20 min before first dose of abx, then q6h × 4 days.
- **Adult:** ceftriaxone 2 g IV q12h (4 g max).
- Cefotaxime 2 g IV q4–6h (12 g max).
- Use ampicillin [2 g IV q4h] if sensitive.
- Beta-lactam alternative: ciprofloxacin 400 mg IV q8h or other FQ.
- **Pediatric:** cefotaxime <7 days, <2 kg: 50 mg/kg IV q12h; >2 kg: 50 mg/kg IV q8h; >7 days: >2 kg: 50 mg/kg IV q6–8h; Children: 200 mg/kg/day IV divided q6h.
- Ceftriaxone: <7 days old, >2 kg: 50 mg/kg IV q24h; >7 days old, >2 kg: 75 mg/kg IV q24h; Children: 100 mg/kg IV divided q12–24h.
- In pediatric studies, at 24 hrs, clinical condition and mean prognostic score significantly better in dexamethasone treated pts. F/u exams demonstrated significant decrease in audiologic and neurologic sequelae.
- Antibiotic duration: 10–14 days.

Severe infections: Adults
- Examples: pneumonia, epiglottis, severe cellulitis, septic arthritis.
- Ceftriaxone 1–2 g IV q24 or dosed q12h.
- Cefotaxime 2 g IV q6h.
- PCN alternative: ciprofloxacin 400 mg IV q8h or other FQ.
- Use ampicillin [2 g IV q6h] if sensitive.
- See specific diagnosis modules for details of nonantimicrobial management.

Prevention
- *Haemophilus influenzae* type b (Hib) vaccine—series of four immunizations: 2, 4, 6, and 12–15 mos.
- Catch-up schedule (if >1 mo. behind schedule): 0, 4 and 8 wks final [total of 3 if >12 mos at start].
- 3 conjugate vaccines licensed, if PRP-OMP used (Pedvax HIV or ComVax) dose at 6 mos not required. DTaP/Hib should not be used at 2, 4, or 6 mos, but can be used as booster thereafter.
- Some groups respond poorly to immunization, e.g., Native Alaskans.
- Absent spleen places host at increased risk for invasive *H. influenzae*. Hib immunization recommended prior to elective splenectomy.
- Otherwise Hib generally not recommended for those >5 yrs. age, but could be considered for those with chronically weakened immune system (including iatrogenic), cancer, and chemotherapy.
- Post-meningitis exposure prophylaxis: rifampin 600 mg PO once daily × 4 days (*MMWR* 1982, 31(50):672).
- Contact defined as spending at least 4 h/day for 5–7 days preceding hospitalization of index case. Rifampin only effective if taken within 7 days of index hospitalization.
- Chemoprophylaxis not recommended if all household contacts under 48 mos have completed Hib immunizations, unless child is immunocompromised.

OTHER INFORMATION
- The childhood vaccination campaign using protein-conjugated *H. influenzae* antigens has virtually eliminated invasive *H. influenzae* type B infections in children in the U.S.
- Adults usually infected with non-typeable *H. influenzae*, hence reason Hib immunization not recommended after age 5.

- Most *H. influenzae* treated empirically, since cx's not obtained for sinusitis, AECB, OM etc. Significance of beta-lactamase production or empiric use of amp/amoxicillin unclear in these settings.
- A pt with suspected epiglottitis should never be left unattended (e.g., for x-rays etc.)—it is better to forgo the test than to leave the pt alone.

BASIS FOR RECOMMENDATIONS

Murphy, TF. Haemophilus infections. *Principles and Practice of Infectious Diseases, 6th ed.* 2005; Vol. Chap 222; p. 2661.
Comments: Overview of diagnosis and management of all haemophilus infections including *H. influenzae*.

Red Book Immunization Recommendations: ages 0–6. *http://aapredbook.aappublications.org/resources/2007Imm Sched06.pdf*
Comments: Recommendations for Hib immunization, 2007.

KLEBSIELLA GRANULOMATIS/CALYMMATOBACTERIUM GRANULOMATIS/GRANULOMA INGUINALE/DONOVANOSIS

Noreen A. Hynes, MD, MPH

PATHOGENS

MICROBIOLOGY

- *Klebsiella granulomatis* is the proposed and preferred reclassification name of the organism *Calymmatobacterium granulomatis* and is a member of the family *Enterobacteriaceae*; reclassification is based upon nucleotide relatedness to other *Klebsiella* spp. especially to *K. rhinoscleromatis*, another tropical infection (nasal).
- Pleomorphic, intracellular (macrophages>neutrophils), Gram-negative bacillus surrounded by a well-defined bipolar staining capsule (seen with Wright, Giemsa, or Leishman stain) giving the organism a safety-pin appearance.
- Organism is difficult to demonstrate microbiologically because it does not grow on any standard microbiological laboratory media.
- Culture has been achieved in the research setting using peripheral blood mononuclear cells cultivated with fetal calf serum after exposure to vancomycin and metronidazole for decontamination; culture also has been successful on cyclohexamide-treated Hep-2 cell monolayers in RPMI 1640 medium, supplemented with fetal calf serum, penicillin, and vancomycin.

CLINICAL

- Causes the disease known as granuloma inguinale or donovanosis; the mode of transmission is uncertain but is believed to be sexually transmitted based on a history of sexual exposure prior to appearance and location of lesions; in ulcerative disease, transmission is likely via organisms in ulcers contacting microabraded skin or in non-ulcerative forms via transepithelial elimination of the organism to the skin surface with subsequent transmission via contact with microabraded skin. Rarity of the disease in very young children or sexually inactive persons further supports sexual contact as primary mode of transmission. Congenital transmission has been reported.
- Presence of infection increases risk of HIV acquisition at the time of sexual contact with an HIV-infected person.
- **History:** incubation period is unknown but estimated to be 1 to 3 wks; uncommon to see in developed, temperate countries. In endemic areas this is a disease of poverty and coinfection with other STDs is common. Important to ascertain history in pt with suspect infection of recent sexual contact while travelling in endemic areas in Southeast Asia, Papua New Guinea, KwaZulu/Natal (South Africa), India, Brazil, the Caribbean, and Australian aboriginal peoples.
- **Physical findings:** The first sign of infection occurring 8 days to 14 wks after exposure (median 2 wks), regardless of ultimate clinical presentation is a firm papule or subcutaneous nodule that later ulcerates. One of 4 clinical presentations (below) are seen; clinical diagnosis alone difficult due to pleomorphic presentation and atypical presentations. Systemic symptoms are rare. Differential diagnosis includes syphilis, lymphogranuloma venereum, chancroid, mycobacterial infections.
- **Ulcerogranulomatous presentation:** most common form seen; non-tender, single or multiple exuberant beefy red ulcer that bleeds when touched; autoinoculation may account for

lesions on adjacent skin. Prior to ulceration, there may be a soft, non-tender nodule, at times mistaken for a bubo that eventually ulcerates to the form described.

- **Hypertrophic or verrucous presentation:** an ulcer with an irregular, raised edge; lesion can be hard and look somewhat like a walnut. May mimic large condylomata acuminata secondary to human papillomavirus.
- **Necrotic presentation:** foul smelling, deep ulcer with underlying tissue destruction; tissue destruction can be rapid in this form of infection.
- **Sclerotic or cicatricial presentation:** rare form of infection; dry, non-bleeding ulcers are noted and suggests hematogenous spread and an increase risk of death. Ulcers spread to form plaques with subsequent fibrous band scarring. Lymphedema may accompany this form. Complications included stenosis of the vagina, urethra, or anus and requires surgical intervention.
- **Complications of untreated infection:** pseudoelephantiasis is most common complication (females [up to 5%] > males) and requires surgical intervention; hematogenous dissemination is unusual and may be fatal; autoinoculation can cause "kissing lesions on adjacent skin, also oral cavity and gastrointestinal tract involvement have been reported. A reported association with squamous cell carcinoma of the penis is suggested but unproven.
- **Diagnosis:** clinical suspicion is key to diagnosis! Direct microscopy—most practical and reliable; direct visualisation of intracytoplasmic bipolar staining inclusion bodies (Donovan bodies). To collect and make the smear, cleanse the lesion thoroughly using saline soaked gauze followed by patting dry with a dry gauze. Collect the sample by either deep punch biopsy within the ulcer or using a scalpel or curette, collect scrapings from the edge of the lesion. Biopsy samples should be sent to pathology with a request for *K. granulomatis,* chancroid, lymphogranuloma venereum and syphilis identification. Material collected by scraping should be spread between 2 clean microscope slides; allow the slide to air dry and provide to the laboratory with a request to look for Donovan bodies. Repeated sampling may be needed. Culture—isolation is difficult and impractical and is usually available only in research laboratories. Nucleic acid based tests—a polymerase chain reaction assay has been developed but is not commercially available. Serologic tests—a indirect immunofluorescent antibody test for *K. granulomatis* is insufficiently sensitive or specific for confirmatory diagnosis. Serological tests for syphilis and HIV should be collected.

SITES OF INFECTION

- **Male genitalia:** penis, scrotum, glans penis.
- **Female genitalia:** labia minora, fourchette, mons, cervix (10% of reported cases).
- **Extragenital sites:** occurs in ~5% of cases; autoinoculation sites include the gastrointestinal tract and oral cavity; spread via the hematogenous route include liver, spleen, bones, orbit.

TREATMENT

Genital and Mucocutaneous Infection

- Doxycycline 100 mg PO twice daily for at least 3 wks and until all lesions are healed (CDC recommended treatment).
- Alternative treatments: all for at least 3 wks and until all lesions are healed: azithromycin 1 m PO q wk or ciprofloxacin 750 mg PO twice daily or erythromycin base 500 mg PO 4 times a day or trimethoprim-sulfamethoxazole 1 double-strength (160 mg/800 mg) tab PO twice daily.

Genital and Mucocutaneous Infection in Pregnant and Lactating Women

- Erythromycin base 500 mg PO four times a day for at least 3 wks and until all lesions are healed. Some experts would add gentamicin 1 mg/kg IV q8h to this regimen.
- Erythromycin ethylsuccinate 800 mg PO four times a day for at least 3 wks and until all lesions are healed. Some experts would add gentamicin 1 mg/kg IV q8h to this regimen.

Genital and Mucocutaneous Infection in HIV-infected Persons

- Doxycycline 100 mg PO twice daily for at least 3 wks with gentamicin 1 mg/kg IV q8h until all lesions are healed.
- Alternative treatments: as for non-HIV infected, non-pregnant or lactating women along with gentamicin 1 mg/kg IV q8h.

Complicated Infection Secondary to Hematogenous Spread
- Manage in consultation with an expert.

OTHER INFORMATION
- The first description of granuloma inguinale was in 1882 by McLeod, a surgeon, at the Medical College of Calcutta, India. The causative organism was initially described by Donovan in 1905 while also working in India.
- Studies from Durban, South Africa had identified an association between infection and HLA-B57 as well as a trend toward resistance to infection among those who are HLA-A23.
- Efficiency of transmission has been reported to be between 2% and 50%, the latter reported among marital partners.
- Granuloma inguinale was successfully treated in the pre-antibiotic era with antimonial compounds. The first antibiotic shown to cure infection was streptomycin (in 1947) and was first used extensively in India, particularly for treating large lesions, for which long-term daily dosing was required.
- Other drugs that may have activity against *K. granulomatis* include chloramphenicol and high dose ceftriaxone (1–2 g/day).

BASIS FOR RECOMMENDATIONS
Centers for Disease Control and Prevention, Workowski KA, Berman SM. Sexually transmitted diseases treatment guidelines, 2006. *MMWR Recomm Rep*, 2006; Vol. 55; pp. 1–94.

Comments: These STD guidelines were developed by CDC after consultation with a group of professionals knowledgeable in the field of STDs. The information in this report updates the *Sexually Transmitted Diseases Treatment Guidelines, 2002*. The new guidelines include only one recommended regimen for the treatment of granuloma inguinale (GI)—doxycycline whereas in the 2002 guidelines trimethoprim sulfamethoxazole was also a first line choice but appears only as an alternative regimen in these new guidelines. These guidelines available electronically at: http://www.cdc.gov/std/treatment/

KLEBSIELLA SPECIES

Lisa A. Spacek, MD, PhD and Joseph Vinetz, MD

MICROBIOLOGY
- Gram-negative, aerobic bacilli of *Enterobacteriaceae* family. Human pathogens: *K. pneumoniae*, *K. oxytoca*, *K. rhinoscleromatis*, and *K. granulomatis*.
- Forms highly mucoid colonies w/ polysaccharide capsule, a virulence factor that inhibits phagocytosis. Easily cultured on non-selective media for sterile specimens or MacConkey's agar for contaminated specimens.
- Beta-lactamases are constitutive, usually produced at low levels, and provide resistance against ampicillin, amoxicillin, and ticarcillin. Few klebsiellae lack these beta-lactamases.
- Extended-spectrum beta-lactamases (ESBLs) are plasmid-mediated, confer multidrug resistance (TEM or SHV types), and are detected by *in vitro* resistance to ceftazidime and aztreonam. CTX-M type ESBLs, which hydrolyze ceftazidime much less than other 3rd and 4th generation cephalosporins, are becoming more prevalent.
- *Klebsiella pneumoniae* carbapenemases (KPC) confer broadest resistance and are detected by modified Hodge test.

CLINICAL
- Causes pneumonia and UTIs in immunocompetent hosts.
- Pneumonia due to *K. pneumoniae*, known as "Friedlander's disease" is seen in alcoholic or diabetic pts, involves upper lobes, and is associated with "currant jelly" sputum and abscess/cavity. CXR with classic "bowed fissure sign."
- Nosocomial infections include: pneumonia, sepsis, intra-abdominal infections (biliary tract infections and peritonitis), meningitis, and surgical wound infections.
- Primary pyogenic liver abscess due to *K. pneumoniae* described in diabetic pts in Korea, Taiwan, Singapore, and Indonesia.
- Risk factors for ESBL infection include recent hospitalization, residence in long-term care facility, and recent abx use.

PATHOGENS

SITES OF INFECTION
- Pulmonary: pneumonia, either nosocomial or community-associated.
- GU: UTI often catheter or instrumentation-related.
- HEENT: rhinoscleroma, due to *K. rhinoscleromatis,* is a chronic granulomatous infection of the upper and lower respiratory tract, endemic in E. Europe and Central America. Bx shows Mikulwicz cells, foamy macrophages with ingested bacilli.
- GI: peritonitis and biliary tract infection. Liver involvement primary monomicrobial pyogenic liver abscess due to *K. pneumoniae,* may also involve metastatic foci.
- Bacteremia: associated with primary organ system infection, peripheral, or central venous catheters.
- Ocular: endophthalmitis (rare), in association with liver abscess, diabetes.
- Chronic genital ulcerative disease, due to organism known previously as *Calymmatobacterium granulomatis,* now classified as *K. granulomatis.*

TREATMENT
Severe, nosocomial infection
- Initiate broad coverage to minimize risk of treatment with therapy to which organism is resistant. Once susceptibility is known, narrow coverage.
- For hospital-acquired, ventilator-associated pneumonia as per IDSA guidelines: cefepime 2 g IV q8h or ceftazidime 2 g IV q8h or imipenem 500 mg IV q6h or meropenem 1 g IV q8h or piperacillin-tazobactam 4.5 g IV q6h **plus** aminoglycoside or respiratory fluoroquinolone.
- For coverage of ESBLs in pneumonia, sepsis, complicated UTI or intra-abdominal infxn use carbapenems: imipenem 500 mg IV q6h or meropenem 1 g IV q8h. Ertapenem 1 g IV q24h and doripenem 500 mg IV q8h FDA-approved for complicated UTI or intra-abdominal infxn.
- In ESBLs, inconsistent activity seen with aminoglycosides, fluoroquinolones, and piperacillin-tazobactam. Avoid cephalosporins.
- Carbapenemase producers (KPCs) are resistant to carbapenems, penicillins, cephalosporins, fluoroquinolones, and aminoglycosides. Treatment options usually limited to colistin (preferred for UTIs) and tigecycline.
- Important to consider drug penetration at infection site, e.g., lung tissue penetration in pneumonia and urine concentration in UTIs. For liver abscess, percutaneous drainage for single, large abscess.

Mild to moderate, community-acquired infection
- Uncomplicated UTI: levofloxacin 250 mg PO once daily, ciprofloxacin 250 mg PO twice daily, or nitrofurantoin 100 mg PO four times daily or nitrofurantoin macrocrystals (Macrobid) 100 mg twice daily.
- Choose antimicrobials based on susceptibility.

BASIS FOR RECOMMENDATIONS
Mandell LA, Wunderink RG, Anzueto A, et al. Infectious Diseases Society of America/American Thoracic Society consensus guidelines on the management of community-acquired pneumonia in adults. *Clin Infect Dis,* 2007; Vol. 44 Suppl 2; pp. S27–72.
Comments: Guidelines regarding treatment of pneumoniae, community-acquired.

Solomkin JS, Mazuski JE, Baron EJ, et al. Guidelines for the selection of anti-infective agents for complicated intra-abdominal infections. *Clin Infect Dis,* 2003; Vol. 37; pp. 997–1005.
Comments: Guidelines regarding management of complicated intra-abdominal infections.

LACTOBACILLUS

Paul G. Auwaerter, MD

MICROBIOLOGY
- Gram-positive, facultative anaerobic rod.
- Normal flora of GI/GU tract.
- Produces lactic acid from glycogen providing for a low vaginal pH.

CLINICAL
- Rarely a human pathogen.
- Isolation usually indicates a contaminant. If pathogen, has a low level of virulence unless comorbidities present.

- Occasionally associated with polymicrobial bacteremia (often w/ streptococci, candida, Gram-negative enteric bacteria).
- Actual infection usually a marker of serious underlying disease, such as chronically ill, debilitated or immunosuppressed pts with overall mortality rate greater then 50% at 1 yr.
- Liver transplantation with roux-en-y choledochojejunostomy is a major risk factor for infection.
- Selective bowel decontamination, especially with vancomycin another major risk factor for infection.
- Other risk factors include: abdominal surgery, HIV, transplantation, neoplasm, immunosuppression, diabetes, and valvular disease.
- Portals of entry include: GI Tract, oropharynx, and female reproductive tract. No intravenous catheter related infections have been reported.

SITES OF INFECTION
- Dental: caries and periodontal abscesses.
- Abscesses: intraabdominal, splenic, hepatic.
- Bacteremia: frequently seen as part of polymicrobial process.
- Endocarditis (rare): few reports of pts with abnormal valves, following dental manipulation.
- Urinary tract infection: dominant organism of the female GU tract. Numbers usually fall with UTI or vaginal infection. May be a contaminant. Treat only with repeated isolation and appropriate symptoms.
- Chorioamnionitis/endometriosis: seen postpartum as complication of delivery.
- Meningitis: few case reports in neonates.

TREATMENT
Endovascular Infection
- Penicillin G 20 Million units/day for serious infections. Typical duration, 6-wk course.
- Gentamicin 1.3 mg/kg IV q8h (trough <1.5 mg/L) in combination with PCN often administered for pts with endocarditis.
- Resistance to vancomycin typical.

Odontogenic Infection
- Clindamycin 450 mg PO q6h.
- Extraction and drainage essential.

Intrabdominal Abscess
- Penicillin G 20 Million units/day divided q4h.
- Drainage of abscess cavity and necrotic debris necessary.

Probiotic Prophylaxis
- Effective dose 10^9–10^{11} microorganisms.
- Administration routes include direct inoculation or oral ingestion of yogurt or freeze dried preparations.
- Role unclear. Some studies using certain products may decrease rates of antibiotic associated diarrhea, *C. difficile* associated diarrhea or recurrent UTI in woman.

OTHER INFORMATION
- Often a component of probiotic therapy. No reports of associated infection, although therapy should probably be avoided in high-risk pts. See "detailed information" below.
- AIDS pts with lactobacillus infection noted to be late stage. CD4 <50, polymicrobial infections and other risk factors such as vancomycin therapy or GI manipulation.
- Treatment associated with clearance in most cases of serious disease. However, if true infection occurs, there is a relationship documented with high in-hospital and 1 yr mortality.

DETAILED INFORMATION
Other 1
Probiotic therapy: various mechanisms ascribed to benefit in both urogenital and gastrointestinal prophylaxis. Direct instillation to restore vaginal flora has proven to be beneficial in preventing urinary tract infection. Ingestion of organisms has also shown to be beneficial to restore vaginal flora. Menopausal state associated with depletion of vaginal lactobacilli spp. May be beneficial in preventing and decreasing the duration of certain diarrheal illness although debated

PATHOGENS

with recent contradictory literature in the prevention of vulvovaginal candidiasis and post operative bacterial complications.

BASIS FOR RECOMMENDATIONS

Author opinion.

Comments: No guidelines exist for treatment of lactobacillus infection. Main issues usually circle about whether recovery of organism represents actual infection or colonization.

LEGIONELLA SPECIES

John G. Bartlett, MD

MICROBIOLOGY

- Gram-negative aerobe, cause of legionellosis or Legionnaires' disease.
- Common environmental organism, found in warm water sources (e.g., 32°–45°C temperature range as in warm ponds, air chillers, or industrial air conditioning systems).
- At least 50 species and 70 serogroups, most common human pathogen: *L. pneumophila*.
- Side chain carbohydrate groups (O antigen determinants), thought to most contribute to serological classification of this species.
- Laboratory growth best achieved when using buffered charcoal yeast extract (bCYE). L-cysteine and ferric iron essential.

CLINICAL

- **Legionellosis:** disease caused by *Legionella*—mainly serious pneumonia (Legionnaires' disease), self-limited febrile disease (Pontiac fever) and miscellaneous, rare extrapulmonary infections—see sites of infection.
- Human pathogens: *Legionella pneumophilia* (most common) then *L. micdadei*, *L. bozemanae*, *L. dumoffii* and *L. longbeachae*.
- Habitat: water; most common outbreak source—cooling towers, evaporative condensers, hot and cold water supplies and spas.
- Epidemics: hospitals, hotels, spas.
- Risk factors for pneumonia: age >50, smoking, compromised CMI (steroids, etc.) and point source exposure.
- Diagnosis: urinary antigen (detects only *L. pneumophila* serogroup, causes 70–80% of total cases) and culture that requires special media (bCYE) and requires 3 days for growth with many false negatives due to technical reasons. Sputum DFA has fallen out of favor due to low sensitivity and specificity.

SITES OF INFECTION

- Lung: pneumonia (may be lobar, patchy, interstitial).
- Systemic: Pontiac fever, no pulmonary infiltrate but flu-like symptoms including fever, headache, myalgia. Usually described in epidemics, and self-limiting course.
- Miscellaneous sites (rare): prosthetic valve endocarditis, sternal wound infections, sinusitis, pericarditis, peritonitis, dialysis shunt infections abscesses.

TREATMENT

Pneumonia

- Preferred: levofloxacin 750 mg PO or IV once daily × 7–10 days, moxifloxacin 400 mg PO or IV once daily × 7–10 days or azithromycin 500 mg PO or IV once daily × 7–10 days.
- Rifampin 300 mg PO or IV twice daily (optional) + any other agent listed.
- Alternatives: erythromycin 1 g IV q6h, then 500 mg PO four times a day 7–10 days total.
- Ciprofloxacin 400 mg IV q12h, then 750 mg PO twice daily 7–10 days total.

Other sites

- Pontiac Fever: no abx (self-limited, and usually only diagnosed by delayed serologic testing).
- Endocarditis: fluoroquinolone (see above pneumonia) + rifampin 300 mg PO twice daily × 4–6 wks. Valve replacement usually required.

Outbreaks

- Most outbreaks are in hospitals, hotels or spas. However, most cases are sporadic.
- Identify water source by culture (50% of all water sources yield *Legionella* spp.).

- Match water source and clinical strains by species/serogroup and location.
- Sterilization interventions: (1) copper-silver ionization, (2) superheat to 60–77°C and flushing, (3) ultraviolet light for localized areas.

OTHER INFORMATION
- Natural habitat is water—all water.
- *Legionella* causes one common and important potentially fatal infection—Legionnaires' disease, also causes Pontiac fever and, rarely, endocarditis.
- Legionnaires' disease may be epidemic or sporadic, nosocomial or community acquired. Typical host: >40 yrs, smoker, compromised CMI (chemotherapy, organ tx, steroids).
- An intracellular pathogen, effective drugs in animal models include fluoroquinolones, macrolides, TMP-SMX, rifampin, and doxycycline.

BASIS FOR RECOMMENDATIONS
Mandell LA, Wunderink RG, Anzueto A, et al. Infectious Diseases Society of America/American Thoracic Society consensus guidelines on the management of community-acquired pneumonia in adults. *Clin Infect Dis,* 2007; Vol. 44 Suppl 2; pp. S27–72.
Comments: Basis for recommendations regarding treatment of pneumonia.

Stout JE, Yu VL. Legionellosis. *N Engl J Med,* 1997; Vol. 337; pp. 682–7.
Comments: General review. The authors claim the following are clinical clues to *Legionella* infection: high fever, CNS manifestations, LDH >700 units/mL and severe disease.

LEPTOSPIRA INTERROGANS

Joseph Vinetz, MD and Paul G. Auwaerter, MD

MICROBIOLOGY
- One of 4 spirochetes pathogenic for humans (others being *Borrelia burgdorferi* causing Lyme Disease, relapsing fever Borreliae, *Treponema pallidum* (syphilis).
- Zoonotic disease, transmitted by domestic animals (dogs, cattle, pigs, and more) and rodents (rats, mice).

CLINICAL
- In U.S., Hawaii endemic for leptospirosis; worldwide infection due to contact with contaminated body fluids of infected animals.
- Transmitted in inner cities, suburban and rural areas.
- Risk factors include farming, slaughterhouse work, walking in alleys, swimming in fresh water (triathletes, kayaking), flood victims.
- Consider dx in pts with fever, elevated bilirubin, transaminases ~5–7-fold above normal, elevated creatinine.
- Hx: abrupt onset fever, rigors, headache, severe leg muscle aches, in appropriate epidemiological context.
- May be biphasic illness: septicemic phase then immune phase (fever, meningitis).
- Complications: renal failure, hemorrhage, myocarditis; mortality can be as high as 25% if untreated.
- Diagnosis uncommon, depends on serology or culture in specialized laboratory.
- Diagnosis: two FDA-approved commercially available kits available, an indirect hemagglutination (MRL) and a dipstick test (PanBio). Dipstick test is better performer.
- In U.S., definitive testing (culture and microagglutination test (MAT) only available at CDC through state health labs, and at Vinetz lab at the U. of Cal San Diego (joseph_vinetz@ hotmail.com). Blood should be inoculated into Fletcher's media immediately for subsequent transport to specialized lab for culture.

SITES OF INFECTION
- Systemic illness with protean manifestations; multi-organ involvement possible.
- Weil's disease: acute fever, jaundice, splenomegaly, and nephritis. Severe infection includes bleeding manifestations including in lung.
- Liver: jaundice, transaminases can be normal or elevated typically no more than 5–7-fold above normal.

PATHOGENS

- Renal: acute renal failure usually resolves, but may require dialysis; ATN, interstitial nephritis; RBCs, WBCs, protein seen in urine; IV fluids may obviate need for dialysis.
- Pulmonary: hemorrhage; atypical pneumonia, scattered patchy infiltrates, or ARDS.
- Cardiac: EKG abnormalities common; myocarditis; heart failure.
- CNS: aseptic meningitis (CSF WBCs 10–1000); hyporeflexia and axonal motor weakness.
- GI: diarrhea, intestinal hemorrhage (rare); elevated lipase, amylase mimicking pancreatitis; mimics cholecystitis leading to surgery.
- Eye: conjunctival suffusion (dilated small vessels, in up to 50%), hypopyon, uveitis.
- Derm: non-specific rash can occur, not typical.

TREATMENT

Penicillin
- 1.5 million units IV q6hr for hospitalized pts × 5–7 days.

Doxycycline
- 100 mg twice daily IV or PO × 5–7 days.

CEFTRIAXONE
- 1 g IV q day × 5–7 days.

PROPHYLAXIS
- Doxycycline 200 mg PO once per wk when unavoidable exposure to environments at high risk for leptospirosis (e.g., swimming through jungle waters, kayaking in developing countries).
- Should be part of pre-travel medicine advice.

OTHER INFORMATION
- Cultures should be obtained prior to abx (inoculated into Fletcher's media); some commercial blood culture systems do not kill leptospires, and such specimens should be sent expeditiously to CDC or UCSD for specific leptospiral cultures.
- Epidemiology: leptospirosis can be transmitted to humans from vaccinated animals (e.g., cattle or dogs)—the vaccine may prevent animal illness but not the chronic carrier/transmission state.
- Case fatality rates can be as high as 10–15% in hepato-renal or pulmonary forms.
- Doxycycline has been shown to reduce clinical illness and mortality.

BASIS FOR RECOMMENDATIONS

Panaphut T, Domrongkitchaiporn S, Vibhagool A, et al. Ceftriaxone compared with sodium penicillin g for treatment of severe leptospirosis. *Clin Infect Dis,* 2003; Vol. 36; pp. 1507–13.

Comments: Important open label clinical trial comparing the use of ceftriaxone vs. penicillin for the treatment of severe leptospirosis; the two were equivalent, but late initiation of Rx does not always forestall death in severe cases.

LISTERIA MONOCYTOGENES

John G. Bartlett, MD

MICROBIOLOGY
- Small Gram-positive rod.
- Isolated from environmental sources such as water, sewerage, and foodstuffs.
- Grows on routine media. Micro labs may occasionally confuse with frequent contaminant diphtheroids.
- Main human pathogen is *Listeria monocytogenes.* Rarely, *L. ivanovii* has been described.
- Ability to grow in wide range of temperatures 4°C–37°C likely accounts for hardiness and ability to leave many foods in refrigerator capable of causing infection.

CLINICAL
- Colonizes colon in 5% of adults.
- Important cause of foodborne disease in vulnerable populations: pregnancy, compromised cell-mediated immunity, elderly.
- Important cause meningitis in compromised host (organ transplants, cancer therapy, steroids, lymphoma) and persons >50 yrs.
- Dx: culture from normally sterile site (CSF, blood, etc.). Serology (listeriolysin O antibody) helpful in the investigation of foodborne outbreaks.

SITES OF INFECTION
- CNS: meningitis, brain abscess, rhomboencephalitis (rare)
- Septicemia
- Pregnancy: bacteremia with stillbirth and/or premature delivery
- Gastroenteritis
- Endocarditis
- Focal infections: lymphadenitis, cellulitis, pneumonia, osteomyelitis, septic arthritis, conjunctivitis (all rare)

TREATMENT
Infections
- Principles: most common serious forms—meningitis, especially w/ defective cell-mediated immunity and age >50, also 3rd trimester pregnancy.
- Meningitis (preferred, consensus choice): ampicillin 2 g IV q4–6h +/– gentamicin 1.7 mg/kg IV q8h × ≥ 3 wks.
- Meningitis (alternative, pen allergy): TMP-SMX 3–5 mg/kg (trimethoprim) q6h IV × ≥3 wks.
- Bacteremia: use meningitis options × 2 wks.
- Brain abscess or rhomboencephalitis: use meningitis options × 4–6 wks.
- Gastroenteritis: usually no antibiotic treatment, but consider with susceptible host using amoxicillin or TMP-SMX × 7 days.

General Prevention Measures
- Thoroughly cook animal source food.
- Thoroughly wash raw vegetables.
- Avoid unpasteurized milk and food from unpasteurized milk.
- Wash hands, utensils, and cutting boards used with uncooked food.
- Keep ready-to-eat food cold.

Prevention: High Risk Persons
- High risk groups: pregnant women, CMI compromise (organ transplants, chronic steroids, infliximab or other TNF-antagonists, cancer chemotherapy, elderly).
- Avoid soft cheeses: Mexican style, feta, brie, camembert, blue cheese.
- Leftover foods and ready-to-eat foods should served only steaming hot.
- May wish to avoid food from delicatessen counters.

OTHER INFORMATION
- Major risks: (1) compromised CMI (steroids, transplants, cancer chemo Rx, AIDS); (2) 3rd trimester pregnancy; (3) occasional cases: age >50 yrs, diabetes, ulcerative colitis, antacids, cirrhosis.
- Mortality: meningitis 20%; endocarditis 50%; pregnant women 20% stillbirths.
- Major source: ingestion unpasteurized milk, fresh cheeses (especially imported, soft, ripened), ice cream, raw vegetables, fermented raw sausages, raw/cooked poultry, raw meats, smoked fish, deli meats, and hot dogs.
- Think Listeria when: "diphtheroids" in CSF, meningitis in compromised host or >50 yrs, fever 3rd trimester, foodborne outbreak w/ negative cultures.

BASIS FOR RECOMMENDATIONS
Rados C. Preventing Listeria contamination in foods. *FDA Consum*, 2004; Vol. 38; pp. 10–1.

Comments: Keep ready-to-eat food cold.

Tunkel AR, Hartman BJ, Kaplan SL, et al. Practice guidelines for the management of bacterial meningitis. *Clin Infect Dis*, 2004; Vol. 39; pp. 1267–84.

Comments: IDSA Guidelines for meningitis: For *L. monocytogenes* meningitis—preferred is Penicillin G or ampicillin (consider adding gentamycin). Alternatives are TMP-SMX or meropenem. Doses: Amp—12 g/day, gent 5 mg/kg/day, TMP-SMX 10–20 mg/kg (TMP)/day.

No authors listed. *Medical Letter*, 2004; Vol. 2; p. 22.

PATHOGENS

LYMPHOGRANULOMA VENEREUM (LGV)

Noreen A. Hynes, MD, MPH

MICROBIOLOGY

- *Chlamydia trachomatis* L1, L2, and L3 serovars (distinct from other chlamydia serovars causing either common genital chlamydial disease or trachoma).
- All chlamydia, including those serovars causing LGV, are obligate intracellular Gram-negative microorganisms but LGV serovars are lymphotrophic and are considered to cause systemic disease rather than superficial mucosal infection.
- The L2 serovar (and L2b strain) is the major cause of LGV outbreaks in the North America and Europe.

CLINICAL

- LGV is a re-emerging STD in developing countries, particularly among MSM with high-risk behaviors, among whom outbreaks have been recently reported. Co-infection with HIV and other STDs is a common feature in this risk group. LGV remains a risk among all sexually-active travelers to endemic areas especially Subsaharan Africa, India, Southeast Asia, Papua New Guinea, and some of the Caribbean Islands.
- Three stages have been described: primary, secondary, and tertiary. LGV enhances the acquisition and transmission of HIV infection.
- **Primary LGV:** may take one of four forms—a papule, an ulcer or erosion, a herpetiform (small) lesion, or non-specific <u>urethritis</u>. Manifests 3-30 days after sexual exposure; this stage is missed in 50–90% by both pt and provider; the lesions heal rapidly and without scarring.
- **Secondary LGV:** an inguinal syndrome characterized by acute lymphadenitis with bubo formation and/or anogenital syndrome characterized by acute hemorrhagic <u>proctitis</u>. Both forms are associated with fever and other constitutional symptoms associated with systemic infection including inflammation and swelling of lymph nodes and surrounding tissue. In heterosexual men tender inguinal and/or femoral painful unilateral <u>lymphadenopathy</u> is seen in 2/3 of cases; one node or the entire chain may be involved with our without bubo formation. Areas overlying nodes/buboes may ulcerate, discharge pus from >1 point and create chronic fistulae. "Groove sign" is noted when both inguinal and femoral chains are involved simultaneously, seen in 15–20% of cases. Complications of this stage include febrile arthritis, pneumonitis, and (rarely) perihepatitis. This stage usually occurs 2–6 wks after initial infection. Most pts do not progress beyond this stage.
- **Tertiary LGV:** very uncommon, seen predominantly in women. Results from the persistence of infection or progression into adjacent tissue leading to chronic inflammation and destruction of tissue in the involved area. Resulting clinical syndromes include proctitis, fistulae, acute proctocolitis (mimics Crohn's disease), esthiomene of the vulva (chronic granulomatous condition resulting in an "eaten away" appearance), rectal stricture, anal fistula, perirectal abscesses, lymphorrhoids, frozen pelvis. Infertility may result in women.
- **Differential diagnosis:** primary LGV—syphilis, chancroid, genital herpes, granuloma inguinale; secondary LGV—cat scratch disease, granuloma inguinale, secondary syphilis; tertiary LGV—rectal strictures secondary to carcinoma, Crohn's disease.
- **Diagnosis:** clinical suspicion is key; other etiologies of the presenting syndrome need to be excluded. Specimens should be collected for testing (if available). Genital or lymph node specimens (lesion swab or bubo aspirate) may be tested for *C. trachomatis* by culture (30–85% sensitivity), direct immunofluorescence, or nucleic acid detection. Nucleic acid amplification tests (NAAT) are the tests of choice for all chlamydia strains including LGV; importantly NAAT are not FDA cleared for detection of *C. trachomatis* from rectal specimens.
- Genotyping is not widely available and should be requested through the local state health department (CDC may assist the health department).
- Chlamydia serology (complement fixation test, single L-type immunofluorescence, or microimmunofluorescence) may support the clinical diagnosis but is not a definitive diagnostic test; four-fold rise of IgM and IgG antibody is diagnostic of active infection. A single IgM antibody >1:64 or single IgG >1:256 are considered positive for invasive disease. Interpretation of results is not standardized for LGV and validity in LGV proctitis is unknown. Serology has low sensitivity early in disease, but high titers alone without clinical signs/

symptoms does not confirm infection with LGV. Histology of collected biopsy specimens is not specific; the Frei test is no longer used.

- **Additional testing:** all pts with suspect LGV should be tested for other STDs including syphilis, chancroid, granuloma inguinalelink to donovaniasis module, herpes simplex, HIV, other genital chlamydia, gonorrhea, and trichomoniasis link.

SITES OF INFECTION

- **Primary LGV in men:** coronal sulcus → frenum → prepuce → penis → glans penis → scrotum. If intraurethral infection, a non-specific urethritis is seen with a thin, mucopurulent discharge. Uncommonly balanitis may be seen; extragenital lesions have been reported including in the oral cavity (tonsil).
- **Primary LGV in women:** posterior vaginal wall → the fourchette → the posterior lip of the cervix → the vulva. Cervicitis and urethritis may be more common than reported due to mischaracterization as common genital chlamydial infection. Extragenital lesions have been reported including in the oral cavity (tonsil).
- **Secondary LGV:** site determined by lymphatic drainage of the primary site of infection. Penis, anterior urethra → superficial and deep inguinal nodes; posterior urethra → deep iliac, perirectal nodes; vulva → inguinal nodes; vagina, cervix → deep iliac, perirectal, retrocrural, lumbosacral nodes; anus → inguinal nodes; and rectum → perirectal, deep iliac nodes.
- **Tertiary LGV:** anus, rectum, pelvis, vulva, perineum, colon.

TREATMENT

Recommended Regimen

- Doxycycline 100 mg PO twice daily × 21 days or until signs and symptoms have resolved, whichever is longer.

Alternative Regimen

- Erythromycin base 500 mg PO four times daily × 21 days or until signs and symptoms have resolved, whichever is longer.

Pregnant or Lactating Women

- Erythromycin base 500 mg PO four times daily × 21 days or until signs and symptoms have resolved, whichever is longer.
- There are **no** published data available regarding the safety and efficacy of azithromycin in the treatment of LGV in pregnancy; doxycycline is contraindicated in pregnancy.

HIV Infected Persons

- Use the same regimen (doxycycline or erythromycin) as in HIV-negative persons.
- Prolonged therapy may be needed due to delay in resolution of lesions.

Surgical Considerations

- Except for diagnostic specimen collection by lymph node aspiration (if indicated), surgical treatment should be avoided when possible. Surgical extirpation of buboes can lead to postoperative elephantiasis of the genitals.
- Surgery may be required in tertiary LGV where rectal strictures are present.
- Other indications for surgery include: bowel obstruction, persistent rectovaginal fistula, gross destruction of the anal canal, anal sphincter, or/and perineum.
- Antibiotic treatment must be given before, during, and following surgery.
- Consultation with an infectious disease specialist with expertise in STD complications is indicated in all cases requiring surgical intervention.

FOLLOW UP

General Recommendations

- Buboes may relapse in up to 20% after treatment.
- Re-examine the pt every 7 days until full resolution of all signs and symptoms; pts who demonstrate no improvement after 2 wks of adequate treatment should be referred to an infectious disease specialist with expertise in management of complicated STDs.
- Pts should refrain from sexual intercourse until treatment is completed and all sexual contacts evaluated and treated.

PATHOGENS

Management of Sexual Partners

- Persons with sexual contact with LGV pt within the 60 days before onset of pt's symptoms should be examined, tested for urethral or cervical chlamydial infection.
- For partners without clinical infection, treatment at the time of presentation should be for standard genital chlamydia.
- Treat with either doxycycline 100 mg orally twice a day for 7 days or azithromycin 1 g orally one time.

IMPORTANT

- Primary lesions in men: may be associated with lymphangitis of the dorsal penis leading to the formation of a large, tender lymph-like nodule—the bubonulus. The bubonuli can rupture and when this occurs sinus tracts may form as well as fistulous tracts communicating with the urethra. Fibrotic scars may form and phimosis may be noted.
- Primary lesions in women: may be associated, infrequently, with genital swelling.

BASIS FOR RECOMMENDATIONS

Centers for Disease Control and Prevention, Workowski KA, Berman SM. Sexually transmitted diseases treatment guidelines, 2006. *MMWR Recomm Rep,* 2006; Vol. 55; pp. 1–94.

Comments: The CDC treatment guidelines provide clinicians with a readily available reference for STD treatments recommended by a panel of national and international experts in STD diagnosis, treatment, prevention and control. These guidelines available electronically from cdc: http://www.cdc.gov/

Clinical Effectiveness Group of the British Association for Sexual Health and HIV (CEG/BASHH). 2006 National Guideline for the Management of Lymphogranuloma Venereum (LGV). *http://www.bashh.org/guidelines.asp,* 2006.

Comments: Comprehensive lymphogranuloma clinical, diagnostic and treatment guideline for the United Kingdom. This guideline is based upon the original UK guideline for LGV "Management of LGV", published in 1999 in Sex Transm Infect and then revised in 2001 and 2003 and the current UK Health Protection Agency guidance on the diagnosis of LGV.

MORAXELLA CATARRHALIS

John G. Bartlett, MD

MICROBIOLOGY

- Gram-negative diplococcus, appears identical to *N. gonorrhoeae.*
- Grows easily on blood chocolate agar.
- Colonizes upper airways in 5–15% of population, found only in humans.

CLINICAL

- Respiratory pathogen causing disease by contiguous spread: otitis, sinusitis, acute exacerbations of chronic bronchitis.
- Rare cause of invasive disease.
- Frequencies: pneumonia <1%, bacterial sinusitis 10%, bacterial exacerbations chronic bronchitis 20–30%.

SITES OF INFECTION

- Bacterial sinusitis (10–20%)
- Acute otitis media
- Acute exacerbations of chronic bronchitis: responsible for 10–20% of exacerbations, second only to *H. influenzae*
- Pneumonia (<1%)
- Bacteremia (<100 reported cases)
- Endocarditis (rare)
- Eye: keratitis

TREATMENT

Treatment

- Nearly all antibiotics commonly used for URIs are active except amoxicillin.
- TMP-SMX 1DS PO twice daily.
- Macrolides: erythromycin 500 mg PO four times a day, clarithromycin 500 mg twice daily or XL 1 g daily PO or azithromycin 500 mg × 1 then 250 mg PO daily.
- Tetracyclines: doxycycline 100 mg PO/IV twice daily.
- Parenteral cephalosporins: cefuroxime, cefotaxime, ceftriaxone.

- Oral cephalosporins: cefprozil (Cefzil) 200–500 mg twice daily, cefpodoxime (Vantin) 200–400 mg twice daily, cefuroxime (Ceftin) 250–500 mg twice daily, cefdinir (Omnicef) 300 mg twice daily.
- Fluoroquinolones: moxifloxacin (Avelox) 400 mg IV/PO daily, levofloxacin (Levaquin) 500 mg IV/PO daily.
- Penicillins: amoxicillin-clavulanate (Augmentin) 875/125 mg PO twice daily or XL 2000/125 PO twice daily.

OTHER INFORMATION

- Respiratory tract pathogen in sinusitis, otitis, AECB. Only a rare cause of pneumonia.
- Commonly produces beta-lactamase, 95% of strains resistant to amoxicillin.
- Nearly every abx except penicillin and amoxicillin work (TMP-SMX, cephalosporins, macrolides, doxycycline).
- Looks like meningococcus and gonococcus on Gram-stain. Causes contiguous disease, not invasive disease.

BASIS FOR RECOMMENDATIONS

Medical Letter, 2004; Vol. 2; p. 22.

Comments: Suggested drugs taken from this source.

MORGANELLA

PATHOGENS

Aimee Zaas, MD

MICROBIOLOGY

- Facultative anaerobic Gram-negative rod. Non-lactose fermenter in the same family as Proteus.
- Morganella only has single member in its genus *M. morganii*, and two subspecies: *M. morganii* and *M. sibonii*, which differ only in trehalose fermentation.
- Naturally resistant to penicillin, 1st–2nd generation cephalosporins, macrolides, sulfamethoxazole.
- Generally sensitive to aminoglycosides, piperacillin, ticarcillin, 3rd–4th gen cephalosporins, carbapenems, quinolones.
- Tigecycline not reliably effective due to ArcAB efflux pump, although may show synergy *in vitro* with other antimicrobials.

CLINICAL

- Environmentally ubiquitous, part of normal colonic flora.
- Rare cause of human infection, most commonly UTIs.
- Risk factors: old age, immune compromise, prolonged hospital stay, urinary catheter.
- "Urea splitter," but stones seen less frequently than Proteus due to less effective urease enzyme.
- Extended-spectrum beta-lactamases, inducible beta-lactamases and fluoroquinolone resistance reported.
- Beta-lactamase is inducible, chromosomal AmpC type. May confer resistance to imipenem in some isolates.

SITES OF INFECTION

- Urinary tract infection (most common): urea splitter, look for elevated urine pH.
- Bacteremia (rare): one report related 11/19 bacteremic cases related to surgical wounds. Also described secondary to urinary or hepatobiliary pathology.
- Bacteremia is polymicrobial in 40% (described in single series).
- Surgical wound infections, nosocomial spread reported.
- Meningitis, endophthalmitis, pericarditis (case reports).
- Septic arthritis (rare): usually in damaged joint.
- Neonatal sepsis and chorioamnionitis.

TREATMENT
Preferred Treatment
- Imipenem 500 mg IV q6h or meropenem 1.0 g IV q8h, adjust dose if necessary for renal function.
- Carbapenems are considered first line therapy due to inducible cephalosporinases, and presence of extended-spectrum beta-lactamases in some isolates.
- One *in vitro* study has shown 20 isolates of Morganella to be susceptible to ertapenem.
- Duration of treatment UTI (generally complicated): 7 days.
- Duration of treatment bacteremia: 14 days.
- Tigecycline is not reliably effective.

Alternative Treatments
- Decided based upon susceptability profile.
- Cefepime 2.0 g IV q8–12h.
- Ciprofloxacin 500 mg PO/400 mg IV q12, has best *in vitro* activity of all quinolones.
- Piperacillin 3 g IV q6 or ticarcillin 3g IV q4.
- Aminoglycosides can be used alone for treatment of UTI; dose gentamicin or tobramycin 1 mg/kg IV q24; 3 mg/kg/day amikacin.

OTHER INFORMATION
- Surveillance of ICU's report 16–27% resistance to 3rd generation cephalosporins. Fluoroquinolone resistance reported in Taiwan.
- Failure of therapy after initial success indicates possible inducible beta-lactamase.
- Skin and soft tissue infections described with snake bites. *M. morganii* found commonly in oral flora of snakes. Has been described as causing human abscesses after the bite of Bothrops (venomous pit vipers mostly seen in Central and South America).

BASIS FOR RECOMMENDATIONS
Author opinion.
Comments: No guideline recommendations exist that focus specifically on Morganella spp.

MYCOBACTERIUM ABSCESSUS

Paul G. Auwaerter, MD

MICROBIOLOGY
- Human pathogen, occasional environmental contaminant. Present in water, sewerage, vegetation.
- Considered among the most pathogenic and chemotherapy-resistant of rapid-growing mycobacterium.
- Formerly part of "*M. chelonae*-complex," but important to distinguish as antimycobacterial therapy more difficult with *M. abscessus senso strictu*.
- Occasionally confused with *Corynebacterium* spp. (described as diphtheroid growing in broth systems).

CLINICAL
- Southeastern U.S. (Texas-Florida) considered endemic, but reported throughout U.S.
- Community-acquired and health-care-associated disease.
- Relatively antibiotic resistant.
- Diagnosis by AFB culture +/– compatible histopathology and stains.
- ATS criteria for Pulmonary disease: The minimum evaluation of suspected of nontuberculous mycobacterial (NTM) lung disease: (1) chest radiograph or, in the absence of cavitation, chest high-resolution computed tomography (HRCT) scan; (2) three or more sputum specimens for acid-fast bacilli (AFB) analysis; and (3) exclusion of other disorders, such as tuberculosis (TB). Clinical, radiographic, and microbiologic criteria are equally important and all must be met to make a diagnosis of NTM lung disease. ATS states that criteria apply to symptomatic pts with radiographic opacities, nodular or cavitary, or an HRCT scan that shows multifocal bronchiectasis with multiple small nodules. These criteria fit best with Mycobacterium avium complex (MAC), *M. kansasii*, and *M. abscessus*. There is not enough known about most other NTM to be certain that these diagnostic criteria are universally applicable for all NTM respiratory pathogens.

- Microbiologic criteria: positive culture results from at least two separate expectorated sputum samples or at least one bronchial wash or lavage, or transbronchial or other lung biopsy with mycobacterial histopathologic features (granulomatous inflammation or AFB) and positive culture for NTM or biopsy showing mycobacterial histopathologic features (granulomatous inflammation or AFB) and one or more sputum or bronchial washings that are culture positive for NTM.
- Pts who are suspected of having NTM lung disease but who do not meet the diagnostic criteria should be followed until the diagnosis is firmly established or excluded.

SITES OF INFECTION

- Pulmonary disease (most common): risk factors bronchiectasis, cystic fibrosis, gastroesophageal disorders; older women without apparent underlying pulmonary disease or immunosuppression.
- Health-care-associated disease: surgical wound infections (mammoplasty, facial plastic surgery, cardiac surgery), post-injection abscesses.
- Cutaneous: post-traumatic wound infections after break in skin followed by contact w/ contaminated soil or water, localized (cellulitis/abscess) or may develop sporotrichoid appearance of ascending lymphadenitis.
- Lymphadenitis: rare.
- Disseminated disease (mostly immunosuppressed w/ corticosteroids): rare, usually presents w/ multiple draining erythematous cutaneous nodules.
- Bacteremia/endocarditis: described in hemodialysis pts.

TREATMENT

Limited, localized extrapulmonary disease

- Macrolides only compounds with reliable *in vitro* susceptibility.
- Clarithromycin alone (500 mg PO twice daily).
- Acquired mutational resistance has not been observed when treating localized infections with macrolide monotherapy.
- Amikacin (10–15 mg/kg/day IV) may be added, most active aminoglycoside. Use levels to adjust dosing. Some use 25 mg/kg three times weekly.
- Amikacin can be combined with high dose cefoxitin (12 g/day) typically for two wks until clinical improvement in severe cases.
- Imipenem 500 mg IV q6–8h may be substituted for cefoxitin.
- Duration guided by clinical response; typically 4 mos. Osteomyelitis 6-mo minimum recommended.
- Infected foreign bodies should be removed.
- Surgical: indicated for abscesses, extensive disease, when drug therapy is limited by resistance or adverse effects, and in localized pulmonary disease poorly responsive to medical therapy.

Pulmonary or serious extrapulmonary disease

- *In vitro* data has not yielded effective regimen for treating pulmonary disease. May not achieve sputum culture negativity even with 12 mos of therapy. Lung disease should be considered a chronic, incurable infection. Susceptibility testing should guide therapy in case of macrolide-resistance. Goal is to limit progression and control symptoms.
- Combination therapy always recommended: clarithromycin 500 mg PO twice daily plus amikacin (15 mg/kg/day IV) plus either cefoxitin (2 g q4hr IV) or imipenem (1 Gram-q6hr) IV.
- Duration: combination therapy w/ injectable agents + clarithromycin at least 2–4 mos but duration often limited by adverse effects, then switch to oral clarithromycin 500 mg PO twice daily or 1000 mg xr once daily or oral azithromycin 250 mg PO once daily ("suppressive treatment") indefinitely.
- Tigecycline 100 mg IV load then 50 mg IV q12h. Little reported clinical data but may be *in vitro* susceptable and could be substituted as one of the injectables. Often poorly tolerated due to GI distress.
- Linezolid (600 mg q12h) is potentially useful oral agent (combined with clarithromycin) in pts in whom parental tx not tolerated or feasible; no clinical studies to guide this practice, and long-term risks exist (neuropathy, optic neuritis, cytopenias). Some use 600 mg once daily to reduce risk of toxicities.

PATHOGENS

- For refractory or macrolide-resistant pulmonary disease consider periodic 1–2 wk courses of parenteral agents as tolerated.
- Treatment duration: 6 mos for extrapulmonary, at least 12 mos for pulmonary (see above).
- Often not considered a medically curable condition, but rather that antibiotics contain the infection from spreading.
- Not infrequent that sputum remains culture positive while on drug therapy (with clarithromycin for example) and the isolate remains reported as susceptible to macrolides *in vitro*.
- Surgery, if feasible, is only known predictably curative strategy.

OTHER INFORMATION

- Of rapidly growing mycobacteria, *M. abscessus* is most virulent respiratory pathogen. Pulmonary disease is often incurable medically, and careful consideration should be weighed as whether surgery can render a cure (consider referral to center with significant experience).
- Clinical significance of a positive culture should be carefully evaluated (see ATS diagnostic criteria).
- Drug susceptibility testing should be used to guide antibiotic therapy. *M. abscessus* is resistant to first-line tuberculosis drugs (isoniazid, rifampin, pyrazinamide, ethambutol).
- Almost all isolates resistant to tetracycline, doxycycline, ciprofloxacin. 5–10% of isolates susceptible to gatifloxacin and moxifloxacin.
- Cluster of pts with *M. abscessus* infection after cosmetic injections by nonmedical practitioners in New York City area in 2002.

BASIS FOR RECOMMENDATIONS

Griffith DE, Aksamit T, Brown-Elliott BA, et al. An official ATS/IDSA statement: diagnosis, treatment, and prevention of nontuberculous mycobacterial diseases. *Am J Respir Crit Care Med*, 2007; Vol. 175; pp. 367–416.
Comments: Guideline reviews evaluation and treatment recommendations presented in this module.

MYCOBACTERIUM AVIUM-COMPLEX (MAC, MAI, NON-HIV)

Susan Dorman, MD and Christopher J. Hoffmann MD, MPH

MICROBIOLOGY

- *M. avium* and *M. intracellul* are slow growing mycobacteria (10–21 days on solid media).
- *M. intracellulare* is principally causes pulmonary disease. *M. avium* principally causes disseminated disease (among immunocompromised people).
- Environmental sources, especially water, are the reservoir for most human infections.

CLINICAL

- *M. avium* complex (*M. avium* and *M. intracellulare*) strains are frequent causes of mycobacterial lung disease in the USA.
- No convincing evidence for person-to-person spread of MAI.
- **ATS criteria (2007):** The minimum evaluation of suspected of nontuberculous mycobacterial (NTM) lung disease: (1) chest radiograph or, in the absence of cavitation, chest high-resolution computed tomography (HRCT) scan; (2) three or more sputum specimens for acid-fast bacilli (AFB) analysis; and (3) exclusion of other disorders, such as tuberculosis (TB). Clinical, radiographic, and microbiologic criteria are equally important and all must be met to make a diagnosis of NTM lung disease. ATS states that criteria apply to symptomatic pts with radiographic opacities, nodular or cavitary, or an HRCT scan that shows multifocal bronchiectasis with multiple small nodules. These criteria fit best with Mycobacterium avium complex (MAC), *M. kansasii*, and *M. abscessus*. There is not enough known about most other NTM to be certain that these diagnostic criteria are universally applicable for all NTM respiratory pathogens.
- **Microbiologic criteria:** positive culture results from at least two separate expectorated sputum samples or at least one bronchial wash or lavage, or transbronchial or other lung biopsy with mycobacterial histopathologic features (granulomatous inflammation or AFB) and positive culture for NTM or biopsy showing mycobacterial histopathologic features (granulomatous inflammation or AFB) and one or more sputum or bronchial washings that are culture positive for NTM.

- Commercially available nucleic acid probe test can identify cultured mycobacteria as MAI. No PCR or other rapid test is FDA-approved for direct use on sputum or blood.
- Antimicrobial susceptibility testing: correlation between *in vitro* susceptibility testing and clinical response is only clear for macrolides. Macrolide susceptibility should be assessed before initiating therapy and in the setting of treatment failure. There is no clear role for using susceptibility results for other agents as *in vitro* susceptibility results do not appear to correlate with rifampin, ethambutol, and aminoglycoside clinical response. *In vitro* susceptibility and clinical response fluoroquinolones is unclear (absence of prospective study). Macrolides should not be used in treating macrolide resistant disease and fluoroquinolones probably provide little benefit in fluoroquinolone-resistant disease.

Sites of Infection

- Pulmonary—two major manifestations: a) cavitary, b) nodular with bronchiectasis. Cavitary disease can have upper lobe location (like TB). Associated conditions/risk factors: cystic fibrosis, silicosis, tobacco smoking, bronchiectasis, pectus excavatum/thoracic scoliosis.
- Pulmonary—"hot tub lung:" acute, diffuse lung disease with cough/fever/hypoxia due to high inhalation inoculum. Non-necrotizing granulomatous inflammation +/– interstitial pneumonia. Pathogenesis unclear-"infection" vs. hypersensitivity.
- Extrapulmonary localized (skin, soft tissue, joints, tendons, bones): less common than pulmonary disease, but may occur after trauma or environmental exposure.
- Cervical lymphadenitis: typically in children ages 1–5 yrs. May occur in immunocompetent children.
- Disseminated: rare except in AIDS pts. Typically occurs in immunocompromised hosts (exogenous immunosuppression, SCID, IFN gamma or IL–12 pathway disorders).

Treatment

Pulmonary MAI Disease

- **Severe or cavitary disease:** macrolide (clarithromycin 500 mg PO twice daily or azithromycin 500 mg PO daily) plus ethambutol 15 mg/kg/day PO plus rifampin 600 mg PO daily. Initial 2 mos of higher dose ethambutol 25 mg/day no longer recommended. Note: use of ethambutol and rifampin reduces emergence of macrolide resistance.
- **Nodular (non-cavitary) disease:** macrolide (clarithromycin 1000 mg tiw or azithromycin 500 mg PO tiw) plus ethambutol 25 mg/kg PO tiw plus rifampin 600 mg PO tiw Note: intermittent therapy not recommended for pts with cavitary lung disease. Use of ethambutol and rifampin reduces emergence of macrolide resistance.
- **Aminoglycoside choice:** sometimes used adjunctively in severe disease or treatment refractory infections. Amikacin (15 mg/kg/dose, max 1 g, 3 times per wk IV) most active against MAI, and the traditional choice. Alternative: streptomycin 15 mg/kg/dose (max 1 g) 3 times per wk IM. Severity of MAI disease, immunosuppression, toxicities important in balancing when considering use of aminoglycoside. Macrolide resistant-MAI: aminoglycoside with ethambutol, rifampin and possibly, isoniazid. Moxifloxacin may also have a role. Fluoroquinolones have activity against MAI but prospective studies are lacking to guide optimal use.
- Clinical expectations of treatment: symptomatic and radiographic improvement within 2–6 mos, and conversion of sputum culture from positive to negative within approximately 6 mos. Outcome usually better with noncavitary (compared with cavitary) disease.
- **Duration:** not definitively established. Typical duration is 18–24 mos total, including 12 mos after sputum culture becomes negative for MAI. Monitor sputum smear and culture monthly.
- Rifabutin is alternative to rifampin. No demonstrated superiority of rifabutin vs rifampin (rifampin usually better tolerated). No head to head comparisons of clarithromycin vs azithromycin for pulmonary MAI; though azithromycin has fewer drug-drug interactions, and is often better tolerated, especially if used tiw.
- **Adjunctive treatment:** bronchial hygiene (inhaled beta agonists, mucus-clearing devices) and antibiotic treatment as needed for nonmycobacterial pulmonary superinfection.
- **Role of surgery:** no randomized studies, typically reserved for pts with poor response to medical therapy and who are good surgical candidates, generally localized/cavitary disease. Should be performed in centers with extensive experience. Surgical resection of a solitary pulmonary nodule is considered curative.

PATHOGENS

- **Monitoring for drug adverse reactions:** hepatotoxicity (rifampin, rifabutin), uveitis (rifabutin), ocular toxicity (ethambutol), nephrotoxicity and/or ototoxicity (aminoglycosides).
- Withholding treatment is acceptable in pts with close follow-up to determine if disease is significant (e.g., continue to collect sputa for culture) or who have mild disease and poorly tolerate therapy. In both cases close follow-up (including CT imaging) is needed. Of note, pts with upper lobe fibrocavitary disease tend to progress rapidly and withholding therapy is not recommended.

Hot Tub Lung
- Discontinuation of exposure necessary.
- No consensus opinion about role of corticosteroids and/or antibiotics. Anecdotal reports of rapid improvement after stopping exposure (no steroids or antibiotic).

Cervical Lymphadenitis in Children
- Excisional surgery without chemotherapy (success rate of >95%).
- If surgical risk high (e.g., facial nerve involvement), macrolide-containing multidrug regimen is reasonable, but limited experience, optimal duration unknown.
- Incisional biopsy, or use of non-macrolide-containing regimens often associated with persistent clinical disease including sinus tract formation.

Extrapulmonary localized disease
- Surgery (excisional or debridement) plus macrolide-containing multidrug regimen (same doses as for pulmonary disease).
- Optimal duration unknown, but usually follow pulmonary guidelines.

Disseminated disease
- Macrolide-containing multidrug regimen as for cavitary pulmonary disease.
- Optimal duration unknown and dependent on clinical response and predisposing factors.

FOLLOW UP
- For pulmonary disease, monthly sputum for AFB stain and culture recommended monitoring.
- Clinical expectations of treatment: symptomatic and radiographic improvement within 2–6 mos, and conversion of sputum culture from positive to negative within approximately 6 mos. Outcome usually better with noncavitary (compared with cavitary) disease.
- Macrolide-resistant infection: aminoglycoside plus high dose ethambutol 25 mg/kg/day PO plus rifabutin 300–600 mg/day PO. Surgery should be considered. Clinical outcome poor; most pts who remain culture positive die of progressive pulmonary disease with respiratory failure (Griffith DE et al. *Am J Respir Crit Care Med* 2006;174:928).
- Pts respond best to therapy the first time it is administered, therefore multidrug therapy (not clarithromycin monotherapy) is important to initiate the first time pts receive therapy for MAC pulmonary disease.

OTHER INFORMATION
- Interpretation of a single positive respiratory culture for MAI should take into account the possibility of environmental contamination.
- MAI lung disease is typically associated with persistently positive respiratory cultures, with heavy MAI growth. Most experts recommend a thoracic CT as part of diagnostic workup for pulmonary MAI.
- For pulmonary MAI disease, ATS diagnostic criteria (see "Clinical" information above) are guidelines and applicability in specific pts should be carefully considered by an experienced clinician.
- For pts with positive MAI respiratory cultures in whom decision is made not to treat MAI, long-term close followup is essential (symptoms, repeat sputum exams, thoracic CT scans).
- Monitoring for drug toxicity is essential given the long duration of therapy and typical older age of affected individuals: rifampin (hepatitis), rifabutin (uveitis especially when used with macrolide, hepatitis, polyarthralgias), ethambutol (retrobulbar neuritis manifest by decreased visual acuity or red-green color discrimination), amikacin (ototoxicity, nephrotoxicity), clarithromycin (GI upset), azithromycin (reversible hearing loss, GI upset).

BASIS FOR RECOMMENDATIONS

Griffith DE, Aksamit T, Brown-Elliott BA, et al. An official ATS/IDSA statement: diagnosis, treatment, and prevention of nontuberculous mycobacterial diseases. *Am J Respir Crit Care Med*, 2007; Vol. 175; pp. 367–416.

Comments: Comprehensive document that is the basis of recommendations in this module. It is also well worth reading for pts with MAC not responsive to initial therapy for additional detailed information.

MYCOBACTERIUM CHELONAE

Susan Dorman, MD and Christopher J. Hoffmann MD, MPH

MICROBIOLOGY

- Rapidly growing, hardy, ubiquitous mycobacterium commonly found in municipal tap water.
- Results of *in vitro* drug susceptibility tests should be used to guide antimicrobial therapy (though susceptibility is unpredictable).
- Lab should differentiate from *M. abscessus* with which it can be confused, since this organism is more difficult to treat.

CLINICAL

- May cause soft tissue infections, including post-surgical or deep infections/disseminated disease in both immunocompetent and immunocompromised hosts.
- *M. chelonae* may be a pathogen or environmental contaminant. Careful clinical evaluation may be required to determine significance of a positive culture, especially from respiratory secretions.
- Nosocomial pseudo-outbreaks related to contaminated bronchoscopes have been reported.
- Physical exam: disseminated skin lesions typically erythematous subcutaneous nodules on extremities, but may also cause cellulitis or abscesses.
- Histopathology of skin lesions: usually granulomatous inflammation, but can be neutrophilic predominance with abscess formation. AFB stain positive in 25% of cases. Send biopsy specimens for AFB stain, AFB culture, and histopathology. No rapid diagnostic tests (for use on primary specimen) FDA-approved or commercially available.

SITES OF INFECTION

- Localized, community-acquired infections (cellulitis, abscess, osteomyelitis) may occur or follow medical procedures in immunocompetent persons. (*M. fortuitum* is more likely pathogen after soft tissue trauma such as with a motor vehicle collision.).
- Disseminated skin disease: most common manifestation, typically in immunosuppressed hosts on corticosteroids (unusual in HIV/AIDS pts).
- Nosocomial: wound infections following surgery, liposuction, needle injection (botulinum toxin injection), and catheter-related infections (intravenous catheter most common; hemodialysis shunts and chronic peritoneal dialysis catheters also reported).
- Ocular: keratitis after LASIK procedures increasingly reported (*Ophthalmology* 2003;110:276). Slit lamp exam: typical appearance is "cracked windshield" pattern. Obtain specimen for AFB stain/microscopy and mycobacterial culture; avoid ophthalmic steroids.
- Pulmonary: rare cause of disease (unlike related *M. abscessus*).

TREATMENT

Localized infections

- Clarithromycin monotherapy (500 mg PO twice daily) typically adequate. There is less clinical experience with azithromycin but response is likely similar.
- Surgical debridement is often a helpful adjunct to antibiotic treatment.
- Acquired resistance to clarithromycin has not been observed when clarithromycin has been used as monotherapy for localized disease.

Disseminated or extensive disease

- Clarithromycin monotherapy (500 mg PO twice daily) resulted in 100% response rate and low relapse rate in small prospective study of disseminated skin disease (*Ann Intern Med* 1993;119:482).
- During initial treatment, multidrug therapy may prevent development of acquired resistance: clarithromycin 500 mg PO twice daily **plus** either tobramycin 5 mg IV/kg/day or imipenem 0.5–1 g IV q6h or linezolid 600 mg IV/PO twice daily for 4–8 wks.
- Treatment duration: typically 6 mos.

PATHOGENS

- Moxifloxacin (400 mg daily), and linezolid (600 mg twice daily) have activity *in vitro* against most *M. chelonae* isolates. Clinical experience for *M. chelonae* is limited.
- Cefoxitin not active against *M. chelonae*.

Keratitis (LASIK-related)

- Clarithromycin 500 mg PO twice daily plus topicals (tobramycin 0.3%, 2 gtts q4h plus either gatifloxacin 0.3%, 1 gtt q4h or moxifloxacin 0.5%, 1 gtt q4h).
- Topical ophthalmic moxifloxacin 0.5% or topical ophthalmic gatifloxacin 0.3% may be more effective than other fluoroquinolones or ciprofloxacin ophthalmic for *M. chelonae* keratitis.
- Avoid use of ophthalmic fluoroquinolone monotherapy without concomitant systemic clarithromycin.
- Surgical debridement may shorten course (*Ophthalmology* 2003;110:276).
- Avoid ophthalmic corticosteroids.

BASIS FOR RECOMMENDATIONS

Griffith DE, Aksamit T, Brown-Elliott BA, et al. An official ATS/IDSA statement: diagnosis, treatment, and prevention of nontuberculous mycobacterial diseases. *Am J Respir Crit Care Med*, 2007; Vol. 175; pp. 367–416.

Comments: Although this organism does not commonly cause lung disease, pulmonary or deep infections are recommended to be treated with combination therapy for periods of 4–12+ mos.

Hamam RN, Noureddin B, Salti HI et al. Recalcitrant post-LASIK Mycobacterium chelonae keratitis eradicated after the use of fourth-generation fluoroquinolone. *Ophthalmology*, 2006; Vol. 113; pp. 950–954.

Comments: Case report and review of recent literature on LASIK keratitis. Newer ophthalmic fluoroquinolones (gatifloxacin and moxifloxacin) have increased activity against *M. chelonae* compared with older fluoroquinolones.

Wallace RJ, Tanner D, Brennan PJ, et al. Clinical trial of clarithromycin for cutaneous (disseminated) infection due to *Mycobacterium chelonae. Ann Intern Med*, 1993; Vol. 119; pp. 482–6.

Comments: Prospective, open, noncomparative trial of clarithromycin as single drug therapy for cutaneous disseminated *M. chelonae* infection. 14 pts (10 with disseminated disease enrolled), treated with clarithromycin monotherapy, typically 500 mg bid for 6 mos. Response rate 100%, with approximately 10% relapse rate (1 pt stopped therapy after 3.5 mos and relapsed with clarithromycin resistant strain).

MYCOBACTERIUM FORTUITUM

Paul G. Auwaerter, MD

MICROBIOLOGY

- Rapidly growing mycobacterium.
- Typically takes 3 to 7 days for clinical cultures to become positive, but may require longer incubation.
- Reservoirs: soil, water, animals, marine life. Worldwide distribution.
- *M. fortuitum* group includes *M. peregrinum, M. houstonese, M. boenickei, M. mageritense, M. senegalense,* and *Mycobacterium setense* sp. nov. Differentiation only by molecular testing.

CLINICAL

- Most commonly causes skin, bone and joint disease in both immunocompetent and immunosuppressed. True pulmonary infections are rare.
- Cases recently related to manicures, pedicures using contaminated soaks/baths.
- Nosocomial disease outbreaks (e.g., sternal wound infections, plastic surgery wound infections, postinjection abscesses) have been reported.
- Pseudo-outbreaks related to contaminated bronchoscopes or hospital water supplies have been reported.
- No strong evidence of human to human spread.
- **Diagnostic criteria (nonpulmonary):** recovery of organism from wound or tissue without alternative explanation.
- **ATS criteria (pulmonary disease):** The minimum evaluation of suspected of nontuberculous mycobacterial (NTM) lung disease: (1) chest radiograph or, in the absence of cavitation, chest high-resolution computed tomography (HRCT) scan; (2) three or more sputum specimens for acid-fast bacilli (AFB) analysis; and (3) exclusion of other disorders, such as tuberculosis (TB). Clinical, radiographic, and microbiologic criteria are equally important and all must be met to make a diagnosis of NTM lung disease. ATS states that criteria apply to symptomatic

pts with radiographic opacities, nodular or cavitary, or an HRCT scan that shows multifocal bronchiectasis with multiple small nodules. These criteria fit best with *Mycobacterium avium* complex (MAC), *M. kansasii,* and *M. abscessus.* There is not enough known about most other NTM to be certain that these diagnostic criteria are universally applicable for all NTM respiratory pathogens.

- Microbiologic criteria: positive culture results from at least two separate expectorated sputum samples or at least one bronchial wash or lavage, or transbronchial or other lung biopsy with mycobacterial histopathologic features (granulomatous inflammation or AFB) and positive culture for NTM or biopsy showing mycobacterial histopathologic features (granulomatous inflammation or AFB) and one or more sputum or bronchial washings that are culture positive for NTM.
- Pts who are suspected of having NTM lung disease but who do not meet the diagnostic criteria should be followed until the diagnosis is firmly established or excluded.

Sites of Infection

- Cutaneous disease (cellulitis, abscesses, ulcers): common manifestation of infection; usually associated with trauma, and can occur in immunocompetent and immunocompromised persons.
- Typically starts as small erythematous papule(s) and after wks or mos progresses to large, fluctuant, painful violaceous boil(s) which can ulcerate. Lymphadenitis rarely encountered.
- Osteomyelitis and/or joint disease: may result from local extension of posttraumatic wound infection (more common) or from hematogenous spread (less common).
- Pulmonary disease: rare (*M. abscessus* more common), except in pts with esophageal achalasia, lipoid pneumonia, diseases characterized by chronic vomiting and aspiration.
- Since pulmonary *M. fortuitum* disease is uncommon, and *M. fortuitum* can be a contaminant, careful clinical evaluation is required to determine the significance of a pulmonary *M. fortuitum* isolate.
- Catheter-related infections.
- Otitis media: rare.
- Keratitis: rare.
- CNS infection: rare.
- Dissemination: rare.

Treatment

General Comments

- Disease typically chronic, progressive; rare spontaneous resolution has been reported.
- Results of antimicrobial susceptibility testing should be used to guide treatment.
- Typically susceptible to amikacin, cefoxitin, levofloxacin, sulfonamides, imipenem, linezolid. Most isolates susceptible to clarithromycin, 50% are susceptible to doxycycline.
- Linezolid: excellent *in vitro* activity but limited clinical experience for treatment of *M. fortuitum.*
- Caution advised if using macrolides. Inducible erythromycin (*erm* gene) resistance described and may develop resistance in the 80% of isolates deemed initially susceptible to clarithromycin.

Limited, localized wound infections

- Oral monotherapy with sulfonamide (trimethoprim-sulfamethoxazole 1 DS twice daily), doxycycline (100 mg qday), or clarithromycin (500 mg twice daily). Acquired resistance to these drugs not yet reported.
- Oral monotherapy with quinolones has been associated with acquired resistance and treatment failure. Quinolones should therefore be used in combination with another antimicrobial agent.
- Surgical excision or debridement typically not necessary for limited skin disease, except when chemotherapy is limited by toxicity.
- Duration of therapy typically 3–4 mos but depends on pace of improvement.

Severe skin/soft tissue/bone infections or pulmonary disease

- Combination therapy recommended with at least two agents with *in vitro* activity.
- Amikacin (15 mg/kg IV q24h, adjust if renal dysfunction) plus either a beta-lactam (cefoxitin 2 g IV q6h or imipenem 1 g IV q6h) or quinolone (levofloxacin 500 mg or moxifloxacin 400 mg qday) for initial therapy.

PATHOGENS

293

- When clinically improved on one of above initial regimens, oral therapy can be initiated with at least 2 drugs (based on susceptibility testing).
- Frequently used oral agents: clarithromycin (500 mg PO twice daily), doxycycline (100 mg PO twice daily), trimethoprim-sulfamethoxazole (1 DS PO twice daily), levofloxacin (500–750 PO mg qday).
- For skin and soft tissue infections, surgical excision or debridement may be beneficial for extensive disease, abscess formation, or when chemotherapy is limited by toxicity.
- Infected or potentially infected foreign bodies (e.g., intravenous catheters, breast implants) should be removed.
- Duration of therapy depends on extent of disease and immunosuppression; 6 mos minimally required to prevent relapse.

BASIS FOR RECOMMENDATIONS

Griffith DE, Aksamit T, Brown-Elliott BA, et al. An official ATS/IDSA statement: diagnosis, treatment, and prevention of nontuberculous mycobacterial diseases. *Am J Respir Crit Care Med*, 2007; Vol. 175; pp. 367–416.

Comments: Document provides diagnostic and treatment considerations slanted toward pulmonary aspects.

MYCOBACTERIUM KANSASII

Paul G. Auwaerter, MD and Christopher J. Hoffmann MD, MPH

MICROBIOLOGY

- Slow grower, photochromogen.
- DNA analysis suggests there may be 5–7 subspecies.
- Subtype I appears to be responsible for most human infection.

CLINICAL

- Second most common cause of nontuberculous mycobacterial pulmonary disease in most parts of USA, and 2nd most common cause of nontuberculous mycobacterial disease in HIV/AIDS pts.
- Water is major environmental reservoir; infection probably occurs via aerosol route.
- Risk factors for pulmonary disease: chronic obstructive pulmonary disease, pneumoconiosis, cystic fibrosis, prior mycobacterial lung disease, malignancy, alcoholism, HIV/AIDS.
- *M. tuberculosis* and *M. kansasii* can occur together: cultures positive for *M. kansasii* should be incubated for prolonged periods to exclude *M. tuberculosis*, which grows slightly slower than *M. kansasii*.
- Dx: suspect in chronic pulmonary infections +/– bronchiectasis, cavitation resembling TB or MAC. Order AFB stains/culture by expectorated sputa or BAL.

SITES OF INFECTION

- **Pulmonary:** most frequent site in immunocompetent and immunocompromised pts.
- Clinical presentation and clinical course similar to tuberculosis. Upper lobe cavitary infiltrates common, but noncavitary or nodular/bronchiectatic pulmonary disease also occurs.
- Natural history of untreated cavitary (and probably non-cavitary) lung disease is progression of disease.
- In HIV-infected pts, cavitation on chest x-ray is common with high CD4 counts and middle/lower lung fields more commonly affected; interstitial infiltrates and hilar adenopathy without pulmonary cavitation may occur with low CD4 counts.
- **Disseminated disease:** (Typically occurs in the setting of advanced lung disease). Can occur in AIDS and in severely immunocompromised HIV-negative persons (e.g., organ transplant recipients).
- **Lymphadenitis :** rare
- **Cutaneous:** rare
- **Osteomyelitis/arthritis:** rare

TREATMENT

Pulmonary disease, HIV-negative, or HIV-positive without HAART

- Rifampin (10 mg/kg/day or 600 mg max PO daily) + isoniazid (5 mg/kg/day or 300 mg max PO daily plus pyridoxine 50 mg PO daily) + ethambutol (15 mg/kg/day). Two mos of initial ethambutol 25 mg/kg/day no longer recommended.
- Clinical response: with effective therapy, expect conversion to negative sputum culture by 6 mos (*RID* 1981;3:1028–34, 1035–39).

- Monitor sputum AFB smear and culture monthly until at least 3 consecutive negative monthly cultures.
- Duration of therapy 12 mos after sputum culture negativity (often total of 18–24 mos).
- Currently recommended regimens based on available information using older "anti-tuberculosis" drugs. Clarithromycin and moxifloxacin appear very active *in vitro*, and possible that (as part of combination therapy) they could be as or more effective than current rifampin-based regimens, but insufficient clinical information exists.

Pulmonary disease, HIV-positive on HAART

- If not on HAART, then above recommendations for HIV-negative pts apply.
- Rifampin may be used with efavirenz (increase of EFV dose to 800 mg/day), but switching to rifabutin is preferred.
- Rifampin should not be used in pts receiving indinavir, nelfinavir, amprenavir, darunavir, tipranavir, saquinavir, fosamprenavir, delavirdine. Rifabutin is alternative, with dose adjustments. Avoid rifabutin + delavirdine combination.
- Clarithromycin 500 mg twice daily + rifabutin (see drug module for dose adjustment with PIs and NNRTIs) + isoniazid 300 mg once daily (plus pyridoxine 50 mg once daily) + ethambutol 15 mg/kg/day, max 2.5 g/day). Consider streptomycin or moxifloxacin (good *in vitro* data but little clinical experience) as alternatives or for severe dz.
- Monitor closely for adverse effects, including uveitis from rifabutin.
- Duration of therapy: generally total of 18 mos including 12 mos of sputum culture negativity.
- Immune reconstitution syndrome can occur after starting mycobacterial or HIV therapy; consider steroids if severe/life-threatening signs or symptoms.
- Intermittent clarithromycin-based regimens not evaluated in HIV positive persons.

Treatment of disseminated disease

- Regimens described above for various pt groups are suitable for treatment of disseminated disease.
- Rifamycins play critical role, hence all regimens should be based upon one of the drugs except when resistance is documented.

Non-rifamycin-containing regimen

- Rifamycins are cornerstone of *M. kansasii* therapy and should be included unless isolate is rifamycin resistant or pt is rifamycin-intolerant.
- Rifampin-resistant disease: may include clarithromycin 500 mg PO twice daily or azithromycin 250 mg PO once daily, moxifloxacin 400 mg PO once daily, ethambutol 15 mg/kg/day, sulfamethoxazole 1 mg PO three times a day or streptomycin 0.5–1.0 g IM q24 × 1–3 mos then thrice weekly.
- Duration of therapy: 12 mos of sputum culture negativity.

OTHER INFORMATION

- ATS diagnostic criteria for pulmonary *M. kansasii* disease (see "Detailed Information") are guidelines; applicability in specific pts should be carefully considered by an experienced clinician.
- In pts with cavitary pulmonary dz, and in HIV-infected pts, a single positive respiratory culture may be adequate for diagnosis, although no consensus. If not treated, follow pt closely.
- Acquired resistance to isoniazid, rifampin, and ethambutol has been documented and is associated with treatment failure or relapse. Avoid addition of a single drug to a failing regimen.
- *M. kansasii* is typically inhibited by rifampin, rifabutin, isoniazid, ethambutol, ethionamide, amikacin, streptomycin, clarithromycin, and newer quinolones at concentrations achievable in serum.
- Susceptibility testing to rifampin should be performed; results of susceptibility testing to other agents of unclear clinical relevance. *M. kansasii* is resistant to pyrazinamide and capreomycin.

MORE INFORMATION

Diagnostic criteria for pulmonary M. kansasii disease (*Am J Respir Crit Care Med* 2007;175: 367–416).

PATHOGENS

ATS criteria: The minimum evaluation of suspected of nontuberculous mycobacterial (NTM) lung disease: (1) chest radiograph or, in the absence of cavitation, chest high-resolution computed tomography (HRCT) scan; (2) three or more sputum specimens for acid-fast bacilli (AFB) analysis; and (3) exclusion of other disorders, such as tuberculosis (TB). Clinical, radiographic, and microbiologic criteria are equally important and all must be met to make a diagnosis of NTM lung disease. ATS states that criteria apply to symptomatic pts with radiographic opacities, nodular or cavitary, or an HRCT scan that shows multifocal bronchiectasis with multiple small nodules. These criteria fit best with Mycobacterium avium complex (MAC), *M. kansasii*, and *M. abscessus*. There is not enough known about most other NTM to be certain that these diagnostic criteria are universally applicable for all NTM respiratory pathogens.

Microbiologic criteria: positive culture results from at least two separate expectorated sputum samples or at least one bronchial wash or lavage, or transbronchial or other lung biopsy with mycobacterial histopathologic features (granulomatous inflammation or AFB) and positive culture for NTM or biopsy showing mycobacterial histopathologic features (granulomatous inflammation or AFB) and one or more sputum or bronchial washings that are culture positive for NTM.

BASIS FOR RECOMMENDATIONS

Griffith DE, Aksamit T, Brown-Elliott BA, et al. An official ATS/IDSA statement: diagnosis, treatment, and prevention of nontuberculous mycobacterial diseases. *Am J Respir Crit Care Med,* 2007; Vol. 175; pp. 367–416.

Comments: Current American Thoracic Society guidelines for diagnosis and treatment.

MYCOBACTERIUM LEPRAE

Paul G. Auwaerter, MD and Joseph Vinetz, MD

MICROBIOLOGY

- AFB morphologically resembles tubercle bacillus.
- Slow growing obligate intracellular pathogen, average doubling time ~2 wks. Cannot culture in microbiology lab.
- Armadillos and immunocompromised mice used to grow *M. leprae* for research purposes.

CLINICAL

- Etiological agent of leprosy (some prefer term Hansen's Disease): chronic, progressive skin, neurological disorder of high morbidity and stigma.
- Most U.S. cases in immigrants from developing world, especially Africa, India, Pacific Islands. Three million people infected worldwide.
- Indigenous leprosy in LA, TX, Hawaii.
- Transmission: most likely from nasal discharge of lepromatous leprosy pts not from skin contact.
- Incubation period: 2–5 yrs, rarely decades.
- Rare nosocomial transmission; infection requires sustained exposure.
- Clinical manifestations due to host response.
- Natural history and treatment complicated by reversal reactions and erythema nodosum leprosum (ENL).
- Accurate classification fundamental for establishing treatment and prognosis (see Other Information below).
- Clinical diagnosis based on (1) hypopigmented/reddish skin lesions, (2) involvement of peripheral nerves—thickening and associated loss of sensation, (3) skin-smear positive for acid-fast bacilli.

SITES OF INFECTION

- Eye: iridocyclitis (acute or chronic), corneal changes due to exposure, lagophthalmos (VII cranial nerve palsy), cataracts.
- Skin: hypopigmented, anesthetic macules, plaques, nodular lesions, infiltrated thickened lesions—can appear as "chronic dermatitis." Many mimics.
- Neurologic: peripheral involvement only. Great auricular classic, also supraclavicular, ulnar, antebrachial, radial/median nerves at wrist, femoral cutaneous, common peroneals, posterior tibial. Early and late anesthesia, tingling.
- Systemic: fever, arthralgia, arthritis usually in context of ENL.
- Kidney: glomerulonephritis due to ENL.

- Musculoskeletal: trophic changes due to nerve destruction, claw-hand, ulcerations, deformity of feet.
- HEENT: nasal discharge, airway blockage, ulceration, septum perforation, saddle-nose deformity; nodules on lips, tongue, palate, larynx; edema of glottis as part of reversal rxn.

TREATMENT

Multibacillary Leprosy (Skin smear positive)

- Adults: dapsone 100 mg/day + rifampin 600 mg q4 wks + clofazimine 50 mg/day supplemented by monthly loading dose of 300 mg of clofazimine.
- Others: dapsone 1–2 mg/kg/day, rifampin 450 mg <35 kg, 300 mg <20 kg, 150 mg <12 kg.
- Length of treatment: 12–24 mos.

Paucibacillary Leprosy (Skin Smear negative)

- Rifampin 600 mg once monthly × 6 mos + dapsone 100 mg/day for 6 mos.

Erythema Nodosum Leprosum (ENL)

- Continue anti-leprosy drugs throughout.
- Mild: rest affect limb, analgesics, f/u q2wks, check for iridocyclitis; chloroquine, aspirin may be useful.
- Severe reactions defined: numerous nodules + fever, ulcerating/pustular ENL, visceral involvement, nodules + neuritis, recurrent ENL.
- Severe (WHO guideline, http://www.paho.org/English/AD/DPC/CD/who-enl-guidelines.htm): prednisolone 30–40 mg/day (not to exceed 1 mg/kg) × 1–2 wks, then taper over 12 wks.
- If unresponsive to corticosteroids or if risk of corticosteroids prevent administration: start clofazimine 100 mg three times a day for maximum of 12 wks. Complete the standard course of prednisolone, if given. Taper the dose of clofazimine to 100 mg twice a day for 12 wks and then 100 mg once a day for 12–24 wks.
- If anti-leprosy drugs completed, no reason to restart therapy.
- Some use pentoxyfylline as adjunctive therapy.
- WHO does not recommend thalidomide due to teratogenicity concerns; however, useful under strict supervision, if not contraindicated: thalidomide 200–400 mg/day, reduced to 50–100 mg/day after 1–2 wks.

Reversal Reaction

- Goal is to prevent nerve damage.
- Prednisolone: start with 40 mg/day then taper by 10 mg q2wks over about 12 wks.

Eye Complications

- Lagophthalmos (VII palsy): goggles, sunglasses, saline eye drops, night-time eye closure, surgery (lateral tarsorrhaphy).
- Iridocyclitis: topical atropine, corticosteroids; chronic forms may need chronic therapy.

Prophylaxis

- Although studies with dapsone not helpful, recent large study using single dose rifampin suggests benefit household contacts.
- Rifampin, single dose, oral: 600 mg for adults weighing 35 kg and over, 450 mg for adults weighing less than 35 kg and for children older than 9 yrs, and 300 mg for children aged 5 to 9 yrs.

MORE TREATMENT

For treatment purposes:

- **Paucibacillary:** Skin smear neg, usually. TT, BT, I
- **Multibacillary:** Skin smear pos, usually. BB, BL, LL

Classic Ridley-Jopling classification

- **Tuberculoid (TT):** single or few anesthetic macules or plaques; borders well define; peripheral nerve involvement common; Bacillary density in skin: Rare; Lepromin skin test strongly pos.
- **Borderline tuberculoid (BT):** lesions similar to TT but more of them; borders less distinct; satellite lesions around larger lesions; peripheral nerve involvement common; Bacillary density in skin: Scanty; Lepromin skin test pos.
- **Borderline (BB):** more lesions than BT; vague borders; satellite lesions often seen; peripheral nerve involvement common; Bacillary density in skin: moderate; Lepromin skin test neg or weakly pos.
- **Borderline lepromatous (BL):** numerous lesions, similar to BB; some nerve damage; Bacillary density in skin: heavy; Lepromin skin test neg.

- **Lepromatous (LL):** multiple, non-anesthetic, macular or papular, symmetrically distributed; no neural lesions until late; Late complications: leonine facies, testicular damage, etc.; Bacillary density in skin: heavy; Lepromin skin test neg.
- **Indeterminate (I):** vaguely define hypopigmented or erythematous macule; Bacillary density in skin: rare or scanty; Lepromin skin test neg or weakly pos.

OTHER INFORMATION

- Physical findings: observe anesthetic patches, nerve trunk thickening (e.g., great auricular nerve), deformities, paralysis; histopath exam of skin bx; exam of skin smears for bacilli.
- Dx: obtain skin smears from 6–8 sites; bx edge of lesions for histopath to classify disease. Fite stain essential to demonstrate organisms.
- For consultation expertise, inquire to the U.S. Public Health Service Hansen's Disease Program: http://www.hrsa.gov/hansens/—accessed 8/18/09.
- Ambulatory Hansen's Disease Program maintains a national referral list: 800-642-2477. Hawaii Hansen's Disease Program: (808)-733-9831.
- Lepromin skin testing reagent produced by WHO; contact National Hansen's Disease Center to discuss obtaining it.

MORE INFORMATION

Immune Reactions Requiring Special Treatment in Leprosy

Reversal Reactions: increased cell-mediated immunity mediated by specific T cell responses to *M. leprae* antigens, moving towards TT form; lesions become erythematous, edematous, with concomitant acute neuritis; may cause severe sensory loss and paralytic deformities such as clawhand, footdrop. LL pts probably do not experience these reactions spontaneously; treated with watchful waiting, analgesics, and corticosteroids for paresis or muscle paralysis **Erythema Nodosum Leprosum (ENL):** immune complex-mediated seen only in lepromatous, border-line lepromatous pts; half of LL pts have ENL after a few mos of drug therapy; characterized by rapid onset of tender subcutaneous and intracutaneous nodules that become erythematous; accompanied by fever, sometimes synovitis, iridocyclitis, glomerulonephritis, secondary amyloi-dosis; treated with analgesics; severe cases with thalidomide, sometime clofazimine; iridocyclitis requires topical steroids.

BASIS FOR RECOMMENDATIONS

Ooi WW, Moschella SL. Update on leprosy in immigrants in the United States: status in the yr 2000. *Clin Infect Dis*, 2001; Vol. 32; pp. 930–7.

Comments: This article describes the clinical presentation and management of leprosy pts as approached in the U.S. There is focus on differential diagnosis, clinical presentations, reasons to suspect the diagnosis of leprosy, and treatment approaches.

7th WHO Expert Committee on Leprosy June 1997. **Major conclusions and recommendations**.

Comments: These are the major international policy recommendations on control and treatment of leprosy.

MYCOBACTERIUM MARINUM

Paul G. Auwaerter, MD

MICROBIOLOGY

- Slow growing pigmented AFB. Grows best at 30–33°C.
- Reservoir: water and marine organisms. Worldwide distribution. Survives in fresh or salt water.

CLINICAL

- Causes soft tissue, bone infections ("fish tank granuloma," "fish tuberculosis," "swimming pool granuloma").
- Infection follows trauma (which can be minor) in aquariums, swimming pools, other bodies of water, or associated with fish spines, crustaceans, shellfish.
- Higher incidence in males than females, presumably related to more frequent exposure in males.
- Incubation period typically 2–4 wks but can be longer.
- Disease may occur in immunocompetent or immunosuppressed persons. Immunosuppression may increase susceptibility, severity of disease.

- Alert laboratory so that appropriate culture conditions used if clinical suspicion for *M. marinum*.
- Susceptibility testing not routinely performed, generally only indicated for treatment failure.
- Diagnosis: appropriate material from active lesion should be evaluated by AFB smear, AFB culture, and histopathology.
- AFB smear rarely positive. Granulomas on histopathology in 3/4 of cases.

SITES OF INFECTION

- **Soft tissues:** upper extremities most common site of trauma and cutaneous disease (>75% fingers, hands, forearm, olecranon bursa > upper arm), but localized disease can occur at any site of trauma. Many cases without known trauma.
- Initial cutaneous lesion typically papular or nodular including sporotrichoid appearance often subcutaneous, and may acquire a blue-purple color. Ulcers, abscesses, pustules are less common.
- Spread of disease is typically by local extension or lymphatics.
- **Deep infection:** involvement of tendon, joint or bone is typically due to extension of overlying skin infection.
- **Disseminated disease:** unusual, but has been reported in immunosuppressed and apparently immunocompetent persons.

TREATMENT

Antibiotic Treatment

- No prospective studies, no strong consensus to guide antimicrobial treatment, but 2-drug combination therapy probably optimal.
- Isolates typically susceptible to rifampin/rifabutin, ethambutol, clarithromycin, minocycline, doxycycline, and sulfonamides. Resistant to isoniazid, pyrazinamide, ciprofloxacin, ofloxacin, levofloxacin.
- Preferred oral regimens: clarithromycin 500 mg twice daily + ethambutol 15 mg/kg/day, clarithromycin 500 mg twice daily + rifampin 600 mg every day. Rifampin containing regimen preferred by some for osteomyelitis or deep structure involvement.
- Other active oral agents: minocycline 100 mg twice daily doxycycline 100 mg twice daily, trimethoprim-sulfamethoxazole 1 DS twice daily.
- Treatment duration: rate of response variable and can be delayed. For immunocompetent persons stopping antibiotics 4–6 wks after clinical resolution may be considered; typical minimum duration 3 to 4 mos.
- Longer duration of therapy may be required if spread of infection from skin to deeper structures, and in immunocompromised pts.
- Linezolid has good *in vitro* activity, but limited published clinical experience.

Surgical Treatment

- Surgery not clearly beneficial for most infections limited to skin/soft tissue. Surgery may be beneficial for infections involving closed spaces of hand, refractory tendon involvement, or disease poorly responsive to antibiotics.

FOLLOW UP

- New nodules may develop in the first 8–12 wks of therapy, especially with extensive infection. This doesn't usually mean treatment failure but may wish to order susceptibility testing.

OTHER INFORMATION

- Susceptibility testing not routinely recommended; reserve for cases of treatment failure.
- Spontaneous remission has been described in immune competent individuals.

BASIS FOR RECOMMENDATIONS

Griffith DE, Aksamit T, Brown-Elliott BA, et al. An official ATS/IDSA statement: diagnosis, treatment, and prevention of nontuberculous mycobacterial diseases. *Am J Respir Crit Care Med*, 2007; Vol. 175; pp. 367–416.

Comments: Guideline includes mention of soft tissue *M. marinum*, but no comparative trials exist for basis of recommendations.

PATHOGENS

MYCOPLASMA PNEUMONIAE

Paul G. Auwaerter, MD

MICROBIOLOGY

- Aerobic, fastidious organism. Believed to be a frequent cause of atypical pneumonia but secure diagnosis difficult with current diagnostic assays.
- Organism lacks cell wall. Member of Mollicutes class, among the smallest known free-living bacteria, indicate acute infection.
- *M. pneumoniae* culture difficult. Growth often requires 7–21 days, successful in 40–90% of cases.
- Erythromycin resistance has not been described.

CLINICAL

- Peaks late summer/fall, most frequent in children/young adults but also elderly; may cause epidemics (schools, barracks).
- *Mycoplasma pneumoniae* onset often gradual with dry cough, prominent headache, fever, malaise and sore throat. Cough may last 4–6 wks.
- Exam may show erythematous posterior pharynx. Lung exam may be normal early in infection, but later with rales, rhonchi or wheezing. In general, pts appear non-toxic.
- Extrapulmonary abnormalities frequently associated with infection (see sites of infection).
- Cold agglutinin ABs occur in 50–70%, but nonspecific. These anti-I IgM ABs are directed against rbc antigen; may be associated w/ hemolysis, renal failure, Raynauds. Peak 2–3 wks, last 2–3 mos.
- **Dx:** if sputum produced see PMN's without bacteria (lacks cell wall so does not pick up Gram-stain). Cold agglutinin titer 1:32 or greater supportive but non-specific. Bedside cold agg. if + = equiv. titer 1:64.
- Most labs do not perform mycoplasma Cx routinely. Need special transport media and cx methods, then 1–2 wks to show characteristic mulberry colonies on culture.
- Mycoplasma IgM more specific, but commonly negative first 7–10 days. DNA detection by GenProbe or PCR on sputum ~89–95% sens./specificity compared to culture/serology. Throat swabs results worse. Serology no longer recommended for pneumonia diagnosis.

SITES OF INFECTION

- Respiratory (1): may appear like routine URI with 5–10% developing tracheobronchitis or pneumonia. Often with headache. Distinguish from virus by gradual progression of sx over 1–2 days (vs. abrupt onset w/ influenza).
- Resp. (2): dry cough, nontoxic ("walking pneumonia"). Often minimal exam findings compared to CXR. Pleural effusion 5–20%.
- HEENT: bullous myringitis **very rare** w/ native infection. Frequent association only with experimental inoculation.
- Derm: erythema multiforme in 7% especially children. Also Steven-Johnson syndrome, macular or morbilliform or papulovesicular rashes.
- Cardiac: arrhythmias, CHF in up to 10%. EKG changes common, especially conduction abnormalities.
- Neuro: meningoencephalitis, aseptic meningitis, Guillain-Barre, ataxia, transverse myelitis, peripheral neuropathy. Association based on serology making true causation uncertain.
- Heme: hemolytic anemia (rarely clinically significant).
- Rheum: occasional arthritis, transient Raynauds phenomenon.

TREATMENT

Pneumonia

- Often not severe, rather mild and self-limited. Antibiotics may shorten duration, though cough may linger for wks. Beta-lactams ineffective since organism lacks cell wall.
- Usual dose duration is 7–14 days, but this is not based on prospective study.
- Erythromycin 250 mg PO four times a day or doxycycline 100 mg PO twice daily are traditional and inexpensive choices.
- Newer, more expensive drugs with excellent *in vitro* MIC's include: azithromycin 250 mg PO once daily, clarithromycin 250 mg PO q12h, levofloxacin 500 mg PO once daily, moxifloxacin 400 mg PO once daily.

- New drugs not superior over older; however, definitive dx of mycoplasma rare at time of treatment decision.
- Dosing of FQ and advanced macrolides are typically only $\sim\frac{1}{2}$ of usual empiric pneumonia doses, as *M. pneumoniae* very sensitive to these drugs.

Upper Respiratory Tract Infections
- Most go undiagnosed.
- Supportive care, antimicrobials not required as infection self-limited.

Extrapulmonary Disease
- Effect of antibiotics unknown, but using 10–14 days of a drug listed in the pneumonia section likely prudent.

Prevention
- Outbreaks described in the military, families and long-term care facilities.
- Prophylaxis: azithromycin 500 mg day 1 then 250 mg day 2–5 (Zpack) may reduce secondary attack rate.

OTHER INFORMATION
- Problematic diagnosis since culture difficult, serology insensitive at time of pt presentation. Sputum GenProbe or PCR probably best for rapid, accurate diagnosis but availability limited.
- Normal WBC # and clear chest exam despite pneumonia on CXR should prompt consideration of atypical pneumonias, esp. Mycoplasma.
- Bedside cold agglutinin test: draw blood into anticoagulant test tube, cool to 4°C and formerly smooth adherence of rbcs to glass display macroscopic agglutination that reverses with warming.
- *M. pneumoniae* often severe in sickle cell pts w/ overwhelming infection—severe cold agglutinin disease causing digital necrosis.
- Cold agglutinin ABs are insensitive and nonspecific for *M. pneumoniae* dx. Complement fixation AB and anti-IgM AB more specific, but arise later in infection therefore less helpful since frequently negative at presentation.

BASIS FOR RECOMMENDATIONS

Mandell LA, Wunderink RG, Anzueto A, et al. Infectious Diseases Society of America/ American Thoracic Society consensus guidelines on the management of community-acquired pneumonia in adults. *Clin Infect Dis*, 2007; Vol. 44 Suppl 2; pp. S27–72.

Comments: Guideline states atypical agents of pneumonia a common cause, especially of outpt pneumonia, but acknowledge that except for Legionella, agents such as Mycoplasma are hard to diagnose in routine practice. Doxycycline or macrolide therapy advocated for outpatient CAP without risk factors for drug-resistant *S. pneumoniae*. Fluoroquinolones are listed as an alternative if *M. pneumoniae* specifically identified as the causal pathogen.

Baum, S. *Mycoplasma pneumoniae* and Atypical Pneumonia *Mandell, Bennett, and Dolin: Principles and Practice of Infectious Diseases*, 6th ed., 2005 Churchill Livingstone, Chap 181.

Comments: Latest overview of Mycoplasma re: diagnosis and treatment.

NEISSERIA GONORRHOEAE

Noreen A. Hynes, MD, MPH

MICROBIOLOGY
- Gram-negative diplococci, oxidase and catalase positive. Grows best on blood agar medium or chocolate medium (blood heated at 176–194°F).
- Always considered pathogenic when identified.
- Infects surfaces lined with columnar epithelial cells: endocervix, urethra, anogenital and oropharyngeal mucous membranes, conjunctiva.
- Has a loose capsule and pili. Antigenic variation of pili can be used for epidemiological characterization.
- Strains with nutrient requirements for arginine, hypoxanthine, or uracil are more likely to cause asymptomatic infection.

CLINICAL
- Gonorrhea is the second most commonly reported infectious disease in the United States with 355,991 cases reported in 2007. It is substantially under diagnosed and under reported, and approximately twice as many new infections are estimated to occur each yr beyond those

PATHOGENS

reported. _N. gonorrhoeae_ resistance rates to fluoroquinolone antibiotics have increased to >25% in some U.S. cities and are no longer recommended for use in treatment of gonococcal infections at any site.

- In men, usually causes symptomatic urethritis, **but** up to 25% of infections asymptomatic; circumcision does not decrease the risk of incident gonorrhea. Epididymitis is most frequent complication of GC in men. Less common complications in men include "bull headed clap," urethral stricture, and prostatitis.
- MSM should be screened at least once annually for urethral and rectal and chlamydia gonorrhea and pharyngeal gonorrhea and every 3 to 6 mos for MSM with multiple or anonymous sexual partners, have sex in conjunction with illicit drug use, use methamphetamines, or have a sex partner who participates in these activities.
- Up to 50% of infections in women are asymptomatic. In women, accessory gland infections, perihepatitis, perinatal morbidity, PID can occur.
- In both sexes anorectal infection, pharyngitis, conjunctivitis and disseminated infection may occur.
- Incubation period is 3–7 days in men; unclear incubation period in women but maybe 10 days.
- Disseminated gonococcal infection (DGI) including gonococcal tenosynovitis is increasingly rare. Severe DGI (meningitis or endocarditis) should be managed w/ help from an ID consultant.
- **Gram-stain**: (1) Use for urethral and accessory gland secretions (~95% sensitive) without further testing needed, (2) inadequate alone for female cervical secretions (~50%). (3) Don't Gram-stain pharyngeal secretions due to confusion with _N. meningitidis_. Test all sites (oral, anal, genital) to increase yield.
- **Nucleic acid amplification tests (NAATs):** (1) can be used routinely for vaginal, penile, and ocular secretion testing; use culture only for dx from pharyngeal or rectal secretions unless the laboratory has conducted internal validation of the method to be used by a verification study which will allow use of the tests for a non-FDA-cleared purpose (Laboratory Corporation of America and Quest Diagnostic have completed these verifications), (2) more sensitive and specific than non-amplification nucleic acid based tests, (3) more rapid than culture, (4) more specific than rapid point-of-care immunoassays.
- **Culture**: (1) diagnostic standard for ALL sites of infection, (2) only diagnostic modality for determining antibiotic sensitivity, (3) empiric treatment often needed as results not available for 24–48 hrs, (4) preferred use when dx unclear, when rx failure is a concern, or legal issues are present such as in possible rape cases.

SITES OF INFECTION
- Urethra: urethritis
- Cervix: cervicitis
- Epididymis: epididymitis
- Fallopian tubes: PID; accessory glands (Skene's, Bartholin's)
- Endometrium: endometritis
- Glisson's capsule of the liver: (Fitz-Hugh-Curtis syndrome)
- Throat: pharyngitis
- Conjunctiva: conjunctivitis
- Anorectum: proctitis
- Dissemination: skin lesions, arthralgia, tenosynovitis, septic arthritis, hepatitis, myocarditis, endocarditis, meningitis

TREATMENT
Uncomplicated infection of cervix, urethra, rectum
- Standard of care = 2 drug regimen that will treat gonorrhea and chlamydia if chlamydia infection not ruled out. **Fluoroquinolones are no longer recommended for treatment due to high prevalence of fluoroquinolone resistance in _N. gonorrhoeae_.**
- Cefixime 400 mg PO × 1 plus antichlamydial if chlamydia not ruled out (azithromycin 1 g PO × 1 or doxycycline 100 mg twice daily PO × 7 days).
- Ceftriaxone 125 mg IM × 1 plus antichlamydial if chlamydia not ruled out (azithromycin 1 g PO × 1 or doxycycline 100 mg PO twice daily × 7 days).

- **Alt regimens**: Spectinomycin 2 g IM × 1 plus antichlamydial if chlamydia not ruled out (azithromycin 1 g PO × 1 or doxycycline 100 mg twice daily PO × 7 days). Spectinomycin is not currently available in the U.S. If spectinomycin unavailable, consultation with a specialist recommended for allergy testing and desensitization, if needed, prior to treatment with a cephalosporin.
- Ceftizoxime 500 mg IM × 1 plus antichlamydial if chlamydia not ruled out (azithromycin 1 g PO × 1 or doxycycline 100 mg twice daily PO × 7 days). Cefoxitin 2 g IM × 1 w/ probenecid 1 g PO × 1 plus antichlamydial if chlamydia not ruled out (azithromycin 1 g PO × 1 or doxycycline 100 mg twice daily PO × 7 days). Cefotaxime 500 mg IM × 1 plus antichlamydial if chlamydia not ruled out (azithromycin 1 g PO × 1 or doxycycline 100 mg twice daily PO × 7 days).

Severe or Disseminated Gonococcal Infections (DGI)
- Ceftriaxone 1 g IV q24h (recommended).
- **Alt:** cefotaxime 1 g IV q8h, or ceftizoxime 1 g IV q8h. or spectinomycin 2 g IM q12h.
- All of the preceding regimens should be continued for 24–48 hrs after improvement begins, at which time therapy may be switched to one of the following regimens to complete at least 1 wk of antimicrobial therapy.
- **Oral regimens (post-improvement):** cefixime 400 mg PO twice daily.
- Fluoroquinolones are no longer recommended for treatment due to high prevalence of fluoroquinolone resistance in *N. gonorrhoeae*.
- **Meningitis:** ceftriaxone 1–2 g IV q12h × 10–14 days.
- **Endocarditis:** ceftriaxone 1–2 g IV q12h × at least 4 wks.
- Allergy/intolerance to cephalosporins: spectinomycin 2 g q12h. Spectinomycin is not currently available in the U.S. If spectinomycin unavailable, consultation with a specialist recommended for allergy testing and desensitization, if needed, prior to treatment with a cephalosporin.

Uncomplicated pharyngeal infections
- Standard of Care = 2 drug regimen to Rx gonorrhea and chlamydia if chlamydia infection not ruled out.
- Ceftriaxone 125 mg IM × 1 plus antichlamydial if chlamydia not ruled out (azithromycin 1 g PO × 1 or doxycycline 100 mg twice daily × 7 days).

Gonococcal conjunctivitis
- Ceftriaxone 1 g IM once (plus saline lavage).

Special Patient Situations
- HIV: should receive the same treatment as HIV-uninfected persons.
- Pregnancy: use any regimen above except quinolones or tetracyclines. Use erythromycin and amoxicillin in presumptive or definitive Rx.
- Allergy, intolerance, adverse reactions: if truly intolerant of cephalosporins, use spectinomycin. If used for possible pharyngeal infection, test of cure needed at 3–5 days post Rx. Spectinomycin is not currently available in the U.S. If spectinomycin unavailable, consultation with a specialist recommended for allergy testing and desensitization, if needed, prior to treatment with a cephalosporin.
- Test of cure: routinely **not** needed for anogenital infection. Routinely needed for following treatment of pharyngeal gonorrhea. Other situations when a test of cure should be considered: (1) persistent symptoms, and (2) when antibiotic resistance suspected.

FOLLOW UP
- Pts who have documented or suspect pharyngeal gonorrhea should have a test of cure 3–5 days after treatment.

OTHER INFORMATION
- Dual therapy for gonorrhea and chlamydia is the **standard of care** if chlamydia infection has not been ruled out at the time of treatment.
- Pharyngeal and anorectal infection appear to be associated with DGI.
- Severe DGI should be treated in consultation with an infectious disease expert.
- Spectinomycin currently unavailable in the U.S. (2006).

BASIS FOR RECOMMENDATIONS
Bignell C, IUSTI/WHO. 2009 European (IUSTI/WHO) guideline on the diagnosis and treatment of gonorrhoea in adults. *Int J STD AIDS,* 2009; Vol. 20; pp. 453–7.

PATHOGENS

Comments: These is the most recently published clinical practice guideline on the diagnosis and treatment of gonorrhea (GC) in adults. These guidelines incorporate recent any recent findings through January 2008 and build upon both the Centers for Disease Control and Prevention (CDC) STD Treatment Guidelines of 2006 (www.cdc.gov/std/) and the CDC 2007 update on treatment of gonorrhea and the British Association for Sexual Health and HIV Guideline (http://www.bashh.org/) published in 2005. These European guidelines underscore the recommendations made by the other bodies.

Centers for Disease Control and Prevention (CDC) Update to CDC's sexually transmitted diseases treatment guidelines, 2006: fluoroquinolones no longer recommended for treatment of gonococcal infections. *MMWR Morb Mortal Wkly Rep,* 2007; Vol. 56; pp. 332–6.

Comments: Fluoroquinolones (FQ) have been used in the U.S. for the treatment of gonorrhea since 1993. Since, 2000 FQ resistance among *Neisseria gonorrhoeae* isolates reported by the Centers for Disease Control and Prevention (CDC)-sponsored sentinel surveillance system, the Gonococcal Isolate Surveillance System (GISP) has been steadily increasing. Data available from the GISP for 2005 and preliminary data from 2006 demonstrate FQ resistant gonorrhea continues to increase among heterosexuals as well as men who have sex with men. Rates among heterosexual men are now as high as 26.6% in some cities. Therefore, on 13 April 2006, the CDC revised its 2006 *Sexually Transmitted Diseases Treatment Guidelines* and no longer recommend the use of any FQ for the treatment of proven or suspect gonorrhea at any site of infection.

Centers for Disease Control and Prevention Sexually transmitted diseases treatment guidelines 2006. Centers for Disease Control and Prevention. *MMWR Recomm Rep,* 2006; Vol. 55; pp. 1–100.

Comments: The CDC treatment guidelines provide clinicians with a readily available reference for STD treatments recommended by a panel of national and international experts in STD diagnosis, treatment, prevention and control. These guidelines available electronically from: http://www.cdc.gov/std/treatment/default.htm.

NEISSERIA MENINGITIDIS

John G. Bartlett, MD

MICROBIOLOGY
- Aerobic, Gram-negative diplococcus.
- Grows in blood or chocolate agar or selective media, e.g., Thayer Martin.
- Capsule dictates 13 serogroups: most important are A, B, C, W135, X and Y.

CLINICAL
- Epidemics usually due to A, B or C serogroups.
- Usual pathogenesis: oropharynx (carriage/infection) then bacteremia, then meningitis and/or fulminant meningococcemia.
- Usual presentation: fever + leukocytosis, HA, altered mental status (if meningitis) then petechial rash, then purpura fulminans + shock.
- Diagnosis by culture: blood, CSF and skin (rash).
- Vaccines mix serogroups A, C, Y, and W135 (no licensed vaccine for B).

SITES OF INFECTION
- Meningitis
- Bacteremia
- Rash: petechial, pustular. May be confused with disseminated GC
- Respiratory tract infection: pneumonia (often acute/fulminant), otitis, epiglottitis
- Focal infection: pericarditis, urethritis, arthritis, conjunctivitis
- Chronic meningococcemia (complement deficiency in many)

TREATMENT
Meningococcal Meningitis or Bacteremia
- Preferred: ceftriaxone 2 g IV q24h or cefotaxime 2 g IV q4–6h × 7–10 days.
- Alternatives: chloramphenicol 4–6 g/day × 7–10 days, penicillin 18–24 mil units/day IV, ampicillin 12 g/day IV; aztreonam 6–8 g/day IV or moxifloxacin 400 mg/day IV.
- Steroids: dexamethasone 10 mg IV q6h × 2–4 days starting before or with first dose.

Prevention
- Respiratory isolation for suspected meningococcal meningitis × 24 hrs.
- **Chemoprophylaxis:** any household or intimate contact, medical personnel with contact w/ oral secretions. Use rifampin 600 mg PO twice daily × 2 days or ciprofloxacin 500 mg PO × 1 dose or ceftriaxone 250 mg IM × 1.

- **Immunization:** conjugated vaccine (Menactra) with more durable immunity then old polysaccharide version. Target population immunize all children at 11–12 yrs or anyone over 2 yrs of age w/ risk factors for infection such as travel to high risk areas (sub-Saharan Africa), college freshmen in dorms, military recruits, asplenia, occupational.
- Polysaccharide vaccine: available for yrs, A, C, Y, W135 for outbreaks and international travel to endemic areas (meningitis belt of Africa). Now mainly used for pts >65 yrs or as an alternative to conjugated vaccine.
- Neither vaccine has coverage for serogroup B.

OTHER INFORMATION
- Penicillin resistance is increasing but is not yet relevant in U.S.—penicillin is preferred drug.
- Virulence is determined by serogroup and serotype.

BASIS FOR RECOMMENDATIONS

van de Beek D, de Gans J, McIntyre P, et al. Corticosteroids for acute bacterial meningitis. *Cochrane Database Syst Rev,* 2007; Vol. CD004405.

Comments: Supports administration of corticosteroids in conjunction with the first dose of an antibiotic for meningitis for adults. Data supported this approach in children from high-income countries but not children from low-income countries.

Bilukha OO, Rosenstein N, National Center for Infectious Diseases, Centers for Disease Control and Prevention (CDC). Prevention and control of meningococcal disease. Recommendations of the Advisory Committee on Immunization Practices (ACIP). *MMWR Recomm Rep,* 2005; Vol. 54; pp. 1–21.

Comments: ACIP recommendations of the tetravalent conjugated meningococcal vaccine: (1) children age 11–12 yrs, (2) travel to endemic area, (3) military recruits, (4) asplenia, (5) college freshmen living in dorms.

NOCARDIA

John G. Bartlett, MD

PATHOGENS

MICROBIOLOGY
- Gram-positive branching, beaded, filamentous rod.
- Weakly acid fast.
- Grows on special media (Thayer-Martin) in 3–5 days.
- 12 species: *N. asteroides* 90% (lung +/– CNS disease), *N. brasiliensis* = mycetoma (tropics), *N. farcinica* (bad prognosis).
- More recently detected species include *N. nova, N. cyriacigeorica* and *N. farcinica.*

CLINICAL
- Suspect in pts with CMI defect (AIDS, steroids, CGD, organ transplant) + indolent lung +/– CNS disease.
- Looks like Actinomycetes spp., but acid fast, aerobic and seen mostly in compromised hosts.
- Smears and cx positive in only 1/3rd of cases; send multiple specimens and warn lab of suspected dx.
- Dx: Gram-stain + AFB stain + sputum cx; rarely seen as colonization (take [+] sputum culture seriously).
- No person-person transmission.

SITES OF INFECTION
- Lung: indolent pneumonia, abscess, fibronodular infiltrates
- Brain: abscess or granulomas
- Disseminated: 20–30% of cases in immunosuppressed hosts including bones, heart, renal, joints, retina, skin, CNS, peritonitis, endocarditis
- Primary cutaneous: sporotrichoid (non-tropics) or mycetoma (madura foot, tropics)
- Ocular: keratitis, endophthalmitis

TREATMENT
Sulfonamide-based therapies
- Principles: treat based on host, site of disease and *in vitro* activity; sulfas usually preferred, must treat for 6–12 mos. Preferred drugs for resistant strains—amikacin and/or imipenem.
- Two categories: seriously ill usually treated w/ IV imipenem or sulfa or cefotaxime all potentially combined w/ amikacin; less seriously ill treated with oral agents—especially TMP-SMX or minocycline.

- Pulmonary: TMP-SMX 10 mg/kg/day (TMP) in 2–4 doses IV × 3–6 wks, then PO (2 DS twice daily) × >5 mos.
- Pulmonary alternatives: sulfisoxazole, sulfadiazine, trisulfapyrimidine 3–6 g/day PO 2–4 doses or TMP-SMX 2 DS twice daily up to 2 DS three times a day.
- CNS (AIDS, severe or disseminated disease): TMP-SMX 15 mg/kg/day (TMP) IV × 3–6 wks, then PO (3 DS twice daily) × 6–12 mos.
- CNS alternatives: imipenem 1000 mg IV q8h or ceftriaxone 2 g IV q12h or cefotaxime 2–3 g IV q6h + amikacin.
- Severe disease, compromised host, multiple sites: TMP-SMX IV (above doses) + amikacin 7.5 mg/kg q12h (adjust per levels) or oral sulfas 6–12 m/day.
- Sporotrichoid (cutaneous): TMP-SMX 1 DS twice daily × 4–6 mos.
- Sensitivity *N. asteroides*: sulfas (e.g., TMP-SMX)-95%, minocycline-90%, imipenem-85%, amikacin-90%, cefotaxime-80%, amoxicillin/clavulanate-50%, ciprofloxacin-40%, ampicillin-30%.
- Rx duration: immunocompetent-6 mos; immunosuppressed-12 mos. Immunosuppressed and continued immunosuppression—low dose abx indefinitely.

Sulfa alternatives
- Oral: minocycline 100 mg twice daily × > 6 mos (initial treatment of local disease or maintenance).
- Oral alternative if *in vitro* activity shown: amoxicillin/clavulanate 875/125 mg twice daily, doxycycline, erythromycin, clarithromycin, linezolid or fluoroquinolone or combinations × >6 mos.
- Severe disease, AIDS: imipenem 1000 mg IV q8h or meropenem (CNS) 2 g q8h, each + amikacin 7.5 mg/kg q12h IV.
- Severe disease: cefotaxime 2–3 g q6–8h or ceftriaxone 2 g/day IV +/– amikacin.

Miscellaneous
- Chronic granulomatous disease pts: should get gamma interferon + sulfa prophylaxis.
- Surgical debridement or drainage, consider for extrapulmonary lesions.
- *In vitro* sensitivity tests important, especially if considering non-sulfa therapy.
- Sulfa intolerance (esp AIDS): consider desensitization.
- Sulfa therapy: some get sulfa levels, 2 hrs post oral dose. Expect peak of 100–150 mg/L.
- Decrease/reduce immunosuppression if possible.

FOLLOW UP
- Monitor for relapse × 1 yr post-treatment.

OTHER INFORMATION
- 60% pts are compromised: chronic steroids—<u>major</u> risk; also diabetes, steroids, organ tx, cancer chemo Rx, AIDS; TMP-SMX/dapsone prophylaxis prevents.
- Rx is normally long (6–12 mos) and hard (high dose sulfa, imipenem/amikacin etc.); less serious—can use oral sulfa or minocycline from the start.
- Cure rates: soft tissue-100%, pulmonary-90%, disseminated-60%, CNS-50%.
- Dx: Pulmonary +/– CNS, indolent course, Low CMI, filamentous branching, beaded, Gram pos rod. CNS in 40%; if pul disease—get brain MRI.

MORE INFORMATION
- **Classification:** Aerobic actinomycetes.
- **Species:** 12; most important clinically are *N. asteroides* complex (includes *N. farcinica* and *N. nova*) accounting for 90% of extracutaneous disease; *N. brasiliensis*— mycetoma. Epidemiology: soil, worldwide. Most common—mycetoma in tropics. Most common outside tropics—pulmonary +/– disseminated, esp. CNS in host with decreased CMI.
- **Clinical:** (1) Mycetoma—tropics, local inoculation, *N. brasiliensis*, progressive destructive lesions, distal external sinuses. Also caused by Streptomyces and Actinomadura; (2) Sporotrichoid—lymphocutaneous, local inoculation. N. asteroides; (3) Pulmonary— inhaled, N. asteroides, indolent, X-ray—infiltrate nodule, cavity, multiple nodules; (4) Disseminated—pulmonary first, *N. asteroides* 90%, CNS 40%—abscess or granuloma; other sites—eye, renal, joints, bone, heart.
- **Diagnosis:** Warn lab. GS shows highly characteristic beaded filamentous Gram-positive rod that is weakly acid-fast; grows on routine media (blood agar) requires up to 3 wks, usually 3–5 days.

- **Rx:** Sulfa are best by *in vitro* tests and clinical experience; TMP-SMX is formulation preferred. Alternatives—amikacin + imipenem (best in animal models) or ceftriaxone/cefotaxime +/– amikacin for "induction" Rx of serious disease or minocycline (less serious disease or "maintenance").

BASIS FOR RECOMMENDATIONS

Lerner PI. Nocardiosis. *Clin Infect Dis,* 1996; Vol. 22; pp. 891–903; quiz 904–5.

Comments: Emphasizes that "*N. asteroides* complex" has 3 species: *N. asteroides, N. farcinica,* and *N. nova.* Importance is that *N. farcinica* is resistant to tobramycin and third generation cephalosporins; in some studies it is the predominant species in the complex. For treatment: Sulfonamides preferred, TMP-SMX is most common form used (but need for TMP is ?), relevance of *in vitro* tests is questioned, minocycline data look good, the best *in vitro* synergy data for parenteral agents is amikacin + imipenem.

PASTEURELLA MULTOCIDA

Paul G. Auwaerter, MD

PATHOGENS

MICROBIOLOGY

- Aerobic to facultatively anaerobic, nonmotile small Gram-negative bacillus.
- Common inhabitant of feline > canine oral flora. Common cause of illness in rabbits.
- Often part of polymicrobial aerobic and anaerobic flora of domestic pet bite wound infections.
- Animal bites or scratches may result in cellulitis +/– bacteremia.
- Pasteurella usually susceptible to penicillins, tetracyclines or chloramphenicol.

CLINICAL

- Most commonly associated with cat bite infections resulting cellulitis +/– bacteremia. May also result from scratch or lick.
- Occasionally associated with dog bite infections.
- Occasional cause of pneumonia.
- Rare cause of bacteremia or endocarditis.
- Cat bites have less crush injury and trauma than dog bites, but more often result in osteomyelitis and septic arthritis. The thought is that cats have sharper teeth and more deeply penetrating bites.
- Diagnosis based on culture (swab, blood, body fluid).

SITES OF INFECTION

- Skin and soft tissue: cellulitis, abscesses—most often following cat bite.
- Bone/joint infections: osteomyelitis, tenosynovitis—following penetrating cat bites; septic arthritis—knee most common, especially pts with RA, OA, or prosthetic joint.
- Respiratory: may cause lobar pneumonia +/– abscess or empyema. May also cause URTI: sinusitis, otitis media, mastoiditis, epiglottitis, and pharyngitis.
- Bloodstream: bacteremia may be primary or secondary to a bite.
- Endocarditis: rare.
- Other: metastatic seeding of internal organs from bacteremia.
- CNS: meningitis (rare), most often in young children or the elderly. May be confused with *Haemophilus* or *Neisseria* spp. on Gram-stain.

TREATMENT
Antibiotics

- Amoxicillin/clavulanate 500 mg PO q8h or 875 mg PO twice daily with food (also preferred empirical coverage of animal bite wounds).
- Ampicillin/-sulbactam 3 g IV q6h.
- Penicillin 500 mg PO q6h or 4 million units IV q4h (use only if isolate known to be susceptible).
- Ciprofloxacin 500 mg PO or 400 mg IV q12h or levofloxacin 500 mg PO or IV q24h.
- Doxycycline 100 mg PO twice daily or TMP-SMX DS PO twice daily are also alternatives for beta-lactam allergic pts.
- First generation cephalosporins (e.g., cephalexin [Keflex] and clindamycin) ineffective.
- Occasional strains produce beta-lactamases making then penicillin resistant.

General Management
- Bite infections are frequently polymicrobial and thus amoxicillin/clavulanate usually recommended to provide broad-spectrum empirical coverage.
- For infections of limbs, keep involved extremity elevated. Involve a hand surgeon early w/ hand bite infections.

FOLLOW UP
- *P. multocida* associated with bite wounds are most commonly complicated by abscesses and tenosynovitis.
- Suspect septic arthritis or osteomyelitis especially if incorrect antibiotics are initially employed.

OTHER INFORMATION
- *Pasteurella multocida* does not cause "cat scratch disease", (rather that entity caused by *Bartonella henselae*).
- *Pasteurella multocida* can be a cause of rapidly progressive infections similar to Group A strep or *vibrio* spp. (i.e., pt may present within a few hrs of a cat bite with established severe infection).
- Pts with endocarditis often have no history of animal contact (11/17 cases).

BASIS FOR RECOMMENDATIONS
Stevens DL, Bisno AL, Chambers HF, et al. Practice guidelines for the diagnosis and management of skin and soft-tissue infections. *Clin Infect Dis*, 2005; Vol. 41; pp. 1373–406.
Comments: Guidelines include comments on animal bite wound infections.

PEPTOSTREPTOCOCCUS/PEPTOCOCCUS

John G. Bartlett, MD

MICROBIOLOGY
- Anaerobic Gram-positive cocci, normal flora of the mouth, GI tract, genital tract, and skin.
- Heterogeneous group of "anaerobic strep" now classified in 5 groups.
- Small, may be seen on Gram-stain in short chains, pairs. GPC seen may appear identical to aerobic streptococci (chains) or staphylococci (clusters).
- Peptostreptococcus and Peptococcus account for nearly all anaerobic GPC except *Finegoldia magna* (formerly *Peptostreptococcus magnus*).
- Most common and important: *Finegoldia magna, P. asaccharolyticus.* Less common: *P. micros, P. anaerobius.*

CLINICAL
- Common in mixed anaerobic infections at all anatomical sites.
- Requires uncontaminated specimen (blood, sterile body fluid, etc.) and anaerobic culture for clear-cut diagnosis.
- Pathogenesis: endogenous infection, no pt-to-pt transmission. Does not have predilection for compromised hosts.
- Clinical clues: putrid discharge (Gram-stain often with both GPC + GNB), abscess (mixed infection).
- Alert: microaerophilic streptococci like *Streptococcus milleri* group are pathogenic, often important in mixed infections. They are not Peptostreptococci and are not sensitive to metronidazole.

SITES OF INFECTION
- Nearly always part of mixed infection except for rare cases of endocarditis.
- All abscesses: brain, liver, lung, abdominal, pelvic, dental, tubo-ovarian, etc.
- Intraabdominal sepsis: part of mixed infection
- Lung: aspiration pneumonia, lung abscess, empyema
- Female genital tract: part of mixed infection
- Dental infection: part of mixed infection
- Musculoskeletal: ulcers, cellulitis, fasciitis, soft tissue +/− osteomyelitis
- Endocarditis: <1% endocarditis cases
- Bacteremia: <1% bacteremias

TREATMENT
Antibiotics
- Principles: nearly always part of mixed infections. Peptostreptococcus is rarely cultured. Sensitive to many abx. Treatment usually empiric for mixed flora.
- Best abx: penicillin, amoxicillin, clindamycin, imipenem, beta-lactam/beta-lactamase inhibitors (e.g., amoxicillin/clavulanate, piperacillin/tazobactam, ampicillin/sulbactam). Resistance to beta-lactams and clindamycin recently reported in 4–7% of strains.
- Also active: vancomycin, quinolones (moxifloxacin, levofloxacin), linezolid, daptomycin.
- Variable activity: metronidazole, doxycycline, macrolides (erythromycin/ azithromycin/clarithromycin), ceftazidime.
- No activity: TMP-SMX, norfloxacin, aztreonam, aminoglycosides.
- Caution: metronidazole not active vs. microaerophilic strep which are important in mixed infections.

Treatment–Other
- Abscesses: require drainage except lung and tubo-ovarian + some brain or hepatic abscesses.
- No pt-pt transmission risk, normal flora of everyone.
- Host defenses—less important; not disease of compromised host.
- *In vitro* sensitivities: rarely done except for endocarditis, persistent bacteremia or osteomyelitis. *In vitro* testing results may be deceptive.

OTHER INFORMATION
- Most infections: Peptostreptococci found with other anaerobes + streptococci +/− coliforms.
- Suspect organism with Gram-stain showing mixed flora, putrid states. Endogenous infection capable of being found in any abscess.
- Culture: requires uncontaminated specimen + anaerobic cx (rarely achieved).
- ABX: nearly always empiric. Metronidazole generally active vs. Peptostreptococci but not active vs. aerobic streptococci, including *S. anginosus (S. milleri)* complex, etc. **Be careful** not to narrow treatment to include strict anaerobic coverage only.

BASIS FOR RECOMMENDATIONS
Author opinion.

Comments: No published guidelines exist regarding specific therapy for this pathogen.

PLESIOMONAS

Paul G. Auwaerter, MD

MICROBIOLOGY
- *P. shigelloides* is a facultative, anaerobic, Gram-negative rod weakly related to the species of Enterobacteriaceae and Vibrionaceae.
- Ubiquitous environmentally, it can be isolated from soil, water, and a wide range of animal species.
- Many reports linking organism to gastroenteritis, but remains controversial whether true human pathogen. Rare reports of bacteremia.
- Mechanism of diarrhea due to *Plesiomonas shigelloides* is unknown. It is capable of producing a cholera-like enterotoxin, thermostable enterotoxin, and also a thermolabile enterotoxin.

CLINICAL
- *P. shigelloides* not always pathogenic but may be transient part of intestinal flora. Sometimes isolated from healthy individuals (0.2–3.2% of population).
- Uncommon cause of gastroenteritis; children > adults, especially in tropical and sub-tropical climates.
- Associated w/ drinking untreated water, eating uncooked shellfish, or travel to underdeveloped countries.
- *P. shigelloides* may cause both sporadic cases as well as outbreaks. Increasing incidence in summer mos.
- Infection typically characterized by self-limited watery diarrhea w/ blood or mucus, abdominal pain, emesis, and fever.
- Sx usually occur within 48 hrs of exposure.

PATHOGENS

- Although normally self-limited, up to 30% may develop more persistent diarrhea and abdominal pain lasting >3 wks.
- Prevalence of *P. shigelloides* among pts w/ infectious diarrhea estimated from 0–8%.
- Highest incidence reported in traveler's returning to Japan where ~75% of microbiologically confirmed cases of traveler's diarrhea in 1999 due to *P. shigelloides*.
- Dx: stool culture.

SITES OF INFECTION
- Gastrointestinal: if caused by Plesiomonas, limited to GI tract causing diarrheal illness.
- Dissemination: bacteremia/sepsis, such infection is more common in immunocompromised hosts—associated w/ high mortality.
- CNS: meningitis (rare)
- Musculoskeletal: osteomyelitis, septic arthritis (all rare)
- Ocular: endophthalmitis (rare)

TREATMENT
Immunocompetent Hosts: Mild Infection
- Illness usually self-limited, lasting <2–4 days.
- Antibiotic rx not usually indicated.

Immunocompetent Hosts or Severe Infection
- Severe/protracted diarrhea or extra-intestinal disease: rx empiric antibiotics until culture and sensitivity available.
- Abx shown to shorten the duration of symptoms.
- Plesiomonas chronic diarrhea (sx >3 wks), abx resolve sx.
- Isolates frequently express beta-lactamases, therefore PCN-resistant.
- **Preferred:** ciprofloxacin 500 mg PO twice daily or 400 mg IV q12h.
- **Alt:** ofloxacin 300 mg PO, norfloxacin 400 mg PO; TMP-SMX DS PO (if susceptible), all twice daily × 3 days.
- Ceftriaxone (1–2 g IV once daily) used successfully in severe cases.

Immunocompromised Hosts
- Greater likelihood of dissemination and severe infections, empiric antibiotics recommended for pts w/ AIDS or other immunocompromised pts.
- **Preferred:** ciprofloxacin 500 mg PO twice daily × 3 days.
- **Alt:** ofloxacin 300 mg PO, norfloxacin 400 mg PO; TMP-SMX DS PO (if susceptible), all twice daily × 3 days.
- Ceftriaxone: (1–2 g IV once daily) used successfully in severe cases.

OTHER INFORMATION
- *P. shigelloides* is the most common species of Plesiomonas reported to cause human disease. Previously known as *Aeromonas shigelloides*.
- Approximately 15% of cases cultured w/ a co-pathogen in addition to Plesiomonas.

BASIS FOR RECOMMENDATIONS
Guerrant RL, Van Gilder T, Steiner TS, et al. Practice guidelines for the management of infectious diarrhea. *Clin Infect Dis*, 2001; Vol. 32; pp. 331–51.
Comments: IDSA guidelines for diarrhea suggest using TMP-SMZ DS PO twice daily × 3 days (if susceptible), fluoroquinolone (e.g., 300 mg ofloxacin, 400 mg norfloxacin, or 500 mg ciprofloxacin twice daily × 3 days). Guidelines note that the data supporting the pathogenicity of *Plesiomonas* is weaker than for it's *cousin Aeromonas*.

PROPIONIBACTERIUM SPECIES

Paul G. Auwaerter, MD

MICROBIOLOGY
- Gram-positive pleomorphic rod that grows best anaerobically.
- Usually inhabits human skin, sebaceous glands, nasopharynx, GI/GU tracts.
- Generally sensitive to beta-lactams and resistant to aminoglycosides.

CLINICAL
- Most common, non-spore forming anaerobic rod found in clinical specimens.
- Frequent blood culture contaminant. *P. acnes* is the species most often isolated.

- Commonly associated w/ acne vulgaris.
- Most frequent serious infection: CNS shunt infections.
- Also growing reports implicating medical-device infections. The problem is distinguishing between common surgical contaminant vs. actual pathogen.
- Low virulence, and slow growth—often requiring 5–10 days for significant growth in cxs (often from broth). Request microbiology lab perform extended cultures if suspecting.

SITES OF INFECTION

- **Skin:** associated with acne conditions, soft tissue infection (occasional)
- **CNS:** shunt infections, meningitis (post-operative), brain abscess, subdural empyema
- **Renal:** infectious shunt-related glomerulonephritis described, CAPD catheter infection and peritonitis
- **Cardiac:** endocarditis (rare)
- **Ocular:** endophthalmitis (usually post-cataract surgery)
- **Bone:** prosthetic joint infection (especially shoulder), osteomyelitis (rare)
- **Dental:** caries, abscesses

MORE SITES OF INFECTION

P. acnes Antimicrobial Resistance:

Information mainly gleaned from isolates in refractory cases of acne vulgaris, so correlation with the much less common systemic infections are unclear.

Resistance approximately: erythromycin (50%), clindamycin (35%), and tetracycline (25%). Erythromycin and clindamycin resistance often occur in tandem.

Tetracycline is often used if disease breaks through erythromycin or clindamycin therapy.

Minocycline may still have effect when either tetracycline or doxycycline-resistant strains of *P. acnes* are suspected.

Fun Fact: related *P. freudenreichii* is responsible for both flavor and the characteristic holes during Swiss cheese manufacture.

TREATMENT

Systemic infection

- Routine anaerobic bacterial abx sensitivity testing often unavailable and problematic due to lack of standardization. Choice often empiric.
- *P. acnes* often susceptible to PCN, tetracyclines, chloramphenicol, erythromycin, and vancomycin (including teicoplanin)—but resistance increasing likely due to widespread abx use for acne vulgaris.
- Preferred: penicillin G 2mU IV q4h.
- Alt: clindamycin 600 mg IV q8h, vancomycin 15 mg/kg IV q12h.
- Shoulder prosthesis infection: 1-stage or 2-stage joint replacement plus amoxicillin + rifampin for 3–6 mos.
- Consider removal of foreign bodies. Some success w/ retention of shunts, prostheses but no clear data to guide.
- Duration: 2–4 wks, may be able to switch to oral meds in some circumstances (soft tissue infections).
- Note: metronidazole or tinidazole w/o activity against Propionibacterium species.

Acne Vulgaris

- See Acne vulgaris module.

OTHER INFORMATION

- *P. acnes* mostly a contaminant, especially from blood cxs. Clinician must carefully weigh clinical situation to judge culture results.
- Do not routinely dismiss as contaminant if isolated (especially repeatedly) from CSF shunts and sterile medical devices.
- Slow growing organism, so blood and other specimen cxs often only positive after 3–5 days incubation.
- Most eubacteria such as *P. acnes* are resistant to nitroimidazoles such as metronidazole—preferred choices: penicillins, clindamycin.

BASIS FOR RECOMMENDATIONS

Viraraghavan R, Jantausch B, Campos J. Late-onset central nervous system shunt infections with Propionibacterium acnes: diagnosis and management. *Clin Pediatr (Phila)*, 2004; Vol. 43; pp. 393–7.

PATHOGENS

Comments: Authors suggest high dose PCN IV therapy, externalization of shunt and then complete removal as best approach. Some may try salvage with medical therapy alone for this relatively avirulent pathogen.

Author opinion.

Comments: No guideline statements exist for deep infection with *P. acnes*.

PROTEUS SPECIES

Paul G. Auwaerter, MD

MICROBIOLOGY
- Aerobic, Gram-negative, urease-splitting rod.
- "Swarms" on moist agar (many flagella per organism).
- Second most commonly isolated Enterobacteriaceae after *E. coli* in many series.
- Most common species: *P. mirabilis* (indole negative), causes 90% of infections. Other *Proteus* spp. are indole positive, e.g., *P. vulgaris* and *P. penneri*.
- *P. mirabilis* usually resistant to tetracycline, and 10–20% are resistant to ampicillin or cephalexin. *P. vulgaris* usually resistant to ampicillin or cephalexin/cefazolin.

CLINICAL
- Causes ~10% of uncomplicated UTIs.
- May also cause wound infections, bacteremia and nosocomial pneumonia.
- Organism splits urea, raising urinary pH (>8.0) and can cause struvite stone formation.
- Struvite stones can be nidus of chronic renal infection or obstruction. Suspect anatomical problem or stones if recurrent Proteus isolated.
- Dx: urine, blood, body fluid or swab culture.
- Generally inherently resistant to tetracycline and nitrofurantoin. About 10–20% isolates resistant to ampicillin and 1st generation cephalosporins.

SITES OF INFECTION
- **GU:** UTI, pyelonephritis
- **Abdomen:** intra-abdominal infection
- **Skin:** burn wound infections, surgical site infections
- **Other:** pneumonia (usually nosocomial), bacteremia, line sepsis, prosthetic device or bronchoscope infections, endocarditis (rare).

TREATMENT
Proteus mirabilis
- Base choices upon susceptibility profiles. Other agents may be used dependent upon profile.
- Ampicillin: 500 mg PO four times a day or 2 g IV q6h.
- Cefuroxime: 250 mg PO twice daily or 750 mg IV q8h.
- Ciprofloxacin 250–500 mg PO twice daily or 400 mg IV q12h.
- Levofloxacin 500 mg PO once daily or 500 mg IV q24h.
- Duration: uncomplicated UTI 3 days, pyelonephritis 7–14 days, complicated UTI 10–21 days. Bacteremia 7–14 days.

Indole positive Proteus species
- Ceftriaxone 1 g IV q24h.
- Imipenem 500 mg IV q6h.
- Ciprofloxacin 400 mg IV q 12h or 250–500 mg PO twice daily. Levofloxacin 500 mg IV/PO q24h.
- Other agents effective per susceptibility testing.

OTHER INFORMATION
- Reservoir often pt's own GI tract.
- Need urology for management of struvite stones.
- Most nosocomial Proteus infections due to indole + strains (not *P. mirabilis*).
- Consider evaluation for struvite stones if alkaline urine detected.

BASIS FOR RECOMMENDATIONS
Warren JW, Abrutyn E, Hebel JR, et al. Guidelines for antimicrobial treatment of uncomplicated acute bacterial cystitis and acute pyelonephritis in women. Infectious Diseases Society of America (IDSA). *Clin Infect Dis*, 1999; Vol. 29; pp. 745–58.

Comments: Used for uncomplicated UTI and pyelonephritis recommendations.

Author opinion.

PROVIDENCIA

Paul G. Auwaerter, MD

MICROBIOLOGY

- Member of Enterobacteriaceae.
- Motile, Gram-negative, facultative aerobic rod.
- Same tribe as *Proteus* and *Morganella* spp.
- Common constituents of normal GI flora in both humans and animals.
- 5 species: *P. alcalifaciens*, *P. heimbachae*, *P. rettgeri*, *P. rustigianii*, *P. stuartii*.

CLINICAL

- *Providencia stuartii* most common *Providencia* isolate causing infections in humans.
- Isolates can recovered from urine, throat, perineum, axillae, stool, blood, and wound culture specimens.
- Described more commonly in nosocomial and long-term care facility infections than community-acquired GU tract infections.
- *P. stuartii* and *P. rettgeri* are common causes of Gram-negative bacteremia in nursing home pts. Elderly pts w/ chronic indwelling catheters at especially high risk.
- Over 50% of *P. stuartii* infections in one academic hospital setting found to be ESBL-multidrug resistant strains.
- Increasing age, underlying neoplasm, and previous hospitalization and antibiotic therapy a risk for ESBL multidrug resistance for *P. stuartii* infections.
- Although usually a commensal organism, *P. alcalifaciens* implicated as an agent of enteroinvasive gastroenteritis. Most studies in children. Overseas travel may increase risk.
- Dx: culture of urine, blood, wound, or other sterile site.

SITES OF INFECTION

- GU: UTI, most commonly catheter-associated.
- Bacteremia (rare): associated with older age and chronic indwelling catheters.
- Nosocomial: reports of highly resistant *P. rettgeri* UTI outbreaks associated with chronic indwelling catheter and exposure to multiple abx.
- Pulmonary: endotracheal intubation or suctioning may confer a higher risk for pneumonia.

TREATMENT

Preferred agents

- Often a cause of complicated UTI as opposed to uncomplicated bacterial cystitis. Regimens for cUTI, pyelonephritis or urosepsis. May narrow once susceptibilities known. Prostatitis similar drugs but would favor FQ if susceptible.
- Ciprofloxacin 500–750 mg PO q12h or 400 mg IV q8–12h.
- Levofloxacin 500 mg IV/PO q24h.
- Piperacillin-tazobactam: 3.375 mg IV q6h.
- Ceftriaxone 1–2 g IV q24h (do not use if ESBL suspected or critically ill).
- Meropenem 1 g IV q8h (consider if critically ill or ESBL suspected).
- Amikacin 7.5 mg/kg IV q12h. Gentamicin or tobramycin acceptable if susceptible but many species are resistant.
- Duration (UTI): 7 days common or 3–5 days after defervescence or control/elimination of complicating factors e.g., removal of foreign material (e.g., catheter).
- Duration (bacteremia): 10–14 days or 3–5 days after defervescence or control/elimination of complicating factors.
- Duration for acute prostatitis (2 wks) shorter than chronic prostatitis (4–6 wks).

Alternative regimens

- TMP-SMX (Bactrim) DS 1 PO q12h for 10–14 days or 5–10 TMP/kg/day IV divided q6h.
- As a rule, multiple resistance profiles have been reported for *Providencia* spp. and antimicrobial testing is extremely important.

OTHER INFORMATION

- Treatment failures: may carry chromosomal gene encoding extended-spectrum beta-lactamase (ESBL), usually induced in the presence of some but not all beta-lactam antibiotics.
- *P. rettgeri* can hydrolyze urea, unlike the other *Providencia* spp. Look for elevated urinary pH.

PATHOGENS

- *P. alcalifaciens* and *P. rustigianii* tend to be the most susceptible of the *Providencia* spp.
  P. stuartii generally is the least susceptible species to antibiotic therapy.

BASIS FOR RECOMMENDATIONS

Naber KG, Bergman B, Bishop MC, et al. EAU guidelines for the management of urinary and male genital tract infections. Urinary Tract Infection (UTI) Working Group of the Health Care Office (HCO) of the European Association of Urology (EAU). *Eur Urol*, 2001; Vol. 40; pp. 576–88.

Comments: Basis for duration recommendations for various GU infections; however, doesn't specifically address Providencia (but rather "other Enterobacteriaceae").

Author opinion.

Comments: In critically ill pts, would favor use of carbapenem given multiple resistance profiles often seen with Providencia including ESBL. Once susceptibilities known, can narrow drug choice if possible.

PSEUDOMONAS AERUGINOSA

Khalil G. Ghanem, MD

MICROBIOLOGY

- Gram-negative bacillus, motile, aerobic, lactose nonfermenter.
- Laboratory dx: culture of sputum, urine, blood, abscess fluid, joint fluid, or CSF.
- Inhabits moist environments including soil, water (hot tubs, sinks, water faucets, respirators, disinfectants), plants and animals.

CLINICAL

- Primarily a nosocomial pathogen.
- Cause of pneumonia (usually nosocomial), UTI, bacteremia, post-neurosurgical meningitis and skin-soft tissue, post-surgical infections.
- Risk factors include neutropenia, diabetes, skin burns, cystic fibrosis, and AIDS.

SITES OF INFECTION

- Respiratory: pneumonia (nosocomial, CF, AIDS) and lung abscesses.
- CV: endocarditis (IVDU); bacteremia (primary and secondary due to indwelling catheters).
- Skin: ecthyma gangrenosum (neutropenia); cellulitis (DM, IVDU, post-operative); folliculitis; abscesses; noma neonatorum (infants).
- GU: UTI/pyelonephritis (DM and hospitalized pts w/ indwelling catheters).
- ENT: otitis externa and malignant otitis externa (DM); chronic otitis media; sinusitis (AIDS).
- CNS: brain abscesses; meningitis especially post-neurosurgical manipulation.
- Bone/joint: vertebral, sternoclavicular or pelvic bone infections (IVDU); osteochondritis of foot (following penetrating injuries through tennis shoes).
- Eye: keratitis; endophthalmitis.
- GI: diarrhea; necrotizing enterocolitis "typhlitis" (young children and neutropenia).

TREATMENT

General principles

- Isolation of infected pts, hand-washing by staff and visitors, and vigilant infection control measures may help prevent nosocomial transmission.
- In pts w/ chronic lung disease (e.g., CF), good pulmonary toilet (mucolytic agents, chest PT, postural drainage) are important adjunctive treatment measures.
- Double coverage using high doses of synergistic antibiotic combinations (B-lactam + aminoglycoside) possibly recommended, especially empirically for serious infections with known organism susceptability profiles.
- Rx of AIDS-related pseudomonas infections may require a more prolonged course of therapy to prevent chronic infections/relapses.
- Multiple resistance mechanisms occur; increasing resistance especially in CF wards and ICUs; chemotherapy based on susceptibility testing.
- Multi-drug resistant strains may be susceptible to colistin or polymyxin B.
- Pseudomonas endocarditis may require surgical intervention in addition to chemotherapy.
- Pts with CF, pregnancy, burns, and critical illnesses may require higher doses of aminoglycosides. Serum drug levels should be monitored carefully.

Chemotherapy

- Use susceptibilities to guide final choices.
- Cefepime 2 g IV q8h or ceftazidime 2 g IV q8h.
- Piperacillin 3–4 g IV q4h (no benefit for pseudomonas from beta-lactamase inhibitor).
- Ticarcillin 3–4 g IV q4h (no benefit for pseudomonas from beta-lactamase inhibitor).
- Imipenem 500 mg—1 g IV q6h; meropenem 1 g IV q8h or doripenem 500 mg IV q8h (carbapenemase-producing strains are increasing).
- Ciprofloxacin 400 mg IV q8h or 750 mg PO q12h (for less serious infections); may not be wise single empiric choice due to rising resistance.
- Aztreonam 2 g IV q6–8h.
- Colistin 2.5 mg/kg IV q12h.
- Polymyxin B 0.75–1.25 mg/kg IV q12h
- Gentamicin or tobramycin 1.7–2.0 mg/KG IV q8h or 5–7 mg/kg IV every day or amikacin 2.5 mg/kg IV q12h. Usually used in combination w/ other antimicrobials (preferably beta-lactams). Note: amikacin > tobramycin > gentamicin with respect to *P. aeruginosa* susceptibility percentages at most institutions.

Follow Up

- Left-sided pseudomonas endocarditis may require surgical intervention.

Other Information

- Ecthyma gangrenosum (skin lesion w/ hemorrhage, necrosis, and surrounding erythema) is a clue to Pseudomonas bacteremia in the neutropenic host.
- Suspect malignant otitis externa in pts with DM, otalgia and facial nerve palsy (may have bilateral infections).
- Pseudomonas keratitis can complicate prolonged corneal exposure in ICU pts.
- Advanced AIDS predisposes to *P. aeruginosa* pneumonia, bacteremia, endocarditis, sinusitis, skin infections, and malignant otitis externa.
- Many clinicians now feel that monotherapy is adequate for treatment of most all *P. aeruginosa* infections with known susceptibility profiles. The main exception is monotherapy with an aminoglycoside has been shown to be correlated with worse outcomes and higher mortality—hence should be avoided if possible.

Basis for Recommendations

Paul M, Benuri-Silbiger I, Soares-Weiser K, et al. Beta lactam monotherapy versus beta lactam-aminoglycoside combination therapy for sepsis in immunocompetent pts: systematic review and meta-analysis of randomised trials. *BMJ*, 2004; Vol. 328; p. 668.

Comments: 64 trials with 7586 pts were included. There was no advantage to combination therapy among pts with Gram-negative infections (1835 pts) or *P. aeruginosa* infections (426 pts). This meta-analysis highlights the controversy in non-neutropenic pts regarding double coverage.

RHODOCOCCUS EQUI

Aimee Zaas, MD

Microbiology

- Pleiomorphic, nonmotile Gram + coccobacillus.
- Ubiquitous in environment. Inhalation, local inoculation or ingestion are modes of acquisition.
- Variable acid-fast staining; salmon-pink colonies at 4–7 days.
- Lab may dismiss as "diphtheroids" (then considered a "contaminant"). Make lab aware of clinical history.
- Can also be confused with Micrococcus, Bacillus (all common contaminants) or Mycobacteria species.

Clinical

- Typically infects persons with impaired cell-mediated immunity (AIDS, corticosteroids, organ transplant).
- 10–15% of Rhodococcus infections in immunocompetent pts.
- Pulmonary infection (cavity, nodules, bronchopneumonia) most common manifestation.
- HIV: pts often co-infected with other pathogens at presentation.

PATHOGENS

- Social Hx: exposure to animals, particularly horses.
- Chest CT appearance includes consolidation +/– cavities, ground glass, nodules and tree-in-bud. Effusions and lymph node enlargement unlikely.
- Dx: sputum/blood cx; may need CT guided biopsy culture or bronchoscopy. HIV + pts often bacteremic at time of bronchopneumonia.
- Case report of infection after anti-CD52 immunotherapy (alemtuzumab).

SITES OF INFECTION

- **Pulmonary:** most commonly necrotizing pneumonia/abscess/cavitation.
- Cavities tend to be thick-walled; air-fluid levels distinguish from tuberculosis/nocardia.
- Local spread may occur to chest wall, mediastinal lymph nodes.
- **Dissemination (hematogenous):** brain, bone, subcutaneous tissue.
- Relapse after treatment often at sites of hematogenous dissemination.
- **Other infections:** wound, ocular, bacteremia, peritonitis, osteomyelitis, brain abscess, abdominal organ abscess.

TREATMENT
Antibiotic Therapy

- Treatment (induction) lengthy: at least 4 wks or until infiltrate disappears.
- Some authors recommend at least 8 wks in immunocompromised pts.
- Combination therapy with intracellular activity recommended (see below).
- Suppressive therapy 3–6 mos in non HIV, often lifelong in HIV; no data on stopping if immune reconstitution on HAART.
- **First line:** vancomycin 1 g IV q12h (15 mg/kg q12 for >70 kg) **or** imipenem 500 mg IV q6h **plus**.
- Rifampin 600 mg PO once daily **or** ciprofloxacin 750 mg PO twice daily **or** erythromycin 500 mg PO four times a day.
- **Oral/maintenance therapy (after infiltrate clears):** ciprofloxacin 750 mg PO twice daily **or** erythromycin 500 mg PO four times a day.
- Avoid penicillins/cephalosporins due to development of resistance.
- Linezolid effective *in vitro*; no clinical reports of use.
- Other agents reported with activity: azithromycin, TMP-SMX, chloramphenicol, clindamycin.

Surgical

- Resection of large abscesses/necrotizing pneumonias adds to success in combination with abx.

OTHER INFORMATION

- If relapse occurs on maintenance therapy, beware of resistant organisms.
- Notify lab if suspicious of Rhodococcus—otherwise an isolate may be dismissed as a contaminant.
- Mortality 20%, up to 50% in pts with AIDS.
- Histopathology: often shows malakoplakia—plump epithelioid histiocytes with eosinophilic, homogenous, or granular cytoplasm.
- Many drug interactions may occur if rifampin used (especially with HAART).

BASIS FOR RECOMMENDATIONS

Stiles BM, Isaacs RB, Daniel TM, et al. Role of surgery in Rhodococcus equi pulmonary infections. *J Infect*, 2002; Vol. 45; pp. 59–61.
Comments: Successful surgical/medical treatment of severe rhodococcus equi necrotizing pneumonia.

Verville TD, Huycke MM, Greenfield RA, et al. Rhodococcus equi infections of humans. 12 cases and a review of the literature. *Medicine (Baltimore)*, 1994; Vol. 73; pp. 119–32.
Comments: Author recommends minimum of 8 wks therapy in immunocompromised hosts.

Nordmann P, Ronco E. *In vitro* antimicrobial susceptibility of Rhodococcus equi. *J Antimicrob Chemother*, 1992; Vol. 29; pp. 383–93.
Comments: Highlights rifampin (rif)-erythromycin(ery), rif-minocycline(min), ery-min, and imipenem-amikacin as synergistic combinations.

RICKETTSIA RICKETTSII

Paul G. Auwaerter, MD and Joseph Vinetz, MD

MICROBIOLOGY

- Obligately intracellular, Gram-negative agent of Rocky Mountain Spotted Fever.
- Tick-transmitted, late spring to early fall. (common brown dog tick) may transmit in Arizona and West Coast.
- American dog tick (*Dermacentor variabilis*) and Rocky Mountain wood tick (*Dermacentor andersoni*) primary arthropods vectors in U.S. Brown dog tick (*Rhipicephalus sanguineus*) also reported as a vector in Arizona. *Amblyomma cajennense* may carry *R. rickettsii* in Central and South America.

CLINICAL

- Potential for rapidly lethal illness, can be difficult to diagnose. Must start presumptive Rx (doxycycline) in the right setting.
- Endemic areas: East of Rocky Mountains, most common in Oklahoma, Carolinas, Virginia, Maryland. Also present in Montana, Wyoming, and Arizona. Has occurred in all lower 48 states.
- Typically 400–1500 cases reported annually in U.S.
- Most (90%) but not all cases present with rash, usually after 3–5 days prodrome of constitutional symptoms such as malaise, myalgia, headache and fever.
- Severity ranges from undifferentiated febrile syndrome to hypotension and multiorgan failure.
- Classic triad: fever, headache, rash. Occurs mostly May to September in endemic areas.
- General lab findings: nl to low WBC, thrombocytopenia characteristic, occasionally mild anemia, abnormal liver function tests and coagulopathy (DIC). Hyponatremia in 50% while high CK, LDH may be seen with tissue injury in severe cases.
- Ddx: other tick-borne infections including Ehrlichia, Anaplasma, other Rickettsial spp., bacterial sepsis including *N. meningitidis*, *N. gonorrheae*, viral infections (enterovirus, influenza), drug reactions.
- Dx: skin bx w/ direct fluorescent antibody (DFA rapid, but not available routinely in many places) or serum indirect fluorescence assay (IFA) to detect acute/convalescent antibodies to spotted fever group *Rickettsia*. PCR on skin bx (not blood) useful in qualified labs; culture not routinely done—hazardous (BSL3 agent).
- IFA often negative early in course of illness.

SITES OF INFECTION

- General: fever, myalgia, sepsis syndrome.
- Skin: petechial rash (although early rashes may be more nonspecific in nature/ maculopapular), begins on extremities, moves towards trunk (centripetal); endothelial cell dysfunction leads to edema of hands and feet. 50% of rashes begin after 3 days of fever.
- Neuro: vasculitis; headache, focal neuro deficits, deafness, meningismus (sometimes with CSF mononuclear/polymorphonuclear pleocytosis), delirium, abnormal EEG (diffuse slowing).
- Renal: acute renal failure—ATN and/or intravascular volume depletion, may require hemodialysis.
- Pulmonary: pneumonia (alveolar infiltrates), non-cardiogenic pulmonary edema, hyaline membrane dz (ARDS).
- Cardiac: myocardial dysfunction unusual.

TREATMENT

Doxycycline

- Important to treat empirically upon clinical suspicion rather than weight for confirmatory testing.
- Drug of choice in children as well as adults given potential fatal outcome.
- Adult: 200 mg load (severe disease) and then 100 mg PO/IV twice daily × 7 days or 3 days after defervescence.
- Treatment with doxycycline or tetracycline recommended in children for 2 reasons: (1) RMSF can be life threatening; (2) a brief course of Rx is unlikely to lead to tooth problems or staining.

PATHOGENS

- Children: 2–4 mg/kg/day (up to 200 mg/day) divided and given every 12 hrs.
- Adjunctive steroids not recommended.
- Don't use in pregnancy.

Tetracycline
- Child: 25 to 50 mg/kg/day PO in 4 divided doses.

Alternatives
- Chloramphenicol: Adult, 500 mg PO four times a day, 7 days or stop 3 days after defervescence. Child, 50–75 mg/kg/day PO in 4 divided doses.
- Useful in pregnancy or severe tetracycline allergy.

Prevention
- Wear light-colored clothing, tuck your pant legs into socks.
- DEET commonly recommended repellent applied to skin, use lower % sprays for children. Permethrin-containing repellents can be sprayed on boots and clothing.
- Perform a full body check after visiting tick-infested areas.
- No well-accepted recommendations exist for antibiotic prophylaxis following tick bite.
- No vaccine available.

FOLLOW UP
- Infection is believed to confer long-lasting immunity to *R. rickettsii*.
- Overall mortality rate in modern era is now <2% but can range to 9% in the elderly even with antibiotic treatment.

OTHER INFORMATION
- It is better to treat empirically in appropriate setting (endemic region, spring-summer) even if diagnosis not confirmed (but only suspected), rather that wait to prove diagnosis and then treat.
- RMSF can occur in fall or winter, primarily in Southern states.
- Fewer than 20% of RMSF cases have history of known tick bite (since often pediatric cases).
- Up to 10% of RMSF cases may lack a rash, especially early in course of infection.

BASIS FOR RECOMMENDATIONS
Holman RC, Paddock CD, Curns AT, et al. Analysis of risk factors for fatal Rocky Mountain Spotted Fever: evidence for superiority of tetracyclines for therapy. *J Infect Dis*, 2001; Vol. 184; pp. 1437–44.

Comments: The major point of this paper is that RMSF deaths continue to occur because of delayed dx and failure to initiate timely, appropriate Rx. Chloramphenicol was inferior to tetracyclines. Risk factors for death included non-use of tetracyclines, older pts treated w/ chloramphenicol only, initiation of appropriate abx ≥5 after onset of sxs.

RICKETTSIA SPECIES

Paul G. Auwaerter, MD and Joseph Vinetz, MD

MICROBIOLOGY
- Obligately intracellular, Gram-negative rod. Expanding number of species causing human infection.
- Transmitted by a variety of hematophagous arthropods: ticks, mites, chiggers.
- Divided into spotted fever group (SFG) and typhus group (TG) (see below section under Clinical).
- Organisms infected endothelial cells, whose dysfunction leads to severe manifestations of disease.
- For Rocky Mountain Spotted Fever, see *Rickettsia rickettsii* module.

CLINICAL
- Two major groups of obligately intracellular, Gram-negative bacteria: (1) Spotted fever group, (2) Typhus group.
- Generic syndrome: fever, headache, rash, in appropriate epidemiological context (i.e., tick bite). Since lab diagnosis difficult, should start empiric treatment before diagnosis established.
- Suspect in febrile travelers returning from Africa, South America, Mediterranean region and Asia, with rural—especially brush—exposure; look for skin lesions.

- Spotted fever group [SFG]: *R. conorii* (Mediterranean spotted or Boutonneuse fever)—tick-borne, tache noire (eschar at site of tick bite); *R. africae* (tick-borne, African tick fever), *R. akari* (mite-borne; rickettsialpox; found in U.S.) and many others.
- SFG infections usually non-fatal; serious illness can occur with RMSF-like syndrome (esp. *R. conorii* infection).
- Tache noir (ulcerated, necrotic lesion at site of infectious tick bite/black eschar) characteristic of *R. conorii* (usually), *R. africae* (may be many), *R. akari* (but not RMSF). *R. parkeri* described in U.S. (Gulf coast, Chesapeake Tidewater region), may be misdiagnosed as RMSF, has similar rash but has eschar at site of tick bite; may cross react with RMSF serologies.
- SFG: African Tick Bite Fever—emerging dz caused by *R. africae*; acute febrile illness with HA, tache noire w/ regional adenitis, vesicular rash, aphthous ulcers; cattle tick vector.
- Scrub typhus, caused by *Orientia tsutsugamushi* (formerly *R. tsutsugamushi*), transmitted by chiggers in southeast Asia; associated with inoculation eschar. Can be tetracycline resistant.
- Typhus group: *R. prowazekii* (epidemic typhus; louse borne; associated w/ poor sanitation, e.g., Burundi, Peru); *R. typhi* (endemic/murine typhus, fleas; in U.S., especially border w/ Mexico, also Hawaii).
- Lab diagnosis: serologic (indirect immunofluorescence assay), direct immunofluorescence on skin biopsy, polymerase chain reaction (all done in reference labs).

SITES OF INFECTION
- General: fever, headache, myalgia reflective of disseminated infection, shock (especially possible with epidemic, endemic or scrub typhus).
- Skin: inoculation eschar, "tache noire"; may be multiple especially with *R. africae*; also maculopapular or vesicular rash; peripheral gangrene in advanced cases (except for RMSF and typhus).
- HEENT: occasional oral aphthous ulcers.
- Heart: myocarditis (RMSF and typhus forms).
- Pulmonary: noncardiogenic pulmonary edema, ARDS (with typhus; spotted fever rickettsioses usual do not lead to serious disease except for RMSF).
- Liver: elevated transaminases 5–10 × normal; normal or moderately elevated alkaline phosphatase; jaundice rare unless there is shock.
- Neurological: delirium, coma, focal infarction, manifested pathologically as glial nodule (with typhus; spotted fever rickettsioses usual do not lead to serious disease except for RMSF).
- Heme: thrombocytopenia, leukocytosis, leukopenia (less common).

TREATMENT
Doxycycline
- 100 mg PO twice daily for 5–10 days or ≥3 days after cessation of fever; this applies to non-severe cases.
- For severe cases, use 200 mg IV loading dose, then 100 mg IV q12 hrs up to 24 hrs after defervescence, followed by 2–3 days more of oral doxycycline as above.
- Drug of choice for typhus forms whether child or adult; optimal treatment balancing risks and benefits for less severe rickettsial infection of children unclear.

Tetracycline
- 500 mg PO q6h on empty stomach for 5–10 days or ≥3 days after cessation of fever.

Chloramphenicol
- 500 mg PO q6hr for 5–10 days or ≥3 days after cessation of fever.
- 50–100 mg/kg IV in 4 divided doses for severe cases in which other antimicrobials are contraindicated.

Ciprofloxacin
- 500 mg PO twice daily for 5–10 days or ≥3 days after cessation of fever.
- Second-line choice with limited data, but some prefer for *R. conorii* infections.

OTHER INFORMATION
- Laboratory diagnosis assistance: CDC Division of Viral and Rickettsial Diseases (404)-639-1075; also contact state health departments.
- In the U.S., suspect murine/endemic typhus in south Texas, California; rickettsialpox in New York City in pts with fever, eschar, papulovesicular rash; transmitted by mites from house mice.

PATHOGENS

- Suspect African tick-bite fever, Boutonneuse fever, scrub typhus in pts with fever, tache noire, returning from travel to Africa, Mediterranean, Middle East, Thailand.
- Look for skin lesions, especially on legs, suggestive of inoculation eschar, which may be papules or ulcerated (tache noire).
- Maculopapular rash may appear late in the course of illness, after fever develops.

DETAILED INFORMATION

Other 1

Laboratory Diagnosis: General (non-specific) laboratory findings: elevated transaminases, thrombocytopenia, leukopenia or leukocytosis. Specific diagnosis: indirect immunofluorescence assay (IFA); direct immunofluorescence assay on skin biopsy polymerase chain reaction on skin biopsy, or white cells from peripheral blood (reference laboratory).

Other 2

Rickettsial species and associated arthropod vectors: *R. rickettsia* (RMSF), tick (*Dermacentor* spp., dog and wood ticks). *R. prowazekii* (epidemic typhus), body louse (*Pediculus humanus* var. *corporis*). *R. typhi* (murine/endemic typhus), rat flea (*Xenopsylla cheopsis*) and cat flea (*Ctenocephalides felis*). *R. akari* (Rickettsialpox), mite (*Lioponyssoides sanguineus*, ectoparasite of house mice) *R. parkeri* (spotted fever syndrome in United States), Gulf Coast tick (*Amblyomma maculatum*). *R. africae* (African tick-bite fever), tick (*Amblyomma hebraeum*, *A. variegatum*). *R. conorii* (Mediterranean spotted fever), dog tick (*Rhipicephalus* and *Haemaphysalis genera*).

BASIS FOR RECOMMENDATIONS

Watt G, Chouriyagune C, Ruangweerayud R, et al. Scrub typhus infections poorly responsive to antibiotics in northern Thailand. *Lancet*, 1996; Vol. 348; pp. 86–9.

Comments: This landmark paper reports data that have proven true, that scrub typhus in southeast Asia can be resistant to treatment with doxycycline.

SALMONELLA SPECIES

John G. Bartlett, MD

MICROBIOLOGY

- Aerobic, Gram-negative rod, 2–4 × 0.4–0.6 μm.
- Grows on standard media from stool source, but need fresh specimen.
- Non-typhoid *Salmonella* spp. are the major bacterial cause foodborne infection, formerly primarily from poultry and eggs and now from diverse sources.
- *S. typhi* only acquired from human sources shedding to water, food or waste.

CLINICAL

- *S. typhi* (typhoid fever) colonizes humans only, seen mostly in developing countries; 15% mortality. In U.S., 400 cases/yr, many cases of travelers returning to visit family, India especially.
- *Salmonella* spp. (non-typhoid) one of top 2 bacterial enteric pathogens (*C. jejuni* is other).
- Nontyphoid *salmonella*: 1–3 million cases/yr in U.S. Common bacterial cause of foodborne diarrhea; usual sources: meat, poultry, eggs, dairy products. Multistate outbreaks are often due to wide distribution from a common local source (e.g., large outbreak due to commercial peanut paste in U.S. 2008–2009).
- Clinical spectrum: ranges from colon colonization to acute gastroenteritis to enteric fever (without diarrhea) and focal infections.
- Dx: culture of blood, urine or stool. Outbreaks link source strain by PFGE. Serology not useful. Bone marrow said to be most sensitive sample for recovery of *S. typhi.*

SITES OF INFECTION

- Typhoid fever (enteric fever of *S. typhi* only): high fevers 103°–104°F (39°–40°C) typical with malaise, abdominal pain, headaches. Diarrhea may occur, but not common. Rash, if present, is macular rose-colored spots. Relative bradycardia is classical finding. Hepatosplenomegaly possible. Leukopenia with relative lymphocytosis may be seen. LFT abnormalities common. Rare in U.S. and rare in U.S. travelers.
- GI: <u>acute gastroenteritis</u> (nausea/vomiting, abdominal cramps, diarrhea +/– bloody. Incubation 8–48 hrs with sx often self-limiting within 3–7 days), <u>enteric fever</u> (*S. typhi* or non-typhoidal strains of *Salmonella*: incubation period 5–21 days, often diarrheal symptoms

may resolve and then reoccur—fever, abdominal pain, malaise, constipation. Progressive infection often evolves with delirium.
- Vascular infection: aortitis, graft infections.
- Osteomyelitis: sickle cell pts more prone to *salmonella* osteomyelitis than others.
- Septic arthritis.
- Endocarditis.
- Meningitis (mostly infants).
- Reactive arthritis.
- Carrier state.

TREATMENT

Gastroenteritis
- Usually no treatment necessary for uncomplicated diarrheal illness.
- Indications to treat: severe disease, >50 yrs, prosthesis, presence of valvular heart disease or severe atherosclerosis, cancer, uremia, immunosuppression.
- Immunocompetent (preferred, if tx is indicated): TMP-SMX DS PO twice daily, ciprofloxacin 500 mg PO twice daily or ceftriaxone 2 g IV/day all × 5–7 days.
- Immunosuppressed (preferred): above choices × ≥14 days.

Other infections, including Typhoid fever
- Typhoid fever: ceftriaxone 1–2 g IV q24h then cefixime (Suprax) 400 mg PO daily × 10–14 days total antibiotic therapy or ciprofloxacin 400 mg IV q12h or 500 mg PO twice daily.
- Non-typhoid (serious infection): 3rd generation cephalosporin (ceftriaxone/cefotaxime) or fluoroquinolone (ciprofloxacin, levofloxacin). Use sensitivity testing to guide therapy.
- Bacteremia: ceftriaxone 2 g IV q24h or cefotaxime 2 g IV q6–8h × 7–14 days or ciprofloxacin 400 mg IV q12h × 7–14 days.
- Vascular prosthesis infection: ceftriaxone, cefotaxime or fluoroquinolone (above doses) × 6 wks + early removal of prosthesis or give suppressive therapy life-long.
- Osteomyelitis: ceftriaxone 2 g IV q24h, cefotaxime 2 g IV q6–8h or ciprofloxacin 750 mg PO twice daily × ≥ 4 wks + remove sequestra.
- Arthritis: ceftriaxone 2 g IV q24h or cefotaxime 2 g IV q6–8h × 6 wks.
- Endocarditis: ceftriaxone 2 g IV q24h or cefotaxime 2 g IV q6–8h × 6 wks.
- UTI: ceftriaxone, cefotaxime or ciprofloxacin IV × 1–2 wks, then oral ciprofloxacin or TMP-SMX × 6 wks + remove any GU obstructions.
- HIV + salmonellosis: IV cephalosporin or IV fluoroquinolone, then oral FQ (ciprofloxacin 500–750 mg PO twice daily etc.) × 4 wks. If relapse occurs within 6 wks give life-long abx or until immune recovery post-ART.

Prevention
- Avoid use of raw or undercooked eggs.
- Time-temperature standards for food preparation.
- Health care workers or food handlers who are long term carriers are at low risk to transmit.
- Stool surveillance for food handlers is not recommended.
- Food handlers—personal hygiene prevents transmission.
- Typhoid fever vaccine: recommended for travel to developing countries, especially with rural travel and prolonged exposure.
- Available typhoid vaccines in U.S.: (1) oral, live attenuated vaccine (Vivotif Berna vaccine/Ty21 a strain) given 1 dose every other day × 4 doses, (2) Vi capsular polysaccharide given IM × 1. Either has 50–80% efficacy.

FOLLOW UP
- Carrier state (use sensitivity tests to guide rx): ciprofloxacin 500 mg PO twice daily × 4–6 wks or TMP-SMX 1 DS twice daily PO × 6 wks or amoxicillin 500 mg PO three times a day × 6 wks + cholecystectomy if stones present.

OTHER INFORMATION
- Common sources: undercooked food from animals—meat, poultry, eggs.
- Abx for most gastroenteritis unnecessary. Antibiotic therapy associated with prolonged carrier state and represents abx abuse.
- Abx resistance is big problem: chloramphenicol, TMP-SMX and ampicillin—more recently cephalosporins and fluoroquinolones. Need sensitivity tests to treat properly.

PATHOGENS

BASIS FOR RECOMMENDATIONS

Guerrant RL, Van Gilder T, Steiner TS, et al. Practice guidelines for the management of infectious diarrhea. *Clin Infect Dis,* 2001; Vol. 32; pp. 331–51.

Comments: Basis, in part, for recommendations made in this module regarding *Salmonella* gastroenteritis.

No authors listed. The choice of antibacterial drugs. *Med Lett Drugs Ther,* 2001; Vol. 43; pp. 69–78.

Comments: Recommendations used for non-gastroenteritic *Salmonella* infections.

SERRATIA SPECIES

Paul G. Auwaerter, MD

MICROBIOLOGY

- Aerobic, Gram-negative rod of Enterobacteriaceae family, Klebsiella tribe.
- Only *S. marcescens* is a routine cause of human disease, others (*S. liquefaciens, S. rubidaea, S. dorifera*) rare.

CLINICAL

- Common cause of nosocomial infection, as often colonizes respiratory or GU tracts with GI less common except in neonates.
- Hand-to-hand spread implicated mostly in transmission.
- Infections described in heroin-using addicts.
- May cause nosocomial outbreaks especially in neonatal units or related to contaminated equipment.
- Inherently resistant to ampicillin, macrolides, and first-generation cephalosporins.

SITES OF INFECTION

- Bacteremia: usually catheter associated.
- UTI: often w/ catheter or instrumentation association.
- Wound infection: post-operative complications.
- Endocarditis: rare, mostly IDU populations.
- Osteomyelitis: rare, mostly IDU populations.
- Pneumonia: usually nosocomial with history of intubation, or invasive procedures. May occur as "community-acquired" pathogen in the elderly or nursing home resident.
- Septic arthritis: described after intra-articular injections.
- Ocular: conjunctivitis, keratitis.

TREATMENT

Bacteremia, Pneumonia or Serious Infections

- Organisms frequently drug resistant. Amikacin susceptibility usually maintained and often capable of synergy w/ antipseudomonal penicillins.
- Often plasmid-mediated resistance to third-generation cephalosporins, but also described with fourth-gen cephs (cefepime) and carbapenems. ESBL strains reported (SEM1/SEM2). Fluoroquinolone resistance described.
- Cefepime 1–2 g IV q8h or imipenem 0.5–1.0 g IV q6h or ciprofloxacin 400 mg IV q8h. Sensitivities should guide choices.
- Aztreonam, gentamicin or amikacin, piperacillin/tazobactam also often effective.
- Duration depends on clinical response, usually 7–14 days.

Endocarditis

- Choice dictated by sensitivities.
- 4- to 6-wk duration of parenteral therapy.

Osteomyelitis

- Choice dictated by sensitivity profile.
- Treat for 6–12 wks depending upon response. Use IV treatment until stable/clinically improved (10–14 days min) then may convert to PO therapy if appropriate.

UTI

- Fluoroquinolones often sensitive but in seriously ill pt consider empiric coverage with two drugs (e.g., beta-lactam + aminoglycoside or FQ + carbapenem) until susceptibilities known.
- Ciprofloxacin 250 mg PO twice daily or 400 mg IV q12h or levofloxacin 250 mg PO every day or 500 mg IV q24h.

OTHER INFORMATION
- Important nosocomial pathogen implicated as both cause of actual outbreaks due to contaminated equipment as well as pseudo-outbreaks due to inability to sterilize contaminated instruments.
- Mostly likely a cause of hospital-acquired UTI, pneumonia, or bacteremia. IVDUs prone to endocarditis or osteomyelitis.

BASIS FOR RECOMMENDATIONS
Author opinion.
Comments: No guidelines exist for treatment of this specific pathogen.

SHIGELLA DYSENTERIAE

Khalil G. Ghanem, MD

MICROBIOLOGY
- Aerobic, Gram-negative bacillus.
- Constitute group A of the 4 Shigella groups (see *Shigella species* module).

CLINICAL
- *Shigella dysenteriae* type 1 (SD1) serotype is responsible for pandemics and for the most severe clinical illness of *Shigella species*.
- Diagnosis of SD predominates in the developing world; in the U.S., it is rare and typically diagnosed in returning travelers.
- Only SD1 elaborates true Shiga toxin: a neurotoxin and enterotoxin that is associated with the Hemolytic Uremic Syndrome (HUS). All *Shigella* spp. secrete enterotoxins responsible for the watery diarrhea.
- Sx: [see *Shigella species* module] SD1 has longer incubation period (6–8 days vs. 2–4 days) and clinical symptoms are similar to other species but **more severe.**
- Dx: the same diagnostic modalities apply to SD as to other *Shigella species* [see *Shigella species* module].

SITES OF INFECTION
- **GI:** small intestine (watery voluminous diarrhea), large intestine (tenesmus, urgency, smaller volume diarrhea).
- **Rheum:** sero-negative arthritis, Reiter's Syndrome (especially HLA-B27 + pts).
- **CNS:** seizures in children.
- **Heme/Renal:** HUS (microangiopathic hemolytic anemia, renal failure, and thrombocytopenia).
- Bacteremia occurs in young, often malnourished children in the developing world.

TREATMENT
Antibiotics
- It is recommended that cases of SD1, as all other cases of Shigella, be treated with antibiotics.
- Antibiotic regimens same as with other *Shigella species* (see *Shigella species* module).
- Increasing fluoroquinolone resistance in SE Asia.

Prevention
- Same as other *Shigella species* (see *Shigella species* module).

OTHER INFORMATION
- Cases of SD1 diagnosed in the U.S. with no exposure history (travel or exposure to returned traveler) should prompt consideration of possible bioterrorism.

BASIS FOR RECOMMENDATIONS
Zimbabwe, Bangladesh, South Africa (Zimbasa) Dysentery Study Group. Multicenter, randomized, double blind clinical trial of short course versus standard course oral ciprofloxacin for Shigella dysenteriae type 1 dysentery in children. *Pediatr Infect Dis J*, 2002; Vol. 21; pp. 1136–41.
Comments: A multicenter, randomized, double blind, controlled clinical trial. Children between 1 and 12 yrs of age with SD1 dysentery were randomized to receive oral ciprofloxacin suspension 15 mg/kg every 12 hrs for 3 days followed by placebo for 2 days or ciprofloxacin suspension for 5 days. The success rates were 65 and 69% for short and standard course ciprofloxacin, respectively. All pts had bacteriologic cure, and all SD1 isolates were susceptible to ciprofloxacin. No bacteriologic relapses occurred during the study period.

SHIGELLA SPECIES

Khalil G. Ghanem, MD

MICROBIOLOGY

- Aerobic Gram-negative rod (non-motile, non-spore forming), family Enterobacteriaceae.
- Four groups: A (*S. dysenteriae*), B (*S. flexneri*), C (*S. boydii*), and D (*S. sonnei*).
- See module *Shigella dysenteriae* for discussion on Group A.
- In clinical microbiology laboratories, MacConkey or EMB agar in addition to Shigella-Salmonella agar yields best growth.

CLINICAL

- Causes spectrum of illness: watery diarrhea to dysentery.
- As few as 10 organisms can cause disease, hence person-to-person transmission is common especially w/ crowding. Invades mucosa but generally not beyond that, hence blood cx are usually negative.
- Predilection for children 6 mos–10 yrs, adults infected from kids. Person-to-person mostly, but water (wells contaminated w/ feces) and food (20% of cases in U.S.) more common vectors in developing countries.
- 60–80% of cases in the U.S. are caused by *S. sonnei*.
- Classic sx: fever (30%) + abdominal cramps then voluminous stool [small intestinal phase]. 48 hrs later, stools more frequent, less fever, tenesmus + blood (40%) and mucus (50%) [colonic phase].
- Dx: stool cx in first 48 hrs of sx with highest yield. Use MacConkey or EMB agar in addition to Shigella-Salmonella agar. Gram-stain stool may see sheets of PMN (~40% cases). Serology used for epidemiology studies, underline not clinically diagnostic.
- If no abx used, fecal excretion lasts 1–4 wks. Longer term carriage documented. Amount excreted usually low hence person-to-person spread in carriers less likely.
- Duration of illness without abx lasts from 1–30 days (mean of 7 days). Complications rare except w/ *S. dysenteriae*.

SITES OF INFECTION

- **GI:** small intestine (abdominal pain, watery diarrhea and fever), colon (diarrhea, tenesmus, mucus and blood)
- **Ocular:** keratoconjunctivitis
- **Joints:** arthritis and post-shigella Reiters syndrome (post-infectious spondyloarthropathy) in pts especially HLA-B27 positive
- **Pulmonary:** pneumonia, usually in immunocompromised host

TREATMENT

Therapy

- Appropriate rehydration in cases of severe fluid losses.
- **All infections should be treated.** Use of antimicrobials shortens duration of illness and shedding, decreases risk of transmission since person-to-person is common route.
- If known sulfa sensitive: TMP(160 mg)/SMX(800 mg) PO q12h × 3–5 days. Pediatric dosing TMP 5 mg/ SMX 25 mg/kg PO twice daily.
- If TMP/SMX resistant or in area of high resistance (SE Asia, Africa, S. America) or unknown susceptibility: ciprofloxacin 500 mg, norfloxacin 400 mg, ofloxacin 200 mg all PO twice daily × 3–5 days.
- Alternatives (usual duration 5 days): ceftriaxone (1 g IV q24h), azithromycin (500 mg PO day 1, then 250 mg PO days 2–4), nalidixic acid (250 mg PO four times daily or pediatric dose 55 kg/day), ampicillin (500 mg PO four times daily) depending on susceptibility patterns. In southeast Asia, growing resistance seen to fluoroquinolones, azithromycin may be preferred.

Prevention

- Safe water supply (chlorination and effective sewage treatment).
- Routine garbage collection.
- Regular hand washing.
- Appropriate refrigeration and cooking of food.

- Isolating and treating cases of diarrhea.
- Contact precautions are very effective in decreasing spread.

OTHER INFORMATION

- With bloody diarrhea **Do not use motility agents**. Increased risk of toxic dilatation of colon and increased Shigella carriage time.
- Specific diagnosis by stool culture is recommended.
- Empiric treatment for Shigella is recommended in an outbreak situation or w/ increased index of suspicion.
- It is recommended to treat pts with suspected shigella infection with antibiotic therapy in view of **multiple** randomized trials clearly showing benefit.
- Antibiotic resistance patterns vary: resistance to TMP/SMX is increasing; quinolones are favored when susceptibility is unknown; quinolone resistance increasing in the Far East.

BASIS FOR RECOMMENDATIONS

Guerrant RL, Van Gilder T, Steiner TS, et al. Practice guidelines for the management of infectious diarrhea. *Clin Infect Dis,* 2001; Vol. 32; pp. 331–51.

Comments: IDSA recs: Any diarrheal illness lasting >1 day, especially if accompanied by fever, bloody stools, systemic illness, recent use of antibiotics, day-care center attendance, hospitalization, or dehydration (defined as dry mucous membranes, decreased urination, tachycardia, symptoms or signs of postural hypotension, or lethargy or obtundation), should prompt evaluation of a fecal specimen. Pts with febrile diarrheal illnesses, especially w/ moderate to severe invasive disease, empirical treatment considered after fecal specimen is obtained. Rx of Shigella Class A1 rec [highest rec].

STAPHYLOCOCCI, COAGULASE NEGATIVE

John G. Bartlett, MD

MICROBIOLOGY

- Coagulase negative staphylococci (CNS) are aerobic, Gram-positive coccus, occuring in clusters. Frequently found on skin and mucous membranes.
- Catalase positive, coagulase negative. Major pathogen is *S. epidermidis*, colonies typically small, white-beige (about 1–2 mm in diameter).
- Over forty recognized species of CNS, with other major entities including *S. lugdunensis, S. haemolyticus*. Susceptibility to the novobiocin distinguishes *S. epidermidis* from other common coagulase negative organisms. *S. saprophyticus* is phosphatase negative, urease and lipase positive.
- Many strains with propensity to produce biofilm, allowing for adherence to medical devices.
- Usually resistant of penicillin and methicillin.

CLINICAL

- Nearly always a nosocomial pathogen. Source is skin flora. Pathogen primarily associated with foreign bodies and biofilm.
- *Staphylococcus epidermis*—the major pathogen of the coagulase negative staphylococcus category.
- #1 cause of nosocomial bacteremia, but also #1 contaminant.
- #1 infection of plastic/metal: lines, artificial valves, joints, pacemakers, and central nervous system shunts, etc.
- Diagnosis by cultures: need at least 2 positive blood cultures, or heavy growth in presence of, e.g., foreign body.
- Outbreaks in hospitals, ICUs, oncology centers may represent clonal spread.
- *S. lugdunensis* infections more similar in type to *S. aureus* than other coagulase-negative staphylococci. After *S. epidermidis*, second leading cause of CNS endocarditis. May be cause of aggressive infection. Organism often susceptible to methicillin, only ~25% of strains produce beta-lactamase.
- *S. haemolyticus* is second leading cause of CNS neonatal bloodstream infections. Often has reduced susceptibility to glycopeptide abxs (teicoplanin > vancomycin).
- *S. saprophyticus*: often listed as second leading cause of UTI (after *E. coli*) in young, sexually active women.

PATHOGENS

SITES OF INFECTION
- Bacteremia: most often due to IV lines, vascular grafts, cardiac valves (30–40% of all coag-neg staph infections)
- CSF shunt: meningitis
- Peritoneal dialysis catheter: peritonitis
- Prosthetic joint: septic arthritis
- Prosthetic or natural cardiac valve: endocarditis
- Post-sternotomy: osteomyelitis
- Implants (breast, penile, pacemaker) and other prosthetic devices: local infection
- Post-ocular surgery: endophthalmitis
- Surgical site infections

TREATMENT
General principles
- Most common cause of infection with any foreign material. Pathophysiology is based on biofilm on plastic or metal by relatively avirulent bacterium. Treat bacteremia only if ≥2 positive blood cultures (preferably from peripheral sources) or heavy/repeated growth from device.
- Abx: >80% are beta-lactamase positive and methicillin-resistant. Most active: vancomycin, linezolid, daptomycin. Rifampin often added.
- Standard for deep infection: vancomycin 15 mg/kg IV q12h +/– rifampin 300 mg q8h IV/PO. Gentamicin 3 mg/kg/day IV divided q8h added to vancomycin + rifampin for prosthetic valve IE.
- Alt (MRSE): linezolid 600 mg IV/PO twice daily, daptomycin IV 6 mg/kg/day. Each +/– rifampin.
- Alt (methicillin-sensitive): oxacillin/nafcillin 1.5–3 g IV q6h, cefazolin 1–2 g IV q8h, ciprofloxacin 400 mg IV q12h, clindamycin 600 mg IV q8h, TMP-SMX. Use sensitivities to guide choice. Note, only assume methicillin susceptible if multiple isolates are so identified.

Site specific recommendations
- Prosthetic valve: consider valve replacement, abx × 6 wks. See prosthetic valve endocarditis module.
- Peripheral line: remove line, abx × 5–7 days.
- Central line: may often keep line and systemic abx × 2 wks + abx lock.
- Prosthetic joint: typically remove joint (two stage more common than single stage replacement), abx × 6 wks. If very early infection (less than 3 wks post-op, debridement and retention an option).
- Dialysis catheter: keep catheter (at least for first effort) and IV vanco (usually 2 g IV/wk and redose when level <15 mcg/mL) + abx lock ×10–14 days.
- Vascular graft: remove graft, abx × 6 wks.
- CSF shunt: shunt removal usually recommended but variable. IV vancomycin 22.5 mg/kg q12h and PO/IV rifampin plus possible intraventricular antibiotics: vancomycin 20 mg/day +/– gentamicin 4–8 mg/day.

S. saprophyticus UTI
- When occuring in males, suggestive of anatomic abnormality or history of catheterization.
- High incidence of failure with single dose antibiotic regimens.
- Variably susceptible to vancomycin.
- See "Bacterial Cystitis, Acute, Uncomplicated" module for details on multiple regimens.

OTHER INFORMATION
- Most common cause of bacteremia, but also the most common contaminant in all specimens.
- CDC: "Never treat a single positive blood culture for *Staphylococcus epidermidis*."
- Major cause of all foreign body infections: lines, joints, implants, shunts, valves, etc.
- Usually need foreign body plus 2 positive cultures or heavy growth to implicate as causative pathogen.

BASIS FOR RECOMMENDATIONS
No authors listed. Choice of antibacterial drugs. *Treat Guidel Med Lett,* 2007; Vol. 5; pp. 33–50.
Comments: Basis for recommendations in this module.

Archer G. *Staphylococcus epidermidis* and other coagulase-negative *staphylococci*; *Chapter 184 in Principles and Practice of Infectious Disease, Mandell JL, Bennett JE and Dolin R (Editors) Churchill Livingston Phil 5th Ed*, 2000; pp. 2092–2100.

Comments: Coagulase neg. staph include 32 species with 15 indigenous to humans. The value for routine speciation is unclear. Most pathogenic in humans are *S. epidermidis* (foreign bodies) and *S. saprophyticus* (UTI's). Other less common pathogens- *S. haemolyticus*, *S. lugdunensis*, and *S. scheiferi*. Nearly all *S. epidermidis* infections are nosocomial and come from pt or HCW indigenous flora.

STAPHYLOCOCCUS AUREUS

Sara E. Cosgrove, MD

MICROBIOLOGY

- Gram-positive cocci in clusters.
- Easily grown on blood agar or other conventional media.
- Coagulase positive and thermonuclease positive.
- Penicillin resistance conferred by penicillinase production which can be overcome by the addition of a beta-lactamase inhibitor (e.g., ampicillin/sulbactam) or use of a penicillinase-resistant penicillin (e.g., oxacillin, nafcillin). Methicillin resistance conferred by presence of mecA gene which encodes penicillin binding protein 2a, an enzyme that has low affinity for beta-lactams and thus leads to resistance to methicillin, oxacillin, nafcillin, and cephalosporins.
- Community-acquired MRSA (CA-MRSA) isolates often maintain susceptability to tetracyclines and TMP-SMX. Clindamycin susceptibilities vary geographically. If isolate is erythromycin resistant, must confirm clindamycin susceptibility with D-test.

CLINICAL

- Carried in anterior nares by 20–30% of population. Higher carriage rates seen in diabetics, injection drug users (IDU), HIV or dialysis pts. Carriers have > risk of subsequent infection.
- Risk factors: skin disease, venous catheters, other foreign bodies (e.g., prosthetic joints, pacemakers), IDU, hemodialysis, recent surgical procedure.
- Dx: positive cx from sterile site (blood, joint, CSF), abscess or wound. Positive cx from nares = colonization, not infection.
- Methicillin resistance increasing. MRSA traditionally associated w/ healthcare system interaction; CA-MRSA has emerged as significant pathogen, especially in children, prisoners, IDU's (although rates also increased rates in adults with no clear risk factors).
- CA-MRSA causes mostly skin/soft tissue infections. Most infections are relatively benign with good response to IandD ± antibiotics although recurrent disease can occur and rarely there is serious disease with pyomyositis or necrotizing fasciitis.
- CA-MRSA also a cause of necrotizing pneumonia. Consider diagnosis in persons presenting with severe pneumonia with evidence of cavitation/necrosis, particularly after influenza-like illness.
- Staphylococcal toxic shock syndrome (see separate module) caused by TSST-1 or other enterotoxin producing strains = fever, low BP, red rash and multiorgan failure. Risks: tampon use, nasal packing, surgical wounds.
- Diarrhea: ingestion of preformed Staphylococcal enterotoxin causes acute, self-limited gastroenteritis. Incubation 2–6 hrs.

SITES OF INFECTION

- Bloodstream: primary risk is presence of intravascular catheter, which should be removed. Community-onset bacteremia has worse prognosis.
- Skin/soft tissues: folliculitis, cellulitis, furuncle, carbuncle, abscess, impetigo (often in combination with *Streptococcus pyogenes*). Breast: mastitis.
- Abscesses: liver, spleen, kidney, epidural space; results from hematogenous seeding from bacteremia.
- Cardiac: endocarditis occurs in 6–25% of *S. aureus* bacteremia; native and prosthetic valves.
- Bone: osteomyelitis (*S. aureus* leading cause, most common is vertebral secondary to bacteremia/discitis).
- Prosthetic devices: pacemaker leads and pocket, prosthetic joints.

PATHOGENS

- Lung: nosocomial pneumonia or following influenza. Septic pulmonary emboli (associated with right-sided endocarditis).
- Mucosal surfaces: related to release of TSST-1 and subsequent toxic shock syndrome.
- GI: toxin-associated gastroenteritis.
- CNS: post-operative meningitis, meningitis or cerebritis associated with bacteremia/endocarditis

TREATMENT

Bacteremia

- Perform detailed history and physical to detect source and metastatic spread. Consider infectious diseases consultation.
- Remove foci of infection whenever possible.
- Rule out endocarditis with echocardiography (TEE preferred).
- MSSA (preferred): oxacillin or nafcillin 2 g IV q4h. Alternative for non-life threatening PCN allergy: cefazolin 2 g IV q8h. Cefazolin can be given to hemodialysis pts: 2 g after dialysis if next dialysis in 2 days and 3 g after dialysis if next dialysis in 3 days.
- Consider oxacillin/nafcillin desensitization for life-threatening PCN allergy (hives/anaphylaxis only).
- MRSA or life-threatening PCN allergy: vancomycin 15–20 mg/kg q12h. Consider loading dose of 25–30 mg/kg for severe infections.
- Vancomycin alternatives for allergy or treatment failure (infectious disease consult recommended for optimization of regimen): daptomycin 6 mg/kg IV daily (FDA approved for *S. aureus* bacteremia and right-sided endocarditis, preferred in most instances); some experts recommend higher doses 8–12 mg/kg daily for severe infections) or linezolid 600 mg IV/PO q12h (not FDA approved for *S. aureus* bacteremia), quinupristin-dalfopristin 7.5 mg/kg IV q12h. (not FDA approved for *S. aureus* bacteremia), TMP/SMX 5 mg/kg IV q8–12h (not FDA approved for *S. aureus* bacteremia).
- Duration of therapy: 28 days is the standard course of therapy (42-day minimum for concomitant osteomyelitis/epidural abscess); 14 days can be considered if the pt meets the following criteria: endocarditis is ruled out with transesophageal echocardiography, the pt has no implanted prostheses (e.g., prosthetic valves, cardiac devices, or arthroplasties), blood cultures drawn 2–4 days after the initial cultures were negative, the pt defervesces within 72 hrs of appropriate therapy, and metastatic disease has been ruled out.

Endocarditis, native valve

- Perform detailed history and physical to detect source and metastatic spread.
- Remove foci of infection whenever possible. Obtain brain and CNS vessel imaging if neurologic symptoms or persistent headache present.
- Consult w/ cardiac surgery if pt has persistently positive blood cultures, evidence of heart failure or embolic disease.
- Obtain spine imaging if back pain present.
- MSSA, native valve, left-sided: oxacillin or nafcillin 2 g IV q4h for 4–6 wks with optional addition of gentamicin 1 mg/kg IV q8h for 1st 3–5 days. Alternative for non-life threatening PCN allergy: cefazolin 2 g IV q8h with optional addition of gentamicin 1 mg/kg IV q8h for 1st 3–5 days. Use of synergistic gentamicin does not improve mortality but is associated with nephrotoxicity-avoid in pts with baseline decreased CrCl, diabetes, advanced age.
- MSSA, native valve, right-sided involvement only w/o AIDS, vascular prosthesis or embolic dz other than septic pulmonary emboli: oxacillin or nafcillin 2 g IV q4h ± gentamicin 1 mg/kg IV q8h for 14 days. Use of synergistic gentamicin does not improve mortality but is associated with nephrotoxicity-avoid in pts with baseline decreased CrCl, diabetes, advanced age.
- Alt (oral regimen only for IDU, TV endocarditis): ciprofloxacin 750 mg PO twice daily **plus** rifampin 300 mg PO twice daily for 28 days, if isolate proven susceptible to both agents.
- Alt (if life-threatening penicillin allergy): desensitize to oxacillin/nafcillin or vancomycin 15–20 mg/kg IV q12h (consider loading dose of 25–30 mg/kg).
- MRSA, native valve, right or left sided involvement: vancomycin 15–20 mg/kg IV q12h for 4–6 wks.
- Alt: daptomycin 6 mg/kg IV daily for 4–6 wks; some experts recommend higher doses 8–12 mg/kg daily.

Soft Tissue Infections

- Surgical drainage for any collection. Antibiotics indicated for severe/rapidly progressive infections, signs and symptoms of systemic illness, diabetes or other significant immunosuppression, advanced age, location of abscess in an area where complete drainage is difficult, lack of response to initial IandD (also assess for need for additional IandD), extensive-associated cellulitis.
- IV antibiotics generally not needed unless severe infection, concomitant bacteremia or systemic toxicity.
- IV antibiotic choices same as for bacteremia (except daptomycin dose is 4 mg/kg IV daily).
- MSSA (oral): cephalexin 500 mg PO four times a day, dicloxacillin 500 mg PO four times a day, clindamycin 300–450 mg PO three times a day, amoxicillin/clavulanate 875 mg PO twice daily.
- MRSA (oral—check susceptibilities): clindamycin 300–450 mg PO three times a day, TMP-SMX 1–2 DS tabs PO twice daily, minocycline 100 mg PO twice daily or linezolid 600 mg PO twice daily.
- Duration of therapy: depends on extent of disease, range 5–10 days.
- Recurrent soft tissue infections: education regarding hand hygiene and personal hygiene (e.g., regular bathing, no sharing of personal items, clean personal sporting equipment, avoid shaving).
- Consider decolonization for recurrent soft tissue infections: 2% mupirocin ointment to nares twice daily for 5 days +/− Hibiclens washes; efficacy of this strategy is unproven.
- Some clinicians add rifampin to oral agents for MRSA for pts with recurrent soft tissue infections; rifampin should never be used as monotherapy; efficacy of this strategy is also unproven.

Endocarditis, prosthetic valve

- TEE recommended for all cases of bacteremia if TTE doesn't show vegetation in pts with prosthetic valves.
- MSSA, prosthetic valve: oxacillin or nafcillin 2 g IV q4h for 6 wks **plus** gentamicin 1 mg/kg IV q8h for 1st 2 wks **plus** rifampin 300 mg PO q8h for 6 wks after blood cultures have cleared; confirm susceptibility to all agents.
- MRSA, prosthetic valve: vancomycin 15–20 mg/kg IV q12h for 6 wks (consider loading dose of 25–30 mg/kg) **plus** gentamicin 1 mg/kg IV q8h for 1st 2 wks plus rifampin 300 mg PO q8h for 6 wks after blood cultures have cleared; confirm susceptibility to all agents.

Toxic Shock Syndrome

- See Staph TSS module for details.
- Remove focus of staphylococcal colonization or infection.
- Stabilize blood pressure w/ aggressive hydration +/− pressors.
- MSSA: oxacillin or nafcillin 2 g IV q4h plus clindamycin 600 mg IV q8h.
- MRSA: vancomycin 15–20 mg/kg IV q12h **plus** clindamycin 600 mg IV q8h (if susceptible) or linezolid 600 mg IV/PO q12h.
- Consider intravenous immunoglobulin infusions.

Pneumonia

- Antibiotic choices same as for bacteremia except daptomycin cannot be used for pulmonary infections because it is inactivated by pulmonary surfactant.
- Duration of therapy: depends on severity; many cases of ventilator associated pneumonia can be treated for 8 days; necrotizing pneumonia usually requires longer courses ≥14 days; bacteremic pneumonia requires at least 14 days.

Meningitis

- Refractory infections: consider intrathecal vancomycin, 5–20 mg daily.
- MRSA: vancomycin 15–20 mg/kg IV 12 hrs (consider loading dose of 25–30 mg/kg). Strive for trough level ~20 μg/mL.
- Alt: linezolid 600 mg IV q12h (less).
- MSSA: nafcillin or oxacillin 2 g IV q4h.
- Alt (use susceptibilities to guide data): TMP/SMX 4–5 mg/kg (of trimethoprim component) q8h.

PATHOGENS

FOLLOW UP
- For pts with bacteremia or endocarditis, follow up blood cultures should be obtained to document clearance of bacteremia.
- Endocarditis treatment failure: alternative antibiotic regimens as for bacteremia; ID and cardiac surgery consults recommended.
- For pts with serious *S. aureus* infections treated with vancomycin, trough levels should be 15–20 mcg/ml (20 mcg/ml for CNS infection and severe pneumonia).
- Severe MRSA infections with vancomycin MIC 1.5–2.0 not responding to therapy, consider alternative agent (e.g., daptomycin). Several studies have worse clinical outcomes with vancomycin in these settings.

OTHER INFORMATION
- Mortality associated with *S. aureus* bacteremia is 20–40%.
- *S. aureus* bacteremia is associated with heart valve involvement in 25% when studied with transesophageal echo (TEE). Clinicians must rule out endocarditis before treating *S. aureus* bacteremia with short (i.e., 2 wks) course antibiotics.
- All pts with *S. aureus* bacteremia should undergo at least an "adequate" transthoracic echo (TTE). TEE is preferred for pts with prosthetic valves or with inadequate TTE.
- Be alert for the development of metastatic abscess formation w/ any *S. aureus* bacteremia. *S. aureus* in urine cx should alert to the possibility of associated bacteremia.
- Pts with MRSA colonization or infection should be placed on contact precautions.

BASIS FOR RECOMMENDATIONS
Rybak MJ, Lomaestro BM, Rotscharfer JC, et al. Vancomycin therapeutic guidelines: a summary of consensus recommendations from the infectious diseases Society of America, the American Society of Health-System Pharmacists, and the Society of Infectious Diseases Pharmacists. *Clin Infect Dis,* 2009; Vol. 49; pp. 325–7.
Comments: New guidelines for vancomycin dosing and monitoring.

Stevens DL, Bisno AL, Chambers HF, et al. Practice guidelines for the diagnosis and management of skin and soft-tissue infections. *Clin Infect Dis,* 2005; Vol. 41; pp. 1373-406.
Comments: Latest set of guidelines from the Infectious Diseases Society of American, incorporating recommendations for CA-MRSA.

Baddour LM. et al. AHA scientific statement on infective endocarditis. Diagnosis, antimicrobial therapy, and management of complications. *Circulation,* 2005; Vol. 111; pp. e394–e434.
Comments: Guidelines for the management of infective endocarditis.

STENOTROPHOMONAS MALTOPHILIA

John G. Bartlett, MD

MICROBIOLOGY
- Non-fermenting Gram-negative rod, easily grown on standard media. Formerly called *Xanthomonas maltophilia*.
- Ubiquitous—found in water, soil, plants.

CLINICAL
- Usually acquired from nosocomial sources: distilled water, nebulizers, dialysates, contaminated disinfectants, etc.
- Risks: foreign bodies (catheters), neutropenia, broad spectrum abx, cystic fibrosis.
- Often seen as multiply resistant pathogen in critically ill pt.

SITES OF INFECTION
- Nosocomial pneumonia
- Sinopulmonary infection, especially cystic fibrosis pts
- Bacteremia +/– septic shock and DIC
- Plastic: IV lines, CSF shunts, catheters
- Skin and soft tissue: wound, burns, metastatic nodules
- Urinary tract infection
- Ecthyma gangrenosum (rare)
- Ocular: corneal transplant, contact lens users, HSV keratitis

TREATMENT

Treatment

- Preferred: TMP-SMX 15–20 (TMP component) mg/kg/day IV/PO in three divided doses.
- Alternatives: ceftazidime 2 g IV q8h or ticarcillin/clavulanate 3.1 g IV q4h or tigecycline 100 mg IV × 1, then 50 mg IV q12h.
- Alternative (fluoroquinolones): ciprofloxacin 500–750 mg PO/ 400 mg IV q12h, moxifloxacin 400 mg PO/IV every day, levofloxacin 750 mg PO/IV every day (limited clinical experience; development of resistance with treatment observed *in vitro*).
- Some experts recommend coverage with TMP/SMX plus ticarcillin/clavulanate due to concern for resistance.
- Multiply-resistant: colistin 2.5 mg/kg q12h IV.
- Remove catheter in catheter-related bacteremia.
- Treatment duration uncertain, but usually ≥14 days.

Prevention

- Judicious abx use
- Hand washing
- Barrier precautions
- Surveillance
- For nosocomial outbreaks, identify common source: water, equipment

OTHER INFORMATION

- Risks—hospitalization, plastic, multiple abx, trauma, neutropenia, cancer, carbapenem use (imipenem, meropenem).
- **Outbreaks**—waterborne, equipment, solutions.
- Resistant to most abx including imipenem, aminoglycosides, cefepime.

BASIS FOR RECOMMENDATIONS

No author listed. The choice of antibacterial drugs. *The Medical Letter*, 2001; Vol. 43; pp. 69–78.

Comments: Recommendations for treatment in this module.

STREPTOBACILLUS MONILIFORMIS

Khalil G. Ghanem, MD

MICROBIOLOGY

- Pleomorphic, nonencapsulated Gram-negative bacillus.
- A major cause of **Rat Bite Fever** [RBF—the other species, *Spirillum minus* occurs mostly in Asia].

CLINICAL

- Normal commensal of rodent oropharynx also in ferrets, weasels, gerbils.
- Risk factors for acquisition: crowded urban dwellings (especially kids), lab workers. Transmission: bite/scratch from rat, mice, squirrels—also cats, dogs, pigs.
- Symptoms: incubation ~10-day fever, chills, HA, N/V, migratory arthralgias, leukocytosis (~30 K). Days 2–4 days: nonpruritic maculopapular, petechial, or pustular rash (palms soles, extremities). May be purpuric/confluent.
- In 50% pts, polyarthritis (even septic arthritis) with or after onset rash (knees>ankles>elbows>hips). Most sx resolve within 2 wks (even if no abx). Arthritis can persist ~2 yrs.
- Nonzoonotic transmission (orally): aka Haverhill Fever (similar manifestations as RBF). Rodent excrement contaminating water, milk, turkey meat. Milk contamination associated w/ epidemics.
- DDx: rash on palms/soles consider RMSF, syphilis. Arthritis: disseminated gonorrhea, Lyme, brucella, endocarditis, rheumatological dz, and rheumatic fever.
- Dx: Gram or Giemsa stain blood, joint fluid, pus. Perform Cx using TSA or blood agar. ELISA or agglutinins (sero-negative within 5 mos–2 yrs); PCR.

SITES OF INFECTION

- **Joints:** migratory arthropathy and arthritis
- **GI:** diarrhea, especially kids. Liver or spleen abscess

- **Systemic:** undifferentiated fever
- **Cardiac:** endocarditis, myocarditis, pericarditis
- **CNS:** meningitis, brain abscess
- **Heme:** anemia
- **Pulmonary:** pneumonia
- **Pregnancy:** amnionitis
- **GU:** renal abscess

TREATMENT

Therapy

- IV PCN G (preferred): uncomplicated disease—2.4–4.8 mU/day IV divided q6h. If better after 1 wk, switch to oral amoxicillin or PCN Vk complete 14 days.
- Complicated (endocarditis or CNS): PCN 20 mU/day IV divided q4h. Optimal duration?—recommendation for IE is 4 wks.
- Alternatives: cephalosporins (ceftriaxone), clindamycin, erythromycin, chloramphenicol and streptomycin.

Prevention

- Eradication of rats.
- Pasteurize milk.
- Avoid contaminated water.
- Use gloves when handling rodents in lab (can also be carried by hamsters and other laboratory rodents).
- If bitten: oral PCN (2 gs) × 3 days **may** be beneficial. No clinical data available.

FOLLOW UP

- Relapse may be due to L-forms which have no cell wall.
- Some advocate initial use of PCN followed by tetracycline or streptomycin as these drugs that do not require a cell wall for activity.

OTHER INFORMATION

- 25% pts with RBF have false positive RPR making it more difficult to r/o syphilis. Check FTA/MHA-TP which should be negative.
- Handling of dead rat has been reported to cause RBF, or bite may occur at night hence no history given by pt of exposure. Bite may have healed by the time sx begin.
- RBF caused by *Spirillum minus* occurs in Asia, similar to streptobacillary form but with lymphadenopathy and ulceration of bite. Not orally transmitted.
- Haverhill Fever: same as RBF but more vomiting and pharyngitis (1st 10 days).

BASIS FOR RECOMMENDATIONS

Elliott SP. Rat bite fever and *Streptobacillus moniliformis*. *Clin Microbiol Rev*; 2007; Vol. 20; pp. 13–22.

Comments: The clinical and biological features of rat bite fever and *Streptobacillus moniliformis* are reviewed in this paper, as are the latest treatment recommendations.

STREPTOCOCCUS PNEUMONIAE

John G. Bartlett, MD

MICROBIOLOGY

- Aerobic, Gram-positive diplococcus with capsule.
- Grows on blood agar.
- Capsular swelling w/ application of Quelling sera.
- Serotypes: immunity is serotype-specific. Abx resistance is often serotype-specific. Serotype 19A has emerged as predominant pathogen.
- Minimum Inhibitory Concentration (MIC) (mcg/mL) breakpoints: Susceptible (2), Intermediate (4) and Resistant (8). Previously S = 0.06, I = 0.12–1.0 and R = 2. Susceptible breakpoint for meningitis caused by S. pneumoniae remains unchanged (0.06 mcg/mL).

CLINICAL

- Most common bacterial pathogen of otitis, sinusitis and pneumonia, but usually not cultured in any of these.
- Ecologic niche: nasopharynx in 5–10% adults, 20–40% of children.

- Abx resistance best predicted by abx exposure within prior 3 mos and exposure to children, especially day care centers.
- Penicillin resistance: now ~5% with new definition; serotypes 6A, 6B, 9V, 14, 19A, 19F and 23F—all from children.
- Serotype 19A has emerged "replacement strain"—not in Prevnar vaccine, now epidemic and has reduced sensitivity to antibiotics.
- Dx: proven by positive culture of body fluid (blood, CSF, joint, etc.); supportive dx if positive Gram-stain or cx from respiratory specimen and/or urine antigen test in adult.
- Risk for bacteremia: splenectomy, HIV, smokers, black race, multiple myeloma, asthma.

MORE CLINICAL

	Sensitivity	Specificity
Urine antigen	81%	98%
Gram-Strain	58%	—
Immunochromatic test	74%	94%

SITES OF INFECTION

- Lung (pneumonia)
- Sinuses (sinusitis)
- Middle ear (otitis media)
- Bronchi (acute exacerbation of chronic bronchitis)
- CNS (meningitis)
- Peritoneum (spontaneous bacterial peritonitis)
- Pericardium (purulent pericarditis)
- Skin (cellulitis)
- Eye (conjunctivitis)

TREATMENT

Respiratory tract

- Pneumonia (community-acquired, ATS/IDSA 2007 guidelines, preferred PCN sensitive (MIC ≤2):Pen G: 1–2 mil U q6h IV or ceftriaxone 2 g IV q24h or cefotaxime 1–2 g IV q6–8h.
- Oral agents: Pen V 500 mg PO four times a day, amoxicillin 500–1000 mg PO three times a day, cefpodoxime 200 mg PO twice daily, cefprozil PO 500 mg twice daily, cefditoren 400 mg PO twice daily, cefdinir 300 mg PO twice daily, or doxycycline 100 mg PO twice daily.
- PCN-resistant (PCN MIC >8): levofloxacin (Levaquin) 750 mg or moxifloxacin (Avelox) 400 mg either IV/PO q24h, telithromycin (Ketek) 800 mg PO once daily, ceftriaxone IV, cefotaxime IV, vancomycin 15 mg/kg IV q12h or linezolid 600 mg IV/PO q12h.
- Sinusitis (empiric): amoxicillin 500–1000 mg PO three times a day or amoxicillin/clavulanate 875/125 mg PO twice daily.
- Acute exacerbations of chronic bronchitis : amoxicillin 2–3 PO g/day or doxycycline 100 mg PO twice daily.

Meningitis

- Empiric, preferred: vancomycin 30–45 mg/kg/day in 2 divided doses IV plus ceftriaxone 2 g IV q12h or cefotaxime 2 g IV q4h or 3 g q6h.
- Pen sensitive (MIC ≤0.06): ceftriaxone 2 g IV q12h, or cefotaxime 2 g IV q4h or 3 g IV q6h.
- Pen resistant (MIC ≥0.12) or beta-lactam hypersensitivity: vancomycin 30–45 mg/kg/day IV.
- Dexamethasone 0.15 mg/kg q6h IV × 2–4 days starting 10–20 min before antibiotic.

Prevention (Adult)

- Pneumovax (23-valent) prevents bacteremia; impact on rates of CAP are modest or nil.
- Prevnar vaccine for children <2 yrs age: prevents invasive pneumococcal infection in adults by herd effect. Impact is impressive with rates of invasive pneumococcal infection down 80% in peds and 20–40% in adults.
- Risk for bacteremia: splenectomy, HIV, smokers, black race, multiple myeloma, asthma.

OTHER INFORMATION

- Best abx without meningitis: ceftriaxone, cefotaxime, amoxicillin (95% sensitive). For high level PCN-resistance: use fluoroquinolones, telithromycin.

PATHOGENS

- Penicillin resistance in U.S. is now lower than previous citations in the literature due to re-established breakpoints. PCN-resistant strains often resist to macrolides (>60%), cephalosporins, doxycycline, TMP-SMX.
- Abx active vs 98–100% *S. pneumoniae* strains: vancomycin, fluoroquinolones (except ciprofloxacin), linezolid, telithromycin, daptomycin (but don't use daptomycin in pneumonia as drug rendered inactive by surfactant).

BASIS FOR RECOMMENDATIONS

Mandell LA, Wunderink RG, Anzueto A, et al. Infectious Diseases Society of America/American Thoracic Society consensus guidelines on the management of community-acquired pneumonia in adults. *Clin Infect Dis,* 2007; Vol. 44 Suppl 2; pp. S27–72.

Comments: IDSA guidelines for community acquired pneumonia used here.

Tunkel AR, Hartman BJ, Kaplan SL, et al. Practice guidelines for the management of bacterial meningitis. *Clin Infect Dis,* 2004; Vol. 39; pp. 1267–84.

Comments: IDSA guidelines for pyogenic meningitis used here.

Snow V, Lascher S, Mottur-Pilson C, et al. Evidence base for management of acute exacerbations of chronic obstructive pulmonary disease. *Ann Intern Med,* 2001; Vol. 134; pp. 595–9.

Comments: This is the ACP/ASIM 2001 recommendations for treatment of **exacerbations of acute exacerbations of chronic bronchitis**. *S. pneumoniae* and *H. influenzae* are commonly implicated, but most studies do not provide convincing evidence that bacterial infections account for a substantial number; most are viral infections, allergies, smoking, etc. There is marginal support for antibiotic treatment of severe exacerbations and the recommended agents are amoxicillin, doxycycline and TMP-SMX.

STREPTOCOCCUS PYOGENES (GROUP A)

John G. Bartlett, MD

MICROBIOLOGY

- Group A Streptococcus (GAS), beta-hemolytic—grows on blood agar, best in anaerobic conditions.
- Gram-positive cocci in chains.
- Ecologic niche is pharynx. 2–3% of adults colonized, 15–20% school children.
- Virulence depends on proteins that represent toxins, mimic host macromolecules and after immune responses.

CLINICAL

- Common infections: bacterial pharyngitis and cellulitis.
- Rare but devastating: toxic shock syndrome, necrotizing fasciitis.
- Dx: recovery from normally sterile site, ASO antibody response (rheumatic fever), anti-DNAase B (pyoderma). Supportive: (+) throat culture or rapid strep antigen test.
- Cellulitis: <u>very</u> hard to detect Gr A strep by culture (needle aspiration or blood culture).
- Macrolide resistance: U.S. = 7%, Europe = 2–32%; penicillin—<u>always</u> active and preferred.

SITES OF INFECTION

- Pharynx: pharyngitis
- Skin: erysipelas, lymphangitis, cellulitis
- Soft tissue: fasciitis
- Muscle: myositis
- Endometrium: puerperal sepsis
- Lung: pneumonia +/− early bloody effusion
- Bacteremia
- Cardiac: endocarditis (very rare in antibiotic era)
- Toxin mediated: Scarlet fever, Toxic shock syndrome
- Non-suppurative complications: acute rheumatic fever, glomerulonephritis

TREATMENT

Pharyngitis

- Principles: **Gas** only causes 10–20% of adult pharyngitis, most cases are viral (including EBV and HIV). Treatment criteria are clinical (Centor criteria) or antigen detection. Drug = penicillin.
- **Preferred (Amer Heart Assoc, Am Acad Peds, IDSA, Med Letter):** PCN—benzathine penicillin 1.2 mU IM × 1 or penicillin VK 500 mg PO twice daily or three times a day × 10 days.

- **Alternatives:** amoxicillin 750 PO twice daily or three times a day × 10 days.
- Pen allergy: erythromycin 500 mg PO twice daily or three times a day × 10 days. Alt: azithromycin 500 mg, then 250 mg × 5 days, clarithromycin (Biaxin) 1 g XR/day or 500 mg twice daily × 10 days. Note: 5–10% isolates are macrolide resistant.
- Cefpodoxime proxetil (Vantin) 200 mg twice daily × 5 days.
- Cefdinir 300 mg twice daily PO × 5 days.
- Cefadroxil 500 mg twice daily PO × 5 days.
- Loracarbef 200 mg PO twice daily × 5 days.

Soft tissue infections or sepsis

- **Preferred:** clindamycin 600 mg IV q8h + penicillin G 4 mU IV q4h. (clindamycin to stop toxin production).
- **Alternatives:** Penicillin G 2–4 mU IV q4h.
- Clindamycin 600 mg IV q8h.
- Cefazolin 1–2 g IV q6–8h.
- Cefotaxime 2–3 g IV q6–8h or ceftriaxone 2 g/day IV.
- Vancomycin 15 mg/kg IV q12h.

Special considerations

- Necrotizing fasciitis: surgical consultation for emergent fasciotomy and debridement; repeat debridements usually necessary.
- Myositis: debridement.
- Toxic shock syndrome: IVIG 2 or more doses, massive IV fluids (10–20 L/day), albumin if <2 g/dL, debridement of necrotic tissue.
- Prophylaxis: rheumatic fever: benzathine penicillin 1.2 mu IM q mo, pen V 250 mg PO twice daily, erythro 250 mg PO twice daily until >5 yrs post-ARF and age in 20's.
- Prophylaxis (recurrent cellulitis, chronic lymphedema): clindamycin 150 mg PO once daily or TMP-SMX 1 DS PO once daily or "stand-by therapy" immediate treatment with pen V or amox 500–750 mg PO twice daily at onset of sx.

OTHER INFORMATION

- Diverse and sometimes devastating: pharyngitis, non-suppurative (ARF, Scarlet fever, nephritis); soft tissue (erysipelas, myonecrosis, lymphangitis, impetigo, fasciitis); toxic shock; misc (endocarditis, pneumonia, puerperal sepsis).
- All *S. pyogenes* sensitive to penicillin. >5% resistant to erythromycin, rare strains resistant to clindamycin.
- Clindamycin is superior to penicillin in animal models of fasciitis/myonecrosis.
- Predisposing factors: soft tissue (IDU, diabetes, surgery, trauma, varicella, vein donor, lymphedema); pneumonia (influenza), contacts w/ **gas** (pharyngitis and fasciitis).

BASIS FOR RECOMMENDATIONS

Gerber MA, Baltimore RS, Eaton CB, et al. Prevention of rheumatic fever and diagnosis and treatment of acute Streptococcal pharyngitis: a scientific statement from the American Heart Association Rheumatic Fever, Endocarditis, and Kawasaki Disease Committee of the Council on Cardiovascular Disease in the Young, the Interdisciplinary Council on Functional Genomics and Translational Biology, and the Interdisciplinary Council on Quality of Care and Outcomes Research: endorsed by the American Academy of Pediatrics. *Circulation,* 2009; Vol. 119; pp. 1541–51.
Comments: Official recommendations of strep infections and sequelae including rheumatic fever.

Stevens DL, Bisno AL, Chambers HF, et al. Practice guidelines for the diagnosis and management of skin and soft-tissue infections. *Clin Infect Dis,* 2005; Vol. 41; pp. 1373–406.
Comments: Skin/soft tissue infection guidelines from IDSA include impetigo, cellulitis and necrotizing fasciitis.

Bisno AL, Gerber MA, Gwaltney JM, et al. Practice guidelines for the diagnosis and management of group A streptococcal pharyngitis. Infectious Diseases Society of America. *Clin Infect Dis,* 2002; Vol. 35; pp. 113–25.
Comments: Guidelines for managing pharyngitis in adults from IDSA. The main difference with the ACP/CDC guidelines is that the IDSA guidelines accept only group A strep as the cause only if it is detected by culture or rapid antigen test. The concern with the more liberal ACP/CDC guidelines which accept clinical criteria that appear to overtreat about 50% of cases. The authors argue that overtreating is unnecessary and undertreating is not terrible because: (1) Rheumatic fever has nearly disappeared; (2) clinical response is modest/nil; (3) adults do not pose a public health problem; (4) quincy has become rare.

Stevens DL, Madaras-Kelly KJ, Richards DM. *In vitro* antimicrobial effects of various combinations of penicillin and clindamycin against four strains of Streptococcus pyogenes. *Antimicrob Agents Chemother,* 1998; Vol. 42; pp. 1266–8.
Comments: The authors show the absence of antagonism with **Clindamycin Plus Penicillin** vs. *Strep pyogenes in vitro.* The relevance is for the use of this combination in deep strep infections.

PATHOGENS

STREPTOCOCCUS SPECIES

Michael Melia, MD and Paul G. Auwaerter, MD

MICROBIOLOGY

- Clinical labs classify streptococci by hemolytic characteristics on 5% sheep blood agar (e.g., beta-hemolysis), Lancefield Group antigens and other biochemical tests.
- Nomenclature and taxonomy of streptococci confusing because of many historical efforts at describing the class.
- Often described by blood agar hemolysis (1902) or Lancefield carbohydrate group antigens (1933). Organization into 4 groups by hemolysis, Lancefield and phenotype testing (1937): 1. Pyogenic (beta-hemolytic) including Groups A, B, C, E, F, and G, 2. Viridans 3. Lactococci (generally not human pathogens) and 4. Enterococci.
- 16S rRNA gene sequencing (1990s) yield true phylogenetic relationships. Facklam classification presented here.
- Viridans streptococci produce alpha (green-hence viridans) hemolysis on blood agar.

CLINICAL

- Group A Strep, *S. pyogenes* (see separate pathogen module).
- Group B Strep (*S. agalactiae*): neonatal sepsis/meningitis, puerperal sepsis, chorioamnionitis; also bacteremia (often without clear source), skin and soft-tissue infections, septic arthritis. Found in GI/GU tracts. More common in adults >65 and those w/ comorbidities.
- Groups C, F, G Strep: bacteremia, endocarditis, septic arthritis, osteomyelitis.
- Group D Strep (non-enterococcal), e.g., *S. bovis*: associated with colonic malignancy. Cause of endocarditis.
- *S. intermedius/S. anginosus/S. constellatus* group (microaerophilic strep; "*S. milleri*" no longer appropriate): propensity for invasion, meningitis, abscess production (e.g., head and neck infections), bacteremia. Rarely "contaminants" when present in blood cultures.
- *S. suis*: zoonotic pathogen associated with pig farming or exposure to contaminated pork products. Most prevalent in southeast Asia, where it is a common cause of meningitis, hearing loss, cutaneous lesions, and bacteremia.
- *Streptococcus viridans:* oropharynx/GI tract usual niche. Common cause of dental infections, subacute bacterial endocarditis, bacteremia. If isolated from CSF or respiratory sections, usually contaminants, but occasionally are responsible for disease. May also be common bloodstream contaminant, but need to clinically correlate.
- *Abiotrophia* and *Granulicatella* spp. (formerly known as nutritionally variant streptococci): endocarditis.
- *Streptococcus pneumoniae* (see separate pathogen module).

SITES OF INFECTION

- Blood: primary bacteremia, especially with neutropenia or malignancy
- Cardiovascular: endocarditis
- Head and neck: dental infections, deep neck space infections (including submandibular, retropharyngeal, and lateral neck)
- Lung: pneumonia (rare) associated with oropharyngeal aspiration, abscess and empyema
- Abdomen: abscesses, cholangitis, visceral infections, GU tract
- Shock syndrome (low BP, rash, ARDS) due to viridans strep (e.g., *S. mitis*) described in cancer pts
- CNS: brain abscess, meningitis
- Musculoskeletal: septic arthritis, cellulitis

TREATMENT

Viridans Streptococci

- Cause of primary bacteremia, but up to 80% of cultures may represent contaminants or transient bacteremia. Don't dismiss in cancer pts. on chemotherapy. Continuous bacteremia = suspect endocarditis.
- Viridians group responsible for declining amt of endocarditis compared to "enteric" strep such as *S. bovis* and enterococci—probably due to aging population and less rheumatic heart disease.

- For endocarditis see Diagnosis section endocarditis–pathogen specific therapy for regimen.
- Tetracyclines, macrolides, clindamycin with 25–50% isolates resistant; TMP-SMX >75%. Increasing resistance to beta-lactams, esp. S. mitis (>40%).
- Penicillin G 2–4 million IV q4h +/– gentamicin for synergy 1.0 mg/kg/q8h IV.
- Ceftriaxone 2 g IV once daily.
- Vancomycin 15 mg/kg q12h with dose to achieve trough of 15–20 mcg/mL (if PCN allergic).
- Duration 10–14 days (not endocarditis).

Streptococcus anginosus group

- Group comprises 3–15% of streptococcal isolates of endocarditis. See Diagnosis section for Endocarditis module for management, follow viridans Streptococci recommendations.
- Dental abscesses, sinusitis, fasciitis of head and neck: can be life threatening and require aggressive surgical management. See appropriate HEENT module for specific management.
- Bacteremia often associated with deep-seated abscess. Investigate for abscess—most often intraabdominal. Drainage is usually recommended.
- Brain abscesses often polymicrobial, but *S. intermedius* found in 50–80%. See Brain abscess module for management.
- Implicated in aspiration pneumonia, lung abscess and empyema.
- Penicillin G 2–4 million U IV q4h preferred.
- Alt: ceftriaxone 2 g IV once daily; clindamycin 600–900 mg IV q8h or 300–450 mg PO four times a day or vancomycin 15 mg/kg IV q12h (PCN-allergic).

Group B Streptococcus (S. agalactiae)

- Bacteremia, soft tissue infections: PCN G 10–12 million units/day × 10 days [e.g., give 2 MU q4h or six divided doses/day].
- Meningitis (Adult): PCN G 20–24 million units/day × 14–21 days.
- Osteomyelitis: PCN G 10–20 million units/d × 21–28 days.
- Endocarditis: PCN G 20–24 million units/day × 4–6 wks and gentamicin 1 mg/kg q8h for first 2 wks.
- PCN allergic: may substitute vancomycin 15 mg/kg IV q12h for PCN. Clindamycin can be considered, but rates of resistance vary. Consider confirming absence of inducible clindamycin resistance (typically associated with macrolide resistance) before using as monotherapy.
- Some use gentamicin (1 mg/kg q8h IV) additionally for any serious GBS infection.

Group D Streptococci

- Penicillin high-level resistance not described, some strains resistant to clindamycin.
- Bacteremia: PCN 12–18 million units/day IV × 10–14 days.
- Endocarditis: PCN 14–18 million units/day IV × 4 wks, may consider gentamicin 1 mg/kg q8h to shorten duration to 2 wks, **or** use if PCN MIC >0.1, and definitely if MIC >0.5 and <2 (rare).

Group C, E, F Streptococci

- Bacteremia, cellulitis, septic arthritis or other serious infection: PCN 12–18 million units/day IV × 10–14 days.
- Endocarditis: See the Endocarditis module on p. 19 using viridans streptococci recommendations for specifics.

Abiotrophia and Granulicatella spp

- Mainly a cause of endocarditis.
- Many isolates with some PCN resistance.
- See Diagnosis section for Endocarditis module (p. 19) using viridans Streptococci recommendations, though would not use 2 wks "short-course" therapy.

General Considerations Regarding Streptococcal Endocarditis

- Criteria favoring 2-wks short course beta-lactam + aminoglycoside combination for endocarditis:
- PCN sensitive oral viridans Streptococci or *S. bovis* (PCN MIC <0.125 mg/L).
- Native valve endocarditis.
- No heart failure, aortic insufficiency or conduction abnormality.
- No metastatic infectious foci.
- Quick clinical response and afebrile within 7 days.

PATHOGENS

Streptococcus suis
- Meningitis: Ceftriaxone 2 g IV q12h × 14 days; also consider penicillin G 24 million units/day × 10–14 days.
- Pts who relapse after two wks of therapy should received prolonged treatment (4–6 wks).
- Dexamethasone 0.4 mg/kg q12h × 4 dis standard recommendation for confirmed bacterial meningitis among adults in Southern Vietnam as morbidity and mortality has been shown to be reduced with administration.

Streptococcus pyogenes (Group A Strep)
- See specific modules for Streptococcus pyogenes (Group A), cellulitis, pharyngitis, acute rheumatic fever, etc.

Streptococcus pneumoniae (Pneumococcus)
- See modules *Streptococcus pneumoniae*, pneumonia-community acquired, chronic bronchitis-acute exacerbations, otitis media, sinusitis-acute, etc.

OTHER INFORMATION
- A high proportion of blood cultures growing viridans streptococci may be due to cutaneous contamination, or transient oral bacteremia.
- Penicillin-resistance w/ viridans streptococci not due to beta-lactamase production (hence no benefit from using agents such as ampicillin-sulbactam).
- *S. anginosus* group especially confusing as can be either beta-hemolytic or nonhemolytic. Penicillin resistance is not an issue for the *S. intermedius* group.
- Recurrent invasive Group B Streptococcal infection described in 4% of nonpregnant adults within 1 yr of first episode.
- Nutritionally variant strains (Abiotrophia/Granulicatella) consider in "culture negative" endocarditis; special media historically required, though many modern broth micro systems should recover.

BASIS FOR RECOMMENDATIONS
Baddour LM, Wilson WR, Bayer AS, et al. Infective endocarditis: diagnosis, antimicrobial therapy, and management of complications: a statement for healthcare professionals from the Committee on Rheumatic Fever, Endocarditis, and Kawasaki Disease, Council on Cardiovascular Disease in the Young, and the Councils on Clinical Cardiology, Stroke, and Cardiovascular Surgery and Anesthesia, American Heart Association: endorsed by the Infectious Diseases Society of America. *Circulation*, 2005; Vol. 111; pp. e394–434.
Comments: Endocarditis treatment recommendations are based upon this document.

TREPONEMA PALLIDUM (SYPHILIS)

Noreen A. Hynes, MD, MPH

MICROBIOLOGY
- *Treponema pallidum*, a spirochete, is the sole causative agent of syphilis.

CLINICAL
- 4 adult stages: primary, secondary, latent, tertiary. This is a systemic infection. High index of suspicion needed! Signs and sx are protean. Lesions of primary and secondary syphilis resolve without treatment although person remains infected. Time course through stages may be more rapid in HIV-infected persons.
- **Primary syphilis:** chancre occurs at point of introduction/contact 10–90 days (avg 3 wks) after exposure. Begins as a papule, quickly ulcerates to form a single (usually), painless, clean-based ulcer with indurated edges with the consistency of a man's oxford shirt collar buttonhole. Untreated, it will spontaneously heal in 3–6 wks without a scar. Chancre often missed if occurring on the cervix or if intraanal. Screening syphilis serology (a non-treponemal test such as the RPR [Rapid Plasmin Reagin] test) often negative until later in this stage of disease. Darkfield microscopy or direct fluorescent antibody of air dried ulcer secretions on slide provide definitive diagnosis. Pt is highly infectious at this time.
- **Secondary syphilis:** highly varied lesions in appearance and location. Classic rash is the so-called "copper penny" macular lesions on the palms and/or soles. Rash can be generalized or focal as well as macular, papular, pustular or a combination. Mucous-membrane related lesions include condylomata lata (papillomatous-appearing, heaped-up lesions) and mucous patches occuring in the mouth, vagina, on the glans penis. Lymphadenopathy is often seen.

Onset up to 6 mos following exposure, usually after primary lesions have healed. During this stage the pt is highly infectious. The lesions (not the infection) will heal spontaneously even if untreated. The RPR is positive in 100% of pts with secondary syphilis. A reflex treponemal test will provide confirmation of the diagnosis.

- **Early latent syphilis:** asymptomatic period from the spontaneous resolution of the lesions of primary and secondary syphilis to the end of the first yr following the exposure. During this period, 25% will have a relapse of secondary stage signs. Dx by serology—both non-treponemal and treponemal tests are positive. During this stage, pts are considered to be infectious due to the possibility of unrecognized relapse. The early latent period is extended to 4 yrs for pregnant women who can transmit to the fetus during this time and cause congenital syphilis.

- **Late latent syphilis:** the period of asymptomatic infection. The pts are considered non-infectious. Evaluate for clinical evidence of tertiary disease and syphilitic ocular disease. Dx is made by serology but over time, the non-treponemal test may revert to normal but the treponemal test usually remains positive. CSF exam needed if there are neurologic or ophthalmologic signs/sx, evidence of active tertiary disease such as aortitis or gumma, treatment failure (as assessed by failure to note a 4-fold decline in RPR titer 6 mos after treatment), HIV infected persons with late latent syphilis or syphilis of unknown duration.

- **Neurosyphilis:** CNS involvement can occur during any stage of syphilis. May be asymptomatic. Signs include cognitive impairment, motor or sensory deficits, ophthalmologic or auditory symptoms, cranial nerve palsies, signs and symptoms of meningitis, syphilitic eye disease (uveitis, iritis, optic neuritis, neuroretinitis) is considered a subset of neurosyphilis for management purposes. CSF examination and serology on all suspect cases. Clinical findings need to be evaluated along with laboratory (serology and CSF) findings.

- **Tertiary syphilis:** late manifestations of syphilis including gumma, cardiovascular, and neurologic syphilis.

- Preventing congenital infection is **key**! Up to 70% of untreated woman can transmit to fetus for up to 4 yrs. Pregnant women should be screened at the first prenatal visit, at 28 wks, and at the time of delivery in areas with high rates of syphilis.

- Consider in differential DDX of all genital ulcers and generalized rashes especially in IDUs or those who exchange sex for drugs or money. Treat before lab results reported in high risk persons who may not return for results. This is a reportable disease, local health department (in U.S.) should be notified to carry out contact tracing activities.

MORE CLINICAL
Clinical Findings in Syphilis
Primary syphilis

- Most common location of lesions: penis (heterosexual men) and men engaging in anal insertive intercourse; in women most commonly seen on labia and on cervix.
- Usually a single chancre but may be multiple; in women, opposing genital labial skin surfaces may produce "kissing" lesions.
- "Hidden" lesions on the cervix and intra-anal area can lead to delayed diagnosis because lesions are asymptomatic. Presentation during secondary stage is more common when chancre is at this site.
- Chancre occurs at the site of innoculation therefore can be seen in many locations: anal canal, mouth, eyelid, etc.
- Regional lymphadenopathy, unilateral or bilateral, is often found if sought. Inguinal adenopathy, when present, is usually discrete, firm-to-rubbery in character, mobile, and painless, without overlying skin changes. Dark field microscopy of lymph node aspirate is positive and diagnostic.

Secondary syphilis

- The lesions do **not** reflect the location of the innoculation as is systemic at this stage.
- Rash is usually symmetrical, non-pruritic, painless. May be macules, papules, pustules, or mixed.
- Generalized lymphadenopathy is usually present at this stage. Dark field microscopy of lymph node aspirate is positive and diagnostic.
- Condylomata lata are most commonly seen in warm, moist area of the body—intertriginous zones. These lesions are teaming with spirochetes.

PATHOGENS

- Mucous patches can be found on any mucosal surface and also team with spirochetes.
- Constitutional symptoms: fever, headache, general malaise, sore throat, anorexia, and occasionally, meningismus.
- Less common manifestations: proctitis, hepatitis, nephritis, arthritis, uveitis and other eye findings, meningitis, acute presbycusis.

Tertiary syphilis

- Onset of symptoms can be as early as 1 yr and as late as 50 or 60 yrs following infection.
- Gummas, grouped or coalescing granulomatous lesions, can affect any organ but usual location is bone, skin, mucus membranes.
- Cardiovascular syphilis: large arteries are invaded by the spirochetes leading to endarteritis, particularly the aorta in which ortitis and ultimately aortic aneurysm occurs.
- Neurosyphilis can occur at any stage of syphilis and is traditionally thought of as a tertiary or late manifestation of disease.
  - All neurosyphilis requires parenteral treatment preferably with non-benzathine containing penicillin at concentrations that cross the blood-brain barrier.
  - Meningitis and eye disease may occur during primary or secondary syphilis as well as during the first 5–10 yrs of untreated infection.
  - Meningovascular disease may present as a stroke.
  - After 15–20 yrs the "classic" manifestations of late untreated infection—tabes dorsalis and paresis may be seen.
  - CSF findings in neurosyphilis: pleocytosis, elevated protein, decreased glucose, or a reactive CSF Venereal Disease Research Laboratory (VDRL).

SITES OF INFECTION

- **Skin:** chancre of primary syphilis, rash of secondary syphilis, patchy bald spots on the head (alopecia areata) in secondary syphilis.
- **Mucus membranes:** condylomata lata, mucous patches.
- **CNS:** asymptomatic, meningitis (1–2 yrs after infection), meningovascular (5–7 yrs), general paresis and tabes dorsalis (10–20 yrs), gummatous neurosyphilis.
- **Cardiovascular system:** aortitis (ascending).
- **Bone:** arthritis, osteitis, periostitis.
- **Liver:** hepatitis.
- **Eye:** iritis, uveitis, iridocyclitis, Argyll-Robertson pupils.
- **Constitutional symptoms:** fever may be seen; can be the first manifestation in secondary syphilis.

TREATMENT

Primary and Secondary Syphilis in Adults

- Recommended: benzathine penicillin (PCN) G 2.4 million units IM × 1.
- PCN allergy (non-pregnant, preferred): doxycycline 100 mg PO twice daily × 14 days **or** tetracycline 500 mg PO four times a day × 14 days, requires well-documented close f/u.

Latent Syphilis in Adults

- Early latent [<1 yr infection duration] (w/ normal CSF exam, if done): benzathine penicillin G (BPG) 2.4 million units IM × 1.
- Early latent with PCN allergy: doxycycline 100 mg PO twice daily × 14 days, requires well-documented close f/u.
- Late latent or latent of unknown duration (w/ normal CSF exam, if done): benzathine penicillin G 2.4 mil units qwk × 3 wks. If any dose >2 days late, must recommence RX from 1st dose.
- Late latent or latent of unknown duration with PCN allergy (not for pregnant women) (1) doxycycline 100 mg PO twice daily × 4 wks or (2) tetracycline 500 mg PO four times a day × 4 wks. Requires well-documented close follow-up.

Neurosyphilis or Ocular Syphilis in Adults

- Recommended: aqueous crystalline penicillin G 18–24 million units/day IV, administer as 3–4 million units IV q4h × 10–14 days.
- Alternative: Procaine penicillin 2.4 million units IM daily, PLUS probenecid 500 mg PO four times a day × 10–14 days.

- Penicillin allergic persons ideally should be desensitized and treated with a penicillin regimen (above). However in non-pregnant pts with non-IgE mediated PCN allergy ceftriaxone can be used. Some specialists recommend ceftriaxone 2 g q24h IM or IV × 10–14 days. Very close follow-up is required.

Syphilis in HIV-Infected Persons

- Penicillin is the highly preferred regimen for all stages of syphilis in HIV-infected persons.
- Primary, secondary and early latent syphilis: use benzathine penicillin G as for non-HIV persons; some experts recommend 3 weekly doses (i.e., as for late latent syphilis).
- PCN-allergic HIV + w/ primary, secondary or early latent syphilis: can be treated as allergic HIV-neg person (although **not** the ideal).
- Late latent syphilis or syphilis of unknown duration requires a LP to rule out neurosyphilis. PCN-based treatment is strongly preferred. Desensitization required.
- Limited clinical studies suggest that ceftriaxone might be effective but optimal dose and duration is unknown.

Syphilis in Pregnancy

- Only penicillin is currently recommended. Treatment during pregnancy should be the penicillin regimen appropriate to the stage of syphilis dx'd; desensitization required for PCN-allergic preg pts.
- Some experts recommend a second dose of benzathine PCN G 2.4 million units IM 1 wk after the initial dose for primary, secondary, early latent syphilis in pregnancy.

MORE TREATMENT

(1) Parenteral penicillin G is the preferred drug for RX of all stages of syphilis. It's the **only** documented efficacious therapy for neurosyphilis and in pregnancy. (2) Jarisch-Herxheimer reaction: an acute febrile reaction, often accompanied by headache, myalgia, and rash may occur within 24 hrs of RX; most often in early syphilis. May induce premature labor or cause fetal distress but is **not** a contraindication to treatment and should **not** delay RX.

(3) Pharmacologic data suggest that ceftriaxone should be effective in treating primary and secondary syphilis. But, data are limited. Optimal dose and duration has **not** been established. Single dose **not** effective. May try 1 g once daily for 8 to 10 days.

(4) There are increasing reports of documented treatment failures when azithromycin is used to treat primary or secondary syphilis or their contacts. Azithromycin should be avoided in most pts with incubating or infectious syphilis. It should not be used treatment of **any** pregnant or HIV-infected pts. Closed follow-up is required for penicillin-allergic non-HIV infected, non-pregnant pts treated with this antibiotic.

(5) Follow-up using quantitative non-treponemal tests should be done based upon stage of syphilis.

FOLLOW UP

Follow-up using quantitative non-treponemal tests should be done based upon stage of syphilis.

OTHER INFORMATION

Diagnostic Considerations

Definitive diagnosis: requires direct identification of the organism. This can be done by darkfield microscopy (sensitivity = 74–86%, specificity = 85–100%) or direct fluorescent antibody testing (sensitivity = 73–100%, specificity = 89–100%) of a sample collected from a site usually free of any spirochetal lesions including the vaginal, penis, lymph nodes (aspirate), skin rash, condylomata lata in intertriginous areas. Samples from the mouth are not useful as non-treponemal spirochetes can be found there.

Presumptive diagnosis: uses 2 types of serological tests—non-treponemal (such as the RPR and VDRL) and treponemal tests (such as the FTA-ABS or the *T. pallidum* particle agglutination (TP-PA). Use of only 1 type of test is insufficient to establish a presumptive diagnosis because the non-treponemal tests can give false positive results due to other medical conditions. Therefore, the positive screening test (non-treponemal) needs to be confirmed with a treponemal assay. Because the treponemal tests are positive for many yrs in the absence of a positive screening test, a positive test cannot usually be used as an indicator of current infection.

* Primary syphilis: the first tests to be positive: FTA-19S IgM (sensitivity 90%, and not commonly available), VDRL (sensitivity 44–76%), T. pallidum hemagglutination test-TPHA (sensitivity 50–83%) and FTA-ABS (sensitivity 75–92%).

* Secondary syphilis: RPR and VDRL are 98–100% sensitive.

* Biologic false positives: can be transient or chronic. Transient causes include acute bacterial, viral and malaria infections and some pregnant women; lasts for <6 mo. Chronic causes include chronic infections (including HIV), autoimmune diseases, rheumatic disorders, some malignancies, some elderly; lasts >6 mo.

* Prozone phenomenon: associated with secondary syphilis; false negative result on undiluted serum (with a reported negative test result); seen in cases often with large amounts of antibody. May be seen more often in HIV-infected person. Dilution of the serum with retesting converts the test to positive.

Use of non-treponemal antibody tests (NTAT) to follow disease activity. Antibody titers using NTAT correlate well with disease activity. A 4-fold change in titer, the equivalent of 2 dilutions (e.g., from 1:8 to 1:32) is considered to be a clinically significant change between 2 NTAT provided the tests the same type of NTAT was used, and preferably carried out by the same laboratory. Although the VDRL and RPR are equally valid NTAT, their titers are not precisely equivalent and therefore cannot both be used in the same pt to follow disease activity over time. RPR titers tend to be slightly higher than VDRL titers. NTAT usual revert to non-reactive over time. However, some pts can have persistent low-level titers for life. This is referred to as serofast.

Treponemal EIA tests: some blood banks have begun to use this modality for screening. The test identifies both previously treated and untreated persons. Persons testing positive need to be retested with a non-treponemal test to determine the current active infection status. If the NTAT is negative a different treponemal test should be performed to confirm the blood bank's finding. If the 2nd test is positive, then management of the pt should be in consultation with a specialist.

HIV infected persons: may have unusually high, unusually low, or fluctuating titers. When the serologic tests do not correlate with the clinical syndromes of primary, secondary, or early latent syphilis other tests such as biopsy or direct tests (see above) should be used.

Neurosyphilis: no single test can usually diagnose. Hence, use various combination of serologic test results, CSF cell count (>5 WBC/mL) or protein, or a reactive VDRL-CSF with or without clinical manifestations. A reactive CSF VDRL alone in the absence of blood contamination is considered diagnostic of syphilis. VDRL on CSF is highly specific (i.e. few false positives) but is very insensitive (many false negatives). The CSF FTA-ABS is very non-specific but highly sensitive and some specialists believe that a negative test excludes neurosyphilis. CSF WBC can be used as a sensitive measure of rx effectiveness.

BASIS FOR RECOMMENDATIONS

Centers for Disease Control and Prevention, Workowski KA, Berman SM. Sexually transmitted diseases treatment guidelines, 2006. *MMWR Recomm Rep,* 2006; Vol. 55; pp. 1–94.

Comments: The CDC treatment guidelines provide clinicians with a readily available reference for STD treatments recommended by a panel of national and international experts in STD diagnosis, treatment, prevention and control. These guidelines available electronically from: www.cdc.gov

TROPHERYMA WHIPPLEI

Paul G. Auwaerter, MD

MICROBIOLOGY
- Agent of Whipple's disease (WD), distant relationship to actinomyces by 16 s rDNA sequence.
- Detected in multiple environmental samples, including soil and sewerage.
- Fastidious organism, 0.25 μm rods may appear Gram-positive upon staining.

CLINICAL
- Epidemiology not well-known, male:female 8:1. Typical pt said to be Caucasian male, >40 yrs living in rural environment.
- Rare infection, worldwide incidence estimated 12 cases annually—but rate may increase with improved diagnostics (PCR).
- WD may cause chronic GI illness, CNS or ocular problems, lymphadenopathy, FUO (fever of unknown origin) are the more common presentations.
- Ddx: Crohn's, lymphoma, celiac disease, Still's disease, amyloidosis, atypical mycobacteria.
- Dx(1): traditional dx by duodenal biopsy demonstrating PAS-staining large foamy macrophages in lamina propria.
- Dx(2): PAS staining macrophages in LN, brain or other tissue; electron microscopy demonstrating rod-shaped bacteria with unique trilaminar membrane, now rarely performed.

- Dx (3): PCR of fluid or tissue (sensitivity/specificity unknown and false positive described; use for first-line screening in saliva or stool), culture (difficult, only specialized laboratories).
- Dx (4): immunostains for histopathology are recent discoveries and not widely available but offer better sensitivity than PAS staining. Serology unhelpful clinically due to low specificity.
- Note: carriage in healthy individuals described in saliva, subgingival plaques, intestinal biopsies, and stool specimens.

SITES OF INFECTION

- GI: "classical presentation"—wt. loss, fever, diarrhea (steatorrhea), abdominal pain, lymphadenopathy, arthralgia (may precede GI sx for yrs).
- CNS: dementia (reversible) without other cause, personality change, hemiparesis, sz, ophthalmoplegia.
- Ocular: uveitis; oculomasticatory or oculofacial-skeletal myorhythmia (nystagmus with rhythmic movement of other facial muscles or jaw movement) rare but considered pathognomonic of WD if present.
- Cardiac: culture-negative endocarditis, myocarditis, pericarditis.
- Less common: skeletal muscle, arthralgia, pulmonary, renal involvement.

MORE CLINICAL

Video example of oculofacial-skeletal myorhythmia (OFSM) can be viewed at this URL [http://www.neurology.org/cgi/content/full/69/11/E12/DC1], permission may be required.

TREATMENT

Initial Therapy

- Initial therapy usually parenteral to eradicate 1° disease and some advocate to be certain the CNS is primarily treated even if no indication of active disease (duration: usually 10–14 days).
- PCN G 6–24 mU IV per day in divided dose (q4h).
- Alt: procaine PCN 1–2 million units IM once daily.
- Alt: ceftriaxone 2 g IV q24.
- PCN allergic: TMP-SMX DS PO twice daily **plus** streptomycin 1 g IM once daily.
- Steroids occasionally added for CNS disease, severe constitutional sx or granulomatous process. In 1950s, steroids commonly used alone without abx in WD. They helped some, but many worsened.
- Lack of good clinical trials to guide treatment, given rarity. Current recommendations garnered from case series and retrospective analysis.
- In stable pt (usually without CNS disease), exclusive oral therapy can be used.

Relapsed Initial Therapy

- Ceftriaxone 2 g IV q24h
- Penicillin G 4 million units IV q4h

Long-Term Therapy

- 1 yr (or longer) total duration often suggested to prevent relapses seen with shorter term therapy.
- Co-trimoxazole (TMP-SMX) DS PO twice daily × 1 yr (preferred for CNS involvement).
- Sulfadiazine 2 g–4 mg total dose orally daily. Used by some especially with CNS disease in place of TMP-SMX, especially as *T. whipplei* is intrinsically resistant to trimethoprim.
- Doxycycline 100 mg PO twice daily Plus hydroxychloroquine 200 mg PO three times a day (preferred if no proven CNS involvement or sulfa-allergic).
- Other abx used: chloramphenicol, clarithromycin, fluoroquinolones.
- Some physicians follow duodenal biopsies and treat only until PAS negative.
- Recent *in vitro* studies suggest cephalosporins, aztreonam, and fluoroquinolones were not active. Doxycycline and hydroxychloroquine judged to be bactericidal combination.

Relapse Maintenance Therapy

- TMP-SMX DS PO twice daily.
- Doxycyline 100 mg PO twice daily **plus** hydroxychloroquine 200 mg PO three times a day. Use only if certain no active CNS disease.

FOLLOW UP

- Clinical improvement often seen within 7–21 days. Most pts completely recover, although neurological sequelae in some persist.
- Duration of maintenance antibiotic therapy not well-defined.

PATHOGENS

- Relapses described with shorter courses, therefore 1 yr often recommended. Some clinicians maintain treatment indefinitely especially with CNS disease.
- CSF PCR useful to follow; negative results suggestive of sufficient antibacterial therapy.

OTHER INFORMATION

- Clinical pearls: pts. w/ hyperpigmentation and relative hypotension may be confused with Addison's; granulomatous adenopathy may be confused with sarcoid.
- Macrophages containing MAI in pts with HIV may be confused w/ Whipple's on PAS stain.
- Arthralgia very common (>90%) and may precede GI sx in one-third. Joint complaints tend to be intermittent, migratory and transient generally of peripheral joints.
- Anemia common (90%) and may be due to B12 deficiency secondary to malabsorption.
- PCR of CSF, blood is decreasing need to obtain brain or other organ tissue for PAS staining.

BASIS FOR RECOMMENDATIONS

Schneider T, Moos V, Loddenkemper C, et al. Whipple's disease: new aspects of pathogenesis and treatment. *Lancet Infect Dis,* 2008; Vol. 8; pp. 179–90.

Comments: Most recent and excellent review by a leading researcher in the clinical diagnostics of intracellular pathogens. Updates latest pathophysiology, diagnostics and treatment suggestions. For proven non-CNS involvement (including negative CSF PCR), group favors use of both doxycycline and hydroxychloroquine due to treatment failures when using co-trimoxazole due to genetic mutations within T. whipplei genome.

VIBRIO CHOLERAE

Joseph Vinetz, MD and Paul G. Auwaerter, MD

MICROBIOLOGY

- Aerobic, Gram-negative, comma-shaped bacillus.
- Water-borne pathogen, humans acquire infection through ingesting contaminated water or food.
- *V. cholerae* serogroup O1, biotype El Tor, originated in Asia but has caused pandemic infection throughout Africa and South America for ~40 yrs.
- Newer serogroup O139 described in SE Asia in 1992 now endemic.
- Isolates described with resistance to ampicillin, tetracycline, ampicillin, aminoglycosides, sulphonamides, and trimethoprim.

CLINICAL

- Cause of the secretory diarrheal syndrome, cholera.
- Epidemic and endemic cause of massive diarrhea.
- Most commonly found in Africa, South America, south and east Asia, eastern Europe.
- Usually a non-invasive organism that causes diarrhea by elaboration of a toxin.
- Along U.S. Gulf coast, transmission occurs but is rare, sporadic.
- Incubation time usually 18–40 hrs, followed by nausea, abdominal rumbling followed by the onset of massive, watery diarrhea.
- Most infections mild-moderate, ~1 in 20 develop severe disease.
- Morbidity and mortality due to dehydration so severe as to elicit hypotension, shock and multi-organ failure. Many deaths occur within the first day.
- Dx: stool cx, biochemical ID on isolate; specialized laboratories can diagnose by serological techniques, PCR.
- Rarely a cause of skin/soft tissue infection, bacteremia, disseminated infections, which are usually caused by non-cholerae vibrios.

SITES OF INFECTION

- Small intestine: cholera toxin induces secretion of Na and bicarbonate-rich non-inflammatory fluid, so-called "rice water" stools.
- Skin/soft tissue (rare): non-epidemic strains of *V. cholerae.*

TREATMENT

Fluid Replacement (Priority)

- Rapid replacement of water and electrolyte deficits, major goal to avoid mortality.
- Maintenance fluids to replace ongoing measured losses.
- IV replacement until oral hydration therapy can keep up with losses.
- Severely dehydrated pts should have 10% of bodyweight repleted within 2–4 hrs.

- IV replacement fluid: Ringer's lactate with extra K+.
- If unavailable, normal saline may be used but avoid dextrose water solutions as not with sufficient electrolyte characteristics to compensate for loses.
- Oral rehydration solutions (ORS): use commercially prepared if available. To prepare, for 1L purest available water, add 2.6 g sodium chloride, 2.9 g trisodium citrate, 1.5 g potassium chloride, and 13.5 g glucose (or 50 g boiled and cooled rice powder).
- A rice-based ORS solution, in combination with tetracycline, is effective but not as good as a glucose-based ORS.

Antibiotics
- Reduces diarrhea duration, volume. Selection should be guided by knowledge of local susceptibility pattern of *V. cholerae* in circulation.
- Administer antibiotic as soon as vomiting ceases.
- Tetracycline 500 PO four times daily.
- Doxycycline 100 mg PO twice daily.
- Azithromycin 1000 mg PO × 1 dose.
- Erythromycin 250 mg PO four times daily × 5 days.
- TMP/SMX 160 mg/800 mg (DS) PO twice daily.
- Ampicillin 500 mg PO four times daily.
- Ciprofloxacin 250 mg PO once to twice daily.
- Duration of antibiotic 1–3 days.

FOLLOW UP
- Without treatment, case-fatality rate is 50%.
- As soon as able, pts should eat food without restriction.

OTHER INFORMATION
- Avoid trimethoprim/sulfamethoxazole if causative agent *is V. cholerae* serovar O139, due to resistance.
- Tetracycline or other abx useful for prophylaxis among close contacts.
- Cholera vaccine (Dukoral from SBL Vaccines) not available in the U.S. (low efficacy, but improved from prior vaccine).

BASIS FOR RECOMMENDATIONS

Sack DA, Sack RB, Nair GB, et al. Cholera. *Lancet*, 2004; Vol. 363; pp. 223–33.

Comments: Authors recommend rehydration with ORS, or parenteral rehydration if clinically with severe dehydration. Antibiotics are secondary, and mainly to assist with shortening duration of diarrhea, hence duration recommended of only 1–3 days.

VIBRIO SPECIES (NONCHOLERA)

John G. Bartlett, MD

MICROBIOLOGY
- Aerobic, Gram-negative, comma-shaped rod (1–3 × 0.5–0.8 μm). Vibrio species usually divided into cholera and noncholera groups.
- *Vibrio parahaemolyticus* is the most common noncholera species, while *V. vulnificus* is less common but more lethal. Occasional Vibrio species causing human infection also include: *V. fluvialis, V. fumissii, V. hollisae, V. alginolyticus, V. damsela, V. cincinnatiensis.*
- Easily grown on routine media but identification from stool cultures requires use of selective media: thiosulfate-citrate-bile salts-sucrose (TCBS).
- Common in warm marine environs, e.g., brackish waters, estuaries and coastal bays.
- Cholera caused by *V. cholerae* (see this module for details).

CLINICAL
- Cause of severe skin/soft tissue infections, sepsis and gastroenteritis. Occurrence rates *V. vulnificus:* wound infection = sepsis → gastroenteritis; *V. parahaemolyticus*: gastroenteritis → wound infection → sepsis.
- *Vibrio vulnificus* (and other vibrio) part of normal marine flora in temperate climates: Gulf of Mexico (50% of oyster beds), East/West Coasts. Most U.S. cases: FL, LA, TX.
- Disease acquired from ingestion (especially raw oysters) or salt water contact with skin lesion. May also cause gastroenteritis (as do other vibrio spp., e.g., *V. parahaemolyticus*).

PATHOGENS

- Predisposed: men >50 yrs (estrogen protects), liver disease, alcoholism, chronic hemolytic anemia, hemochromatosis (iron overload conditions), diabetes, renal failure, adrenal insufficiency.
- Clinical presentation: contact with seawater or raw seafood + susceptible host + sepsis ± necrotic skin lesions.
- Dx: recovery from blood or necrotic lesions = medical emergency.
- Microbiology: cx-blood (sepsis), wound (wound infection), stool (gastroenteritis).
- Notify micro lab if suspected as cause of gastroenteritis to use special selective media (TCBS). Some labs in endemic areas routinely use this media as part of stool culture protocol.

SITES OF INFECTION

- Wound infection (cellulitis, may spread rapidly with bullae, features of myonecrosis or fasciitis)
- Blood (primary septicemia)
- GI tract (gastroenteritis)

TREATMENT

Sepsis or Soft Tissue Infection Antibiotic Management

- Sepsis or soft tissue infection: doxycycline 100 mg IV q12h + ceftazidime 2 g IV q8h or fluoroquinolone. Do not delay abx. May need fasciotomy for necrotizing fasciitis.
- Alt: cefotaxime 2 g IV q6h IV plus ciprofloxacin 400 mg IV q12h (synergistic *in vitro*) or moxifloxacin 400 mg IV q24 or levofloxacin 750 mg IV q24.
- Alt: cefotaxime plus minocycline (synergistic *in vitro*).

Surgery

- Necrotizing fasciitis: obtain urgent surgical consultation for consideration of rapid fasciotomy, surgical debridement, and/or amputation.

Gastroenteritis

- Most cases self-limiting.
- Maintain hydration: oral or parenteral routes.
- Role of doxycycline or fluoroquinolones unclear, does not appear to shorten duration of non-cholera gastroenteritis.
- Consider whether sporadic or worth considering investigation for food-borne illness by notifying public health authorities.

OTHER INFORMATION

- Causes 90% of seafood-related deaths in U.S., especially due to raw oyster ingestion. Coastal areas afflicted April–Oct. Men w/ liver disease most at risk.
- Predisposing factor for sepsis: liver disease (80%); less common: diabetes, immunodeficiency, iron overload conditions.
- Pathogenesis for sepsis: eat raw oysters → fever/chills in 3–7 days → shock + necrotic/hemorrhagic bullae in 50–75%. Considerable mortality, ~55%.
- Pathogenesis for wound infection: (secondary to bacteremia) or prior/new wound + estuarine water contact. Clinical course: fever, chills and painful extremity → then for (*V. vulnificus*) bacteremia in 30%, mortality = 24%.

BASIS FOR RECOMMENDATIONS

Kuo YL, Shieh SJ, Chiu HY, et al. Necrotizing fasciitis caused by *Vibrio vulnificus*: epidemiology, clinical findings, treatment and prevention. *Eur J Clin Microbiol Infect Dis,* 2007.

Comments: Host susceptibility: Liver disease, diabetes, chronic renal insufficiency, adrenal insufficiency. Clinical features in 67 cases-contact with seawater or raw seafood (100%), most common site-arm (75%). Survival improved with early fasciotomy (<24 hrs) (5% vs 23%).

No authors listed. Choice of antibacterial drugs. *Treat Guidel Med Lett,* 2007; Vol. 5; pp. 33–50.

Comments: Partly used as basis for recommendations in this module.

YERSINIA PESTIS

John G. Bartlett, MD

MICROBIOLOGY

- Aerobic, Gram-negative bipolar rod ("safety pin" appearance upon staining, Giemsa preferred). Member of the *Enterobacteriaceae* family.
- Must warn lab of suspicion.
- Grows on standard media.
- Culture at 28° and 35°C.
- May take up to 6 days to identify.

CLINICAL

- Usually acquired by bite of rodent flea carrying *Y. pestis* or handling infected animal.
- Three forms: bubonic (lymph nodes), pneumonic and septicemic. U.S. bubonic plague: ~10 cases/yr usually in NM, AR, CO, CA. Pneumonic plague: 1 case per 10 yrs in U.S.
- Presentations: a) Bioterrorism: epidemic of pneumonia with critically ill, previously healthy adults; need to r/o tularemia and anthrax. Clue is hemoptysis. b) Lymphadenitis/bubo: most common form, usually painful and fever present. Chills, headache, fatigue common. Ask if hx of exposure to rodents, rabbits or fleas. Incubation period: 2–6 days. c) Sepsis: usually evolves from untreated bubo. High mortality. d) Pneumonic: severe, often with hemoptysis and marked dyspnea. High mortality.
- Always significant when recovered.
- Dx: culture, DFA and serology EIA for F1 capsular antigen. Antigen and PCR are other methods.
- Mortality pneumonic plague, 50–60%; bubonic, 5–15%.
- Prophylaxis is nearly 100% effective.

SITES OF INFECTION

- Bubonic plague (enlarged, tender to fluctuant lymphadenopathy—distribution inguinal → axillary → cervical or epitrochlear): 85% of *Y. pestis* infections
- Bacteremia: 13%. Sepsis can lead to DIC, acral cyanosis/necrosis ("Black death")
- Pneumonic plague: 2%
- Cutaneous: rare
- Meningitis: rare

TREATMENT

General recommendations

- Indication to treat empirically in an outbreak: persons with temperature >38.5°C or new cough.
- Preferred: streptomycin 1 g IM twice daily or gentamicin IV 5 mg/kg/loading dose, then 1.7 mg/kg q8h × 10 days.
- Alt: doxycycline 100 mg PO or IV twice daily or ciprofloxacin 400 mg IV q12h or chloramphenicol 1 g IV four times a day × 10 days.
- Pregnancy: gentamicin 5 mg/kg/day × 10 days. Alt: doxycycline or ciprofloxacin × 10 days.
- Meningitis: chloramphenicol 1 g IV q6h.
- Animal data: levofloxacin may be the best.

Bioterrorism Suspect: Notifications

- Notify hospital infection control and state/local health departments.
- Definitive dx of *Y. pestis*: Ft. Collins 970-221-6400.
- **Confirmed case**: compatible clinical **and** (1) isolation of *Y. pestis* **or** (2) 4 × increase in titer of Ab to F1 antigen.
- **Presumptive case**: compatible clinical **and** Ab to F1Ag **or** positive FA to F1 Ag.

Prevention and Infection Control Measures (Bioterrorism)

- Pneumonic plague can be transmitted from person-person, but this is rare.
- Indications for prophylaxis: household, hospital or other close contact (definition: within 2 meters of case who has been treated <48 hrs).
- Preferred: doxycycline 100 mg PO twice daily × 7days or ciprofloxacin 500 mg PO twice daily × 7 days or levofloxacin 750 mg PO daily × 7 days.
- Alt: chloramphenicol 1 g PO four times a day × 7 days.

PATHOGENS

- Pregnancy: doxycycline 100 mg PO twice daily × 7 days or ciprofloxacin 500 mg PO twice daily × 7 days or levofloxacin 750 mg PO daily × 7 days.
- Infection control: surgical mask, gowns, gloves and eye protection until case treated >48 hrs.
- Other: isolate or cohort pts.
- Warn lab: biosafety level 2 pathogen.

OTHER INFORMATION
- Bioterrorism (pneumonic): aerosol—incubation 2–4 days, fever, cough +/– hemoptysis, dyspnea → DIC → death day 2–6.
- Bubonic plague: flea bites, incubation 2–8 days, fever, tender bubo, bacteremia +/– DIC.
- Clinical clues bioterrorism: many healthy persons w/ pneumonia +/– hemoptysis and rapid death, also r/o anthrax.

BASIS FOR RECOMMENDATIONS
Inglesby TV, Dennis DT, Henderson DA, et al. Plague as a biological weapon: medical and public health management. Working Group on Civilian Biodefense. *JAMA*, 2000; Vol. 283; pp. 2281–90.
Comments: Article covers naturally occurring plague, bioterrorism clues and treatment recommendations.

YERSINIA SPECIES (NON-PLAGUE)

Khalil G. Ghanem, MD

MICROBIOLOGY
- Gram-negative coccobacilli of family Enterobacteriaceae.
- 3 species cause human disease: *Y. pestis, Y. enterocolitica,* and *Y. pseudotuberculosis.*
- Other *Yersiniae: fredrikensii, intermedia, kristensenii, bercovieri, mollaretti, rhodei, ruckeri, aldovae* **may** cause gastroenteritis and soft tissue infections in humans.

CLINICAL
- Transmission: contaminated food/water/blood. Reservoirs: farm (pigs, cattle, sheep, chicken), mammals, pets (dog/cat), birds, environmental.
- Virulence factors: plasmid and chromosomal.
- Dx: blood cxs (virulence confirmed); stool (biotype or serotype to ascertain virulence, e.g., 1A biogroup avirulent); mesenteric LN bx and cx; pharyngeal exudate cx; serological (limited use); PCR.
- Prevention: focus on animal reservoirs. Avoid undercooked meats, screen blood bank donors for acute symptoms (fevers, diarrhea).

SITES OF INFECTION
- **Y. enterocolitica:** GI (colitis, "pseudoappendicitis," mesenteric adenitis, rectal bleeding, ileal perforation). Skin: erythema nodosum (30%).
- Joints: Reiter's reactive arthritis in 30%, onset 2–30 days after diarrhea. HLA-B27 risk. sx last >1 mo in 66%. Knees, ankles, toes, fingers; synovial fld: 25,000 WBC with 60–90% PMNs.
- **Other Yersiniae:** possible cause GI (enteritis) and skin (soft tissue infxn). Pathogenicity still debated.

TREATMENT
Y. enterocolitica
- Enterocolitis and adenitis usually self-limited. No treatment unless clinically indicated.
- Septicemia: gentamicin 5 mg/kg IV q24h or divided doses. Other abxs: fluoroquinolones, chloramphenicol, doxy, TMP/SMZ.
- Some isolates resistant to cephalosporins. **Avoid** in sick pts unless susceptibility known.

Y. pseudotuberculosis
- Clinically ill pts and septicemia: ampicillin 100–200 mg/kg/day; others: gentamicin; tetracycline.

OTHER INFORMATION
- Iron overload syndromes (esp. use of deferoxamine), raw oyster ingestion and chitterlings classically associated w/ increased risk of infection with Yersiniae.
- Contaminated blood products described in cases of *Y. enterocolitica* and *Y. pseudotuberculosis* septicemia. Mortality in sepsis despite proper Rx: enterocolitica = 50%, pseudotuberculosis = 75%.

- Enterocolitica resistant to PCNs whereas pseudotuberculosis sensitive. Resistance to 3rd gen cephalosporins w/ enterocolitica emerging.
- Reiter's syndrome (conjunctivitis, urethritis, and arthritis) associated with *Y. enterocolitica* infection.

BASIS FOR RECOMMENDATIONS

Butler T. Yersinia species, including plague. *Mandell, Douglas and Bennett's Principles and Practice of Infectious Diseases, VIth edition; Churchill Livingston,* 2005; pp. 1406–1413.

Fungi

ASPERGILLUS

John G. Bartlett, MD

Microbiology

- Hyphae 2–4 µm wide, usually septate, 40 degree angle branching.
- Ubiquitous mold present worldwide in soil, plants, cellars, marijuana, etc.
- Dominant species: *A. fumigatus* > *A. flavus, A. terreus, A. niger.*

Clinical

- Major pathogen in following conditions: marrow failure (acute leukemia, aplastic anemia), allogenic stem cell transplants, solid organ transplants, AIDS with CD4 <400 cells/ml, chronic granulomatous disease and preexisting structural lung disease.
- Aspergillus spp. commonly colonize the respiratory tract and are often laboratory contaminants, so positive cultures need to be interpreted carefully.
- Diagnosis usually by combination of host status, imaging and mycological findings. Culture often false negative (blood rarely yields positive culture) and sensitivity with BAL culture is <50%.
- Dx: culture in right context or histopathology (show dichotomously branching, septate hyphae but may be confused with other species) or body fluids w/ evidence of mold or fungal invasion (may culture negative). Important to recognize that widely acknowledged lung-CT w/ halo/crescent sign only described in neutropenic populations. Clinical specimens.
- Galactomannan: constituent of fungal cell wall, serum assay may assist with detection of invasive aspergillosis or use for early diagnosis in BAL specimens. False positives may occur due to the fungal infections or administration of an antibiotic derived from fungus (e.g., piperacillin/tazobactam).

Sites of Infection

- Pulmonary (four forms): (1) allergic bronchopulmonary (ABPA), (2) invasive or semi-invasive, (3) fungus ball (aspergilloma), and (4) tracheobronchitis. Airways: also laryngeal forms.
- Sinusitis: allergic, fungus ball, invasive.
- Otitis externa.
- CNS: abscesses, meningitis.
- Bone: osteomyelitis (often vertebral).
- Cutaneous: burns, wounds.
- Ocular: endophthalmitis.
- Other (rare): catheter and shunts infections, urinary tract infection, endocarditis.

Treatment
Pulmonary

- Invasive pulmonary: voriconazole 6 mg/kg q12h PO/IV × 2 doses, then 4 mg/kg q12h, then when stable 200–300 mg twice daily (300 mg twice daily for severe disease).
- Some consider the non-loading voriconazole dosing as too low for some pts/conditions. Consider therapeutic monitoring to avoid toxicities (possibly with peak levels >5.5 mg/L) and perhaps enhance efficacy (maintain trough levels >2 mg/L).
- Invasive pulmonary (alt): amphotericin B 1 mg/kg/day IV or liposomal amB (preferred amB product) 5 mg/kg/day.
- Invasive (alt): caspofungin 70 mg IV × 1 dose then 50 mg/day IV (has FDA salvage indication) or micafungin 100–150 IV/day or posaconazole 200 mg PO q6h × 7 days, then 400 mg PO q8–12hrs (take with food).
- Failure with voriconazole: consider amphotericin products, posaconazole, caspofungin or micafungin. Role of combination antifungal use unclear but often done.
- Aspergilloma: no consensus on whether anti-fungal treatment effective—main concern is hemoptysis.
- Aspergilloma resection: consider if adequate pulmonary function plus if pt w/ sarcoidosis, immunocompromise, increasing IgG or recurrent hemoptysis.

- Aspergilloma-other approaches: observe (most cases), bronchial artery embolism (temporizing, especially for hemoptysis), intracavitary amB (1 positive report), oral itraconazole (anecdotal successes), amB (not usually recommended).
- Allergic bronchopulmonary aspergillosis (ABPA): prednisone 0.5 mg/kg/day × 1 wk then 0.5 mg/kg every other day × 5 wks or itraconazole 200 mg PO twice daily +/– prednisone or voriconazole 200 mg PO twice daily +/– prednisone.
- Costs (AWP, max dose × 21 days): voriconazole PO-$1500; voriconazole IV-$3800; amphotericin B-$16; liposomal amphotericin B (AmBisome)-$28,000; caspofungin-$7,500; itraconazole PO-$382.

ENT Infections

- Sinonasal, acute invasive, compromised host: surgery + amB lavage + correction of host defect (increase WBC, decrease steroids as feasible, etc.).
- Sinonasal chronic invasive, healthy host: surgical debridement +/– voriconazole, posaconazole, or amphotericin.
- Sinus fungus ball: surgical removal.
- Sinusitis, allergic fungal: surgical drainage + corticosteroids (inhaled or systemic) + antibacterials (role of antifungals controversial).
- Otic infection, immunocompetent: topical cresylate, alcohol, boric acid, 5–FC ointment, clotrimazole, etc.
- Otic infection, compromised host: voriconazole 200 mg PO twice daily or posaconazole 200 mg PO q6h or itraconazole 200 mg PO twice daily.

Other Infections

- Brain abscess: surgical drainage plus amB 1–1.5 mg/kg/day and 5FC 100–150 mg/kg/day PO; role unclear for voriconazole, echinocandins and lipid AmB products. Poor CNS penetration with echinocandins.
- Meningitis: AmB 1–1.5 mg/kg/day IV + intrathecal dosing (usually 0.1 mg/day via Ommaya reservoir).
- Bone: surgical debridement + voriconazole, polyene (amphotericin products), caspofungin, micafungin or posaconazole.
- Endocarditis: valve replacement + liposomal amphotericin 5 mg/kg IV q24.
- Hepatosplenic: lipid amphotericin formulation 5 mg/kg/day and/or voriconazole.
- Catheter-associated: remove line.

OTHER INFORMATION

- Voriconazole and caspofungin are replacing AmB as preferred treatment for they are less toxic agents. RCT suggests voriconazole is more effective than AmB (see Herbrecht et al).

BASIS FOR RECOMMENDATIONS

Walsh TJ, Anaissie EJ, Denning DW, et al. Treatment of aspergillosis: clinical practice guidelines of the Infectious Diseases Society of America. *Clin Infect Dis*, 2008; Vol. 46; pp. 327–60.

Comments: 2008 IDSA Guidelines for treatment of aspergillosis. This is the source document used here.

Pascual A, Calandra T, Bolay S, et al. Voriconazole therapeutic drug monitoring in pts with invasive mycoses improves efficacy and safety outcomes. *Clin Infect Dis*, 2008; Vol. 46; pp. 201–11.

Comments: This study is based on 181 measurements of voriconazole levels and showed, despite standard dosing, 31% showed levels considered potentially toxic and 25% showed levels considered subtherapeutic.

Herbrecht R et al. Voriconazole versus amphotericin B for primary therapy of invasive aspergillosis. *N Engl J Med*, 2002; Vol. 347; pp. 408–15.

Comments: Large multicenter study of 144 pts with invasive aspergillosis randomized to receive voriconazole or amphotericin B. Voriconazole was superior in rates of success (53% vs 32%), survival (71% vs 58%) and reduced adverse effects.

BLASTOMYCES DERMATITIDIS

John G. Bartlett, MD

MICROBIOLOGY

- Dimorphic fungus: mycelial in nature (room temperature) and yeast in tissue (37°C).
- Yeast—8×30 micron, broad-based budding differentiates (histoplasma, narrow-based budding).
- Fungus especially found in moist, acid soils in forests.

CLINICAL

- Epidemiology: found in N. and S. America. Also Europe, Africa, Asia. In U.S., southeastern and southcentral states that border Mississippi and Ohio Rivers, Midwest and southern Canadian provinces bordering the Great Lakes. Wisconsin typically reports the most cases annually in the U.S.
- Most cases: manual laborers, hunters, farmers. Usually sporadic. Epidemics sometimes associated with activities around rotting/decayed wood.
- Pathogenesis: inhalation leads to pneumonia (range: acute, chronic, asymptomatic) +/– dissemination, especially to skin, bone/joints, GU tract. Incubation period is 30–45 days.
- Dx: large yeast w/ broad based bud upon wet mount w /KOH (e.g., skin, CSF, urine, BAL). For tissue, use PAS, GMS, or silver stains. Cx: Sabouraud media at 30°C, slow growth often contributes to delay in diagnosis. Serology usually not useful.
- *B. dermatitidis* antigen assay available from MiraVista Labs (866-647-2847). May help speed diagnosis if not apparent by histopathological methods.
- Sensitivity of diagnostic tests: antigen assay 90%, cytology 50–93%, KOH 30–80%, histopathology 85%, culture 66–75%, serology poor.
- Urine assay for blastomyces antigen: 90% sensitive and 80% specific (MiraVista Lab).

SITES OF INFECTION

- Pulmonary (70–75% cases): acute forms may resemble bacterial pneumonia. More indolent disease may mimic malignancy, tuberculosis. In immunosuppressed, may quickly progress to ARDS-like picture.
- Pulmonary forms: asymptomatic (50% cases, most common), acute, chronic pulmonary and disseminated chronic pulmonary.
- Disseminated (10–20%): skin, bones, and prostate are most common.
- Cutaneous: most common extrapulmonary site. Papules typically evolve verrucous or ulcerative lesions. Some become pustules/cold abscesses. Often accompanied by systemic symptoms.
- Bone/Joint: arthritis, osteomyelitis (typically lytic lesions in long bones).
- GU: primarily prostate/prostatitis, also epididymitis.
- CNS: meningitis or brain abscess. Rare except in immunosuppressed pts such as AIDS.

TREATMENT

Pulmonary

- Moderate-severe infection: lipid amphotericin B 3–5 mg/kg/day or amphotericin B 0.7–1 mg/kg/day × 1–2 wks or until improvement, then itraconazole 200 PO mg three times daily × 3 days then twice daily × 6–12 mos.
- Mild-moderate infection: itraconazole 200 mg PO three times daily × 3 days, then 200 mg PO twice daily × 6–12 mos.

Osteoarticular, CNS and disseminated infections

- **Disseminated disease**: as above for moderate-severe pulmonary dz, with itraconazole for ≥12 mos.
- If disseminated infection is only of mild-moderate severity, use itraconazole as above for 6–12 mos.
- **Osteoarticular**: treat ≥12 mos.
- **CNS**: lipid amphotericin B 5 mg/kg/days × 4–6 wks, then: (1) itraconazole 200 mg 2–3 ×/day or (2) fluconazole 800 mg/days or (3) voriconazole 200–400 mg twice-daily × ≥12 mos and until CNS cleared.

Treatment—Immunosuppressed

- Regimen recommended for severe pulmonary infection as above with itraconazole × ≥12 mos then ± lifetime itraconazole 200 mg/day if immune suppressive state persists.

OTHER INFORMATION

- Most cases should be treated—usually with itraconazole.
- Ampho B preferred treatment for immunosuppressed, CNS infections, life-threatening disease, and azole failures. Itraconazole—preferred azole (monitor itraconazole levels).
- Most common clinical presentation is chronic pulmonary infection (infiltrates, nodules, cavitation).

BASIS FOR RECOMMENDATIONS

Chapman SW, Dismukes WE, Proia LA, et al. Clinical practice guidelines for the management of blastomycosis: 2008 update by the Infectious Diseases Society of America. *Clin Infect Dis*, 2008; Vol. 46; pp. 1801–12.

Comments: Source document for recommendations.

CANDIDA ALBICANS

Paul Auwaerter, MD and Dionissis Neofytos, MD, MPH

MICROBIOLOGY

- Budding yeast, capable of >10 diseases. Causes ~100% oropharyngeal (OPC), 90% vulvovaginitis candidiasis.
- Normal commensals of skin, GI and GU tracts. Difficulty is often separating invasive disease from asymptomatic colonization.
- *C. albicans*: germ-tube (early hyphal-like extensions at 24 hrs of culture) positive (note ~5% may be initially called germ-tube negative). *C. dubliniensis* may other yeast routinely germ-tube positive. All other *Candida* spp. germ tube negative.

CLINICAL

- Common risk factors for candidemia: prior abx use, immune suppression (hematologic malignancy, organ or hematopoietic stem cell transplantation, chemotherapy), malignancy, diabetes, malnutrition, post-abdominal surgical, catheters, acute renal failure, TPN.
- Clinical manifestations: range from local mucous membrane involvement (local overgrowth and invasion) to dissemination (hematogenous spread).
- Candidemia sources include: lines and GI track (e.g., translocation s/t severe mucositis s/t chemo).
- *C. albicans:* most commonly isolated spp. in pts with candidemia; however, collectively non-albicans *Candida* spp. more common.
- Dx: culture normally sterile site; mucosal—typical lesion and positive KOH/Gram-stain.
- Blood cultures positive in 50–70% of candidemia cases. Antigen (e.g., beta-D-glucan) and PCR assays hold promise for diagnosis of candidemia. PNA-FISH testing on a positive blood cx: rapid detection of *C. albicans.*
- Empiric anti-fungal treatment should be considered in seriously ill pts with risk of candidemia.

SITES OF INFECTION

- Cutaneous: diaper dermatitis, monilia, intertriginous infections, balanitis, vulvitis, paronychia.
- Chronic mucocutaneous candidiasis: persistent infections of the skin, nails, and mucous membranes; most pts have T-cell dysfunction/disorder.
- Oropharyngeal/esophageal: thrush, esophagitis. Very common with advanced HIV infection.
- Vulvovaginal: vaginitis—most common in women of childbearing age.
- Blood/cardiovascular: candidemia, often catheter-related; endocarditis—prosthetic and native valves.
- Genitourinary: candiduria common in catheterized pts (often not significant), renal abscess, fungal balls.
- GI: hepatosplenic candidiasis (often in setting of resolving neutropenia, malignancy or GI disease), peritonitis.
- Musculoskeletal: septic arthritis, osteomyelitis, myositis.
- Ocular: endophthalmitis; screening recommended for pts with documented candidemia.
- Neurological: meningitis.

TREATMENT

Treatment-General comments

- *C. albicans* is generally susceptible to all major antifungal categories: azoles, echinocandins, amphotericin B. Azole resistance seen mostly in HIV with OPC.
- *Candida* speciation is reasonably predictive guide to therapy (see below and *Candida* spp. module).
- *Candida* susceptibility testing not widely performed; however, some centers do routinely test candidemia isolates. Most helpful for guiding therapy with non-albicans *Candida* or if resistance suspected especially with hx of prior azole use.

PATHOGENS

Mucocutaneous Candidiasis

- Cutaneous candidiasis: maintain dry skin surface (frequent diaper changes), control hyperglycemia. Topicals: clotrimazole, miconazole, nystatin, ketoconazole 2% all twice daily for 3–5 days.
- Oropharyngeal candidiasis (OPC): clotrimazole oral troches 10 mg 5×/day, nystatin [suspension 400,000–600,000 U four times a day or 200,000 U pastilles 1–2 used 4 or 5×/day]; fluconazole 100 mg daily PO. Duration 7–14 days.
- OPC (alt): itraconazole 200 mg/day PO (use solution, ~66% response rate for fluconazole-resistant OPC), AmB 0.3 mg/kd/day IV, caspofungin 70 mg IV load then 50 mg q24h, micafungin 100–150 mg IV q24h, anidulafungin 200 mg IV × 1 (load, d1), then 100 mg IV q24h or voriconazole 200 mg PO twice daily. All for 7–14 days.
- OPC (alt): AmB 1ml oral suspension PO four times a day (no longer commercially available in U.S.).
- Esophageal: fluconazole 200 mg PO/IV daily to improvement then 100 mg/day PO (14–21 days total) or maintenance if recurrent. Alt: voriconazole 200 mg PO/IV twice daily, AmB 0.3–0.7 mg/kg/day IV, caspofungin 70 mg IV load then 50 mg q24h, micafungin 100–150 mg IV q24h, anidulafungin 200 mg IV × 1 (d1, load), then 100 mg IV q24h.
- Vulvovaginal: suppositories/topical [OTC: clotrimazole, butoconazole, miconazole, tioconazole], use short course (1–3 days) for mild sx, >7–14 days if severe, recurrent or abnormal host.
- Vulvovaginal: systemic fluconazole 150 mg PO single dose (wait 3 days for response), topical nystatin 100,000 U/day × 7–14 days. Boric acid 600 mg gel capsule intravaginal daily × 14 days effective especially for non-albicans species.
- Chronic mucocutaneous candidiasis: azoles (fluconazole) or amphotericin B effective.
- Relapses not uncommon, esp AIDS. Long-term suppression w/ fluconazole 200 mg PO daily works for OPC; however, try to avoid due to the development of resistance.

Candiduria

- Presence not necessarily equating renal tract infection as colonization common even w/ pyuria. Some exceptions: renal transplantation, pregnancy, neutropenic pts, urology pts with hardware in place or undergoing a procedure.
- Catheter-related infection often resolves without therapy (40%). Urine cx post catheter removal can help determine need for treatment. Catheter change alone rarely effective.
- Upper tract disease (fever/leukocytosis) requires systemic therapy. Any hardware such as stents may need to be removed for eradication.
- Persistence/recurrence or suspect source of sepsis should prompt GU tract studies. Fungal balls likely require surgical removal.
- If treatment required (preferred): fluconazole 400 mg load followed by 200 mg PO/IV daily × 7–14 days.
- Alt: ampho B 0.5 mg/kg/day IV × 7–14 days.
- Alt: 5-FC 25 mg/kg PO four times a day × 7 days. One of the only indications for 5-FC monotherapy. Effective but be wary of initial or emerging resistance w/ therapy. Myelosuppressive, need to monitor drug levels if used >7 days.
- Alt: amphotericin B bladder washings, 50 mg/1L sterile water @ 40 ml/hr × 5 days. Never a favorite with pts or nurses, now mostly reserved for localization purposes.
- Limited experience with caspofungin (and other echinocandins) or voriconazole: all with poor urinary levels.

Candidemia/Invasive Candidiasis

- Nonneutropenic hosts: fluconazole 800 mg IV/PO load then 400 mg q24h (only if clinically stable), caspofungin 70 mg IV load then 50 mg q24h, micafungin 100–150 mg IV q24h, anidulafungin 200 mg IV × 1 (d1 load) the 100 mg IV q24h, amB 0.6–1.0 mg/kg/day IV.
- Neutropenic hosts: limited data available. caspofungin 70 mg IV load then 50 mg q24h, micafungin100–150 mg IV q24h, anidulafungin 200 mg IV × 1 (d1 load), then 100 mg IV q24h, amB 0.7–1.0 mg/kg/day or LFAmB 3–5 mg/kg/day IV. Alt: fluconazole 6–12 mg/kgIV/PO q24h: only for stable pts without prior azole exposure.

- Duration of treatment: 14 days after last (+) cx and sx resolution; treat longer if complications present (e.g., endophthalmitis, endocarditis, septic arthritis or osteomyelitis, etc.).
- Chronic disseminated candidiasis: follow neutropenic recommendations, but conversion to fluconazole (200–400 mg PO daily) usual after 1–2 wks. Duration of rx totals 3–6 mos. or calcification of radiologic lesions.
- Remove all percutaneous lines if suspected, although controversial in neutropenic host (as GI tract is likely source).
- All pts w/ candidemia need to undergo ophthalmological exam to r/o endophthalmitis. Onset of disease rare after otherwise successful course of therapy.

Endocarditis

- Replacement of infected valve almost always required.
- AmB 0.6–1.0 mg/kg or LFAmB 3.0–6.0 mg/kg IV q24h plus 5-FC 25–37.5 mg/kg PO four times a day.
- Alt (less clinical experience): fluconazole 6–12 mg/kg IV/PO q24h or caspofungin 70 mg IV load then 50 mg q24h, micafungin 150 mg IV q24h, anidulafungin 200 mg IV × 1 (d1 load), then 100 mg IV q24h.
- Duration: at least 6 wks after valve replacement; post-op chronic suppressive treatment with fluconazole may be of benefit (more so for prosthetic heart valve endocarditis as rates of relapse often high in these pts).
- Success w/ long-term fluconazole suppression reported in pts unable to undergo valve surgery.
- Histopathologic examination and culture of the valve can confirm the diagnosis and allow resistance testing.

Prevention

- Neutropenia: limited good data until recently; fluconazole 400 mg, or posaconazole (200 mg PO three times a day) in pts at high-risk of invasive candidiasis (prolonged severe neutropenia in pts with acute leukemia or following intensive myelosuppressive chemotherapy). Duration rx unclear, but minimum should be for period of neutropenia.
- HSCT recipients: fluconazole 400 mg for first 75 days post-HSCT or posaconazole 200 three times a day during acute or chronic GVHD/treatment with steroids. Voriconazole has been studied but data yet to be published.
- Solid-organ transplants: best evidence for high-risk liver transplant pts, use fluconazole 400 mg/day.
- ICU: controversial, some evidence that units w/ high rates of *candida* infection may benefit if oral fluconazole 400 mg/day employed.

MORE TREATMENT

- **Endophthalmitis:** uncomplicated small lesions in pts otherwise at low risk may be initially managed with fluconazole 6–12 mg/kg/day IV/PO; poor response (e.g., progression or lack of a response) should prompt change to AmB 0.7–1.0 mg/kg IV q24h or fluconazole 6–12 mg IV/PO q24 and early vitrectomy. Alt: voriconazole 400 mg IV/PO q12 × 2 doses then 200–300 mg IV/PO q12. Duration: 6–12 wks. Intravitreal amphotericin B controversial, dose is 5–10 μg. Caspofungin or other echinocandins may be but not well studied. There is a concern regarding ocular penetration of caspofungin.
- **Central Nervous System (meningitis):** Am B (0.7–1.0 mg/kg IV q24 +/– 5-FC (25 mg/kg PO four times a day); consider fluconazole(400–800 m IV) in low risk pts. Treat minimum 4 wks. Shunt removal usually required.
- **Peritonitis:** AmB or fluconazole (see candidemia recommendations) and surgical exploration/drainage in pts suspected of perforation and/or secondary peritonitis or abscess. Pts on CAPD should have dialysis catheter removed, treat 2–3 wks. Wait 2 wks minimum before replacing catheter.
- **Bone and Soft Tissue Infections:** surgical debridement + AmB 0.5–1.0 mg/kg/day (better studied) × 6–10 wks or fluconazole 6 mg/kg/day × 6–12 mos. Can add AmB to bone cement. Many start with AmB 2–3 wks then change to fluconazole.

PATHOGENS

OTHER INFORMATION

- See *Candida* spp. module for non-albicans specifics.
- Rarely a laboratory contaminate from a sterile specimen. Clinical correlation of *in vitro* susceptibility patterns is not firmly established for most species, especially for systemic *Candida* infections.
- Isolation from respiratory tract rarely represents actual infection. *Candida* pneumonia should only be diagnosed with biopsy-proven evidence.
- "Chronic candidiasis" (The Yeast Connection) unproven as cause of chronic fatigue, non-specific sx. No benefit to stool cx or GI eradication in these pts.

General Patterns Susceptibility (*CID* 2004;38:161)

Candida species	F	I	V	5-FC	AmB	Cand
C. albicans	S	S	S	S	S	S
C. tropicalis	S	S	S	S	S	S
C. parapsilosis	S	S	S	S	S	S**
C. glabrata	S*-R	S*-R	S*-R	S	S^	S
C. krusei	R	S*	S^	R	S^	S
C. lusitaniae	S	S	S	S	S-R	S

F = fluconazole, I = itraconazole, V = voriconazole
AmB = amphotericin B, Cand = echinocandins, e.g., caspofungin
S = generally susceptible
S* = dose dependent susceptibility (needs higher azole dose)
S^ = susceptible to intermediate susceptibility
R = resistant
**Higher MICs

BASIS FOR RECOMMENDATIONS

Cornely OA, Maertens J, Winston DJ, et al. Posaconazole vs. fluconazole or itraconazole prophylaxis in pts with neutropenia. *N Engl J Med*, 2007; Vol. 356; pp. 348–59.
Comments: In pts undergoing chemotherapy for acute myelogenous leukemia or the myelodysplastic syndrome, posaconazole prevented invasive fungal infections more effectively than did either fluconazole or itraconazole (2% vs. 8%; P<0.001) and improved overall survival (P = 0.04).

Pappas PG, Rex JH, Sobel JD, et al. Guidelines for treatment of candidiasis. *Clin Infect Dis*, 2004; Vol. 38; pp. 161–89.
Comments: Source document for most of current recommendations. Some important points include that Fluconazole 400 is generally viewed as equivalent to AmB (0.5–0.6 mg/kg/day). However, since many decisions for starting medication are done without knowledge of positive cultures or the specific *Candida* spp., for pts more likely to have non-albicans isolates and/or for those very ill—clinicians may not wish to depend on fluconazole initially.

Slavin MA, Osborne B, Adams R, et al. Efficacy and safety of fluconazole prophylaxis for fungal infections after marrow transplantation—a prospective, randomized, double-blind study. *Clin Infect Dis*, 1995; Vol. 171; pp. 1545–52.
Comments: Landmark antifungal prophylaxis trial in allogeneic HSCT recipients. 400 mg/day fluconazole administered during the first 75 days after marrow transplantation resulted in significantly less systemic fungal infections (7% vs. 18%; P = .004) and better survival (P = 0.004) compared to placebo. There were no *Candida albicans* infections in fluconazole recipients compared with 18 in placebo recipients (P < .001).

Rex JH, Bennett JE, Sugar AM, et al. A randomized trial comparing fluconazole with amphotericin B for the treatment of candidemia in pts without neutropenia. Candidemia Study Group and the National Institute. *N Engl J Med*, 1994; Vol. 331; pp. 1325–30.
Comments: The first randomized trial to compare therapeutic options for the treatment of invasive candidiasis: AMB-d vs. FLU, in non-neutropenic hosts. Survival and clinical outcome were comparable between the two study arms. The authors concluded: "fluconazole and AMB are not significantly different in their effectiveness in treating candidemia".

CANDIDA SPECIES

John G. Bartlett, MD

MICROBIOLOGY

- Yeast, seen as 4–6 μm, pseudomycelia.
- One of few fungi that grow on blood agar and in blood culture.
- Common non-albicans spp: *C. glabrata, C. guilliermondii, C. krusei, C. kefyr, C. lusitaniae, C. parapsilosis, C. tropicalis.*
- See previous module for *Candida albicans*.

CLINICAL

- Most infections: endogenous from colonization of GI, GU tract or skin. Also environmental sources.
- Dx: positive culture of normally sterile site. Mucosal: typical lesion and positive KOH/Gram-stain.
- Evidence of need to treat: Culture source, symptoms, concentration (e.g., heavy growth), multiple cultures, host, evidence seen on stains, no other likely pathogen.
- Need care with interpreting some cultures: 1/3 sputum and 1/5 BAL yield Candida spp. In absence of severe neutropenia or immunosuppressive disease, Candida pneumonia is very rare.
- For prevention in high-risk populations see "Fever and Neutropenia" module.

SITES OF INFECTION

- Mucocutaneous: thrush, esophagitis, vaginitis and paronychia
- Disseminated, Candidemia
- Chronic disseminated candidiasis (formerly called "hepatosplenic candidiasis")
- Urinary
- Pneumonia (rare)
- Osteomyelitis
- Peritoneal, gallbladder
- Endocarditis
- Endophthalmitis
- Meningitis

TREATMENT

Invasive or non-mucosal Infections

- Principles: establish Candida as causal pathogen. Rx: remove any foreign bodies. Use Echinocandin or azole primarily. Be wary if using fluconazole for non-albicans species that may have significant rates of azole-resistance (e.g., *C. glabrata, C. krusei*). Neutropenia; echinocandin preferred.
- Regimens: ampho B 0.6–1.0 mg/kg/d IV, lipid ampho 3–5 mg/kg/day IV, caspofungin 70 mg IV × 1, then 50 mg IV/day or anidulafungin 200 mg IV × 1, then 100 mg/day; fluconazole 800 IV/PO × 1, then 400 mg qd.
- Remove all lines. Use Ampho B or fluconazole until cx negative × 14 days.
- **Candidemia and neutropenia:** remove all lines, use amphotericin B, lipid formulation amphotericin, echinocandin (e.g., caspofungin), or voriconazole.
- **Genitourinary:** urine often culture positive but not pathogenic. Remove catheter if present. Indications to treat: symptoms, neutropenia, prior to GU surgery or hardware implant or pregnancy. If treatment needed: fluconazole 200 mg PO/IV daily × 7–14 days or amphotericin B (alt.).
- **Osteomyelitis:** debride nonvital bone. Lipid amphotericin × 6–10 wks, some use fluconazole with success. Alt: Amphotericin B or Echinocandin.
- **Intra-abdominal:** remove catheters. Amphotericin B or fluconazole × 2–3 wks.
- **Endocarditis:** remove valve. Treat with amphotericin B or lipid formulation amphotericin B (5 mg/kg/day) + 5FC 25 mg/kg PO q6h × 4–6 wks. Echinocandin can be considered.
- **Meningitis:** remove any shunt/device. Lipid amphotericin 5 mg/kg IV q24h plus 5FC 25 mg/kg PO q6h until signs resolved >4 wks.
- **Endophthalmitis:** early vitrectomy combined with amphotericin B 0.7–1.0 mg/kg IV q24 or fluconazole 6–12 mg/kg IV/PO daily. Alt: voriconazole 400 mg IV/PO q12 × 2 doses then

PATHOGENS

200–300 mg IV/PO q12. Intravitreal amphotericin B controversial (usual dose 5–10 µg). Caspofungin may be useful, but not well studied and ocular penetration uncertain. Ambisome can be considered.

Mucosal Candidiasis

- **Thrush:** clotrimazole 10 mg 4–5 ×/day, nystatin 2–400,000 U 5 ×/day or fluconazole 100–200 mg daily PO × 7–14 days.
- Alt: itraconazole 200 mg PO daily, caspofungin IV or amphotericin B 0.3–0.7 mg/kg/d IV.
- **Esophagitis:** fluconazole 200–400 mg IV/PO daily × 14–21 days post improvement.
- Alt: posaconazole 400 mg daily (also FDA approved for refractory esophageal candidiasis in HIV at 400 mg PO twice daily until resolution of symptoms) or voriconazole 4 mg/kg IV/PO twice daily or caspofungin 70 mg × 1 then 50 mg IV/d (or micafungin or anidulafungin) or amphotericin B 0.3–0.7 mg/kg.
- **Vaginitis:** topical (butoconazole, miconazole, tioconazole, terconazole) applied × 1–7 d or fluconazole 150 mg PO × 1 dose.
- **Vaginitis-recurrent:** fluconazole 150 mg q wk, itraconazole 100 mg every other day or topical agent. All × 6 mos.

Treatment Options/Issues for certain Candida Species

- Most resistant species is *C. glabrata* (some centers 30–40% azole-resistant). Also *C. krusei* (azole-resistant, intrinsic), *C. lusitaniae* (amB resistant, intrinsic), *C. tropicalis* (some azole resistance, ~5%).
- Topical Ampho B: rarely indicated.
- Costs per 7 days treatment: amB–$6, Ambisome–$7,000, fluconazole PO–$55, IV–$700–1,800, caspofungin–$3,000, micafungin–$1,500, anidulafungin–$1,300.

OTHER INFORMATION

- Candida is common contaminant: consider culture source, Gram-stain findings, concentrations, and host before considering whether it is a true pathogen (especially pulmonary, GU sources).
- Blood cultures for candida merit a minimum 14 days of antifungal therapy.
- Candidiasis and foreign bodies: must remove foreign body for cure.
- Antifungals: Ampho always active, azoles usually preferred.
- Fungal sensitivity testing recommended for deep, refractory, and recurrent infections and/ or history of antifungal therapy.

BASIS FOR RECOMMENDATIONS

Pappas PG, Rex JH, Sobel JD, et al. Guidelines for treatment of candidiasis. *Clin Infect Dis*, 2009; Vol. 48; pp. 503.
Comments: IDSA guidelines for treatment of candidiasis. These guidelines are the basis of recommendations used here.

Benson CA, Kaplan JE, Masur H, et al. Treating opportunistic infections among HIV-infected adults and adolescents: Recommendations from the CDC, the National Institutes of Health and the HIV Medicine Association of the IDSA. *Clin Infect Dis*, 2005; Vol. 40; pp. S131.
Comments: These are the recommendations given here.

Medical Letter Consultants. Antifungal drugs. *Treat Guidel Med Lett*, 2005; Vol. 3; pp. 7–14.
Comments: These are the recommendations given here which are identical to those from the CDC/NIH/IDSA.

Spellberg BJ, Filler SG, Edwards JE. Current treatment strategies for disseminated candidiasis. *Clin Infect Dis*, 2006; Vol. 42; pp. 244–51.
Comments: Fluconazole is best drug based on efficacy, cost and safety. Exceptions are resistant strains *of C. krusei* and possibly *C. glabrata*. For serious cases of candidemia they suggest empiric treatment with echinocandins, voriconazole and polyenes. For *C. glabrata* or *C. krusei* the best choices are echinocandins or high dose polyenes.

COCCIDIOIDES IMMITIS

John G. Bartlett, MD

MICROBIOLOGY

- Dimorphic fungus: large spherule 15–75 µm diameter often containing endospores 2–5 µm in diameter at 37°C.
- Prefers warm but dry environs; low deserts.
- *C. immitis* found only in San Joaquin Valley while closely related *C. posadasii* is found elsewhere in desert regions of southwest U.S., Mexico, and Central/South America.
- Grows readily on standard fungal media.

CLINICAL
- Endemic in CA, AZ, TX, NM, Mexico, S. America.
- Most common presentation: acute or subacute pneumonia. Acute infections often with fever and constitutional complaints.
- Incubation period for acute infection: 7–21 days. Sx: cough (25–50%), fever, infiltrate (50%). Chronic pulmonary disease in 4% (nodule or cavity) or dissemination (0.5%).
- Risk for severe disease: low CMI (AIDS, organ tx, steroids), 3rd trimester pregnancy, large inoculum; race: Black, Filipino, populations from Oceania.
- Always pathogenic when seen on histopathology or cultured.
- Dx: (1) identify spherule, (2) culture fungus, (3) positive serology w/ blood or body fluid.
- Diagnostic stains: H&E, PAS, KOH, calcofluor (Gram-stain not useful).
- Serology: complement fixation titer ($\geq$1:16 = likely disseminated infection); serial tests immunodiffusion, EIA (need confirmation). Negative tests don't exclude diagnosis. l g positive in 90% with acute disease of at least 3 wks duration.
- Seroconversion (skin test) 3%/yr in highly endemic areas.

SITES OF INFECTION
- Pulmonary: lobar consolidation possible or effusions. Spectrum: ranges from acute pneumonia to chronic nodular, cavitary disease. May be asymptomatic with positive radiographic findings.
- Skin: erythema nodosum classic over anterior tibia, but these painful lesions may occur anywhere, including maculopapular findings; onset typically 3 days–3 wks after end of initial fever +/– eosinophilia. E. multiforme or vesicles also described.
- Bone/joints: vertebral infection, mono- or polyarticular joint involvement. Predilection for bone. Arthralgia commonly associated with E. nodosum presentations.
- CNS: meningitis usually subacute-chronic.

TREATMENT
General
- Azoles active: fluconazole, itraconazole, posaconazole, voriconazole.
- Follow clinical features and serology q2–4 mos.
- Treatment duration: may range from 1 mo to lifetime.
- It's commonly said that only 5% of cases require treatment.

Acute Pulmonary Infection
- Most cases resolve without treatment, though fatigue and flu-like symptoms may persist.
- Treat if high risk (AIDS, steroids, organ txp pt, 3rd trimester pregnancy) or if severe (wt loss >10%, intense night sweats >3 wks, infiltrates >½ lung, CF titer >1:16, prominent or persistent hilar adenopathy).
- Rx: itraconazole 200 mg PO twice daily or fluconazole 400 mg PO daily × 3–6 mos. In pregnancy use amphotericin B 0.5–0.7 mg/kg IV q24.
- Bilateral reticulo-nodular or severe unilateral infiltrates: amphotericin B 0.7–1 mg/kg IV q24h until stable, then itraconazole 200 mg PO twice daily or fluconazole 400 mg PO daily × >1 yr.
- ARDS presentation: antifungals + corticosteroids such as prednisone 60–80 mg PO daily until improved, then taper.

Chronic Pulmonary Infection
- Pulmonary nodule: no antifungals and no surgery, observe.
- Cavitary and asymptomatic: usually observe. Consider surgery if persists >2 yrs, progresses >1 yr or near pleura.
- Cavitary, symptomatic: resection or azole therapy such as itraconazole 200 mg PO twice daily or fluconazole 400 mg PO daily × 8–12 mos.
- Ruptured cavity: lobectomy + decortication + antifungal agents.
- Chronic fibrocavitary: itraconazole 200 mg PO twice daily or fluconazole 400 mg PO daily × >1 yr.
- Posaconazole has been used for refractory cases.
- Consider surgery for relative treatment failures with significant hemoptysis and lesions that are well localized.

PATHOGENS

Extrapulmonary Infection
- Non-meningeal (preferred): itraconazole 200 mg PO twice daily or fluconazole 400 mg PO daily, doses up to 1200 mg/day have been used.
- Non-meningeal (alt): amphotericin B 0.5–0.7 mg/kg IV q24h.
- Ampho B preferred for pregnancy, lesions that worsen rapidly or are in critical loci, e.g., spinal column disease.
- Meningitis: fluconazole 400–1000 mg IV/PO q24h. May give intrathecal amphotericin B as initial treatment in combination with azole therapy. Alternative: itraconazole 400–600 mg daily. After clinical improvement, continue fluconazole 400 mg PO forever.
- Meningitis (failure to respond to azoles or IV AmB): intrathecal amphotericin, 0.1–1.5 mg.
- Hydrocephalus usually requires neurosurgical consultation for shunt placement.

Follow Up
- Monitor itraconazole serum levels (goal: >1 mcg/ml).
- Indefinite azole therapy recommended with CNS infection, or disseminated disease in hosts with predilection to relapse (African-Americans, Filipino, Oceanic populations).

Other Information
- Fluconazole and itraconazole are considered best azoles for coccidioides. Amphotericin B products: usually reserved for respiratory failure, rapidly progressive disease, and pregnancy.

Basis for Recommendations
Galgiani JN, Ampel NM, Blair JE, et al. Coccidioidomycosis. *Clin Infect Dis*, 2005; Vol. 41; pp. 1217–23.
Comments: This is the source document for the recommendations used here.

CRYPTOCOCCUS NEOFORMANS

John G. Bartlett, MD

Microbiology
- Yeast-like round fungus, 5–10 μm with polysaccharide capsule.
- Reproduces by narrow-based budding.
- Epidemiology: worldwide in soil, high levels in pigeon droppings (but relevance is questionable).
- *C. neoformans*: four serotypes (A to D) described based upon the capsule components. Three varieties described as causing human disease *C. neoformans v. neoformans* (most common), *v. gattii*, and *v. grubii* (recently established).
- *C. neoformans* most common, usually afflicting immunocompromised hosts while *C. gattii* is most common in immunocompetent host—treated like *C. neoformans*.

Clinical
- Common cause of disease with reduced CMI, e.g., lymphoma, chronic steroid use, transplant pts, AIDS w/ CD4 <100 (most common). Approximately 20–30% pts are apparently immunologically normal hosts.
- Pathogenesis: inhaled, then pneumonia, then meningitis +/– skin, bone, prostate infection.
- Clinical: most common presentation is meningitis which may be asymptomatic w/o fever or meningismus.
- Dx: serum cryptococcal antigen positive in 80–95% w/ meningitis and 20–50% w/ non-meningeal presentations. May also be grown in culture (blood agar). Sensitivity of cryptococcal antigen in CSF 99%, while traditional India ink stain only yields 65%.
- Diagnosis in pulmonary infection: positive sputum culture or serum antigen plus clinical/x-ray findings.

Sites of Infection
- CNS: meningitis, meningoencephalitis.
- Lung: pneumonitis.
- GU: prostatitis (may be asymptomatic infection).
- Disseminated: fungemia.
- Cutaneous: nodules/vesicles (reflects dissemination).
- Rarer forms: colitis, osteomyelitis, septic arthritis, myocarditis, hepatitis, pancreatitis, adrenal gland, ocular disease, and brain abscess.

TREATMENT

Meningitis AIDS patients

- **Induction phase:** Amphotericin B 0.7 mg/kg IV + flucytosine 25 mg/kg PO four times a day × 2 wks, then fluconazole 400 mg PO once daily × 8 wks, then 200 mg PO once daily until CD4 >200 × >6 mos.
- Monitor 5-FC levels and CBC to avoid bone marrow suppression.
- Alternative: above without flucytosine, but need to treat for 4–6 wks of ampho B or ~12 wks of fluconazole 1200 mg/day (especially if neutropenic).
- Alternative: fluconazole 800–1200 mg/day IV/PO + flucytosine 25 mg/kg PO four times a day.
- Fluconazole alternative: itraconazole (not as effective). Ampho B alternative: liposomal AmB 4–6 mg/kg/day IV.
- **Maintenance phase:** fluconazole 200 mg PO once daily life long or discontinue maintenance fluconazole when CD4 >200 × 6 mos and completed 10 wks rx minimum and asymptomatic.
- CSF pressure OP > 250 mm H_2O: remove CSF fluid until pressure drops 50%, then daily LP with same rule until OP <200 mm H_2O.
- Fluconazole failures: limited but favorable experience with posaconazole 400 mg PO twice daily.

Non-AIDS meningitis

- Ampho B 0.7 mg/kg/day IV + flucytosine 25 mg/kg PO four times a day × 2 wks then fluconazole 400 mg PO once daily × 8 wks.
- Alt: ampho B 0.7–1.0 mg/kg/day IV + flucytosine 25 mg/kg PO four times a day × 6–10 wks.
- Duration: as above, but then maintain on fluconazole PO (200 mg/day) until immunocompetent, then D/C.
- CSF Pressure management: as above.

Non-CNS Infections (AIDS or non-AIDS)

- Must do LP to r/o meningitis.
- AIDS + pneumonia + neg LP: fluconazole 400 mg/day or itraconazole 200–400 mg/day both life-long or until CD4 > 200 × 6 mos.
- AIDS + pneumonia + neg LP alternative: fluconazole 400 mg/day + flucytosine 25 mg/kg four times a day × 10 wks.
- Non-AIDS, pulmonary/symptomatic + neg LP: fluconazole 400 mg/day PO × 3–6 mos.
- Non-AIDS + severe pulmonary dz: ampho B 0.4–0.7 mg/kg/day IV to 1–2 g total, when improved can switch to oral fluconazole to complete course.
- Non-AIDS, pulmonary, mild-mod sx + neg LP: fluconazole 400 mg/day PO × 3–6 mos.
- Antigenemia or positive urine cx and neg LP: fluconazole 400 mg/day × 3–6 mos.

OTHER INFORMATION

- This fungus has great tropism for CNS; LP to r/o meningitis with any lab evidence of *C. neoformans.*
- Often very quiet (asymptomatic) including meningitis, but meningitis is 100% fatal w/o treatment.
- Dx: meningitis—blood antigen 95% sensitive, CSF >99% sensitive, near 100% specific.
- Biggest management mistake is failure to reduce intracranial pressure when OP is >200; may need daily LP drainage.

BASIS FOR RECOMMENDATIONS

Benson CA, Kaplan JE, Masur H, et al. Treating opportunistic infections among HIV-exposed and infected children: recommendations from CDC, the National Institutes of Health, and the Infectious Diseases Society of America. *MMWR Recomm Rep*, 2004; Vol. 53; pp. 1–112.

Comments: CDC/IDSA guidelines for treating OIs in pts with HIV infection. Recommendations are those provided here.

Saag MS, Graybill RJ, Larsen RA, et al. Practice guidelines for the management of cryptococcal disease. Infectious Diseases Society of America. *Clin Infect Dis*, 2000; Vol. 30; pp. 710–8.

Comments: Guidelines from the IDSA for managing cryptococcosis which is the basis for recommendations here. AIDS: Pul—fluconazole, itraconazole or fluconazole + flucytosine lifelong; CNS: Ampho B + flucytosine—fluconazole lifelong. Non-AIDS: Pul—fluconazole or itraconazole × 6–12 mos or Ampho B 1000–2000 mg total dose, CNS: AmphoB + flucytosine then fluconazole × 6–10 wks.

PATHOGENS

DERMATOPHYTES

Khalil G. Ghanem, MD and Dionissis Neofytos, MD, MPH

MICROBIOLOGY

- Filamentous fungi (molds) able to digest nutrients from keratin, living tissue usually not invaded. 3 genera: *Microsporum*, *Trichophyton*, and *Epidermophyton* species.
- Dermatophytes can be zoophilic (cats, dogs, horses, pigs, etc.), geophilic (soil), or anthropophilic (natural pathogens of humans).
- Transfer from soil, animals or humans via arthrospores (very hardy vegetative cells). Direct contact is not necessary to acquire infection.
- *Microsporum* most common species: *M. canis*. *Epidermophyton* most common species: *E. floccosum*.
- *Trichophyton* most common species: *T. tonsurans, T. rubrum, T. mentagrophytes*.

CLINICAL

- Causative agents of: (a) skin and hair infections [e.g., tinea capitis, tinea corporis, etc] and (b) nail infections [onychomycosis].
- Deep infections: rarely in immunocompromised hosts (dermis and deep organs), invasion via lymphatics (Squeo RF et al. 1998. *J Am Acad Dermatol*. 39:379–80; Seddon ME et al. 1997. *Clin Infect Dis*. 25:153–154).
- Microscopic diagnosis sufficient to guide therapy in most cases; tissue (skin, hair follicle, nail) scraping for KOH.
- Dx(1): Wood's lamp-Microsporum = green (Trichophyton—usually no fluorescence).
- Dx(2): microscopy—preliminary ID of genus. Cx in Sabouraud's media may be helpful, but not great sensitivity and results may take 2–4 wks.
- Dx(3): onychomycosis: culture in dermatophyte test medium (DTM) may be used instead of Sabouraud's medium—cheaper, easy to perform, faster results (3–7 days).

SITES OF INFECTION

- **Tinea capitis:** children > adults, "endothrix" infection (conidia within the hair shaft), two forms: (a) "gray patch" (*M. canis,* cat and dog exposure, secondary staphylococcal infections) and (b) "black dot" (*T. tonsurans*, common in African-American children) [see *T. capitis/ T. barbae* on p. 45].
- **Tinea pedis** (athlete's foot): (a) acute (*T. mentagrophytes*, self-limited/recurrent, vesicles/ bullae on soles and between toes) and (b) chronic (*T. rubrum*, lesions between toes, but can extend to involve soles, sides of feet) [see *T. pedis* on p. 48].
- **Tinea corporis:** adults caring for children with T. capitis, *T. tonsurans* and *M. canis/ T. rubrum*, underlying disease (DM, HIV). **T. corporis gladiatarum:** athletes (e.g., wrestling) [see *T. corporis/T. cruri* on p. 46].
- **Tinea cruris** (jock itch): inner thigh patches, *T. rubrum/T. mentagrophytes*, men/women [see *T. corporis/T. cruri* on p. 46].
- **Tinea incognito:** T. pedis, T. corporis and T. cruris that look differently when inappropriately treated w/ steroids.
- **Onychomycosis:** due to dermatophytes (toenails) vs. yeasts (fingernails), prevalence: 4–18%, risk factors (older age, *T. pedis*, swimming, swimming, presence in family, psoriasis), white vs. yellow vs. brown nail discoloration, *T. rubrum/T. mentagrophytes*.

TREATMENT

General Principles

- Usual approach is to Rx with topical agents.
- Most nail infections, all hair infections, and widespread infections should be treated with systemic therapy.
- Very few comparative trials for the topical antifungals to yield firm recommendations.
- Treatment failure and relapse of infections may happen in 30–50% of cases.
- Tinea capitis: (a) gray patch: identify and treat infected pets with *M. canis* and (b) black dot: identify asymptomatic carriers and consider treating them with selenium sulfide shampoo or oral therapy.

Therapeutic agents

- **Topicals:** (a) keratolytics: Whitfield's ointment = salicylic and benzoic acid, used for soles/palms. (b) antifungals: azoles (miconazole, clotrimazole, ketoconazole, oxiconazole etc.) or others (terbinafine, butenafine).
- **Oral agents:** griseofulvin, terbinafine, itraconazole and fluconazole.

Therapeutic regimens

- See *T. corporis*, *T. cruris*, *T. capitis*, *T. barbae*, and *T. pedis* on pp. 45–50.
- Onychomycosis ddx includes Fusarium, Acremonium, Aspergillus, Scopulariopsis as some may not respond to typical oral rx; need to examine microscopically to get fungal ID.
- Onychomycosis should be treated with oral antifungal agents if possible (Crawford F; Cochrane Database Syst Rev. 2007;(3):CD001434).
- Onychomycosis: itraconazole 200 mg twice daily × 1 wk/mo × 2 mo for fingernails. Toenails 200 mg/day × 12 wk or 200 mg PO twice daily × 1 wk/mo × 3–4 mo or terbinafine 250 mg/day × 6 wks (fingernails), 12 wks (toes).
- Onychomycosis (alternate): fluconazole 150 mg q wk × 6 mos. [Fluconazole 150 mg q wk was less effective than itraconazole or terbinafine (*J Dermatolog Treat* 2002;13(1):3–9)].
- Deep Infections: data from case reports only. Consider antifungals: itraconazole 200 mg PO twice-daily or fluconazole 400 mg IV/PO once-daily.

FOLLOW UP

- If source of ringworm is household pet, **remember**, in order to avoid re-infection, **must treat pet.**
- Suspected onychomycosis not getting better on appropriate treatment: consider alternative diagnosis (e.g., psoriasis, eczema, trauma, lichen planus).

OTHER INFORMATION

- For scalp infection: important to ID causative organism. If zoophilic, usually not spread from person to person. If anthropophilic, higher rates of person to person spread.
- Tinea versicolor is caused by *Malassezia* species which are yeasts. They are not dermatophytes [see Tinea Versicolor on p. 50].
- Other skin infections: Tinea nigra (*Phaeoannellomyces werneckii*) palms and soles in tropics. White piedra (Trichosporon, yeasts) white/yellow on hair shaft; tropics. Black piedra (Piedrae, yeast) tropical.

BASIS FOR RECOMMENDATIONS

Foster KW, Ghannoum MA, Elewski BE. Epidemiologic surveillance of cutaneous fungal infection in the United States from 1999 to 2002. *J Am Acad Dermatol*, 2004; Vol. 50; pp. 748–52.

Comments: Dermatophytes remain the most commonly isolated fungal organisms except from clinically suspected finger onychomycosis, in which case *Candida* species comprise >70% of isolates. Trichophyton rubrum remains the most prevalent fungal pathogen, and increased incidence of this species was observed in finger and toe onychomycosis, tinea corporis and tinea cruris, tinea mannum, and tinea pedis. As the causal agent of tinea capitis, *T. tonsurans* continues to increase in incidence, especially in the U.S.

Author opinion.

Comments: No guideline recommendations exist for treatment of deep dermatophyte infection.

FUSARIUM

Aimee Zaas, MD

MICROBIOLOGY

- Filamentous nonpigmented (hyaline) septated fungi with acute angle branching.
- Ubiquitous in environment.
- Major species: *F. oxysporum* and *F. solani*.

CLINICAL

- Most common in immunocompromised hosts, with neutropenia as strongest risk factor. Median time between transplant and diagnosis was 48 days in one large series evaluating fusariosis in stem cell transplant pts.
- Typically presents as fever refractory to broad-spectrum antibacterial agents.
- Characteristic feature is skin lesions: erythematous, nodular, ulcerated—often with central eschar. Skin lesions occur before fungemia, therefore always biopsy any new skin lesion in immunocompromised pts.

PATHOGENS

- Local or disseminated infection can also occur in solid-organ transplant pts.
- Infection tends to spread rapidly in immunocompromised pts, while in immunocompetent pts, infections may remain localized.
- High mortality once disseminated. Survival in immunocompromised pts is 0% if neutropenia does not reverse. 30–50% of pts with recovery of neutropenia survive.
- Dx: skin or tissue biopsy with cx (positive blood cx if immunocompromised).
- Histologically indistinguishable from aspergillus, therefore **culture** in addition to pathology is imperative for proper dx.

SITES OF INFECTION

- **Immunocompromised pts:** skin, respiratory tract, venous catheters, GI tract are portals of entry.
- 50% of disseminated fusariosis occur in acute leukemia pts.
- Angioinvasiveness and adventitious sporulation (fungal growth in bloodstream) lead to disseminated infections.
- 88% of Fusarium infections in immunocompromised pts have skin lesions.
- Skin lesions: painful, multiple, erythema +/– central necrosis. Tend to develop over days; will find various stages of development.
- 50% of pts have positive blood cx.
- Classic portal of entry: paronychia (nailbed inflammation) in immunocompromised pt.
- **Immunocompetent pts:** area of skin or eye trauma is portal of entry.
- Localized skin lesion or eye lesion (keratitis). Outbreak of keratitis has been associated with a certain contact lens solution. Thought to be due to improper storage of solution at manufacturing plant.

TREATMENT

Immunocompromised Patients

- Recovery from neutropenia imperative (many authors recommend G-CSF, whereas WBC transfusions are controversial).
- Voriconazole, amphotericin B, or amphotericin B lipid products are commercially available choices.
- Voriconazole: 6 mg/kg IV q12 day 1, then either 4 mg/kg IV twice daily or 200–300 mg PO twice daily. Use IV until pt is stable.
- Alt: lipid formulation amphotericin B (Abelcet, Ambisome or Amphotec) 5 mg/kg IV every day.
- Alt: amphotericin B 1.0–1.5 mg/kg IV every day.
- Fusarium intrinsically resistant to many antifungals (including itraconazole, 5-flucytosine, fluconazole, echinocandins such as caspofungin, and in some isolates—amphotericin B).
- New antifungals (not FDA approved for this indication): posaconazole effective *in vitro*; salvage therapy effective in 48% of hematologic malignancy pts (10/21) who received 400 mg PO twice daily for refractory disease.
- New antifungals (not FDA approved): ravuconazole not effective *in vitro*. Experimental advanced generation isavuconazole has variable activity against *Fusarium* spp.
- Treatment duration: prolonged, no firm recommendations but most would continue therapy 6 mos after recovery of neutropenia.
- Surgical debridement of large single lesions and removal of infected catheters recommended.

Immunocompetent Patients: Skin Lesion

- Surgical debridement.
- Topical antifungals (natamycin) can be used.
- Voriconazole 200 mg PO twice daily for 6 mos after lesion is resolved.

Ocular involvement

- Ocular involvement can involve cornea, retina and vitreous humor.
- **Immunocompromised:** secondary infection due to dissemination.
- Intra-ocular antifungals and vitrectomy usually ineffective.
- Voriconazole and posaconazole may be active in the eye.
- **Immunocompetent:** keratitis occurs after trauma or corneal surgery (LASIK), contact lens wearer.
- Topical: natamycin drops, referral to ophthalmology for keratoplasty and close follow-up.

- Alt: topical 2% voriconazole 7 times/day used in 2 case reports of keratomycosis treatment.
- Systemic: reports of successful treatment with voriconazole and posaconazole.
- Combination topical and systemic therapy reported w/ excellent success. Systemic therapy duration short (14 days) in immunocompetent.
- Corneal transplant may be required in severe cases of keratitis.

TREATMENT REGIMEN DETAILS
- Posaconazole has best *in vitro* activity against Fusarium. Author prefers voriconazole to amphotericin B/lipid amphotericin B. *In vitro*, sensitivities have been variable for voriconazole and posaconazole.

OTHER INFORMATION
- Immunocompromised pts: consider fusarium if fever refractory to antibacterial agents, paronychia, positive blood cultures for "mold", skin lesions with necrotic centers.
- Immunocompromised pts: neutrophil recovery is critical to survival.
- Keratitis: think fusarium when traditional topical agents fail; prompt referral to ophthalmology essential.
- Consider posaconazole in refractory cases (not FDA approved for this indication but evidence suggests efficacy).

BASIS FOR RECOMMENDATIONS
Author opinion.

Comments: No guidelines statements exist for treatment of this infection.

HISTOPLASMA CAPSULATUM

John G. Bartlett, MD

MICROBIOLOGY
- Dimorphic fungus, yeast at 37°C.
- Endemic in Ohio and Mississippi River valleys, also Central America, Asia, and Africa.
- Present in soil, associated with birds and bats.

CLINICAL
- Infection by inhalation of mycelia.
- Disease may be acute or reactivation of latent focus.
- Spectrum of acute infection ranges from asymptomatic to fulminant. Pulmonary most common, but extrapulmonary infection occurs, especially in hosts with defective cell mediated immunity.
- Common exposures: work on surface soil, chicken coops, areas with bird droppings, cave exposure, demolition of old buildings.
- No human-to-human transmission documented.
- Hx: exposure, then fever + pulm sx. CXR either clears or chronic pulmonary disease develops or dissemination. Severity of acute disease depends upon exposure inoculum and immune response.
- Dx: positive culture (diagnostic), antigen (urine (preferred) or blood), serology by complement fixation assay >1:8 or 4× rise. Tissue stains, e.g., PAS, GM, Giemsa (see Wheat 2007 reference for more details).
- Antigen assay (urine or blood): specificity >95%, sensitivity depends upon disease burden. Source MiraVista Lab (T: 866-647-2847 or http://www.miravistalabs.com/). Sensitivity in AIDS pts with disseminated infection—urine 95%, serum 85%.

SITES OF INFECTION
- Pulmonary (acute): pneumonia
- Pulmonary (chronic): reticulonodular, cavitary; may resemble tuberculosis
- Disseminated: predilection for bone marrow (cytopenias), liver, spleen, GI involvement
- CNS: meningitis, abscesses
- Mediastinitis: granulomatous form
- Mediastinitis: fibrosing (low organism burden, actual organisms rarely identified or cultured)
- Pericarditis
- Ocular

PATHOGENS

TREATMENT
Pulmonary
- **Acute and severe:** liposomal amphotericin B 3 mg/kg × 2 wks or until clinically improved, then itraconazole 200 mg three times a day × 3 days then 200 mg daily × 12 wks.
- Alternative: ampho B 0.7 mg/kg/day IV if pts are low risk for nephrotoxicity.
- Less severe: itraconazole 200 mg/day.
- **Mild-moderate infection:** treatment usually unnecessary as infection self-limiting. May use itraconazole 200 mg PO three times daily × 3 days then 200 mg PO twice daily if symptoms do not resolve within one mo.
- **Chronic cavitary:** itraconazole 200 mg PO three times a day × 3 days then 200 mg PO twice daily ≥1 yr.
- **Pulmonary nodule:** no treatment.

Extrapulmonary/Mediastinal
- Pericarditis and rheumatologic syndromes: (1) NSAIDs or (2) prednisone 0.5–1 mg/kg/day with taper over 1–2 wks plus itraconazole 200 mg PO three times a day × 3 days, then 200 mg PO twice a day × 6–12 wks.
- Mediastinal lymphadenitis: (1) no rx usually needed or (2) itraconazole (above doses) × 6–12 wks ± prednisone 0.5 mg/kg/day with taper over 1–2 wks with severe cases.
- Mediastinal granulomata: (1) no Rx usually, (2) itraconazole (above doses) × 6–12 wks if especially symptomatic.
- Mediastinal fibrosis: (1) no treatment usually needed or apparently effective, (2) intravascular stent for sclerosing causing pulmonary vessel obstruction or (3) itraconazole (above doses) if unable to distinguish fibrosis and granuloma.
- CNS: liposomal amphotericin B 5 mg/kg/day IV to total dose 175 mg/kg in 4–6 wks, then itraconazole 200 mg twice daily or three times a day PO for ≥1 yr.
- Disseminated: (1) severe: liposomal amphotericin B 3 mg/kg q24h × 1–2 wks then itraconazole 200 mg PO three times a day × 3 days then 200 mg PO twice daily ≥1 yr or alternative lipid amphotericin (5mg/kg) if necessary; (2) moderate: itraconazole above doses × ≥1 yr possibly life long if immunosuppression cannot be reversed.

FOLLOW UP
- Itraconazole levels (2 hr peak, >1.0 μg/mL) should be obtained if using drug >2 wks to ensure adequate drug exposure.

OTHER INFORMATION
- Histoplasma antigen (urine): good test for disseminated disease (blood Ag test less specific). Titer indicates antigen burden, and should show response to treatment and relapse. Pts with disseminated disease—measure at baseline, 2 wks, 1 mo and q3mo for 6 mo after treatment stopped. Decline in antigen should be seen within 2–12 wks after initiation of therapy.
- Itraconazole—best azole. Concerns: absorption, drug interactions and toxicity (hepatitis, CHF). Metabolite is hydroxy-itraconazole is also active. Measure levels, expect >1.0 μg/mL.
- Voriconazole and posaconazole are active vs >99% isolates *in vitro*.

BASIS FOR RECOMMENDATIONS
Wheat LJ, Freifeld AG, Kleiman MB, et al. Clinical practice guidelines for the management of pts with histoplasmosis: 2007 update by the Infectious Diseases Society of America. *Clin Infect Dis*, 2007; Vol. 45; pp. 807–25.
Comments: Clinical Practice Guidelines for the management of pts with histoplasmosis.

Antifungal drugs. *Treat Guidel Med Lett*, 2005; Vol. 3; pp. 7–14.
Comments: Another source used for developing guidelines presented in this module.

Benson CA, Kaplan JE, Masur H, et al. Treating opportunistic infections among HIV-infected adults and adolescents: recommendations from CDC, the National Institutes of Health, and the HIV Medicine Association/Infectious Diseases Society of America. *MMWR Recomm Rep*, 2004; Vol. 53; pp. 1–112.
Comments: Specifically for HIV infected pts with *H. capsulatum*.

PSEUDALLESCHERIA BOYDII

Aimee Zaas, MD

MICROBIOLOGY

- Thin-walled, septate, branching hyphae; 2.5–5 microns.
- Ubiquitous; typically found in soil, sewage, brackish/polluted water.
- *P. boydii* is the sexual form of *Scedosporium apiospermum.*

CLINICAL

- Emerging infection in immunocompromised hosts.
- Immunocompromised pts at risk: hematologic malignancy/BMT, solid organ transplants > AIDS pts
- Angioinvasive tendencies.
- Presentation/appearance similar to Aspergillus and Fusarium.
- Immunocompromised: mortality 77% (100% if disseminated).
- Important to diagnose *securely since P. boydii* is likely ampho B resistant.
- Best stained with Gomori methenamine silver; obtain fungal cx and histopath on all biopsies.

SITES OF INFECTION

- **Immunocompetent:** mycetoma at site of trauma/surgery, sinusitis, fungus ball.
- Classic: brain abscess or pneumonia after near-drowning.
- Endocarditis, endophthalmitis, osteomyelitis, septic arthritis (case reports).
- Sinusitis in immunocompetent is more likely allergic/hypersensitivity-related than infectious; analogous to ABPA.
- **Immunocompromised:** pneumonia or fungus ball, disseminated, brain abscess, skin lesions.
- Portal of entry: inhaled or via skin trauma.
- Skin lesions may be pustular, nodular, or necrotic.
- Isolation from bronchoalveolar lavage specimen in lung transplant recipients should prompt thorough investigation.

TREATMENT

Immunocompetent

- Non-pulmonary mycetoma: debridement combined with antifungals (see below).
- Pulmonary fungus ball: no standardized regimen; surgical resection alone is reasonable if symptomatic (hemoptysis).
- Brain abscess: surgical drainage plus voriconazole (see below) for 6–12 mos.
- Sinusitis: usually allergic not infectious; corticosteroids, decongestants are mainstay.
- No data to support antifungal use *for P. boydii* allergic fungal sinusitis.
- Voriconazole dose (IV = PO bioavailability): 6 mg/kg IV q12 on day 1 then 4 mg/kg IV twice daily or 200–300 mg PO twice daily.
- May increase voriconazole dose to 300 mg PO twice daily if needed for slow/insufficient clinical response.

Immunocompromised

- General note: 85% of isolates resistant to amphotericin B.
- Combined medical and surgical approach for localized lesions.
- Fungus ball/abscess (pulmonary or CNS): surgical resection plus voriconazole.
- Voriconazole: FDA-approved for refractory/ampho-intolerant pts; experts feel this is drug of choice.
- Voriconazole dose (IV = PO bioavailability): 6 mg/kg IV q12 on day 1 then 4 mg/kg IV twice daily or 200–300 mg PO twice daily.
- May increase voriconazole dose to 300 mg PO twice daily if clinical response judged slow/insufficient. No information regarding voriconazole serum levels and clinical efficacy against *P. boydii.*
- Posaconazole: has *in vitro* activity; case reports of successful treatment; not FDA-approved for this indication.
- Traditional azoles: antifungal activity against *P. boydii*—miconazole, ketoconazole, itraconazole.

PATHOGENS

- Duration: recommend prolonged therapy with any azole: 6–12 mos guided by clinical resolution (e.g., obtaining serial imaging of affected areas).
- Sinusitis: infectious if not allergic; combined surgical debridement and voriconazole for 6–12 mos.

OTHER INFORMATION
- Fungal culture is imperative as histopathology is indistinguishable from aspergillus.
- *In vitro*, caspofungin shows activity against *P. boydii.*

BASIS FOR RECOMMENDATIONS
Author opinion.
Comments: No guideline recommendations exist for the treatment of this pathogen.

SPOROTHRIX SCHENCKII

John G. Bartlett, MD

MICROBIOLOGY
- Thermally dimorphic fungus, world-wide distribution.
- Growth at 37°C yields cigar-shaped 1–3 × 3–10 μm yeast, while growth at 25°C produces septate hyphae and conidia.

CLINICAL
- Endemic fungus seen globally. Present in soil and on plants, most famously in rose thorns, sphagnum moss and recently from cats.
- Most cases are lymphocutaneous with inoculation injury leading to slow spread by lymphatic system producing nodules (sporotrichoid). Fungus likes cold which explains its distribution.
- Most cases are occupational or vocational, e.g., farming, gardening. Cases also attributed to zoonotic spread (infected cats, armadillos). First signs usually take 1–12 wks from inoculation. Infection usually remains localized in the immunocompetent.
- Dx: definitively by culture fungus, may need multiple biopsies. Positive culture = diagnosis. Yeast forms may be seen in tissue.
- Differential (cutaneous): *M. marinum* (marine exposure), *Nocardia brasiliensis,* pyoderma, foreign body reaction, blastomycosis, Leishmania and Tularemia.

SITES OF INFECTION
- Lymphocutaneous (most common): skin inoculation (soil) → skin nodule (extremity) → regional nodes that develop over mos–yrs.
- Cutaneous: inflammatory nodules spreading proximally in lymphatic distribution from initial skin infection.
- Pulmonary: pneumonia or chronic cavitary. Among others, described in alcoholics.
- Musculoskeletal: osteoarticular infections, granulomatous tenosynovitis.
- Meningitis.
- Sinusitis.
- Disseminated (rare, mostly immunocompromised, AIDS).

TREATMENT
Lymphocutaneous/cutaneous–Adult
- Indications to treat: nearly all pts.
- Preferred: itraconazole 200 mg PO once daily. Duration: use daily until 2–4 wks after all lesions have resolved.
- If using itraconazole, monitor levels (1–2 hrs post oral dose) to assure absorption, expect >1 mcg/ml.
- For unresponsive lesions: use higher dosage of itraconazole 200 mg PO twice daily.
- Alternatives: terbinafine 500 mg orally twice daily or saturated solution of potassium iodide (SSKI), initiated at a dosage of 5 drops (using a standard eye-dropper) 3 times daily and increasing, as tolerated, to 40–50 drops 3 times.
- Alt: fluconazole 400–800 mg PO daily only if the pt cannot tolerate itraconazole, terbinafine or SSKI.
- Adjunctive therapy: local hyperthermia with pocket warmer, infrared or far-infrared heater. Heat to 42°C daily × 2–3 mos. Especially useful for pregnant or nursing pts who cannot use drug regimen.

Extracutaneous Infections—Adult

- Pulmonary (severe, life-threatening: lipid formulation amB 3–5 mg/kg IV daily, or amB deoxycholate 0.7–1.0 mg/kg IV daily for initial therapy. After improvement, switch to itraconazole 200 mg PO twice daily to complete a minimum of 12 mos of therapy.
- Pulmonary (less severe): itraconazole 200 mg PO twice daily × 12 mos.
- Osteoarticular (preferred): itraconazole 200 mg PO twice daily for 12 mos, at a minimum.
- Osteoarticular (alternative): lipid formulation amB 3–5 mg/kg IV daily, or amB deoxycholate 0.7–1.0 mg/kg IV daily for initial therapy. After improvement, switch to itraconazole 200 mg orally twice daily to complete a minimum of 12 mos of therapy.
- Meningitis (preferred): lipid formulation amB 5 mg/kg IV daily × 4–6 wks as initial therapy, then switch to itraconazole 200 mg PO twice daily to complete 12 mos. For AIDS pts or others with continued immunosuppression after first 12 mos of treatment, itraconazole 200 mg PO daily recommended to prevent relapse.
- Meningitis (alt): amB 0.7–1.0 mg/kg IV daily × 4–6 wks then switch to itraconazole 200 mg PO twice daily to complete 12 mos.
- Disseminated (preferred): use regimen as described above for meningitis.
- If using itraconazole, monitor levels after 2 wks of use (take level 1–2 hrs post oral dosing) to assure absorption, expect >1 mcg/ml.

Pregnancy

- Use lipid formulation amB 3–5 mg/kg IV daily, or amB deoxycholate 0.7–1 mg/kg IV daily for severe sporotrichosis that must be treated.
- Azoles should be avoided.
- Hyperthermia can be used for localized lymphocutaneous dz.

Children

- Cutaneous, lymphocutaneous: itraconazole 6–10 mg/kg, 400 mg max PO orally daily. Alt: SSKI, start at 5–10 drops (using a standard eye-dropper) 3 times daily, increasing, as tolerated, up to a maximum of 1 drop per kg of body weight or 40–50 drops 3 times daily, whichever is lowest.
- Disseminated sporotrichosis: amB 0.7 mg/kg IV daily initially then itraconazole PO (6–10 mg/kg, up to a maximum of 400 mg daily) as step-down therapy.

MORE TREATMENT

- Heat: works because organism is temperature sensitive. Warm cutaneous lesions to 42–43° degrees C with topical treatments. This is usually an adjunctive treatment to SSKI or itraconazole.
- New azoles (voriconazole, posaconazole) active *in vitro*; less published clinical experience.

FOLLOW UP

Prognosis

- Lymphocutaneous: benign and responds to treatment.
- Extracutaneous: morbid and hard to treat.

BASIS FOR RECOMMENDATIONS

Kauffman CA, Bustamante B, Chapman SW, et al. Clinical practice guidelines for the management of sporotrichosis: 2007 update by the Infectious Diseases Society of America. *Clin Infect Dis*, 2007; Vol. 45; pp. 1255–65.

Comments: This document is the basis for recommendations here: Sporotrichosis rarely spontaneously resolves—need to treat nearly all pts. lymphocutaneous—easy to treat. Disseminated, pulmonary, osteoarticular, meningeal are hard to treat. Best azole—itraconazole.

ZYGOMYCETES

Aimee Zaas, MD

MICROBIOLOGY

- Wide (6–16 μm), aseptate, ribbon-like, nonpigmented fungi with wide angle branching.
- Classically called "mucormycosis."
- *Mucor, Rhizopus, Rhizomucor, Absidia, Cunninghamella, Saksanea* species all belong to the class "Zygomycetes."
- Mucor causes <10% of all infections (Rhizopus causes 90%).

CLINICAL

- Syndromes: rhinocerebral, pulmonary, disseminated, GI, cutaneous, allergic.
- Risk factors: ketoacidosis, neutropenia, iron overload, iron chelation drug use, IDU, immunosuppression (e.g., prednisone).
- Emerging risk factor for zygomycosis is long term therapy with voriconazole either as prophylaxis for or treatment of invasive fungal infections in hematopoeitic stem cell transplantation or pts with hematologic malignancies.
- Acquisition: mainly inhalation; also skin trauma and ingestion.
- Defenses: macrophages (kill spores); neutrophils (kill germinating hyphae).
- Mortality: (range 11–100%); nearly 100% for disseminated disease or in those for whom immunosuppression cannot be corrected.
- Send tissue for histopathology (silver stain) and culture; blood cultures are unhelpful (never positive).
- Mincing of tissue during specimen preparation can disrupt fungal structure, impairing diagnosis. Inform microbiology laboratory that zygomycosis is a concern so that tissue can be processed appropriately.
- Prophylaxis options in haematopoietic stem cell transplantation and treatment of high-risk hematologic malignancies (AML, MDS) with posaconazole achieves coverage for zygomycetes.

SITES OF INFECTION

- Rhinocerebral: invasive sinusitis; classic palate eschar, proceeds to involve skull base + cranial nerve palsies.
- Rhinocerebral: MRI with gadolinium of head/skull base to define extent of disease is crucial.
- Pulmonary: localized infiltrate; angioinvasion leads to infarct/cavitation with hemoptysis (may mimic PE).
- Disseminated: multi-organ failure, tissue infarctions due to angioinvasion.
- Cutaneous: at sites of trauma; can have nailbed infections; ranges from erythema to pustules to necrotizing fasciitis.
- Gastric (rare): necrotic gastric ulcers in immunocompromised pts consuming fermented food.
- Allergic: hypersensitivity pneumonitis without invasion; exposure in malt workers, farmers.
- External otitis: noninvasive superficial crusting otitis.
- GI basidiobolomycosis: emerging infection in Arizona; abdominal pain, leukocytosis, inflammatory mass on imaging.

TREATMENT

Rhinocerebral

- Aggressive surgical debridement; consult otorhinolaryngologist promptly.
- Lipid preparation amphotericin B 5 mg/kg IV q24h for prolonged (>6 wks) period.
- Posaconazole (200 mg PO q6h or 400 mg PO q12) reported effective in open label salvage therapy studies.
- Fluconazole and voriconazole not effective.
- Echinocandins (e.g., caspofungin) not effective.
- Hyperbaric oxygen helpful in case reports.
- Correct underlying predisposition (acidosis, neutropenia, steroids).
- Combination therapy with caspofungin and polyene (ABLC) showed improved outcomes over historical cohort treated with polyene monotherapy.

Pulmonary

- Surgical resection of uni-lobar disease recommended.
- Surgical resection can be helpful if massive hemoptysis present.
- Lipid preparation amphotericin B 5 mg/kg IV q24h for prolonged period.
- Correct underlying predisposition (acidosis, neutropenia, steroids) and stop iron chelating meds.
- Posaconazole reported effective in salvage therapy studies.

Cutaneous

- Surgical resection to bleeding, uninvolved margin necessary.
- Lipid amphotericin B 5 mg/kg IV q24.
- If infection is superficial in immunocompetent pt, can try topical natamycin (5% opthalmic suspension) or ketoconazole.

Gastrointestinal

- Basidiobolomycosis: treat with resection and itraconazole liquid 200 mg PO twice daily for >3 mos.
- Surgical resection of involved areas imperative.
- Lipid preparation of amphotericin B 5 mg/kg IV q24h.
- Correct underlying predisposition.
- When using itraconazole, should document absorption and monitor itraconazole levels.

OTHER INFORMATION

- Interesting emerging data regarding specific risk of developing zygomycosis when using desferoxamine as an iron chelator.
- Interesting emerging data regarding use of non-desferoxamine chelators as adjunctive therapy for zygomycosis.

BASIS FOR RECOMMENDATIONS

Rogers TR. Treatment of zygomycota: current and new options. *J Antimicrobial Chemotherapy,* 2008; Suppl 1; pp. 135–40.
Comment: No guidelines exist, but this review is a reasonable commentary on treatment options.

PATHOGENS

Other

LICE

Noreen A. Hynes, MD, MPH

Microbiology

- Lice are ectoparasites that cause an infestation rather than infection. They live off of their human hosts by feeding on blood after piercing the skin and injecting saliva, which causes pruritus. They can survive away from the human host for up to 10 days, after which time they die of starvation.
- 3 species infests humans: *Phthirus pubis* (crab louse), *Pediculus humanus* (body louse), *Pediculus humanus capitis* (head louse).
- Life cycle: female lives 1–3 mos; lays up to 300 eggs (nits); nits hatch in 6–10 days; give rise to nymphs; become adults in 10 days.

Clinical

- Transmission: by direct contact and fomite. Pruritis common in all infested locations. Secondary bacterial infection of excoriated areas can occur. The body louse can transmit infections.
- Lice serve as a marker for the presence of other possible infections. Pubic lice: suspect other STDs. Body lice seen among displaced and homeless persons and can serve a vectors of infectious diseases. Head lice are seen in children of all socioeconomic groups. Dual infestation with scabies is not uncommon.
- **Pubic lice:** #1 louse infestation in U.S. adult; maculae ceruleae (blue spots) seen on trunk, thighs, upper parts of arms. Pubic lice can also infest head, eyelashes (nits or crusts), axillae; transmission is **not** prevented by condom use.
- **Body lice:** only louse type that can transmit infections including epidemic typhus (often found in refugee camps), trench fever (may be found among urban homeless), and epidemic relapsing fever (in the Western U.S.) caused by *Rickettsia prowazekii, Bartonella quintana,* and *Borrelia recurrentis,* respectively. Find body lice in seams of clothes rather than on skin.
- **Head lice:** most commonly seen in children, ages 3–12 yrs in U.S.
- Diagnosis: both adult lice and their eggs (nits) are easily visible with the naked eye.

Sites of Infection

- Head: an infestation of head hair. Nits seen more often than lice; scalp hair grows 0.4 mm/day, nits hatch within 9 days, most nits within 5 mm of the scalp surface.
- Body: infestation of clothing seams; can transmit infectious diseases with blood meal.
- Pubis: an infestation of pubic/axillary/head/eyelash hair. Pubic lice may seem to be scabs of a "scratch area" but if crust removed and placed on slide, it walks away before cover slip added. Pubic lice can also infest head, eyelashes (nits or crusts), axillae.

Treatment

Phthiriasis or Pediculosis pubis (pubic lice, crabs)

- **Recommended:** permethrin 1% cream rinse, apply to affected areas and washed off after 10 minutes.
- Pyrethrins (0.33%) with piperonyl butoxide (4%), apply lotion to affected DRY hair and skin. Wash off out in no longer than 10 minutes.
- **Alternatives:** malathion 0.5% lotion applied for 8–12 hrs and washed off. Use when treatment failure with recommended regimen is believed to be due to resistance. Odor makes this a less attractive treatment than others listed.
- Ivermectin 250 micrograms/kg PO and repeated in 2 wks.
- Lindane is no longer recommended as a recommended treatment and should only be used as a secondary alternative due to its toxicity (seizures and aplastic anemia). If used remove after 4–minute application to decrease absorption and toxicity.

Pediculosis corporis (body lice)

- Treat clothes, not person! Body lice found in seams of clothes rather than on skin.
- Machine wash clothes on hot cycle then iron seams.

Pediculosis capitis
- Benzyl alcohol lotion, 5%. For short hair (0–4 inches): apply up to one 8–ounce bottle to dry hair for 10 minutes, then rinse. Repeat in 7 days. For hair >16 inches: apply up to six 8–ounce bottles to dry hair for 10 minutes, then rinse. Repeat in 7 days.
- Permethrin 1% cream rinse applied topically once for 10 minutes, then washed off. Nit removal with 1:1 solution of water and vinegar applied to hair then run vinegar-dipped fine tooth comb through hair.
- Pyrethrins (0.33%) with piperonyl butoxide (4%): apply lotion to cover affected DRY hair and scalp. Shampoo out in no longer than 10 minutes.
- Malathion 0.5%: **use only if resistant to all other** RX! Apply to hair, let dry naturally. (**Do not use any electric products while hair drying—highly flammable**). Wash off after 8–12 hrs. Repeat 7–10 days.

Phthiriasis palpebarum (eyelash lice)
- Petroleum jelly applied to the lids twice daily × 10 days.
- Yellow oxide of mercury 1% applied four times a day × 14 days.

FOLLOW UP
- Pubic lice serve as a marker for other STDs—therefore test for them.
- Treat ALL contacts of persons with pubic lice.
- Secondary cutaneous bacterial infection, usually due to *S. aureus*, seen when extensive excoriations occur in setting of uncontrolled pruritis.

OTHER INFORMATION
- 2003 FDA public health advisory on lindane use; note increased risk of neurologic side effects in the elderly, persons weighing <50 kg, and children. Use other products when possible in these groups.
- Head lice in an adult, usually means child in home.
- Hydroxyzine 25–50 mg PO three times a day/four times a day may be needed to control itch in addition to lice-specific RX. Topical steroids may be needed as well.

BASIS FOR RECOMMENDATIONS
Centers for Disease Control and Prevention, Workowski KA, Berman SM. Sexually transmitted diseases treatment guidelines, 2006. *MMWR Recomm Rep*, 2006; Vol. 55; pp. 1–94.
Comments: The CDC treatment guidelines provide clinicians with a readily available reference for STD treatments recommended by a panel of national and international experts in STD diagnosis, treatment, prevention, and control. These guidelines available electronically from: http://www.cdc.gov/

Frankowski BL, Weiner LB. Committee on School Health the Committee on Infectious Diseases. American Academy of Pediatrics. Head lice. *Pediatrics*, 2002; Vol. 110; pp. 638–43.
Comments: This is a statement of the AAP attempting to clarify issues of diagnosis and treatment of head lice and makes recommendations for dealing with head lice in the school setting. Permethrin, 1% is the treatment of choice in this setting; combing to remove nits is not needed; exclusion from school due to "nits" is discouraged.

SARCOPTES SCABIEI VAR. HOMINIS (SCABIES)

Noreen A. Hynes, MD, MPH

MICROBIOLOGY
- *Sarcoptes scabiei*, a mite.
- Mites burrow into the skin and lay their eggs; new mites hatch and form new burrows.

CLINICAL
- Scabies is a hypersensitivity reaction to the mite feces in skin capillaries. Generalized itch may take up to 4–6 wks to develop after initial exposure.
- **Classic scabies:** intensely pruritic rash (including nocturnal) with excoriations; papules and silvery linear and serpiginous burrows that may contain the mites and their eggs (nearly pathognomonic) in characteristic distribution in the interdigital folds, the belt line, under breasts, on penis. May have a somewhat cryptic presentation in the elderly, often with only intense pruritis. Cyclical epidemics often in long-term care facilities. Occurs in 2% to 4% of pts with HIV infection; unusual presentations common in this group. Pruritis may persist for

1–2 wks after curative therapy. Clothes, bed linens decontaminated by machine washing at 60°C. Insecticidal spray or powder applied to items which cannot be washed.

- **Nodular scabies:** reddish to brown pigmented, intensely pruritic, firm, nodules approximately 0.5 cm or larger found exclusively on covered parts of the bodies, such as the scrotum, penis, buttocks, groin, axillary folds, and upper back. Nodules do not contain mites; thought to be a hypersensitivity reaction; seen in 7% of scabies cases. Often delayed diagnosis due to somewhat cryptic presentation.
- **Crusted scabies:** also known as Norwegian scabies; an aggressive form especially in immunodeficient, debilitated, or malnourished persons; if generalized, hospitalize and get ID consult. Highly contagious form especially for care providers. Hyperkeratotic plaques and crusts, far less pruritic (50% report no itching) than the typical inflammatory papules and burrows of classic scabies. May have a generalized distribution and the tracks of classic scabies are not seen. Clothes, bed linens decontaminated by machine washing at 60°C. Insecticidal spray or powder applied to items which cannot be washed. Predominant CD8+ T lymphocytes found in the dermis with few CD4+ cells seen and no B cells explain, in part, the failure of the skin immune system to mount a needed response. Elevated levels of IgE, IgG, IgG1, IgG3, and IgG4 also noted.
- Definitive dx by microscopic identification of the mite, eggs, or its feces. Scrape under fingernails or the end of a burrow.
- Relapse may be more common than previously thought. Urticaria can be seen even w/ small number of mites.
- Infestation of other household members is common.

SITES OF **I**NFECTION
- Sites seen in **Classical Scabies:** interdigital web spaces of hands
- Flexor surfaces of the wrists and elbows
- Axillae
- Male genitalia
- Female breasts and inframammary folds
- Belt line
- Buttocks
- Sites in **Crusted Scabies:** generalized dermatitis
- Face, scalp

TREATMENT
Recommended Regimens
- Permethrin cream (5%): apply to all areas of body from the neck down and washed off after 8–14 hrs.
- Ivermectin 200 micrograms/kg PO × 1; repeat again in 2 wks.

Alternative Regimens
- Lindane (1%): apply 1 oz. of lotion or 30 g of cream thinly to all areas of the body from the neck down. Thoroughly wash off after 8 hrs. Avoid use in the elderly and those <50 kg; contraindicated in children.

Crusted scabies in Immunodeficient Persons
- Manage in consultation with a specialist. Ivermectin 200 micrograms/kg once combined with Permethrin cream (5%) (**not** lindane). Repeat, if needed, after 2 wks.

Pregnant and lactating women
- Permethrin cream (5%): apply to all areas of body from the neck down and washed off after 8–14 hrs.
- Lindane and ivermectin are contraindicated.

FOLLOW **U**P
- Inform pts that the rash and pruritis may persist up to 2 wks after treatment.
- If sx persist >2 wks after treatment consider: a. treatment failure due to resistance to scabicide, b. treatment failure due to faulty application of scabicide, c. in crusted scabies there may have been poor penetration into thick, scaly skin with mite persistence,

    d. reinfestation by fomites in the home, e. persistence or worsening sx due to allergic dermatitis.

- If the decision is to retreat because the pt has not responded to a recommended regimen, retreat with an alternate regimen.

OTHER INFORMATION

- Common findings: papules, burrows, excoriations, nodules, vesicles, pyoderma, eczema. In nodular scabies the mildly pigmented, pruritic nodules may be present for mos before dx.
- Uncommon presentations: crusts, urticaria, vasculitis, attenuated or exaggerated lesions.
- Generalized crusted scabies requires hospitalization and ID consultation.
- Mites that have left the body will die within 72 hrs.

BASIS FOR RECOMMENDATIONS

Centers for Disease Control and Prevention, Workowski KA, Berman SM. Sexually transmitted diseases treatment guidelines, 2006. *MMWR Recomm Rep*, 2006; Vol. 55; pp. 1–94.

Comments: The CDC treatment guidelines provide clinicians with a readily available reference for STD treatments recommended by a panel of national and international experts in STD diagnosis, treatment, prevention, and control. These guidelines available electronically from: http://www.cdc.gov/

PATHOGENS

Parasites

ACANTHAMOEBA

Lisa A. Spacek, MD, PhD and Khalil G. Ghanem, MD, PhD

MICROBIOLOGY

- Acanthamoeba spp (>20 species) most prevalent protozoa; 1 of 4 genera associated with disease: *Acanthamoeba* spp, *Naegleria fowleri*, *Balamuthia mandrillaris* and *Sappinia diploidea*.
- 2 stage life cycle: (1) actively feeding and dividing trophozoite; (2) dormant cyst (double-walled wrinkled cyst) which are resistant to chlorine and antibiotics. Encystation occurs under stress.

CLINICAL

- Ubiquitous, isolated worldwide from soil, air, fresh and salt water. Serologic surveys detected antibodies in 50–100% of healthy people.
- Causes keratitis in immunocompetent pts and granulomatous amoebic encephalitis (GAE), disseminated acanthamebiasis, pneumonitis, sinusitis, osteomyelitis, leukocytoclastic vasculitis, and painful, ulcerated nodules in immunocompromised pts.
- **Diagnosis:** in GAE-wet mount of CSF (trophozoites look like macrophages); fixed specimens with H and E staining; can also grow in special growth medium or cell cultures. Calcofluor white fluorescently stains cysts and trophozoites in tissue section.
- Immunofluorescent staining with monoclonal antibodies very useful; transmission electron microscopy has also been used successfully. Real time PCR assays validated for diagnosis of keratitis.
- In GAE, space occupying or ring-enhancing lesions on CT and MRI.
- In GAE, if lumbar puncture is deemed safe (i.e., no increased ICP), the CSF has low glucose, high protein, and elevated WBCs with lymphocyte predominance.
- Keratitis: scrapes or biopsy of chronic corneal ulcers that have not responded to routine antibiotic therapy.

SITES OF INFECTION

- **Eye:** keratitis (AK) is painful, vision-threatening infection associated with amoeba-contaminated saline solution or lens case (contact lens users); consider when chronic corneal ulcers are unresponsive to routine abx; corneal scrapes or bx needed for dx; may also culture contact lenses and saline solution. **Will lead to visual loss if rx delayed**.
- **CNS:** GAE-chronic CNS infection associated w/ confusion, stiff neck, HA, irritability over wks to mos; can be associated with pulmonary symptoms. Portal of entry is either lungs or skin.
- GAE can present as multifocal lesions in midbrain, brain stem, and cerebellum; rarely abscess-like; cyst-like lesions can occur.
- GAE occurs in immunocompromised hosts: ETOH, steroids, chemotherapy, organ transplantation, AIDS; rarely in immunocompetent host.
- **Skin:** most common in pts with AIDS; reported in transplant recipients; painful ulcerated nodules on trunk or extremities; 73% mortality rate. Leukocytoclastic vasculitis reported.
- **Bone:** osteomyelitis reported; usually from cutaneous focus.
- **Disseminated** acanthamebiasis involving skin, bone, lungs, and CNS reported in immunocompromised pts.

TREATMENT

CNS, skin, lung, and disseminated disease

- Combination therapy for skin, CNS and disseminated disease is the rule. Diamidine derivatives (propamidine, pentamidine, dibromopropamidine) have greatest activity. Other active drugs: ketoconazole, fluconazole, sulfadiazine, TMP-SMX, 5-flucytosine, rifampin.
- Test for drug sensitivity. All non-ocular treatment regimens are based on case reports; no prospective studies available.
- Drugs must be cysticidal to prevent recurrence from dormant cysts.
- TMP-SMX + ketoconazole + rifampin used in 2 pediatric pts with CNS disease (Singhal, 2001).

- IV pentamidine + topical chlorhexidine + topical ketoconazole successful for cutaneous disease without CNS involvement.
- Fluconazole + sulfadiazine + surgery in AIDS pt with localized CNS involvement.
- Mortality rate is very high because dx is delayed. Combination Rx often results in serious toxicities.
- There is no formal recommendation that can be made. In most instances, any previously described successful combination regimen should be started and surgical intervention considered.

Keratitis

- Earliest sign, dendriform pattern on corneal epithelium.
- Aggressive surgical and medical management include debridement and high concentration of topical drugs.
- Test for drug sensitivity to guide therapy; do not wait for results; initiate therapy, then modify based on results.
- Early infection: 0.1% propamidine isethionate topically + 0.15% dibromopropamidine given for prolonged periods (6 mos–1 yr). Chlorhexidine and propamidine topically successful in a series of 12 pts.
- Successful regimen for AK: polyhexamethylene biguanide 0.02% +/– chlorhexidine 0.02% +/– propamidine isethionate and dipropamidine (Brolene) 0.1% +/– hemamidine 0.1% (Perez-Santonja, 2003).
- Penetrating keratoplasty has been used in combination with chemotherapy, especially in more advanced disease.
- Reserve topical steroids for severe pain or inflammation.

OTHER INFORMATION

- The diagnosis can be very difficult because of the resemblance of trophozoites to macrophages/histiocytes in tissue specimens. A high level of suspicion is necessary.
- There are no prospective controlled trials for therapeutic options: combination therapy is the rule; tailor to individual pts based on toxicity profile.
- Mortality for non-ocular disease is >70% in most cases despite aggressive combination Rx.
- AK occurs in pts who use contact lenses. Immediate ophthalmology consultation warranted.

BASIS FOR RECOMMENDATIONS

Hammersmith KM. Diagnosis and management of Acanthamoeba keratitis. *Curr Opin Ophthalmol*, 2006; Vol. 17; pp. 327–31.

Comments: Comprehensive up to date review of the management of *Acanthamoeba keratitis.*

Pérez-Santonja JJ, Kilvington S, Hughes R, et al. Persistently culture positive acanthamoeba keratitis: in vivo resistance and in vitro sensitivity. *Ophthalmology*, 2003; Vol. 110; pp. 1593–600.

Comments: Retrospective study of 11 pts, 87% were diagnosed after 1 mo of symptoms. Nearly 5% developed recurrent episodes of corneal and scleral inflammation with viable Acanthamoeba in the cornea despite prolonged treatment with biguanides and/or diamidines. There was no correlation between *in vitro* drug sensitivities and the *in vivo* response for biguanides.

BABESIA SPECIES

John G. Bartlett, MD

MICROBIOLOGY

- Transmitted by Ixodes (hard bodied) ticks, mostly from May to September.
- Malaria-like protozoan infection, infects erythrocytes. Common, global zoonosis (domestic and wild animals) may rarely infect humans.
- Greater than 70 species worldwide, most human infections due to the rodent strain *B. microti* in U.S. while *B. divergens* and *B. bovis* cattle strains cause human illness in Europe and elsewhere.
- Strain WA-1 described in California and Washington state. Strain MO-1 described in Missouri. The importance is that standard babesia serology will not detect these infections.

CLINICAL

- Tick-borne, protozoal cause of potentially lethal, undifferentiated febrile syndrome, especially in splenectomized pts.
- Usually transmitted in focal costal areas of northeast U.S. from NJ to MA, also in the upper Midwest and Washington State.

- May also be seen in co-infection along with Lyme disease (*Borrelia burgdorferi*) and the agent of human granulocytic anaplasmosis (*A. phagocytophilum*) as all three are transmitted by the *Ixodes scapularis* (deer) tick.
- In non-immunocompromised people, illness typically asymptomatic or mild, but parasitemia can be prolonged as detected by molecular tests.
- Symptoms: flu-like, febrile illness typical. Severe complications include CHF, renal failure, ARDS. Laboratory findings may include anemia (with hemolytic features), thrombocytopenia.
- Severe illness seen more in older ages, immunosuppressed or splenectomy pts.
- Severe illness: parasitemia >10%, severe hemolysis or renal, hepatic, or pulmonary compromise.
- Diagnosis: obtain thick/thin blood smears with Giemsa or Wright-Giemsa stains. May be confused with Plasmodium ring forms, but Babesia do not have brownish pigment in cells and morphology of Plasmodium gametocytes differs from Babesia.
- Characteristic babesial Maltese cross/tetrads are rare. Diagnosis: indirect fluorescence antibody test available (IFA IgM >1:64 diagnostic), serology, PCR (not widely available, but may be most sensitive test).
- *B. microti* serology will not detect WA-1 strain or MO-1 strain, so need to order those specific Babesia serologies if suspicious.

SITES OF INFECTION
- Red blood cells

TREATMENT
Combination antimicrobial regimens

- Preferred: atovaquone 750 mg twice daily PO × 7 days, plus azithromycin 500 mg–1 g IV/PO × 1 dose, then 250 mg PO daily × 7 days.
- Alt: clindamycin 600 mg PO three times daily or 300–600 mg IV q6h × 7 days plus quinine 650 mg PO three times daily × 7 days.
- Clindamycin regimen is tolerated better if it can be administered with quinine (or IV quinidine).
- Critical illness: clindamycin regimen preferred. Give IV and consider exchange blood transfusion to decrease parasitemia.
- Response to therapy: mild-moderate disease should begin improvement within 48 hrs, resolve in 3 mos.
- Severe disease: monitor hematocrit and percent parasitized cells daily until <5%.
- Longer courses than 7 days may be required with persistent symptoms and persistent parasitemia.
- For persistent/recurrent parasitemia: treat with one of the above regiments for >6 wks and >2 wks after the parasitemia has resolved.

OTHER INFORMATION
- LFT abnormalities and leukopenia (including atypical lymphocytes) may also be commonly seen.
- Evidence of Howell-Jolly bodies on blood smear may indicate absence of spleen (and therefore be a risk factor for severe infection).
- Differential diagnosis: malaria, HGA, HME, Lyme disease (mild infection), Rocky Mountain Spotted Fever, Typhoid fever, thrombotic thrombocytopenic purpura (TTP).

BASIS FOR RECOMMENDATIONS

Krause PJ, Gewurz BE, Hill D, et al. Persistent and relapsing babesiosis in immunocompromised pts. *Clin Infect Dis*, 2008; Vol. 46; pp. 370–6.
Comments: Comparison of 14 case pts also had substantial morbidity with persistent *Babesia microti* infection despite treatment were compared to 46 controls who had this parasitic infection and responded to treatment. The case pts were all immunosuppressed, most had B cell lymphomas and were asplenic or received rituximab. Case pts had persistence with 2–10 courses of treatment and 3 died. The recommendation is to treat these pts for ≥6 wks and ≥2 wks after the parasitemia has resolved.

Wormser GP, Dattwyler RJ, Shapiro ED, et al. The clinical assessment, treatment, and prevention of lyme disease, human granulocytic anaplasmosis, and babesiosis: clinical practice guidelines by the Infectious Diseases Society of America. *Clin Infect Dis*, 2006; Vol. 43; pp. 1089–134.
Comments: IDSA Guidelines—source document for recommendations given here.

CRYPTOSPORIDIA

John G. Bartlett, MD

MICROBIOLOGY

- *Cryptosporidium parvum.*
- *C. hominis.*
- *C. meleagridis.*
- Time from acquisition to symptoms ranges 2–10 days, average 7 days.
- Sporulated oocysts (with four sporozoites) are spread through fecal material from infected host. Mostly acquired through drinking contaminated water with infective oocysts.

CLINICAL

- Epidemiology: major cause of epidemic diarrhea from contaminated water, severe diarrhea in AIDS pts with low CD4 cell counts and sporadic diarrhea in immunocompetent pts. The cause is ingestion of oocysts after person-person contact or contaminated food or water. Risks are children attending day care centers, child care workers, travelers or backpackers/hikers/ swimmers. May also be found in shallow, contaminated water wells.
- Symptoms: acute or subacute large volume secretory diarrhea, often with nausea, cramps, vomiting, weight loss. Fever found in one third.
- Course: self-limited in the immune competent, but often lasts 2–3 wks. In AIDS pts, it causes severe diarrhea lasting >2 mos in 60% of cases.
- Diagnosis: oocyst detection exam with AFB stain, IFA (most sensitive and specific) or EIA stains. Routine O and P does not detect. Request detection of Cryptosporidia specifically on O and P specimen. A single specimen is usually adequate, occasionally multiple specimens required.

SITES OF INFECTION

- Intestine, small intestine most commonly.
- Rarely extraluminal, e.g., pulmonary.

TREATMENT

Antimicrobials

- Immunocompetent pt: no clear benefit with trials testing >28 antimicrobials including macrolides, paromomycin, etc.
- Nitazoxanide 500 mg PO three times a day × 3 days shown effective for immune competent treatment (and FDA approved).
- Advanced HIV (only proven treatment): HAART with immune reconstitution. Even minor increases in CD4 count often work.
- AIDS (possibly effective): nitazoxanide or 0.5–1.0 g PO twice daily with food × 14 days.

Antiperistaltic agents

- Loperamide 4 mg PO, then 2 mg PO with each loose stool up to 16 mg/day max.
- Lomotil 2.5 mg PO four times a day.
- Codeine 15–60 mg (usually 30 mg) PO q3–6h prn.
- Deodorized tincture of opium (DTO) 0.3–1 ml (usually 0.6 ml) PO 3–4 ×/day prn.

Non-specific treatment

- Diet: frequent, small feedings, low-fat, lactose-and caffeine-free, high fiber, bland foods.
- Fluid support, losses may be up to 10 L/day with AIDS.
- Oral feedings to replace $NaHCO_3$, K^+, Mg^{++}, PO_4^-, glucose.
- Non-specific agents: NSAIDs, bismuth subsalicylate (PeptoBismol).
- Food supplements for AIDS pts: Vivonex, TEN, etc.
- Octreotide: not effective.

Prevention

- Avoid contaminated water/food.
- Maintain good hand hygiene.
- Boil water × 3 minutes or filter (www.nsf.org or 800-673-6275) or use bottled water. Remember that ice may also be a source.
- Safe: nationally distributed bottled water, canned carbonated soft drinks, frozen fruit concentrates, and pasteurized drinks.
- Avoid exposure to fecal material during sexual activity.

PATHOGENS

OTHER INFORMATION
- Healthy host may have self-limited disease lasting 2–3 wk; compromised hosts (CD4 <100) may have very severe and debilitating chronic diarrhea.
- Supportive care: rehydration and antiperistaltics.

BASIS FOR RECOMMENDATIONS

Benson C, Holmes K, Masur H. Guidelines for Prevention and Treatment of Opportunistic Infections in HIV-Infected Adults and Adolescents (http://AIDSinfo.nih.gov/), 2008.
Comments: Source document for recommendations given here. This is the June 2008 edition.

Benson CA, Kaplan JE, Masur H, et al. Treating opportunistic infections among HIV-infected adults and adolescents: recommendations from CDC, the National Institutes of Health, and the HIV Medicine Association/Infectious Diseases Society of America. *MMWR Recomm Rep*, 2004; Vol. 53; pp. 1–112.
Comments: **prevention of cryptosporidiosis**: (1) Avoid contact with human/animal stool; (2) Lakes, rivers, salt water beaches and swimming pools may be contaminated; avoid them or at least avoid drinking; (3) Municipal water supplies may be contaminated. During "boil water advisory" boil × 1 min, use submicron personal use water filter (1 µm filter) or use bottled water; (4) Avoid raw oysters; (5) For filters call 800-673-8010.

Rossignol JF, Ayoub A, Ayers MS. Treatment of diarrhea caused by Cryptosporidium parvum: a prospective randomized, double-blind, placebo-controlled study of Nitazoxanide. *J Infect Dis*, 2001; Vol. 184; pp. 103–6.
Comments: Nitazoxanide (500 mg twice daily × 3 days) vs placebo in 100 HIV-negative pts with cryptosporidiosis. **There was a superior response in the nitazoxanide group** (80% vs 51%).

CYCLOSPORA CAYETANENSIS

Joseph Vinetz, MD and Paul G. Auwaerter, MD

MICROBIOLOGY
- Single celled coccidian parasite, first reported causing human disease in 1979.
- 8–10 µm in diameter, can be responsible for water or food-borne outbreaks.

CLINICAL
- Protozoal cause of diarrhea, worldwide, more common in tropical settings.
- Cause of prolonged diarrhea in travelers, often remitting and relapsing for wks to mos, ultimately self-limited (7–9 wks typical).
- Associated with food-borne outbreaks in the U.S., e.g., raspberries from Guatemala.
- Associated with water-borne outbreaks in U.S., developing world (especially Nepal).
- Incubation period ~7 days, often with antecedent flu-like illness, then nausea, anorexia, abd cramps, watery diarrhea. Fatigue and malaise may be prominent.
- In AIDS, can range from asymptomatic to severe, ascending biliary tract infection (rare).
- Dx: direct exam of stool; 8–10 µM variably acid fast oocysts; iodine stain and autofluorescence under UV improves sensitivity.
- Note: may be missed on routine exam or mistaken for *Cryptosporidium*, MUST request specifically from lab to assist proper identification.

SITES OF INFECTION
- GI: small intestine (acute and chronic inflammation can persist after cure), biliary tract (rare), gall bladder (rare).
- Systemic: Reiter's syndrome (inflammation, inflammatory oligoarthritis, sterile urethritis) can develop in setting of prolonged diarrheal illness.

TREATMENT
Preferred treatment
- Sulfa-containing regimen preferred.
- TMP-SMX 160 mg/800 mg (1 DS tab) PO twice daily × 7–10 days.
Alternate regimens
- Ciprofloxacin 500 mg PO twice daily × 7 days (less effective than TMP-SMZ).
- Nitazoxanide 500 mg PO q6–12h × 7 days. Only case report information available on efficacy.
Secondary prophylaxis (AIDS)
- TMP-SMX 160 mg/800 mg (1 DS) tab three times a wk offers secondary prophylaxis, prevention of relapse.

OTHER INFORMATION

- Different from many enteric infections since organisms are not infectious when passed from human stool. Cyclospora needs days–wks after leaving bowels to become infectious. Therefore, this is unlikely to be an agent of person-person transmissible infection.
- Can be particularly important cause of diarrhea in travelers to specific locales such as Nepal.
- Transmission associated also with basil, salad greens especially mesclun lettuce.
- Does not cause fever, inflammatory diarrhea or eosinophilia.
- In HIV/AIDS, associated cases, but not particularly severe disease.

BASIS FOR RECOMMENDATIONS

Verdier RI, Fitzgerald DW, Johnson WD, et al. Trimethoprim-sulfamethoxazole compared with ciprofloxacin for treatment and prophylaxis of Isospora belli and Cyclospora cayetanensis infection in HIV-infected pts. A randomized, controlled trial. *Ann Intern Med*, 2000; Vol. 132; pp. 885–8.

Comments: This is an important clinical trial in which TMP-SMZ is shown to be superior to ciprofloxacin for treatment and prophylaxis of *Cyclospora* in HIV-infected people in Haiti; ciprofloxacin, while having a somewhat lower clinical and parasitological cure rate, was still useful.

Hoge CW, Shlim DR, Ghimire M, et al. Placebo-controlled trial of co-trimoxazole for *Cyclospora* infections among travellers and foreign residents in Nepal. *Lancet*, 1995; Vol. 345; pp. 691–3.

Comments: Demonstration of efficacy of TMP-SMZ for treatment of *Cyclospora* infection in travelers and expatriates who developed infection in Nepal.

ECHINOCOCCUS

Joseph Vinetz, MD

MICROBIOLOGY

- Cestode parasite, most common *E. granulosus*; less common, *E. multilocularis.*
- *E. granulosus*: intermediate hosts are sheep, cattle, pigs, camels, goats; definitive hosts are dogs and other canids that eat internal organs of intermediate host. Humans infected by ingestion of eggs indirectly from canid feces via environmental contamination of food/water.
- *E. multilocularis*: intermediate hosts are rodents, domestic pigs, wild boars, dog, monkey; definitive hosts are foxes, dogs, cats.
- *Echinococcus vogeli* (very rare): rodents intermediate host, while bush dogs definitive host in central, south America.

CLINICAL

- Cestode parasite: *E. granulosus*, cause of hydatid disease—most common. *E. multilocularis*, cause of alveolar echinococcosis—less common. *E. vogeli, E. oligarthus*, rare human pathogens.
- Epidemiology: highest prevalence in Mediterranean, Russian Federation and neighboring countries, China, central Asia, north and east Africa, Australia, South America especially in Andean highlands.
- *E. granulosus*: humans infected by ingesting infectious forms from feces of definitive hosts (primarily dogs that are infected from eating viscera of infected intermediate hosts, e.g., sheep, cattle.
- Organs involved by *E. granulosus* of cervid (cattle, moose, elk, deer) strains predominantly localize in lung, with a more benign clinical course.
- Organs involved by *E. granulosus* of sheep-infecting strain, by frequency: liver (65%), lung (25%), spleen heart, kidney, bone, brain, eye (less common).
- *E. multilocularis*: humans infected by ingesting infectious forms from feces of foxes, who are infected from wild animals such as rodents.
- *E. multilocularis* acts like invasive tumor; primarily found in liver, can metastasize to other organs, including brain, with disastrous effect. Invariably fatal if not treated.
- Clinical manifestations variable, depending on organ involved. Can involve mass effect, allergic manifestations from cyst leakage, chronic cough/hemoptysis from pulmonary cyst.
- Often detected only incidentally radiographically as space-occupying lesions in lungs, liver (hydatid disease). Initial phase of infection asymptomatic.
- Diagnosis supported by typical radiological signs. Microscopic detection of protoscolices or hydatid membranes in cyst aspirate is definitive. Serology can be useful if done in reference labs (ELISA, Western blot).

SITES OF INFECTION

- Brain (*E. granulosus*): slowly progressive, space-occupying lesions, symptomatically manifesting as local mass effect, symptoms of intracranial hypertension.
- Brain (*E. multilocularis*): invasive, tumor-like, often multifocal, symptoms of intracranial hypertension, seizures, mass effect.
- Lung: may be detected incidentally in asymptomatic infection or slowly progressive with cough (salty cyst contents), hemoptysis, chest pain.
- Liver: may be incidental (by ultrasound), or manifest by hepatomegaly, dull RUQ pain, local mass effect depending on location of cyst(s)—including biliary compression, jaundice, cholangitis.
- Disseminated: rare multi-organ involvement (any combination of liver, lung, brain, heart, spine, etc.).
- Systemic: anaphylaxis or allergic symptoms such as urticaria in case of spontaneous cyst rupture at any site. Biliary sepsis due to ductal compression.

TREATMENT

Surgical: Hydatid Disease

- Percutaneous aspiration-injection-reaspiration drainage (pair) plus albendazole effective, safe, and less complex (see references) than surgery.
- Primary surgical therapy indicated primarily for isolated hepatic lesions.
- Open excision of large hepatic cysts historical mainstay, only favored now in cases of excessive risk for standard aspiration (pair).
- Risks of pair: hemorrhage, mechanical lesions of other tissues, infection, anaphylaxis/allergic reactions, chemical cholangitis, biliary fistula, systemic toxicity.
- Pair should be performed in centers with experience and ability to deal with complications of the technique.
- Secondary echinococcosis from rupture, leakage possible.
- Likely only useful for *E. granulosis* but not *E. multilocularis*.

Surgical: Alveolar Disease

- Preferred choice in operable cases: radical surgical research of entire parasitic lesion from liver, or other affected organs.
- Albendazole recommended for limited duration after radical surgery.
- Long-term (yrs) albendazole mandatory after incomplete resection.

Albendazole

- 10–15 mg/kg PO in two divided doses (typically 400 mg twice daily) in three to six 4-wk cycles, each cycle separated by 14 days.
- Most effective in combination with surgical or drainage procedure.
- When combined with pair (see below), 7 days of pre-pair Rx and 28 days post-pair.
- Toxicities with prolonged use remain rare: monitor liver function tests, complete blood count q2wks.
- Existing hepatic dysfunction predisposes to toxicity.

Praziquantel

- Limited role, perhaps useful in case of ruptured cysts to prevent intraabdominal or intrathoracic spread of daughter cysts.
- Anecdotal evidence of utility in combination therapy with albendazole.
- Used as adjunct agent at dose of 50 mg/kg PO either once weekly or every 2 wks during primary therapy.

Mebendazole

- 40–50 mg/kg PO per day in three divided doses, taken with fatty meals.
- Best combined with surgical or percutaneous drainage procedure.
- Less effective than albendazole.
- Toxicities with prolonged use remain rare: monitor liver function tests, complete blood count q2wks.

OTHER INFORMATION

- Diagnosis: ultrasonography or other imaging plus serology (commercially available EIA, consult CDC for advanced tests) or observation of protoscolices w/ hooklets in cyst fluid (ascertain viability).

- Serological dx: not all pts have antibodies, depending on characteristics and location of cysts. EIA or IHA used to screen w/ positives confirmed by immunoblot; may cross-react w/ cysticercosis.
- Staging based on ultrasound examination (see detailed information below for classification).

More Other Information

Hydatid Disease: staging classification based on ultrasound examination (summarized in DP McManus, *Lancet* 2003;362:1429).

CL: active, nonfertile, no visible cyst wall, early stage of development (additional tests required to establish diagnosis of cystic echinococcosis).

CE1: active, fertile, visible cyst wall, unilocular, anechoic or "snowflake sign."

CE2: active, fertile, visible cyst wall, multiseptate and multivesicular, daughter cysts present.

CE3: transitional, fertile, visible cyst wall, anechoic content with detached laminated membrane ("waterlily sign"). Decreased intracystic pressure. Cyst starting to degenerate.

CE4: inactive, infertile, no visible cyst wall, heterogeneous hyperechoic or hypoechoic contents, no visible daughter cysts (additional tests required to establish diagnosis of cystic echinococcosis).

CE5: inactive, infertile, calcified cyst wall, thick, variably calcified wall producing a cone-shaped shadow. Usually no viable protoscolices (additional tests required to establish diagnosis of cystic echinococcosis).

Staging system for human alveolar echinococcosis.

P: primary localization of cyst(s) to liver.

PX: primary lesion unable to be assessed.

P0: no detectable liver lesion.

P1: peripheral lesions without biliary or proximal vascular involvement.

P2: central lesions with biliary or proximal vascular involvement of one lobe.

P3: central lesions with biliary or proximal vascular involvement of both lobes or two hepatic veins or both.

P4: any lesion with extension along the portal vein, inferior vena cava, or hepatic arteries.

N: extrahepatic involvement of neighboring organs.

M: presence of distant metastases.

BASIS FOR RECOMMENDATIONS

Smego RA, Sebanego P. Treatment options for hepatic cystic echinococcosis. *Int J Infect Dis*, 2005; Vol. 9; pp. 69–76.

Comments: This is a well-written article on treatment approaches to the treatment of the most common form of Echinococcus infection, that involving the liver.

Khuroo MS, Wani NA, Javid G, et al. Percutaneous drainage compared with surgery for hepatic hydatid cysts. *N Engl J Med*, 1997; Vol. 337; pp. 881–7.

Comments: A landmark article describing a prospective trial of 50 pts assigned either to pair or surgical excision for treatment of hepatic hydatid disease. Percutaneous drainage plus albendazole was found to be effective and safe for the treatment of uncomplicated hydatid cyst disease.

ENTAMOEBA HISTOLYTICA

Lisa A. Spacek, MD, PhD and Joseph Vinetz, MD

MICROBIOLOGY

- Protozoan species in the genus *Entamoeba*.
- Mature cysts ingested, followed by excystation in the distal ileum. Motile trophozoites are released and migrate to the large intestine. Both trophozoites and cysts are excreted in stool.
- Trophozoites exist only in host and fresh feces. Cysts remain viable outside host in water, soil, and sewage for wks or mos.
- *E. histolytica* must be distinguished from *E. dispar*, a morphologically identical parasite that does not cause disease.

CLINICAL

- Clinical syndromes include asymptomatic, intraluminal infection, invasive intestinal disease (dysentery, colitis, appendicitis, toxic megacolon, amebomas) and invasive extraintestinal disease (abscesses in liver, lung, or brain; peritonitis, cutaneous or genital lesions).

PATHOGENS

- Occurs primarily in developing countries, but immigrants, travelers, MSM diagnosed with infection in U.S. Fulminant colitis may occur in immunocompromised, malnourished, pregnant women, or pts on corticosteroids.
- Amebic colitis characterized by abdominal pain, tenesmus, frequent, small volume stool with mucus +/– blood.
- Dx: stool smear and stain (e.g., trichrome) to visualize by microscopy.
- Dx: serology highly sensitive for extraintestinal disease, e.g., liver abscess; moderately sensitive for intestinal disease; and poorly sensitive for asymptomatic infection. Antibodies persist for yrs after effective treatment and may provide false positive results.
- Dx: stool and serum antigen tests can distinguish *E. histolytica* from *E. dispar*, PCR also available. Both better than O and P.
- Colonoscopy: biopsy or scraping at margin of colonic mucosal ulcer, parasite may be seen. H and E shows necrosis, classic flask-shaped ulcers.
- Imaging: U/S, CT scan and MRI to visualize cystic liver lesions and guide aspiration.
- Liver abscess aspiration yields anchovy paste-like material. Most amebas reside at edge of cyst and may be missed in aspirate. For dx, aspirate can be antigen tested. Peritoneal spillage of contents increases mortality. May drain to bronchial tree and cause cough productive of abscess material.

SITES OF INFECTION

- Colon: dysentery, colitis, ameboma (tumor-like lesion of colonic lumen that can be confused radiographically with cecal cancer), toxic megacolon
- Liver: abscess, rupture can cause peritonitis
- Lung: empyema (right sided, direct extension from liver)
- Heart: pericarditis (direct extension from liver)
- Brain: abscess (by hematogenous spread, rare)
- Skin: usually perineal, genital
- GU: recto-vaginal fistula

TREATMENT

Asymptomatic, intraluminal infection

- Luminal agents used to treat intraluminal infection and clear cysts, include: iodoquinol, paromomycin and diloxanide furoate.
- Iodoquinol 650 mg PO three times a day × 20 days, take after meals.
- Paromomycin: 25–35 mg/kg/day PO in 3 divided doses × 7 days, take with meals.
- Diloxanide furoate 500 mg PO three times a day × 10 days, may be difficult to obtain in U.S.

Diarrhea/dysentery, mild to moderate infection

- Metronidazole 500–750 mg PO three times a day × 10 days followed by luminal agent, e.g., paromomycin 500 mg PO three times a day × 7 days or iodoquinol 650 mg PO three times a day × 20 days.
- Tinidazole 2 g PO once daily × 3 days followed by luminal agent, paromomycin 500 mg PO three times a day × 7 days or iodoquinol 650 mg PO three times a day × 20 days.
- Nitazoxanide 500 mg PO twice daily × 3 days (not FDA-approved for this indication).

Extrahepatic or severe intestinal disease

- Metronidazole 750 mg IV or PO three times a day × 10 days followed by luminal agent as above.
- Tinidazole 2 g PO qd × 5 days followed by luminal agent.
- Liver abscess: aspiration not necessary for treatment.

More Treatment

Treatment guidelines published in *The Medical Letter* available through CDC website at: http://www.dpd.cdc.gov/dpdx/HTML/PDF_Files/MedLetter/Amebiasis.pdf

BASIS FOR RECOMMENDATIONS

Abramowicz, M, Editor. Drugs for Parasitic Infections. *Medical Lett Drugs Ther*, 2007; pp. 3–4.
Comments: U.S.-based guidelines for treatment of amebiasis.

Rossignol JF, Kabil SM, El-Gohary Y, et al. Nitazoxanide in the treatment of amoebiasis. *Trans R Soc Trop Med Hyg*, 2007; Vol. 101; pp. 1025–31.
Comments: This report of two prospective, randomised, double-blind, placebo-controlled studies conducted in pts with intestinal amebiasis in Egypt showed nitazoxanide is effective in treating invasive intestinal amebiasis and eliminating *E. histolytica* colonization.

GIARDIA LAMBLIA

Lisa A. Spacek, MD, PhD and Joseph Vinetz, MD

MICROBIOLOGY

- *Giardia lamblia*, also known as *G. intestinalis*, is a flagellated enteric protozoan, most common intestinal parasite in North America.
- Life cycle includes trophozoite and cyst forms, ingestion of 15–25 cysts can lead to infection. Following excystation, trophozoites multiply and colonize the upper small intestine.
- Trophozoites have flat ventral surface allowing adherence at brush border of enterocytes and contributing to malabsorption.
- Transmitted by contaminated water, food, person-to-person, fecal-oral contact. Surface water easily contaminated by cysts shed from mammalian hosts such as beavers, sheep, cattle, dogs, or cats.

CLINICAL

- Occurs worldwide, specifically in settings of day care centers, exposure to contaminated surface water, and fecal-oral sexual contact.
- Incubation period: 1–2 wks.
- Presentations include: asymptomatic cyst passage, acute diarrhea, and chronic diarrhea with malabsorption.
- Sxs include abdominal pain, nausea, vomiting, anorexia, and bloating. Stools large volume, watery, foul-smelling and greasy. Chronic diarrhea with malabsorption accompanied by weight loss, lactase deficiency, and steatorrhea. Fever is unusual.
- Mucosal invasion is rare; blood, pus and mucus absent from stool.
- Dx: stool O and P exam for cysts/troph forms. Pear-shaped, trophozoites with flagella seen with iodine and trichrome staining. Concentration and repeat samples may increase sensitivity. Stool antigen detection with immunofluorescence and ELISAs offer improved sensitivity/specificity over O and P. PCR available.
- Dx: duodenal aspirate or bx for trophozoites in cases of malabsorption.

SITES OF INFECTION

- GI: upper small bowel, adherent to enterocytes.

TREATMENT

Preferred agents

- Tinidazole 2 g PO × 1, take with food.
- Nitazoxanide 500 mg PO twice daily × 3 days, take with food.
- Metronidazole 250 mg PO three times a day × 5–7 days.

Alternative agents

- Paromomycin 25–35 mg/kg/day PO divided into 3 doses × 5–10 days, take with food.
- Furazolidone 100 mg PO four times a day × 7–10 days.
- Quinacrine 100 mg PO three times a day × 5 days, take with liquids after meal.
- Albendazole 400 mg PO once daily × 5 days.

Pregnancy

- Paromomycin recommended in pregnancy due to poor absorption.
- Paromomycin 25–35 mg/kg/day PO divided into 3 doses × 5–10 days, taken with food.

FOLLOW UP

Refractory Giardiasis

- Usual cure rate is >90% with most regimens. Pts who fail two rounds of conventional therapy may be considered to have "refractory" giardiasis.
- Consider using quinacrine 100 mg three times daily PO plus metronidazole 250 mg PO three times daily × 21 days.

OTHER INFORMATION

- Treatment guidelines published in the Medical Letter available through CDC website at: http://www.dpd.cdc.gov/dpdx/HTML/PDF_Files/MedLetter/Giardiasis.pdf

PATHOGENS

FILARIASIS

Paul G. Auwaerter, MD and Joseph Vinetz, MD

MICROBIOLOGY

- Nematode parasite transmitted by mosquitoes.
- Most disease caused by three species of tissue-dwelling nematodes: *Wuchereria bancrofti* (Asia, Africa, Latin America, Pacific islands), *Onchocerca volvulus* (Africa >> Latin America, Middle East), *Brugia malayi* (South-east Asia).
- See loa loa or *Onchocerca volvulus* modules for information on these filarial parasites. Other less common species involved include *Mansonella perstans*, *M. streptocerca*, *M. ozzardi*, and *Brugia timori* (few Indonesian islands, may cause lymphatic filariasis).
- Transmitted by night or day biting mosquitoes (*Anopheles, Culex*).

CLINICAL

- Asymptomatic microfilaremia most common.
- Acute: filarial fever (lymphadenitis, fever, chills), lasting ~1 wk, may recur (w/ bacterial lymphangitis) up to 1 yr, +/– epididymo-orchitis (uni- or bilateral).
- Tropical pulmonary eosinophilia: seen more commonly in Asia with paroxysmal cough/ wheezing, worse at night; extreme eosinophilia (>3000/uL). Responds to DEC. No visible microfilaremia but positive antigen test.
- Chronic manifestations: hydrocele +/– acute pain/swelling (most common); classic elephantiasis due to *Wuchereria bancrofti* (uni- or bilateral) of leg (most common), scrotum/ vulva (common), arm (less common).
- Other syndromes: acute monoarthritis; hematuria, proteinuria, endomyocardial fibrosis (in presence of marked eosinophilia).
- Species vary regionally by diurnal or nocturnal periodicity, making timing of blood examination to detect microfilaria important.
- Diagnosis: parasitological (obtain blood to seek microfilaremia at peak time of day/night, depending on region of infection, e.g., within 2 hrs of midnight for nocturnally periodic forms). Improved sensitivity can be gained by using concentration techniques such as Knott's technique (blood lysis centrifugation using 2% formalin), or Nucleopore® filtration.
- Dx: (1) serological-antigen detection by commercially available card test; IgG4 antibody (not filaria species specific and may cross react with other helminths); in U.S. contact NIH (see below).
- Dx: (2) special maneuvers-DEC provocative days test (induce microfilaremia with dose of DEC); polymerase chain reaction (reference labs only).
- Dx: (3) skin snips (detect *Onchocerca volvulus*, *Mansonella streptocerca*). Ultrasonography can detect adult *W. bancrofti* worms in scrotal lymphatics.

MORE CLINICAL

Skin snip technique (from CDC): skin snips can be obtained using a corneal-scleral punch, or more simply a scalpel and needle. The sample must be allowed to incubate for 30 minutes to 2 hrs in saline or culture medium, and then examined for microfilariae that would have migrated from the tissue to the liquid phase of the specimen.

SITES OF INFECTION

- General: filarial fever includes fever, chills, malaise during acute or recurrent episode.
- Lymph: localized lymphadenitis, may be painful (red, warm) or painless, unilateral or bilateral groin swelling. May be due to adult worm or complicating bacterial infection.
- Derm: pruritus, dermatitis, subcutaneous nodules.
- Genital: scrotal or vulvar swelling/hydrocele; may be able to visualize adult *W. bancrofti* worm by ultrasound.
- Extremities: unilateral or bilateral swelling, acute or chronic. May be extreme (classic elephantiasis) or mild. May be associated w/ recurrent bacterial cellulitis (abrupt onset of redness, fever).
- Lungs: tropical pulmonary eosinophilia (miliary pattern on CXR, nocturnal paroxysmal cough, wheezing, accompanied by marked eosinophilia, responds to DEC, usually amicrofilaremic).
- Renal: chyluria, hematuria (rupture of dilated lymphatics into urinary excretory system). May see weight loss, hypoproteinemia, lymphopenia, anemia.

- Musculoskeletal: acute monoarthritis (knee > ankle) which responds to DEC, tenosynovitis (rare), thrombophlebitis (rare).

TREATMENT

Filariasis: *Brugia malayi, B. timori* or *Wuchereria bancrofti*

- Diethylcarbamazine (DEC) preferred: 2 mg/kg PO three times daily × 12 days (may be accompanied by systemic reaction to dying worms, local reactions include lymphadenitis, transient lymphedema).
- Scaled dose DEC escalation recommended to reduce reactions: day 1–50 mg, day 2–50 mg three times a day, day 3–100 mg three times a day, day 4 through 14–6 mg/kg in 3 doses.
- Corticosteroids or antihistamines may be needed to treat allergic reactions that develop as a consequence of dying microfilariae.
- Treatment of endosymbiont Wolbachia (bacteria) may help clear infection: doxycycline 100 mg once or twice daily × 6–8 wks in lymphatic filariasis although effect may be more important for co-infecting pathogens such as Wuchereria or Onchocerca than loa loa [Taylor et al, *Lancet* 2005;365:2116].
- To obtain DEC, CDC access number 404-639-3670.
- Retreatment for microfilaremia often necessary q6–12 mos as demonstrated by repeat blood smear or antigen testing.
- Note: do not use DEC due in *Onchocerca volvulus* to increased risks of precipitating blindness.

Wuchereria bancrofti

- Most symptoms with this parasite are due to the adult worm.
- Combination single dose regimen of albendazole 400 mg PO PLUS either ivermectin 200 mcg/kg PO or DEC 6 mg/kg may reduce or suppress microfilariae; however, this will not affect adult worms.

General management: lymphatic filariasis

- Foot care to reduce fungal and bacterial infection in presence of lymphedema.
- Surgical: after DEC treatment, chronic hydroceles require excision and eversion of sac. Removal of grossly elephantoid skin in scrotal/vulvar involvement useful.
- Surgery for extremity elephantiasis usually unsuccessful.

OTHER INFORMATION

- Drug treatment only kills microfilaria not adult worms; retreatment necessary q6–12 mos when microfilaremia recurs. May need to use antigen detection test to diagnose.
- Microfilaremia may not be present for a variety of reasons (low organism load, early in infection, time of day when blood sample obtained for testing, concentration by nucleopore filtration not done).
- In U.S., diagnostic assistance (antibody detection, antigen detection, PCR) through NIH Laboratory of Parasitic Diseases: 301-496-5398.
- Antibody testing for IgG4 anti-recombinant microfilarial antibody may be useful for diagnosis; it is species specific.
- Eosinophilia and elevated IgE levels are supportive of filarial diagnosis.

BASIS FOR RECOMMENDATIONS

No authors listed. Drugs for Parasitic Infections. *Med Lett Drugs Ther*, 2007; Volume 5; pp. e1–e14.

Comments: Download available at http://medlet-best.securesites.com/html/parasitic.htm

MALARIA

Lisa A. Spacek, MD, PhD and Joseph Vinetz, MD

MICROBIOLOGY

- Malaria is caused by *Plasmodium* parasites belonging to the *Apicomplexa* group of protozoa, transmitted by night-time or pre-dawn biting mosquitoes.
- Species causing human malaria include: *P. falciparum, P. vivax, P. ovale,* and *P. malariae. P. knowlesi,* a monkey malaria parasite, noted to cause human malaria in Southeast Asia and morphologically resembles *P. malariae.*
- Life cycle: anopheline mosquito bites human host and injects sporozoites, which invade hepatocytes and become schizonts. Hepatocytes rupture and release merozoites that invade

PATHOGENS

RBCs. In RBCs, merozoites develop from ring forms into trophozoites then schizonts, followed by rupture of RBCs and a new cycle of RBC invasion.

- *P. vivax* and *P. ovale* can persist in hepatocytes as hypnozoites for mos to yrs. Eradication requires treatment for both liver and blood stages. *P. vivax* preferentially invades reticulocytes.
- *P. falciparum* invades RBCs of all ages, causes most severe and lethal illness as RBCs sequester in microvasculature, and damage heart, brain, kidney, lung, placenta.

CLINICAL

- Presents as acute febrile illness. Headache, spiking fevers, abdominal complaints common. Classic malaria paroxysm (chills, fever, and sweats at regular intervals usually in the semi-immune resident of an endemic region as opposed to a traveler) occurs with release of blood schizonts.
- Suspect in any febrile traveler who visited malarial endemic area in prior 3 mos.
- Prompt evaluation necessary; untreated *P. falciparum* malaria rapidly progresses, often fatal if untreated. Disease course is unpredictable in nonimmune individuals.
- Severe malaria: hypoglycemia, anemia, thrombocytopenia, metabolic acidosis, encephalopathy, seizure, hyperparasitemia ($>5\%$ of RBCs, defined as $>10\%$ in endemic areas), pulmonary edema, renal failure. Rarely presents with splenic rupture.
- Uncomplicated malaria: symptomatic parasitemia without signs of severity or evidence of organ dysfunction.
- Dx: light microscopy, Giemsa-stained thick smears used to screen for presence of parasites and to determine parasitemia, RBCs lyzed in process, and parasites seen outside RBCs. Thin blood smears used to determine species and degree of parasitemia. Repeat blood smear every 12 hrs to detect parasitemia that may lag behind clinical presentation.
- Dx: rapid diagnostic tests employ lateral flow immunochromatographic technology with capture and detection antibodies. Diagnostic targets are malaria antigens conserved across all species or antigens specific to *P. falciparum* or *P. vivax*.

SITES OF INFECTION

- RBCs: in case of *P. falciparum* parasitized RBCs cause disease by sequestering in post-capillary venules of heart, brain, placenta, lung, kidney, gut.
- Liver (dormant stages): *P. vivax, P. ovale* only.
- Spleen.

TREATMENT

General Principles

- Consider disease severity, geographic origin of infection, parasite species.
- Hyperparasitemia, CNS symptoms are medical emergencies requiring IV therapy.
- Guidelines for treatment of malaria in the U.S. available at the CDC website: http://www.cdc.gov/malaria/pdf/treatmenttable.pdf.

Uncomplicated P. falciparum or species unidentified

- In chloroquine—resistant or unknown resistance, choose one of following four options. Consider only if certain that PO can be tolerated. Use mefloquine as last choice due to neuropsychiatric reactions seen at treatment doses.
- Atovaquone/proguanil (Malarone 250/100) 4 tabs PO once-daily for 3 days, taken with milk or fatty meal.
- Artemether-lumefantrine (Coartem) adult dose (>65 kg) 4 tab PO initial dose (wt-based dosing, see www.hopkins-abxguide.org), then 4 tab PO 8 hrs later, then 4 tab PO twice daily × 2 days.
- Quinine sulfate 650 mg PO q8h × 3–7 days plus doxycycline 100 mg PO twice-daily × 7 days or tetracycline 250 mg PO q6h × 7 days or clindamycin 20 mg base/kg/day PO divided q8h (average dose 450 PO q8h) × 7 days.
- Mefloquine 750 mg PO initial dose, then 500 mg 6–12 hrs later.
- For known chloroquine-sensitive *P. falciparum* (Central America west of Panama Canal, Haiti, Dominican Republic and Middle East): chloroquine phosphate 1 g salt (600 mg base) PO once, then 500 mg salt (300 mg base) 6 hrs, 24 hrs and 48 hrs later.
- Pregnancy: use chloroquine or hydroxychloroquine (for chloroquine-sensitive species) or quinine sulfate + clindamycin (for chloroquine-resistant species).

- Quinine associated with cinchonism (reversible tinnitus and reversible high-tone hearing loss).

Complicated *P. falciparum*

- For quinine-based therapy, use IV quinidine gluconate + doxycycline or tetracycline or clindamycin, admit to telemetry unit. Monitor for QTc prolongation, QRS widening, ventricular arrhythmia, hypotension and hypoglycemia. If significant QRS widening, slow or hold infusion. Hypotension common with quinidine/quinine (may be due to drug or the infection itself). Treat hypotension with judicious use of fluids.

- Quinidine gluconate IV 10 mg salt/kg loading dose (max 600 mg) in saline over 1–2 hrs, then infuse 0.02 mg salt/kg/min for at least 24 hrs. Once parasitemia <1% and oral meds tolerated treat with quinine PO; maximum duration of parenteral treatment is typically 1–2 days. Do not use loading dose of quinidine in pts with hx of mefloquine or quinine derivative in prior 12 hrs.

- For quinidine availability, call CDC Malaria Hotline 770-488-7788 or Eli Lilly 800-821-0538.

- Alternative: artemisinin-based therapy, artesunate 2.4 mg/kg/dose IV × 3 days at 0, 12, 24, 48, and 72 hrs. For quinine—resistant *P. falciparum*, combine with tetracycline or mefloquine. Use of artemisinin derivative avoids quinine—associated hypoglycemia. Available through a treatment IND in the U.S. (call the CDC: 1-770-488-7788 or after hrs: 770-488-7100).

- Consider exchange transfusion for parasitemia >10%, coma, ARDS or kidney failure. Early hemofiltration and mechanical ventilation may improve survival.

- Treat severe malaria aggressively with IV antimalarials in pregnancy.

P. vivax, P. ovale, P. malariae

- Chloroquine phosphate 1 g salt (600 mg base) PO once, then 500 mg salt (300 mg base) 6 hrs, 24 hrs and 48 hrs later.

- Treatment of liver forms (*P. vivax/ovale* only): primaquine 30 mg (base) PO once-daily × 14 days. May cause hemolytic anemia due to G6PD deficiency—test first. Contraindicated in pregnancy/breastfeeding.

- Primaquine treatment is not mandatory. Some prefer to wait for the low risk of relapse rather than face potential side-effects of the drug.

- Chloroquine—resistant *P. vivax* acquired in Papua New Guinea and Indonesia is treated with quinine sulfate + doxycycline or tetracycline + primaquine or atovaquone/proguanil + primaquine or mefloquine + primaquine.

Prophylaxis

- General recommendations for U.S. adults: most malaria-endemic regions (i.e., where chloroquine resistance is known or likely to be present).

- Atovaquone/proguanil (Malarone): 1 tab PO daily. Take with food or milky drink. Start 1–2 days before entry to malarial region, discontinue 7 days after leaving.

- Mefloquine 250 mg (Lariam) 1 tab PO q wk. Start 1 wk prior to travel and continue weekly, always on the same day each wk, preferably after the main meal, until 4 wks after return.

- Doxycycline 100 mg PO daily. Optimally taken in evening. Start 1–2 days before travel, until four wks after travel. Photosensitivity risk >3%, avoid sun, use sunscreen.

- Central America north of Panama Canal (only): chloroquine 300 mg PO qwk. Start 1 wk before, continue 4 wk after.

- Mosquitoes bite at any time of day but *Anopheles* bite mainly at night with most activity at dawn and dusk. Use insecticide-treated bed netting, sprays (DEET) and screens.

- Terminal prophylaxis with primaquine 30 mg base PO daily × 14 days at end of malaria exposure period, may be considered to prevent *P. vivax* and *P. ovale* malaria. Some clinicians do not use terminal prophylaxis, and reserve treatment for confirmed *P. vivax* or *P. ovale* episodes. Screen for G6PD deficiency prior to treatment.

MORE TREATMENT

- A recently developed malaria vaccine RTS,S (GlaxoSmithKline Biologicals and the Walter Reed Army Institute of Research) targets the circumsporozoite protein of *P. falciparum* during the preerythrocytic stage of the life cycle. Two adjuvant systems, AS01B (liposomal-based) and AS02A (oil-in-water emulsion), are undergoing evaluation.

OTHER INFORMATION

- CDC Malaria Hotline: 770-488-7788 or 770-488-7100 (after hrs). CDC website (http://www.cdc.gov/malaria/index.htm) provides treatment guidelines and map of malaria

PATHOGENS

risk areas for travelers. WHO document available at: http://apps.who.int/malaria/docs/TreatmentGuidelines2006.pdf.
- IV quinine not available in U.S. Quinidine gluconate may not be available in some hospital pharmacies.
- Even if *P. vivax* diagnosed, consider possibility of co-infection with *P. falciparum*.
- Consider bacterial meningitis and Gram-negative bacteremia in setting of suspected severe malaria.
- Malaria in pregnancy is more severe with greater frequency of hypoglycemia and pulmonary compromise due to relative immunosuppression and parasite sequestration. Chloroquine, quinine, quinidine, and clindamycin are safe in pregnancy. Proguanil requires folate supplementation. Mefloquine is thought to be safe in second half of pregnancy. Tetracycline, doxycycline and primaquine are contraindicated in pregnancy. Artemisinin derivatives are contraindicated during first trimester and should be used cautiously in 2nd and 3rd trimesters.

BASIS FOR RECOMMENDATIONS

Griffith KS, Lewis LS, Mali S, et al. Treatment of malaria in the United States: a systematic review. *JAMA,* 2007; Vol. 297; pp. 2264–77.
Comments: Useful, comprehensive up-to-date review from the CDC.

Abramowicz M, Editor. Drugs for Parasitic Infections. *Medical Lett Drugs Ther,* 2007; Vol. pp. 32–44.
Comments: U.S.-based guidelines for treatment and prevention of malaria.

STRONGYLOIDES STERCORALIS

Paul G. Auwaerter, MD and Joseph Vinetz, MD

MICROBIOLOGY
- Helminthic parasite, common worldwide but especially in warmer climes.
- Larvae live in soil. Human infection by contact with contaminated soil.
- Filariform larvae penetrate skin and enter lymphatics → lung alveoli. Migration from lung to trachea to GI tract/small intestine. Females yield to parthenogenic reproduction with eggs that turn to rhabditiform larvae within the intestine. Immunosuppression can yield increased organisms by result of autoinfection.
- Larvae are typically seen ~1 mo after exposure.

CLINICAL
- Widely distributed in tropics; estimated prevalence up to 4% in U.S. South, Appalachian regions.
- May cause enteric symptoms especially diarrhea, abdominal pain/bloating.
- Infection can asymptomatically last decades, activated by immune suppression.
- Hyperinfection syndrome seen in pts given corticosteroids, HTLV-I infection, occasionally in HIV/AIDS (likely due to steroids, inanition, HTLV coinfection).
- Common scenario for hyperinfection syndrome: immigrant from developing country given high dose steroids, develops pulmonary infiltrates and possibly Gram-negative sepsis, meningitis, sometimes in presence of eosinophilia (usually not).
- Can cause Loeffler-like syndrome (transient pulmonary infiltrates plus eosinophilia).
- Diagnosis may be difficult because few organisms may be present.
- Diagnosis of intestinal infection: observation of larvae on direct stool smear (insensitive); Baermann test (larval concentration, specialized labs only); serology (possible problems with cross-reactivity and may be falsely negative in immunocompromised pts).
- Diagnosis of CNS or pulmonary infection: observation of larvae on direct wet mount examination of centrifuged CSF or BAL specimen.
- Mortality rate in immunocompromised with disseminated infection may be >60–85%, pts with multi-organ system failure.

SITES OF INFECTION
- GI: nausea, vomiting, cramping, diarrhea, epigastric pain/burning, weight loss. Eosinophilia is typical but usually asymptomatic with chronic infection.
- Lung: Loeffler-like syndrome. In presence of immunocompromise, may have overwhelming larval invasion plus Gram-negative bacterial infection.

- CNS: larval invasion in superinfection syndrome, accompanied by Gram-negative bacterial meningitis; may be associated with peripheral and/or CSF eosinophilia.
- Skin: generalized or localized urticaria. Larva currens syndrome (larvae migrating to perianal area, flank, with pruritic, serpiginous or linear urticarial lesions).
- Systemic: Gram-negative sepsis with pulmonary infiltrates, in pt given steroids, and recent or distant immigration from strongyloidiasis-endemic region.

TREATMENT
Ivermectin
- Drug of choice.
- 200 microgram/kg/day PO × 1–2 days.
- May need to be repeated or prolonged in pts with hyperinfection syndrome.

Thiabendazole
- 50 mg/kg/day PO in 2 doses (max. 3 g/days) × 2 days.
- Toxicity at this dose common: confusion, diarrhea, hallucinations, irritability, loss of appetite, nausea and vomiting, numbness/tingling in hands/feet.

BASIS FOR RECOMMENDATIONS
Abramowicz, M, Editor. Drugs for Parasitic Infections. *Medical Lett Drugs Ther*, 2007; vol. 3–4 pp. 32–44.
Comments: U.S.–based guidelines for treatment and prevention of malaria.

TAENIA SOLIUM

Joseph Vinetz, MD and Paul G. Auwaerter, MD

MICROBIOLOGY
- Cestode parasite also known as the pork tapeworm.
- Pigs are intermediate hosts; humans acquire intestinal tapeworm by eating undercooked pork.
- Humans acquire disseminated cysticercosis by ingesting eggs (oncospheres) transmitted to environment then to food/water by human tapeworm carriers.

CLINICAL
- Cestode (helminth parasite) that causes cysticercosis.
- Disease endemic throughout Latin America, Balkans, East Africa, India, China, Indonesia; often imported to U.S. yrs after primary infection.
- Transmitted by oncospheres human to human through fecal-oral route; after ingestion of undercooked meat of intermediate host such as pigs leads to intestinal infection in humans.
- Intestinal infection in humans causes few if any symptoms but leads to transmission to other humans.
- Calcified CNS lesions are dead parasites that can be epileptogenic foci.
- Important cause of late onset seizures (focal or generalized), chronic headache, symptomatic hydrocephalus, or radiological discovery of asymptomatic brain lesions.
- Can present as calcified nodules in other parts of body, demonstrable through plain x-rays.
- Dx: typical neuroimaging in pt with endemic risk, excision of cyst, serology (95% sensitive but cross-reaction may occur from other parasitic infections, especially particularly echinococcus; Western blot may enhance specificity ~100%).
- Definitive diagnosis depends on the observation of the scolex or membranes of *T. solium* from tissue samples. Stool: proglottid uterus when stained, *T. solium* with 5–10 uterine branches per side distinguishes from *T. saginata* (>12 branches).
- More commonly, diagnosis based on clinical signs and symptoms, radiologic testing, with biopsy reserved for only the most diagnostically vexing cases.

SITES OF INFECTION
- CNS, active: parenchymal (CT/MRI shows one or more rounded hypodense areas of variable size, no enhancement) or extraparenchymal (subarachnoid or ventricular).
- CNS, transitional: parenchymal (hypodense lesions with enhancement, edema); encephalitic (diffuse cerebral edema, multiple small enhancing lesions); meningeal (CSF changes and serologic evidence).

PATHOGENS

- CNS, inactive: parenchymal (one or more calcifications); meningeal (hydrocephalus with normal CSF and calcifications).
- Ocular: live parasites can be directly visualized, surgical removal recommended.
- Spinal cord: surgical removal recommended along with chemotherapy for spinal subarachnoid disease; with degenerating intramedullary parasites, steroids + chemotherapy.
- Somatic: manifests as calcified lesions on plain radiographs, no intervention required.
- Intestinal: humans definitive host for *T. solium* tapeworms; oncospheres excreted infectious to humans (auto-infection or transmission to others) leading to systemic dissemination of cysticerci.

TREATMENT

Active parenchymal neurocysticercosis

- Anti-convulsant drugs in standard doses, titrate to effect.
- Albendazole: 15 mg/kg/day or 800 mg/day PO in 2 divided doses, usually for 28 days (duration with variable recommendations).
- Praziquantel: 50–100 mg/kg/day PO in 3 divided doses for 14 days +/– cimetidine 400 mg PO 3 times a day to increase PZQ levels.
- Corticosteroids: some use dexamethasone 6–12 mg/day in divided doses prior to initiation of specific chemotherapy to reduce inflammatory response to parasites dying from drug.
- Cimetidine 400 mg PO twice daily or 3 times a day to increase PZQ or ABZ levels.

Inactive parenchymal disease

- Phenytoin or carbamazepine in standard doses, titrated to effect, may need to be long-term in presence of calcifications for control of seizures, but perhaps short-term if lesions disappear by CT.
- Anti-helminthic treatment (praziquantel or albendazole) not recommended.
- Surgical intervention (shunt), if required, to relieve intracranial hypertension.

Extra-parenchymal disease

- Ventricular: symptoms resulting from hydrocephalus require shunt; not all cysts require surgery; surgery may be necessary for removal of 3rd/4th ventricle cysts; ependymitis may lead to clogged shunt.
- With shunt in the setting of ventricular disease, ABZ or PZQ associated with better outcome; unknown whether chemotherapy alone is effective.
- Subarachnoid: anticonvulsants as needed; surgery for giant cysts in Sylvian fissure; corticosteroids for involvement of basilar cisterns, meningitis; shunting.
- Spinal and ocular: surgical removal of subarachnoid lesions; chemotherapy +/– corticosteroids for inflamed intramedullary lesions.

OTHER INFORMATION

- Diagnosis and management should be in consultation with an expert in the field.
- In the U.S., neurocysticercosis may be in differential diagnosis of malignant brain tumor.
- Serological diagnosis remains experimental and not generally available in the United States. Contact the Centers for Disease Control in Atlanta for definitive Western blot testing which can test serum and spinal fluid; 770-488-4056.
- In the U.S., neurocysticercosis may be in differential diagnosis of malignant brain tumor.

BASIS FOR RECOMMENDATIONS

Garcia HH, Pretell EJ, Gilman RH, et al. A trial of antiparasitic treatment to reduce the rate of seizures due to cerebral cysticercosis. *N Engl J Med*, 2004; Vol. 350; pp. 249–58.

Comments: It has been unclear whether anti-helminthic therapy directed against *T. solium* is beneficial for neurocystic-ercosis, the most common cause of acquired epilepsy in the world, because of spontaneous, immune-mediated killing of parasites within the brain resulting in calcification. Treatment of calcified lesions is widely thought to have little or no important clinical effect. These authors carried out a double-blind, placebo-controlled trial in which 120 pts with living cysticerci in the brain and seizures treated with antiepileptic drugs were randomly assigned to receive either 800 mg of albendazole per day and 6 mg of dexamethasone per day for 10 days (60 pts) or two placebos (60 pts). They found that In pts with seizures due to viable parenchymal cysts, antiparasitic therapy decreases the burden of parasites and is safe and effective, at least in reducing the number of seizures with generalization.

TOXOPLASMA GONDII

Joseph Vinetz, MD

MICROBIOLOGY

- Protozoan parasite, transmitted either through ingestion of undercooked meat or oocysts in cat feces.

CLINICAL

- Protozoan parasite with major morbidity in immunocompromised, pregnant women/fetus.
- Transmitted from undercooked meat (usually beef or pork in Western countries) and from infectious oocysts in cat feces.
- Seroprevalence varies by region. United States ~15%, France 50–75%.
- Primary infection usually subclinical in the immune competent, but can produce mono-like syndrome w/ painless lymphadenitis (usually cervical)—most commonly single but can be multiple or generalized.
- Acute disease in normal, non-pregnant host generally self-limited, not requiring treatment.
- Isolated ocular disease most commonly in otherwise healthy teenagers, young adults.
- Toxoplasma encephalitis (TE), ring-enhancing lesions in AIDS (mostly CD4 <50 cells/mm^3, arising from reactivation of latent cysts). Usual presentation is headache, focal neurological signs, weakness, and confusion. Also other immunocompromised pts: also causes chorioretinitis, systemic infection, myocarditis, pneumonitis.
- Congenital disease: arises by transplacental infection of fetus, causes severe CNS sequelae, chorioretinitis, systemic disease.
- Dx (acute): antibody detection-seroconversion or 4-fold rising titers necessary to confirm new infection, IgM can last >1 yr; demonstration of organisms in tissue (rare).
- Dx: direct detection of parasite by microscopy of affected tissue; culture of blood or tissue—especially immunocompromised (rarely done, expensive), PCR (for TE, specificity is good (96%–100%), but sensitivity is low (50%). For TE, typical CT or MRI show multiple ring-enhancing lesions with surrounding edema, classically in basal ganglia region. Occasionally TE can present as a single lesion, and ddx includes primary CNS lymphoma, TB, cryptococcosis, brain abscess, PML and Chagas disease. PET or SPECT scans can help distinguish between toxo and primary CNS lymphoma.

SITES OF INFECTION

- CNS: encephalitis, seizures, coma. Visualized typically as multifocal lesions on contrast brain CT or MRI, especially affecting basal ganglia. Radiographic appearance + therapeutic response = most diagnoses.
- Eye: chorioretinitis, can be necrotizing, important to distinguish from CMV or VZV (PORN) in AIDS.
- Lymph node: isolated, multiple or generalized lymphadenopathy.
- Heart: myocarditis, in the severely immunocompromised.
- Lung: pneumonitis, in the immunocompromised, particularly bone marrow transplant pts.
- Systemic: wide dissemination particularly in congenital infection.

TREATMENT

Primary Infection

- Acute disease in immunocompetent, non-pregnant pts usually requires no treatment, as self-limiting.
- Consider treatment (as below) if visceral disease exists or symptoms are severe or persistent.

Immunocompromised/reactivation Infection

- TE often treated empirically looking for clinical and radiographic response within 2 wks of initiation of anti-toxo therapy to "confirm" diagnosis.
- Treatment (AIDS, preferred): 200 mg × 1 load pyrimethamine 50–100 mg/day + leucovorin 10–20 mg/day + sulfadiazine 1–1.5 g four times a day all PO × 6 wks after resolution of signs/symptoms including resolution of enhancement on MRI imaging; followed by pyrimethamine 25 mg/day + leucovorin 15 mg/day + sulfadiazine 500 mg PO four times a day indefinitely (or until immune reconstitution).
- Folinic acid (leucovorin) 15–20 mg PO daily prevents bone marrow suppressive effect of pyrimethamine.

PATHOGENS

- Alternatives: pyrimethamine load 200 mg × 1, then 50–100 mg/day + leucovorin 10–20 mg/day + clindamycin 600 mg four times a day (PO or IV).
- TMP-SMX possible option if pts unable to tolerate sulfadiazine + pyrimethamine.
- Atovaquone 750 mg PO q6h + pyrimethamine + leucovorin or sulfadiazine (or if unable to tolerate sulfa or pyrimethamine, as single agent); azithromycin 1200–1500 mg PO daily plus pyrimethamine plus leucovorin.
- Other regimens examined in small studies: clarithromycin 500 mg twice daily plus pyrimethamine; 5-fluorouracil plus clindamycin; dapsone plus pyrimethamine plus leucovorin; minocycline or doxycycline combined with either pyrimethamine plus leucovorin, sulfadiazine, or clarithromycin.
- If pt unable to take PO, little data exist regarding parenteral options. Consider TMP-SMX IV or clindamycin IV + oral pyrimethamine.
- If corticosteroids needed for CNS mass effect, use shortest duration possible.

Secondary Prophylaxis After Treatment of TE in AIDS
- Preferred: pyrimethamine 25–50 mg plus sulfadiazine 500–1000 mg four times a day (50% of acute dose) plus leucovorin 10–25 mg daily (also protects against PCP).
- May give total dose of sulfadiazine either twice or four times daily.
- Alt: pyrimethamine 25–50 mg plus clindamycin 600 mg PO three times a day (lower doses have higher failure rates, not protective against PCP) or atovaquone 750 mg q6–12h + pyrimethamine 25 mg + leukovorin 10 mg daily.

Pregnancy
- Spiramycin 3–4 g/day in three divided doses in first trimester. Prevent transmission.
- Treatment of the pregnant pt for toxoplasmosis is the same as above usually with pyrimethamine + leukovorin + sulfonamide or clindamycin.

Primary Prophylaxis
- All HIV-infected pts should be checked for toxo IgG antibody. Repeat antibody testing advised if CD4 <100 cell/mm³ if not taking a PCP prophylactic regimen known to be active against toxo (e.g., aerosolized pentamidine).
- HIV-infected, seronegative pts should be advised to avoid eating raw/undercooked meats and have others handle kitty litter.
- HIV only if CD4 <100 cells/mm³, toxo IgG seropositive.
- TMP-SMX DS PO daily.
- Alternatives: TMP-SMX DS three times/wk, dapsone 50 mg PO daily + pyrimethamine 50 mg PO q wk + leucovorin 25 mg PO q wk (also effective against PCP).
- Monotherapy with dapsone, pyrimethamine, azithromycin or clarithromycin not recommended.
- Can discontinue maintenance or prophylaxis if effective HIV virologic control on HAART, CD4 >200 cells/mm³ × 6 mos.

Follow Up
- Consider brain biopsy for pts who fail to respond to anti-toxo therapy for TE.
- If LP performed, EBV positive PCR highly suggestive of primary CNS lymphoma in pts with AIDS and CNS mass lesion(s).
- Reports of immune reconstitution in setting of toxoplasmosis exist.

Other Information
- Rx of seroconversion in pregnancy not always effective in preventing congenital dz or sequelae.
- Risk of toxoplasmosis in HIV-infected pts seronegative for *T. gondii* is low.
- Human-to-human spread impossible since spread occurs from ingesting oocysts excreted by animals or ingesting undercooked meat.

Basis for Recommendations
Kaplan JE, Benson C, Holmes KH, et al. Guidelines for prevention and treatment of opportunistic infections in HIV-infected adults and adolescents: recommendations from CDC, the National Institutes of Health, and the HIV Medicine Association of the Infectious Diseases Society of America. *MMWR Recomm Rep,* 2009; Vol. 58; pp. 1–207; quiz CE1–4. **Comments:** Guidelines for treatment of toxoplasma encephalitis used here.

Montoya JG, Liesenfeld O. Toxoplasmosis. *Lancet,* 2004; Vol. 363; pp. 1965–76.

Comments: This is a very useful recent summary of the state-of-the-art of diagnosis of toxoplasmosis by leading experts in the field. Of importance, an update on management of pts with acute infection, pregnant women who acquire infection during gestation, fetuses or infants who are congenitally infected, those with ocular disease, and immunocompromised individuals is provided. Controversy about the effectiveness of primary and secondary prevention in pregnant women is discussed.

TRICHOMONAS VAGINALIS

Noreen A. Hynes, MD, MPH

MICROBIOLOGY

- *Trichomonas vaginalis* (TV) is a 5–15 µm, pear-shaped, motile, flagellated protozoan parasite that exists in the trophozoite stage only.
- Facultative anaerobe, divides by binary fission; optimal growth in moist milieu at a pH of 4.9–7.5 and a temperature of 35°C–37°C.
- Trichomonads gather in clusters on the stratified urogenital epithelium, covering only a small surface area; invade the superficial epithelium causing damage directly beneath the clustered trichomonads; non-specific inflammatory response is noted in the lamina propria with plasma cells, lymphocytes, and neutrophils present. Superficial ulceration of the epithelium can occur.
- Can survive up to 45 minutes on clothing, washcloths, and in bath water.

CLINICAL

- The most common non-viral STD in the U.S. with 7.3 million estimated new cases each yr; U.S. prevalence among women is ~3.1% (1.2% in non-Hispanic white women, 13.%% in non-Hispanic black women). Risk factors in U.S. include being born in the U.S., age >20 yrs, lower educational level, poverty, vaginal douching, having a greater number of lifetime sexual partners, non-Hispanic black race/ethnicity.
- Increases risk of acquisition and transmission of HIV by disruption of epithelium, increase in the number of CD4+ lymphocytes in vaginal, cervical, or urethral secretions; increases HIV RNA concentration in the seminal plasma of HIV-infected men with urethritis caused by *T. vaginalis,* or lymphocyte activation.
- Co-existing infection with other STDs very common therefore test for other treatable STDs.
- **Spectrum of disease in women:** ranges from asymptomatic infection (approximately 50%) to severe infection with complicating pelvic inflammatory disease.
- **Common findings in symptomatic women:** discharge—profuse, sometimes frothy, yellow-green to grey, homogeneous, with or without a mild fishy odor; vulvovaginal area—usually erythematous; cervix—ectocervical erythema, colpitis macularis ("strawberry cervix") caused by punctate hemorrhages is pathognomonic but infrequently seen (2–5% of infections); pruritis—occasional complaint; some may complain of dysuria; lower abdominal tenderness may be noted (up to 10%) signals possible salpingitis and need to manage for pelvic inflammatory disease (See Vaginal Discharge module and Pelvic Inflammatory Disease module).
- **Infection in pregnant women:** infection (definitely) and treatment (possibly) is associated with perinatal morbidity, therefore risks and benefits need to be discussed with the pt.
- **Spectrum of disease in men:** ranges from asymptomatic infection (up to 75%) to severe infection with complicating epididymitis or prostatitis.
- **Common findings in symptomatic men:** non-gonococcal urethritis with mucoid to purulent discharge in 30–50% of men occurring ≤10 days from exposure; local inflammation including balanitis or balanoposthitis may be seen.
- **Point of care diagnosis:** includes clinical exam findings and pH of discharge >4.5 (sensitivity = 56%, specificity = 50%); saline wet preparation of vaginal or urethral discharges, prostatic secretions, and urine sediments—motile trichomonads (60–70% sensitive compared with culture) and increased PMNs (ratio of PMNs to vaginal epithelial cells >1:1 but can also be seen in gonorrhea, chlamydia, and HSV discharge). 10% KOH slide yields positive "whiff" test (increase in foul fishy odor upon the addition of 10% KOH to vaginal discharge sample) in some cases. Other non-microscopy based FDA-cleared point of care diagnostics are >83% sensitive and >97% specific and include: OSOM Trichomonas Rapid Test (Genezyme Diagnostics, Cambridge, MA) which takes 10 minutes (83% sensitivity, 98.8% specificity).

PATHOGENS

Culture using Diamond's media and commercially available culture based tests such as the InPouch system are 90–95% sensitive and >95% specific.

- **Laboratory-based diagnosis:** Culture is considered the diagnostic gold standard; Nucleic acid detection techniques include both direct detection probes and amplification methods. The Affirm VPIII (Becton Dickinson and Co, Sparks, MD) is a direct DNA probe test for detection of organisms collected using vaginal swabs testing for bacterial vaginosis, *Candida albicans,* and *T. vaginalis.* The sensitivity of the *T. vaginalis* component of the assay is 90% and the specificity is 98%. Nucleic acid amplification tests such as polymerase chain reaction are not available commercially at this time.

SITES OF INFECTION

- Female urogenital epithelium: vagina, cervix, urethra, bartholin glands, Skene's ducts, bladder, fallopian tubes.
- Male urogenital epithelium: urethra, epididymis, prostate, bladder; semen.
- Neonatal infection: up to 17% of female infants born to infected mothers develop vaginal infections due to influence of maternal estrogen on neonatal vaginal epithelium; pneumonia may also occur following passage through infected birth canal.

TREATMENT
Uncomplicated Urogenital Infection in Men and Non-pregnant Women

- Metronidazole 2 g PO once.
- Tinidazole 2 g PO once.
- Alternative treatment: metronidazole 500 mg PO q12h × 7 days.

Treatment of Uncomplicated Urogenital Infection in Pregnant and Lactating Women

- Metronidazole 2 g PO × 1 may be used. If post-partum and breastfeeding, do not breastfeed for 12–24 hrs following treatment.
- Pregnant women should be advised of the risk and benefits to treatment as infection (definitely) and treatment (possibly) associated with perinatal morbidity. Consider deferring treatment until >37 wks gestation.

Cystitis

- **Women:** Metronidazole or tinidazole 500 mg PO q12h × 7 days.
- **Men:** Metronidazole or tinidazole 500 mg PO q12h × 7 days followed by test of cure and urinary tract evaluation in consultation with a specialist.

Prostatitis

- Metronidazole 500 mg PO twice daily × 28 days followed by test of cure. If cure not acheived, further management should be in consultation with a specialist.
- Tinidazole 500 mg PO twice daily × 28 days followed by test of cure. If cure not acheived, further management should be in consultation with a specialist.

Pelvic Inflammatory Disease (in the presence of *T. vaginalis*)

- **Outpatient regimens:** ceftriaxone 250 mg IM × 1 plus doxycycline 100 mg PO twice daily × 14 days plus metronidazole 500 mg PO twice daily × 14 days or cefoxitin 2 g IM plus probenecid 1 g PO × 1 plus doxycycline 100 mg PO twice daily × 14 days plus metronidazole 500 mg PO twice daily × 14 days or other parenteral 3rd generation cephalosporin plus doxycycline 100 mg PO twice daily × 14 days plus metronidazole 500 mg PO twice daily × 14 days.
- **Inpatient regimens:** cefoxitin 2 g IV q6h plus doxycycline 100 mg IV or PO q12h plus metronidazole 500 mg PO or IV q12h for at least 24 hrs after clinical improvement, then outpatient regimen to complete 14 days or Clindamycin 900 mg IV q8h plus gentamicin loading dose IV/IM (2 mg/kg), then 1.5 mg/kg q8h or 5 mg/kg once daily plus metronidazole 500 mg PO or IV q12h for at least 24 hrs after clinical improvement, then change to outpatient regimen to complete 14 days.

Epididymitis

- Metronidazole 500 mg PO q12h × 10 days.
- Adjunctive treatment: bed rest; scrotal elevation; analgesics until fever and local inflammation subside. Reexamine every pt within 72 hrs to assess original DX and RX. Failure to improve by this time requires reevaluation of diagnosis and treatment. Swelling and tenderness persisting after completion of antibiotics should be evaluated comprehensively with a differential diagnosis considering: (1) tumor, (2) abscess, (3) infarction, (4) testicular cancer, (5) TB, and (6) fungi.

Treatment of Patients with Metronidazole or Tinidazole Hypersensitivity

- Consult the Division of STD Prevention at the U.S. Centers for Disease Control and Prevention for metronidazole desensitization protocols (oral and intravenous) and other possible treatment options at 404-639-1898.

FOLLOW UP

- All current sexual partners of infected pts should be treated to prevent pt reinfection; non-current sexual partners with whom there has been sexual contact in the past 90 days should be referred for evaluation and possible treatment.
- All pts should be tested for co-infection with other STDs including HIV, chlamydia, gonorrhea (in populations with high prevalence) and syphilis (in populations with high prevalence).
- Advise pts to avoid sexual intercourse until treatment is complete and partner(s) have been treated and both pt and partners are free of symptoms.
- Retreat pts with uncomplicated infections with the 7-days regimen rather than the single-dose regimen should the infection not resolve; insure that all partners have been identified and treated. Pts failing retreatment should be managed in consultation with an expert.
- Pt education regarding infection avoidance, including use of male latex or female condoms should be stressed.
- Woman with PID or who are pregnant need follow-up during and following treatment.
- Men with cystitis, epididymitis, or prostatitis need follow-up during and following treatment.

OTHER INFORMATION

- The majority of infections are asymptomatic. This along with the organism's role in the transmission and acquisition of HIV infection underscores the importance of routine testing for this pathogen amongst pts who are not in long-term mutually monogamous sexual relationships.
- *T. vaginalis* induces local production of secretary IgA in women but rarely in infected men. Antibodies to the IgG class of antibodies becomes undetectable after treatment.
- Despite the repeated isolation of the organism from fomites, non-sexual transmission is rare.
- Factors that may play a role in treatment failure of vaginal trichomoniasis: adherence to the treatment regimen if other than single-dose therapy; vomiting after taking the drug thereby preventing therapeutic level from being attained; re-infection from an untreated or incompletely treated sexual partner; inactivation of metronidazole by aerobic or anaerobic vaginal bacteria; low plasma zinc level (rare).
- Metronidazole resistance has been documented in 2.5% to 9.6% of clinical isolates; resistance is defined as an aerobic minimal lethal concentration (MLC) of ≥ 50 micrograms/mL. Most resistance is considered to be mild, i.e., MLC of 50–100 micrograms/mL meaning they can be cured with either a higher dose of metronidazole or tinidazole therapy.

BASIS FOR RECOMMENDATIONS

Centers for Disease Control and Prevention, Workowski KA, Berman SM. Sexually transmitted diseases treatment guidelines, 2006. *MMWR Recomm Rep*, 2006; Vol. 55; pp. 1–94.

Comments: The information in this report updates the *Sexually Transmitted Diseases Treatment Guidelines, 2002.* Included in these updated guidelines are an expanded diagnostic evaluation for trichomoniasis; new antimicrobial recommendations for trichomoniasis; discussion of the role of trichomoniasis in urethritis/cervicitis and treatment-related implications. These guidelines available electronically at: http://www.cdc.gov/std/treatment/

PATHOGENS

Viruses

ADENOVIRUS

Lisa A. Spacek, MD, PhD and Khalil G. Ghanem, MD, PhD

MICROBIOLOGY

- Non-enveloped virus w/ double-stranded DNA, 52 known serotypes. Similar viruses found in monkeys, bovine species, and birds.
- Mostly respiratory spread; also person-to-person, water, fomites and instruments.
- May remain infectious at room temperature up to 3 wks; high potential for transmission.
- Stable at low pH, resistant to gastric and biliary secretions. Virus can replicate to high viral load in gut.
- Can remain latent in lymphoepithelial tissue.

CLINICAL

- Epidemiology: ubiquitous, worldwide. Endemic in pediatric population. Crowding is a risk factor for acute infection (military personnel at high risk).
- Respiratory and conjunctival infections most common. Mild pharyngitis/tracheitis in children. Bronchiolitis and pneumonia in infants. Mild tracheobronchitis in adults is the norm, but atypical pneumonia also occurs.
- Broad spectrum of disease due to serotype and tissue tropisms. Both T-cell-mediated and humoral immunity important for control.
- Children: URI (associated serotypes 1, 2, 4–6), diarrhea (2, 3, 5, 40, and 41), hemorrhagic cystitis (7, 11, and 21), pharyngo-conjunctivitis (3 and 7), and meningo-encephalitis (2, 6, 7, and 12).
- Adults: URI (3, 4, and 7), pneumonia and keratoconjunctivitis (8, 19, and 37) common. Adenovirus 14 causes very serious pneumonia in previously healthy young adults (Louie JK. *CID* 2008;46:421).
- Immunocompromised hosts: may develop disseminated infection, most commonly involves lungs, liver, and urinary tract: pneumonia (5, 31, 34, 35, and 39), UTI/hemorrhagic cystitis, intestinal infection (42–47) and meningoencephalitis (7, 12, and 32).
- Solid-organ transplant recipients: disease site is usually transplanted organ. In pediatric liver transplant, incidence 4–10% with 53% mortality. Renal transplant, hemorrhagic cystitis and pneumonia with 17% mortality. Adenovirus detected in 50% pediatric lung or heart-lung transplant with bronchiolitis or graft loss.
- Dx: growth in tissue culture (2–7 days), PCR (rapid and sensitive), real-time PCR for viral quantification Ag by immunofluorescence or ELISA, four-fold rise in serum antibodies, acute and convalescent serum required.
- Serotyping mostly a tool for outbreak investigations, research.

SITES OF INFECTION

- Fatal disseminated infections in neonates (serotypes 3, 7, 21, and 30 frequently involved).
- Coryza/pharyngitis in infants (1, 2, and 5).
- Pharyngoconjunctival fever occurs in children: fever, conjunctivitis, pharyngitis, rhinitis, and cervical adenitis. Associated w/ type 3 infection.
- Eyes: epidemic keratoconjunctivitis in adults (types 8, 19, and 37). Conjunctivitis may last 1 to 4 wks. Keratitis may last several mos. Secondary spread to household contacts occurs in 10% of cases.
- Genitourinary: hemorrhagic cystitis in children and immunocompromised adults. Duration of symptoms ~7 days.
- Gastrointestinal: infantile diarrhea-watery, associated w/ fever, 1–2 wks duration. Intussusception in children. A preceding or concurrent respiratory illness is common.
- CNS: acute encephalitis or meningo-encephalitis especially in children and immunocompromised adults. Chronic meningoencephalitis reported in pts w/ hypogammaglobulinemia.

TREATMENT

Prevention

- Hand washing is an effective means of prevention for all adenoviral infections.
- In an epidemic, the Standard Precautions (hand washing, antiseptic solutions, respiratory isolation) plus cohorting of both pts and staff has been effective in controlling nosocomial transmission.
- Effective prevention was shown with an oral vaccine used successfully in the military. Production of the oral vaccine ceased in 1996, no vaccine is currently FDA approved.
- Oral vaccine contained live, non-attenuated adenovirus types 4 and 7, which produce protective antibody responses.

Chemotherapy

- Most adenoviral infections in immunocompetent hosts are self-limited and do not require therapy.
- Drugs that are FDA-licensed for other indications (e.g., cidofovir, ribavirin) are used to treat severe adenoviral infections. Preemptive therapy and reduced immunosuppression used in cases of viremia and severe lymphocytopenia.
- Cidofovir used in stem cell and solid organ transplant; significant side effects are nephrotoxicity, myelosuppression, and uveitis. All serotypes susceptible *in vitro*.
- Ribavirin used with mixed results, serotypes susceptible to ribavirin may be limited (1, 2, 5, and 6).
- Immune recovery, CD4 increase, and serotype-specific neutralizing antibodies correlate with viral clearance.

OTHER INFORMATION

- Associations between serotypes and clinical syndromes exhibit some geographic variation.
- Complement-fixing Abs are group-specific and disappear within a yr. Neutralizing and hemagglutination-inhibiting Abs are type-specific and may persist for ~10 yrs or longer.

BASIS FOR RECOMMENDATIONS

Echavarría, M. Adenoviruses in immunocompromised hosts. *Clin Microbiol Rev*, 2008; Vol. 21; pp. 704–715.
Comments: Current review of literature with focus on pathogenesis and molecular diagnostic methods.

Ison MG. Adenovirus infections in transplant recipients. *Clin Infect Dis*, 2006; Vol. 43; pp. 331–339.
Comments: An excellent review highlighting that clinical presentations range from asymptomatic viremia to respiratory and gastrointestinal disease, hemorrhagic cystitis, and severe disseminated illness.

CYTOMEGALOVIRUS

Lisa Spacek, MD, PhD

MICROBIOLOGY

- Member of the betaherpesvirus group with envelope and dsDNA; establishes lifelong latency.
- Transmitted sexually or by close contact (family members, daycare), blood or tissue exposure, perinatally. Cultured from urine, blood, throat, tears, stool, cervix, semen, breast milk.
- Seroprevalence increases with age and varies throughout the world; adult seroprevalence rates range from 40–100% and are highest in developing countries.
- Exhibits slow growth in cultured cells (can be up to 6 wks until cytopathic effect is detected in tissue culture) and cytopathology is characterized by large cells with nuclear (Cowdry owl's eye) and cytoplasmic inclusions.
- Isolation of virus or detection of viral proteins or nucleic acid defines CMV infection. Presence of signs/symptoms of end organ disease + CMV infection = CMV disease.

CLINICAL

- Immunocompetent adult: ranges from asymptomatic infection to heterophile-negative mononucleosis syndrome, characterized by protracted fevers, lassitude, and possibly a rash with absolute lymphocytosis, atypical lymphocytes and elevated transaminases.
- Transplant pts (especially between 30–100 days post txp): risk depends on type of transplant (lung > kidney), CMV serostatus of donor and recipient (D+/R–, CMV-seropositive donor/CMV-seronegative recipient), type (>> risk with antilymphocyte ab tx) and depth/duration of immune suppression. Active disease may range from asymptomatic to CMV syndrome (fever, neutropenia or thrombocytopenia, detection of CMV in blood), or signs and symptoms related to end-organ disease.

PATHOGENS

- Without prophylaxis, 80–100% D+/R– solid organ txp pts will develop CMV infection, and 50–70% of these develop CMV disease.
- HIV/AIDS: most cases of CMV disease occur in setting of advanced immunosuppression, CD4 < 50.
- Congenital: 90% of newborns with congenital infection are asymptomatic at birth; 10% will have microcephaly, seizures, abnormal neurologic exam, sensorineural hearing loss, feeding difficulties. Greatest risk with primary infection of mother during pregnancy: first trimester (2% risk to fetus) to third trimester (28% risk).
- Dx of CMV disease is made by the combination of appropriate clinical syndrome + detection of CMV in blood, plasma, or tissue in the absence of other likely microbial etiology.
- Dx: culture in human fibroblasts (time consuming); shell vial (monoclonal ab to early CMV ag in cultured cells, 2–3 days); serology (IgM/IgG-used in dx of primary infection only in immunocompetent host); antigenemia (ag detection in neutrophils w/ ab against CMV matrix protein pp. 65); PCR using primers for early antigens or for CMV DNA polymerase, PCR can be qualitative or quantitative. PCR assays have largely replaced antigen studies in clinical practice.
- CMV antigenemia and quantitative PCR assay may be negative despite significant disease involving the GI, pulmonary or CNS systems.

Sites of Infection

- Organ specific manifestations of CMV are rare in immunocompetent pts, however, pneumonia, colitis, myocarditis, meningoencephalitis have been reported. Elevated liver enzymes are frequently encountered in pts with symptomatic CMV infection. Guillain-Barre syndrome also has been associated with CMV.
- **Transplant:** the allograft is a "privileged" site for CMV replication given MHC mismatch; pneumonitis (especially lung transplant and BMT; up to 84% mortality in BMT); hepatitis (especially liver txp); nephritis; esophagitis, gastritis, colitis (GI disease common among all solid organ transplants), meningoencephalitis, myocarditis, pancreatitis. CMV chorioretinitis is a rare manifestation of CMV disease in txp recipients.
- **Transplant:** effects of CMV disease include indirect immunomodulatory effects, higher rates of bacterial and invasive fungal infections, posttransplant lymphoproliferative disease, acute allograft rejection, chronic allograft rejection, and allograft loss.
- **Congenital:** small infant size, jaundice, hepatosplenomegaly, petechial/purpuric rash, microcephaly, chorioretinitis.
- **Perinatal** (via milk or cervical secretions): asymptomatic; subtle effects on hearing and intelligence possible long-term.
- AIDS: retinitis (CD4 < 50), polyradiculopathy and meningoencephalitis, esophagitis, colitis. CMV as a sole cause of pneumonia is not common, but can occur in very late stages of HIV disease.

Treatment (in Transplant Recipients)
Prevention

- The provision of CMV negative bone marrow, stem cells, or solid organs to CMV-negative recipients is recommended, if possible.
- Giving CMV-negative or leukocyte-depleted blood products to txp recipients is highly effective.
- Txp pts who are sexually active and not in long-term monogamous relationships should use latex condoms during sexual contacts.
- Handling or changing diapers or wiping oral secretions from toddlers represents a potential risk for CMV transmission to seronegative individuals and should be avoided.

Prophylaxis vs Pre-emptive Therapy

- Prophylaxis = treat all D+ or R+ pts (universal prophylaxis); high risk solid organ txp: D+/R– pts or R+ pts treated with antilymphocyte antibodies (ATG, thymoglobulin, OKT3 or similar); or high risk BMT: D+ or R+, mismatched or unrelated txp, GVHD.
- Solid organ prophylaxis: ganciclovir IV (5 mg/kg/day) or valganciclovir (900 PO mg/day) × 3–6 mos. Optimal duration uncertain, depends on depth of immunosuppression.
- Pre-emptive tx: only treat pts w/ evidence of CMV infection (in blood or lungs) detected by viral surveillance monitoring (+CMV antigenemia or PCR) after txp to prevent active disease. Prophylaxis and pre-emptive both effective in preventing CMV disease.

- Pre-emptive tx against early CMV (<100 days after txp) for allogeneic txp is preferred for D+/R– given low attack rate if screened or filtered blood product support is used: IV ganciclovir 5 mg/kg IV twice daily for 14 days then 5 mg/kg/day for 5 days/wks until day 100 posttransplant or until antigenemia or PCR is negative. Foscarnet (90 mg/kg IV twice daily for 2 wks followed by 90 mg/kg IV once daily 5 days per wk for 2 wks) as effective as ganciclovir for allogeneic BMT recipients. Combination not more effective and more toxic.
- In D+/R– kidney, liver, pancreas, heart: oral ganciclovir, valganciclovir, or valacyclovir (in kidney) for 3 mos, or IV ganciclovir for 1–3 mos. Pre-emptive therapy **not** preferred. CMV Ig maybe added.
- In R+ kidney, liver, pancreas, heart: oral ganciclovir, valganciclovir, or valacyclovir (in kidney) for 3 mos, or IV ganciclovir for 1–3 mos, or pre-emptive therapy, or clinical observation in low risk pts.
- In D+/R– or D+/R+ lung, heart-lung: IV gancyclovir or oral valganciclovir for 3 mos, oral ganciclovir can be used in R+, CMV Ig may be used, prophylaxis may be extended to 6 mos (esp in D+/R–).
- FDA cautions against use of valganciclovir in liver recipients because of greater incidence of invasive disease detected in a valganciclovir vs. oral ganciclovir study. However, many experts cite a study bias and recommend valganciclovir.
- In the setting of treatment of acute rejection (high dose steroids, antilymphocyte antibody therapy, or OKT3), consider prophylactic valganciclovir.

Therapy
- Immunocompetent host: usually self-limited; no specific antiviral therapy necessary.
- Solid organ txp, invasive end-organ disease and or high viral loads: ganciclovir 5 mg/kg IV q12h induction × 14–21 days or until documented clearance of viremia and/or significant clinical improvement.
- CMV IV Ig often used for severe interstitial pneumonitis, relapsing or resistant CMV infections. No good prospective data in these populations.
- HSCT pneumonia: IV ganciclovir 5 mg/kg q12 × 21 days then 5 mg/kg q24 × 3–4 wks **plus** IV Ig (500 mg/kg) or CMV-IG (150 mg/kg) 2 ×/wk × 2 wks then qwk for 4 wks.
- HSCT w/ CMV GI or retinitis: ganciclovir 5 mg/kg q12 × 14–21 days then q24 × 3–4 wks or until day 100. Substitute foscarnet 90 mg/kg q12h for ganciclovir in case of BM suppression.
- Cidofovir has documented effectiveness in cases of CMV retinitis. Cross-resistance to ganciclovir-resistant strains relatively common, especially w/ high-level ganciclovir resistance. Limited use in txp pts.
- Consider valganciclovir 900 mg PO twice daily for induction therapy in the absence of tissue invasive disease, because of excellent bioavailability. Some experts treat asymptomatic viremia or mild disease (clinical symptoms present—CMV syndrome) with valganciclovir for a minimum of 21 days or longer until viremia clears.
- Valganciclovir approved for the treatment of CMV retinitis in pts with AIDS.
- Discontinue or decrease dose of antimetabolite (azathioprine or mycophenolate mofetil) during treatment of CMV disease. The severity of disease and risk of rejection dictate when/if to restart the antimetabolite.

FOLLOW UP
- Risk factors for late (after day 100) CMV disease in HSCT include unrelated or T-cell depleted transplants, chronic GVHD, steroid use, CD4 counts <50, and CMV infection before day 100.
- Risk for CMV relapse in allogeneic BMT if mismatched unrelated donor and GVHD.
- BMT: if antigenemia/positive PCR persists > 4 wks or levels increase after 3 wks, assume resistance; discontinue ganciclovir, begin foscarnet.
- Solid organ: factors associated with the development of clinically significant ganciclovir resistance: D+/R– serostatus, prolonged exposure to ganciclovir, potent immunosuppression, suboptimal ganciclovir levels, and high virus load.
- Solid organ: If quantitative PCR does not decrease by 50% 2 wks into treatment, suspect viral resistance and re-assess recipient immunocompetence.
- Continue treatment for one wk after finding a negative CMV PCR and after resolution of organ specific signs/symptoms of infection.
- Consider secondary prophylaxis for an additional 3 mos after initial treatment of CMV infection/disease, especially in those at high risk for recurrence (D+/R–).

PATHOGENS

OTHER INFORMATION

- CMV (21%) vs. EBV (79%) causing mono-like sx: CMV associated with less tonsillopharyngitis, lymphadenopathy, splenomegaly; more systemic symptoms ("typhoidal") and hepatitis.
- Late CMV infections: early use of antiviral therapy at time of engraftment delays immune reconstitution against the virus, placing the pts at risk for late (>100 days) disease when prophylaxis discontinued.
- Valganciclovir (pro-drug of ganciclovir) has 60–70% oral bioavailability. Effective in AIDS CMV retinitis. Clinical use in txp pts increasing.
- Cross resistance between ganciclovir and valganciclovir. Cross-resistance between ganciclovir and foscarnet uncommon.
- Because resistance testing is time consuming, dx of resistance is made clinically based on clinical evidence of Rx failure. Modify Rx while awaiting resistance test.

BASIS FOR RECOMMENDATIONS

Griffiths P, Whitley R, Snydman DR, et al. Contemporary management of cytomegalovirus infection in transplant recipients: guidelines from an IHMF workshop, 2007. *Herpes*, 2008; Vol. 15; pp. 4–12.

Comments: These guidelines suggest that baseline pre-emptive therapy with oral valganciclovir should be the comparator for new drug evaluation because it is widely used in clinical practice in many groups of txp pts.

Preiksaitis JK, Brennan DC, Fishman J, et al. Canadian society of transplantation consensus workshop on cytomegalovirus management in solid organ transplantation final report. *Am J Transplant*, 2005; Vol. 5; pp. 218–27.

Comments: Partly the basis for recommendations in this module.

Paya C, Humar A, Dominguez E, et al. Efficacy and safety of valganciclovir vs. oral ganciclovir for prevention of cytomegalovirus disease in solid organ transplant recipients. *Am J Transplant*, 2004; Vol. 4; pp. 611–20.

Comments: A phase III randomized, prospective, double-blind, double-dummy study that compared the efficacy and safety of valganciclovir with PO ganciclovir (administered through 100 days after txp) for prevention of CMV disease in high risk (D+/R–) kidney, kidney-pancreas, heart, and liver txp recipients. The incidence of CMV disease was similar in the valganciclovir and ganciclovir study groups at 6 and 12 mos after transplant. The safety profile was similar for both drugs.

Centers for Disease Control and Prevention, Infectious Disease Society of America, American Society of Blood and Marrow Transplantation. Guidelines for preventing opportunistic infections among hematopoietic stem cell transplant recipients. *MMWR Recomm Rep*, 2000; Vol. 49; pp. 1–125, CE1–7.

Comments: Partly the basis for recommendations in this module.

ENTEROVIRUS

Paul G. Auwaerter, MD

MICROBIOLOGY

- Member of Picornaviridae, (+) single strand RNA virus.
- Formerly classified as belonging to four groups (Echoviruses, Coxsackie A, Coxsackie B, and polioviruses), but now non-polio enteroviruses separated into Coxsackie A, Coxsackie B, echovirus and others (newly discovered enteroviruses named by consecutive number: e.g., EV70).
- Ubiquitous virus, totalling 62 non-polio enterovirus types: Group A Coxsackieviruses (1–22, 24), Group B Coxsackieviruses (1–6), Echoviruses (1–9, 11–21, 24–27, 29–33) and Enteroviruses (68–71).
- Believed to be second most common cause of human viral infection after rhinoviruses.

CLINICAL

- Enteroviruses spread mostly by fecal-oral route, but also found in respiratory secretions.
- Peak acquisition typically in late summer and early fall. Often spread in schools, daycare centers, and/or by contact with infected infants/toddlers during diaper changes.
- Incubation period typically 3–5 days, but for CNS may be up to 12 days after acquisition of infection.
- CSF findings may include PMN predominance early in infection that then changes to mononuclear cell pleocytosis.
- Dx: isolation of virus by culture or PCR from normally sterile fluid/tissue diagnostic. PCR superior to culture (in CSF PCR >80% yield vs. 30% for culture methods).

- Note isolation from stool, especially in children given frequency of infection, is not sufficient to offer a definitive (but can be a supportive) diagnosis. Stool carriage of enterovirus may go on for over 8 wks from initial infection.
- Serology available, but acute and convalescent specimens needed to secure diagnosis. Rarely helpful for acute diagnosis.

SITES OF INFECTION

- Most infections (estimated 90%) are asymptomatic or only cause mild illness.
- General viremia.
- Skin: many manifestations. Non-specific maculopapular rashes are most common, but petechial and purpuric rashes can also be seen. Hand, foot, and mouth (HFM) disease (oral vesicles on tongue or buccal mucosa plus hands/feet) is typically due to Coxsackie A virus. Herpangina (tonsillar and posterior pharyngeal vesicles with associated severe sore throat) also typically due to Coxsackie A.
- Nervous system: most common cause of aseptic meningitis (with enteroviruses accounting for perhaps 50% of cases in adults); also acute flaccid paralysis (polio, non-polio enteroviruses especially EV 71), meningoencephalitis, encephalitis.
- Cardiac: pericarditis, myocarditis.
- Ocular: acute hemorrhagic conjunctivitis.
- Respiratory: upper respiratory tract infections ("head colds," acute viral bronchitis), pleurodynia (epidemic pleurodynia sometimes called Bornholm's disease, usually Coxsackie B).
- Neonatal infection: may be disseminated and fulminant, resulting in death.

TREATMENT
General recommendations

- Most infections are self-limiting, with only supportive care needed.
- Exceptions: severely immunodeficient pts (e.g., x-linked agammaglobulinemia), severe acute myocarditis, some cases of meningitis.

Meningoencephalitis

- Treatment usually reserved for pts with severe immunodeficiency or persisting infection.
- IVIG: data is mixed with reports of both successes and failures. Most try it for severe cases, typical dose is 1–2 g/kg IV infused over 24 hrs.
- Pleconaril, an experimental antiviral drug, appeared to have some benefit, but is no longer available.

Myocarditis

- Severe cases in neonatal infants, children, and adults have been treated with IVIG, with two trials showing some benefit (e.g., improved LV function).
- IVIG: typical dose is 2 g/kg IV infused over 24 hrs.

FOLLOW UP

- Most infections are without sequelae.
- Severe infections can occasionally result in paralysis or other neurologic sequelae or, for cardiac cases, dilated cardiomyopathy.
- Immunity is specific to a given serotype.

OTHER INFORMATION

- Enteroviruses may play role in autoimmunity, provoking Type I, juvenile-onset diabetes mellitus.

BASIS FOR RECOMMENDATIONS

Lee BE, Davies HD. Aseptic meningitis. *Curr Opin Infect Dis*, 2007; Vol. 20; pp. 272–7.

Comments: Frequent problem in Emergency departments and hospital wards; PCR enterovirus diagnostics help avoid unnecessary antibiotics and/or hospital admission if done on a timely basis. Despite the advances and the frequency of enteroviral infections, the main issue is to rule-out bacterial infections due to their life-threatening nature. Supportive care remains the norm for enteroviral infection.

PATHOGENS

EPSTEIN-BARR VIRUS

Paul G. Auwaerter, MD

MICROBIOLOGY
- Human herpesvirus (HHV-4), establishes latent infection.

CLINICAL
- Subclinical infection typical (90%), especially children. Infection more prevalent in lower socioeconomic groups. EBV mostly spread by asymptomatic salivary shedding.
- 95% eventually infected by age 40, 30–50% college freshman uninfected.
- Primary symptomatic infection = infectious mononucleosis (IM peaks in teens and early 20s) with 30–70% adolescents/adults experiencing sx.
- Ddx mononucleosis syndrome: includes Gr. A Strep pharyngitis, acute CMV, acute HIV, toxoplasmosis, influenza, viral hepatitis, rubella, drug reactions.
- Elevated WBC (10–18 K), lymphocytosis (40–>60%) common. Atypical lymphocytes usually 10–30% of circulating lymphocytes.
- Dx: heterophile antibody (+) 90% [Monospot], negatives may turn (+) on repeat. 10% remain (−), use EBV- specific ABs: EBV capsid IgM and IgG (+) with negative EBNA diagnostic of acute infection if performed <4–6 wks from onset of symptoms.
- Positive EBNA in pts suspected of IM (<4–6 wks sx) strongly argues that capsid IgM/IgG titers indicate remote infection therefore NOT supportive of EBV as cause of mono-like syndrome.
- False (+) heterophile rare: lymphoma, hepatitis, SLE, HIV.
- EBV PCR most helpful for diagnosis of EBV-driven lymphoma, especially for CNS lymphoma in HIV (+) pts. Sensitivity reported as high as 97%, specificity 98% but may be less. Also useful with EBV-related meningoencephalitis.
- Do not check EBV titers merely as evaluation of fatigue. EBV is not an explanation as currently understood, for chronic fatigue syndrome.

SITES OF INFECTION
- Classic triad **infectious mononucleosis**: fever, pharyngitis, lymphadenopathy (especially posterior cervical).
- Common: elevated LFTs (ALT usually <300), splenomegaly (50%), hepatomegaly, rash (10%). Rash following amoxicillin occurs >98–100% with IM.
- Uncommon: hemolytic anemia, cytopenias, pneumonitis, carditis, seizures, palsies, Guillain-Barr, encephalitis (late).
- Pts. >35 yrs. with IM have atypical presentations with less pharyngitis, LN. These older pts instead present as hepatitis, FUO (fever of unknown origin) or uncommon complications.
- **HEENT:** oral hairy leukoplakia (HIV), nasopharyngeal carcinoma.
- **HEME:** cause of Burkitt's lymphoma, implicated in other lymphomas, especially HIV-related, post-transplant lymphoproliferative disorder.
- EBV not an acknowledged cause of Chronic Fatigue Syndrome.
- True, **chronic active EBV** (rare): pancytopenia, chronic LN, pneumonitis, abnl LFT's >8 wks. Prove by repeated positive EBV blood cx/PCR studies.

TREATMENT
Infectious Mononucleosis
- IM usually self-limited <3 wks average, rest and supportive care.
- Athletes w/ IM: no training, sports × 3 wks from onset; if contact sport e.g., football, no sports × 4 wks from onset and no splenomegaly (preferably by imaging such as ultrasound).
- Corticosteroids (prednisone 40–60 mg/day) indicated for airway obstruction, severe thrombocytopenia or hemolytic anemia. Some give for severe pharyngitis or constitutional sx (controversial).
- Acyclovir/ganciclovir: no role in IM. Reduces viral shedding in mouth, but no clinical benefit.

FOLLOW UP
- Fatigue may persist after IM in 10–20% >1 mo.
- Some information suggestive that IM is associated with subsequent increased risk of Hodgkin's lymphoma.

- By age 40, an estimated 95% of adults are infected.
- Spleen size may be normally increased in some taller individuals (3–7% see *Br J Sports Med.* 2006;40(3):251–254).

OTHER INFORMATION
- Pharyngitis and abnl LFT's tip-off toward IM rather than GAS pharyngitis.
- Roommates, household contacts no increased risk IM routinely.
- Life threatening IM complications: tonsillar airway obstruction (early), splenic rupture (1–2 wks), encephalitis (typically >1 mo after onset of sx).
- EBV-specific ABs helpful especially if heterophile (–) IM. EBV capsid IgM and IgG (+) with neg. EBNA = IM-if sx <4–6 wks. Acute EBV excluded if (+) EBNA since EBNA only expressed >6 wks acute infection as latency established.
- EBV is not a cause of chronic fatigue syndrome (although can cause a post-infectious fatigue after IM). **Don't** draw serologies for chronic fatigue sx.—no data to support as cause.

BASIS FOR RECOMMENDATIONS

Candy B, Hotopf M. Steroids for symptom control in infectious mononucleosis. *Cochrane Database Syst Rev*, 2006; Vol. 3; pp. CD004402.

Comments: Although this evidenced-based Cochrane review found insufficient literature to derive any recommendations for the use of corticosteroids to control common symptoms of IM, it should be noted that available RCTs were few in number, heterogeneous in design, and frequently underpowered to reach conclusions. Where this report leaves clinicians is less than clear: the use of corticosteroids for symptom control remains in the "art" rather than the science of medicine. Further, practitioners need to consider that most individuals will be improved in less than 4 wks regardless of interventions, and that corticosteroids could abet the transformative fires stoked by EBV, leading to future health problems.

Tynell E, Aurelius E, Brandell A, et al. Acyclovir and prednisolone treatment of acute infectious mononucleosis: a multicenter, double-blind, placebo-controlled study. *J Infect Dis*, 1996; Vol. 174; pp. 324–31.

Comments: The combination of corticosteroid and acyclovir offered no clinical benefit in IM.

HANTAVIRUS

Paul G. Auwaerter, MD and Joseph Vinetz, MD

MICROBIOLOGY
- Segmented, negative sense RNA virus.
- Member of Bunyaviridae. Rodent-borne viruses associated with specific reservoirs. For the U.S., in the Southeast deer mice, cotton, and rice rats may carry while in the Northeast the white-footed mouse has been associated.
- Transmission to humans through inhalation of aerosolized saliva, urine, or feces of reservoir host.
- Hantaviruses (Sin Nombre virus) known to cause hantavirus pulmonary syndrome (HPS) carried by the New World rats and mice, family Muridae, subfamily Sigmodontinae; these rodents are not found in urban sites.
- Hantaan virus infection may cause hemorrhagic fever with renal syndrome (HFRS). Puumala virus, a hantavirus carried in bank voles, may cause Nephropathia epidemica in humans.

CLINICAL
- Two major syndromes in humans: Hantavirus pulmonary syndrome [HPS-restricted to New World] and hemorrhagic fever with renal syndrome [HFRS-Asia, Europe].
- In U.S., most common pathogenic Hantavirus is Sin Nombre virus, cause of acute cardiopulmonary syndrome; mostly in southwestern U.S. (four corner states, mainly Arizona, Colorado); also elsewhere (Vermont, Central, and South America).
- Initially manifests as undifferentiated febrile illness, with fulminant progression to ARDS-like picture typically in previously healthy young adults. Other characteristic features include hemoconcentration.
- Early symptoms are non-specific, with cardiopulmonary sxs developing 4–10 days after the initial set.
- High case fatality rate (30–50%).
- In Old World: nonspecific febrile prodrome, signs of endothelial and hematological dysfunction, hemorrhage, back pain, retroperitoneal fluid, hypotension, shock, oliguric renal failure.

PATHOGENS

- Diagnosis: serology (hantavirus-specific (HS) IgM or rising titers of HS IgG), HS RNA by PCR or HS antigen seen on immunohistochemistry, rarely viral isolation.

SITES OF INFECTION
- Lung: pulmonary edema, respiratory failure.
- Renal: U.S.-may complicate shock but usually not primary renal disease: Old world disease, Hantaan-type virus in Asia or Puumula virus in Europe; renal failure in association with hemorrhagic fever.
- Cardiac: the pulmonary edema in U.S. Hantavirus disease can be cardiogenic associated with myocardial depression associated with viral infection of the heart.
- Heme: hemoconcentration; thrombocytopenia; severe left shift with myelocytes, promyelocytes characteristically seen on peripheral smear, important for early clinical suspicion and diagnosis.

TREATMENT
Supportive therapy
- Early recognition important for directing intensive care.
- Management of fluid status critical to reduce risk of respiratory failure.

Antiviral drugs
- None demonstrated to be clinically effective.
- Ribavirin has anti-viral activity *in vitro*.
- Ribavirin has significant toxicities and has not been shown in clinical trials to be effective.

OTHER INFORMATION
- Very important for early diagnosis is to examine peripheral smear for evidence of severe left shift; presence of thrombocytopenia, myelocytes, hemoconcentration, and hypocapnia strongly suggest HPS.
- CDC (9/96) HPS case definition: temp >38.3°C, bilateral diffuse interstitial infiltrates resembling ARDS, oxygen requirement w/i 72 hrs of hospitalization.
- Rodent infestation of home remains leading risk factor, especially cleaning uninhabited trailer, cabin or residence in SW U.S.

BASIS FOR RECOMMENDATIONS
Mertz GJ, Miedzinski L, Goade D, et al. Placebo-controlled, double-blind trial of intravenous ribavirin for the treatment of hantavirus cardiopulmonary syndrome in North America. *Clin Infect Dis*, 2004; Vol. 39; pp. 1307–13.
Comments: As the authors note, ribavirin was well tolerated, but it was probably ineffective in the treatment of HCPS by the time severe disease in the cardiopulmonary stage occurs.

HEPATITIS A

Paul G. Auwaerter, MD

MICROBIOLOGY
- Piconarvirus (RNA virus). Incubation period typically 15–50 days, average 28 days.
- More heat stable than most RNA viruses, for complete inactivation heat food to >85°C for at least 1 minute.

CLINICAL
- Virus acquired from exposure to high risk source often person-person: contaminated food/water, travel-endemic areas, undercooked shellfish, institutionalized pts, daycare, homosexual men, floods/water disasters, IDU. Most often spread among family members, child care settings or similar.
- Usually abrupt onset of acute hepatitis: dark urine, jaundice, fever, malaise, nausea, vomiting, abdominal pain, arthralgia, acolic stools. Usually self-limited, ~3 wks.
- Clinical sxs: may range from asymptomatic to hepatomegaly, splenomegaly, bradycardia, elevated ALT/AST, elevated bilirubins, lymphocytosis, atypical mononuclear cells. ALT returns to normal in about 7 wks.
- Complications: cholestasis, relapsing disease, fulminant hepatitis, chronic active autoimmune hepatitis, autoimmune extrahepatic disease, depression.
- Unusual to be fulminant. Mortality 0.3–0.6% but increases to ~2% for ages >50 yrs, pts with chronic liver disease.
- Ddx: clinical sx of HAV non-specific, cannot distinguish from other common causes.

- Dx: Antibody testing: HAV IgM antibody by radioimmunoassay, may be positive 5–10 days prior to onset of sx. IgM anti-HAV remains elevated for 3–12 mos. Reports of persisting anti-HAV IgM positivity >1 yr correlate with likely false-positive result.
- Total anti-HAV test detects both IgM and IgG, so if positive, may reflect prior exposure.
- HAV IgG remains lifelong following infection; positive in 20–80% of asymptomatic U.S. adults.

SITES OF INFECTION

- Liver.
- Virus excreted in bile, with high concentrations in feces.
- Will grow in epithelial cells, *in vitro*.

TREATMENT

Acute Infection

- Supportive care: bed rest, fluids.
- Approximately 10–15% of symptomatic cases of HAV infection require hospitalization.
- Acute HAV may be severe in persons with underlying liver disease (e.g., hepatitis C).

Pre-Exposure Prophylaxis: routine and international travel

- Per 2006 recommendations, routine vaccination now recommended for all children, targeting 12–23 mos for receiving the vaccine. Previously, target populations were children in states and communities with high rates HAV.
- **Active immunization:** inactivated hepatitis A vaccine, given into deltoid muscle. Forms: VAQTA (for 12 mos–18 yrs give 25U per dose, for >18 yrs 50U per two dose schedule), HAVRIX (for 12 mos–18 yrs give 720El.U per dose, for >18 yrs 1440El.U per two dose schedule) and TWINRIX (>18 yrs only, combines hepatitis A and hepatitis B vaccines in three dose schedule (0, 1, 6 mos or accelerated four dose schedule 0, 7, 21–30 days followed by booster at 12 mos).
- Protective antibody responses seen in 94–100% of adults after 1st vaccine dose. Antibody response ~100% post second dose.
- For adults (recommended): at-risk international travelers, high-risk geographic populations or individuals at risk during outbreaks/close personal contacts, MSM, frequent blood/plasma recipients, chronic liver disease (including. Hep B and C), high risk employment, IDUs.
- **International travel:** give Hepatitis A vaccine, one dose adequate anytime prior to departure: VAQTA or HAVRIX give 1 mL IM into deltoid muscle, with 1 mL IM booster within 6–12 mos. Need for booster dose currently unknown, but expected >10 yr duration of prophylaxis.
- Older adults, immunocompromised pts, chronic liver dz pts, other chronic conditions, or departure ≤2 wks: give initial dose of vaccine and simultaneous Ig (0.02 mL/kg) at separate site.
- If pt elects not to receive vaccine (or cannot, e.g., age <12 mos, etc.), the single Ig dose provides protection for 3 mos.
- When using pooled human immunoglobulin, duration of coverage is 3 mos with 0.02 mL/kg IM, some advocate longer-term coverage 3–5 mos using 0.06 mL/kg and repeat q5 mos for continued exposure risk.

Post-Exposure Prophylaxis

- ACIP recommends hepatitis vaccine alone for healthy individuals ages 1–40 for post-exposure prophylaxis.
- All others should receiving passive immunization: pooled human immunoglobulin. If unavailable, give vaccine for adults greater than age 40. For children <12 mos, immunocompromised, pts with chronic liver disease or have vaccine contraindications, use Ig.
- Immunoglobulin should be administered within 2 wks of exposure. Use IG 0.02 mL/kg IM into gluteus muscle.
- Immunoglobulin prophylaxis: point source outbreaks, close contacts of index cases, daycare center contacts, institutional contacts.

FOLLOW UP

- Viral shedding in stool highest in 2 wks prior to onset of jaundice. Children shed > adults, up to 10 wks.
- Most symptoms resolve within 8 wks.
- Prolonged or relapsing symptoms described in 10–15% that may last up to 6 mos.

PATHOGENS

OTHER INFORMATION
- Hepatitis A rates declining in the U.S. since 1996 introduction of hepatitis A vaccine. Cases declined from >20 cases/100,000 to 1.9 cases/100,000 or 5683 U.S. cases in 2004.

BASIS FOR RECOMMENDATIONS

Advisory Committee on Immunization Practices (ACIP) Centers for Disease Control and Prevention (CDC). Update: Prevention of hepatitis A after exposure to hepatitis A virus and in international travelers. Updated recommendations of the Advisory Committee on Immunization Practices (ACIP). *MMWR Morb Mortal Wkly Rep*, 2007; Vol. 56; pp. 1080–4.
Comments: Update regarding post-exposure prophylaxis and international travel. Key update: vaccine suggest for post-exposure prophylaxis in group age 1–40.

Advisory Committee on Immunization Practices (ACIP), Fiore AE, Wasley A, et al. Prevention of hepatitis A through active or passive immunization: recommendations of the Advisory Committee on Immunization Practices (ACIP). *MMWR Recomm Rep*, 2006; Vol. 55; pp. 1–23.
Comments: Useful recommendations from ACIP and CDC for active or passive prophylaxis of Hepatitis A infection.

HEPATITIS B

David Thomas, MD, MPH

MICROBIOLOGY
- Enveloped, double stranded DNA virus.
- Family: Hepadnaviridae. Genus: Orthohepadnavirus.

CLINICAL
- Infection may be self-limiting or become chronic. Infection spread by contaminated body fluids. Risk factors: multiple sex partners, STD hx, MSM, sex contacts of infected persons, IDU, household contacts of chronically infected persons, infants born to infected mothers, infants/children of immigrants from areas with high rates of HBV infection, health care, and public safety workers, hemodialysis pts.
- Clearance of infection is lowest in very young (infants) and very old (>60 yrs of age). Infants have <5% chance of clearing after vertical transmission.
- Acute infection associated with typical signs of hepatitis: jaundice, fatigue, fever, pruritus, dark urine, nausea/vomiting, anorexia.
- **Clinical syndromes** related to HBV include: acute infection, resolved infection, chronic hepatitis B (which can be e antigen positive or negative), inactive hepatitis B, and hepatitis B flares. Over time, transitions may occur between states and accurate diagnoses may require integrating several test results and long-term follow-up (see Diagnosis below).
- **Acute hepatitis B:** symptoms of acute hepatitis B occur 60–110 days after inoculation (incubation). May begin with flu-like symptoms or immune-complex presentation (maculopapular rash, urticaria, arthralgia, fever, symmetric distal joint arthritis). Jaundice and right upper quadrant pain may follow, with acholic stools, dark urine, and pruritus. Laboratory abnormalities include marked elevation (>10×) of ALT and AST, elevated direct and total bilirubin, moderate elevation in alkaline phosphatase. Fulminant hepatitis may occur and be fatal, especially if accompanied by HDV infection.
- **Resolved hepatitis B:** refers to period >6 mos after acute HBV infection when infection is controlled as indicated by resolution of symptoms, normalization of liver enzymes, and clearance of HBsAg in association with anti-HBs. The incidence of resolution is greatest in the first yr after acute infection, but may occur at any time. Acute hepatitis B resolves in >95% of adults but <10% of infants. (Resolution is a clinical diagnosis as there is evidence that in many persons very small amounts of HBV DNA can continue to be detected and relapses have occurred in persons with resolved infection who subsequently were immunosuppressed by cancer chemotherapy. This state, detection of HBV DNA without HBsAg, is called occult hepatitis B.)
- **Chronic hepatitis B:** defined as persistence of HBsAg >6 mos, is further classified as to whether it is e antigen positive or negative and by whether there is liver necroinflammation. Chronic hepatitis B begins as e antigen positive, usually with very high levels of HBV DNA and necroinflammation. That state may transition (spontaneously or with treatment) into one of 3 conditions: resolved hepatitis B, inactive hepatitis B, or e antigen negative chronic hepatitis B. In each instance, e antigen is cleared and anti-HBe detected. Resolved and inactive hepatitis B

are described above and below, respectively. With e antigen negative chronic hepatitis B, HBsAg and HBV DNA are still detected, although DNA levels are generally lower than when e antigen positive. In this instance, after anti-HBe seroconversion an HBV mutant emerges that prevents or diminishes e antigen expression even though the infection remains chronic. Although each of these two forms of chronic hepatitis B (e antigen negative and e antigen positive) can cause cirrhosis, end stage liver disease, and liver cancer, the incidence is highest in e antigen positive persons with the highest HBV DNA levels and those who have had the disease the longest.

- **Inactive hepatitis B:** Once called the 'healthy carrier state', inactive (normal liver enzymes) hepatitis B is defined as persistence of HBsAg for >6 mos without any evidence of necroinflammation. HBV DNA levels are <2,000 IU/mL. Transmission to others is still possible but the incidence of cirrhosis, end stage liver disease, and liver cancer are much less than with e antigen positive or e antigen negative chronic hepatitis B.

- **Hepatitis B flares:** (exacerbation): refers to >10× elevations in liver enzymes in persons with chronic hepatitis B. IgM anti-HBc may also be positive, making the condition difficult to distinguish from acute hepatitis B. Can herald transition to e antigen negative, inactive hepatitis B, or even resolution. However, the cumulative impact of repeated "unsuccessful" flares is thought to contribute to more rapid liver disease progression.

- **Necroinflammation:** refers to the process through which HBV causes liver disease by protracted inflammation. Necroinflammation is a *criterion for treatment* of chronic hepatitis B and its absence is the basis for classification as *"inactive"* or "immunotolerant" hepatitis B. There is debate among experts as to whether necroinflammation should be documented by liver biopsy or by liver enzymes like ALT. Most treatment guidelines allow either and define disease as persistent or intermittent elevation in ALT or biopsy necroinflammatory score of 4 or more. Biopsy is invasive, expensive, and less precise because of observer and sampling bias. Liver enzymes don't show how much damage has already occurred (liver fibrosis) but are readily available and can be followed over a long period. Liver enzymes should be interpreted in light of true "normal" ranges that are usually much lower than thresholds reported by individual laboratories.

SITES OF INFECTION

- **Acute hepatitis B:** HBsAg positive, Anti-HBc IgM positive.
- **Resolved hepatitis B:** HBsAg negative, Anti-HBs positive, Anti-HBc IgG positive, Anti-HBc IgM negative, HBV DNA undetectable, ALT normal.
- **Chronic hepatitis B (e antigen positive):** HBsAg positive >6 mos, Anti-HBs negative, HBeAg positive, Anti-HBe negative, Anti-HBc IgG positive. HBV DNA >20,000 IU/mL, ALT elevated +/− biopsy necroinflammation score >4.
- **Chronic Hepatitis B (e antigen negative):** HBsAg positive >6 mos, HBeAg negative, Anti-HBe positive, HBV DNA >20,000 IU/mL, ALT elevated +/− biopsy necroinflammation score >4.
- **Inactive HBsAg carrier:** HBsAg positive >6 mos, Anti-HBs negative, Anti-HBc IgG positive, HBeAg negative, Anti-HBe positive, HBV DNA <2,000 IU/mL, persistently normal ALT +/− liver biopsy necroinflammation score <4.
- **HBV vaccination:** Anti-HBs positive and other markers negative (check 2 mos after 3rd dose, once seroconversion documented, no need for booster dose. If anti-HBs neg yrs after vaccination, test for HBsAg to exclude chronic hepatitis B and consider booster with repeat anti-HBs 2 mos after).
- **Hepatitis B flare:** HBsAg positive, Anti-HBc IgM positive, HBV DNA detected, ALT elevated.

TREATMENT

Treatment criteria (see definitions above):

- If jaundice or decompensated, consider referral to specialist. If HIV positive, see below. Otherwise,
- **Chronic hepatitis B (e antigen positive)**
- ALT >2× ULN; confirm ALT and HBeAg in 1–3 mos, then treat (below).
- ALT <1× ULN; follow ALT and HBeAg q3–6 mos.
- ALT 1–2× ULN; follow ALT and HBeAg q3–6 mos, consider biopsy if persistent or >40 yrs; treat based on biopsy.

PATHOGENS

- **Chronic hepatitis B (e antigen negative)**
- ALT >2× ULN and HBV DNA >20,000 IU/mL; confirm ALT in 1–3 mos, then treat (below).
- ALT <1× ULN and HBV DNA <2,000 IU/mL, follow ALT and HBV DNA q3–6 mos.
- ALT 1–2× ULN and HBV DNA 2,000–20,000 IU/mL, follow ALT and HBV DNA q3–6 mos, consider biopsy if persistent or >40 yrs; treat based on biopsy.

Treatment goals
- Reduce risk of end stage liver disease and cancer
- Sustained suppression of HBV DNA
- HBsAg clearance (transition to resolution)
- Decrease necroinflammation (transition to inactive hepatitis B)
- Reduce transmission

Standard interferon alfa 2b
- Dose: 5 million U SQ q24h or 10 million U SQ thrice weekly × 16–24 wks for HBeAg positive and × ≥ 12 mos for HBeAg negative.
- Side effects: fever, myalgia, bone marrow suppression, depression, thyroid abnormalities. Thrombocytopenia, granulocytopenia, fatigue, and depression may respond to dose adjustment.
- Outcomes: sustained loss of HBeAg (33%), HBV DNA (37%), and HBsAg (~15%). Histologic improvement is seen more often in those with sustained HBV DNA suppression. ALT normal in ~25%.
- Response predictors (pretreatment): HBV DNA <100,000 IU/mL, AST, and ALT >100 U/L, liver biopsy with active necrosis and active inflammation.
- Resistance notes: not affected by or a cause of HBV resistance mutations.
- Cost per course: ~$7000.
- Comments: do not use with Child-Pugh B or C cirrhosis.

Peginterferon alfa 2a
- Dose: 180 mcg subcutaneous injection per wks × 48 wks.
- Side effects: similar to standard interferon but lower intensity.
- Outcomes, *e antigen positive* (48 wks treat, 24 wks follow-up): loss of HBeAg 32% (vs 19% for LAM), HBV DNA <20,000 IU/mL 32% (vs 22% for LAM), and HBsAg clearance 3% (vs 0 for LAM). Histologic improvement in 38% (vs 34% for LAM).
- Outcomes, *e antigen negative* (48 wks treat, 24 wks follow-up): HBV DNA <4,000 IU/mL 43% (vs 29% for LAM), and HBsAg clearance 4% (vs 0 for LAM). Histologic improvement in 48% (vs 40% for LAM).
- Resistance notes: not affected by or a cause of HBV resistance mutations.
- Cost per course: ~$16,000.
- Response predictors: ALT >3× ULN, HBV DNA <2 × 10^6 IU/mL.
- Comments: **Do not use** with Child-Pugh B or C cirrhosis. High toxicity and cost constrain applicability, but may have use in persons with high response likelihood and few contraindications.

Lamivudine (LAM)
- Dose: 100 mg PO daily for six mos after HBeAg conversion to Anti-HBe occurs, or lifelong.
- Side effects: same as placebo except HBV resistance, which makes LAM a second-line choice in many settings. Hepatitis B flare can occur after withdrawal of therapy.
- Outcomes, *e antigen positive* (52 wks treat, 16-wk follow-up): loss of HBeAg 32% (vs 11% placebo), HBV DNA <20,000 IU/mL 44% (versus 16% placebo), and HBsAg (0–3%), but may not be sustained. Histologic improvement in 52% (vs 23% with placebo).
- Outcomes, e antigen negative (48 wks treat, 24-wk follow-up): HBV DNA <4,000 IU/mL 29% (vs 43% for peginterferon), and HBsAg clearance 0% (vs 4% for peginterferon). Histologic improvement in 40% (vs 48% for peginterferon).
- Response predictors (pretreatment): HBV DNA <100,000 IU/mL, AST, and ALT >100 U/L, liver biopsy with active necrosis and active inflammation.
- Resistance notes: mutations in polymerase occur ~15% per yr with viral rebound and sometimes disease flare. Fitness of resistant virus probably attenuated. Reversion to wild-type virus occurs with discontinuation.
- Cost per yr: ~$2200.

- Comments: proven clinical benefit with Child-Pugh B or C cirrhosis. High rate of resistance makes some avoid in settings where alternatives exist.

Adefovir

- Dose: 10 mg PO daily; duration unclear but for HBeAg positive, consider stopping 24–48 wks after anti-HBe conversion.
- Side effects: equal to placebo at this dose (renal toxicity seen with higher doses in phase 2). Resistance may occur with long term use.
- Outcomes, *e antigen positive* (48 wks treatment): loss of HBeAg 24% (vs 11% placebo), HBV DNA < detect 21% (vs 0 for placebo), and HBsAg clearance (0–3%). Histologic improvement in 64% (vs 33% placebo). With continued use 5 or more yrs, higher response rates are seen for all outcomes.
- Outcomes: *e antigen negative* (144 wks treatment): HBV DNA <1000 c/mL at 96 wks 71% (vs 8% when ADV stopped after 48 wks), and HBsAg clearance (<2%). Histologic improvement in 89% (vs 50% of those who stopped ADV after 48 wks). With continued use 5 or more yrs, higher response rates are seen for all outcomes.
- Resistance notes: resistance is uncommon (~3.9%) at 3 yrs; novel mutation rtN236T in the D domain of HBV RT confers resistance to adefovir *in vitro* and *in vivo*. LAM remains active, while ADV is active against LAM resistant HBV. Resistance overlaps with tenofovir.
- Cost per yr: ~$6000.
- Comments: less potent than entecavir, telbivudine, and tenofovir but relatively high resistance threshold. For e antigen negative, improvements were lost when use not continued beyond 48 wks.

Entecavir

- Dose: 0.5 mg PO daily (1.0 mg daily if lamivudine experienced); duration unclear but for HBeAg positive, consider stopping 24–48 wks after anti-HBe conversion.
- Side effects: similar to lamivudine.
- Outcomes, *e antigen positive* (48 wks): loss of HBeAg 22% (vs 20% for LAM), HBV DNA <300 c/mL 67% (vs 36% for LAM), and HBsAg clearance 2% (vs 1% for LAM). Histologic improvement in 72% (versus 62% with LAM).
- Resistance notes: little to no resistance apparent at 5 yrs.
- Cost per yr: $7200.
- Comments: more potent than lamivudine and much less resistance risk, but higher cost. Use 1.0 mg if pt has ever had LAM.

Telbivudine

- Dose: 600 mg PO daily, duration unclear but for HBeAg positive, consider stopping 24–48 wks after anti-HBe conversion.
- Side effects: muscle pain and elevated CK in 12 pts (9%) (vs 8 [3%] for LAM) at 104 wks in one study.
- Outcomes: *e antigen positive* (104 wks): loss of HBeAg 35% (vs 29% for LAM), HBV DNA < detect 56% (vs 39% for LAM), and HBsAg clearance 2% (vs 1% for LAM). Histologic improvement in 72% (versus 62% with LAM).
- Resistance notes: key issue is early potency since resistance develops in >75% when HBV DNA >1000 c/mL at 24 wks; M204I resistance mutation in HBV polymerase sequence observed in all individuals with confirmed virologic breakthrough on telbivudine.
- Cost per yr: $7305.
- Comments: too early to tell its role but resistance is clearly an issue; possible role in those who rapidly respond.

Tenofovir disoproxil fumerate

- Dose: 300 mg daily, duration unclear but, for HBeAg positive, consider stopping 24–48 wks after anti-HBe conversion.
- Side effects: Fanconi syndrome and renal insufficiency occur at a low incidence; risk may be greater in pts with other renal risk factors like diabetes.
- Outcomes: Compared to adefovir in registration trials—HBeAg positive: HBV DNA <69 IU/mL 76% vs. 13%; normal ALT 68% vs. 54%; histologic improvement 74% vs. 68%; HBsAg loss 3% vs. 0. HBeAg negative: HBV DNA <69 IU/mL 93% vs. 63%; normal ALT 76% vs. 77%; histologic improvement 72% vs. 69%; HBsAg loss 0 vs. 0.

PATHOGENS

- Resistance notes: low rate of resistance detected in first 3 yrs. Activity is decreased for ADV-resistant mutants but not LAM resistance.
- Truvada and Atripla: tenofovir can be purchased coformulated with emtricitabine, which although not FDA approved for chronic hepatitis B, has activity (and resistance issues) comparable to LAM.
- Cost per yr: $7200 per yr; as Truvada $10,500.
- Comments: like entecavir, is a potent oral agent with low resistance. Combined formulation with emtricitabine is not FDA approved for HBV but has attractive features for those who chose dual oral agent therapy.

Prevention

- Immunization: HBV vaccine for those with increased risk (hemodialysis, HIV infected, sexual contacts and household members, group home residents, health care workers, risky sex behaviors, injection drug users). Check anti-HBs titer 2 mos after last dose. Consider double dose for hemodialysis, HIV infected, and those who fail initial series.
- Postexposure prophylaxis: Specific for type of exposure, host characteristics and source characteristics. Follow CDC guidelines for HBIG and HBV vaccination (see vaccine, drug modules).

OTHER INFORMATION

- Hepatocellular carcinoma associated w/ chronic HBV, especially in endemic Southeast Asia, Japan, sub-Saharan Africa, Greece, Italy, and Oceania. Found especially in perinatally acquired infection. Higher HBV DNA levels associated with higher risk. Screening recommended.
- **If HIV positive,** determine if antiretroviral therapy is needed. If so, consider using tenofovir and FTC as part of HAART (e.g., Atripla or Truvada). If antiretroviral therapy not needed, consider peginterferon, adefovir, or starting tenofovir-based, fully HIV- suppressive antiretroviral therapy.

BASIS FOR RECOMMENDATIONS

No author listed. NIH consensus development statement on management of hepatitis B. *NIH Consensus State Sci Statements*, 2009; Vol. 25; pp. 1–29.
Comments: An independent assessment of which pts should be treated.

European Association For The Study Of The Liver. EASL Clinical Practice Guidelines: management of chronic hepatitis B. *J Hepatol*, 2009; Vol. 50; pp. 227–42.
Comments: The European analog to the AASLD guidelines.

Lok AS, McMahon BJ. Chronic hepatitis B. *Hepatology*, 2007; Vol. 45; pp. 507–39.
Comments: AASLD (and IDSA cosponsored) HBV Treatment guidelines.

HEPATITIS C

Mark Sulkowski, MD

MICROBIOLOGY

- Enveloped, single-stranded, positive sense RNA virus.
- Member of the Flaviviridae.
- Spread by blood-borne transmission. Other routes (vertical transmission, sexual) less common.

CLINICAL

- Risks: exposure to blood/organs before July, 1992; hx IDU at any time; elevated ALT; hemodialysis; other exposure (sexual-multiple partners, or infected partner, both with lower risk).
- Most (80%) have no signs or symptoms of active hepatitis C infection.
- Clinical: acute—20% jaundice; chronic—most asymptomatic until liver failure; extrahepatic findings—cryoglobulinemia +/– vasculitis and glomerulonephritis; porphyria cutanea tarda.
- Diagnostic tests: (1) screen with HCV antibody, >99% sensitivity. (False negatives if <70 days since exposure, dialysis, HIV positive), (2) confirm with HCV RNA (need repeated negative to exclude active infection).

- Evaluation: ALT/AST, albumin, PT, total bilirubin, platelet ct. HCV genotype and viral load helps predict treatment response. Liver biopsy; best indicator of disease stage.
- Supplemental tests (exclude other liver diseases): iron levels, autoimmune (ANA), HBV, alpha-1 antitrypsin deficiency, Wilson's. Consider TSH, alpha-feto protein if cirrhotic.
- Mortality rate of chronic HCV: 1–5%, mostly due to cirrhosis and complications.

Sites of Infection

- Liver: 55–85% develop chronic infection, of those chronically infected, up to 70% may develop significant liver disease.

Treatment

HCV Treatment

- Standard of care: pegylated IFN alfa-2b 1.5 mcg/kg (wt-adjusted) or PEG alfa-2a 180 mcg (fixed) SC injection wkly + Ribavirin (RBV) PO.
- Indications: + HCV RNA and necroinflammation and fibrosis on biopsy. Biopsy: indicated-genotype 1; controversial-genotypes 2/3. Normal ALT and HIV + are candidates for RX based on biopsy findings.
- Contraindications (some relative): severe psychiatric disease, decompensated liver disease, poor adherence, severe cytopenia (wbc, plt, Hgb), pregnancy possible, severe comorbid disease.
- HIV coinfection does not contraindicate therapy for HCV.
- Pre-tx work-up: hx (comorbidity); PE (decompensation); CBC w/plt, ALT/AST, PT, PTT, TBili, TSH, HCV viral load, HCV genotype; liver biopsy—for many pts; consider no biopsy with genotypes 2/3.
- Tx objectives: 1. HCV eradication (cure); 2. slow fibrosis progression—prevent end-stage liver disease, hepatocellular CA, etc.
- Outcomes: sustained viral response (SVR)—negative HCV RNA at end of tx (EOT) and 6 mo post; Relapse—neg HCV RNA EOT but + HCV RNA after d/c; Non-response—HCV RNA not negative during tx.
- Response indicators: SVR rare (<2%) if by wk 12—HCV RNA still + and <2 log drop or by wk 24—HCV RNA still +. Consider d/c Rx if viral failure at wk 12.
- Cure rate: PEG alfa-2a/alfa-2b + RIBA, overall 54–56%; genotype 1—42/46% for 48-wk tx; genotypes 2/3—76/82% for 24-wk tx. RCT (the IDEAL study) involving 3070 HCV genotype 1–infected pts in the U.S. demonstrate similar SVR with both PEG alfa-2a and alfa-2b + RIBA (McHutchison et al, *New Eng J Med* 2009).
- FDA-approved regimens—IFN monotherapy: IFN alfa 2a, 2b, alfacon-1 (consensus), PEG-IFN alfa-2b, PEG-IFN alfa-2a; Combination therapy: IFN alfa-2b + RBV, PEG-IFN alfa-2b + RBV.

Pegylated IFN +/– Ribavirin

- Response to PEG + RIBA strongly influenced by host genetic polymorphism near IL28B gene, encoding interferon—3 (IFN—3). CC genotype is associated with a twofold greater rate of SVR than the TT genotype CC both among pts of European ancestry and African Americans. Because the CC genotype is more common in European than African populations, this genetic polymorphism also explains ~56% of the lower response observed in African—Pegylated +/– Ribavirin (Ge, *Nature* 2009).
- Pegylated interferon: long half life, once weekly injection. Two types PEG alfa-2b—12 kd, linear PEG, wt-based dosing; PEG alfa-2a—40 kd, branched PEG, fixed dosing. Both FDA approved +/– RIBA.
- PEG-IFN alfa-2b dosing (weight-based): monotherapy use 1.0 mcg/kg/wk; PEG alfa-2b + RIBA combination use 1.5 mcg/kg/wk; PEG alfa-2a (fixed dose) 180 mcg/wk for both mono and combo with RIBA.
- Both PEG IFN alfa-2a and 2b monotherapy—approx. twofold higher sustained response rate (SVR) compared to standard IFN alone; similar side effects.
- PEG IFN monotherapy indicated for pts with contraindication to RBV (heart, lung, hemoglobinopathy). Long-term low dose monotherapy does not prevent progression of liver disease in pts with significant fibrosis/cirrhosis and is not indicated (Di Bisceglie et al, *N Engl J Med* 2008).
- Combo PEG alfa-2b or PEG alfa-2a + RBV is the most effective therapy; standard of care for HCV 2004. (Ghany et al. *Hepatology* 2009). Standard regimen: PEG alfa-2b (1.5 mcg/kg/wk) or

PEG alfa-2a (180 mcg/wk) + RIBA 1000 mg/day (<75 kg) or 1200 mg/day (>75 kg) for geno 1 (48 wks Rx) and RBV 800 mg/day all pts with geno 2/3 (24 wks Rx).

- Wt <40 kg (88 lbs): PEG2b = vial size 100 mcg—use 0.5 mL/wk; RBV 800 mg/day.
- Wt = 40–50 kg (88–110 lbs): PEG2b = vial size 160 mcg—use 0.4 mL/wk; RBV 800 mg/day;
  Wt = 51–64 kg (112–141 lbs): PEG2b = vial size 160 use 0.5 mL/wk; RBV 800 mg/day.
- Wt = 65–75 kg (142–166 lbs): PEG2b = vial size 240 mcg—use 0.4 mL/wk; RBV 1000 mg/day;
  Wt = 76–85 kg (167–187 lbs): PEG2b = vial size 240 use 0.5 mL/wk; RBV 1000 mg/day.
- Wt = 86–105 kg (188–231 lbs): PEG2b = vial size 300 mcg—use 0.5 mL/wk; RBV 120 mg/day;
  Wt >105 kg (>231 lbs): PEG2b = vial size 300 use 0.5 mL/wk; RBV 1400 mg/day.

Experimental and Future HCV Treatment Options

- HCV serine protease inhibitors: 2 drugs in phase 2 clinical trials for the treatment of chronic HCV genotype 1 in combination with PEG alfa + RIBA: Telaprevir (Vertex) and Boceprevir (Schering). Phase 2 data indicate significantly increased SVR rate in HCV genotype 1 with protease inhibitor PO q8hrs + PEG + RIBA (63–75%) compared to PEG + RIBA (~40%), (McHutchison et al. New Eng J Med 2009). Side effects: anemia (both), rash (severe ~7% for telaprevir), GI toxicity.
- HCV polymerase inhibitors: multiple drugs in phase 1/2 development. Phase 2 RCT—R7128 orally available + PEG alfa-2a +; achieve 1–2 log10 reduction in HCV RNA in genotype 1 pts—IFN naïve.
- Combination HCV polymerase and protease inhibitor: Proof of concept INFORM-1 study of two agents—ITMN-191/R7227(Intermune/Roche) in combination with polymerase inhibitor R7128 (Roche/Pharmasset).
- Iron reduction: not effective; phlebotomy indicated only with iron overload (hemochromatosis or HCV-related porphyria).

Prevention

- Transmission primarily through repeat exposure or large inoculum of blood.
- Average rate of seroconversion after accidental needlestick from HCV+ pt: 1.8%.
- Rare transmission through mucous membranes or intact skin.
- No recommendations regarding post-exposure treatment; no drugs, no immune globulin.
- Advise to follow carefully for onset of infection (though viral PCR) to diagnose early and consider treatment.
- CDC algorithm: baseline testing to include anti-HCV AB, ALT performed within 7–14 days of the exposure, Follow-up testing for anti-HCV and ALT should be performed 4–6 mos after exposure to assess seroconversion, preferably arranged as part of discharge planning; HCV RNA testing should be performed at 4–6 wks if an earlier diagnosis of HCV infection is desired; and positive anti-HCV with low signal-to-cutoff value should be confirmed using a more specific supplemental assay before communicating the results to the pt; and persons who are tested or are identified as a candidate for testing regarding exposure to HCV while undergoing evaluation or treatment in immediate response to a mass-casualty event should be discharged with a referral for follow-up and written information on pre-discharge treatment.

OTHER INFORMATION

- PEG-IFN side effects: "flu-like"—respond to NSAIDs, tylenol; fatigue; depression and irritability—respond to SSRIs; insomnia—responds to trazodone (avoid benzos); thyroid (hypo-5%/hyper-1%).
- PEG-IFN—neutropenia (<500 cells in 1%)—respond to decrease dose PEG; consider G-CSF (filgrastim) 300 mcg SC injection 2–3× per wk.
- Ribavirin side effects: dyspepsia—responds to antacids; dry cough; gout; anemia— dose-related, reversible hemolytic anemia—develops 2–4 wks; avg drop 2.5–3 g Hb.
- Anemia due to PEG (bone marrow) + Riba (hemolytic)—respond rHu-EPO 40,000 IU SC weekly; avg increase 2.8 g over 4 wks; maintain RBV dose. Caution with rHu-EPO due to cases of pure red blood cell aplasia reported in pts taking rHu-EPO in combination with PEG + RIBA.
- HCV Genotype 1a or 1b.
- PEG-IFN alfa-2b (1.5 mcg/kg/wk) or PEG-IFN alfa-2a (180 mcg/wk) Plus.
- Ribavirin (Wt <64 kg 800 mg/day; 64–85 kg 1000 mg/day; 86–105 kg 1200 mg/day; >105 kg 1400 mg/day) Duration: 48 wks.

- PEG-IFN alfa-2b 1.5 mcg/kg/wk or PEG IFN alfa-2a 180 mcg/wk Standard IFN alfa-2b (3 MIU TIW) plus Ribavirin (<75 kg 1000 mg/day; >75 kg 1200 mg/day).
- HCV Genotype 2 or 3 Same drugs but Duration: 24 wks and RVB dose 800 mg/day.

BASIS FOR RECOMMENDATIONS

Ghany MG, Strader DB, Thomas DL, et al. Diagnosis, management, and treatment of hepatitis C: an update. *Hepatology*, 2009; Vol. 49; pp. 1335–74.

Comments: Review address current areas of concern as well as view toward how drugs in pipeline may alter approach to future care.

Chapman LE, Sullivent EE, Grohskopf LA, et al. Recommendations for postexposure interventions to prevent infection with hepatitis B virus, hepatitis C virus, or human immunodeficiency virus, and tetanus in persons wounded during bombings and other mass-casualty events—United States, 2008: recommendations of the Centers for Disease Control and Prevention (CDC). *MMWR Recomm Rep*, 2008; Vol. 57; pp. 1–21; quiz CE1–4.

Comments: Post-exposure recommendations for large exposures.

HEPATITIS D

Paul G. Auwaerter, MD

PATHOGENS

MICROBIOLOGY
- Defective RNA virus.
- HDV requires active hepatitis B virus (HBV) for replication.

CLINICAL
- Infection occurs either as coinfection (acute hepatitis B) or superinfection (upon chronic hepatitis B), both with increased morbidity. Globally, of with chronic HBV, 5% are believed to be coinfected with HDV.
- Symptoms are typical of hepatitis: jaundice, abdominal pain, anorexia, fatigue, nausea/vomiting, arthralgia.
- Evaluation for hepatitis virus D (HDV) should be undertaken in pts with severe acute hepatitis B or during an exacerbation of chronic hepatitis B who have traveled to a HDV endemic region.
- HDV should also be considered if hepatitis B surface antigen negative but IgM antibody to hepatitis B core antigen positive hepatitis.
- The only FDA-approved assay is for total antibody to HDV—it does not distinguish between acute, chronic, or resolved infection unless seroconversion is documented (indicating acute infection).
- Research assays are available to detect HDV RNA or antigen in the serum or liver or IgM anti-HDV; the latter usually persists in chronic infection and thus is not specific for acute infection.
- Risk of severe disease increased with HDV; risk of acute liver failure increased 2–20% compared to HBV alone. Risk of cirrhosis also likely increased.

SITES OF INFECTION
- Liver

TREATMENT
Treatment of acute HDV infection (coinfection)
- No evidence of benefit giving interferon alpha for acute HDV coinfection or superinfection.
- Mostly care is considered supportive.
- Orthotopic liver transplantation should be considered in pts with fulminant acute hepatitis D.

Treatment of chronic HDV infection
- May be from superinfection (more likely) or coinfection.
- Interferon alpha has shown benefit in chronic HDV infection.
- Early treatment of chronic disease appears to result in improved response
- High dose IFN-alpha 2b (4–5 million units/day, or 9–10 million units three times/wk) improves serum transaminases, liver histopathologic changes, and/or serum HDV RNA levels in nearly one-half of pts. Pegylated IFN can likely be substituted for long-term therapy, but no actual data exists.
- One-third have sustained reduction of their transaminase levels.

- Other forms of treatment—immunosuppressives (corticosteroids, azathioprine), immunomodulatory drugs (levamisole), ribavirin, and lamivudine (3-thiacytidine) have not proven effective.
- Lamivudine and other drugs such as adefovir, entecavir. telbuvidine do have proven benefit for treating chronic hepatitis B, but do not tend to impact hepatitis D.
- Orthotopic liver transplantation should be considered in pts with end-stage chronic disease.

Prevention

- HDV coinfection is effectively prevented by HBV vaccination as well as other HBV preventive measures.
- There is no HDV vaccine to protect HBV carriers from superinfection.

FOLLOW UP

HDV Therapy

- If hepatitis B virus surface antigen becomes repeatedly undetectable, risk of relapse is low and interferon alpha treatment can likely be discontinued.
- If after 3 mos a decline of 50% in transaminases is not achieved (within 1.5 times the upper limit of normal) consideration should be given to discontinuing interferon.
- Otherwise, treatment should be continued for 1 yr as tolerated. Yearly treatment interruptions should be scheduled to assess for relapse.

IMPORTANT POINTS

- Fulminant hepatitis occurs at higher incidence during coinfection than during acute hepatitis B, though fewer (<5%) develop chronic infection.
- Most pts with superinfection, however, develop chronic HDV hepatitis (up to 95%).
- Pts with elevated transaminases, histopathologic evidence of chronic hepatitis, and HDV antigen in the liver should be considered for treatment with interferon alpha.
- HDV RNA decline and improving/stabilizing histopathologic changes are also consistent with a response but their absence does not imply failure.
- Post-transplant survival for pts with chronic hepatitis B may be higher when they are also infected with HDV.

BASIS FOR RECOMMENDATIONS

Lok AS, McMahon BJ, Practice Guidelines Committee, American Association for the Study of Liver Diseases (AASLD) Chronic hepatitis B: update of recommendations. *Hepatology,* 2004; Vol. 39; pp. 857–61.
Comments: I Guidelines point out that higher dose IFN therapy is only one that can be supported based upon one study × 1 yr.

Farci P, Chessa L, Balestrieri C, et al. Treatment of chronic hepatitis D. *J Viral Hepat,* 2007; Vol. 14 Suppl 1; pp. 58–63.
Comments: Review highlights: 1. difficult to treat. 2. alpha-interferon (IFN) remains only documented therapy for chronic HDV. 3. Sustained responses are unusual and are accompanied by the clearance of serum hepatitis B virus surface antigen (HBsAg), seroconversion to anti-HBs and improvement of liver histology. Authors state that pegylated–IFN could reasonably be substituted for long-term treatment required for chronic hepatitis D but that rates of cure are low, and relapse high.

HERPES SIMPLEX VIRUS

Noreen A. Hynes, MD, MPH

MICROBIOLOGY

- Herpes simplex virus 1 and 2 (HSV-1 and HSV-2) are members of the Herpes DNA virus family, *Herpesviridae*, also known as Human Herpes Virus 1 and 2 (HHV-1 and HHV-2).
- After primary infection, virus establishes latency in neurons leading to the potential for reactivation usually near site of initial acquisition.

CLINICAL

- Most infections are asymptomatic. HSV-1: 50%–80% of adults are seropositive, HSV-2 20–40% of adults are seropositive. HSV-1: herpes labialis most common form of recurrent HSV-1, **but** 30% of genital HSV is HSV-1.
- **Primary infection:** asymptomatic in 2/3 of both HSV-1 and 2. Primary gingivostomatitis (fever, sore throat, cervical lymphadenopathy, oral cavity vesicular enanthem), mononucleosis syndrome with pharyngitis, fever, cervical lymphadenopathy (common in primary infection of adolescents). Most HSV is acquired from an infected, **asymptomatic** source of infection.

Neonatal infection risk 40% in primary genital HSV but only 2%–5% if post primary shedding at delivery. Serotype specific serology is useful to confirm seroconversion in primary infection; role in non-primary infection diagnosis is poorly defined. Also <u>genital infection</u> (see below).

- **Genital herpes:** classically presents as small number of painful clustered vesicles with an erythematous base; increased pain is noted when ulcers rupture and leave shallow, ulcers that heal spontaneously without treatment over 4–10 days (without treatment). Primary infection may be associated with constitutional symptoms, often with urinary retention (in women), with or without aseptic meningitis (30% women; 10% men) and takes longer to resolve than recurrent disease. HSV-2 accounts for 70–80% of cases; HSV-1 for 20–30% of cases. HSV-2 is more likely to have clinical recurrences. Genital ulcer disease, including that caused by genital HSV increases the risk of acquisition <u>and transmission of HIV infection</u>. Clinical dx of is both insensitive and nonspecific; lab dx needed—viral cx is gold standard but sensitivity less than HSV DNA PCR (not FDA cleared for this use). See "Genital Ulcer Disease" module. The psychological impact of genital HSV cannot be overstated; 60% report being "devastated" when first told their dx. Recurrent genital herpes (>9 episodes/yr) in non-immunosuppressed may be due to persistently lower levels of IgG1, IgG3, and complement compared with infected persons without recurrent disease.
- **CNS HSV infections:** HSV-1 leading cause of <u>sporadic encephalitis</u> in U.S. adults with early onset of seizures and characteristically localizing signs suggesting temporal >>frontal lobe involvement. Benign recurrent lymphocytic meningitis (at least 3 episodes of fever and meningism lasting 2–5 days with spontaneous recovery) can follow recurrence of genital HSV by 5–7 days and will resolve without treatment although if frequent recurrences, some would give suppressive anti-viral therapy.
- **Ocular herpes:** *Ocular infections are potentially sight-threatening and should be referred to an ophthalmologist for initial management.* <u>Acute follicular conjunctivitis and kerato-conjunctivitis</u>—foreign body sensation, lacrimation, photophobia, conjunctival hyperemia followed by vesicular blepharitis, ulceration, blurring of vision secondary to keratitis, and ultimate healing without scarring. <u>Recurrent herpes keratitis</u> (dendritic keratitis) begins with foreign body sensation, lacrimation, photophobia and decreased vision that is slow to heal; repeated recurrences can lead to scarring. Can also be sight threatening. <u>Herpes retinitis</u>—rare, can lead to acute retinal necrosis secondary to occlusive vasculitis, sight threatening.
- **Infections in immunocompromised persons:** <u>HIV-infected persons</u>—60–70% in USA are infected with HSV-2; disseminated infection with visceral involvement can be seen when CD4 count <200 cells/mL and is potentially life-threatening. <u>Pregnant women</u> may also develop disseminated infection with primary infection during pregnancy. <u>Acute immunosuppression</u>: may reactivate HSV within 2 wks of onset of immunosuppression. <u>HSV esophagitis</u>: often seen in immunocompromised pts and must be differentiated from other causes of esophagitis including CMV and candida. Approximately 5% of isolates from HIV-infected persons and 10–12% from bone marrow transplant recipients are acyclovir resistant, most due to thymidine kinase deficient strains.
- **Severe, recurrent ano-genital herpes:** sx commonly seen in pts with AIDS with low CD4 counts (<200 cells/mL) and high viral loads. HIV-infected, esp w/ AIDS need longer treatment and/or higher dose for episodic cutaneous HSV.
- **HSV tracheobronchitis:** most common in elderly and intubated pts. **HSV esophagitis** in immunocompromised pts must be differentiated from other causes.
- **Dermatological herpes:** <u>Herpes dermatitis</u>—may be seen in athletes (herpes gladiatorum), health care workers (herpetic whitlow) and in pts with eczema who become superinfected with HSV (Kaposi's varicelliform eruption). <u>Orolabial HSV (cold sores)</u>—may reactivate after exposure to sunlight, wind, cold, with emotional stress or late stage of menstrual cycle. 15% of erythema multiforme follows recurrent symptomatic HSV.
- **Neonatal herpes:** occurs in 1 in 3,000 to 1 in 20,000 live births. Vertical transmission is most likely to occur during passage through the birth canal amongst women with active lesions. Primary infection in the mother during the 3rd trimester is associated with 10-fold increase in transmission risk. Elective caesarean section and suppressive therapy needed to decrease risk of transmission in women with genital lesions.

PATHOGENS

MORE CLINICAL

Recurrent benign lymphocytic meningitis (RBLM, Mollaret's meningitis)

- >2 recurrences of fever and meningism lasting 2–5 days with spontaneous recovery.
- Usually HSV-2 but history of clinical genital herpes is not common; approximately 2 times more frequent in females; mean age = 35 yrs.
- Recurrences usually become less frequent over time.
- Syndrome: fever, headache (can be severe), photophobia, meningism; symptoms reach max in a few hrs.
- 50% have transient neurologic signs/symptoms including cranial nerve palsies, diplopia, hallucinations, seizures, altered consciousness thus RBLM must be a dx of exclusion.
- CSF findings: lymphocytic pleocytosis (may begin with polymorphonuclear pleocytosis), mild protein elevation, normal glucose; hallmark is large granular plasma cells seen by Papanicolaou stain during the 1st 24 hrs or illness only but they may be absent (also seen in other viral meningitis including in West Nile Virus meningoencephalitis).
- CSF PCR is the gold standard for diagnosis; 85% sensitivity; culture is usually negative.
- Resolves spontaneously but in those with many recurrences, suppressive therapy recommended by some experts as for genital herpes.

Ocular herpes simplex

- Approximately 50,000 new and recurrent ocular HSV/yr in the U.S.; a leading cause of corneal opacification and infection-related visual loss.
- Spectrum of ocular effects includes: dendritic keratitis, uveitis, blepharoconjunctivitis, necrotizing keratitis.
- Recurrent disease can result in damage to the cornea and uvea with scarring and vision loss; recurrence rate is 20% by 2 yrs; 40% by 5 yrs; 67% by 7 yrs; the Herpetic Eye Disease Study Group has shown that oral acyclovir suppression following initial ocular herpes decreases recurrence by 45% in the 1st yr; the greatest suppressive effect may be seen in those with concommitant history of atopy.
- HSV keratitis causes reactivation of virus previously dormant in the trigeminal ganglia and centrifugal migration of virus with replication of virus in the cornea; pts with atopy may have unusually severe keratitis as those with atopy have been shown to have impaired cell-mediated immunity. These pts often respond very poorly to topical antivirals.

Herpes labialis

- Mostly due to HSV-1.
- Mean duration of recurrence (vesicles to healing of lesions) is 7–8 days.
- Mean duration of viral shedding is approximately 60 hrs (measured by PCR) with a peak viral load during the vesicle/ulcer stage.

SITES OF INFECTION

- Oro-facial: primary gingivostomatitis; recurrent stomatitis; herpes labialis
- Genital: genital ulcer disease
- Eye: follicular conjunctivitis, keratitis, acute retinal necrosis syndrome, endophthalmitis
- Other skin areas: eczema herpeticum; herpetic whitlow, herpes gladiatorum
- Central nervous system: sporadic encephalitis, meningoencephalitis, aseptic meningitis; sacral radiculopathy, aseptic meningitis, benign recurrent lymphocytic meningitis (Mollaret's meningitis)
- Esophagus: esophagitis
- Respiratory system: pneumonia, tracheobronchitis
- Liver: hepatitis
- Rectum: proctitis
- Multiple organs: disseminated infection

TREATMENT

Mucocutaneous Infections

- Genital HSV and proctitis—1st clinical episode: treatment for 7–10 days. Acyclovir 400 mg PO q8h or acyclovir 200 mg PO 5 ×/day or famciclovir 250 mg PO q8h or valacyclovir 1 g PO twice daily.

- Genital HSV and proctitis (HIV negative)—episodic rx: acyclovir 400 mg PO q8h × 5 days **or** acyclovir 800 mg PO twice daily × 5 days **or** acyclovir 800 mg PO q8h × 2 days **or** famciclovir 125 mg PO twice daily × 5 days **or** famciclovir 1000 mg PO twice daily × 1 day **or** valacyclovir 500 mg PO twice daily × 3 days **or** valacyclovir 1.0 g PO daily × 5 days.
- Genital HSV and proctitis (HIV positive)—episodic rx: acyclovir 400 mg PO q8h × 5–10 days **or** famciclovir 500 mg PO twice daily × 5–10 days **or** valacyclovir 1.0 g PO twice daily × 5–10 days.
- Genital HSV or proctitis (HIV negative)—suppressive daily therapy for recurrent disease: acyclovir 400 mg PO twice daily **or** famciclovir 250 mg PO twice daily **or** valacyclovir 500 mg PO daily **or** valacyclovir 1 g PO daily.
- Genital HSV and proctitis (HIV positive)—suppressive daily therapy for recurrent disease: acyclovir 400–800 mg PO q8–12h **or** famciclovir 500 mg PO twice daily **or** valacyclovir 500 mg PO twice.
- Genital HSV or proctitis (severe): acyclovir 5–10 mg/kg IV q8h × 5–7 days or until clinical resolution. Suppressive therapy thereafter, if indicated.
- Genital HSV in pregnancy: acyclovir per above regimen w/ initial HSV or highly symptomatic recurrent HSV. Give IV w/ life-threatening infection.
- Stomatitis: acyclovir 400 mg PO q8h × 7–10 days **or** acyclovir 200 mg PO 5 ×/day × 7–10 days **or** famciclovir 250 mg PO q8h × 7–10 days **or** valacyclovir 1 g PO twice daily × 7–10 days.
- Herpes labialis prophylaxis: acyclovir 400 mg PO twice **or** famciclovir 250 mg PO twice daily **or** valacyclovir 250 mg PO twice daily **or** valacyclovir 500 mg PO daily or Valacyclovir 1000 mg PO daily.
- Esophagitis regimens: acyclovir 400–800 mg PO 5 ×/day × 7–10 days **or** acyclovir 5 mg/kg IV three times a day × 7–10 days.

Central Nervous System Infection

- Encephalitis: acyclovir 10 mg/kg IV q8h × 14–28 days.
- Acute meningitis: acyclovir 10 mg/kg IV q8h × 7–10 days.
- Benign recurrent lymphocytic meningitis: acyclovir 10 mg/kg IV q8h × 7–10 days followed consideration of daily suppressive therapy.

Ocular Infection

- Requires ophthalmological consultation.
- Follicular conjunctivitis: trifluridine or acyclovir and/or corticosteroids.
- Keratitis: trifluridine or acyclovir and/or corticosteroids.
- Endophthalmitis: topical acyclovir and steroids.

Immunosuppressed Persons

- Prophylaxis for acute immunosuppression in organ and bone marrow seropositives: initiation—acyclovir 5 mg/kg IV q8h × 7 days. Follow-up—acyclovir 200–400 mg PO 3 to 5× per day × 1–3 mos.
- Episodic rx of recurrent infection in HIV-infected: acyclovir 200 mg PO 5 ×/day or acyclovir 400 mg PO q8h or famciclovir 500 mg PO twice **or** valacyclovir 1 g PO twice (all for 5–10 days).
- Daily suppressive rx in HIV-infected: acyclovir 400–800 mg PO q8–12h **or** valacyclovir 500 mg daily **or** famciclovir 500 mg twice daily.
- Burn pts: acyclovir 5 mg/kg IV q8h × 7 days then 200 mg PO 5 ×/day × 7–14 days.

Acyclovir-resistant strains

- Foscarnet 40 mg/kg IV q8h until clinical resolution.
- Topical cidofovir gel 1% for genital or perirectal lesions daily × 5 days may be tried (local pharmacy must compound).
- Parenteral cidofovir can be another consideration for treatment of resistant systemic HSV infection.

FOLLOW UP

- Acyclovir resistance: uncommon, disease progression limited to almost exclusively to compromised hosts. If no clinical response and lab-confirmation of HSV infection obtained, change treatment (see acyclovir-resistant recommendations above). Resistance testing not routinely recommended.

OTHER INFORMATION
- HSV suppressive therapy does NOT decrease risk of HIV acquisition among HSV-infected, HIV-uninfected woman.

BASIS FOR RECOMMENDATIONS
Centers for Disease Control and Prevention, Workowski KA, Berman SM. Sexually transmitted diseases treatment guidelines, 2006. *MMWR Recomm Rep*, 2006; Vol. 55; pp. 1–94.
Comments: The CDC treatment guidelines provide clinicians with a readily available reference for STD treatments recommended by a panel of national and international experts in STD diagnosis, treatment, prevention, and control. These guidelines available electronically from: http://www.cdc.gov/

Stevens DL, Bisno AL, Chambers HF, et al. Practice guidelines for the diagnosis and management of skin and soft-tissue infections. *Clin Infect Dis*, 2005; Vol. 41; pp. 1373–406.
Comments: These 2005 Infectious Disease Society of America (IDSA) guidelines for skin and soft tissue infections include recommendations for herpes simplex virus infections, including infections in immunocompromised persons.

ACOG. ACOG practice bulletin. Management of herpes in pregnancy. Number 8 October 1999. Clinical management guidelines for obstetrician-gynecologists. *Int J Gynaecol Obstet*, 2000; Vol. 68; pp. 165–73.
Comments: Clear description and rationale for the recommendation for HSV management in pregnancy.

Cinque P, Cleator GM, Weber T, et al. The role of laboratory investigation in the diagnosis and management of pts with suspected herpes simplex encephalitis: a consensus report. The EU Concerted Action on Virus Meningitis and Encephalitis. *J Neurol Neurosurg Psychiatry*, 1996; Vol. 61; pp. 339–45.
Comments: An excellent summary of the role of the laboratory in the diagnosis of herpes simplex encephalitis.

HHV-8

Joel Blankson, MD, PhD

MICROBIOLOGY
- Human herpesvirus-8 (HHV8): human gammaherpes virus, also known as Kaposi's sarcoma herpesvirus (KSHV).
- 20–30% of homosexual males HHV8 seropositive vs 1% of HIV-1 negative blood donors. Associated with receptive anal intercourse and number of partners.
- An unknown cofactor may be involved in transmission.
- HHV-8 gene products promote spindle cell proliferation and angiogenesis and may therefore eventually lead to tumor transformation.

CLINICAL
- Probable cause of HIV-associated Kaposi sarcoma (KS); typically characterized by violaceous vascular lesions on skin, mucous membranes and/or viscera (e.g., GI tract, and lungs).
- HHV-8 is the probable cause of classic KS (non HIV-associated). This variant is usually limited to skin and typically affects elderly Mediterranean and East European men.
- Probable cause of endemic African KS. Presentation varies from skin lesions only to aggressive systemic disease.
- Associated with multicentric Castleman's disease, a lymphoproliferative disorder mostly seen in HIV+ pts: characterized by B type symptoms, lymphadenopathy, hypergammaglobulinemia.
- Associated with primary effusion lymphoma; a non-Hodgkin's Disease B cell lymphoma mostly seen in HIV+ pts. Presents with body cavity based effusions in the absence of a solid tumor.
- Has been associated with KS as well as a febrile illness with bone marrow failure in transplant pts.
- HIV-associated KS is seen mostly in homosexual men. HHV-8 found in saliva and semen.
- Pulmonary KS typically presents with dyspnea, cough, chest pain, or hemoptysis.
- Gastrointestinal KS can cause abdominal pain, intestinal obstruction or hemorrhage.

SITES OF INFECTION
- Mucocutaneous sites: skin, oropharynx. Endothelial and spindle cells w/ HHV-8 DNA.
- Visceral organs.
- Lung.
- Gastrointestinal tract.
- HHV-8 DNA saliva, semen, viremia (in HIV and transplant pts), B cells of primary effusion lymphoma, and lymphoid tissue of multicentric Castleman's disease.

TREATMENT

Kaposi Sarcoma (local disease <25 lesions)

- Cryotherapy, radiation therapy, surgery.
- Topical alitretinoin has been shown to have an approximately 35% partial response. 0.1% gel applied to affected site 2–4 ×/day.
- Intralesional injections with vinblastine has 60–90% clinical response rate. 0.2–0.3 mg/mL: 0.1 mL/0.5 cm^2 lesion.

Kaposi Sarcoma (Systemic Disease)

- First line of therapy should probably be HAART in HIV infected pts or reduction of immunosuppressive therapy in transplant pts.
- A survival benefit has been demonstrated in a retrospective study in pts treated with protease inhibitor based antiretroviral therapy and chemotherapy versus chemotherapy alone.
- Protease inhibitors have antiangiogenic effects and have been effective in treating KS in animal models. Relapse of disease has been seen in pts when PIs were replaced with NNRTIs in 2 small studies.
- Combination chemotherapy often suggested.
- Paclitaxel 100 mg/m² every 2 wks was associated with a 59% response rate.
- Pegylated liposomal doxorubicin 40 mg/m² q2wk has been shown to be more effective than chemotherapy with 58% response rate.
- Alpha interferon and antiretroviral therapy: in one study, DDI 200 mg twice-daily with alpha interferon at either 1 million units or 10 million units sc daily was associated with 40% or 55% response rate respectively.
- Angiogenesis inhibitors are being used in clinical trials with some success. In one study thalidomide 200–1000 mg (median dose 600 mg) daily resulted in a 40% partial response rate.

Multicentric Castleman's Disease

- Combination chemotherapy, consult oncology. Rituximab (375 mg/mm², once weekly for 4 wks) has been shown to be very effective.
- Alpha-interferon at 5 million units three times a wk was reported to cause prolonged remission in a case report.
- Anti-IL6 antibody has been useful in alleviating symptoms due to IL-6 overproduction (one of HHV-8 genes encodes a viral variant of this cytokine).
- Ganciclovir at 1.25 mg/kg qday or 5 mg/Kg IV twice daily or valganciclovir at 900 mg PO twice daily caused remission of disease in a report of 3 HIV+ pts.
- A case series showed that the initiation of HAART did not prevent relapse of disease, but may prolong survival.

Primary febrile illness with BM failure

- A reduction in immunosuppressive therapy in conjunction with foscarnet 80 mg/kg twice daily × 2 wks was successful on a case report basis in a transplant pt.

OTHER INFORMATION

- HHV-8 mostly causes disease in immunocompromised individuals.
- Treatment with PI-based HAART has been associated with decreased mortality in pts receiving chemotherapy for systemic KS.
- Protease inhibitors may have direct effect on KS due to antiangiogenic properties. It may therefore be beneficial to include this class of drugs in HAART regimens when treating pts with KS.
- Interferon-alpha probably is effective in KS because it has both antiviral and immunomodulatory effects.
- Pulmonary KS can be life threatening and should be treated immediately.

BASIS FOR RECOMMENDATIONS

Sullivan RJ, Pantanowitz L, Casper C, et al. Epidemiology, Pathophysiology, and Treatment of Kaposi Sarcoma-Associated Herpesvirus Disease: Kaposi Sarcoma, Primary Effusion Lymphoma, and Multicentric Castleman Disease. *Clin Infect Dis*, 2008; Vol. 47; p. 1209.

Comments: Recent review of HHV-8 associated diseases.

Leitch H, Trudeau M, Routy JP. Effect of protease inhibitor-based highly active antiretroviral therapy on survival in HIV-associated advanced Kaposi's sarcoma pts treated with chemotherapy. *HIV Clin Trials*, 2003; Vol. 4; pp. 107–14.

Comments: Retrospective study looking at the role of PI based HAART in pts getting chemotherapy for systemic KS. Mortality was 21% in pts getting HAART and chemotherapy versus 70% in those receiving chemotherapy alone.

PATHOGENS

HTLV I/II

Joel Blankson, MD, PhD

MICROBIOLOGY
- Human Type C Retrovirus.

CLINICAL
- **HTLV-I** endemic in Caribbean, Southern Japan, parts of Africa, South America; transmitted by breast feeding, contaminated blood products, IDU, sexual contact.
- Most infections are asymptomatic.
- HTLV-I infection has 5% life time risk of Adult T cell leukemia (ATL). ATL presents with type B symptoms, lymphadenopathy. Skin involvement (plaques, nodules) common. Hypercalcemia a common tipoff.
- HTLV-I infection has 0.5–2% lifetime risk of HTLV-I associated myelopathy/tropical spastic paraparesis (HAM/TSP): progressive disease with leg stiffness, weakness, low back pain, bladder dysfunction.
- HTLV-I infection may result in immunosuppression, associated with strongyloides hyperinfection, and decreased reactivity to PPD.
- HTLV-1 may accelerate the progression to AIDS in HTLV/HIV-1 coinfected pts.
- Transplant recipients of organs from asymptomatic HTLV-1 seropositive pts have developed HAM/TSP.
- **HTLV-II** endemic in IDUs. Most infections believed to be asymptomatic.
- HTLV-II not definitively been shown to cause human disease.
- Virological diagnosis most often made by serology.

SITES OF INFECTION
- CD4+ T cells are the main target of HTLV-I infection.
- In ATL, circulation of monoclonal transformed CD4+ T cells bearing HTLV-I provirus.
- HTLV-II infects peripheral blood mononuclear cells.

TREATMENT

Adult T cell leukemia
- Obtain oncology consultation. Conventional chemotherapy.
- Small prospective phase II trial showed encouraging results with AZT (1 g PO qday) and alpha interferon (9 million units SQ q24h).

HAM/TSP
- Corticosteroids, cyclophosphamide, alpha-interferon, IVIG, plasmapheresis, and danazol have been used with inconsistent results.
- AZT (1–2 g daily) or 3TC (150 mg twice daily) alone, or AZT (250 mg twice daily) and 3TC (150 mg twice daily) used in three small studies. While decreases in proviral HTLV-I load were seen, symptoms did not improve in most pts.

Asymptomatic HTLV-I/II infection
- No evidence for treatment.

OTHER INFORMATION
- >95% of pts seropositive for HTLV-I will not develop disease.
- HTLV-II has not been definitively shown to cause a disease process.
- CDC recommends that pts with asymptomatic infection not breast feed, donate blood, or share needles. Latex condoms should be used.
- Asymptomatic infections probably should not be treated. HTLV genome is integrated into host DNA, therefore it is probably impossible to eradicate infection.
- Higher proviral loads have been associated with development of HAM/TSP.

MORE INFORMATION
While ATL and HAM/TSP are thought to be due mostly to clonal expansion of CD4+ T cells with integrated provirus, the decrease of proviral loads in response to reverse transcriptase inhibitors (AZT, 3TC) suggest that active viral replication may also play a role. Studies looking at the response of both disease processes to sustained highly active antiretroviral therapy are needed especially given the high relapse rate of ATL after treatment with interferon and AZT.

BASIS FOR RECOMMENDATIONS
Centers for Disease Control and the U.S.P.H.S. Working Group. Guidelines for counseling persons infected with human T-lymphotropic virus type I (HTLV-I) and type II (HTLV-II). Centers for Disease Control and Prevention and the U.S.P.H.S. Working Group. *Ann Intern Med*, 1993; Vol. 118; pp. 448–54.
Comments: A practical set of guidelines from the CDC.

HUMAN PAPILLOMAVIRUS (HPV)

Noreen A. Hynes, MD, MPH

MICROBIOLOGY

- Non-enveloped DNA virus.
- The HPVs are widespread worldwide.
- >80 types recognized as capable of causing human infection with specific clinical manifestations.
- Papillomaviruses use skin or mucosal linings (such as oral, genital, anal, or respiratory) to replicate.
- Some types have oncogenic potential.

CLINICAL

- **Anogenital warts** (condylomata acuminatum): flesh to gray colored; sessile or with short, broad peduncle; smooth to jagged, acuminate lesions caused by "low risk" (non-oncogenic) virus types. <u>Men</u>: uncircumcised—85–90% located in preputial cavity; circumcised—most on penile shaft; 1–25% involve initial 3 cm of urethral meatus. Perianal warts common in MSM where internal warts also seen. <u>Women</u>: locations variable including posterior introitus, labia majora, labia minora, clitoris. Overall, perineum, vagina, anus, cervix, urethra. <u>Dx</u>: by visible inspection with biopsy confirmation in certain settings including when diagnosis uncertain such as when lesions are unresponsive to or progress on treatment, the pt is immunocompromised, pigmented warts, or warts that are ulcerated, fixed, bleeding or indurated. New HPV DNA tests should not be used for diagnosis of visible warts. Applying 3%–5% acetic acid usually turns HPV infected mucosa whitish but the sensitivity and specificity of this procedure as a screening method is undefined. Screen high risk STD pts for syphilis in area where this STD is present as warts and secondary syphilis lesions (condylomata lata) may look similar.
- **Uterine cervical infection without visible warts:** usually no clinical signs of infection. "High risk" (oncogenic) virus types responsible for 99.7% of all cervical cancer but most infections do not lead to cervical cancer. New interim screening guidelines recommend use of HPV DNA testing (Hybrid Capture-2™ High Risk DNA Test, Digene, Gaithersburg, MD) in target populations combined with cytology as a screening modality in women >29 yrs of age and all women with ASCUS (atypical squamous cells of undetermined significance) on cytology, screening subsequent to colposcopy, and previous treatment of cervical intraepithelial neoplasia stage 3 (CIN-3).
- **Perianal and intraanal HPV infection without visible warts:** Oncogenic HPV-16 and HPV-18 account for most cases of anal intraepithelial neoplasia (AIN) and squamous cell carcinoma of the ano-rectal area. The cellular transition zone of the anal verge is at higher risk of infection than other mucosal surfaces in the perirectal area. Annual screening for anal neoplasia using anal Pap smears in high risk groups is not currently recommended but may be of use.
- **Cutaneous warts** (common, plantar, flat): mostly seen in children/adolescents but may be occupational hazard in butchers, fish handlers, and meat packers. Caused by non-oncogenic genotypes of HPV (HPV-1, -2, -4, and -27 are most common). Usually asymptomatic except if at weight-bearing, frequent friction site. Spontaneous resolution of 50–90% within 1–5 yrs. Pts with warts lasing >18 mos despite attempts at treatment are more likely to be HLA-type DQA1*0301.
- **Common warts** (verruca vulgaris): most common type of cutaneous wart, most prevalent in young children. Usually on the hands. Brown, exophytic, hyperkeratotic papule. Spontaneous resolution of wart seen in 50–90% within 1–5 yrs.

PATHOGENS

- **Plantar warts** (verruca plantaris): 2nd most common wart; most common in adolescents/ young adults. Thrombosed capillaries upon paring down distinguish from callus. Spontaneous resolution of 50–90% within 1–5 yrs.
- **Flat warts** (verruca plana): most common in children. Occurs on face, neck, chest, flexor surfaces of forearms and legs. Spontaneous resolution of 50–90% within 1–5 yrs.
- **Recurrent respiratory papillomatosis:** a disease primarily of larynx. Two forms: juvenile onset (transmitted from HPV-infected mother during passage through birth canal) and adult-onset, believed to be an STD. Detection is usually following complaints of changes in voice or, in rapidly growing lesions, secondary to difficulty breathing.
- **Other uncommon forms:** Buschke-Lowenstein tumors (giant condylomas), Bowenoid papulosis (flesh colored to reddish papules outside the anogenital area), Bowen's disease (gradually enlarging, well-demarcated, usually solitary (multiple in 10–20%) erythematous plaque with an irregular border and surface crusting or scaling of the skin, often of the lower leg), Erythroplasia of Queyrat on the glans penis (similar in morphology to Bowen's disease lesions) have oncogenic potential. Suspect cases should be referred to a dermatologist for management.

MORE CLINICAL

Anogenital Warts: genital HPVs are most common STD worldwide; 500,000 persons/yr in U.S. acquire symptomatic warts; visible warts usually not associated w/ oncogenic type. **Natural hx of visible anogenital warts:** 3 courses

a. Spontaneous regression: 10–30% regression in 3 mos.

b. Remain unchanged.

c. Progress to dysplasia **DDX of anogenital warts:** includes condylomata lata (secondary syphilis), molluscum contagiosum, seborrheic keratosis, lichen planus, "pink pearly penile papules", and neoplastic lesions **Recurrent Respiratory Papillomatosis:** Can lead to obstructive, life-threatening respiratory compromise in infants/children. Adult form usually not as aggressive as that seen in infants/children. Caused by non-oncogenic HPV genotypes, most frequently HPV-6 and HPV-11.

Uncommon conditions associated with HPV

- **Epidermodysplasia verruciformis:** rare; probably autosomal recessive (sex-linked also reported); disseminated (the trunk, the hands, the upper and lower extremities, and the face are characteristic) flat to warty eruptions and reddish-brown pigmented plaques beginning early in life with frequent malignant transformation to squamous cell carcinomas (SCC), after age 30 yrs, first on sun-exposed areas. Multiple HPV types often present simultaneously. HPV-5 and HPV-8 have been isolated in more than 90% of associated SCC. Pts with suspect disease should be referred to an oncologic dermatologist for definitive diagnosis and management. DDX includes SCC, common warts, flat warts, tinea versicolor, benign papillomas.
- **The giant condyloma of Buschke-Lowenstein (GCBL):** slow growing verrucous lesion that is highly destructive to contiguous tissue; most commonly found on glans penis seldom metastasizes. Most commonly located on the glans penis in (usually uncircumcised men) > other anogenital mucosal surfaces, including the vulva, vagina, rectum, scrotum, and bladder. HPV is suspect cause with types 6 and 11 commonly found and types 16 and 18 occasionally found; type 54 rarely found. In U.S. accounts for 5–24% of penile cancers and 0.3–0.5% of all male malignancies. GCBL located outside the penis are much more infrequent. Bladder lesions have been associated with schistosomiasis (i.e., *Schistosoma haematobium*). Pts with suspect GCBL should be referred for diagnosis and treatment to a dermatologist.
- **Bowenoid papulosis (BP):** HPV (usually type 16)-induced papules with a distinctive histopathology (called Bowen's disease when occuring outside the anogenital region and also seen in erythroplasia of queyrat) of focal epidermal hyperplasia and dysplasia and evidence of squamous cell carcinoma (SCC) in situ. No racial, gender preferences; found in sexually active young adults with mean age of 31 yrs.
- **Bowen's disease (BD):** a gradually enlarging well demarcated, usually solitary (multiple in 10–20%) erythematous plaque with an irregular border and surface crusting or scaling of the skin. BD may occur at any age in adults but is rare before the age of 30 yrs

(6th and 7th decade most common). Affected sites include lower leg (60–85%); other sites (15–40%). Women account for up to 85% of cases. Pts with suspect BD should be referred to a dermatologist for management. HPV is suspected but not proven as the etiological agent of some or all of the cases.

- **Erythroplasia of Queyrat (on the glans penis):** lesions are morphologically similar to those of Bowen's disease and occur on the glans penis and under the prepuce, almost exclusively in uncircumcised men. The histopathology is intraepithelial neoplasia. Pts with suspect BD should be referred to a dermatologist for management. HPV is suspected but not proven as the etiological agent of some or all of the cases.

SITES OF INFECTION

- Cutaneous surfaces: plantar warts, common warts.
- Mucosa: genitalia in areas of coital friction, perianal/anal area, mouth, cervix.
- Larynx: respiratory papillomatosis.

TREATMENT

External Anogenital Warts – Common Treatments

- Response to treatment is variable and no single pt-applied or provider-applied treatment is considered better than another. For a single pt, different options may need to be tried.
- Pt-applied: podofilox 0.5% solution or gel. Apply w/ cotton swab (solution) or finger (gel) to visible warts twice-daily × 3 days, then no treatment × 4 days. Repeat cycle up to 4 cycles. Not to exceed 0.5 mL/day. Treatment area not to exceed 10 cm^2.
- Pt-applied: imiquimod 5% cream. Apply w/ finger qhs, 3 ×/wk for up to 16 wks. Wash Rx area 6–10 hrs after with mild soap and water.
- Provider-applied: trichloroacetic acid (TCA) or bichloroacetic acid (BCA) 80%–90%. Apply small amount to warts, then air dry. Powder area with talc or sodium bicarb to remove unreacted acid. Repeat weekly.
- Provider-applied: cryotherapy with liquid nitrogen or cryoprobe. Repeat q1–2wks.
- Provider-applied: podophyllin resin 10–25% in compound tincture of benzoin. Place small amounts on each wart and allow to air dry. Limit to 0.5 mL solution or 10 cm^2 warts per session. Pt to wash off in 1–4 hrs.
- Provider-applied: surgical removal by tangential scissor or shave excision, curettage, or electrosurgery.
- Alternative provider-applied: intralesional interferon.
- Alternative provider-applied: laser surgery.

Anogenital-Related Warts – Special Considerations

- **Pregnant women:** liquid nitrogen only recommended Rx. Avoid imiquimod, podophyllin, and podophylox.
- **Cervical warts:** must be managed in consultation with an expert. High-grade squamous intraepithelial lesions (SIL) must be excluded before treatment started.
- **Vaginal warts:** TCA or BCA 80–90% applied only to warts in small amounts, let dry to white "frosting" appearance, then powder w/ talc or Na bicarb to remove unreacted acid. Repeat q wk prn.
- **Immunosuppressed pts:** use same Rx as for non-immunosuppressed. May need longer or more frequent treatment due to lower response or non-response.
- **Subclinical genital HPV infection without exophytic warts:** routine use of 3–5% acetic acid to identify these areas not recommended. In absence of coexistent SIL, treatment **not** recommended.
- **Squamous cell carcinoma in SITU:** refer to an expert for Rx.
- **Urethral meatal warts:** provider-applied (cryotherapy or podophyllin resin 10–25%) or Pt-applied (podofilox 0.5% solution or gel or imiquimod 5% cream) can be tried as for anogenital warts (limited data).
- **Oral warts:** provider-applied cryotherapy or surgical removal only.

Cutaneous Warts

- Most will resolve spontaneously.
- Hand warts: self application of salicylic and lactic acid collodion at 1:1:4, daily for up to 12 wks (cure rate about 70%).
- Hand warts: cryotherapy q wk × 3 (70% cure).

PATHOGENS

- Plantar warts: 40% salicylic acid tape kept in place × several days followed by debridement while the wart is still damp followed by cryotherapy or caustics application (30–70% trichloroacetic acid).
- Plantar warts: direct destruction using carbon dioxide laser, acids. Snipping or curettage of filiform warts are alternatives.
- Flat warts: tretinoin (retinoic acid cream 0.05%) daily w/ or w/o topical 5% benzoyl peroxide or topical 5% salicylic acid cream until cured.
- Flat warts: topical 5-fluorouracil cream (1% or 5%) daily until resolved.

Referral for Management

- Cervical warts, rectal mucosal warts, oral warts, suspected laryngeal warts.
- Suspected cancerous lesions.
- Epidermodysplasia verruciformis.
- Bowen's disease and Bowenoid papulosis.
- Buschke-Lowenstein tumors.
- Erythroplasia of Queyrat.

OTHER INFORMATION

- No one RX for anogenital HPV is better than another; recurrences common after RX. Topical therapies for anogenital warts should **not** be used if wart burden exceeds 10 cm^2.
- Interim cervical cancer screening guidelines: may add HPV DNA test (HDT) to cervical cytology (CC) in women >29 yr rescreen using both tests; if both tests neg rescreen in 3 yrs. Rescreen in 6–12 mos if CC neg, HDT positive for high risk types. Colposcopy if either positive on repeat or ASCUS on initial pap. Women <30 should be screened annually beginning 3 yrs after sexual debut or beginning at 21 yrs, whichever occurs first. The American Cancer Society recommendations recommend biannual screening if liquid-based media is used for Pap smear due to its increased sensitivity.

MORE INFORMATION

Anogenital Warts and Oncogenic HPV Types

- >30 types of HPV can infect the genital tract.
- Visible warts are usually caused by HPV types 6 or 11 and are not strongly associated with neoplasia. No data support use of type-specific HPV nucleic acid tests for routine dx of visible warts. Therefore, wart treatment is largely cosmetic; recurrence rates are high. Treating visible warts does not alter risk for the development of cervical cancer.
- Other HPV types (16, 18, 31, 33, 35) in the anogenital region that have been associated with neoplasia are much less likely to cause visible warts. Occasionally these types cause visible findings of the vulva, penis and anus with neoplastic changes on biopsy.

Interim Cervical Cancer Screening Guidelines

- Similar guidelines offered by 3 groups: American Cancer Society, American College of Obstetricians and Gynecologists, and the U.S. Public Health Service Prevention Guidelines. (www.acs.org; www.acog.org; www.cancer.org).

The Use of Quadrivalent Hpv Vaccine (Gardasil®)

- **Vaccine composition:** Gardasil®, protects against four HPV types, which are responsible for 70% of cervical cancers (high risk type 16 and type 18 virus) and 90% of genital warts (low risk type 6 and type 11 virus).
- **Prevention strategy:** Ideally, the vaccine should be administered before sexual debut and these females should receive full immunization. However, females who are sexually active also may benefit from vaccination. Females who already have been infected with one or more HPV type would still get protection from the vaccine types they have not acquired. Few young women are infected with all four HPV types in the vaccine. Currently, there is no test available for clinical use to determine whether a female has had any or all of the four HPV types in the vaccine. The HPV vaccine can be given to females who have an equivocal or abnormal Pap test, a positive Hybrid Capture II® high risk test, or genital warts. However, women should be advised that data do not indicate that the vaccine will have any therapeutic effect on existing Pap test abnormalities, HPV infection or genital warts. Lactating women can receive the HPV vaccine. Immunocompromised females, either from disease or medication, can receive this vaccine; however, the immune response to vaccination and vaccine efficacy might be less than in immunocompetent females. **The HPV vaccine is**

not recommended for use in pregnancy at this time. The vaccine has not been causally associated with adverse outcomes of pregnancy or adverse events to the developing fetus. However, data on vaccination in pregnancy are limited. Any exposure to vaccine in pregnancy should be reported to the vaccine pregnancy registry (800-986-8999). **The HPV vaccine is contraindicated for persons with a history of immediate hypersensitivity to yeast or to any vaccine component.**

- **Recommended for:** a) 11–12 yr-old girls (but can be administered to girls as young as 9 yrs of age) and b) 13–26 yr-old females who have not yet received or completed the vaccine series.
- **Mode of administration:** 1 dose × 3 IM with dosing at mo 0, mo 2, and mo 6. Can be administered at the same visit as other age-appropriate vaccines, such as Tdap, Td, MCV4, and hepatitis B vaccines.
- **Cervical cancer screening in vaccinated women: Cervical cancer screening recommendations have not changed for females who receive the HPV vaccine.**

BASIS FOR RECOMMENDATIONS

American Academy of Pediatrics Committee on Infectious Diseases. Recommended immunization schedules for children and adolescents—United States, 2007. *Pediatrics*, 2007; Vol. 119; pp. 207–8, 3 p following 208.

Comments: The January 2007 American Academy of Pediatrics recommended immunization schedules for children and adolescents for the first time include universal immunization of all females beginning at age 12 yrs (or as early as 9 yrs in some cases) with "catch up" immunization of other girls and women who have not been vaccinated with HPV vaccine (the first was approved by the FDA in November 2006). These recommendations mirror the interim recommendations of the Advisory Committee on Immunization Practices (ACIP) outlined in a press release by CDC in November 2006. No final recommendations have been published.

Centers for Disease Control and Prevention, Workowski KA, Berman SM. Sexually transmitted diseases treatment guidelines, 2006. *MMWR Recomm Rep*, 2006; Vol. 55; pp. 1–94.

Comments: The 2006 CDC treatment guidelines for STDs clearly state that HPV DNA testing for cervical HPV infection should be limited based upon the interim screening recommendation promulgated by the American Cancer Society and others. Treatments for genital warts is clearly outlined and explained. These guidelines were published prior to licensure of the new quadrivalent HPV vaccine (late 2006).

Wright TC, Schiffman M, Solomon D, et al. Interim guidance for the use of human papillomavirus DNA testing as an adjunct to cervical cytology for screening. *Obstet Gynecol*, 2004; Vol. 103; pp. 304–9.

Comments: FDA has approved HPV DNA testing (HDT) as an adjunct to cytology for cervical (CC) CA screening. It is **not** a replacement for CC. The interim consensus guidance was issued from a cosponsored workshop: NIH/NCI, ACS, and ASCCP. The guidance is that clinicians MAY choose to add HDT to CC in women >29 yrs. If both tests negative, repeat screen in 3 yrs; if CC neg and HDT positive for high risk HPV types, repeat both tests in 6–12 mos. If either test positive, proceed to colposcopy. CC with negative HDT should have repeat cytology in 12 mo; Colpo if CC ASCUS w/positive HDT or CC > ASCUS. HPV DNA testing (the Hybrid Capture-2 test) requests should be request high risk virus probes only.

JC/BK VIRUS

Khalil G. Ghanem, MD

MICROBIOLOGY

- BK and JC viruses are DNA polyomaviruses.
- Members of DNA tumor virus family, and both well-known to cause tumors in rodents; however, oncologic potential in humans less certain.

CLINICAL

- Cause of hemorrhagic cystitis (BK virus) and progressive multifocal leukoencephalopathy (PML, JC virus), mainly immunocompromised hosts (AIDS, steroids, transplants).
- Acquired in childhood/adolescence, 60–80% adults seropositive. Virus persists in kidney; asymptomatic viruria in immunosuppression (~50%) and pregnancy (3%). Transmission: saliva, placenta, urine, blood, sex.
- Sx: primary infxn usually asymptomatic. Mild URI sx seen (30%) with BK.
- **Diagnosis:** PCR CSF (JC) or urine (BK and JC). Urine epithelial cell cytology may be suggestive ("decoy Cells"). MRI suggestive (white matter T2 intense for PML); definitive: JC (brain bx), BK (kidney bx with immunohistochemistry).
- Clinical picture (immunocompromised host + symptoms) + radiographic (PML) + suggestive lab finding (PCR/urine cytology). Serology NOT helpful. Renal bx for BK recommended.

- **JC:** CNS [PML: hemiparesis (42%), cognitive (36%), visual (32%), ataxia, aphasia, cranial nerves, sensory]; CNS malignancies, possible link?
- **BK:** GU (hematuria, hemorrhagic cystitis, ureteric stenosis, interstitial nephritis).
- Lung: URI.
- Eye: retinitis.
- Liver: hepatitis.
- CNS or neoplasia link less certain for BK virus.

TREATMENT
BK Virus
- Asymptomatic: no therapy needed. Symptomatic: no effective treatment exists. If possible, decrease immunosuppression.
- Cidofovir: effective in some case reports but nephrotoxicity is an issue.

JC Virus
- Asymptomatic: no treatment. PML: no good therapy exists; in AIDS, antiretroviral medications may help.
- Cidofovir (5 mg/kg baseline, wk 1 then q2 wks) has been used; however, effectiveness unclear (see DeLuca ref, ineffective in AIDS).

OTHER INFORMATION
- For both viruses, a diagnosis should not be made on the basis of PCR data alone. Combine clinical, radiographic, laboratory data.
- Controversy re: optimal therapy for PML. HAART Rx in AIDS favored. Data on cidofovir is observational and conflicting. No prospective randomized trials.
- Association between PML and natalizumab, a monoclonal antibody against alpha4 integrins used for MS and possible association with rituximab.
- Occasionally, apparently immunocompetent individuals are afflicted with PML.

BASIS FOR RECOMMENDATIONS
De Luca A, Ammassari A, Pezzotti P, et al. Cidofovir in addition to antiretroviral treatment is not effective for AIDS-associated progressive multifocal leukoencephalopathy: a multicohort analysis. *AIDS*, 2008; Vol. 22; pp. 1759–67.

Comments: 370 HIV+ PML pts diagnosed from 1996 treated with combination antiretroviral therapy with or without cidofovir were evaluated. In combination antiretroviral therapy-treated PML pts, cidofovir use did not influence PML-related mortality or residual disability (HR 0.93, 0.66–1.32).

Trofe J, Hirsch HH, Ramos E. Polyomavirus-associated nephropathy: update of clinical management in kidney transplant pts. *Transpl Infect Dis*, 2006; Vol. 8; pp. 76–85.

Comments: Review on transplant-associated BK nephropathy with an update on a small series of pts treated with leflunomide, intravenous immune globulin therapy, and fluoroquinolones.

Marra CM, Rajicic N, Barker DE, et al. A pilot study of cidofovir for progressive multifocal leukoencephalopathy in AIDS. *AIDS*, 2002; Vol. 16; pp. 1791–7.

Comments: 24 pts with AIDS and PML received cidofovir 5 mg/kg intravenously baseline, 1 wk a q2wks. Cidofovir did not improve neurological examination scores at wk 8. However, scores were significantly better in subjects who entered with suppressed plasma HIV-1-RNA levels, which could be the result of control of HIV-1 infection itself or cidofovir.

MEASLES

Paul G. Auwaerter, MD

MICROBIOLOGY
- Morbillivirus, RNA virus of paramyxoviridae group, respiratory spread with subsequent viremia.
- Related paramyxoviruses metapneumovirus and Hendra virus newly described agents of resp. illness; Nipah virus cause of encephalitis.

CLINICAL
- Until routine immunization, rubeola virus was the most common and highly infectious of childhood diseases.
- Still a worldwide problem, up to 1 million deaths annually in developing world. Eradication difficult despite WHO efforts.

- Entire illness lasts up to 10 days. Pts usually become afebrile with onset of rash. Pts may also experience diarrhea, vomiting, lymphadenopathy, abdominal pain, pharyngitis, splenomegaly, leukopenia, and thrombocytopenia.
- Diagnosis: usually clinical based on acute febrile illness, characteristic rash and/or Koplik spots (irregular red spots w/ tiny blue-white specks on buccal/lingual mucosa).
- Measles EIA IgM helpful for acute infection, while IgG is used to screen immune status.
- Tissue/secretions may be cultured for virus and/or identified by IFA. Nasopharyngeal aspirate IFA offers rapid dx.
- Secondary complications: otitis media, bronchopneumonia, croup, bronchitis. Most deaths from measles occur in malnourished children succumbing to pneumonia.

SITES OF INFECTION

- **Skin/systemic:** characteristic disease progression—prodrome of fever, cough, coryza, conjunctivitis followed by flat macular rash fusing to form blotches first over chest/trunk then to limbs.
- **Pulmonary:** pneumonitis (giant-cell pneumonia). Atypical measles, now rare, had pneumonitis as hallmark w/ hypersensitivity-like reaction in recipients of killed-measles vaccine exposed to native measles.
- **CNS:** post-infectious encephalitis occurs 1:1000 w/ 15% mortality. Subacute sclerosing panencephalitis (SSPE) very rare, <1:300,000 cases occurring usually many yrs after measles.

TREATMENT

Treatment (Children)

- Most well children may be observed without intervention.
- Supplementation (vitamin A) recommended for children ill enough to be hospitalized (6 mos–2 yrs) or if suffering from neurological/ophthalmological complication, malnutrition or immunodeficiency (>2 yrs).
- Consider vitamin A 200,000 IU PO × 2 days.
- Repeat vitamin A dosing at 4 wks if suffering from eye disease.

Treatment (Adults)

- Supportive care. Disease tends to be more severe than in pediatric populations.
- Some experience w/ ribavirin used parenterally (20–35 mg/kg/day × 7 days) in adults w/ severe pneumonitis [*CID* 1994;19(3):454]. Also available by aerosol, oral routes—but little clinical data for measles.
- Note: IV ribavirin only available from ICN pharmaceutical (only emergency use for hemorrhagic fever): 800-556-1937.

Prevention

- **Children** use two dose schedule in U.S.: routine vaccine w/ MMR at 12 mos (once maternal antibody lost) with booster at ages 4–6 yrs.
- MMR may be administered before age 4–6 yrs, provided more than 4 wks have elapsed since the first dose and both doses are administered at age 12 mos or beyond.
- Measles vaccine does **not** appear to be linked with development of autism, multiple sclerosis, inflammatory bowel disease, etc.
- **Adults** born >1957 should receive at least one dose of measles vaccine unless they have already had measles and are immune. (This vaccine can also be given as measles mumps rubella (MMR) vaccine or measles rubella (MR) vaccine.) Those at increased risk of getting measles—college students, international travelers and health care workers or exposed to a measles outbreak—should receive two doses, provided they are given no less than 1 mo apart.
- Birth prior to 1957, believed immune because of native acquired infection.
- **Exposure:** if age <1 yr, pregnant, immunocompromised or susceptible prophylax w/ IM standard pooled immune globulin. 0.25 mL/kg healthy individuals or 0.5 mL/kg immunocompromised, max dose 15 mL.
- Suspected exposure [e.g., contact w/ known case] in susceptible: immunize w/ vaccine [if no contraindication] within 72 hrs of exposure = disease prevention.
- If receiving gammaglobulin, immunize 6 mos thereafter to avoid antibody neutralization of vaccine.
- Since vaccines (MMR or Attenuvax) are live attenuated viruses, <u>contraindications:</u> pregnancy, immunodeficiencies, lymphoma/leukemia, AIDS.
- Vaccine can be given to HIV+ if asx (CD4 >200) and immunization warranted.

PATHOGENS

OTHER INFORMATION

- Measles not endemic in U.S. since 1997 as most cases imported, outbreaks do occur. Koplik spots may help differentiate febrile illness (like influenza) as they can be seen in prodrome prior to rash.
- HIV, immune suppression, cancer or vitamin A deficiency/malnutrition all risks for severe measles.
- Measles cases (suspected or confirmed) should be reported promptly to local public health authorities.
- Vaccine immunity may wane, but 95% protection commonly quoted; however since 1989 two dose vaccine schedule used to decrease risk of infection with 2–5% who fail to seroconvert after one dose.
- Multiple studies have not been able to link the MMR vaccine to autism, asthma, etc.

MORE INFORMATION

U.S. had fewest measles cases (537) in its history by 2001. However, measles remains fifth leading cause of death below age 5 yrs worldwide. Estimated 31 million cases worldwide in 2000 with 777,000 attributable deaths. Most measles deaths seen in Africa (452,000), SE Asia (202,000), E. Mediterranean (81,000). WHO striving to decrease measles cases and deaths 50% by 2005. Of note, in 1990's WHO and PAHO both had goal of total eradication of measles by 2000, but this was impossible with current vaccine efforts which necessitates maintaining a cold chain for the vaccine supply making complete immunization difficult and expensive. Current efforts are directed at governments to redouble efforts at immunization, and targeted outbreaks.

BASIS FOR RECOMMENDATIONS

Centers for Disease Control. Recommended Immunization Schedules for Persons Aged 0–18 yrs—United States 2007. *MMWR Recomm Rep*, 2007; Vol. 55; pp. 51 and 52.
Comments: Current immunization schedule.

Watson JC, Hadler SC, Dykewicz CA, et al. Measles, mumps, and rubella—vaccine use and strategies for elimination of measles, rubella, and congenital rubella syndrome and control of mumps: recommendations of the Advisory Committee on Immunization Practices (ACIP). *MMWR Recomm Rep*, 1998; Vol. 47; pp. 1–57.
Comments: Current basis for recommendations.

American Academy of Pediatrics Committee. American Academy of Pediatrics Committee on Infectious Diseases: Vitamin A treatment of measles. *Pediatrics*, 1993; Vol. 91; pp. 1014–5.
Comments: Guidelines based on studies suggesting treatment for very sick children or those suffering from malnutrition, immunodeficiency, or complication of infection all do better with measles infection. Note high dose of Vitamin A may cause temporary headache or nausea.

MOLLUSCUM CONTAGIOSUM

Christopher J. Hoffmann MD, MPH

MICROBIOLOGY

- Molluscum contagiosum virus (MCV) is a large, brick or ovoid-shaped double-stranded DNA virus of the genus Molluscipox within the family Poxviridae.
- Two subtypes, MCV I and MCV II result in indistinguishable lesions.
- Viral particles contained in central core of umbilicated lesion.

CLINICAL

- Three populations affected: (1) self limited disease in children, (2) an STD in adults, (3) pts with AIDS.
- Transmitted by skin-to-skin contact, and to a lesser degree by fomites.
- Increased prevalence noted in warm / tropical climates.
- Sx: 2–3 mm (up to 1 cm), single or multiple, firm, umbilicated, pearly papules with waxy surface. Usually asymptomatic. Infrequently: larger, coalescent lesions (giant molluscum) in immunocompromised hosts.
- Symptoms may include: pruritus and associated dermatitis (especially in individuals with atopy).
- Dx: largely based on clinical grounds. If diagnosis is in question, biopsy/histopathology is definitive. May appear similar to cutaneous cryptococcosis or histoplasmosis in AIDS pts.

- Histopathology: molluscum bodies (Henderson-Patterson bodies) visible in cytoplasm of epithelium.
- Some studies have shown increased prevalence in pts with CD4 nadir $<50/mm^3$, during the first 2 mos of immune reconstitution with HAART, only to resolve when CD4 counts rise above $250/mm^3$.
- Ddx (immunocompetent hosts): consider verrucae (common warts), nevi, papular granuloma annulare, pyogenic granuloma.
- Ddx (AIDS): consider cutaneous cryptococcosis or histoplasmosis.

SITES OF INFECTION

- Limited to skin.
- **Children:** lesions most commonly on skin folds and genital region.
- **AIDS:** typical lesions commonly on face/neck, or may be disseminated.
- Large disfiguring, fungating lesions (Giant molluscum) are possible.
- **Atopic dermatitis pts or immunosuppressed:** lesions may spread within plaques of atopic dermatitis, especially those treated with topical immunosuppressive agents, such as tacrolimus or pimecrolimus.

TREATMENT

Treatment of Children

- Often self-limited and does not need treatment. Most cases resolve in 6–9 mos.
- If treatment is desired: curettage, manual expression, liquid nitrogen, trichloroacetic acid, keratolytics, imiquimod, retinoids, electrodesiccation, tape stripping, laser or cantharidin can be used (multiple treatments may be needed for all modalities).
- Only two controlled studies have demonstrated superior efficacy to placebo. Multiple uncontrolled studies have demonstrated efficacy for most destructive techniques.
- Most studies are based upon small case series and open-label studies of the aforementioned modalities.
- The only double blinded studies have tested imiquimod and podophyllotoxin—both result in significantly improved cure rate versus placebo.
- **Preferred:** Imiquimod 5% cream is applied at night for 12 hrs, three evenings per wk for 4–6 wks, or until clinical clearance. Tretinoin 0.05% cream is applied qHS.
- Recent evidence suggests that BIW application of 12% salicylic acid gel or even dilute preparations of potassium hydroxide (10%) twice daily may be superior to vehicle controls.
- Eczema molluscatum is the development of MCV infection in sites treated with topical calcineurin inhibitors. Withdrawal of either the pimecrolimus or tacrolimus is the first step in treatment.
- Other non-specific destructive methods should be performed as infrequently as possible, such as every other mo.

Treatment of Immunosuppressed Patients

- Uncomplicated molluscum is a common nuisance but may represent a serious cosmetic/quality of life problem in the AIDS population.
- Local destructive methods and immunomodulatory agents used, but main goal is to contain spread.
- Localized, minimal disease: curettage, cryotherapy, electrocauterization, KOH solution, trichloroacetic acid, cantharidin or imiquimod cream, or photodynamic therapy w/ visible light-activated ALA.
- To keep minor lesions under control, regular cryotherapy in the office, followed by pt applied imiquimod is preferred. Larger or clustered lesions, trichloroacetic acid/PDT may be necessary.
- Giant molluscum resistant to all known therapies. Cryotherapy, CO_2 laser, tretinoin, and TCA have all been used, and are generally unsuccessful.
- Lesions usually resolve spontaneously and completely when CD4 counts rise above $200–250/mm^3$ with HAART.
- Dosing schedules for imiquimod may need to be increased from three times per wk to qHS, and destructive treatments should be performed more regularly in order to keep the infection under control.
- For recalcitrant infections, especially in immunosuppressed pts, combining therapeutic modalities may be a superior alternative to any one treatment.

PATHOGENS

FOLLOW UP
- For children, it is critical to reassure the parents that this is a benign condition of childhood that will resolve spontaneously.

OTHER INFORMATION
- In children, treatment is usually unnecessary and aggressive destructive modalities may cause scarring.
- In AIDS pts, disseminated cryptococcosis and histoplasmosis may also present as firm umbilicated papules, similar to Molluscum.
- In AIDS pts, it is important to keep lesions under control as if they evolve into giant molluscum, it then is very recalcitrant to treatment.
- In-office curettage/cryotherapy is preferred initial treatments for most cases of molluscum (adults). Adjunctive use of imiquimod at home improves outcomes and may be necessary if many lesions appear.

BASIS FOR RECOMMENDATIONS
van der Wouden JC, Menke J, Gajadin S, et al. Interventions for cutaneous molluscum contagiosum. *Cochrane Database Syst Rev*, 2006; Vol. CD004767.

Comments: Cochrane review of treatments for MCV in non-AIDs pts concludes that no intervention has been shown superior. Only a limited number of studies fit into RCT (137 pts) include 5 total studies of which 3 examined homeopathic remedies, and others looked at salicylic acid, providone iodine + salicylic acid, and potassium hydroxide.

Silverberg N. Pediatric molluscum contagiosum: optimal treatment strategies. *Paediatr Drugs*, 2003; Vol. 5; pp. 505–12.

Comments: This is a fairly thorough review of the treatment options available and a very common-sense approach to the treatment (or no treatment) of molluscum in the pediatric population.

MUMPS

Paul G. Auwaerter, MD

MICROBIOLOGY
- Paramyxovirus (Rubulavirus, ssRNA) spread by respiratory transmission, sx onset 12–25 days post-exposure.
- Acute viral illness, respiratory spread.

CLINICAL
- Average < 300–1000 cases/yr in U.S. until 2006 epidemic. Most cases ages 5–14 yrs, but increasing rates in young adults/college students.
- Adolescent and adult males may experience testicular pain/orchitis (~30%).
- Likely endemic in many developing countries worldwide. Epidemic in U.K. 2004–06. Outbreak in Midwest U.S. from 12/05 mostly in 18–24 yrs olds w/ vaccinated hx.
- Prodromal sx include low grade fever, malaise, headache, anorexia, cough—then leading to salivary gland swelling (parotiditis mostly).
- Up to $\frac{1}{3}$ remain subclinically infected.
- Serious complications (encephalitis, meningitis) occur in adults > children.
- Ddx (parotiditis): enteroviral infection, parainfluenza 3, influenza A, acute HIV, bacterial (*S. aureus*, Gram-negatives), drug reaction, tumor, Sjogrens, sarcoid.
- Dx (serology most commonly available): positive IgM or 4 × rise IgG acute/convalescent sera. Acute titer or IgM assay should be done within 5 days of illness onset. If negative, delayed responses to IgM have been reported, so recommendations are for repeat IgM assessment 2–3 wks after onset of symptoms.
- Dx: isolation of virus from nasopharynx but parotid duct swab best for culture or PCR. Urine samples are no longer recommended. Many laboratories may not have reagents to confirm identity.
- Negative laboratory tests should not conclusively rule-out mumps in previously vaccinated pts, so those with compatible illness with the case definition may be reported as probable.

SITES OF INFECTION
- Salivary glands: parotids > sublingual, submaxillary. Often painful. Lumpy, hamster-like appearance to face. May occur ipsilaterally, but usually bilateral w/i 2–3 days. Develops in ~30–40% of infected.

- GU: orchitis (7–10 days post-parotiditis), may afflict >30% post-pubertal males, 30% bilateral; subsequent infertility rare. Ovarian inflammation described. Spontaneous abortion risk if acquired in first trimester.
- CNS: meningitis (aseptic, occurs up to 50–60%; adults > children), encephalitis (rare, usually postinfectious, 2/100,000). Onset usually ~1 wk post initial sx.
- GI: pancreatitis.
- Otic: deafness occurs 1:20,000 cases.
- Cardiac: 3–15% w/ EKG changes; significant myocarditis rare. Presternal edema is unusual (6% of cases) but seen in setting of Mumps sialoadenitis.
- Joints: migratory arthritis/arthralgia-small and large joints.

TREATMENT

Treatment
- Self-limited, usually sx duration 10–14 days.
- Narcotics or NSAIDs for parotiditis or orchitis pains. Role of corticosteroids unknown.
- MMR given, as thought to be possibly protective against subsequent exposures.
- Reportable disease, notify local health department.

Prevention
- Pts contagious up to 6 days prior to sx onset to 9–10 days after sx resolution. Respiratory viral shedding also occurs in those who never develop sx.
- Adults born prior to 1957 considered immune.
- MMR usually used as vaccine for mumps (ACIP).
- Infant immunization 12–15 mos typical, w/ 2n dose at 4–6 yrs but no later than 11–12 yrs.
- Single dose MMR = 79–91% response in susceptables >12 mos of age (including adults). Second dose likely boosts response rate, do not give earlier than 28 days from initial MMR vaccine.
- MMR revaccination recommended for travelers leaving U.S. (prior to departure) including women of childbearing age, and pts in high-risk groups (college students, healthcare workers, and military personnel).
- **Changes to 1998 ACIP recommendations (May 2006):** 1. Acceptable presumptive immunity—documentation of 2 doses of MMR in school-aged children or high-risk groups (see above). 2. Routine vaccination for HCW—persons born >1957 (2 doses), HCW born < 1957 one dose of mumps vaccine recommended. 3. For outbreaks—children 1–4 yrs and adults at low risk consider 2nd mumps vaccine dose; for HCW born before 1957 without evidence of immunity strongly consider 2 doses of live mumps vaccine.
- Isolation of persons with mumps (*MMWR*, 2008 Oct 10;57(40):1103–5): maintain isolation for 5 days after onset of parotitis, including community or health-care settings. Both standard and droplet precautions should be followed.

OTHER INFORMATION

- More than 250,000 annual cases in U.S. until 1968 introduction of universal immunization (MMR), now usually <1000 cases annually.
- Fatality rare, less than 1 death/yr seen between 1980–99.
- Common in the developing world, most outbreaks in developed countries linked to groups only receiving 1 dose of MMR.
- Orchitis tends to occur ~1 wk after parotiditis w/ high fever, rigor, headache, N/V and abdominal pain. Sx have been misinterpreted for appendicitis.
- Recent U.S. Mumps outbreak due to serotype G, usually covered by MMR vaccine.

MORE INFORMATION

CDC Case Criteria

Acute illness >2 days w/ swelling of parotid +/or salivary glands and no other apparent explanation.

Confirmed case = case definition + lab confirmation or linked to confirmed case.

Probable case = meets case definition, but no supporting lab testing, and not epidemiologically linked.

PATHOGENS

BASIS FOR RECOMMENDATIONS

Centers for Disease Control and Prevention (CDC). Notice to readers: updated recommendations of the Advisory Committee on Immunization Practices (ACIP) for the control and elimination of mumps. *MMWR*, 2006; Vol. 55; pp. 629–30.

Comments: One dose of MMR 78–91% protective, hence emphasizing two dose requirement. See module for changes recommended regarding immunization from the ACIP.

Centers for Disease Control and Prevention (CDC). Brief report: update: mumps activity—United States, January 1–October 7, 2006. *MMWR*, 2006; Vol. 55; pp. 1152–3.

Comments: The 2006 outbreak peaked in April of 2006 with cases reported from 45 states totaling 5783 confirmed and 2597 probable cases. Current diagnostic recommendations are outlined.

NOROVIRUS

Christopher J. Hoffmann, MD, MPH

MICROBIOLOGY

- Noroviruses are 1 of 5 genuses in the Caliciviridae family. Sapoviruses are another genus in the family that also cause acute gastroenteritis.
- Noroviruses are grouped into genogroups (I, II, and IV cause human infections), further divided into genetic clusters.
- Small, nonenveloped, single-stranded positive-sense RNA virus.
- Previously known as "Norwalk-like viruses."

CLINICAL

- Most common cause of food-borne illness in the U.S. with sporadic cases and epidemics (90% of epidemic gastroenteritis is settings such as restaurants, cruise ships, schools, and healthcare settings) due to contaminated food (oysters, frozen raspberries), ill food preparers or contaminated water supplies (usually well water).
- Extremely contagious: infectious dose is <10–100 particles.
- Transmission: fecal-oral, person-to-person transmission, fomites, and airborne transmission (vomitus); viral shedding can occur from 25 hrs after exposure and up to 2 wks after recovery.
- Short incubation period of 12–48 hrs after exposure, duration of illness self-limited with range 12–60 hrs.
- 30% infections asymptomatic; susceptibility to infection involves genetic resistance to infection and acquired immunity.
- Sx: sudden onset of nausea, vomiting, abdominal cramps, myalgias, and non-bloody diarrhea. Constitutional symptoms of headache, fever, and chills occur among <50% and usually resolve after 24 hrs.
- Diarrhea predominates in both children and adults; vomiting alone or in combination with diarrhea is more commonly seen in children than in adults. Children <1 yr predominantly develop diarrhea.
- Dx: often clinical diagnosis, with appropriate epidemiology and after other potential etiologies ruled out. RT-PCR is most reliable, though usually only available through state health department laboratories or CDC. Also available: serology (acute and convalescent), enzyme-linked immunoassay (low sensitivity).
- Prevention: hand hygiene before meals and avoidance of potentially contaminated food and water are recommended.
- Ddx: other infectious or toxin mediated causes of gastroenteritis such as *Bacillus cereus* (toxin), *Staphylococcus aureus* (toxin), other enteric viruses (rotaviruses, other Caliciviruses, adenoviruses), *Campylobacter* spp, *Clostridium perfringens*, *C. difficile*, *Shigella* spp, enterotoxigenic *Escherichia coli* (ETEC).

SITES OF INFECTION

- Gastrointestinal tract, most likely the epithelial cells at or near the duodenojejunal junction; the mechanisms leading to symptomatic infection are not yet delineated.

TREATMENT
General Recommendations

- Treatment: supportive care only.
- Infants and the elderly are most at risk for severe dehydration and may require oral or intravenous hydration.

- Lack of evidence of benefit from antimotility agents (should avoid antimotility agents in children).

FOLLOW UP
- Immunity: 50% of those infected develop short-term immunity to the particular strain only. No evidence of cross-protection between strains.
- Suspected norovirus cases should be reported to the local health department, and if in the health care setting, to infection control.
- Pts with suspected norovirus infection in an outbreak setting should be placed on contact precautions.
- Norovirus is very stable in the environment (can survive freezing and steaming) and only effectively disinfected with bleach. Decontamination requires rigorous, thorough cleaning of all surfaces and floors with bleach as the primary disinfectant.
- Infectivity can last up to 3 days after the last symptoms occur, and thus it is advisable for food handlers and health care providers with suspected infection to be furloughed until they are no longer contagious.

OTHER INFORMATION
- A particular strain of noroviruses in genogroup II.4 is thought to be responsible for an increase in norovirus outbreaks worldwide.
- Noroviruses bind to histo-blood group antigens (HBGA) on gastroduodenal epithelial cells and saliva, which is believed to lead to infection.
- Human histo-blood group antigens (HBGA) appear to affect susceptibility to noroviruses, with HBGA type B being protective.

BASIS FOR RECOMMENDATIONS
Parashar U, Quiroz ES, Mounts AW, et al. "Norwalk-like viruses". Public health consequences and outbreak management. *MMWR Recomm Rep*, 2001; Vol. 50; pp. 1–17.
Comments: This article gives a summary of noroviruses and recommendations about outbreak management.

Centers for Disease Control and Prevention. Norovirus in Healthcare Facilities Fact Sheet. *http://www.cdc.gov/ncidod/dhqp/id_norovirusFS.html.*
Comments: The CDC website gives recommendations for healthcare facilities.

PARAINFLUENZA VIRUS

John G. Bartlett, MD

MICROBIOLOGY
- RNA enveloped (ss strand, negative sense) virus w/ 5 antigenically distinct types (human parainfluenza virus, HPIV, HPIV-1, HPIV-2, HPIV-3, HPIV-4A/4B).
- Viruses are members of the paramyxovirus family with 2 different genera: HPIV-1, HPIV-3 belong to the Respirovirus genus, and HPIV-2, HPIV-4 belong to the Rubulavirus genus.

CLINICAL
- Affects respiratory tract, especially URIs, seasonal. Responsible for ~40–50% of croup, ~10–15% bronchiolitis in children. Bronchitis common but pneumonia uncommon.
- Most common infects pediatric population; most severe infections affect children and compromised hosts.
- Adults: in healthy host causes ~10% of all URIs; complications seen in pts with immunodeficiency, cystic fibrosis, COLD.
- Type 1: big outbreaks, autumn, odd yrs—'03, '05, '07.
- Type 2: October–November.
- Type 3: April–June.
- Types 4A/4B: thought to be rare.
- Dx: culture (gold standard), PCR may be most sensitive and now available in many labs. DFA and EIA serology also used.

SITES OF INFECTION
- Respiratory tract: URIs, pharyngitis (85% of parainfluenza cases), sinusitis, bronchitis, otitis, pneumonitis.
- Small peribronchial nodules in the compromised host.
- CNS: aseptic meningitis (rare).

PATHOGENS

- Disseminated disease: seen in severe immunodeficiency.

TREATMENT
Treatment

- Most cases are mild, self-limited "viral respiratory tract infections." May cause pneumonia, especially in transplant recipients.
- URI: supportive care, for more information see "Upper Respiratory Infections" module.
- Experimental: aerosolized steroids +/− systemic steroids (effective in pediatric croup).
- Experimental: ribavirin for solid organ/bone marrow transplants w/ severe pneumonia. Has been given by aerosol route and orally (30–45 mg/kg/daily PO). Efficacy uncertain.

OTHER INFORMATION

- Parainfluenza causes only respiratory tract infections commonly. Rarely, aseptic meningitis and disseminated infection occur in compromised hosts.
- Adults accounts for ~10% of URIs. Pneumonia seen in pediatric, elderly, and compromised host populations.
- Transmission has been described as pt-pt in paediatric and oncology/transplant units.
- No specific treatment for routine infections. Dx serological tests are insensitive in adult disease.

BASIS FOR RECOMMENDATIONS

Hall CB. Respiratory syncytial virus and parainfluenza virus. *N Engl J Med*, 2001; Vol. 344; pp. 1917–28.

Comments: Review of paraflu and RSV as important ped respiratory tract viruses. Paraflu causes 60% of adult URIs and 5–10% of pneumonias in elderly or immunocompromised adults—esp marrow and organ tx recipients. Most important are paraflu types 1 and 2 which are seasonal.

PARVOVIRUS B19

Khalil G. Ghanem, MD

MICROBIOLOGY

- Single-stranded DNA virus, member the genus, *Parvoviridae*

CLINICAL

- Causes erythema infectiosum/"fifth disease" (children), acute febrile illness with rash.
- May cause also pure red cell aplasia (sickle cell disease, immunocompromised), arthropathy, hydrops fetalis.
- Transmission: respiratory, blood, mother to fetus; high risk contacts (attack rates): students (50%), teachers (30%), day-care (9%), homemaker(9%), other women (4%). Peaks late winter-early spring.
- Infects erythroid progenitor cells; predominant immune response humoral; (+)IgG antibodies associated w/ protection.
- Dx: IgM (85%+ w/ erythema infectiosum or aplastic crisis; turns negative <3 mos), IgG (seen 2 wks post infection; lifelong), PCR most sensitive (**not** diagnostic alone). Giant pronormoblasts seen in blood or bone marrow suggests dx.
- Serology may be negative in immunocompromised.

SITES OF INFECTION

- **Skin:** erythema infectiosum (fifth disease) causing facial erythema ("slapped cheeks"), circumoral pallor (18 days after infection), reticular rash (trunk/limbs).
- **Joints:** complaints seen in 60% females, 30% males, 10% kids: Joints involved: MCP (75%), knees (65%), wrists (55%), ankles (40%). Immune mediated, may persist >1 mo especially women.
- **Bone marrow:** transient aplasia (pts w/ thalassemia, hemolytic anemia), chronic pure red cell aplasia (immunosuppressed, esp HIV, transplant, sickle cell), hemophagocytic syndrome (mostly seen in immunocompromised).
- **Fetus:** hydrops fetalis (pregnant with acute infection, risk ~1.6%. Highest between 11–23 wks gestation), anemia, thrombocytopenia.
- **Other:** CNS (encephalopathy), liver (hepatitis), cardiac (myocarditis).

TREATMENT
Immunocompetent

- No specific treatment usually needed, supportive care.
- NSAIDs for arthropathy.

- Blood products for transient aplasia.
- Weekly U/S for infected pregnant women. Cordocentesis and intrauterine transfusions for hydrops fetalis.

Immunosuppressed
- Chronic pure red cell aplasia: IVIG 0.4 g/kg/day for 5 days or 1 g/kg/day for 2–3 days.
- May need to repeat monthly.

OTHER INFORMATION
- Once the rash appears, the pt is no longer infectious.
- If pregnant woman exposed, check IgG level. If + reassure pt she is immune. If −, risk small but if infected, follow with weekly ultrasound.
- Pregnant women who work in outbreak setting (teachers, child care) should be sent home.
- Parvo B19 may present with symmetrical arthritis identical to rheumatoid arthritis. Parvo B19 arthritis **not destructive**. RF **may** be positive with B19.
- Presence of B19 DNA **not** diagnostic of acute infection. DNA may persist in blood and joints for mos to yrs. Dx based on clinical findings **and** lab findings.

BASIS FOR RECOMMENDATIONS

Frickhofen N, Abkowitz JL, Safford M, et al. Persistent B19 parvovirus infection in pts infected with human immunodeficiency virus type 1 (HIV-1): a treatable cause of anemia in AIDS. *Ann Intern Med*, 1990; Vol. 113; pp. 926–33.

Comments: Case series of 7 pts with HIV and B19 infection with chronic aplasia: of 6 who got treated with IVIG, 4 were cured and 2 relapsed but were successfully treated with additional doses.

RABIES

Khalil G. Ghanem, MD

PATHOGENS

MICROBIOLOGY
- SS-RNA, enveloped Lyssavirus causes rabies, a uniformly fatal encephalitis of humans, and other mammals.
- Domestic dog main reservoir worldwide. Raccoons, foxes, bats, skunks are infected in U.S.

CLINICAL
- Total U.S. human rabies cases: 1–2/yr. Bats most common source of infection in U.S. 39 cases from bats in last 50 yrs (51% pts have no history of bat bite). Between 4–15% of bats in U.S. infected.
- Incubation: 1–3 mos (range: days–yrs).
- Sx (1) **prodrome** (4–10 days): fever, HA, malaise, personality changes, pain/paresthesia at bite and myoedema.
- Sx (2): 2 forms: **furious** [80%: hydrophobia, delirium, agitation, Sz, aerophobia] and **paralytic** [20%: ascending paralysis, meningismus, confusion].
- Both presentations lead to coma within 2–14 days of first symptoms and then death.
- Dx: DFA bx skin specimen from nape of neck above hairline (50% + 1st wk, higher thereafter). RT-PCR on tissue/saliva. CSF (5–30 lymphs, oligoclonal bands). Neutralizing Ab (50% d8, 100% d15). MRI negative usually early in presentation.
- Ddx: HSV encephalitis, tetanus, strychnine or other toxin poisoning, acute inflammatory polyneuropathy, transverse myelitis, polio, PML.
- Ascending paralysis of rabies may be confused with polio.

SITES OF INFECTION
- CNS: hallucinations, confusion, anxiety, biting, hydrophobia, autonomic dysfunction, SIADH.
- Peripheral nervous system and extremities: pain, paraesthesia, ascending paralysis, myoedema.
- CV: arrhythmias, myocarditis, CHF.
- GI: bleeding, N/V, ileus.

TREATMENT
Pre-exposure prophylaxis
- Vaccination of pets.
- Vaccinating those at high risk of acquiring infection (vets, lab workers, spelunkers, travelers to areas with high prev): 3 (1 mL) IM or intradermal [ID] (days 0, 7, 21, or 28). Booster q2–3 yrs if continued risk.

- 4 licensed rabies vaccines: all equally safe and efficacious. Neutralizing Abs produced 7–10 days after vaccine and last for 2–3 yrs.
- Can check serostatus to guide rebooting schedule. No need to check sero-status after treatment in non-immunocompromised hosts.
- Specific pre-exposure prophylaxis recommendations and vaccine info: CDC/ACIP recommendations at: http://www.cdc.gov/mmwr/preview/mmwrhtml/00056176.htm

Postexposure prophylaxis (PEP)

- Wound care w/ 20% soap solution and irrigation with povidone iodine (risk decreased by 90%).
- Contact public health official immediately. if healthy dog/cat, observe × 10 days. If pet develops sx, sacrifice to check DFA for rabies. If +, Rx pt (see below). If skunk/bat/raccoon **immediate** Rx.
- Main concern in the U.S. is bat bites since nearly all cases in the U.S. are bat variant and bat bites may be unnoticed.
- Bites of squirrels, hamsters, gerbils, guinea pigs, rats, mice, chipmunks, rabbits: almost never require PEP but consult local health official.
- PEP: Rabies Immune Globulin RIG (20 IU/kg) [all at wound site if possible, if not, give IM at site other than vaccine site] **and** vaccine: 1 mL IM deltoid days 0,3,7,14, 28.
- If pt previously vaccinated w/i last 3 yrs, then **do not give** rig; only wound cleansing and vaccine on days 0 and 3. If immune status unsure, treat fully with all three measures.
- **In rabies endemic regions: Minor exposures** (licks of broken skin/minor abrasions w/o bleeding): vaccinate while observing animal). **Major exposures** (licks of mucosa/ transdermal bites): **Both** RIG and vaccine.

Therapy

- Supportive care. No currently approved antivirals. All pts until recently succumb to dz, usually w/i 14 days sx onset despite supportive measures (which may prolong lifespan by 50% i.e., 30 days).
- Vaccine + drug-induced coma/ventilator support and ribavirin without vaccine may be the standard of care based upon report of complete recovery [see *NEJM* reference]; regimen has not yet been effective in 2 other pts with rabies.

MORE TREATMENT

- PEP for rabies-endemic areas from: World Health Organization: Expert Committee on Rabies. Eighth Report. Technical report series 824. Geneva, WHO, 1992.

OTHER INFORMATION

- Very often, no history of bite/scratch/exposure making early dx **very** difficult (usually bat-borne).
- Most cases in U.S. are of bat exposure; all U.S. cases in last 10 yrs from dogs/cats were imported. Transmission via organ transplantation documented (see references).
- Location of bite modifies risk of rabies: facial bites are w/ higher risk than extremity bites. Early suturing may be deleterious (especially facial wounds).
- Rabies virus isolated from human saliva, hence theoretical risk of human to human transmission. PEP recommended if bite/scratch/sexual contact with rabid pt.
- In U.S. intradermal vaccination currently approved for pre-exposure prophylaxis **only**.

BASIS FOR RECOMMENDATIONS

Manning SE, Rupprecht CE, Fishbein D, et al. Human rabies prevention—United States, 2008: recommendations of the Advisory Committee on Immunization Practices. *MMWR Recomm Rep*, 2008; Vol. 57; pp. 1–28.
Comments: No new rabies biologics are presented, and no changes were made to the vaccination schedules. However, rabies vaccine adsorbed (RVA, Bioport Corporation) is no longer available for rabies postexposure or pre-exposure prophylaxis, and intradermal pre-exposure prophylaxis is no longer recommended because it is not available in the United States.

Willoughby RE, Tieves KS, Hoffman GM, et al. Survival after treatment of rabies with induction of coma. *N Engl J Med*, 2005; Vol. 352; pp. 2508–14.
Comments: Survival of a 15-yr-old girl in whom clinical rabies developed one mo after she was bitten by a bat. Treatment included induction of coma while a native immune response matured; rabies vaccine was not administered. The pt was treated with ketamine, midazolam, ribavirin, and amantadine.

World Health Organization. World Health Organization: Expert Committee on Rabies. Eighth Report. Technical report series 824. *Geneva, WHO, 1992.*
Comments: Basis for PEP recommendations.

RESPIRATORY SYNCYTIAL VIRUS

John G. Bartlett, MD

MICROBIOLOGY

- Negative sense, single strand, enveloped RNA paramyxovirus.
- Member of *Paramyxoviridae*, along with measles and mumps. RSV part of subfamily *Pneumovirinae*.

CLINICAL

- Respiratory tract pathogens in humans. Major cause of serious disease in infants and immunosuppressed adults, especially lung transplant.
- Epidemics: annually in peds—Nov to mid-May. Nosocomial—pediatric floors, nursing homes, transplant/oncology wards.
- Pediatrics: major cause of infection: otitis, croup, pneumonia, asthma.
- Adult (healthy): URI +/− fever, sinusitis, asthma, otitis, acute exacerbation of chronic bronchitis.
- Causes ~4% of all adult pneumonia. Increased rate in elderly, transplant, cancer chemotherapy pts, use of TNF inhibitors.
- Dx: viral culture (sensitivity 60–90%, 3–7 days); RT-PCR is preferred and now available in most labs as a component of a respiratory virus panel.

SITES OF INFECTION

- Upper respiratory tract: may occur +/− sinusitis, otitis media
- Bronchi: bronchitis, bronchiolitis, asthma
- Lung: pneumonia
- CNS: meningitis, encephalitis (rare)
- Cardiac: myocarditis (rare)
- Derm: exanthem (rare)

Antiviral therapy

- Supportive care usual for most healthy adults, children.
- Pediatrics and some severely immunocompromised adults: ribavirin used for sickest, sometimes combined with RSV immune globulin (RSVIG) and/or palivizumab.
- Experimental for immunosuppressed adult: ribavirin (30–45 mg/kg/day) PO if started early (experience in stem cell and bone marrow tx is poor).
- Ribavirin: can be delivered by aerosol, PO or IV.
- Experimental: RSVIG 1.5 g/kg IVIG with high RSV Ab titer.

Prevention

- Infection control: handwashing, gown, and gloves.
- Palivizumab (humanized monoclonal antibody) for children is recommended for immunoprophylaxis to eligible infants.

OTHER INFORMATION

- Pneumonia seen in the elderly, organ transplant pts, HIV, cancer chemotherapy.
- Diagnostic tests in adults (culture, DFA, PCR). Preferred is PCR.
- High lethality in oncology and transplant pts—consider ribavirin +/− RSV immune globulin (both experimental).
- Typical epidemiology: staff w/ child or pt w/ URI—transmits to oncology pt, then Onc unit, etc.

BASIS FOR RECOMMENDATIONS

Hall CB. Respiratory syncytial virus and parainfluenza virus. *N Engl J Med,* 2001; Vol. 344; pp. 1917–28.

Comments: Reviews of RSV as major epidemic respiratory tract pathogen in peds: 5–40% of pneumonias, 50–90% of hospitalizations for bronchiolitis. In adults—major diseases are URI (10%) +/− sinusitis, fever, otitis and pneumonia in pts with compromised cell-mediated immunity (organ tx, cancer, chemo Rx) and elderly.

PATHOGENS

RHINOVIRUS

Paul G. Auwaerter, MD

MICROBIOLOGY
- Single-strand, nonenveloped positive sense RNA virus, a member of the *Picornaviridae* family of viruses.
- Over 105 serologic virus types.
- Rhinoviruses gain entry via the upper respiratory tract binding to ICAM-1 (intracellular adhesion molecule −1) receptors on epithelial cells lining the respiratory tract. Chemokines and cytokines cause inflammation as a consequence of viral infection causing local symptoms.
- Incubation period is quick; only 8–10 hrs before symptoms begin.

CLINICAL
- Major cause of the common cold, probably causing >50% of cases.
- Frequency of common colds (rhinoviral) more common in childhood, decreasing in adult likely due to partial immunity.
- Major cause of acute flares in persons with reactive airway disease (asthma) and acute flares of chronic bronchitis (AECB).
- Reactive changes in the linings of the sinuses are common (>80%) in the setting of the common cold.
- Bacterial superinfection possible resulting in acute bacterial sinusitis and otitis media.
- Two modes of transmission: aerosol droplets and hand-to-hand contact.

SITES OF INFECTION
- Upper airway

TREATMENT
- Supportive care. See Upper Respiratory Tract Infections module for further details.
- Pleconaril had some minor efficacy in shortening symptoms related to the common cold, but was never FDA approved.
- No vaccine exists.

OTHER INFORMATION
- Not well established that administration of zinc-containing compounds will hasten resolution of the common cold.
- In volunteers, cold symptoms begin within hrs of experimental inoculation with rhinovirus.
- Multiple infections with different strains of rhinovirus are common over one's lifetime.
- Infection is most common in spring and autumn.
- Secondary attack rates can reach ~75% in the home or day care setting.

BASIS FOR RECOMMENDATIONS
Author opinion.
Comments: No guidelines specifically exist for rhinovirus infection.

RUBELLA

Paul G. Auwaerter, MD

MICROBIOLOGY
- RNA togavirus, genus Rubivirus.
- Worldwide infection, with only human reservoirs known.

CLINICAL
- Also known as German measles, spread by respiratory route causing rash and possibly fever, arthralgia/arthritis, LN, conjunctivitis.
- Less severe than measles, sometimes called "3-day measles."
- Only modestly communicable. Most infectious with rash eruption, but viral shed may persist 7 days after onset.
- Incubation 12–23 days, and 20–50% cases may be subclinical. <u>Main public health risk:</u> congenital rubella syndrome (CRS).
- Since 1993 <300 cases/yr in U.S. with <25 cases/yr since 2001. Most (87%) in 15–39 age range. Most cases occur in young Hispanics born elsewhere without routine immunization.

- Ddx includes measles, scarlet fever, parvovirus, infectious mononucleosis.
- Dx usually w/ anti-rubella IgM demonstration. Virus can be cultured from respiratory tract or CSF.
- False (+) IgM may occur with parvovirus, EBV infections or pts with circulating rheumatoid factor (RF).

SITES OF INFECTION

- Skin: maculopapular rash starting on face moving to foot typical, in children often w/o prodrome. Others w/ fever, malaise, LN and URI Sx. Rash fainter than measles w/o coalescing.
- LN: posterior auricular and post. cervical typical. May start before rash, and persist for wks.
- Oropharynx: soft palate petechiae (Forscheimer spots) seen but not specific for rubella.
- Arthralgia/arthritis: expected in adults, less common in children. 70% adult females afflicted esp. fingers, wrists, knees. Duration usually <1 mo, chronic arthritis rare. Ddx includes parvovirus B19.
- Encephalitis: estimated 1:5000 cases, adults > children, mortality up to 50%. Progressive panencephalitis a rare late complication.
- Hemorrhagic events: possible complication of thrombocytopenia with purpura, GI or CNS bleeding. Children > adults, 1:3000.
- Orchitis.
- Neuritis: optic, also described with rubella immunization.
- Congenital rubella syndrome: infection during 1st trimester most dangerous. May cause fetal death, premature delivery. Deafness most common, also eye, cardiac, neuro defects.

TREATMENT

Prevention

- Rubella vaccine licensed 1969, live-attenuated virus (Meruvax II). No communicability of vaccine virus except w/ breastfeeding.
- Although may be given alone, ACIP recommends MMR whenever any individual component is indicated.
- >95% seropositive after single dose if >12 mos. age. 90% remain seropositive at age 15 yrs. Lifelong protection conferred with single dose.
- Two doses rubella vaccine recommended as part of MMR. Current schedule is first dose MMR at 1 yr, then second dose MMR age 4–6.
- Vaccine indications: infants >12 mos., susceptible adolescents and adults (born after 1957), emphasis on non-pregnant women of childbearing age esp. born outside U.S.
- Most vaccine side effects attributed to measles component of MMR. Fever or rash 5–15%, transient joint sx 25% esp. vaccinated adults.
- Contraindications: prior allergic rxn, pregnancy or planned pregnancy within 4 wks, immune suppression, concurrent severe illness, recent immune globulin.
- Post-exp. prophylaxis pregnant pt: if nonimmune exposed to rubella, and abortion not a consideration if rubella develops, some authorities suggest immunoglobulin therapy, though scant evidence for this rx.

Primary Infection (German Measles)

- Often mild illness that necessitates no therapy.
- Fever, arthritic complaints may be treated with acetaminophen or other NSAID's.

OTHER INFORMATION

- In immunized societies, most cases now seen in teen and young adult yrs in unimmunized populations. In U.S., these pts are mostly Hispanic and cases are imported.
- Birth before 1957 or clinical diagnosis of rubella are unreliable as assessing immune status in women still bearing children, therefore serologic screening recommended.
- CDC has declared that rubella is no longer endemic in the U.S. as of 2004.

BASIS FOR RECOMMENDATIONS

Banatvala JE, Brown DW. Rubella. *Lancet*, 2004; Vol. 363; pp. 1127–37.

Comments: Review highlights current issues with rubella, especially it remaining a significant cause of congenital rubella syndrome in developing countries, as well as an uptick in cases recently in Europe. Newer diagnostic technologies such as RT-PCR and detection of rubella-specific IgG and IgM salivary antibody responses are reviewed.

Centers for Disease Control and Prevention (CDC). Recommended adult immunization schedule—United States, 2002–2003. *MMWR Morb Mortal Wkly Rep*, 2002; Vol. 51; pp. 904–8.

PATHOGENS

VARICELLA-ZOSTER VIRUS

Paul G. Auwaerter, MD

MICROBIOLOGY

- DNA virus member of Herpesviridae family.
- Humans only known reservoir.
- Primary infection spread by respiratory route with latency established in nerves.
- By adulthood 90–95% infected (pre-vaccine era).

CLINICAL

- Primary infection = chickenpox = fever <103° F, malaise may precede rash (maculopapular, vesicles, scabs) occurring in crops. Hallmark is appearance of lesions in all stages.
- Immunosuppressed (e.g., leukemics): increased skin lesions often hemorrhagic. Greater risk visceral disease, dissemination (35–50%).
- CNS complications most feared. Cerebellar ataxia children <15 [1:4000] generally benign. Encephalitis 0.1–0.2%, in adults (5–20% mortality). Pneumonitis more common adults/immunosuppressed.
- Herpes zoster = shingles = reactivation from latency in dorsal root ganglia. 20% lifetime risk, mainly elderly; increased rates if immune suppressed. Dermatomal unilateral eruption, thoracolumbar most frequent.
- Dx for chickenpox or shingles mainly clinical. Ddx includes smallpox (distinguish because VZV has lesions in all stages), impetigo by Gr A strep, HSV; vesiculation due to enterovirus.
- If confusing can perform Tzanck smear of vesicle (multinucleated giant cells), viral cx, immunoflourescence stains of fluid/histopathology, PCR. Varicella IgM w/ primary infection.

SITES OF INFECTION

- Cutaneous (primary or reactivation/secondary).
- CNS: ataxia (primary); encephalitis (primary or secondary); cerebral angitis (secondary); meningitis, transverse myelitis, Reye's.
- Pneumonitis (primary).
- Herpes Zoster Ophthalmicus (CN V) +/– keratitis, iridocyclitis (secondary). Acute retinal necrosis, mainly HIV (secondary). Involve ophthalmology consultation.
- Ramsay Hunt Syndrome: geniculate ganglion = facial palsy, aural vesicles, taste abnormal anterior 2/3 tongue (secondary).
- Disseminated (viscera +/– skin): greater mortality with primary infection than dissemination as a result of secondary reactivation.

TREATMENT

Primary Disease: Varicella (Chickenpox)

- Normal children/adolescents (uncomplicated) require no antiviral treatment. Avoid scratching skin which may precipitate secondary bacterial infection/cellulitis. No ASA [Reye's Syn. risk].
- Normal Adult: treat within 24 hr onset of exanthem for efficacy. Acyclovir 800 mg PO four times a day × 5 days.
- Varicella pneumonia: acyclovir 10–12 mg/kg q8h, or valacyclovir 1 g PO three times a day or famciclovir 500 mg PO three times a day all for 7–10 days.

Varicella/Chickenpox Adult Immunosuppressed

- Acyclovir 10 mg/kg IV q8h × 7–10 days.
- Some clinicians will use more bioavailable oral therapy in stable pts to avoid hospitalization, e.g., valacyclovir 1 g PO three times a day or famciclovir 500 mg PO three times a day 7–10 days.
- Varicella pneumonia: acyclovir 10–12 mg/kg q8h, or valacyclovir 1 g PO three times a day or famciclovir 500 mg PO three times a day all for 7–10 days.

Zoster/Shingles

- Normal host (age ≥50 yrs, moderate to severe pain/rash or nontruncal dermatome involvement): valacyclovir 1 g PO three times a day or famciclovir 500 mg PO three times a day or acyclovir 800 mg PO 5 ×/day or 10 mg/kg IV q8h all × 7–10 days. Best if administered within 72 hrs of rash onset. Most studies suggest that early administration to those with significant zoster may decrease degree of PHN.

- Disseminated Zoster or immunosuppressed host: acyclovir 10 mg/kg q8h × 7 days although some use valacyclovir 1 g PO three times a day or famciclovir 500 mg PO three times a day in stable pt.
- Acyclovir-resistant VZV: Foscarnet 40 mg/kg q8h IV × 10 days. Most acyclovir resistant VZV strains are also resistant to ganciclovir and famciclovir.
- There is little apparent efficacy to treat zoster if beyond 72 hr of presentation in a normal host. Indications for treatment also include pain at presentation, age >50, immunosuppressed host or dissemination.
- Normal host: two studies show benefit up to >2 fold reduction in pain if antivirals used <72 hrs of rash presentation. May add Prednisone 60 mg daily w/ taper over 10–21 days, shown to decrease acute zoster pain, lessened narcotic requirements and faster return to usual activities/uninterrupted sleep in pts not at risk for steroid toxicities.
- Treatment of acute pain can include non-steroidal anti-inflammatory agents (NSAIDs) but will often require narcotic therapy or tramadol.
- **Prevention (Zoster):** zoster vaccine (Zostavax) approved with reduction of the incidence and severity of zoster and PHN. Licensed for age ≥60. Less benefit seen for older ages, 70–80 and >80 yrs, but still helps prevent post-herpetic neuralgia even in the older age groups. Given as single injection. Live attenuated vaccine most remain frozen until administration.
- Prevention in immunocompromised host (e.g., HSCT): acyclovir 800 mg PO 5 ×/day, valacyclovir 1000 mg PO three times daily, famciclovir 500 mg PO three times daily.

Postherpetic Neuralgia

- Defined as pain present >120 days following rash. Pain <30 days = acute herpetic neuralgia; 30–120 days = subacute herpetic neuralgia.
- PHN more likely in elderly, those with severe pain at presentation of rash. 20% pts >50 yrs have pain beyond 6 mos despite early antiviral Rx of shingles.
- Four first-line therapies, none clearly superior and often used in combination but multiple Rx use not well studied and increases adverse reactions.
- Gabapentin: start 100–300 mg qhs or 100 mg three times a day then titrate by 100 mg three times a day as tolerated. Trials suggest 1800–3600 mg daily target for benefit. SE: somnolence, dizziness, gait issues, cognitive impairment. Alt: pregabalin (Lyrica) 75 mg PO twice daily, may titrate to 300 mg twice daily max.
- Lidocaine patch 5% (Lidoderm): Use up to 12 hrs daily, up to three patches. Don't use over open lesions. Minimal lidocaine systemic absorption, mild rash usually only side effect. Relief usually by 2 wks.
- Opioids: published trials used either controlled-release oxycodone (up to 60 mg daily) or morphine (up to 240 mg). Many short or long acting preparations available.
- TCAs: many types but nortriptyline best tolerated in elderly. Start 10–25 mg qhs titrate to 75–150 mg. In one trial, amitriptyline 25 mg once daily × 3 mos starting within 48 hrs of rash onset reduced PNH by 50% (*J Pain Symptom Manage* 1997; 13:327). Multiple SE: cardiac, anticholinergic, uses P450 2D6 pathway. Check levels if dose >100 mg.
- Other options for refractory pts: capsaicin 0.025–0.075% cream four times a day, nerve blocks, spinal cord stimulation, intrathecal methylprednisolone (all non-FDA).

Prevention of Varicella/Chickenpox

- Varicella zoster immune globulin (now VariZIG) only to those at high risk [neonates w/ mothers who have signs/sx of varicella between 5 days prior or 2 days after delivery, premature infants >28 wks gestation who were exposed to VZV in neonatal period and in whom mothers have no immunity, premature infants <28 wks or weigh <1000 g at birth who are exposed to VZV regardless of maternal immune status, leukemics or other immunocompromised pts of any age without immunized, nonimmune pregnant women].
- VZIG unavailable due to cessation of manufacture. VariZIG an alternative available in an expanded access program (see below). Standard pooled IVIG (400 mg/kg × 1 dose) may be an alternative.
- VariZIG, an investigational alternative to VZIG, is available by IND expanded access application. Contact FFF Enterprises (1-800-843-7477).

PATHOGENS

- Risk = exposure to chickenpox/shingles + no hx of prior varicella or negative. serology. Give VariZIG 125U/10 kg (625U, 5 vial max) by 96 hrs preferably <48 hrs. No data suggest effectiveness in Rx of severe disease.
- Post-exposure prophylaxis should be within 3 days exposure and could include acyclovir (40–80 mg/kg) or vaccine (if not contraindicated) that offer efficacy of 70–85% vs 90% for VZIG.
- Varicella vaccine: Adults 0.5 cc SQ × 2 doses, separated 4–8 wks. Protection is 70–90% against infection and 95% against severe disease.
- Indications for susceptibles: healthcare workers, household contacts of immunosuppressed, young adults in dorms or military, nonpregnant women in childbearing yrs, susceptible teens and adults.
- Vaccine contraindications: pregnancy, immunosuppressive conditions, active TB, recent blood products with plasma (passive immunity problems), h/o reactions to gelatin or neomycin.
- Adults often uncertain of prior chickenpox hx. VZV Serology (+) in 70–90% of adults who believe they did not have varicella, so check serology prior to vaccination in suspected non-immune.
- Susceptible staff in hospitals with exposure to VZV including. localized zoster should avoid contact with high-risk pts. for 8–21 days after exposure.

MORE TREATMENT

- Brivudin 125 mg once daily × 7 days option for oral antiviral therapy for herpes zoster (unavailable in U.S.). Drug not recommended for cancer immunocompromised pts due to potential for fatal interaction with 5-fluorouracil or 5-fluoropyrimidines.

OTHER INFORMATION

- No American professional societies have formulated management guidelines for zoster.
- Treatment for zoster has only been shown to have benefit if started <72 hr from initial rash lesion, pain w/ rash, >50 yrs, immunosuppressed or disseminated disease. Rx >72 hrs of uncertain benefit, but may help if new vesicles forming.
- VZIG no longer available. VariZIG suggested. IVIG may be substituted for prophylaxis in high-risk individuals, but limited data exists on efficacy.
- Mortality of primary VZV low in children but higher in adults.
- Topical antiviral therapy lacks efficacy for treatment of zoster or chickenpox, and is not recommended.

MORE INFORMATION

- Maternal varicella may cause congenital varicella; however, maternal zoster has never been documented to cause fetal abnormalities.

BASIS FOR RECOMMENDATIONS

Harpaz R, Ortega-Sanchez IR, Seward JF, et al. Prevention of herpes zoster: recommendations of the Advisory Committee on Immunization Practices (ACIP). *MMWR Recomm Rep,* 2008; Vol. 57; pp. 1–30; quiz CE2–4.

Comments: Provides the first comprehensive guideline recommendations from the ACIP on Zoster prevention. Document also nicely reviews epidemiology, biology, post-herpetic neuralgia as well as therapeutic interventions.

Dworkin RH, Johnson RW, Breuer J, et al. Recommendations for the management of herpes zoster. *Clin Infect Dis,* 2007; Vol. 44 Suppl 1; pp. S1–26.

Comments: Paper outlines treatment of both zoster (including complications and special populations) and post-herpetic neuralgia.

No authors listed. VariZIG for prophylaxis after exposure to varicella. *Med Lett Drugs Ther,* 2006; Vol. 48; pp. 69–70.

Comments: Recommendations for use of VariZIG.

WEST NILE VIRUS

John G. Bartlett, MD

MICROBIOLOGY

- Mosquito-borne flavivirus infection.
- Cause of epidemic encephalitis though now endemic in the United States.
- RNA virus, part of Japanese encephalitis antigenic complex of viruses.

- Humans mainly acquire through bite of infected mosquito in tropical and temperate regions, but virus mainly found in birds, but also dogs, cats, horses, bats, chipmunks, and other rodents.

CLINICAL

- WNV infection: 80% asymptomatic; 20% sx w/ fever, lymphadenopathy, GI sx, myalgia, HA, +/– rash. CNS symptoms only occur in 1/150 WNV infections.
- Risks: endemic area, June–Nov, mosquito exposure. Elderly, immune suppressed, anti-TNF-alpha drugs—prone to neurological complications. Transmission reported by blood transfusion and organ transplantation (blood now screened by nucleic acid testing [NAT]).
- CNS sx (often overlapping): encephalitis (fever, altered mental status, paresis, Parkinson-like sx, seizures) and/or aseptic meningitis, (headache + meningismus) and/or myelitis (flaccid paralysis)
- Asymmetric flaccid weakness described/polio-like; CSF pleocytosis helps distinguish from Guillain-Barre.
- Lab: serum/CSF: EIA IgM +/– plaque reduction neutralization assay; RNA PCR—less sensitive. Typical CSF protein 100–1000 mg/dL, CSF WBC 5–1500 per mm^3 with predominance of lymphs or PMNs.
- **CDC definitions** (see www.cdc.gov/ncidod/dvbid/westnile/index.htm for full information).
- WN fever: 2–6 days post mosquito bite pts develop fever, headache, arthralgia, rash (20%) for 2–7 days.
- **WNV CNS infections:** a) meningitis: fever, headache, stiff neck, CSF WBCs; b) encephalitis: fever, headache, changed mental status +/- paresis, seizures, sensory deficits, abnormal movements.
- Compatible illness (1) WNV IgM by EIA and WNV Ab neutralization or (2) positive WNV antigen or PCR (any specimen).
- Dx CNS infection: (1) IgM by EIA in CSF (diagnostic), (2) 4 × increase in Ab (blood, acute and convalescent specimens), (3) IgM + neutralizing ab (blood), or (4) WNV Ag or PCR (CSF or blood). Note that IgM may persist for mos.

MORE CLINICAL

Lab:

- CBC—nl or low
- CSF—WBC 40–400/mL typical; mostly monos, but PMN's early; elevated protein (100–1000)
- Serology—positive at 2–5 wks; EIA IgG; HA ≥ 1:132 or IgM EIA; CSF IgM EIA or PCR
- Culture: blood (+) first 5 days only (use biosafety)

SITES OF INFECTION

- Viremia (1st wk)
- CNS: encephalitis, meningitis, radiculomyelitis
- Other: diarrhea, rash, lymphadenopathy (cervical usual)

TREATMENT

Neuroinvasive

- Principles: **suspect** w/ epidemic or appropriate season + fever (headache, altered mental status), aseptic meningitis (meningismus) and/or myelitis (acute bulbar or limb flaccid paresis).
- Supportive care only, no antiviral treatment documented to help.
- Dx: serology (IgG and IgM) + virus detection including viral culture, Ag detection or PCR; report positive results to local Health Dept.

Experimental

- Ribavirin (up to 4 g IV/day), interferon alpha 2 b (3 mil units/day) or hyperimmune globulin (available in Israel and NIH trial).
- NIH sponsored hyperimmune globulin treatment: see www.casg.uab.edu.

Prevention

- Mechanisms of transmission: Culex mosquito, blood tx, organ transplant, transplacental, breast feeding.
- Insect repellent with DEET or Picaridin (KBR 3203). DEET protection (strength, %): 24%–5 hrs, 5%–1.5 hrs.
- Spray clothing with permethrin.

PATHOGENS

- Drain standing water.
- Screen blood and organ transplant donors (now routinely done in U.S.).

OTHER INFORMATION

- Recommendations: see CDC for most up-to-date; URL: www.cdc.gov/ncidod/dvbid/westnile for surveillance and control.
- Most infected individuals have asymptomatic seroconversion or self-limiting "flu" sx—fever, HA, myalgia +/- rash; CNS w/encephalitis/ myelitis in 1/150, especially in elderly (but mean age 55 in 2002).
- Clues: epidemiology, sx—fever + confusion and/or paresis, hyporeflexia.
- Must r/o HSV (MRI/CT—temporal lobe involvement?, CSF PCR for HSV)—most should get rapid IV acyclovir awaiting dx; no specific treatment exists for any other viral encephalitis including West Nile Virus.

BASIS FOR RECOMMENDATIONS

Davis LE, DeBiasi R, Goade DE, et al. West Nile virus neuroinvasive disease. *Ann Neurol,* 2006; Vol. 60; pp. 286–300.

Comments: Since 1999, there have been >20,000 confirmed cases of WNV infection in U.S. and probably >1 million total. WNV neurologic disease (meningitis, encephalitis and flaccid paralysis): (1) <u>Neuroimaging</u> may be normal or show changes in basal ganglia, thalamus, cerebellum or brainstem. (2) <u>CSF</u> shows pleocytosis with predominance of PMNs in up to half. (3) <u>Diagnosis</u> is virus-specific IgM in CSF. (4) <u>Treatment</u>—none with proven benefit. (5) <u>Outcome</u>—neuro-recovery may be slow and incomplete.

SECTION 3
MANAGEMENT

Fever

CHRONIC FATIGUE SYNDROME see p. 61 in Diagnosis Section

FEVER AND NEUTROPENIA

Khalil G. Ghanem, MD

DEFINITION

- Fever: single oral temp >38.3°C (101°F) or temp >38°C (100.4°F) for >1 h **and** neutropenia: absolute neutrophil count (ANC) <500 cells/mm³ or <1000 cells/mm³ with predicted decline to <500 cells/mm³ [reference; *CID* 2002].

PATHOGENS

- Gram-negative bacilli (*Pseudomonas* spp., Enterobacteriaceae, etc); consider antibiotic resistant GNB (e.g., ESBLs)
- *Staphylococcus aureus* (including MRSA) and coagulase-negative *Staphylococci*
- *Viridans streptococci* (demonstrated to be serious pathogens especially in pts with malignancy/mucositis)
- *Enterococcus* spp.
- *Corynebacterium jeikeium* (not an infrequent cause of catheter-related infections in this pt population)
- *Bacillus* spp.
- *Propionibacterium* spp.
- Anaerobes: less commonly implicated (e.g., periodontal or perirectal abscess, intra-abdominal infection)
- *Candida* spp.
- *Aspergillus* spp. and other filamentous fungi (e.g., *Fusarium* spp.)

Diagnosis

- Detailed history and PE (see below).
- Obtain 2 sets blood cxs; preferably from peripheral veins × 2 (1 minimum) + catheter lumen(s).
- UA w/ micro, CBC w/ diff; LFTs, electrolytes.
- Sputum for Gram-stain and cx; consider bronchoscopy/BAL if respiratory complaints persist and are significant.
- CXR, scans (CT, US, MRI) as per signs/symptoms.

CLINICAL

- Detailed history, recent exposures, sick contacts.
- Risk factors: degree of neutropenia (ANC severity: <100 <500 <1000), rapid decline in ANC, remission of cancer or not, duration of neutropenia., other comorbidities; existence of central lines.
- Correlate date fever onset to date of cytotoxic therapy to predict duration of neutropenia (nadir count usually 10–14 days after chemo).
- PE: exam especially periodontium, pharynx, lungs, perineum/anus, skin, eyes, vascular access sites, BM bx sites.

TREATMENT

Approach to Treatment

- Proceed with Hx, PE, labs(cx), assess risk of pt, and determine whether to use PO (low risk pt, see below) or IV therapy.
- Begin abx (mono or combo) and continue at least 3–5 days before considering any changes unless new cx data available or clinical deterioration.
- Decide if Gram-positive coverage warranted.
- Persistent fever (day 3–5): clinical re-assessment including cx and scans. Decide if continue abx (if pt stable) or change/add abx (if disease progression, or vancomycin criteria met) or add antifungal.

- Antifungals routinely added after 5 days of febrile neutropenia despite broad antibacterial coverage and no identified cause: ampho B (or lipid formulations); voriconazole or posaconazole (although not adequately studied); caspofungin (other echinocandins anidulafungin, micafungin, but not adequately studied for febrile neutropenia; only caspofungin FDA approved).
- Prior to antifungal initiation, work-up for fungal infection should be complete: assess host and clinical factors, bx any suspicious skin lesions, CT of chest/abdomen, sinuses, nasal endoscopy (if indicated), cx's as appropriate, galactomannan enzyme immunoassay.
- If chest CT with nodular lesions +/− halo sign, amphotericin B products or voriconazole favored.
- Amphotericin B 0.5–1 mg/kg/day IV or ambisome 3 mg/kg/day, voriconazole 6 mg/kg IV q12h × 2 and then 4 mg/kg IV q12h, posaconazole 200 mg PO q6h × 7 days and then 400 mg PO q12h, caspofungin 70 mg IV × 1 and then 50 mg IV q24h.
- Routine antivirals not indicated unless lesions c/w herpes/VZV lesions present (use acyclovir). CMV rare except in BMT pts (use ganciclovir).
- Colony-Stimulating Factors (G-CSF): can shorten duration of neutropenia but **not** duration of fever or decrease infection mortality; routine use **not** recommended.
- Consider use of G-CSF in severely neutropenic pts w/ documented infections that do not respond to appropriate rx, or when prolonged delay in marrow recovery is anticipated.
- If central line present, remove if feasible for positive blood cxs for *S. aureus, Pseudomonas* spp., *Stenotrophomonas* spp., *Corynebacterium JK, Bacillus* spp., *Candida* spp., fast-growing atypical mycobacteria.

Oral Antibiotic Therapy

- Adults who are low risk pts may use: ciprofloxacin + amoxicillin/clavulanate. Make sure pts observed carefully and have access to appropriate medical care 24/7.
- **Lower risk pts:** ANC >100, absolute monocytes count >100, nl CXR, nl LFTs, and creatinine, no clinical IV site tunnel/exit site infection, temp <39°C. Also no abdominal pain, evidence of impending bone marrow recovery, no comorbidities. Neutropenia expected to last<10 days.
- Oral therapy: ciprofloxacin 500 mg PO twice daily and amoxicillin/clavulanate 500 mg PO q8h.

Monotherapy and Combination Parenteral Antibacterial Therapy

- No difference between combination or monotherapy for empirical rx of uncomplicated febrile neutropenia. Monotherapy could potentially increase antibiotic resistance (especially w/ use of cephalosporins).
- Choice of empiric therapy: base upon history and exam, antibiotic allergies, historical culture data (if available), recent antibiotic exposure, institutional resistance patterns.
- **Monotherapy:** cefepime, ceftazidime, or carbapenem (imipenem/meropenem) FDA approved. Carbapenems are preferred if ESBL rate is high (**avoid** cephalosporins).
- **Combination:** aminoglycoside or fluoroquinolone (ciprofloxacin, levofloxacin) + [antipseudomonal PCN (piperacillin/tazobactam) **or** cefepime or ceftazidime or carbapenem]. Two antipseudomonal beta-lactams together (not favored).
- Potential advantages of combination rx: synergistic effects against GNRs and decrease in the emergence of drug-resistance. Balance with the potential for nephro- and ototoxicity.
- Ceftazidime 2 g IV q8h or cefepime 2 g IV q12h **or** imipenem 1 g IV q6h (caution in pts with renal insufficiency in view of seizure potential) ormeropenem 2 g IV q8h.
- Addition of aminoglycoside for combination therapy: gentamicin or tobramycin 2 mg/kg q8h or 5 mg/kg q24h (once daily preferred: less toxicity) **or** amikacin 15 mg/kg/day or divided q8–12h.
- Vancomycin: considered if clinically suspected serious catheter-related infection, known MRSA colonization, positive BC results w/ GPC prior to final identification, or hypotension. Otherwise follow initial cx data and add vancomycin as needed. Linezolid can be an option, but not favored if suspect serious or high-grade bacteremia.
- Other drugs used: vancomycin 15 mg/kg IV q12h, linezolid 600 mg IV/PO q12h, daptomycin 6–8 mg/kg IV q24h.
- Quinolones are **not** recommended as routine initial monotherapy agents due to lack of prospective data, and use of quinolones as routine prophylaxis in many centers may predispose to resistance.

Duration of Treatment

- If an infectious source identified continue targeted abx tx for at least the standard duration of the given infection.

MANAGEMENT

- If pt afebrile in 3–5 days: if ANC >500, may d/c abxs if no infection identified; if ANC <500, continue abx at least 7 days or **ideally** until ANC >500 or suspected source treated (if pt HIGH risk). Consider switch to oral ciprofloxacin + amoxicillin/clavulanate or can D/C abxs if afebrile for >7 days (if pt LOW risk).
- Persistent fever: if ANC >500, d/c abx 4–5 days after ANC >500 and reassess. If ANC <500, continue × 14 days and reassess.
- The most important determinant for successful cessation of abx is neutrophil count recovery.

OTHER INFORMATION

- Less than 50% of febrile neutropenics will have an established infection and 1 of 5 pts with ANC <100 cells/mm[3] will have bacteremia.
- Signs and symptoms (induration, erythema, pustulation, CXR infiltrates, CSF pleocytosis) may be absent in pts with neutropenia.
- Median time to defervescence in adequately treated pts is 5 days (range 2–7 days). **Do not** modify initial abx choice unless clinical deterioration or new cx data dictate it.
- Sinusitis should be aggressively diagnosed and treated as neutropenia is a risk factor for invasive mould infections.

BASIS FOR RECOMMENDATIONS

Walsh TJ, Teppler H, Donowitz GR, et al. Caspofungin versus liposomal amphotericin B for empirical antifungal therapy in pts with persistent fever and neutropenia. *N Engl J Med*, 2004; Vol. 351; p. 1391.

Comments: Important study comparing caspofungin to L-AMB for empirical treatment of febrile neutropenia. This study showed similar overall success rates, breakthrough fungal infections, and resolution of fever.

Hughes WT, Armstrong D, Bodey GP, et al. 2002 guidelines for the use of antimicrobial agents in neutropenic pts with cancer. *Clin Infect Dis*, 2002; Vol. 34; pp. 730–51.

Comments: The most recent update of IDSA guidelines for the diagnosis and management of neutropenic fever.

FEVER OF UNKNOWN ORIGIN (FUO)

John G. Bartlett, MD

DEFINITION

- Modern definition: temperature >38.3°C for >3 wks duration without a diagnosis despite 2 outpt visits or 3 hospital days.

PATHOGENS/CAUSES

- **All cases (classical FUO (fever of unknown origin)):** infection 36%, inflammatory/rheumatological 35%, malignancy 15%, miscellaneous 20%.
- **Special subsets:**
- **Nosocomial or post-operative:** *C. difficile* colitis, drug fever, phlebitis, pulmonary embolism, or infection related to surgery.
- **AIDS** (CD4 <200 cells/mL): MAC, CMV, TB, lymphoma, PCP.
- **Elderly:** malignancy, temporal arteritis/polymyalgia rheumatica.
- **Fever >1 yr:** lymphoma, normal variant (benign hyperthermia or FUO (fever of unknown origin) chronic without specific diagnosis), factitious, granulomatous hepatitis.
- **Other:** factitious fever, fraudulent fever, normal temperature variant, hereditary (periodic fever), pulmonary emboli.

CLINICAL

- Verify fever—defined as core temperature >38°C (100.4°F, some use 38.3°C).
- Normal temperature: median 36.8°C (98.2°F), peak 4–6 PM, nadir 6 am, range +/– 0.9°F (0.5°C).
- Examine thoroughly including mouth, temporal arteries (age >50), abdomen, spleen, liver, skin, lymph nodes.
- Lab initial: CBC, CRP, ESR, chemistry panel, chest x-ray, U/A, ANA, blood culture × 3, HIV.
- Scans: CT chest/abdomen (other: WBC scan?, gallium scan?, ultrasound of biliary tract?). New: FDG-PET/CT scan may be useful.
- Next tests: if abnl LFTs consider liver bx; if abnl CBC, consider bone marrow bx + culture (AFB, fungal), temporal artery bx if >50 yrs.
- In stable pts, avoid empiric trials of antibiotics without a likely diagnosis.

- Trials: lymphoma-naproxen; Stills disease—ASA; endocarditis suspect—nafcillin/oxacillin/ vancomycin + gentamicin; TB—4 drugs (INH, RIF, ETH, PZA).

Infectious Diseases Considerations
- Abdominal abscess: CT scan, abx + drainage.
- TB. atypical mycobacteria: PPD, chest x-ray, AFB sputum cx, LP, liver bx, marrow bx—w/ granulomas. Treat tuberculosis w/ 4 drug regimen.
- Cx negative endocarditis: consider HACEK organisms, nutritionally variant streptococci; *Bartonella*, Q fever, *Legionella*, *Brucella* (serology), fungi. DX: echo (TEE), abx-empiric [see *Endocarditis* module].
- Mononucleosis syndromes: ~80% EBV (atypical lymphocytes + Mono spot); other causes include CMV, toxo, acute HIV.

Granulomatous and collagen vascular diseases
- Temporal arteritis: age >50, ESR >50, wt loss, PMR sx, vision sx. Dx—artery bx. Rx prednisone 60 mg/day ASAP to avoid blindness while getting temporal aa bxp within 1 wk to avoid prednisone rendering biopsy as uninformative.
- Polymyalgia rheumatica: age >50, ESR >50, pain (neck, shoulder, pelvis). Clinical dx. Rx: prednisone 20 mg/day (dramatic abatement of sx w/i 1–2 days is supportive of diagnosis).
- Still disease: arthralgia/arthritis, faint fleeting rash, LN, leukocytosis, anemia, ANA negative, remittent fever, high ESR/CRP, ferritin. Rx ASA/NSAID or corticosteroid responsive.
- Sarcoid: chest x-ray, bx of tissue—documenting usually non-caseating granuloma. R/O TB, lymphoma.
- Crohn's dz: dx by endoscopy + bx.
- Granulomatous hepatitis: ESR >50, increased alk phos, wt loss. Dx: liver bx, r/o TB. Rx steroids.

Tumors/miscellaneous
- "Omas": lymphoma, myeloma, hypernephroma. DX: CT scan, serum immunoglobulins, SPEP/ UPEP, biopsies.
- Hodgkins/non-Hodgkins lymphoma: intermittent fever, LN, liver/spleen enlarged, naproxen response. Dx: LN, liver, or marrow bx.
- Solid tissue tumors: CT scan, LFTs for liver mets. Dx: bx.
- Drug fever: looks well for temperature with relative bradycardia. Occurs typically 1–3 wks post start of drug (phenytoin, sulfa, beta-lactam, barbiturate, clindamycin, dapsone, amB). D/C = response w/i 48 hrs.
- Pulmonary embolism: increased respirations or dyspnea, edema, atelectasis, or effusion. Dx V/Q scan or angiography (chronic PE not well dx by CT method). Rx: anticoagulation.
- Familial Mediterranean Fever: Jews, Armenians, Turks. Attacks of fever and pain w/ no alternative cause +/– serositis, amyloidosis. Rx: colchicine.
- Self-induced: fraudulent behavior, may see polymicrobial bacteremia, often young adult; otherwise appears healthy.
- Factitious: deceit in often healthy young adult, negative labs, ESR nl. No diurnal temp change, urine temp nl. Rx: confrontation.

OTHER INFORMATION
- Most common diagnoses: ID—TB, endocarditis. CVD—Stills dz, GCA/PMR, vasculitis. Tumor—lymphoma. Other—granulomatous hepatitis, drug fever, PE, FMF, factitious.
- No diagnosis found in 20–40%. Prognosis for them is generally good.

BASIS FOR RECOMMENDATIONS

Mackowiak PA, Durack DT. Fever of unknown origin. In Mandell, Douglas, Dolin eds. *Principles and Practice of Infectious Diseases*. Churchill Livingstone, pp. 622–633.

Comments: Review by authorities—emphasizing differences by location, age, host status. Categories includes: Classic: Temp >38 deg C × 3 wk + 2O PD visits or 3 days in hospital; Nosocomial: Temp >38 deg C × 3 days and not present or incubating at admission; Immune-deficient: Temp >38 deg C × 3 days and neg cx at 48 hr; HIV: Temp >38 deg C >3 wks (Outpt) and >3 days hospitalized pts.

Author opinion.

Comments: As one might expect with a heterogenous condition, there are no guidelines or solid algorithms that can be recommended.

MANAGEMENT

Management

OUTPATIENT ANTIBIOTIC THERAPY (OPAT)

James DeMaio, MD

DEFINITION

- Use of parenteral antibiotics outside of the hospital setting. Infusions may be administered by either the pt, family members or professional staff in either a home or ambulatory care environment.

PATHOGENS

- CNS **infections**—OPAT safe once pt medically stable; physician should see pt at least every other day during first 7–10 days of therapy.
- **Endocarditis** (non-enterococcal Strep)—Rx 1 wk in hospital then OPAT.
- **Endocarditis** (*S. aureus*)—higher risk of complications; once-daily or every other day follow-up as outpt recommended for first 2 wks.
- **Osteomyelitis/septic arthritis**—OPAT ideal to avoid long hospitalization; ceftriaxone as good as cefazolin and better than vancomycin for MSSA.
- **Lyme disease**—OPAT with ceftriaxone preferred for CNS disease (except facial nerve palsy) and heart block, 3rd degree. Need for OPAT in late Lyme arthritis, if no response to oral therapy.

Criteria For Patient Selection

- The following criteria must be considered for pt selection:
- Pt must be medically stable; low likelihood of complications. Pt/provider must be physically and mentally able to infuse meds.
- Adequate transportation, phone access and refrigeration should be available.
- No intravenous drug use in the prior 12 mos.
- Inform the pt of the economic impact of therapy. Some pts will have significant co-pays.

TREATMENT

Intravenous Line Selection

- Peripheral lines: require good veins, Rx courses of <2 wks, non-irritative meds, can be left in for 7 days if no erythema or tenderness.
- Midline catheters: useful for Rx courses of 1–3 wks, must be non-irritative meds.
- Peripherally inserted central catheters (PICC lines): useful if poor peripheral access, Rx >2 wks or irritative medications.
- Non-tunneled central catheters (e.g., Hohn): if already in place, can use for Rx courses <4 wks. Offers no advantages over PICC lines.
- Tunneled central venous catheters: may be useful in pts with renal disease to save peripheral veins; requires surgical placement; expensive. Often chosen for durations >4 wks.

Drug Delivery Systems

- Gravity mini-bags: least expensive, easy to learn, can use flow regulators, become too labor intensive if >2 doses/day.
- Elastomeric or mechanical infusion pumps: more expensive, easy to learn, high pt acceptance, labor intensive if >2 doses/day.
- Electronic syringe pumps: easy to learn, only small volume infusions possible (<100 ml), drug must be stable at high concentrations.
- Electronic infusion pumps: allows multiple intermittent or continuous infusions, pumps are expensive, may require special tubing.

Lab Testing and Follow-up

- Physician visits at least weekly. More frequent visits (once-daily or every other day) recommended initially for endocarditis, CNS infections and sepsis.
- CBC: twice weekly for ganciclovir and pentamidine. Once weekly all other meds.
- BMP/Chem-7—twice weekly for acyclovir, aminoglycosides and ampho B. Once weekly all other meds.
- LFTs: once weekly for ampho B, caspofungin and oxacillin.

- CPK: once weekly for daptomycin.
- Mg Level: once weekly for acyclovir and ampho B.
- Vancomycin trough level: prior to 4 th dose; repeat every other wk if renal function stable.
- Aminoglycoside: test peak level weekly for synergistic dosing (gentamicin peak = 3). Test trough (level = 0) weekly for daily dosing.
- Inquire about dizziness/change of hearing/vertigo at each pt visit if on aminoglycoside. Stop drug if a change noted by pt.

DRUG-SPECIFIC COMMENTS

Amphotericin B: Deoxycholate Plain Ampho B and also lipid formulations of Ampho B can be given via OPAT. Check BMP/Chem-7 twice weekly. Check CBC, LFTs and Mg once weekly. I always infuse this in office, never in pts home.

Ampicillin + Sulbactam: Limited stability at room temperature. Difficult to use in OPAT. Pt can pre-mix prior to infusion using ADD-Vantage (Registered trademark) system. However, this is labor intensive.

Aztreonam: Stable enough to be used in syringe pumps or electronic infusion pumps.

Caspofungin acetate: Can be given via OPAT. Check CBC, Chem-7/BMP and LFTs weekly while pt is on the drug.

Cefazolin: Stable at room temperature. Can be infused via syringe pump or electronic infusion pump. Limited evidence suggests it can be dosed daily with probenecid (1 g 1 hr prior to infusion) boosting.

Cefepime: Adequate stability at room temperature to use in syringe pump or electronic infusion pump. Can be dosed once daily if creatinine clearance < 60. This reduced frequency of dosing may offer a once daily option for some pts with *Pseudomonas aeruginosa* infections.

Ceftazidime: Adequate stability at room temperature for use in syringe pumps or electronic infusion pumps.

Ceftriaxone: Ideal for OPAT. Once daily dosing. Highly effective against *Staphylococcus aureus* in osteomyelitis. Available frozen in gravity mini-bags—this formulation avoids the need for mixing prior to use.

Clindamycin: Well absorbed. Rarely needs to be given IV in out-patient setting. If given IV, it is stable enough for use in syringe pumps or electronic infusion pumps.

Daptomycin: Well-suited for OPAT since dosed once daily. Check CPK weekly on med. Expensive —make sure pt's co-pay is not excessive. I hold statins while pt is on this med.

Doripenem: Difficult to use in OPAT. Stable < 8 hrs at room temp. Stable 24 hrs if refrigerated.

Ertapenem: Dosed daily. Provides broad spectrum coverage which may be useful in polymicrobial infections (e.g., abdominal/pelvic abscesses). Remember does not provide coverage for Pseudomonas. In my experience, significant percentage of pts complain of nausea on this med.

Gentamicin: Use of any aminoglycoside requires close lab and clinical follow-up. Check CBC weekly, Chem-7/BMP twice weekly. Check peak level (ideal = 3) for synergistic dosing and trough level (ideal = 0) for daily dosing. Inquire about dizziness/change in hearing at each visit. Due to excess malpractice risk, I avoid aminoglycosides unless they are absolutely necessary.

Imipenem/Cilastatin: Limited stability at room temperature. Difficult to use in OPAT. Pt can pre-mix prior to infusion using ADD-Vantage (Registered trademark) system. However, this is labor intensive.

Levofloxacin: Well absorbed. Rarely needs to be given IV in out-patient setting.

Linezolid: Well absorbed. Rarely needs to be given IV in out-patient setting.

Meropenem: Limited stability at room temperature. Difficult to use in OPAT. Pt can pre-mix prior to infusion using ADD-Vantage (Registered trademark) system. However, this is labor intensive.

Oxacillin: Highly stable at room temperature. Ideal for use in electronic infusion pumps. Significant incidence of neutropenia in pts. given prolonged courses. Check CBC, Chem-7 and LFTs weekly—PICC preferred. Irritative med—PICC preferred.

Penicillin: Adequate stability at room temperature for use in electronic syringe pumps.

Piperacillin + Tazobactam: Adequate stability at room temperature for use in electronic infusion pumps. Due to the number of doses required daily, administration via gravity mini-bags or syringe pumps is usually too labor intensive for pts.

MANAGEMENT

Tigecycline: Limited stability at room temperature. Only stable 24 hrs refrigerated.

Vancomycin: Suitable for OPAT. Should be infused no faster than 1 g per hr. In my experience this has been safe with close monitoring of vanco troughs (target = 15–20 mcg/mL).

OTHER INFORMATION

- OPAT is relatively expensive. Always consider if there is an appropriate/less-expensive oral regimen before beginning OPAT.
- DVTs due to PICC lines are frequently missed. Any pain, swelling or collateral vessels in an extremity with PICC should prompt a Doppler study.
- Vancomycin can be dosed q24h (2 g max) based on limited data. In my experience, this has been safe with close monitoring of vanco troughs (5–10 mcg/mL). Some would use q12h dosing for CNS or pulm dz.
- Avoid probenecid if pt allergic to aspirin, allergic to sulfa, has renal failure or hx of kidney stones/gout.
- For skin and soft tissue infections, cefazolin can be dosed daily if probenecid (1 g one hr prior to infusion) is given.

BASIS FOR RECOMMENDATIONS

Tice AD, Rehm SJ, Dalovisio JR, et al. Practice guidelines for outpatient parenteral antimicrobial therapy. IDSA guidelines. *Clin Infect Dis*, 2004; Vol. 38; pp. 1651–72.

Comments: Latest comprehensive review and guideline recommendations for OPAT.

Andrews MM, von Reyn CF. Pt selection criteria and management guidelines for outpatient parenteral antibiotic therapy for native valve infective endocarditis. *Clin Infect Dis*, 2001; Vol. 33; pp. 203–9.

Comments: Offers a conservative, but well reasoned, approach to OPAT for endocarditis.

FEVER IN THE RETURNED TRAVELER FROM TROPICAL AREAS

Noreen A. Hynes, MD, MPH

PATHOGENS

- Approximately 30% of persons seeking medical care following travel have fever. Of these, 35% have undifferentiated fever without localizing signs, others groups include 15% with acute diarrheal disease, 14% respiratory illnesses, 4% genitourinary illnesses, 4% dermatological conditions, 4% non-diarrheal gastrointestinal disease.
- *Plasmodium* spp. (malaria): the leading cause of fever (21% of all fevers and 59% of undifferentiated fevers) and the leading cause of travel-related hospitalization and death. Species include: *P. falciparum* (high case fatality rate if untreated), *P. vivax, P. ovale, P. malariae, P. knowlesi* (simian malaria found in Southeast Asia, rarely transmissible to humans and potential fatal).
- Diarrhea/dysentery: 7% of all fevers; non-typhoidal *Salmonella* spp., *Shigella* spp., and *Campylobacter* spp. are the most commonly isolated organisms; fever is only seen in 10% of pts with *E. histolytica* (amebic dysentery).
- Dengue virus: 6% of all fever and 18% of undifferentiated fever.
- *Salmonella enterica* serovar Typhi or Paratyphi (enteric fever): 2% of all fever and 6% of undifferentiated fever.
- *Rickettsia* spp: 2% of all fever and 5% of undifferentiated fever; 75% of these infections are tick-borne. *R. africae* (cause of tick-bite fever) especially common after safaris or treks in Southern Africa.
- Urinary tract infection/pyelonephritis: 3% of all fevers.
- Tuberculosis: <1% of all fevers.
- Chikungunya virus, a mosquito-borne disease, originally seen in South Asia, is now increasingly found in South East Asia, East and Central sub-Saharan Africa. It may be associated with a fever/undifferentiated fever but is usually associated with arthralgias, which can be severe.
- Uncommon systemic illnesses are caused by leptospirosis, amoebic liver abscess, viral meningitis, relapsing fever.

CLINICAL

- **History is KEY in the returned traveler.** 23% of returned travelers present with fever; patterns of fever and clinical findings similar for many infections. A detailed travel and exposure history (including modes of possible exposure), vaccination history, and treatment history is essential. Consider malaria for every febrile pt who has been in a malarious area.
- **Physical examination:** seek to identify focal signs and symptoms that may assist you. Undifferentiated fever in the returned traveler poses the greatest challenge. Consider malaria regardless of whether or not there are focal findings if the pt has been in a malarious area. Specific localizing findings should be used to help guide the clinician's evaluation of each pt whenever possible. For example, look carefully for rash, adenopathy, and hepatosplenomegaly.
- **Undifferentiated fever with incubation period <2 wks:** malaria (consider as leading dx if the person has been in a malarious area since falciparum malaria can be fatal in non-immune persons, and chemoprophylaxis is not 100% protective), dengue, spotted fever and typhus group rickettsiae, scrub typhus, typhoid and paratyphoid fevers. Also, consider less common illnesses such as brucellosis, leptospirosis, acute HIV, tick and louse borne-relapsing fevers, tularemia, and non-tropical disease (infectious mononucleosis, endocarditis, lymphoma).
- **Fever with hemorrhage with incubation period <2 wks:** meningococcemia, leptospirosis, dengue, yellow fever, Congo-Crimean hemorrhagic fever, hemorrhagic fevers of South America (Manchupo, Junin, Sabia, and Guanarito viruses), hemorrhagic fevers of Africa (Ebola, Rift Valley Fever, Marburg viruses, lassa fever).

MANAGEMENT

- **Fever with CNS findings with incubation period <2 wks:** malaria, meningococcal meningitis, many bacteria/fungi/viruses, African trypanosomiasis (sleeping sickness), tick-borne encephalitis, Japanese encephalitis, West Nile encephalitis, rabies, polio, *Angiostrongyloides cantonensis*.
- **Fever with pulmonary findings with incubation period <2 wks:** seasonal, avian or pandemic influenza, pneumococcal pneumonia, legionellosis, Q fever, meloidosis, acute histoplasmosis, acute coccidioidomycosis, hantavirus pulmonary syndrome, chlamydia, coronavirus.
- **Undifferentiated fever with incubation 2 wks–2 mos:** malaria (leading dx if the person has been in a malarious area). Many of the other diseases noted above can have incubation >2 wks, including many of the hemorrhagic fevers and fungal infections, brucellosis, typhoid fever, leptospirosis, sleeping sickness, melioidosis, amoebic liver abscess, hepatitis A or E, acute schistosomiasis, acute toxoplasmosis, bartonellosis. Consultation with a tropical medicine/infectious disease expert is recommended.
- **Fever with incubation >2 mos after return:** malaria (leading dx if the person has been in a malarious area), hepatitis B, tuberculosis, filariasis, visceral leishmaniasis, fascioliasis, and many of the infections noted with shorter incubations. Consultation with a tropical medicine/infectious disease expert is recommended.
- **Location of travel (undifferentiated fevers):** <u>subsaharan Africa</u>: malaria—other causes of undifferentiated fever. <u>Southeast Asia</u>: dengue—malaria—other causes of undifferentiated fever. <u>South Central Asia, esp. India</u>: malaria = typhoid/paratyphoid fever (especially if visiting family) = dengue. <u>Latin America/Caribbean</u>: dengue—malaria—other causes of undifferentiated fever.
- **Viral hemorrhagic fevers:** caused 4 distinct families of RNA, enveloped viruses (arenaviruses, filoviruses, bunyaviruses, and flaviviruses). Most are biosafety level 4 agents, if suspicious immediately notify local/state health authorities. Survival of VHF viruses in nature is dependent on an animal or insect host; geographically restricted distribution of diseases is based upon the host. Humans are not the natural reservoir for any of these viruses. Human cases or outbreaks of VHFs occur sporadically and usually are not easy to predict.

MORE CLINICAL

Exposure history provides clues to certain pathogens:

Exposure	Some infections to consider
Animals or their products	Anthrax
	Brucellosis
	Q fever
	Plague
Blood and body fluids	CMV
	Hepatitis A, B, C, or D
	HIV
	Syphilis
Dogs, cats, bats, monkeys (bites and saliva exposure)	Rabies
	Herpes B virus (monkeys)
Fresh water	Leptospirosis
	Schistosomiasis

Exposure	Some infections to consider
Ingestions	
—Raw vegetables and water plants	Fascioliasis
—Raw or undercooked animal meat	Campylobacter
	E. coli O157-H7 (and other STECs)
	Toxoplasmosis
	Trichinosis
Raw or undercooked shellfish	Clonorchiasis
	Hepatitis A
	Hepatitis E
	Paragonimiasis
	Vibrios
Unpasteurized milk/milk products	Brucellosis
	Salmonellosis
	Tuberculosis
Rodents	Hantavirus
	Hemorrhagic fevers including Lassa fever
	Plague
	Rat-bite fever
Hiking in the bush	African tick-bite fever (Southern Africa)
	Scrub typhus (eastern Asia, western Pacific)

DIAGNOSIS

- **Initial evaluation:** malaria thick and thin smear if travel to a malarious area regardless of having taking chemoprophylaxis with serial smears in initial smear negative in at-risk traveler; CDC with differential and platelets, blood cultures; urinalysis (with culture if abnormal sediment); liver enzymes.
- **Malaria:** thick and thin smear in ALL returned travelers from malarious areas regardless of history of having taken chemoprophylaxis; rapid tests (e.g., histidine-rich protein [HRP]-2 antigen detection) are highly specific but not as sensitive as thick and thin smears. Five species infect humans, *P. falciparum* (may be fatal, treatment is urgent), *P. vivax*, *P. ovale, P. malariae, P. knowlesi* (may be fatal; treatment is urgent). *P. knowlesi* usually infects monkeys and rarely humans in SE Asia; can be mistaken for *P. malariae* on smear; suspect if high-level parasitemia ($\geq$2.5% of RBCs infected) and lab reports *P. malariae;* PCR identification needed to confirm dx. Presentation within 2 wks of return in 65% with falciparum malaria present compared with 27% of vivax malaria; 60% of vivax malaria presents >2 mos after return.
- **Dengue suspected** (pt with fever, frontal headache, myalgia with or w/o skin petechial or maculopapular eruption) up to 14 days after return; 66% present within 7 days of return): serology; virus isolation from blood (research labs only), PCR.
- **Rickettsial infections suspected:** eschar/tache noir may be present; culture is the most sensitive and specific method but is restricted to reference laboratories as it is a bio-hazard; PCR detection can be done at specialized laboratories on blood, serum, or tissue biopsies; the inoculation eschar is the best biopsy sample to assay. Agent-specific serology is the most

commonly used in dx but often tests available (i.e., Weil-Felix or immunofluorescence assay) cannot distinguish species due to cross reactivity; Western blot and cross-absorption available only in reference laboratories. Hints of rickettsial species based upon geographic location of acquisition.

- **Enteric fever (typhoid or paratyphoid) suspected:** blood and stool cultures; serologic tests lack sensitivity and specificity; bone marrow culture 90% sensitive and not affected by up to 5 days of antibiotics. Current attenuated and killed typhoid vaccines are only 60–70% effective in preventing *S. typhi* only.
- **Hemorrhagic fever:** several associated pathogens may be transmitted nosocomially! Many are Biosafety Level (BSL)-4 agents. Institute barrier isolation in a private room until communicable agents are ruled out. Any returned traveler with hemorrhagic manifestations requires **urgent** intervention. Obtain an infectious disease consult, inform infection control and contact the Special Pathogens Branch at CDC's Division of Viral Diseases in Atlanta, GA. (404.639.1511) for assistance.
- **Fever and CNS:** malaria thick and thin smears if travel to a malarious area, lumbar puncture, blood cultures. Imaging procedures as indicated.
- **Fever and pulmonary findings:** viral and bacterial cultures of respiratory secretions; CXR.
- **Persistent or relapsing fever:** thick and thin blood smears for malaria and borrelia, blood cultures.
- **Leptospirosis suspect:** serology (MAT preferred, available at CDC), isolate organism from urine, blood, CSF (alert lab, special media [Fletcher's media] needed). **Amoebic liver abscess suspected:** hepatic ultrasound and *E. histolytica* serology. Liver aspirate (usually not done if serology available). Serology has >95% sensitivity. **Viral meningitis suspected:** lumbar puncture, culture and PCR for arboviruses, enteroviruses.

TREATMENT

Uncomplicated *Plasmodium falciparum*, *Plasmodium knowlesi*, or Species Unspecified

- **NB:** treatment for malaria should not be initiated until the diagnosis has been confirmed by laboratory investigations. "Presumptive treatment" without the benefit of laboratory confirmation should be reserved for extreme circumstances (strong clinical suspicion, severe disease, impossibility of obtaining prompt laboratory confirmation). If the pt used malaria chemoprophylaxis, choose a different agent for treatment.
- A different drug/drug combination should be used for treatment in a person who had used an antimalarial chemoprophylactic during for travel proximate to the diagnosis of falciparum malaria due to the possibility of drug resistance.
- Chloroquine sensitive areas (Central America west of Panama Canal; Haiti; the Dominican Republic; and most of the Middle East): chloroquine phosphate (Aralen and generics) 600 mg base (=1,000 mg salt) orally immediately, followed by 300 mg base (=500 mg salt) PO at 6, 24, and 48 hrs. Total dose: 1,500 mg base (=2,500 mg salt).
- Chloroquine-resistant or unknown resistance, **several options:** (1) quinine sulfate plus one of the following: doxycycline, tetracycline, or clindamycin. Quinine sulfate: 542 mg base (=650 mg salt) PO three times daily × 3 to 7 days and doxycycline: 100 mg PO twice daily × 7 days or tetracycline 250 mg PO four times daily × 7 days or clindamycin 20 mg base/kg/day PO divided in three times daily × 7 days **or** (2) atovaquone-proguanil (Malarone adult tab = 250 mg atovaquone/ 100 mg proguanil, 4 adult tabs PO daily × 3 days (taken with milk or a fatty meal) **or** (3) Mefloquine (Lariam and generics) 684 mg base (=750 mg salt) PO as initial dose, followed by 456 mg base (=500 mg salt) PO given 6–12 hrs after initial dose. Total dose = 1,250 mg salt.
- Artemether (20 mg) and lumefantrine (120 mg) in a fixed oral dose tablet (Coartem). This drug was approved in late March 2009. The package insert information is not yet available from the FDA Orange Book. This agent is **not** for the treatment of serious malaria.
- Infections acquired in the Newly Independent States of the former Soviet Union and Korea to date have been uniformly caused by *P. vivax* and should therefore be treated as chloroquine-sensitive infections.
- Middle Eastern countries with chloroquine-resistant *P. falciparum* include Iran, Oman, Saudi Arabia, and Yemen.

Uncomplicated Plasmodium malariae (All regions of the world)

- Preferred: chloroquine phosphate (Aralen and generics) 600 mg base (=1,000 mg salt) orally immediately, followed by 300 mg base (=500 mg salt) PO at 6, 24, and 48 hrs. Total dose: 1,500 mg base (=2,500 mg salt).
- Alternative: hydroxychloroquine (Plaquenil™ and generics) 620 mg base (=800 mg salt) PO immediately, followed by 310 mg base (=400 mg salt) PO at 6, 24, and 48 hrs. Total dose: 1,550 mg base (=2,000 mg salt).

Uncomplicated Plasmodium *vivax* and *P. ovale*

- Chloroquine sensitive regions: chloroquine phosphate 1 g salt (600 mg base) orally once, then 500 mg salt (300 mg base) 6 hrs later, then 500 mg at 24 hrs and 48 hrs. At the end of chloroquine treatment begin primaquine phosphate: 30 mg base PO daily × 14 days. Pt must be tested for G6PD deficiency before treating the liver form of the infection with primaquine which is contraindicated in pregnant or breastfeeding women.
- In areas where chloroquine-resistant *P. falciparum* co-circulates with *P. vivax*, consider treatment with one of the oral treatments outline for uncomplicated *P. falciparum* provided above.
- Chloroquine-resistant *P. vivax* (Papua New Guinea and Indonesia): quinine sulfate plus either doxycycline or tetracycline plus primaquine phosphate **or** mefloquine plus primaquine sulfate. See dosing schedules above.

Uncomplicated Malaria Treatment Options for Pregnant Women

- Chloroquine-sensitive areas: chloroquine is considered safe in pregnancy but can only be used to treat sensitive malaria species. The treatment regimen is the same as for non-pregnant pts.
- Chloroquine-resistant *P. falciparum*: quinine sulfate plus clindamycin. Quinine sulfate: 542 mg base (=650 mg salt) PO three times daily × 3 to 7 days **and** clindamycin: 20 mg base/kg/day PO divided three times daily × 7 days. The quinine duration varies due to where the individual acquired the infection: Southeast Asia = 7 days, for infections acquired elsewhere = 3 days.
- Chloroquine-resistant *P. vivax* (Burma, India): quinine sulfate 650 mg salt PO three times daily tid × 7 days.
- Primaquine is contraindicated in pregnant and lactating women.
- Mefloquine is generally not recommended for treatment in pregnant women due to a possible increase in stillbirths; however, it may be used if it is the only treatment option available and if the potential benefit is judged to outweigh the potential risks.

Complicated/Severe Plasmodium falciparum or Intolerance of Oral Treatment (All regions)

- **Quinidine gluconate** 10 mg salt/kg IV loading dose (max 600 mg) in saline over 1–2 hrs, then constant drip of 0.02 mg quinidine salt/kg/min until parasitemia <1% or oral meds tolerated **plus doxycycline** 100 mg IV or orally twice daily.
- **Important:** use of IV quinidine requires admission to a telemetry unit where the pt can be monitored closely for EKG changes (QT prolongation and ventricular arrhythmia), hypoglycemia and hypotension.
- To determine availability of this drug, call for availability call Eli Lilly Customer Services at 800-821-0538 or 317-276-2000.
- Artesunate (IV) the CDC Malaria Hotline: 770-488-7788 (M-F, 8 a.m.– 4:30 p.m., Eastern Time), or after hrs, call: 770-488-7100, and request to speak with a HHS/CDC Malaria Branch clinician. On June 21, 2007, the Food and Drug Administration (FDA) approved investigational new drug (IND) protocol # 76,725, entitled Intravenous Artesunate for Treatment of Severe Malaria in the United States. This IND makes a new class of antimalarial medication-artemisinins-available in the United States for the first time.
- Artesunate must be followed by one of the following to effect cure: atovaquone-proguanil (Malarone), doxycycline (clindamycin in pregnant women), or mefloquine.
- Consider exchange transfusion if parasitemia >5–10%.

Febrile Diarrhea/Dysentery

- **Non-typhoidal Salmonella spp:** ill and immunocompetent persons with severe diarrhea (9–10 stools/day), high fever, or who require hospitalization for management should receive antibiotics. Diarrhea alone is not an indication for treatment of those with non-typhoidal gastroenteritis.

MANAGEMENT

- Antibiotic resistance patterns should guide treatment or modification of empiric therapy. Fluoroquinolone resistance is increasing worldwide.
- Empiric treatment: ceftriaxone 1–2 g IV once daily **or** cefotaxime 2 g IV every 8 hrs. Change to other agent based on resistance pattern.
- All immunocompromised persons (organ transplant, AIDS, persons received corticosteroids or immunosuppressive therapies), those with sickle cell disease, hemoglobinopathies, cirrhosis, cancer or lymphoproliferative disease) should be treated regardless of severity of symptoms.
- *Shigella* spp: In healthy adults most shigella infections are self-limiting but for public health reasons, all persons with a positive stool culture should be treated to decrease shedding and person-to-person spread. Antibiotic resistance is widespread. Empiric rx should be provided to the following groups before culture results are reported: >64 yrs, malnourished persons, all HIV-infected persons regardless of CD4 count or viral load, bacteremic persons, food handlers.
- Empiric treatment: ciprofloxacin 500 mg orally twice daily × 5 days (consider 7–10 days for immunocompromised pts). Other fluoroquinolones may also be used. Base final treatment on culture and sensitivity results.
- *Campylobacter* spp: those with fever/dysentery are considered to have severe illness and should receive antimicrobials. Those who are >64 yrs, pregnant, immunocompromised should also be treated. Drug resistance is widespread.
- Preferred: erythromycin stearate 500 mg orally twice daily for 5 days or azithromycin.
- **Amebic dysentery/colitis:** metronidazole 500–750 mg orally three times daily for 10 days or tinidazole 600 mg orally twice daily for 5 days and followed by a luminal amebicidal agent active against *E. histolytica* cysts including iodoquinol 650 mg orally three times daily for 20 days or paromomycin 25–35 mg/kg/day orally divided three times daily for 7 days or diloxanide (not available in the U.S.) 500 mg orally three times daily for 10 days.

Enteric Fever (Salmonella enterica serovar Typhi or Paratyphi)

- **Acquired in South Asia or East Asia:** uncomplicated infection use cefixime 10–15 mg/kg orally twice daily for 7–14 days or azithromycin 1 g orally each day for 5 days. Complicated Infection use ceftriaxone 1–2 g IV once daily for 7–14 days or cefotaxime 1–2 g IV every 8 hrs for 7–14 days.
- **Acquired in Eastern Europe, Middle East, South America or Sub-Saharan Africa:** uncomplicated infection use ciprofloxacin 250–500 mg orally twice daily for 7–14 days or ofloxacin 200–400 mg orally every 12 hrs for 7–10 days. Complicated infection use ciprofloxacin 500 mg IV every 12 hrs daily for 10–14 days or ofloxacin 400 mg IV/PO every 12 hrs for 10–14 days.
- **Acquisition location unknown or in Southeast Asia:** ciprofloxacin 250–500 mg orally twice daily for 7–14 days for 7–10 days or ofloxacin 200–400 mg orally every 12 hrs for 7–10 days. Complicated Infection: ceftriaxone 1–2 g IV once daily for 7–14 days or cefotaxime 1–2 g IV every 8 hrs for 7–14 days **plus** ciprofloxacin 500 mg IV every 12 hrs daily for 10–14 days or ofloxacin 400 mg IV every 12 hrs for 10–14 days.
- Dexamethasone use is controversial and may decrease mortality in severe typhoid fever cases where delirium, coma, obtundation or stupor are present.
- An infectious disease specialist should be consulted in all cases of typhoid fever given its low prevalence in the developed world. Consult a surgeon if GI perforation, GI hemorrhage is suspect. Ileal perforation usually occurs in the third wk of febrile illness.
- Relapse of typhoid fever occurs in 1–6% of immunocompetent persons, occurring 2–3 wks following resolution of symptoms.

Dengue

- There are no dengue-specific treatments available.
- Usually, it is a self-limited disease; requires only supportive treatment.
- Avoid NSAIDs, aspirin, and steroids.
- Closely monitor all pts with evidence of hemorrhagic associated symptoms: tachycardia, prolonged capillary refill time, cool or mottled skin, evidence of volume depletion, narrowed pulse pressure, hypotension, rising packed cell volume or falling platelet count. Such pts should be hospitalized for correction of volume deficits and for monitoring.
- If dengue hemorrhagic fever is suspected, consider consult with a specialist.

Rickettsial Infections
- If suspected, begin treatment empirically since diagnostic test results often delayed.
- Preferred (outpatient): doxycycline 100 mg orally twice daily for 5 days or until 48 hrs after defervescence.
- Preferred (severely ill/hospitalized): doxycycline 100 mg IV twice daily for up to 24 hrs after defervescence, then change to oral doxycycline 100 mg twice daily to complete 5 days post defervescence. Consider doxycycline 200 mg loading dose.
- Pregnant women: if life-threatening infection, doxycycline should be used despite being a Category D agent. Consider consultation with an infectious disease expert.

Urinary Tract Infections/Pyelonephritis
- Acute bacterial cystitis: see separate module.
- Pyelonephritis: see separate module.
- Urinary tract infections in pregnant women: see separate module.

TREATMENT REGIMEN DETAILS

Severe Malaria
Persons with a positive blood smear or history of recent possible exposure and no other recognized pathology who have one or more of the clinical criteria listed below are considered to have severe malaria:
- impaired consciousness/coma
- severe normocytic anemia
- renal failure
- pulmonary edema
- acute respiratory distress syndrome
- circulatory shock
- disseminated intravascular coagulation
- spontaneous bleeding
- acidosis
- hemoglobinuria
- jaundice
- repeated generalized convulsions
- parasitemia of >5%
- Severe malaria is practically always due to *P. falciparum*.
- Pts diagnosed with severe malaria should be treated aggressively with parenteral antimalarial therapy.
- Treatment with IV quinidine should be initiated as soon as possible after the diagnosis has been made. Pts with severe malaria should be given an intravenous loading dose of quinidine unless they have received more than 40 mg/kg of quinine in the preceding 48 hrs or if they have received mefloquine within the preceding 12 hrs. **Consultation with a cardiologist and a physician with experience treating malaria is advised when treating malaria with quinidine.** During administration of quinidine, blood pressure monitoring (for hypotension) and cardiac monitoring (for widening of the QRS complex and/or lengthening of the QTc interval) should be monitored continuously and blood glucose (for hypoglycemia) should be monitored periodically. Cardiac complications, if severe, may warrant temporary discontinuation of the drug or slowing of the intravenous infusion. Do **not** delay treatment with quinidine while waiting for parenteral artesunate to arrive from CDC if you have arranged for this to be provided to you.
- Consider exchange transfusion if the parasite density (i.e., parasitemia) is >10% or if the pt has altered mental status, non-volume overload pulmonary edema, or renal complications. The parasite density can be estimated by examining a monolayer of red blood cells (RBCs) on the thin smear under oil immersion magnification. The slide should be examined where the RBCs are more or less touching (approximately 400 RBCs per field). The parasite density can then be estimated from the percentage of infected RBCs and should be monitored every 12 hrs. Exchange transfusion should be continued until the parasite density is <1% (usually requires 8–10 units). IV quinidine administration should not be delayed for an exchange transfusion and can be given concurrently throughout the exchange transfusion.
- Pregnant women diagnosed with severe malaria should be treated aggressively with parenteral antimalarial therapy.

MANAGEMENT

OTHER INFORMATION

- Consider consultation with an infectious disease or tropical medicine expert for any returned traveler with undifferentiated fever, suspect malaria, enteric fever, viral hemorrhagic fever, or neurological findings.

BASIS FOR RECOMMENDATIONS

Centers for Disease Control and Prevention. Treatment of Malaria (Guidelines For Clinicians); http://www.cdc.gov/malaria/pdf/clinicalguidance.pdf; 2007; The malaria treatment guidelines are provided on-line for clinicians and updated as needed by CDC. Last update was Mar 2007.

Comments: This is CDC's most up-to-date malaria treatment guideline from 24 May 2007. Coartem (artemether/lumefantrine combination therapy), although approved for use is not yet available (as of May 2009) and is not included in the recommendations.

Griffith KS, Lewis LS, Mali S, et al. Treatment of malaria in the United States: a systematic review. *JAMA*, 2007; Vol. 297; pp. 2264–77

Comments: This review provides the underlying rationale for the CDC's treatment guidelines utilizing an in-depth Medline review of the literature from 1966–2006. The safety and efficacy of each of the regimens is provided. Basis for recommendation.

Jensenius M, Fournier PE, Raoult D. Rickettsioses and the international traveler. *Clin Infect Dis*, 2004; Vol. 39; pp. 1493–9.

Comments: This is a literature-based review and additional case synthesis by one world experts. There are 15 recognized tick-borne rickettsioses; 8 of the 15 have ben reported in international travelers (African tick-bite fever, Mediterranean spotted fever, Indian tick typhus, Astrakhan fever, Rocky Mountain spotted fever, Queensland tick typhus, *R. aeschlimannii* infection, and North Asian tick typhus. Off the ~400 cases of tick-borne rickettsioses reported among international travelers, most are due to either Rickettsia africae (Subsaharan Africa-African tick-bite fever) or *R. conorii* (North Africa/Mid-East/India—Mediterranean spotted fever). The incidence among travelers appears to be increasing for several possible reasons: increased ecotoursim, increased travel to previously restricted areas (such as to post-apartheid game parks in the Republic of South Africa), and increased diagnostic awareness. Provides recommendations for treatment.

Warren JW, Abrutyn E, Hebel JR, et al. Guidelines for antimicrobial treatment of uncomplicated acute bacterial cystitis and acute pyelonephritis in women. Infectious Diseases Society of America (IDSA). *Clin Infect Dis*, 1999; Vol. 29; pp. 745–58.

Comments: Provides the full IDSA guideline which provides the complete rationale for the current treatment guidelines, using evidence-based decision making. Endorsed by the American Urologic Ass'n and the European Soc for Clin Micro and Infect Disease. A must read for anyone interested in understanding the rationale for current approach. The authors advocate 3-days abx RX of uncomplicated cystitis; the preferred drug is TMP-SMX unless resistance rates in community exceed 20%—then empiric use of a fluoroquinolone recommended.

RESPIRATORY TRACT INFECTIONS: IN THE RETURNED TRAVELER

PATHOGENS

- Viral: rhinoviruses; coronaviruses; parainfluenza viruses; respiratory syncytial virus; adenovirus, influenza A and B viruses; Coxsackie viruses; echoviruses; herpes simplex virus, types 1 and 2; Epstein Barr virus; cytomegalovirus; human metapneumovirus (hMPV); novel human coronavirus (agent of SARS)
- Bacterial: Group A, C, G streptococcal disease; *Mycoplasma pneumoniae*, *Chlamydophila (formerly Chlamydia) pneumoniae*, *Chlamydophila psittaci*, *Neisseria gonorrhoeae*, *Arcanobacterium haemolyticum*, *Corynebacterium diphtheriae*; *Yersinia enterocolitica*; *Y. pestis*; *Burkholderia pseudomallei*; *Francisella tularensis*
- Fungal: *Blastomyces dermatitidis*; *Coccidioides immitis*; *Cryptococcus neoformans*; *Histoplasma capsulatum* var *capsulatum*
- Parasitic: *Ascaris lumbricoides*; *Strongyloides stercoralis*; *Echinococcus granulosis*; *E. multilocularis*; *Paragonimus westermani*; *Entamoeba histolytica*.

CLINICAL RELEVANCE

- Respiratory conditions are the 6th most common cause of illness in returning travelers; 3rd most common cause of febrile illness among returning travelers after systemic febrile illness and acute diarrheal disease. Acute viral rhinitis and acute febrile viral respiratory infections occur throughout the world, including the tropics and are associated with the majority of acute respiratory illnesses in returned travelers and often commence during travel or immediately upon return. Illness is rarely due to a pathogen unique to the tropics.

- Location of travel and exposure history is key for inclusion of uncommon respiratory tract illnesses in differential diagnosis; immunization history needs to be elicited.
- Incubation periods: *Short incubation* (≤7–10 days): acute viral rhinitis-associated infections, diphtheria, acute histoplasmosis, influenza, Legionnaires' disease, measles, melioidosis, meningococcal pharyngitis, pertussis, pneumonic plague, psittacosis. *Intermediate incubation* (within 1 mo): rubella. *Long incubation* (>3 mos): melioidosis, penicilliosis, tuberculosis.
- Acute viral rhinitis: coryza, sneezing, lacrimation, irritation of the nasopharynx; chilliness, malaise lasting 2–7 days; fever very uncommon.
- Acute rhinosinusitis: nasal congestion and obstruction, purulent nasal discharge, facial pain/pressure that worsens with bending over, headache, fever, cough, hyposmia or anosmia, ear fullness/pressure, halitosis. Acute bacterial rhinosinusitis: symptoms ≥7 days and any of the following: purulent nasal discharge, unilateral maxillary tooth or facial pain, unilateral maxillary sinus tenderness, worsening symptoms after initial improvement. Urgent referral/hospitalization for diplopia or blindness, periorbital edema, mental status change.
- Acute pharyngitis: in adults, ~50% due to viruses, 10% due to Group A beta-hemolytic streptococci (GABHS). Suspect GABHS: sudden onset, sore throat, fever, headache, nausea, vomiting, abdominal pain, inflammation of the pharynx and tonsils, patchy and discrete exudate, tender and enlarged anterior cervical lymph nodes. Similar symptoms to GABHS may be seen with mononucleosis, acute HIV infection, oropharyngeal gonorrhea. Suspect a common viral cause: conjunctivitis, coryza, dry cough, occcasional diarrhea.
- Influenza-like illness: cough, fever, rigors or chills, fever, prostration or weakness, widespread, erythematous pharynx and nasal mucous membranes, history of similar illness in close contacts. Retrosternal cough, fever, myalgia or fatigue is most suggestive of influenza virus infection, particularly if other contacts ill. Ddx may include other conditions based on travel history including blastomycosis, coccidioidomycosis, cryptococcosis, histoplasmosis; psittacosis, melioidosis (eco-tourists and adventure travelers) and parasitic infections (either migratory stage or primary site of infection).

MORE CLINICAL

More commonly considered

Group A streptococcus: Key is identification and treatment to prevent the major non-suppurative complication of rheumatic fever. Suppurative complications include tonsillar or peritonsillar abscess.

Groups C and G streptococcus: These streptococci are not associated with acute rheumatic fever.

Chlamydophila pneumoniae: usually pharyngitis with acute bronchitis, occasionally with pneumonitis.

Corynebacterium diphtheriae: gradual onset of mild pharyngitis with pharyngeal erythema that may evolve to the hallmark feature of a tightly adherent grey membrane that bleeds when disrupted on attempt to dislodge it (seen in $\frac{1}{3}$ of cases); pharyngitis, malaise, and low grade fever. Membrane may cause respiratory compromise. Immunization history is key.

Influenza: The most common vaccine-preventable illness in travelers. Important to recognize because amenable to treatment within 48 hrs of onset. Occurs yr-around in the tropics.

Primary HIV: Acute retroviral syndrome often mimics EBV mononucleosis. History of risk activities is key! Fever, weight loss, adenopathy, and splenomegaly are common; lymphopenia and increased transaminases; mono spot is negative; HIV viral load assay with >10,000 copies/mL is diagnostic.

Mononucleosis: The majority of mononucleosis syndromes caused by Epstein-Barr virus (EBV) and cytomegalovirus (CMV). Acute retroviral syndrome due to HIV can cause this. In addition to the pharyngitis with or without exudates (EBV/CMV), there are varying systemic features including lymphadenopathy (tender anterior cervical nodes in EBV), splenomegaly, hepatitis, weight loss. Mononucleosis is a systemic illness that is often associated with splenomegaly, lymphadenopathy, persistent fatigue, weight loss, and hepatitis.

Neisseria gonorrhoeae: rare cause of pharyngitis; treatable but must use antibiotic to which organism is sensitive and that penetrates Waldeyer's ring.

Mycoplasma pneumoniae: usually pharyngitis with acute bronchitis.

MANAGEMENT

Parasitic diseases with respiratory manifestations

Entamoeba histolytica—Acquired by consumption of contaminated food or water; occurs worldwide especially where there is poor sanitation. Suspect in person with hepatic amebiasis with an elevated right hemidiaphragm and "anchovy paste" expectorate due to hepatobronchial fistula. Pleural effusion is a common finding with hepatic abscess and may be sterile (inflammatory reaction) or represent an empyema.

Ascaris lumbricoides—Acquired by consumption of contaminated food or water; occurs worldwide especially where there is poor sanitation. Suspect with fever, cough, expectoration, eosinophilia, patchy alveolar exudates on CXR or chest CT that clear within 10 days; confirmed larvae in sputum +/– eggs in stool.

Strongyloides stercoralis—Can be seen in an immunocompetent person as well as immuno-compromised (more severe illness). Suspect with suspect exposure and fever, eosinophilia (may be absent in immunocompromised person), bronchospasm or bronchitis, abdominal pain, and diarrhea. Ill-defined, patchy, migratory airspace consolidation that resolves in 7–10 days. Definitive diagnosis by finding larvae in sputum. Hyperinfection can lead to overwhelming diseases with ARDS.

Echinococcus granulosus—Occurs wherever there are canines. Long incubation period; may be asymptomatic for yrs. Hydatid cysts found in liver>lung>other organs. Lung disease causes cough, hemoptysis, pneumothorax, lung abscess, bilioptysis, parasite pulmonary embolism. Definitive diagnosis is made by histopathology. Pre-surgical ELISA and abdominal ultrasound are useful. Consult with infectious disease expert and surgeon strongly advised.

E. multilocularis—Exposure history to canines in Mediterranean, Eastern Europe, Turkey, China, South America, Australia, New Zealand, Russia, Japan, Canada, Alaska. Very long incubation of 5–15 yrs. Liver commonly involved. Lung ds. causes cough, fatigue, weight loss, hemoptysis, tumor-like invasion of chest wall, "metastases." Dx by histopathology or serology (available from CDC) plus characteristic appearance on imaging; Consult with infectious disease expert and surgeon strongly advised.

Paragonimus westermani—Exposure in Southeast Asia, Asia, Latin America (primarily Peru), Africa (primarily Nigeria). Lung is the target of this fluke. Fever, chest pain, chronic cough, hemoptysis with eggs found in the sputum, feces and pleural fluid. Often mistaken for TB on CXR. Alert laboratory as acid fast staining for TB will destroy eggs in sputum or pleural fluid.

DIAGNOSIS

- Influenza-like illness: nasopharyngeal swab or aspirate for novel H1N1 and seasonal influenza viruses (culture, RT-PCR or rapid testing), other respiratory viruses; if rare/exotic infections suspect, consider consultation with a tropical medicine expert.
- Productive cough: sputum Gram-stain and culture, chest X-ray; other tests as suggested by travel and exposure history.
- Acute rhinosinusitis: purulent rhinorrhea with nasal congestion or facial pressure/pain. Cultures and radiography usually not indicated.
- Pharyngitis: No pathogen is found in 30% of cases; rapid streptococcal antigen test; throat culture; mononucleosis screen; HIV testing (in the right exposure setting); culture for *N. gonorrheae* (in right exposure setting; requires special media—nucleic acid tests should not be used). Antistreptolysin (ASO), anti-deoxyribonuclease B (DNaseB) or other streptococcal antibody tests not helpful because results available too late.
- Febrile respiratory illness: blood culture; chest X-ray (+/– chest CT); sputum for Gram-stain with culture and sensitivity.
- Productive cough: chest X-ray; sputum for Gram-stain with culture and sensitivity; acid fast sputum smear and mycobacterial culture (in the right epidemiological setting); sputum smear for ova and parasites (if indicated).
- Abnormal auscultatory examination: chest X-ray (or chest CT); eosinophil count in addition to standard laboratory evaluation.
- Consider consultation with an tropical medicine expert if you suspect an unusual/exotic infection.

TREATMENT

General recommendations

- See individual modules (e.g., community-acquired pneumonia) or pathogen-specific therapy based on suspected/proven organism either listed below or in separate module.

BASIS FOR RECOMMENDATIONS

Bisno AL, Gerber MA, Gwaltney JM, et al. Practice guidelines for the diagnosis and management of group A streptococcal pharyngitis. Infectious Diseases Society of America. *Clin Infect Dis,* 2002; Vol. 35; pp. 113–25.

Comments: The 2002 Infectious Disease Society of America guideline for the management of streptococcal pharyngitis makes clear that signs and symptoms are neither sensitive nor specific in the diagnosis of this condition, including in the 10% of adults with this pathogen who have pharyngitis. Importantly, however, the use of a rapid streptococcal antigen test is useful in adults when negative as it virtually rules out infection. A positive test should be confirmed by culture. Notably, the importance of treating GABHS pharyngitis is to prevent both non-suppurative and suppurative complications and to decrease spread in the community.

Centers for Disease Control and Prevention (CDC). Update to CDC's sexually transmitted diseases treatment guidelines, 2006: fluoroquinolones no longer recommended for treatment of gonococcal infections. *MMWR Morb Mortal Wkly Rep,* 2007; Vol. 56; pp. 332–6.

Comments: Report of increasing fluoroquinolone-resistant Neisseria gonorrhoeae in the U.S. leading CDC to modify its 2006 Sexually Transmitted Disease Treatment Guidelines regarding this pathogen. Fluoroquinolones have been dropped from all preferred and alternate regimens. The new guideline outlines the recommended treatments of gonorrhea found at various mucosal sites.

SKIN CONDITIONS IN THE RETURNED TRAVELER

Noreen A Hynes, MD, MPH, DTM and H

PATHOGENS

- **Papular eruptions:** *Sarcoptes scabiei, Onchocerca volvulus;* non-human schistosomes (e.g., avian)*; Edwardsiella lineata* larva (sea anemone)*; Linuche unguinculata* (jellyfish); bedbugs; fleas.
- **Nodules/subcutaneous swellings:** myiasis due to *Cordylobia anthropophaga* larvae, *Dermatobia hominis* larvae, *Tunga penetrans; Loa loa; Trypanosoma bruceii gambiense* and *T.b. rhodesiense* (more common to see nodule in this form)
- **Ulcers:** *Staphylococcus aureus* (MRSA, MSSA-both with or without Panton-Valentine leucocidin); Group A streptococci; *Leishmania (Viannia) braziliensis* complex; *Mycobacterium marinum; Rickettsia conorii; R. africae; Orientalis tsutsugamushi; Haemophilus ducreyi; Chlamydia trachomatis* L serovars; *Klebsiella granulomatis; Treponema pallidum;* Herpes simplex virus.
- **Geographic Migratory and Linear Lesions:** (1) Non-human nematode larvae-*Ancylostoma braziliense, A. caninum, Gnathostoma* spp, zoonotic strongyloides, Spururina spp; (2) Human nematode larvae- *Strongyloides stercoralis;* (3) Migratory maggots; (4) Adult nematodes, *Loa loa; Dracunculus medinensis;* (5) Trematode larvae, *Fasciola giganta;* (6) Mites, *Sarcoptes scabei.*
- **Exanthema:** dengue virus serotypes 1, 2, 3, and 4; chikungunya virus; *Rickettsia africae; R. conorii;* other location-specific arthropod-borne rickettsioses
- Additional systemic infections of travelers associated with skin lesions: (1) *Bartonella bacilliformis* (Oroya fever, Verruga peruana, Carrion disease); (2) Brucella spp; (3) Ehrlichia spp; (4) Enteroviruses; (5) *Neisseria gonorrheae;* (6) Acute HIV infection; (7) Leishmania major (visceral leishmaniasis); (8) Leptospira spp; (9) *Borrelia burgdorferi* (Lyme disease); (10) Measles; (11) *Burkholderia pseudomallei;* (12) *Neisseria meningitidis;* (13) Parvovirus; (14) *Streptobacillus moniliformis* (Rat bite fever); (15) *Spirillum minus* (Rat bite fever); (16) *Borrelia recurrentis* (Louse borne relapsing fever); (17) *Borrelia hermsii* (Tick borne relapsing fever); (18) *Trypanosoma cruzi* (Chagas disease); (19) Coccidioides spp; (20) *Paracoccidioides braziliensis;* (21) Agents of dermatophytoses (fungal infections of the superficial keratinized areas of the body).

CLINICAL

- Leading causes of skin conditions in returned travelers: (1) insect bites (with or without secondary infection), (2) hookworm-related cutaneous larval migrans [HR-CLM, most commonly due to *Ancylostoma duodenale* and *Necator americanus*], (3) allergic skin reactions, (4) skin abscesses, carbuncles and folliculitis.
- Some conditions occur more commonly in certain regions: animal bites—Southeast Asia, HR-CLM—Caribbean cutaneous leishmaniasis—Central and South America, myiasis—Central and South America.

MANAGEMENT

- **Papules:** (1) bedbugs and fleas-very pruritic, linear papules or clusters; (2) scabies-history of sexual contact; (3) sea bather's eruption (*E. lineata,* sea anemone larvae and *L. unguinculata,* thimble jellyfish)-pruritic, erythematous macular or papular dermatitis, with or without urticaria, on skin areas covered by bathing suit swimming exposure in subtropical or tropical salt water; (4) swimmer's itch-pruritic macular-papular eruption caused by avian schistosomiasis soon after exposure in fresh water, (5) *Onchocerca volvulus* (cause of river blindness)—pruritic, papular rash with associated eosinophilia in expatriates and long term travelers to Subsaharan Africa and focal areas of 6 countries in the Americas (Guatemala, Mexico, Venezuela, Brazil, Columbia, Ecuador); symptomatic onchocerciasis usually requires heavy infestations and repeated exposure to Simulium spp (black flies), usually >3 mos; symptoms may occur mos to yrs after leaving the endemic area.

- **Subcutaneous swellings and nodules:** (1) furuncles: painful, raised, erythematous area often occurring in a moist or irritated area, usually Staphylococcal, (2) myiasis-fly larvae including *C. anthropophaga,* the tumbu fly in Africa and *D. hominis,* the botfly in Latin America; lesions are boil-like with central punctal opening (breathing canal) with serosanguineous ooze through which larva may emerge; may be pruritic; pt may sense movement in area, (3) tungiasis caused by *Tunga penetrans,* the female sand flea; invades around toenails and soles in Latin American and Indian travelers; painful, (4) Loa loa-may be seen up to yrs after return of long-term expatriate or immigrant with eyeworm or migratory area of angioedema (Calabar swellings), (5) Acute human African trypanosomiasis (HAT)—painless, indurated, erythematous lesions (Calabar swellings) that may ulcerate and be mistaken for focal cellulitis; evolves to fatal sleeping sickness if untreated, rapidly in the East African form, more slowly in the West African form.

- **Ulcers:** (1) Pyoderma (ecthyma): the most frequent cause of cutaneous ulcer among travelers; painful, purulent, shallow ulcer; often after insect bite or skin trauma; *S. aureus* and group A streptococci are the most common pathogens, (2) cutaneous leishmaniasis: painless, non-pruritic; slowly evolving ulcer with raised margins and crusted or granulomatous base; occasional isolated lymphadenopathy or sporotrichoid-like form. Must speciate if acquired in New World as *L. (Viannia) braziliensis* can evolve to highly destructive mucocutaneous form; (3) small, painless eschars (usually <1 cm) can be seen with the rickettsia-caused African tick fever, Mediterranean spotted fever, or scrub typhus at the site where the arthropod fed; may present as febrile illness and must search for the eschar (tache noir); (4) genital ulcers suggest sexually transmitted infection; painless ulcer with syphilis and 1st stage of lymphogranuloma venereum; painful, ragged, and "dirty" based ulcer seen in chancroid; painful, shallow ulcer more common with genital herpes.

- **Geographic Migratory and Linear Lesions:** (1) HR-CLM is the most common cause of serpiginous skin lesions (creeping eruption) in returned travelers due to animal hookworm larva; seen after direct skin contact with contaminated sand or soil in the tropics/subtropics; 3 mm × 15–20 cm, pruritic, often with local edema; may have vesiculobullous lesions; other sx may include folliculitis, eosinophilic pneumonitis; (2) Larval currens is a rapidly mobile (5 cm per hr) serpiginous track, often perianal and due to *Strongyloides stercoralis;* (3) *Fasciola giganta:* migrating erythematous areas in the skin of the trunk or other areas during ectopic infection.

- **Febrile exanthema:** >60% caused by dengue, chikungunya and African tick bite fever. (1) Classic dengue—mosquito-borne; incubation period 3–14 days; sudden onset of fever, intense headache, myalgia, arthralgia; lymphadenopathy; diffuse, sometimes pruritic, macular or maculopapular eruption with small islands of normal skin, rash most commonly seen in light skinned persons; leukopenia, neutropenia, and thrombocytopenia are common; minor hemorrhagic features including petechiae and epistaxis may be seen; major hemorrhagic features such as melena suggest dengue hemorrhagic fever; (2) Chikungunya—often occurs with a rash similar to that seen in dengue virus infection; also high fever, severe arthralgia, lymphopenia, prominent lymphadenopathy with a prolonged convalescence; incubation period 3–12 days; cases with aphthous-like ulcers and vesiculobullous lesions have been reported; (3) African tick-bite fever (*R. africae*)—multiple, small (2–5 mm) "tache noire" at site of tick bites with surrounding edema; generalized maculopapular or vesicular eruption seen in about 1/2 of cases; aphthous stomatitis not uncommon; fever is less common than in other rickettsioses; incubation period 5–10 days; travel to southern subsaharan Africa and the Lesser Antilles is key; (4) Boutonneuse fever (*R. conorii*): mild to severe illness usually with an eschar and maculopapular rash that involves palms and soles appearing on the 4–5th day of illness; fever for up to 2 days; tick-borne with diverse distribution in Africa, India, Middle East; incubation period usually 5–7 days.

- Other location-specific tick-borne Rickettsioses: (1) Queensland tick typhus: *R. australis*; Australia-Queensland, New South Wales, Tasmania, coastal areas of eastern Victoria; (2) North Asian tick fever: R. sibeirica; North China; Mongolia; Asiatic areas of Russia; (3) Tick-borne lymphadenopathy (TIBOLA): *R. slovaca*; Europe and Asia; (4) Far-Eastern tick-borne rickettsiosis: R. beilongjiangensis; Far East Russia and northern China; (5) Oriental spotted fever: *R. japonica*; Japan; (6) Maculatum infection: *R. parkeri*; Southern South America including Argentina, Uruguay, parts of Brazil; coastal southeaster USA; (7) Thai tick typhus: R. bonei; Thailand, Australia; Tasmania; Flinders Island; (8) Australian spotted fever: *R. marmionii*; Australia

DIAGNOSIS

- Pyogenic lesions including abscess/carbuncle/furuncle: culture and sensitivity of purulent material after incision and drainage or spontaneous drainage. Often caused by *S. aureus* (MSSA or MRSA).
- Rickettsial diseases: Boutonneuse fever-serological test, PCR or immunostains of biopsied tissues; other suspect conditions may cross react with available serological tests and need to consider specialty laboratory testing in an endemic country for confirmation. Rickettsia are considered biohazards and warn the laboratory if you have ordered a culture. If suspected, embark upon empiric doxycycline therapy while seeking confirmation.
- Creeping Eruptions: (1) Hookworm-related CLM—this is a clinical diagnosis; (2) larval currens-identification of *S. stercoralis* larvae in concentrated stool specimens or visualization of motile larvae in freshly passed feces, in the agar plate method, duodenal aspirates, or occasionally in sputum; serological tests based on larval stage antigens are positive in 80–85% of infected persons; (3) *Fasciola giganta*: finding eggs in the feces or in bile aspirated from the duodenum; serology suggests but does not prove the diagnosis.
- Infestations: botfly and tumbu fly myiasis; tungiasis, and scabies are all most commonly clinical diagnoses based upon travel and exposure history. Bot and tumbu flies are diagnosed by the appearance of a furuncular-like lesion with a central punctum with opening which is the orifice of the larva's breathing tube; to identify the effects of the human flea *T. perstans*, direct skin microscopy (dermoscopy) helps identify the typical features: irregular central brown discoloration with a plugged opening in the middle or a grey-blue discoloration; the scabies mite elaborates linear tunnels in digital web spaces that are diagnostic.
- Leishmaniasis (cutaneous and mucocutaneous): The WHO operational case definition is "a person showing clinical signs of leishmaniasis with parasitological confirmation and/ or, for mucosal leishmaniases **only**, serological diagnosis." Microscopic identification of the non-motile, intracellular form (amastigote) in stained specimens of the lesions; culture of the motile, extracellular form (promastigote) on suitable media (such as NNN media ordered from CDC); IFA or ELISA can be helpful in the mucosal form only where antibodies are commonly detectable; speciation is based upon biological, immunological, molecular and biochemical criteria. Consultation with an infectious disease expert with experience in tropical medicine is strongly recommended.
- Loiasis: transient, recurrent calabar swellings in a person with exposure (usually >2 wks) in African rain forests who sustain deer fly bites (*Chrysops* spp), especially in central Africa and the Congo River basin suggest this diagnosis; microfilaria in peripheral blood smear taken during the daytime or stained thick blood smears with eosinophilia; DNA detection in blood in sometimes available as a research tool.
- **Onchocerciasis**: Microscopic examination of a fresh superficial skin biopsy incubated with water or saline with observation of emerging microfilariae; finding adult worms in nodules (if present); antibody detection is of limited value due to antigenic cross reactivity between filaria and other helminths.

MANAGEMENT

- Genital ulcers: depending on the region and exposure history, test for appropriate STIs including syphilis, chancroid, lymphogranuloma venereum, granuloma inguinale or donovanosis (*Klebsiella granulomatis*), and herpes simplex.
- Human African Trypanosomiasis (HAT): finding trypanosomes in blood, lymph or eventually, the CSF. Parasite concentration techniques always needed in *T.b. gambiense*, less so in *T.b. rhodesiense*.

TREATMENT
Pyogenic Infections: Furuncle, Carbuncle, Abscess
- Empiric treatment: Small furuncle—warm compresses to promote drainage are usually sufficient treatment; larger furuncles, all carbuncles, and all abscesses require incision and drainage with material sent for culture and sensitivity. Persons at risk for endocarditis should receive vancomycin 1 g IV 60 minutes before the procedure.
- Empiric oral antibiotics: usually reserved for lesions accompanied by systemic signs such as fever or significant surrounding cellulitis. If needed, assume the presence of MRSA and use one of the following regimens for 7–14 days: First line: TMP-SMX—2 double-strength tablets orally twice daily **or** doxycycline or minocycline—100 mg orally twice daily **or** clindamycin—300 to 450 mg orally every 6 to 8 hrs. Alternative: Linezolid 600 mg orally twice daily.
- Follow-up: Repeat evaluation after 24 to 48 hrs of outpatient empiric oral antibiotic therapy; the clinical response to therapy should guide antibiotic duration; lack of response requires evaluation for possible resistant organism or deeper and more serious infection.

Tick-borne Rickettsioses
- Preferred: tetracycline 500 mg PO four times a day **or** doxycycline 100 mg PO twice daily for 5–7 days.
- Alternatives (only consider in those who cannot take tetracyclines): azithromycin 500 mg PO Q day or clarithromycin 500 mg PO twice daily. (Tetracyclines preferred for Rocky Mountain spotted fever.)
- Chloramphenicol 500 mg PO four times a day for 7–10 days (oral formulation unavailable in U.S.). Do not use for Rocky Mountain spotted fever (increased fatality rate compared to doxycycline).

Infestations
- Furuncular myiasis: tumbu fly—application of lateral pressure may result in spontaneous ejection of the maggot; for both tumbu fly and bot fly suffocation by occlusion of the punctum with mineral oil, petroleum jelly, or bacon fat may result in spontaneous emergence of the maggot after several hrs. If these methods fail, surgical excision is needed.
- Tungiasis: extraction of the gravid flea using a sterile needle is diagnostic and therapeutic; cleanse area after extraction; cover area with topical antibiotic; give tetanus booster if not up-to-date.
- Scabies (preferred): ivermectin 200 mcg/kg orally once [off label] **or** permethrin cream (5%): apply to all areas of body from the neck down and wash off after 8–14 hrs. Alternative: lindane (1%) apply 1 oz. of lotion or 30 g of cream thinly to all areas of the body from the neck down. Thoroughly wash off after 8 h. Avoid use in the elderly, those <50 kg, and those with a seizure history, contraindicated in children.

Creeping Eruptions
- Hookworm-related cutaneous larval migrans: ivermectin 200 micrograms/kg as a single dose **or** albendazole 400–800 mg/day for 3 days.
- Larval currens (*S. stercoralis*, preferred): ivermectin 200 micrograms/kg/day × 2 days [treat all infections regardless of worm burden due to risk of autoinfection]; alternative: albendazole 400 mg once or twice a day for 3 days. Repeated courses may be required.
- *Fasciola gigantica* (preferred): triclabendazole 10 mg/kg orally once or twice (availability problems exist). Alternative: bithionol 10–15 mg/kg on alternate days for 10–15 doses **or** nitazoxanide 500 mg orally twice daily for 7 days.

Cutaneous and Mucocutaneous Leishmaniasis
- Cutaneous (preferred): sodium stibogluconate 20 mg Sb/kg/day IV or IM × 20 days **or** meglumine antimonate 20 mg Sb/kg/day IV or IM × 20 days **or** miltefosine 2.5 mg/kg/day orally (max 150 mg/day) × 28 days [CDC Drug Service can assist in obtaining this drug. Tel: daytime 404.639.3670; evenings, weekends, holidays: 404.770.7100]. Alternatives:

paromomycin topically twice daily for 10–20 days **or** pentamidine 2–3 mg/kg IV or IM daily or every 2nd day for 4–7 days.

- Mucosal: sodium stibogluconate 20 mg Sb/kg/day IV or IM for 28 days **or** meglumine antimonate 20 mg Sb/kg/day IV or IM for 28 days **or** amphotericin B 0.5 mg/kg IV daily or every 2nd day for up to 8 wks **or** miltefosine 2.5 mg/kg/day orally (max 150 mg/day) for 28 days.

Filarial Infections with Dermal Manifestations

- Loiasis: diethylcarbamazine (DEC) 6 mg/kg/day orally in 3 doses for 12 days. There are availability problems for this drug.
- **Onchocerciasis:** ivermectin 150 microgram/kg orally once; repeat every 6–12 mos until asymptomatic.

"Tropical" Genital Ulcer Diseases

- Primary or Secondary (infectious) Syphilis (preferred): benzathine penicillin G 2.4 million units IM once. Alternative (PCN allergic and non-pregnant): doxycycline 100 mg orally twice daily for 14 days.
- **Chancroid:** azithromycin 1 g orally once **or** ceftriaxone 250 mg IM once **or** ciprofloxacin 500 mg orally twice daily for 3 days **or** erythromycin base 500 mg orally 4 times daily for 7 days.
- Lymphogranuloma venereum (preferred): doxycycline 100 mg orally twice daily for a minimum of 21 days. Alternative: erythromycin base 500 mg orally 4 times daily for a minimum of 21 days.
- Donovanosis (Granuloma inguinale): treatment for 3 wks or until the lesion(s) heal using doxycycline 100 mg orally twice daily **or** azithromycin 1 g orally daily **or** ciprofloxacin 750 mg orally twice daily.

Human African Trypanosomiasis

- Begin treatment ASAP based on sx and laboratory results
- See trypanosomiasis module for additional details and consideration of combination drug regimens.
- *T.b. rhodesiense* hemolymphatic stage: suramin, contact CDC Drug Service to receive this Investigation New Protocol drug (Tel: daytime 404.639.3670; evenings, weekends, holidays: 404.770.7100). Early stage: suramin use 100–200 mg test dose IV then 1 g IV on days 1, 3, 7, 14, and 21. Late stage (see below)
- *T.b. gambiense* hemolymphatic stage: first Line, pentamidine isethionate 4 mg/kg/day IM for 7 days. Alternative: suramin—Contact CDC Drug Service to receive this Investigation New Protocol drug (Tel: daytime 404.639.3670; evenings, weekends, holidays: 404.770.7100).
- *T.b. rhodesiense* late disease with CNS involvement: melarsoprol 2–3.6 mg/kg/day IV for 3 days; after 7 days give 3.6 mg/kg/day for 3 days; repeat again after 7 days.
- *T.b. gambiense* late disease with CNS involvement: eflornithine 400 mg/kg/day IV in 4 doses for 14 days (very limited supply; available only directly from WHO) **or** melarsoprol 2.2 mg/kg/day IV for 10 days.

BASIS FOR RECOMMENDATIONS

Abramowicz M (Ed). Drugs for parasitic infections. *The Medical Letter,* 2007; Vol. 5 (Suppl); pp. e1–e15 Available at: http://medlet-best.securesites.com

Comments: This compendium of drugs of choice for parasitic diseases is an up-to-date resource for use by clinicians based upon both FDA recommendations and the medical literature.

Abramowicz M (Ed). Choice of antibacterial drugs. *Treatment guidelines from The Medical Letter,* 2007; Vol. 5; pp. 33–50 Available at: http://medlet-best.securesites.com

Comments: This pathogen-specific reference provides information on the empirical treatment of bacterial infections, trends in antimicrobial resistance, and new drug data. These treatment guidelines are based on clinical trials, susceptibility studies and expert consultants.

MANAGEMENT

SECTION 4
DRUGS

Antibacterial

AMIKACIN

Paul A. Pham, PharmD and John G. Bartlett, MD

INDICATIONS

FDA

- Amikacin sulfate indicated in the short-term treatment of serious infections due to susceptible organisms. [With the exception of uncomplicated UTI, aminoglycosides are generally used in combination for treatment of *Pseudomonas aeruginosa*].
- Bacterial septicemia (including neonatal sepsis)
- Respiratory tract infections
- Bones and joint infections
- Central nervous system infections
- Skin and soft tissue infections
- Intra-abdominal infections
- Burns
- Post-operative infections
- Complicated and recurrent urinary tract infections.

Non-FDA Approved Uses

- Pneumonia, hospital-acquired (in combination with a beta-lactam, beta-lactam/beta-lactamase inhibitor, or a 3rd/4th generation cephalosporin)

FORMS

Brand name (mfr)	Forms	Cost*
Amikacin (generic manufacturers)	IV vial 1000 mg/4 mL; IV vial 100 mg/2 mL; IV vial 500 mg/2 mL	$16.05; $8.13; $8.13

*Prices represents Average Wholesale Price (AWP).

USUAL ADULT DOSING

- **Once daily dosing:** 15–20 mg/kg IV. Therapeutic drug monitoring generally not recommended. Consider trough in pts at risk for nephrotoxicity (ICU pts, elderly, and concomitant nephrotoxin). Target trough <4 mcg/mL. Don't use once daily dosing in pts w/ unstable renal fxn, CrCl <60 mL/min, endocarditis, meningitis, or increased Vd (pregnancy, ascites, edema).
- **Traditional dosing (mild-moderate infections):** 8 mg/kg load, then 7 mg/kg IV q8h **or** 7.5–10 mg/kg IV q12h (goal peak >20–30 mcg/mL and trough <10 mcg/mL).
- **Traditional dosing (severe infections, e.g., Pseudomonas, pneumonia):** 8–12 mg/kg load, then 8 mg/kg IV q8h (goal peak >25–35 mcg/mL and trough <10 mcg/mL).
- Consider a higher loading dose and obtain a peak and trough after 1 dose in severe infections (+/– diffuse edema, ascites, shock, burns, CF pts, and pregnancy) in order to calculate pt-specific pharmacokinetic dose. Doses need to be adjusted based on changing renal function and/or volume status.
- Troughs should be obtained (generally after 3rd dose) immediately before next dose.
- Peak should be obtained 30 mins after the end of a 30 mins infusion (generally after 3rd dose).
- For obese pts: use calculated lean body weight plus 40% of excess fat. Dosing Body Weight (DBW) = Ideal Body Weight (IBW) + 0.4 (Actual body weight-IBW).
- IBW= 50 kg (for males) **or** 45.5 kg (for females) **plus** (2.3 × inches over 5 ft).
- Intraventricular or intrathecal administration: amikacin 15 mg q24h (range 10–50 mg). Note: preservative free amikacin is not available. Sodium bisulfite preservative may increase risk of neurotoxicities (e.g., seizure, aseptic meningitis, and radicular pain). Use IT amikacin only if organism is resistant to gentamicin and tobramycin (both available preservative free).

RENAL DOSING

Dosing for GFR 50–80: Standard loading dose for all levels of renal function. GRF >70 mL/min: Use standard dose. GFR 50–69 mL/min: calculated GFR × 0.18 = "mg/kg" q12h (Ex. for GFR 56 mL/min: 56 × 0.18 = "10" mg/kg q12h). Monitor peak and trough.

Dosing for GFR 10–50: Standard loading dose for all levels of renal function. GFR 40–49 mL/min: calculated GFR × 0.18 = "mg/kg" q12h (Ex. for GFR 45 mL/min: 45 × 0.18 = "8" mg/kg q12h). GFR 20–39: calculated GFR × 0.36 = "mg/kg" q24h. Monitor peak and trough.

Dosing for GFR <10: Standard loading dose for all levels of renal function. GFR <20 mL/min: 10 mg/kg × 1, then redose when level <2 mcg/mL. Monitor peak and trough.

Dosing in hemodialysis: Standard loading dose, then 8 mg/kg post-HD (treatment doses). Peak (measure 2 hrs-post dose, target 25–35 mcg/mL) and trough (before next HD session, depending on residual renal function, expect 12–16 mcg/mL).

Dosing in peritoneal dialysis: 9–20 mg per liter of dialysate exchange per day. Aminoglycosides given for prolonged periods to pts receiving continuous peritoneal dialysis have been associated with high rates of ototoxicity.

Dosing in hemofiltration: CVVH or CVVHD: loading dose 10–12 mg/kg, then 8 mg/kg q24–48 (measure peak 2 hrs-post dose, target 25–35 mcg/mL). Check a 24-hr concentration (redose <10 mcg/mL).

ADVERSE DRUG REACTIONS

Common

- Renal failure (usually reversible): risk factors include older pts, preexisting renal and hepatic disease, volume depletion, traditional q8h dosing, large doses, concomitant nephrotoxic drug (including vancomycin), and length of therapy (most important). Controversial but trough level may be associated with nephrotoxicity.

Occasional

- Irreversible vestibular toxicity (4–6%). Most pts compensate with visual and proprioceptive cues. Monitor for nausea, vomiting, nystagmus, and vertigo (exacerbated in the dark).
- Irreversible cochlear toxicity (3–14%). Risk factors include repeated exposure (cumulative dose and duration of therapy), genetic predisposition, renal impairment, specific aminoglycoside (neomycin>streptomycin>gentamicin>tobramycin>amikacin>netilmicin), elderly, age, bacteremia, hypovolemia, degree of temperature elevation, and liver dysfunction (*JID* 1984;149:23–30). 62% of hearing lost were at frequency above 9 kHz (high pitch) at a mean of 9 days of therapy (*JID* 1992;165:1026–1032).
- Genetic predisposition may be present in some cases of vestibular and cochlear toxicity. Check family hx for aminoglycoside ototoxicity.
- Monitor for ototoxicity in any pts receiving >3 days of aminoglycoside. Vestibular toxicity monitoring: check baseline visual acuity using a Snellen pocket card. After 3 days of aminoglycoside, have pt shake head (side to side) while reading a line. Early sign of ototoxicity if pt loses 2 lines of visual acuity. Check Romberg sign. Cochlear toxicity monitoring: audiology test.

Rare

- Neuromuscular blockade (especially with myasthenia or Parkinsons and rapid infusion of large aminoglycoside doses).
- Allergic reaction (secondary to sulfites in some formulations).

DRUG INTERACTIONS

- Penicillins: *in vitro* inactivation. Do not mix or run in the same tubing.
- Cephalothin: increased risk of nephrotoxicity.
- Nondepolarizing muscle relaxants (atracurium, pancuronium, tubocurarine, gallamine triethiodide): possible enhanced action of nondepolarizing muscle relaxant resulting in possible respiratory depression.
- Loop diuretics (bumetanide, furosemide, ethacrynic acid, torsemide): cochlear toxicity (esp. w/ ethacrynic acid). Avoid co-administration.
- Other nephrotoxic agents (e.g., amphotericin B, foscarnet, cidofovir, and IV contrast dyes): additive nephrotoxicity. Avoid co-administration.
- Vancomycin: increased risk of nephrotoxicity.

SPECTRUM—See Appendix II, p. 797

RESISTANCE

- MIC-sensitive breakpoint for Enterobacteriaceae and Gram-negative non-lactose fermenters including *P. aeruginosa* is 16 mcg/mL.

ANTIBACTERIAL DRUGS

PHARMACOLOGY

Mechanism

Aminoglycosides inhibit protein synthesis by irreversibly binding to 30S ribosomal subunit. Amikacin has an s-4 amino 2-hydroxybutyryl (AHB) side-chain that prevents inactivation by many bacterial enzymes that inactivate other aminoglycosides.

Pharmacokinetic Parameters

- **Absorption** Aminoglycosides are rapidly absorbed after IM administration. Intrapleural and intraperitoneal administration results in rapid absorption. Poor absorption with oral administration.
- **Cmax** 17–25 mcg/mL 1–2 hrs after 7.5 mg/kg dose administration. In addition to the dose, Cmax will be affected by the volume of distribution.
- **Distribution** 0.2–0.4 L/kg (may be higher in pregnancy, ascites, edema, sepsis, and burn pts); distributed in extracellular fluid, abscesses, ascitic fluid, pericardial fluid, pleural fluid, synovial fluid, lymphatic fluid and peritoneal fluid. Not well distributed into bile, aqueous humor, bronchial secretions, abscess, sputum, and CSF.
- **Protein binding** 0–10%.
- **Metabolism/Excretion** Aminoglycosides are not metabolized in the liver, they are excreted unchanged in the urine.
- **T1/2** 2–4 hrs (note: cystic fibrosis pts may have shorter half life of 1–2 hrs; burn and febrile pts may have increased clearance of aminoglycosides).

Dosing for Decreased Hepatic Function

No dose adjustment, but may increase risk of nephrotoxicity and ototoxicity. Use with close monitoring.

Pregnancy Risk

D: No reports linking the use of amikacin to congenital defects have been located. Ototoxicity has not been reported as an effect of in utero exposure to amikacin, however, eighth cranial nerve toxicity in the fetus is well known following exposure to other aminoglycosides (kanamycin and streptomycin) and could potentially occur with amikacin.

Breast Feeding Compatibility

Only a trace amount of amikacin was found in some nursing infants. Due to the poor absorption of aminoglycoside, the systemic toxicity should not occur, but alteration in normal bowel flora may occur in nursing infants.

COMMENTS

Amikacin is an aminoglycoside that is active against many Gram-negative bacteria resistant to gentamicin and tobramycin. In many institutions, drug has the most predictable activity against *P. aeruginosa*. Amikacin should be restricted to infections with organisms resistant to other aminoglycosides. Desired peak 25–35 mcg/mL (high peak for serious, pulmonary, and pseudomonal infections).

SELECTED REFERENCES

American Thoracic Society, Infectious Diseases Society of America. Guidelines for the management of adults with hospital-acquired, ventilator-associated, and healthcare-associated pneumonia. *Am J Respir Crit Care Med*, 2005; Vol. 171; pp. 388–416.

Baron EJ, Young LS. Amikacin, ethambutol, and rifampin for treatment of disseminated Mycobacterium avium-intracellulare infections in pts with acquired immune deficiency syndrome. *Diagn Microbiol Infect Dis*, 1986; Vol. 5; pp. 215–20.

AMOXICILLIN

Paul A. Pham, PharmD and John G. Bartlett, MD

INDICATIONS

FDA

- Bronchopulmonary infections
- Urinary tract infections (cystitis, pyelonephritis)
- Duodenal ulcer caused by *H. pylori* (in combination with clarithromycin and a PPI)
- Acute bacterial sinusitis
- Uncomplicated gonorrhea (currently not the drug of choice)
- Otitis media (*Haemophilus influenzae*, nonbeta-lactamase producer)
- *Proteus mirabilis* infections

- Lower respiratory infection (PCN-sensitive community-acquired pneumonia: CAP)
- Skin and skin structure infections and nose and throat infections

Non-FDA Approved Uses
- Lyme disease
- Enterococcus
- Group A strep pharyngitis

FORMS

Brand name (mfr)	Forms	Cost*
Amoxil (generic)	PO cap 250 mg; PO cap 500 mg;	$0.27; $0.60;
	PO cap 875 mg	$1.00
	PO chew tab 200 mg;	$0.50;
	PO chew tab 400 mg	$0.60
	PO susp 125 mg/5 mL;	$0.11/5 mL;
	PO susp 250 mg/5 mL;	$0.24/5 mL;
	PO susp 400 mg/5 mL	$0.54/5 mL
	IV vial 250 mg, 500 mg, 1000 mg	Not available in the U.S.
*Prices represents Average Wholesale Price (AWP).		

USUAL ADULT DOSING
- CAP: 500 mg PO q8h (for sensitive *S. pneumoniae*); 1000 mg PO q8h (for pts at risk for drug resistant *S. pneumoniae*) **plus** a macrolide.
- Higher doses (3–4 g/day) recommended for some intermediately resistant pneumococcal infections.
- UTI (uncomplicated): 250–500 mg PO q8h (consider 875 mg q12h).
- Skin and soft tissue infections: 250 mg–500 mg PO q8h (consider 875 mg q12h).

RENAL DOSING
Dosing for GFR 50–80: 250–500 mg q8h.
Dosing for GFR 10–50: 250–500 mg q12–24h.
Dosing for GFR <10: 250–500 mg q12–24h.
Dosing in hemodialysis: 250–500 mg q12–24h. On days of HD, dose post-HD or supplement 250–500 mg post-HD.
Dosing in peritoneal dialysis: 250 mg q12h.
Dosing in hemofiltration: No data. Consider 500 mg q12h.

ADVERSE DRUG REACTIONS
General
- Generally well tolerated
Common
- Rash (especially w/ infectious mononucleosis)
Occasional
- Diarrhea
- *C. difficile* colitis
- Hypersensitivity reactions
- Jarisch-Herxheimer reaction with spirochetal infections
- Drug fever
Rare
- Coombs' test positive, hemolytic anemia
- Leukopenia
- Thrombocytopenia
- CNS: seizures and twitching (especially seen with high doses in pts with renal failure)
- Interstitial nephritis
- LFT elevations

DRUG INTERACTIONS
- Allopurinol: may increase the risk of rash with amoxicillin co-administration.
- Tetracyclines: *in vitro* antagonism when co-administered. In 2 studies involving a total of 79 pts with pneumococcal meningitis treated with either penicillin plus tetracyclines or

ANTIBACTERIAL DRUGS

penicillin monotherapy resulted in a higher mortality rate (79–85%) in the combination therapy compared to penicillin monotherapy (30–33%) [*Arch Intern Med* 1951:88:489, *Ann Intern Med* 1961;55:545]. Interaction resulted in higher treatment failure for meningitis but not pneumonia (*Arch Intern Med* 1953;91:197). Do not co-administer PCN with tetracycline.

SPECTRUM—See Appendix II, p. 795

RESISTANCE

- *S. pneumoniae:* PCN resistance rate was 10.3% (using resistance break point MIC of 2 mcg/mL), but only 1.2% (using an MICs of 8 mcg/mL for IV PCN for non-meningeal involvement, *MMWR* 2008;57:1353). Without meningeal involvement, *S. pneumoniae* with MIC of 2 mcg/mL or lower can be treated with high dose of PCN or amoxicillin (3–4 g/day; *CID* 2005;41:139–148).
- *S. pneumoniae* break points (non-meningeal, oral therapy PCN): ≤ 0.06 mcg/mL (sensitive); 0.12–1.0 mcg/mL (intermediate); ≥ 2 mcg/mL (resistant).
- *S. pneumoniae* break points (non-meningeal, parenteral therapy PCN): ≤ 2 mcg/mL (sensitive); 4 mcg/mL (intermediate); ≥ 8 mcg/mL (resistant).
- *S. pneumoniae* break points (meningeal isolates, PCN): ≤ 0.06 mcg/mL (sensitive); ≥ 2 mcg/mL (resistant).
- Risk factors for drug resistant *S. pneumoniae* (DRSP): chronic heart, lung, liver, or renal disease; diabetes mellitus; alcoholism; malignancies; asplenia; immunosuppressing conditions or use of immunosuppressing drugs; use of antimicrobials within the previous 3 mos.

PHARMACOLOGY

Mechanism

Beta-lactam antibiotics inhibit mucopeptide synthesis in the bacterial cell wall, this results in the formation of defective cell walls and osmotically unstable organisms susceptible to cell lysis.

Pharmacokinetic Parameters

- **Absorption** 74–92% absorbed.
- **Cmax** 4–5 mcg/mL after 250 mg dose administration.
- **Distribution** 0.36 L/kg; Distributed to blister fluid, urine, peritoneal fluid, pleural fluid, middle ear fluid, intestinal mucosa, bone, gallbladder, lung, female reproductive tissue, bile, and inflamed meninges.
- **Protein binding** 20%.
- **Metabolism/Excretion** Hepatic metabolism accounts for about 10% of administered dose. Both unchanged drug and metabolites are excreted via glomerular filtration and tubular secretion.
- **T1/2** 1.3 hrs.

Dosing for Decreased Hepatic Function

Usual dose.

Pregnancy Risk

B: Several collaborative perinatal project reports involving over 12,000 exposures to penicillin derivatives during the first trimester indicated no association between penicillin derivative drugs and birth defects.

Breast Feeding Compatibility

Excreted in breast milk at low concentrations. The American Academy of Pediatrics considers amoxicillin compatible with breast feeding.

COMMENTS

Aminopenicillin derivative with comparable Gram-positive and Gram-negative coverage to ampicillin, but better absorption and GI tolerance with oral administration. This is the preferred oral penicillin for all infections w/ possible exception of Group A strep pharyngitis (PCN preferred) and shigellosis (ampicillin preferred). When rash occurs with amoxicillin in setting of infectious mononucleosis, this is not a true allergy and does not preclude future use of drug.

BASIS FOR RECOMMENDATIONS

Mandell LA, Wunderink RG, Anzueto A, et al. Community-Acquired Pneumonia in Adults: Guidelines for Management. *Clinical Infectious Diseases*, 2007; Vol. 44; pp. S27–S72.

Comments: Amoxicillin 1 g q8h **or** amoxicillin-clavulanate 2 g q12h plus a macrolide is the preferred outpatient treatment regimen in pts at risk for drug resistant *S. pneumoniae* (DRSP). Pts with chronic illness, alcoholism, and abx within the last 3 mos are at risk for DRSP.

SELECTED REFERENCES

Doern GV, Richter SS, Miller A, et al. Antimicrobial resistance among Streptococcus pneumoniae in the United States: have we begun to turn the corner on resistance to certain antimicrobial classes? *Clin Infect Dis*, 2005; Vol. 41; pp. 139–48.

AMOXICILLIN + CLAVULANATE

Paul A. Pham, PharmD and John G. Bartlett, MD

INDICATIONS

FDA
- Lymphadenitis
- Mastitis
- Otitis media
- Pharyngitis
- Community-acquired pneumonia (XR formulation)
- Acute bacterial sinusitis (XR and IR formulations)
- Skin and skin-structure infections (carbuncles, cellulitis, subcutaneous abscess)
- Tonsillitis
- Urinary-tract infection

Non-FDA Approved Uses
- Sinusitis, Acute
- Lung Abscess
- Empyema
- Pyomyositis
- Bite wound (human, dog, and cat)

FORMS

Brand name (mfr)	Forms	Cost*
Augmentin (generic)	PO susp 125 mg/31.25 mg per 5 mL;	$1.50 per 5 mL;
	PO susp 250 mg/62.5 mg per 5 mL;	$2 per 5 mL;
	PO susp 400 mg/57 mg per 5 mL;	$3.52 per 5 mL;
	PO susp 600 mg/42.9 mg per 5 mL	$2.95 per 5 mL
	PO chew tab 125:31;	$1.5;
	PO chew tab 250:62	$3
	PO tab 250:125; PO tab 500:125;	$3; $4.39;
	PO tab 875:125	$5
	IV vial 500:100;	Not available in the U.S.;
	IV vial 1000:200	Not available in the U.S.
Augmentin ES (GlaxoSmithKline)	PO suspension 600 mg/42.9 mg per 5 mL (75 mL, 125 mL, 200 mL)	$3.62 per 5 mL
Augmentin XR (GlaxoSmithKline)	Oral tab, XR 1000 mg/62.5 mg	$4.10

*Prices represents Average Wholesale Price (AWP).

USUAL ADULT DOSING
- 250–1000 mg PO three times daily.
- 875/125 mg PO twice daily.
- XR: 2 tablets (2000 mg:125 mg) PO twice daily.

RENAL DOSING
Dosing for GFR 50–80: Usual dose.
Dosing for GFR 10–50: GFR 10–30 mL/min: 0.25 g–0.5 g q12h. GFR >30 mL/min: usual dose.
Dosing for GFR <10: 0.25 g–0.5 g q24h.
Dosing in hemodialysis: 0.25 g–0.5 g q24h (XR product not recommended in HD).
Dosing in peritoneal dialysis: Usual regimen.
Dosing in hemofiltration: No data. Consider 0.5 g q12h.

ADVERSE DRUG REACTIONS
Common
- GI intolerance and diarrhea
- Rash (especially if administered in setting of infectious mononucleosis)

ANTIBACTERIAL DRUGS

Occasional
- *C. difficile* colitis
- Hypersensitivity reactions
- Jarisch-Herxheimer reaction with spirochetal infection
- Drug Fever

Rare
- Coombs' test positive, hemolytic anemia
- Leukopenia and thrombocytopenia
- CNS-seizures and twitching (with high doses in pts with renal failure)
- Interstitial nephritis
- LFTs elevation

DRUG INTERACTIONS
- Allopurinol: may increase the risk of rash
- Oral contraceptives: may decrease the efficacy of OCs. Use an additional form of contraception.
- Tetracyclines: avoid concurrent administration. In 2 studies involving a total of 79 pts with pneumococcal meningitis treated with either penicillin plus tetracyclines or penicillin monotherapy resulted in a higher mortality rate (79–85%) in the combination therapy compared to penicillin monotherapy (30–33%) (*Arch Intern Med* 1951;88:489, *Ann Intern Med* 1961;55:545). However, there was not a higher mortality rate between penicillin monotherapy and penicillin plus tetracycline in the treatment of pneumococcal pneumonia. (*Arch Intern Med* 1953;91:197).

SPECTRUM—See Appendix II, p. 795

RESISTANCE
- *S. pneumoniae:* PCN resistance rate was 10.3% (using resistance break point MIC of 2 mcg/mL), but only 1.2% (using an MICs of 8 mcg/mL for IV PCN for non-meningeal involvement, *MMWR* 2008;57:1353). Without meningeal involvement, *S. pneumoniae* with MIC of 2 mcg/mL or lower can be treated with high dose of PCN or amoxicillin (3–4 g/day; *CID* 2005;41:139–148).
- *S. pneumoniae* break points (non-meningeal, oral therapy PCN): ≤ 0.06 mcg/mL (sensitive); 0.12–1.0 mcg/mL (intermediate); ≥ 2 mcg/mL (resistant).
- *S. pneumoniae* break points (non-meningeal, parenteral therapy PCN): ≤ 2 mcg/mL (sensitive); 4 mcg/mL (intermediate); ≥ 8 mcg/mL (resistant).
- *S. pneumoniae* break points (meningeal isolates, PCN): ≤ 0.06 mcg/mL (sensitive); ≥ 2 mcg/mL (resistant).

PHARMACOLOGY

Mechanism

Beta-lactam antibiotics inhibit mucopeptide synthesis in the bacterial cell wall, this results in the formation of defective cell walls and osmotically unstable organisms susceptible to cell lysis. Clavulanic acid also inhibits beta-lactamases, and when combined with beta-lactam antibiotics, the activity of the combination is extended against beta-lactamase-producing organisms which would otherwise be resistant.

Pharmacokinetic Parameters
- **Absorption** 75% absorbed.
- **Cmax** 12 mcg/mL (amoxicillin)/ 2 mcg/mL (clavulanate) after 875/125 mg dose administration.
- **Distribution** 0.36 L/kg. Distributed to blister fluid, urine, peritoneal fluid, pleural fluid, middle ear fluid, intestinal mucosa, bone, gallbladder, lung, female reproductive tissue, bile, and inflamed meninges.
- **Protein binding** 20% (amoxicillin)/ 30% (clavulanate).
- **Metabolism/Excretion** Hepatic metabolism accounts for about 10% of administered dose. Both unchanged drug and metabolites are excreted via glomerular filtration and tubular secretion.
- **T1/2** 1.3 hrs.

Dosing for Decreased Hepatic Function

No data. Consider standard dose.

Pregnancy Risk

B: in surveillance study of Michigan Medicaid recipients, 556 newborns were exposed to clavulanate/penicillin during the first trimester, there were no associations between birth defects and clavulanate/penicillin.

Breast Feeding Compatibility

No studies with clavulanate.

COMMENTS

Oral beta-lactam w/ activity against common bacteria that produce beta-lactamases, e.g., *H. influenzae*, MSSA, Moraxella, and all PCN-resistant anaerobes. Diarrhea is common due to both clavulanate and amoxicillin. The IDSA recommends amox/clav if anaerobes or *H. influenzae* are suspected [CID 2007 44 Suppl 2:S27–72.]. No advantage using Augmentin XR over amoxicillin 1 g PO q8h for intermediately-resistant *S. pneumoniae* since reduced susceptibility to penicillin by the pneumococcus is mediated by an alteration in the penicillin binding protein (PBP), therefore the addition of clavulanate, a beta-lactamase inhibitor, offers no benefit to high dose amoxicillin.

BASIS FOR RECOMMENDATIONS

Mandell LA, Wunderink RG, Anzueto A, et al. Community-acquired pneumonia in adults: guidelines for management. *Clinical Infectious Diseases*, 2007; Vol. 44; pp. S27–S72.

Comments: Amoxicillin 1 g q8h **or** amoxicillin-clavulanate 2 g q12h plus a macrolide is the preferred outpatient treatment regimen in pts at risk for drug resistant *S. pneumoniae* (DRSP). Pts with chronic illness, alcoholism, and abx within the last 3 mos are at risk for DRSP. For the treatment of PCN-resistant *S. pneumoniae*, there is no advantage of using high dose amoxicillin/clavulanate over high dose amoxicillin, but if anaerobes or *H. influenzae* are suspected amox/clav should be considered.

SELECTED REFERENCES

Henry DC, Riffer E, Sokol WN, et al. Randomized double-blind study comparing 3- and 6-day regimens of azithromycin with a 10-day amoxicillin-clavulanate regimen for treatment of acute bacterial sinusitis. *Antimicrob Agents Chemother*, 2003; Vol. 47; pp. 2770–4.

Siquier B, Sanchez-Alvarez J, Garcia-Mendez E, et al. Efficacy and safety of twice daily pharmacokinetically enhanced amoxicillin/clavulanate (2000/125 mg) in the treatment of adults with community-acquired pneumonia in a country with a high prevalence of penicillin-resistant Streptococcus pneumoniae. *J Antimicrob Chemother*, 2006; Vol. 57; pp. 536–45.

AMPICILLIN

Paul A. Pham, PharmD and John G. Bartlett, MD

INDICATIONS

FDA

- Streptococcal infections (Group A streptococcal pharyngitis, Group B streptococci)
- Otitis media (*Haemophilus influenzae* due to beta-lactamase negative strains)
- Diverticulitis (in combination with metronidazole)
- Gonorrhea (in combination with probenecid, however currently not recommended due to high failure rate)
- Enteric infections (*Proteus mirabilis* infections, salmonellosis, shigellosis)
- Urinary tract infections
- Bacterial vaginosis; endocarditis; meningitis; respiratory tract infections; septicemia

Non-FDA Approved Uses

- Bacterial meningitis, acute, community-acquired (*Listeria monocytogenes*)
- Intra-abdominal abscess (in combination with gentamicin and metronidazole)
- Enterococcal endocarditis (in combination with gentamicin)
- Enterococcus
- Enteric infections (*Vibrio cholerae*)

FORMS

Brand name (mfr)	Forms	Cost*
Ampicillin (Various generic manufacturers)	IV vial 250 mg, 2 g, 3 g, 10 g PO susp 125/5 mL (100 mL) PO tab 500 mg; PO tab 250 mg PO susp 250 mg/5 mL (100 mL and 200 mL); (100 mL) (200 mL)	$4; $9; $17; $67 $5.04 per bottle <$1–2; <$1–2 $7.83; f$14.86
*Prices represents Average Wholesale Price (AWP).		

ANTIBACTERIAL DRUGS

USUAL ADULT DOSING
- Oral: 250–500 mg q6h
- Parenteral (usual dosing): 1–2 g IV q4–6h
- Endocarditis or meningitis: 2 g IV q4h

RENAL DOSING
Dosing for GFR 50–80: 1 g–2 g IV q4–6h.
Dosing for GFR 10–50: 1 g–2 g IV q6–8h, no dose adjustment needed for oral administration.
Dosing for GFR <10: 1 g–2 g IV q8–12h; no dose adjustment needed for oral administration.
Dosing in hemodialysis: 1 g–2 g IV q8–12h. On HD days, give post HD.
Dosing in peritoneal dialysis: 250–2000 mg q12h.
Dosing in hemofiltration: CVVH: 2 g q6–12h. CVVHD: 2 g q6h.

ADVERSE DRUG REACTIONS
Common
- GI intolerance and diarrhea with PO therapy (more common than amoxicillin)
- Rash (especially seen if given in setting of infectious mononucleosis)

Occasional
- Hypersensitivity reaction
- Maculopapular rash (not urticarial)
- Drug fever
- Jarisch-Herxheimer reaction with spirochetal infection
- Phlebitis at infusion sites and sterile abscesses at IM sites

Rare
- Coombs' test positive, hemolytic anemia
- Leukopenia and thrombocytopenia
- CNS: seizures and twitching (especially with high doses in pts with renal failure)
- Interstitial nephritis
- LFTs elevation

DRUG INTERACTIONS
- Allopurinol: incidence of skin rash increased to 14–22% when the 2 are co-administered compared to 6–8% with ampicillin when administered alone or 2% when allopurinol.
- Oral contraceptives: may decrease efficacy of OC. Use an additional form of contraception with co-administration of oral ampicillin.
- Tetracyclines: avoid concurrent administration. In two studies involving a total of 79 pts with pneumococcal meningitis treated with either penicillin plus tetracyclines or penicillin monotherapy resulted in a higher mortality rate (79–85%) in the combination therapy compared to penicillin monotherapy (30–33%) (*Arch Intern Med* 1951;88:489, *Ann Intern Med* 1961;55:545). However, there was not a difference in mortality between penicillin monotherapy and penicillin plus tetracycline in the treatment of pneumococcal pneumonia (*Arch Intern Med* 1953;91:197).

SPECTRUM—See Appendix II, p. 795
RESISTANCE
- Resistant break points for *S. pneumoniae:* ≥0.12 mcg/mL for *S. pneumoniae* meningitis, but ≥2 mcg/mL (PO) and ≥8 mcg/mL (for IV) for *S. pneumoniae* pneumonia and non-meningeal infections.
- Break points for Enterobacteriaceae is 8 mcg/mL.
- Break points for *Enterococci* is 8 mcg/mL.

PHARMACOLOGY
Mechanism
Beta-lactam antibiotics inhibit mucopeptide synthesis in the bacterial cell wall, this results in the formation of defective cell walls and osmotically unstable organisms susceptible to cell lysis.

Pharmacokinetic Parameters
- **Absorption** 40% absorbed.
- **Cmax** 3–6 mcg/mL after 500 g PO dose administration; 47 mcg/mL 1 hr after 2 g IV dose administration.
- **Distribution** 0.29 L/kg; distributed to blister fluid, urine, peritoneal fluid, pleural fluid, middle ear fluid, intestinal mucosa, bone, gallbladder, lung, female reproductive tissue, bile, and inflamed meninges.

- **Protein binding** 20%.
- **Metabolism/Excretion** Hepatic metabolism accounts for about 10% of administered dose. Both unchanged drug and metabolites are excreted via glomerular filtration and tubular secretion. Biliary excretion also occurs accounting for the high biliary concentration.
- **T1/2** 1.0 hr.

Dosing for Decreased Hepatic Function

Usual dose.

Pregnancy Risk

B: several collaborative perinatal project reports involving over 12,000 exposures to penicillin derivatives during the first trimester indicated no association between penicillin derivative drugs and birth defects.

Breast Feeding Compatibility

Excreted in breast milk at low concentrations.

COMMENTS

Oral and parenteral beta-lactam. Due to inferior absorption of ampicillin, oral amoxicillin has replaced oral ampicillin for all infections except shigellosis. IV ampicillin is the drug of choice for infections involving ampicillin-sensitive enterococci.

BASIS FOR RECOMMENDATIONS

Mandell LA, Wunderink RG, Anzueto A, et al. Infectious Diseases Society of America/American Thoracic Society consensus guidelines on the management of community-acquired pneumonia in adults. *Clin Infect Dis*, 2007; Vol. 44 Suppl 2; pp. S27–72.

Comments: Cefotaxime, ceftriaxone, or IV ampicillin **plus** a macrolide is the preferred treatment regimen for CAP in non-ICU inpts.

SELECTED REFERENCES

Bennish ML, Salam MA, Haider R, et al. Therapy for shigellosis. II. Randomized, double-blind comparison of ciprofloxacin and ampicillin. *J Infect Dis*, 1990; Vol. 162; pp. 711–6.

AMPICILLIN + SULBACTAM

Paul A. Pham, PharmD and John G. Bartlett, MD

INDICATIONS

FDA

- Gynecologic infections caused by beta-lactamase producing strains of *E. coli*, and *Bacteroides* spp. (including *B. fragilis*).
- Intra-abdominal infections caused by beta-lactamase producing strains of *E. coli, Klebsiella* spp. (including *K. pneumoniae*), *Bacteroides* spp. (including *B. fragilis*), and *Enterobacter* spp.
- Skin and soft tissue infections caused by *S. aureus* (MSSA), *E. coli, Klebsiella* spp.(including *K. pneumoniae*), *P. mirabilis, B. fragilis, Enterobacter* spp., and *A. calcoaceticus*.

Non-FDA Approved Uses

- Epiglottitis (*H. influenzae*)
- Appendicitis
- Cholecystitis
- Cholangitis (consider in mild disease)
- Diverticulitis
- Peritonitis, spontaneous bacterial and secondary
- Hepatic abscess (consider in mild disease)
- Diabetic foot infection (w/ mild superficial ulcer)
- Aspiration pneumonia
- Bite wounds (*Eikenella corrodens, Pasteurella multocida*)

FORMS

Brand name (mfr)	Forms	Cost*
Unasyn (Roerig)	IV vial 1 g:0.5 g; IV vial 2 g:1 g	$5.00; $10.00
*Prices represents Average Wholesale Price (AWP).		

ANTIBACTERIAL DRUGS

USUAL ADULT DOSING

- Mild to moderate infections: 1.5 g (1 g ampicillin/0.5 g sulbactam) IV q6h.
- Moderate to severe infections: 3 g (2 g ampicillin/1 g sulbactam) IV q6h.
- MDR Acinetobacter: 3 g (2 g ampicillin/1 g sulbactam) IV q4h. Up to 18–24 g ampicillin / 9–12 g sulbactam per day have been evaluated (sulbactam is the active agent against acinetobacter, J Infect. 2008;56:432; Scand J Infect Dis. 2007;39:38).

RENAL DOSING

Dosing for GFR 50–80: 1.5–3 g q6h.

Dosing for GFR 10–50: GFR >30 mL/min: 1.5–3 g q6h; GFR 15–29: 1.5–3 g q12h.

Dosing for GFR <10: GFR <15 mL/min: 1.5–3 g q24h. HD: 1.5 g q12h with 2 g ampicillin post dialysis.

Dosing in hemodialysis: 1.5 g q12h with 2 g ampicillin post dialysis.

Dosing in hemofiltration: CVVH: 3 g q12h; CVVHD 3 g q8h.

ADVERSE DRUG REACTIONS

General

- Generally well tolerated

Common

- Rash (especially if drug administered in w/ infectious mononucleosis due to ampicillin component)

Occasional

- Maculopapular rash (not urticarial)
- Hypersensitivity reaction
- Drug fever
- Jarisch-Herxheimer reaction with spirochetal infection
- Phlebitis at infusion sites and sterile abscesses at IM sites

Rare

- Coombs' test positive, hemolytic anemia
- Leukopenia and thrombocytopenia
- CNS-seizures and twitching (with high doses in pts with renal failure)
- Interstitial nephritis
- LFTs elevation

DRUG INTERACTIONS

- Allopurinol: incidence of skin rash increased to 14–22% when the 2 are co-administered compared to 6–8% with ampicillin when administered alone or 2% when allopurinol is administered alone.
- Tetracyclines: avoid concurrent administration. In 2 studies involving a total of 79 pts with pneumococcal meningitis treated with either penicillin plus tetracyclines or penicillin monotherapy resulted in a higher mortality rate (79–85%) in the combination therapy compared to penicillin monotherapy (30–33%) (*Arch Intern Med* 1951;88:489, *Ann Intern Med* 1961;55:545). However there was not a difference in mortality between penicillin monotherapy and penicillin plus tetracycline in the treatment of pneumococcal pneumonia (*Arch Intern Med* 1953;91:197).

SPECTRUM—See Appendix II, p. 795

RESISTANCE

- Generally not active against *Citrobacter* spp., *Enterobacter* spp., *Proteus* spp., *Pseudomonas aeruginosa,* and *Serratia* species.

PHARMACOLOGY

Mechanism

Beta-lactam antibiotics inhibit mucopeptide synthesis in the bacterial cell wall, this results in the formation of defective cell walls and osmotically unstable organisms susceptible to cell lysis.

Pharmacokinetic Parameters

- **Cmax** 109–150 mcg/mL after 2 g (ampicillin): 1 g (sulbactam) dose administration.
- **Distribution** 0.29 L/kg; distributed to blister fluid, urine, peritoneal fluid, pleural fluid, middle ear fluid, intestinal mucosa, bone, gallbladder, lung, female reproductive tissue, bile, and inflamed meninges.
- **Protein binding** 28% (ampicillin)/38% (sulbactam).
- **Metabolism/Excretion** Hepatic metabolism accounts for about 10% of administered dose. Both unchanged drug and metabolites are excreted via glomerular filtration

and tubular secretion. Biliary excretion also occurs accounting for the high biliary concentration.

- **T1/2** 1.2 hrs.

Dosing for Decreased Hepatic Function

Limited data. Consider standard dose.

Pregnancy Risk

B: several collaborative perinatal project reports involving over 12,000 exposures to penicillin derivatives during the first trimester indicated no association between penicillin derivative drugs and birth defects. The safety of sulbactam has not been evaluated in humans. There was no adverse effect reported in animal data.

Breast Feeding Compatibility

Excreted in breast milk at low concentration.

COMMENTS

Parenteral beta-lactam/beta-lactamase inhibitor. Sulbactam increases the activity of *ampicillin*, but inducible chromosomal B-lactamases produced by Citrobacter, Enterobacter, Proteus, Pseudomonas, and Serratia species are not generally inhibited by sulbactam. Growing rates of resistance with *E. coli*, >50% resistance at some institutions. Active vs. *H. influenzae*, MSSA, most anaerobes (including *B. fragilis*) and many GNB (but resistance rate vary widely). Sulbactam is active against most strains of Acinetobacter. Contains Na+ 5 Meq/1.5 g.

SELECTED REFERENCES

Harkless L, Boghossian J, Pollak R, et al. An open-label, randomized study comparing efficacy and safety of intravenous piperacillin/tazobactam and ampicillin/sulbactam for infected diabetic foot ulcers. *Surg Infect (Larchmt)*, 2005; Vol. 6; pp. 27–40.

Mandell LA, Wunderink RG, Anzueto A, et al. Community-acquired pneumonia in adults: guidelines for management. *CID*, 2007; Vol. 44; pp. S27–S72.

AZITHROMYCIN

Paul A. Pham, PharmD and John G. Bartlett, MD

INDICATIONS

FDA

- Community-acquired pneumonia of mild severity (20%–30% of *S. pneumoniae* strains resistant to azithromycin but clinical significance unknown).
- Pharyngitis/tonsillitis; acute bacterial sinusitis.
- Acute bacterial exacerbations of chronic obstructive pulmonary disease.
- Treatment and prophylaxis of disseminated *M. avium* infection (treatment requires co-administration with ethambutol).
- Uncomplicated skin and skin structure infections.
- Urethritis and cervicitis (caused by GC and *C. trachomatis*).
- Genital ulcer disease.

Non-FDA Approved Uses

- Toxoplasmosis (with pyrimethamine).
- Meningococcal meningitis prophylaxis.

FORMS

Brand name (mfr)	Forms	Cost*
Zithromax (Pfizer)	PO Z-Pak 250 mg × 6 tabs	$47.72 per pack
	PO T ri-pack 6–250 mg tabs (500 mg × 3 days)	$47.72 per pack
	PO tablet 250 mg; PO tablet 500, 600 mg	$8; $16; $19
	IV vial 500 mg	$35.83
	PO powder packet 1 g	$34.50
	PO suspension 100 mg/5 mL; 200 mg/5 mL (15 mL, 22.5 mL and 30 mL);	$44.90
	PO Zmax (SR suspension) 2 g/60 mL	$63.49

ANTIBACTERIAL DRUGS

483

FORMS *(cont.)*

Brand name (mfr)	Forms	Cost*
azithromycin (Generic manufacturers)	PO tablet (pack) 250 mg × 6 tabs; PO tablet 250 mg; PO tablet 500, 600 mg	$46.70 per pack; $7.77; $15.57; $18.68
	IV vial 500 mg; PO powder packet 1 g PO tablet (pack) 3–500 mg (500 mg × 3 days)	$29.94 $24.15 $46.67
	PO suspension 100 mg/5 mL; 200 mg/5 mL (15 mL, 22.5 mL, and 30 mL)	$32.93
*Prices represents Average Wholesale Price (AWP).		

USUAL ADULT DOSING

- CAP: *Z-pack* 500 mg 1st day, then 250 mg once daily × 4 days; 500 mg IV daily or *Zmax* 2 g × 1 **or** *Tri-pak* 500 mg daily × 3 days (not FDA approved but effective; Eur Respir J., 1995, 398–402).
- Acute bacterial sinusitis; acute exacerbation of chronic bronchitis: *Tri-pak* 500 mg PO daily × 3 days or *Z-pack* 500 mg 1st day, then 250 mg every day × 4 days or *Zmax* 2 g × 1.
- MAC prophylaxis: 1200 mg (two 600 mg tabs or suspension) PO every wk.
- MAC treatment: 600 mg daily + ethambutol 15 mg/kg/day.
- Toxoplasmosis: 900–1200 mg PO daily + pyrimethamine 200 mg PO × 1, then 50–75 mg PO daily + leucovorin 10–20 mg daily × 6 wks, then half dose of each until immune reconstitution.
- Gonococcal urethritis or cervicitis: 2 g PO × 1 (poor GI tolerability, second-line therapy).
- Genital ulcer disease (chancroid) or non-gonococcal urethritis (*C. trachomatis*) or cervicitis: 1 g PO × 1.
- Early syphilis: 2 g PO × 1 (poor GI tolerability). High rates of macrolide resistance reported in San Francisco (*CID* 2006;42:337).
- Meningococcal meningitis prophylaxis: 500 mg × 1 (15 yrs or older); 10 mg/kg × 1 (<15 yrs). Due to reports of fluoroquinolone resistance, rifampin, ceftriaxone, and azithromycin is recommended in selected counties in North Dakota and Minnesota (*MMWR* 2008;57:173).
- Obese pts: 500–600 mg/day.

RENAL DOSING

Dosing for GFR 50–80: Usual dose.
Dosing for GFR 10–50: No data. Usual dose likely due to high biliary excretion.
Dosing for GFR <10: No data. Usual dose likely due to high biliary excretion.
Dosing in hemodialysis: HD: no data, but usual dose likely.
Dosing in peritoneal dialysis: Usual regimen.
Dosing in hemofiltration: No data.

ADVERSE DRUG REACTIONS

Common

- GI intolerance: diarrhea, nausea, and abdominal pain in 4% of pts, but may be up to 17% with 2000 mg administration.

Occasional

- Reversible dose-dependent hearing loss in 5% with mean exposure of 59 g.

Rare

- Erythema multiforme
- Vaginitis
- Transaminase elevations
- *C. difficile* colitis

DRUG INTERACTIONS—See Appendix III, p. 808, for table of drug-to-drug interactions.

- Unlike other macrolides, azithromycin does not significantly inhibit CYP3A4. Low likelihood of drug-drug interactions compared to other macrolides.
- No significant interaction with antiretrovirals.

SPECTRUM—See Appendix II, p. 800

RESISTANCE
- Breakpoint for *Haemophilus* spp.: ≥4 mcg/mL.
- Breakpoint for *Streptococcus* spp.: ≤0.5 mcg/mL (sensitive); 1 mcg/mL (intermediate); ≥2 mcg/mL (resistant).

PHARMACOLOGY
Mechanism
Macrolides inhibit protein synthesis by binding to 50S ribosomal subunits, inhibiting translocation of peptidase chain and polypeptide synthesis. The addition of nitrogen at position 9 a of the lactone ring, gives azithromycin improved resistance to acid degradation, improved tissue penetration and activity against Gram-negative organisms, and a longer elimination half-life.

Pharmacokinetic Parameters
- **Absorption** 37% absorbed (although food improves tolerability, 600 mg tab and 1 g powder packet may be taken without regard for food).
- **Cmax** 0.4 mcg/mL 2 hrs after 500 mg PO dose administration (on day 5 of therapy). 3.63 mcg/mL 1 hr after 500 mg IV administration (on day 5 of therapy).
- **Distribution** Distributed throughout the body. Concentrated intracellularly, resulting in tissue concentration 10–100 × those found in serum. Highly concentrated in fibroblasts and phagocytes. Poor CNS penetration.
- **Protein binding** 10–50% (concentration dependent; the lower the serum levels the higher the protein binding).
- **Metabolism/Excretion** Demethylation of 35% of administered dose to inactive metabolites. Up to 10 inactive metabolites identified. Biliary excretion of active drug and inactive metabolites.
- **T1/2** Serum 12 hrs; intracellular: 68 hrs.

Dosing for Decreased Hepatic Function
No dose adjustment (Mazzei T, et al. *J Antimicrob Chemother* 1993;31(Suppl E):57).

Pregnancy Risk
B-Animal studies show no harm to the fetus. No human data available.

Breast Feeding Compatibility
Accumulates in breast milk. The American Academy of Pediatrics considers erythromycin compatible with breast feeding. No recommendation has been made for azithromycin.

COMMENTS
Oral and parenteral macrolide w/ convenient once daily dosing. Expanded spectrum includes improved *in vitro* activity against *H. influenzae* compared to erythromycin and clarithromycin. In contrast to other macrolides, azithromycin is not likely to interact with drugs metabolized by CYP3A4. New Zmax (2000 mg × 1) formulation allows DOT (directly observed therapy) for CAP and acute sinusitis but is associated with a higher incidence of GI side effects. Significance of rising macrolide-resistance in *S. pneumoniae* (~25% U.S. isolates) of uncertain significance for the treatment of ambulatory respiratory tract infections.

SELECTED REFERENCES

D'Ignazio J, Camere MA, Lewis DE, et al. Novel, single-dose microsphere formulation of azithromycin versus 7-days levofloxacin therapy for treatment of mild to moderate community-acquired pneumonia in adults. *Antimicrob Agents Chemother*, 2005; Vol. 49; pp. 4035–41.

Saha D, Karim MM, Khan WA, et al. Single-dose azithromycin for the treatment of cholera in adults. *N Engl J Med*, 2006; Vol. 354; pp. 2452–62.

AZTREONAM

Paul A. Pham, PharmD and John G. Bartlett, MD

INDICATIONS
FDA
- Gram-negative bacterial pneumonia
- Skin and soft tissue infections (caused by Gram-negative bacilli)
- Complicated and uncomplicated urinary tract infections
- Intra-abdominal infections (in combination with metronidazole)
- Septicemia (cause by Gram-negative bacilli)
- Gynecologic infections (in combination with anaerobic coverage)

Non-FDA Approved Uses
- Osteomyelitis (caused by Gram-negative bacilli)
- Diabetic Foot Infection (in combination with anaerobic and Gram-positive coverage)

FORMS

Brand name (mfr)	Forms	Cost*
Azactam (Elan)	IV vial 1000 mg; IV vial 2000 mg	$39.33; $78.50

*Prices represents Average Wholesale Price (AWP).

USUAL ADULT DOSING
- Gram-negative infections: 1–2 g IV q8h
- UTI: 0.5–1 g IV q8h–q12h
- Serious infections and meningitis: 2.0 g IV q6–8h
- For obese pts: consider 2 g IV q6h, but no data exist

RENAL DOSING
Dosing for GFR 50–80: 1 g–2 g q8h.
Dosing for GFR 10–50: GFR: 30–50 mL/min: 2 g IV q12h. GFR: 10–30 mL/min: 1–2 g q12h.
Dosing for GFR <10: 1 g–2 g q24h.
Dosing in hemodialysis: 1–2 g q24h. Dose post-HD on days of dialysis or supplement with 250 mg post-dialysis.
Dosing in peritoneal dialysis: 1–2 g loading dose, then 250–500 mg q8h. May be given by intraperitoneal route: loading dose of 1 g, then 250 mg per liter exchange.
Dosing in hemofiltration: CVVH: 1–2 g q12h. CVVHD: 1 g q8h to 2 g q12h.

ADVERSE DRUG REACTIONS
General
- Generally well tolerated.

Common
- Transient eosinophilia (however, drug can be safely used in PCN allergic pts)

Occasional
- Phlebitis at infusion site
- Rash
- Diarrhea
- Nausea
- LFT elevations

Rare
- *C. difficile* colitis
- Thrombocytopenia
- Seizures
- Altered sense of taste or bad taste

DRUG INTERACTIONS
Probenecid: may increase serum concentrations of aztreonam. Clinical significance unclear. Use standard dosing.

SPECTRUM—See Appendix II, p. 789

RESISTANCE
- MIC breakpoint for *Enterobacteriaceae:* ≤8 mcg/mL (sensitive); 16 mcg/mL (intermediate); ≥32 mcg/mL (resistant).
- MIC breakpoint for Gram-negative non-lactose fermenters including *P. aeruginosa:* ≤8 mcg/mL (sensitive); 16 mcg/mL (intermediate); ≥32 mcg/mL (resistant).
- ESBL producing *Klebsiella* spp. and *E. coli* may be clinically resistant to aztreonam, despite *in vitro* susceptibility.

PHARMACOLOGY
Mechanism
A monobactam antibiotic, inhibits mucopeptide synthesis (by preferentially binding to penicillin-binding protein 3 of susceptible Gram-negative bacteria) in the bacterial cell wall, this results in the formation of defective cell walls and osmotically unstable organisms susceptible to cell lysis.

Pharmacokinetic Parameters
- **Absorption** <1% oral, rapidly absorbed following IM administration.
- **Cmax** 125 mcg/mL after 1 g IV dose administration.
- **Distribution** 0.11–0.22 L/kg; distributed widely throughout the body including aqueous humor, prostatic tissue, inflamed meninges.
- **Protein binding** 56%.
- **Metabolism/Excretion** Hepatic metabolism accounts for only 1–7% of administered dose. Excreted principally via glomerular filtration and tubular secretion as unchanged drug.
- **T1/2** 2 hrs.

Dosing for Decreased Hepatic Function
Some recommend dose reduction of 20–25%, but use standard dose for severe infections.

Pregnancy Risk
B-animal studies show no harm to the fetus. No human data available.

Breast Feeding Compatibility
Excreted in breast milk at low concentration. The American Academy of Pediatrics considers aztreonam to be compatible with breast feeding.

COMMENTS
A parenteral monobactam for infections caused by Gram-negative bacteria that can be used in penicillin-allergic pts. Isolated cross-reactivity described in ceftazidime-allergic pts. Spectrum of activity includes Pseudomonas but no activity against Gram-positive bacteria or anaerobes. Check local susceptibility patterns, before using aztreonam for the empiric treatment of serious *P. aeruginosa* infections due to rising rates of resistance observed in many institutions.

SELECTED REFERENCES
Breedt J, Teras J, Gardovskis J, et al. Safety and efficacy of tigecycline in treatment of skin and skin structure infections: results of a double-blind phase 3 comparison study with vancomycin-aztreonam. *Antimicrob Agents Chemother*, 2005; Vol. 49; pp. 4658–66.

Cavallo JD, Hocquet D, Plesiat P, et al. Susceptibility of Pseudomonas aeruginosa to antimicrobials: a 2004 French multicentre hospital study. *J Antimicrob Chemother*, 2007; Vol. 59; pp. 1021–4.

BACITRACIN

Paul A. Pham, PharmD and John G. Bartlett, MD

INDICATIONS

FDA
- Prevention of infection in minor cuts, scrapes, and burns (topical formulation)
- Superficial eye infections (opthalmic formulation)
- Treatment of infants with pneumonia and empyema (IM bacitracin)

Non-FDA Approved Uses
- Component of irrigation solutions

FORMS

Brand name (mfr)	Forms	Cost*
Bacitracin (Various generic manufacturers)	IM vial 50,000 U Topical oint 500 U/g Ophthalmic oint 500 U/g	$19.80 $0.04–0.24 per g $1.34 per g
*Prices represents Average Wholesale Price (AWP).		

USUAL ADULT DOSING
- **Topical administration:** apply to affected area 1–5 times/day.
- **Oral:** 25,000 units PO q6h (*C. difficile* colitis, not first-line therapy).
- **Parenteral:** 10,000–25,000 units IM q6h (injection may be painful).

RENAL DOSING
Dosing for GFR 50–80: Avoid systemic use.
Dosing for GFR 10–50: Avoid systemic use.
Dosing for GFR <10: Avoid systemic use.

ANTIBACTERIAL DRUGS

Dosing in hemodialysis: No data.
Dosing in peritoneal dialysis: No data.
Dosing in hemofiltration: No data.

ADVERSE DRUG REACTIONS
Common
- Nephrotoxicity with IM use (proteinuria, oliguria, azotemia)
- Pain at injection site with IM use

DRUG INTERACTIONS
Non-depolarizing muscle relaxants (atracurium, vecuronium, pancuronium, tubocurarine): neuromuscular blockade may be enhanced with IM bacitracin.

PHARMACOLOGY
Mechanism
Bacitracin inhibits bacterial cell-wall synthesis by preventing the incorporation of peptidoglycans and lipopolysaccharides.

Pharmacokinetic Parameters
- **Absorption** Not absorbed in GI tract. Rapidly and completely absorbed following IM administration. Systemic absorption following intraperitoneal and mediastinal irrigation.
- **Cmax** Therapeutic concentration of 2 units/mL after IM administration.
- **Distribution** Distributed to all body organ including ascitic and pleural fluid.
- **Protein binding** Low protein binding.
- **Metabolism/Excretion** Excreted in the feces following oral administration. Approximately 10–40% of IM dose is excreted via glomerular filtration.
- **T1/2** 10–40% excreted by GFR within 24 hrs.

Dosing for Decreased Hepatic Function
No data.

Pregnancy Risk
C: One report listed 18 pts exposed to bacitracin (route was not specified) during the first trimester, there was no association with malformation found.

Breast Feeding Compatibility
No data available.

COMMENTS
Bacitracin 25,000 units q6h is a cost-effective alternative to oral vancomycin or metronidazole in the treatment of *C. difficile* colitis, but has not been as well studied as either drug and is no longer available in the U.S. in oral formulation. Often used for topical therapy of wounds, but most authorities are unconvinced that topical antibiotics have established merit in promoting wound healing, preventing infection, or treating infection. Due to severe nephrotoxicity, systemic bacitracin is not recommended.

SELECTED REFERENCES
Freiler JF, Steel KE, Hagan LL, et al. Intraoperative anaphylaxis to bacitracin during pacemaker change and laser lead extraction. *Ann Allergy Asthma Immunol*, 2005; Vol. 95; pp. 389–93.

Leyden JJ, Bartelt NM. Comparison of topical antibiotic ointments, a wound protectant, and antiseptics for the treatment of human blister wounds contaminated with Staphylococcus aureus. *J Fam Pract*, 1987; Vol. 24; pp. 601–4.

CEFACLOR

Paul A. Pham, PharmD and John G. Bartlett, MD

INDICATIONS
FDA
- Otitis media caused by *Streptococcus pneumoniae, Haemophilus influenzae, staphylococci,* and *Streptococcus pyogenes*
- Lower respiratory tract infections including pneumonia caused by *Streptococcus pneumoniae, Haemophilus influenzae,* and *Streptococcus* (author's comment: not a first line agent)
- Pharyngitis and tonsillitis caused by *Streptococcus pyogenes* (PCN is the drug of choice)
- Pyelonephritis and cystitis caused by *Escherichia coli, Proteus mirabilis, Klebsiella* spp., and *coagulase-negative staphylococci* (author's comment: not a first line agent)
- Skin and skin structure infections caused by *Staphylococcus aureus* (MSSA) and *Streptococcus pyogenes*

Non-FDA Approved Uses
• Chronic Bronchitis, Acute Exacerbations

FORMS

Brand name (mfr)	Forms	Cost*
Raniclor (Ranbaxy and other generic manufacturers)	PO tab, chewable 250 mg; PO tab, chewable 375 mg PO tab, SR 500 mg	$1.99; $2.98 $3.79
Ceclor (Various generic manufacturers)	PO pulvules 250 mg; PO pulvules 500 mg PO susp 125 mg/5 mL; PO susp 187 mg/5 mL; PO susp 250 mg/5 mL; PO susp 375 mg/5 mL	$1.99; $3.89 $2.28 per 150 mL; $1.50 per 5 mL; $51.80 per 150 mL; $51.80 per 100 mL

*Prices represents Average Wholesale Price (AWP).

USUAL ADULT DOSING
250–500 mg PO q6–8h (regular release). Sustained release (Ceclor SR): 375 mg or 500 mg PO q12h with food.

RENAL DOSING
Dosing for GFR 50–80: Usual dose.
Dosing for GFR 10–50: Usual dose.
Dosing for GFR <10: 50% of usual dose.
Dosing in hemodialysis: 50% of usual dose plus 250–500 mg post-dialysis.
Dosing in peritoneal dialysis: Usual regimen.
Dosing in hemofiltration: No data. Consider standard dose.

ADVERSE DRUG REACTIONS
General
• Generally well tolerated
Occasional
• Allergic reactions (eosinophilia)
• Diarrhea and *C. difficile* colitis
• Positive Coombs' test (without hemolytic anemia)
• Serum sickness (more common than other cephalosporins)
Rare
• Drug fever
• Neutropenia and thrombocytopenia
• Hepatitis
• Hemolytic anemia (theoretical, case reports with ceftriaxone, cefotetan, cefoxitin, cefamandole, ceftazidime, and cefalothin)
• Anaphylaxis
• CNS: convulsions (high dose with renal failure), confusion, disorientation, and hallucinations

DRUG INTERACTIONS
Probenecid: increase in cephalosporin serum concentration due to inhibition of tubular secretion by probenecid. Monitor closely for ADR in ESRD.

SPECTRUM—See Appendix II, p. 792
RESISTANCE
• ß-lactamase-negative, ampicillin-resistant strains of *Haemophilus influenzae* should be considered resistant to cefaclor despite apparent *in vitro* susceptibility.
• MIC breakpoint for *S. pneumoniae*: 1 mcg/mL.
• MIC breakpoint for *Staphylococcus* spp.: 8 mcg/mL.
• MIC breakpoint for *Haemophilus* spp.: 8 mcg/mL.

ANTIBACTERIAL DRUGS

489

PHARMACOLOGY

Mechanism

Cephalosporins like all beta-lactam antibiotics inhibit mucopeptide synthesis in the bacterial cell wall, this results in the formation of defective cell walls and osmotically unstable organisms susceptible to cell lysis.

Pharmacokinetic Parameters

- **Absorption** 93% absorbed.
- **Cmax** 8–9 mcg/mL after 500 mg PO dose administration.
- **Distribution** Diffuses readily into soft tissue interstitial fluid. Cefaclor attains good therapeutic concentration in the middle ear. Its concentration in sputum is usually low.
- **Protein binding** 25–50%.
- **Metabolism/Excretion** Excreted unchanged in urine.
- **T1/2** 0.8 hr.

Dosing for Decreased Hepatic Function

Usual dose.

Pregnancy Risk

B: Cephalosporins are usually considered safe to use during pregnancy.

Breast Feeding Compatibility

Excreted in breast milk at low concentrations. The American Academy of Pediatrics classifies cephalosporin antibiotics as compatible with breast feeding.

COMMENTS

Oral 2nd generation cephalosporin that has poor activity against *S. pneumoniae* and, therefore, is not an ideal agent in the treatment of respiratory tract infections. This drug is a favorite for pediatricians because it wins the taste test. Higher rate of serum sickness reported compared to the other cephalosporins. Cefaclor SR should be taken with food.

SELECTED REFERENCES

Turik MA, Johns D. Comparison of cefaclor and cefuroxime axetil in the treatment of acute otitis media with effusion in children who failed amoxicillin therapy. *J Chemother*, 1998; Vol. 10; pp. 306–12.

CEFADROXIL

Paul A. Pham, PharmD and John G. Bartlett, MD

INDICATIONS

FDA

- Streptococcal pharyngitis and tonsillitis.
- Skin and soft tissue infections caused by staphylococci and/or streptococci. (author's comment: use in uncomplicated cases only).
- Urinary tract infections caused by *E. coli, P. mirabilis,* and *Klebsiella* species.

Non-FDA Approved Uses

- Furuncle/carbuncle (MSSA)
- Impetigo
- Hidradenitis suppurativa

FORMS

Brand name (mfr)	Forms	Cost*
Duricef (Warner Chilcott, Inc and various generic manufacturers)	PO cap 500 mg PO tab 1000 mg PO susp 250 mg/5 mL; PO susp 500 mg/5 mL	$3.72 $7.14 $30.42 per 50 mL; $63.13 per 75 mL
*Prices represents Average Wholesale Price (AWP).		

USUAL ADULT DOSING

- Uncomplicated soft tissue infection: 0.5 g PO twice daily or 1 g PO once daily.
- Pharyngitis: 0.5 g PO twice daily or 1 g PO once daily × 10 days.
- UTI: 1 g PO once daily or 1 g PO twice daily.

RENAL DOSING

Dosing for GFR 50–80: Usual dose.
Dosing for GFR 10–50: 0.5 g q12–24h.
Dosing for GFR <10: 0.5 g q36h.
Dosing in hemodialysis: 0.5–1.0 g post-dialysis.
Dosing in peritoneal dialysis: 0.5 g/day.
Dosing in hemofiltration: No data.

ADVERSE DRUG REACTIONS

Occasional

- Allergic reactions
- Diarrhea or *C. difficile* colitis
- Eosinophilia
- Positive Coombs' test

Rare

- CNS: confusion, disorientation, and hallucinations
- Drug fever
- Neutropenia and thrombocytopenia
- Hepatitis
- Interstitial nephritis
- Anaphylaxis

DRUG INTERACTIONS

Probenecid: increased in cefadroxil serum concentration due to inhibition of tubular secretion by probenecid (no dose adjustment needed).

SPECTRUM — See Appendix II, p. 792

PHARMACOLOGY

Mechanism

Cephalosporins like all beta-lactam antibiotics inhibit mucopeptide synthesis in the bacterial cell wall, this results in the formation of defective cell walls and osmotically unstable organisms susceptible to cell lysis.

Pharmacokinetic Parameters

- **Absorption** 90% absorbed.
- **Cmax** 16 mcg/mL after 500 mg PO dose administration.
- **Distribution** Widely distributed to tissues and fluids, including pleural fluid, synovial fluid, and bone. Low CNS penetration.
- **Protein binding** 20%.
- **Metabolism/Excretion** 70–90% Excreted unchanged in the urine within 24 hrs.
- **T1/2** 1.5 hrs.

Dosing for Decreased Hepatic Function

No data. Usual dose likely.

Pregnancy Risk

B: Cephalosporins are usually considered safe to use during pregnancy.

Breast Feeding Compatibility

Excreted in breast milk at low concentrations. The American Academy of Pediatrics classifies cephalosporin antibiotics as compatible with breast feeding.

COMMENTS

Oral 1st generation cephalosporin with good oral bioavailability and long half-life allowing for once or twice a day dosing, but more expensive than comparable agents (e.g., cephalexin).

SELECTED REFERENCES

Bucko AD, Hunt BJ, Kidd SL, et al. Randomized, double-blind, multicenter comparison of oral cefditoren 200 or 400 mg BID with either cefuroxime 250 mg BID or cefadroxil 500 mg BID for the treatment of uncomplicated skin and skin-structure infections. *Clin Ther*, 2002; Vol. 24; pp. 1134–47.

Tanriseer B, Santella PJ. Cefadroxil. A review of its antibacterial, pharmacokinetic and therapeutic properties in comparison with cephalexin and cephradine. *Drugs*, 1986; Vol. 32 Suppl 3; pp. 1–16.

ANTIBACTERIAL DRUGS

CEFAZOLIN

Paul A. Pham, PharmD and John G. Bartlett, MD

INDICATIONS

FDA

- Respiratory tract infections due to *S. pneumoniae, S. aureus* (MSSA), and *S. pyogenes*.
- Urinary tract infections due to *E. coli, P mirabilis*; prostatitis and epididymitis due to *E. coli, P. mirabilis*.
- Skin and skin-structure infections due to *S. aureus* (MSSA), *S. pyogenes*, and other strains of streptococci.
- Biliary tract infections due to *E. coli* (MSSA), various strains of streptococci, *P. mirabilis*, and *S. aureus*.
- Bone and joint infections due to *S. aureus* (MSSA).
- Septicemia due to *S. pneumoniae, S. aureus* (MSSA), *P. mirabilis, E. coli*.
- Endocarditis due to *S. aureus* (MSSA) and *S. pyogenes*.
- Perioperative prophylaxis.

Non-FDA Approved Uses

- Parotitis (MSSA)
- Other Staphylococcus aureus (MSSA) infections
- Other Streptococcus pyogenes (Group A) infections

FORMS

Brand name (mfr)	Forms	Cost*
Ancef (GlaxoSmithKline and various generic manufacturers)	IV or IM vial 1 g; IV or IM vial 10 g; IV or IM vial 20 g IV bag 0.5 g/50 mL; IV bag 0.1 g/50 mL	$1.81; $2.62; $3.03 $12.6 per bag; $12.6 per bag

*Prices represents Average Wholesale Price (AWP).

USUAL ADULT DOSING

- Usual adult dose: 0.5–1 g IV q6–8h
- UTI: 1 g IV q12h
- Severe infections: 1–2 g IV q6 hrs
- For obese pts: consider 2 g IV q6h
- Surgical prophylaxis: 2 g IV push just before the procedure, repeat if needed for procedures lasting >4 hrs. For obese pts: a minimum of 2 g IV should be given.

RENAL DOSING

Dosing for GFR 50–80: GFR >35 mL/min: 1–2 g q8h.

Dosing for GFR 10–50: GFR 11–34 mL/min: 0.5 g–1.0 g 12 hrs.

Dosing for GFR <10: 0.5 g–1 g once daily.

Dosing in hemodialysis: 0.5 g–1 g once daily plus 1.0 g post dialysis (or on days of HD dose post-HD). Convenient outpatient treatment: 2 g (approx. 20 mg/kg) post-HD on Monday, Wednesday, and 3 g post-HD on Friday.

Dosing in peritoneal dialysis: 0.5 g q12h.

Dosing in hemofiltration: CVVH: 1–2 g IV q12h; CVVHD: 2 g IV q12h (1 g IV q12h for mild-moderate infections).

ADVERSE DRUG REACTIONS

Occasional

- Minimal phlebitis at infusion sites
- Allergic reactions (eosinophilia)
- Diarrhea and *C. difficile* colitis
- Positive Coombs' test (without hemolytic anemia)

Rare

- CNS: convulsions (high dose with renal failure), confusion, disorientation, and hallucinations
- Drug fever
- Neutropenia and thrombocytopenia

- Hepatitis
- Anaphylaxis reaction
- Hemolytic anemia (theoretical, case reports with ceftriaxone, cefotetan, cefoxitin, cefamandole, ceftazidime, and cefalothin)

DRUG INTERACTIONS

- Probenecid: increase in cephalosporin serum concentration. Monitor for ADR in ESRD.
- Warfarin anticoagulation effect may be enhanced. Monitor INR closely.

SPECTRUM—See Appendix II, p. 792

RESISTANCE

- MIC breakpoint for *Enterobacteriaceae*: ≤8 mcg/mL (sensitive); 16 mcg/mL (intermediate); ≥32 mcg/mL (resistant).
- MIC breakpoint for *S. aureus:* ≤8 mcg/mL (sensitive); 16 mcg/mL (intermediate); ≥32 mcg/mL (resistant).

PHARMACOLOGY

Mechanism

Cephalosporins like all beta-lactam antibiotics inhibit mucopeptide synthesis in the bacterial cell wall, this results in the formation of defective cell walls and osmotically unstable organisms susceptible to cell lysis.

Pharmacokinetic Parameters

- **Absorption** —
- **Cmax** 188 mcg/mL after 1 g IV dose administration.
- **Distribution** Distributed to tissues and fluids, including pleural fluid, synovial fluid, and bone. Therapeutic concentration also attained in wound secretions of toe and heal ulcers due to peripheral vascular disease. Poor CNS penetration.
- **Protein binding** 70–90%.
- **Metabolism/Excretion** 80–100% Excreted unchanged in the urine within 24 hrs.
- **T1/2** 1.9 hrs.

Dosing for Decreased Hepatic Function

No data. Usual dose likely.

Pregnancy Risk

B: Cephalosporins are usually considered safe to use during pregnancy.

Breast Feeding Compatibility

Excreted in breast milk at low concentrations. The American Academy of Pediatrics classifies cephalosporin antibiotics as compatible with breast feeding.

COMMENTS

Parenteral 1st generation cephalosporin with relatively long half-life that can be given IV or IM. This is the preferred cephalosporin for methicillin sensitive *S. aureus* and for many forms of monotherapy surgical prophylaxis with the exception of colorectal procedures where cefotetan, cefoxitin or cefazolin + metronidazole is preferred.

SELECTED REFERENCES

Bratzler DW, Houck PM, Surgical Infection Prevention Guidelines Writers Workgroup, et al. Antimicrobial prophylaxis for surgery: an advisory statement from the National Surgical Infection Prevention Project. *Clin Infect Dis*, 2004; Vol. 38; pp. 1706–15.

Marx MA, Frye RF, Matzke GR, et al. Cefazolin as empiric therapy in hemodialysis-related infections: efficacy and blood concentrations. *Am J Kidney Dis*, 1998; Vol. 32; pp. 410–4.

CEFDINIR

Paul A. Pham, PharmD and John G. Bartlett, MD

INDICATIONS

FDA

- Community-acquired pneumonia (CAP) caused by *H. influenzae, H. parainfluenza, S. pneumoniae* (penicillin-susceptible strains only), and *M. catarrhalis*
- Acute exacerbations of chronic bronchitis (AECB) caused by *H. influenzae, H. parainfluenza, S. pneumoniae* (penicillin-susceptible strains only), and *M. catarrhalis*

ANTIBACTERIAL DRUGS

- Acute maxillary sinusitis caused by *H. influenzae*, *S. pneumoniae* (penicillin-susceptible strains only), and *M. catarrhalis*. Pharyngitis and tonsillitis caused by *Streptococcus pyogenes*
- Uncomplicated skin and skin-structure infections caused by *S. aureus* (MSSA) and *S. pyogenes*
- Acute otitis media caused by *H. influenzae*, *S. pneumoniae* (penicillin-susceptible strains only), and *M. catarrhalis*

FORMS

Brand name (mfr)	Forms	Cost*
Omnicef (Abbott and generic manufacturers)	PO capsule 300 mg PO susp 125 mg/5 mL; PO susp 250 mg/5 mL	$5.11 $51.01 per 60 mL; $80.78 per 100 mL; $99.48 per 60 mL; $157.54 per 100 mL
*Prices represents Average Wholesale Price (AWP).		

USUAL ADULT DOSING
- CAP: 300 mg PO twice daily × 10 days.
- AECB, pharyngitis, and tonsillitis: 300 mg PO twice daily × 5–10 days or 600 mg PO once daily × 10 days.
- Soft tissue infections: 300 mg PO twice daily × 10 days.
- Acute sinusitis: 300 mg PO twice daily × 10 days or 600 mg PO once daily × 10 days.

RENAL DOSING
Dosing for GFR 50–80: Usual dose.
Dosing for GFR 10–50: <30 mL/min: 300 mg q24h.
Dosing for GFR <10: 300 mg q24h.
Dosing in hemodialysis: Removed in dialysis; dose after dialysis.
Dosing in peritoneal dialysis: No data.
Dosing in hemofiltration: No data.

ADVERSE DRUG REACTIONS
General
- Generally well tolerated

Occasional
- Allergic reactions
- Diarrhea
- Eosinophilia
- Positive Coombs' test
- *C. difficile* colitis

Rare
- CNS: confusion, disorientation, and hallucinations
- Anaphylaxis
- Drug fever
- Neutropenia and thrombocytopenia
- Hepatitis
- Interstitial nephritis

DRUG INTERACTIONS
Probenecid: may increase cefdinir serum concentrations (no dosage adjustment needed).

SPECTRUM—See Appendix II, p. 792

RESISTANCE
- MIC breakpoint for *S. pneumoniae*: 0.5 mcg/mL.
- MIC breakpoint for *Staphylococcus* spp.: 1 mcg/mL.
- MIC breakpoint for *Haemophilus* spp.: 1 mcg/mL.

PHARMACOLOGY
Mechanism
Cephalosporins like all beta-lactam antibiotics inhibit mucopeptide synthesis in the bacterial cell wall, this results in the formation of defective cell walls and osmotically unstable organisms susceptible to cell lysis.

Pharmacokinetic Parameters
- **Absorption** 20–25%.
- **Cmax** 1.60 mcg/mL after 300 mg dose; 2.87 mcg/mL after 600 mg dose.
- **Distribution** Distributed to tissues and fluids, including pleural fluid, synovial fluid, and bone.
- **Protein binding** 60–73%.
- **Metabolism/Excretion** Not metabolized. 12–18% excreted unchanged in urine.
- **T1/2** 1.7 hrs.

Dosing for Decreased Hepatic Function
No data.

Pregnancy Risk
B: Cephalosporins are usually considered safe to use during pregnancy.

Breast Feeding Compatibility
Excreted in breast milk at low concentrations. The American Academy of Pediatrics classifies cephalosporin antibiotics as compatible with breast feeding.

COMMENTS
Oral 3rd generation cephalosporin that has activity against many Gram-negative organisms, but is not active against Enterobacter and Pseudomonas. Activity against Gram-positive bacteria is good and is similar to cefpodoxime, including good activity MSSA, and *S. pyogenes,* but up to 23.5% of *S. pneumoniae* are resistant although this is based on older breakpoint criteria.

SELECTED REFERENCES

Doern GV, Richter SS, Miller A, et al. Antimicrobial resistance among *Streptococcus pneumoniae* in the United States: have we begun to turn the corner on resistance to certain antimicrobial classes? *Clin Infect Dis,* 2005; Vol. 41; pp. 139–48.

Tack KJ, Littlejohn TW, Mailloux G, et al. Cefdinir versus cephalexin for the treatment of skin and skin-structure infections. The Cefdinir Adult Skin Infection Study Group. *Clin Ther,* 1998; Vol. 20; pp. 244–56.

CEFEPIME

Paul A. Pham, PharmD and John G. Bartlett, MD

INDICATIONS

FDA
- Pneumonia caused by *S. pneumoniae,* including cases associated with concurrent bacteremia, *P. aeruginosa, K. pneumoniae,* or *Enterobacter* species.
- Febrile neutropenia (empiric therapy).
- Uncomplicated and complicated urinary tract infections including pyelonephritis (+/– bacteremia) caused by *E. coli, K. pneumoniae,* or *P. mirabilis.*
- Uncomplicated skin and skin-structure infections caused by MSSA or *S. pyogenes.*
- Complicated intra-abdominal infections (in combination with metronidazole) caused by *E. coli,* viridans group streptococci, *P. aeruginosa, K. pneumoniae, Enterobacter* species, or *B. fragilis.*

Non-FDA Approved Uses
- Shunt infections, CNS
- Appendicitis (with metronidazole)
- Diverticulitis (with metronidazole)
- Intra-abdominal abscess (with metronidazole)
- Osteomyelitis, acute
- Osteomyelitis, chronic
- Diabetic foot infection (with metronidazole or clindamycin)
- Hardware associated septic arthritis
- Acute exacerbations of chronic bronchitis

FORMS

Brand name (mfr)	Forms	Cost*
Maxipime (Elan)	IV vial 500 mg; IV vial 1000 mg; IV vial 2000 mg	$9; $20.33; $40.36
*Prices represents Average Wholesale Price (AWP).		

ANTIBACTERIAL DRUGS

USUAL ADULT DOSING

Although the manufacturer recommends q12h dosing, with the exception of UTI, the authors recommend q8h dosing due to better pharmacodynamic properties (longer time above the MIC).

- Bacteremia, severe infections: cefepime 1–2 g IV q8h or consider continuous infusion: cefepime 6 g over 24 hrs.
- Pseudomonas: 1–2 g IV q8h.
- CNS infections: 2 g IV q8h.
- Mild to moderate UTI: 0.5–1 g IV or IM q12h.
- Empiric therapy for febrile neutropenia: 2 g IV q8h × 7 days or until resolution of neutropenia.
- Obese pts: consider 2 g IV q8h.

RENAL DOSING

Dosing for GFR 50–80: GFR >60 mL/min: usual dose (1–2 g q8h).

Dosing for GFR 10–50: GFR 30–60 mL/min: 1 g q24h (1 g q12h for Pseudomonas; 2 g q12h for CNS infections); GFR <29 mL/min: 0.5 g q24h (1 g q24h for Pseudomonas; 2 g q24h for CNS infections).

Dosing for GFR <10: GFR <10 mL/min: 0.5 g q24h (1 g q24h for Pseudomonas; 2 g q24h for CNS infections).

Dosing in hemodialysis: 0.5 g q24h (1 g q24h for Pseudomonas; 2 g q24h for CNS infections) plus 1 g post-dialysis (or dose post-HD on days of HD).

Dosing in peritoneal dialysis: 1–2 g q48h.

Dosing in hemofiltration: CVVH: 1–2 g q12h; CVVHD with dialysis flow rate > or = 1.5 L/hr: 1–2 g q12h (2 g q12h for severe and CNS infections). CVVHD with dialysis flow rate <1.5 L/hr: 1–2 g q24h (2 g q24h for severe and CNS infections).

ADVERSE DRUG REACTIONS

General
- Generally well tolerated

Occasional
- Minimal phlebitis at infusion sites
- Allergic reactions (eosinophilia). Cross-allergy to PCN lower than 1st generation cephalosporins
- Diarrhea and *C. difficile* colitis
- Positive Coombs' test (without hemolytic anemia)

Rare
- CNS: convulsions (high dose used with renal failure), encephalopathy, myoclonus, confusion, disorientation, and hallucinations
- Drug fever
- Neutropenia and thrombocytopenia
- Hepatitis
- Anaphylaxis
- Hemolytic anemia (theoretical, case reports with ceftriaxone, cefotetan, cefoxitin, cefamandole, ceftazidime, and cephalothin)

DRUG INTERACTIONS

Probenecid: increase in cephalosporin serum concentration, monitor closely with co-administration (esp w/ renal failure).

SPECTRUM—See Appendix II, p. 792

RESISTANCE
- Resistance development on therapy has been reported with Enterobacter species.
- MIC breakpoint for Enterobacteriaceae and Gram-negative non-lactose fermenters is 8 mcg/mL. Higher mortality rate associated with MIC of 8 mcg/mL [Antimicrob. Agents Chemother. 2007;51:4390] but significance debated. For strains with MIC of 8 mcg/mL, use cefepime 2 g IV q8h (consider continuous infusion and/or co-administer with an aminoglycoside).
- MIC breakpoint for *S. pneumoniae* is ≤0.5 mcg/mL (meningitis) and ≤1 mcg/mL (non-meningitis).
- MIC breakpoint for beta-hemolytic *Streptococcus* spp.: ≤0.5 mcg/mL.
- MIC breakpoint for *S. viridans*: ≤1 mcg/mL (sensitive); 2 mcg/mL (intermediate); ≥4 mcg/mL (resistant).

PHARMACOLOGY

Mechanism

Cephalosporins like all beta-lactam antibiotics inhibit mucopeptide synthesis in the bacterial cell wall, this results in the formation of defective cell walls and osmotically unstable organisms susceptible to cell lysis.

Pharmacokinetic Parameters

- **Absorption** —
- **Cmax** 193 mcg/mL after 2 g IV dose administration.
- **Distribution** Distributed into blister fluid, bronchial mucosa, prostate. Achieves CNS penetration through inflamed meninges in animal study.
- **Protein binding** 20%.
- **Metabolism/Excretion** 85% excreted unchanged in the urine. 7% hepatically metabolized to N-methylpyrrolidine-N-oxide.
- **T1/2** 2.0 hrs.

Dosing for Decreased Hepatic Function

Usual dose.

Pregnancy Risk

B: Cephalosporins are usually considered safe to use during pregnancy.

Breast Feeding Compatibility

Excreted in breast milk at low concentrations. The American Academy of Pediatrics classifies cephalosporin antibiotics as compatible with breast feeding.

COMMENTS

Parenteral 4th generation cephalosporin with activity against *P. aeruginosa* comparable to ceftazidime and also has activity against GPC comparable to cefotaxime. Resistant to hydrolysis by some expanded spectrum beta-lactamases (ESBLs), but carbapenems are preferred for ESBL Gram-negative bacteria. A meta-analysis (see Yahav ref) found a 26% higher all-cause mortality with cefepime compared to other beta-lactams; however, a recent analysis by the FDA did not find an increased risk. For strains with MIC of 8 mcg/mL, use cefepime 2 g IV q8h (consider continuous infusion and/or co-administer with an aminoglycoside).

SELECTED REFERENCES

American Thoracic Society, Infectious Diseases Society of America. Guidelines for the management of adults with hospital-acquired, ventilator-associated, and healthcare-associated pneumonia. *Am J Respir Crit Care Med*, 2005; Vol. 171; pp. 388–416.

Yahav D, Paul M, Fraser A, et al. Efficacy and safety of cefepime: a systematic review and meta-analysis. *Lancet Infect Dis*, 2007; Vol. 7; pp. 338–48.

CEFIXIME

Paul A. Pham, PharmD and John G. Bartlett, MD

INDICATIONS

FDA

- Otitis media caused by *H. influenzae, M. catarrhalis,* and *S. pyogenes.*
- Pharyngitis and tonsillitis caused by *S. pyogenes* (PCN is the drug of choice).
- Acute bronchitis and acute exacerbation of chronic bronchitis (AECB) caused by *S. pneumoniae* and *H. influenzae* (poor *S. pneumoniae* activity).
- Uncomplicated urinary tract infections caused by *E. coli* and *P. mirabilis.*
- Uncomplicated gonorrhea (cervicitis and urethritis).

Non-FDA Approved Uses

- Sinusitis, acute (not a first line agent)
- Septic arthritis, community-acquired (due to GC)
- Sexually-associated reactive arthritis (SARA due to GC)

ANTIBACTERIAL DRUGS

FORMS

Brand name (mfr)	Forms	Cost*
Suprax (Lupin Pharmaceuticals Inc.)	PO susp 100 mg/5 mL (50 mL and 100 mL bottle); PO susp 200 mg/5 mL (50 mL and 75 mL bottle) PO tab 400 mg	$119.43 per 50 mL; $241.88 per 100 mL; $223.04 per 50 mL; $299.36 per 75 mL $11.43

*Prices represents Average Wholesale Price (AWP).

USUAL ADULT DOSING
- 400 mg PO once daily.
- Uncomplicated GC: 400 mg PO × 1 dose.

RENAL DOSING
Dosing for GFR 50–80: Usual dose
Dosing for GFR 10–50: 300 mg/day
Dosing for GFR <10: 200 mg/day
Dosing in hemodialysis: 300 mg/day dose post-HD on days of dialysis
Dosing in peritoneal dialysis: 200 mg/day
Dosing in hemofiltration: No data.

ADVERSE DRUG REACTIONS
General
- Generally well tolerated
Common
- Diarrhea
- Nausea
Occasional
- Allergic reactions (eosinophilia): cross-allergy to PCN lower than 1st generation cephalosporin
- Diarrhea and *C. difficile* colitis
- Positive Coombs' test
Rare
- CNS: confusion, disorientation, and hallucinations
- Drug fever
- Neutropenia and thrombocytopenia
- Hepatitis
- Anaphylaxis reaction
- Interstitial nephritis
- Hemolytic anemia

DRUG INTERACTIONS
Probenecid: increase in cephalosporin serum concentration due to inhibition of tubular secretion by probenecid (no dose adjustment needed).

SPECTRUM—See Appendix II, p. 792
RESISTANCE
- MIC breakpoint for *Haemophilus* spp.: 1 mcg/mL

PHARMACOLOGY
Mechanism
Cephalosporins like all beta-lactam antibiotics inhibit mucopeptide synthesis in the bacterial cell wall, this results in the formation of defective cell walls and osmotically unstable organisms susceptible to cell lysis.

Pharmacokinetic Parameters
- **Absorption** 30–50% absorbed
- **Metabolism/Excretion** 7–41% Excreted unchanged in the urine within 24 hrs. Up to 60% excreted via non-renal route(10% biliary excretion in animal study).
- **Protein binding** 65%
- **Cmax** 3–5 mcg/mL after 400 mg PO dose administration

- **T1/2** 3.1 hrs
- **Distribution** Not well studied, but distributed in gallbladder, tonsillar, maxillary sinus tissue, middle ear, and prostatic fluid. Poor penetration into Waldeyer's ring.

Dosing for Decreased Hepatic Function
No data. Usual dose likely.

Pregnancy Risk
B: Cephalosporins are usually considered safe to use during pregnancy.

Breast Feeding Compatibility
Excreted in breast milk at low concentrations. The American Academy of Pediatrics classifies cephalosporin antibiotics as compatible with breast feeding.

COMMENTS
Oral 3rd generation cephalosporin. Poor activity vs *S. aureus* (MSSA) and *S. pneumoniae*. Therefore a poor agent for empiric use in respiratory tract infection. First line oral agent for uncomplicated GC, but does not attain adequate penetration of the Waldeyer's ring and should not be used to treat gonorrhea in anyone with orogenital exposure.

SELECTED REFERENCES
Portilla I, Lutz B, Montalvo M, et al. Oral cefixime versus intramuscular ceftriaxone in pts with uncomplicated gonococcal infections. *Sex Transm Dis*, 1992; Vol. 19; pp. 94–8.

Raz R, Rottensterich E, Leshem Y, et al. Double-blind study comparing 3-day regimens of cefixime and ofloxacin in treatment of uncomplicated urinary tract infections in women. *Antimicrob Agents Chemother*, 1994; Vol. 38; pp. 1176–7.

CEFOTAXIME

Paul A. Pham, PharmD and John G. Bartlett, MD

INDICATIONS
FDA
- Lower respiratory tract infections including pneumonia
- Genitourinary infections
- Gynecologic infection (including pelvic inflammatory disease, endometritis, and pelvic cellulitis)
- Bacteremia and septicemia
- Skin and skin-structure infections
- Intra-abdominal infections including peritonitis
- Bone and joint infections
- Central nervous system infections including meningitis and ventriculitis

Non-FDA Approved Uses
- Brain abscess (in combination with metronidazole)
- Empyema (in combination with metronidazole)
- Lyme disease: late Lyme arthritis and neuroborreliosis
- STD (*Neisseria gonorrhoeae*)

FORMS

Brand name (mfr)	Forms	Cost*
Claforan (Sanofi aventis U.S.)	IV vial 500 mg; IV vial 1000 mg; IV vial 2000 mg; IV vial 10 g	$7; $10; $20; $88
Cefotaxime (Generic manufacturer)	IV bag 1 g/50 mL; IV bag 2 g/50 mL IV vial 500 mg; IV vial 1 g; IV vial 2 g; IV vial 10 g; IV vial 20 g	$17.90; $31.63 $4.38; $4.89; $6.99; $41.54; $170.00

*Prices represents Average Wholesale Price (AWP).

USUAL ADULT DOSING
- Moderate to severe infections: 1–2 g IV q8h.
- Meningitis and septicemia: 2 g IV q4–6h.
- GC (urethritis and cervicitis): 500 mg IM × 1.

ANTIBACTERIAL DRUGS

499

- GC (rectal in males): 1 g IM × 1.
- GC (rectal in females): 500 mg IM × 1.
- Obese pts: consider 2 g IV q4h.

RENAL DOSING

Dosing for GFR 50–80: Usual dose

Dosing for GFR 10–50: 1 g–2 g q8–12h (moderate to severe infections) or 2 g q8h (CNS infections)

Dosing for GFR <10: 1 g–2 g q12–24h (moderate to severe infections) or 2 g q12h (CNS infections)

Dosing in hemodialysis: 1–2 g once daily (dose post-HD on days of HD or supplement with 1 g post dialysis)

Dosing in peritoneal dialysis: 0.5–2 g once daily

Dosing in hemofiltration: CVVH: 1–2 g q12h; CVVHD: 2 g q12h.

ADVERSE DRUG REACTIONS

General

- Generally well tolerated

Occasional

- Minimal phlebitis at infusion sites
- Allergic reactions (eosinophilia); cross-allergy to PCN lower than 1st generation cephalosporin
- Diarrhea and *C. difficile* colitis
- Positive Coombs' test

Rare

- CNS: convulsions (high dose with renal failure); confusion, disorientation, and hallucinations
- Drug fever
- Neutropenia and thrombocytopenia
- Hepatitis
- Anaphylaxis reaction
- Hemolytic anemia
- Interstitial nephritis

DRUG INTERACTIONS

Probenecid: increase in cephalosporin serum concentration due to inhibition of tubular secretion by probenecid (no dose adjustment needed).

SPECTRUM—See Appendix II, p. 792

RESISTANCE

- MIC breakpoint for *S. pneumoniae* is ≤0.5 mcg/mL (meningitis) and ≤1 mcg/mL (non-meningitis).
- MIC breakpoint for *S. aureus*: ≤8 mcg/mL (sensitive); 16–32 mcg/mL (intermediate); ≥64 mcg/mL (resistant).
- MIC breakpoint for beta-hemolytic *Streptococcus* spp.: ≤0.5 mcg/mL.
- MIC breakpoint for *S. viridans*: ≤1 mcg/mL (sensitive); 2 mcg/mL (intermediate); ≥4 mcg/mL (resistant).
- MIC breakpoint for *Enterobacteriaceae* and other Gram-negative non-Enterobacteriaceae: ≤8 mcg/mL (sensitive); 16–32 mcg/mL (intermediate); ≥64 mcg/mL (resistant).

PHARMACOLOGY

Mechanism

Cephalosporins like all beta-lactam antibiotics inhibit mucopeptide synthesis in the bacterial cell wall, this results in the formation of defective cell walls and osmotically unstable organisms susceptible to cell lysis.

Pharmacokinetic Parameters

- **Cmax** 100 mcg/mL after 1 g IV dose administration.
- **Distribution** Widely distributed to tissues and fluids, including pleural fluid, synovial fluid, wand bone. With inflamed meninges therapeutic concentration can be attained with large doses.
- **Protein binding** 30–50%
- **Metabolism/Excretion** 24% of cefotaxime is metabolized to desacetyl active metabolite. Both active metabolite and unchanged drug is excreted in urine by tubular secretion.
- **T1/2** 1.5 hrs.

Dosing for Decreased Hepatic Function
Usual dose.
Pregnancy Risk
B: Cephalosporins are considered safe to use during pregnancy.
Breast Feeding Compatibility
Excreted in breast milk at low concentrations. The American Academy of Pediatrics classifies cephalosporin antibiotics as compatible with breast feeding.

COMMENTS

A parenteral 3rd generation cephalosporin with reliable CNS penetration when dosed at 2 g IV q4h. Cefotaxime and ceftriaxone are the preferred parenteral cephalosporins for serious pneumococcal infections, but 3–5% of strains are resistant. Although less convenient dosing schedule, cefotaxime is therapeutically equivalent to ceftriaxone.

SELECTED REFERENCES

Garber GE, Auger P, Chan RM, et al. A multicenter, open comparative study of parenteral cefotaxime and ceftriaxone in the treatment of nosocomial lower respiratory tract infections. *Diagn Microbiol Infect Dis*, 1992; Vol. 15; pp. 85–8.

Pfister HW, Preac-Mursic V, Wilske B, et al. Randomized comparison of ceftriaxone and cefotaxime in Lyme neuroborreliosis. *J Infect Dis*, 1991; Vol. 163; pp. 311–8.

CEFOTETAN

Paul A. Pham, PharmD and John G. Bartlett, MD

INDICATIONS
FDA

- Urinary tract infections
- Lower respiratory tract infections
- Skin and skin-structure infections
- Gynecologic infections including PID (not active against *C. trachomatis*)
- Intra-abdominal infections (e.g., appendicitis, cholecystitis, diverticulitis. Author's comment: not recommended; high rates resistance with *B. fragilis*)
- Bone and joint infections (author's comment: generally used for mild infections)
- Surgical prophylaxis (e.g., cesarean section, abdominal, or vaginal hysterectomy, transurethral surgery, biliary tract surgery, and gastrointestinal surgery)

Non-FDA Approved Uses

- Venous sinus thrombosis
- Cholangitis (no longer recommended)
- Surgical wound infections
- *Neisseria gonorrhoeae*
- *Bacteroides fragilis*
- *Klebsiella species*
- *Bacteroides species* (no longer recommended for intra-abdominal infections)

FORMS

Brand name (mfr)	Forms	Cost*
Cefotan (Generic manufacturer [APP Pharmaceuticals])	IV vial 1 g; IV vial 2 g; IV vial 10 g	$14.23; $28.45; $140.86
*Prices represents Average Wholesale Price (AWP).		

USUAL ADULT DOSING

- UTI: 0.5 g to 1 g IV or IM q12h.
- Mild to moderate infections: 1 g IV q12h.
- Severe infections: 2–3 g IV q12h (max 6 g/24 hrs).
- Surgical prophylaxis: administer 2 g IV within 1 hr of procedure.

RENAL DOSING

Dosing for GFR 50–80: Usual dose.
Dosing for GFR 10–50: 1 g–2 g q24h.

ANTIBACTERIAL DRUGS

Dosing for GFR <10: 1 g–2 g q48h.
Dosing in hemodialysis: 0.5–1 g q24 plus 1 g post dialysis.
Dosing in peritoneal dialysis: 1 g once daily.
Dosing in hemofiltration: No data.

ADVERSE DRUG REACTIONS
General
- Usually well tolerated

Common
- Phlebitis at infusion sites

Occasional
- Allergic reactions
- Hypoprothrombinemia
- Diarrhea
- *C. difficile* colitis
- Eosinophilia
- Positive Coombs' test without hemolytic anemia

Rare
- Hemolytic anemia
- Anaphylaxis
- CNS: convulsions (high dose with renal failure), confusion, disorientation, and hallucinations
- Neutropenia and thrombocytopenia
- Drug fever
- Interstitial nephritis
- Hepatitis

DRUG INTERACTIONS
- Ethanol: methyltetrazolethiol moiety inhibits aldehyde dehydrogenase resulting in acetaldehyde accumulation and disulfiram-like reactions. Avoid co-administration.
- Probenecid: may increase cefotetan serum concentrations. Clinical significance unknown; no dose adjustment needed.
- Warfarin: INR may be increased (monitor closely).

SPECTRUM—See Appendix II, p. 792
RESISTANCE
- MIC breakpoint for Enterobacteriaceae is 16 mcg/mL.

PHARMACOLOGY
Mechanism
Cephalosporins like all beta-lactam antibiotics inhibit mucopeptide synthesis in the bacterial cell wall, this results in the formation of defective cell walls and osmotically unstable organisms susceptible to cell lysis.

Pharmacokinetic Parameters
- **Absorption** —
- **Cmax** 124 mcg/mL after 1 g IV dose administration.
- **Distribution** Distributed to tissues and fluids, including pleural fluid, synovial fluid, and bone. Poor CNS penetration.
- **Protein binding** 80–90%
- **Metabolism/Excretion** Not metabolized. 49–81% excreted unchanged within 24 hrs in the urine by glomerular filtration (and to a lesser extent tubular secretion). 20% excreted via biliary route.
- **T1/2** 4.2 hrs.

Dosing for Decreased Hepatic Function
No data. Usual dose likely.

Pregnancy Risk
B: Cephalosporins are usually considered safe to use during pregnancy.

Breast Feeding Compatibility
Excreted in breast milk at low concentrations. The American Academy of Pediatrics classifies cephalosporin antibiotics as compatible with breast feeding.

COMMENTS
Cephamycin 2nd generation cephalosporin w/ anaerobic activity, but up to 44% of *B. fragilis* may be resistant (while 5.8% resistance seen with cefoxitin). Longer half-life allows q12h dosing compared to cefoxitin. Now available again in the U.S. Contains the N-methylthiotetrazole (NMTT) side chain, that may result in prolonged hypoprothrombinemia and disulfiram-like reactions.

SELECTED REFERENCES
Bratzler DW, Houck PM, Surgical Infection Prevention Guidelines Writers Workgroup, et al. Antimicrobial prophylaxis for surgery: an advisory statement from the National Surgical Infection Prevention Project. *Clin Infect Dis*, 2004; Vol. 38; pp. 1706–15.

Snydman DR, Jacobus NV, McDermott LA, et al. National survey on the susceptibility of Bacteroides Fragilis Group: report and analysis of trends for 1997–2000. *Clin Infect Dis*, 2002; Vol. 35; pp. S126–34.

CEFOXITIN

Paul A. Pham, PharmD and John G. Bartlett, MD

INDICATIONS
FDA
- Lower respiratory tract infections including pneumonia and lung abscess
- Urinary tract infections
- Intra-abdominal infections including peritonitis and intra-abdominal abscess (author's comment: for mild infections only)
- Gynecologic infections including endometritis, pelvic cellulitis, and pelvic inflammatory disease
- Septicemia caused by *S. pneumoniae*, *S. aureus* (MSSA), *E. coli*, *Klebsiella* species, and *Bacteroides* species including *B. fragilis* (author's comment: not a preferred agent, should confirm sensitivity)
- Bone and joint infections (author's comment: for mild infections only)
- Skin and skin-structure infections

Non-FDA Approved Uses
- Diabetic foot infection (for mild-moderate infections only)
- Surgical prophylaxis (GI, abdominal hysterectomy, vaginal hysterectomy, Cesarean section)

FORMS

Brand name (mfr)	Forms	Cost*
Mefoxin (Merck and generic manufacturers)	IV vial 1 g/50 mL; IV vial 2 g/50 mL; IV vial 10 g; IV bag 1 g/50 mL; IV bag 2 g/50 mL	$11.23; $22.50; $112.25 $307.44; $564

*Prices represents Average Wholesale Price (AWP).

USUAL ADULT DOSING
- UTI or mild, uncomplicated infections: 1.0 g IV or IM q6–8h.
- Moderate infections: 2 g IV q6h.
- Severe infections (generally not a preferred agent): 2 g IV q4h or 3 g q6h (12 g/day max).

RENAL DOSING
Dosing for GFR 50–80: 1 g–2 g q6h.
Dosing for GFR 10–50: GFR 30–49 mL/min: 1 g–2 g q8–12h. GFR 10–29 mL/min: 1 g–2 g q12–24h.
Dosing for GFR <10: 0.5 g–1 g q24h.
Dosing in hemodialysis: 1 g q24h (dose post-HD on days of HD or supplement with 1 g post-dialysis).
Dosing in peritoneal dialysis: 1 g/day.
Dosing in hemofiltration: CVVHD: 1 g IV q12h.

ANTIBACTERIAL DRUGS

ADVERSE DRUG REACTIONS
General
- Usually well tolerated

Occasional
- Minimal phlebitis at infusion sites
- Allergic reactions (eosinophilia): cross-allergy to PCN lower than 1st generation cephalosporin
- Diarrhea and *C. difficile* colitis
- Positive Coombs' test

Rare
- CNS: convulsions (high dose with renal failure); confusion, disorientation, and hallucinations
- Drug fever
- Hepatitis
- Anaphylaxis reaction
- Hemolytic anemia

DRUG INTERACTIONS
- Probenecid: may increase cefotetan serum concentration. No dose adjustment needed, but monitor closely in ESRD.
- Warfarin: anticoagulation effect may be enhanced (monitor closely).

SPECTRUM — See Appendix II, p. 792
RESISTANCE
- MIC breakpoint for Enterobacteriaceae is 8 mcg/mL.

PHARMACOLOGY
Mechanism
Cephalosporins like all beta-lactam antibiotics inhibit mucopeptide synthesis in the bacterial cell wall; this results in the formation of defective cell walls and osmotically unstable organisms susceptible to cell lysis.

Pharmacokinetic Parameters
- **Absorption** —
- **Cmax** 110 mcg/mL after 1 g IV dose administration.
- **Distribution** Widely distributed to tissues and fluids, including pleural fluid, synovial fluid and bone. Attains therapeutic level in pelvic tissue. Poor CNS penetration.
- **Protein binding** 65–80%
- **Metabolism/Excretion** Only 2% of dose is metabolized to descarbamyl inactive metabolite. Excreted primarily unchanged by glomerular filtration and tubular secretion.
- **T1/2** 0.8 hr.

Dosing for Decreased Hepatic Function
No data. Usual dose likely.

Pregnancy Risk
B: Cephalosporins are usually considered safe to use during pregnancy.

Breast Feeding Compatibility
Excreted in breast milk at low concentrations. The American Academy of Pediatrics classifies cephalosporin antibiotics as compatible with breast feeding.

COMMENTS
Parenteral cephamycin 2nd generation cephalosporin with good anaerobic activity including *B. fragilis* (but 5.8% + or more may be resistant). Preferred over cefotetan for *B. fragilis* coverage but requires more frequent administration.

SELECTED REFERENCES
Snydman DR, Jacobus NV, McDermott LA, et al. National survey on the susceptibility of Bacteroides Fragilis Group: report and analysis of trends for 1997–2000. *Clin Infect Dis*, 2002; Vol. 35; pp. S126–34.

Talan DA, Summanen PH, Finegold SM. Ampicillin/sulbactam and cefoxitin in the treatment of cutaneous and other soft-tissue abscesses in pts with or without histories of injection drug abuse. *Clin Infect Dis*, 2000; Vol. 31; pp. 464–71.

CEFPODOXIME PROXETIL

Paul A. Pham, PharmD and John G. Bartlett, MD

INDICATIONS
FDA
- Upper respiratory tract infections including acute otitis media, pharyngitis, tonsillitis, acute exacerbation of chronic bronchitis (AECB), and acute maxillary sinusitis
- Acute uncomplicated urethral and cervical gonorrhea and ano-rectal gonorrhea (females) caused by *N. gonorrhoeae*
- Uncomplicated skin and skin-structure infections *S. aureus* (MSSA) or *S. pyogenes*.
- Uncomplicated urinary tract infections caused by *E. coli, K. pneumoniae, P. mirabilis, or S. saprophyticus.*
- Community-acquired pneumonia (CAP) caused by *S. pneumoniae or H. Influenzae*

FORMS

Brand name (mfr)	Forms	Cost*
Vantin (Pfizer and generic manufacturers)	PO tab 100 mg; PO tab 200 mg; PO susp 50 mg/5 mL; PO susp 100 mg/5 mL	$4.85; $6.41 $28.75 per 50 mL; $54.72 per 50 mL

*Prices represents Average Wholesale Price (AWP).

USUAL ADULT DOSING
- CAP (mild): 200 mg PO twice daily × 14 days. Some would treat for a shorter course (a minimum of 5 days) when pts have been afebrile × 48–72 hrs.
- Soft tissue infections: 400 mg PO twice daily × 7–14 days.
- Uncomplicated GC: 200 mg PO × 1.
- Pharyngitis and/or tonsillitis: 100 mg Q 12 hrs × 5–10 days.
- AECB: 200 mg Q 12 hrs × 10 days.
- Acute bacterial sinusitis: 200 mg Q 12 hrs × 10 days.

RENAL DOSING
Dosing for GFR 50–80: 200 mg–400 mg q12h.
Dosing for GFR 10–50: 200 mg–400 mg q16–24h.
Dosing for GFR <10: 200 mg–400 mg q24–48h.
Dosing in hemodialysis: 200–400 mg 3×/wk, post-HD only.
Dosing in peritoneal dialysis: 200–400 mg q24h.
Dosing in hemofiltration: No data.

ADVERSE DRUG REACTIONS
General
- Generally well tolerated
Occasional
- Allergic reactions
- Diarrhea and *C. difficile* colitis
- Eosinophilia
- Positive Coombs' test
Rare
- CNS: confusion, disorientation, and hallucinations
- Drug fever
- Neutropenia and thrombocytopenia
- Hepatitis
- Interstitial nephritis
- Anaphylaxis reaction

DRUG INTERACTIONS
Probenecid: increase in cephalosporin serum concentration (no dose adjustment needed).

SPECTRUM—See Appendix II, p. 792

ANTIBACTERIAL DRUGS

- MIC breakpoint for *S. pneumoniae*: 0.5 mcg/mL
- MIC breakpoint for *Staphylococcus* spp.: 2 mcg/mL
- MIC breakpoint for *Haemophilus* spp.: 2 mcg/mL

PHARMACOLOGY

Mechanism

Cephalosporins like all beta-lactam antibiotics inhibit mucopeptide synthesis in the bacterial cell wall, this results in the formation of defective cell walls and osmotically unstable organisms susceptible to cell lysis.

Pharmacokinetic Parameters

- **Absorption** 46% absorbed.
- **Cmax** 3 mcg/mL after 200 mg PO dose administration.
- **Distribution** Distributed to tissues and fluids, including pleural fluid, synovial fluid, and bone.
- **Protein binding** 40%
- **Metabolism/Excretion** Within 12 hrs 29–33% of dose is excreted unchanged in the urine. Also excreted via biliary route.
- **T1/2** 2–3 hrs

Dosing for Decreased Hepatic Function

No data. Usual dose likely.

Pregnancy Risk

B: Cephalosporins are usually considered safe to use during pregnancy.

Breast Feeding Compatibility

Excreted in breast milk at low concentrations. The American Academy of Pediatrics classifies cephalosporin antibiotics as compatible with breast feeding.

COMMENTS

Oral 3rd generation cephalosporin is effective for the management of uncomplicated GC but more extensive clinical data exists with cefixime. Up to 21% of *S. pneumoniae* are resistant, but the clinical significance is unclear.

SELECTED REFERENCES

Doern GV, Richter SS, Miller A, et al. Antimicrobial resistance among *Streptococcus pneumoniae* in the United States: have we begun to turn the corner on resistance to certain antimicrobial classes? *Clin Infect Dis*, 2005; Vol. 41; pp. 139–48.

Mandell LA, Wunderink RG, Anzueto A, et al. Infectious Diseases Society of America/American Thoracic Society Consensus Guidelines on the Management of Community-Acquired Pneumonia in Adults. *Clin Infect Dis*, 2007; Vol. 44 Suppl 2; pp. S27–72.

CEFPROZIL

Paul A. Pham, PharmD and John G. Bartlett, MD

INDICATIONS

FDA

- Upper respiratory tract infections (acute bronchitis, acute exacerbation of chronic bronchitis (AECB), otitis media, pharyngitis, acute sinusitis, tonsillitis)
- Secondary bacterial Infection of acute bronchitis and AECB caused by *S. pneumoniae*, *H. influenzae*, and *M. catarrhalis*.
- Uncomplicated, skin and skin structure infections caused by MSSA and *S. pyogenes*.

Non-FDA Approved Uses

- Community-acquired pneumonia (CAP)

FORMS

Brand name (mfr)	Forms	Cost*
Cefzil (Bristol-Myers Squibb and generic manufacturers)	PO tab 250 mg; PO tab 500 mg; PO susp 125 mg/5 mL; PO susp 250 mg/5 mL	$4.38; $8.92 $41.84 per 100 mL; $75.83 per 100 mL
*Prices represents Average Wholesale Price (AWP).		

USUAL ADULT DOSING
- URTIs and uncomplicated soft tissue infections: 250 mg–500 mg PO q12h × 10 days.
- CAP: 500 mg PO q12h. Treatment suggested for a minimum of 5 days, pts should be afebrile for 48–72 hrs.
- Avoid cefprozil oral solution in pts with phenylketonuria since it contains 28 mg of phenylalanine per 5 mL.

RENAL DOSING
Dosing for GFR 50–80: Usual dose.
Dosing for GFR 10–50: 0.25 g–0.5 g q24h.
Dosing for GFR <10: 0.25 g q12h.
Dosing in hemodialysis: 250–500 mg post-dialysis.
Dosing in peritoneal dialysis: 0.25 g q12–24h.
Dosing in hemofiltration: No data.

ADVERSE DRUG REACTIONS
General
- Generally well tolerated
Occasional
- Allergic reactions
- Diarrhea and *C. difficile* colitis
- Eosinophilia
- Positive Coombs' test
Rare
- CNS: confusion, disorientation, and hallucinations
- Drug fever
- Neutropenia and thrombocytopenia
- Hepatitis
- Interstitial nephritis
- Anaphylaxis reaction
- Phenylketonuria pts: avoid cefprozil oral solution in such pts with since it contains 28 mg of phenylalanine per 5 mL.

DRUG INTERACTIONS
Probenecid: may increase in cefprozil serum concentration (no dosage adjustment needed).

SPECTRUM—See Appendix II, p. 792
RESISTANCE
- MIC breakpoint for *S. pneumoniae*: 2 mcg/mL
- MIC breakpoint for *Staphylococcus* spp.: 8 mcg/mL
- MIC breakpoint for *Haemophilus* spp.: 8 mcg/mL

PHARMACOLOGY
Mechanism
Cephalosporins like all beta-lactam antibiotics inhibit mucopeptide synthesis in the bacterial cell wall, this results in the formation of defective cell walls and osmotically unstable organisms susceptible to cell lysis.
Pharmacokinetic Parameters
- **Absorption** 95% absorbed.
- **Cmax** 10.5 mcg/mL after 500 mg PO dose administration.
- **Distribution** Distributed to tissues and fluids, including pleural fluid, synovial fluid, and bone. Good penetration in tonsillar and adenoidal tissue. Poor CNS penetration.
- **Protein binding** 65%
- **Metabolism/Excretion** 60–70% of dose excreted in the urine.
- **T1/2** 1.3–1.8 hrs
Dosing for Decreased Hepatic Function
No data. Usual dose likely.
Pregnancy Risk
B: Cephalosporins are usually considered safe to use during pregnancy.
Breast Feeding Compatibility
Excreted in breast milk at low concentrations. The American Academy of Pediatrics classifies cephalosporin antibiotics as compatible with breast feeding.

ANTIBACTERIAL DRUGS

COMMENTS

Oral 2nd generation cephalosporin with good activity against *S. pneumoniae*. One of the IDSA-ATS recommended 2nd generation cephalosporin for the treatment of CAP caused by PCN-susceptible *S. pneumoniae*, but not FDA indicated.

SELECTED REFERENCES

Mandell LA, Wunderink RG, Anzueto A, et al. Infectious Diseases Society of America/American Thoracic Society Consensus Guidelines on the Management of Community-Acquired Pneumonia in Adults. *Clin Infect Dis*, 2007; Vol. 44 Suppl 2; pp. S27–72.

CEFTAZIDIME

Paul A. Pham, PharmD and John G. Bartlett, MD

INDICATIONS

FDA

- Lower respiratory tract infections including pneumonia caused by *P. aeruginosa* and other *Pseudomonas* spp.; *H. influenzae*; *Klebsiella* spp.; *Enterobacter* spp.; *P. mirabilis*; *E. coli*; *Serratia* spp.; *Citrobacter* spp.; *S. pneumoniae*; and MSSA. (cefotaxime or ceftriaxone preferred for *S. pneumoniae*)
- Skin and skin-structure infections caused by *P. aeruginosa*; *Klebsiella* spp.; *E. coli*; *Proteus* spp., including *P. mirabilis* and indole-positive Proteus; *Enterobacter* spp.; *Serratia* spp.; MSSA; and *S. pyogenes*
- Complicated and uncomplicated urinary tract infections caused by *P. aeruginosa*; *Enterobacter* spp.; *Proteus* spp., including *P. mirabilis* and indole-positive Proteus; *Klebsiella* spp.; and *E. coli*
- Septicemia caused by *P. aeruginosa, Klebsiella* spp., *H. influenzae, E. coli, Serratia* spp., *S. pneumoniae,* and MSSA (cefotaxime or ceftriaxone preferred for *S. pneumoniae*)
- Bone and joint infections caused by *P. aeruginosa, Klebsiella* spp., *Enterobacter* spp., and MSSA
- Gynecologic infections (endometritis, pelvic cellulitis, and other GYN infections) caused by *E. coli*
- Intra-abdominal Infections, including peritonitis caused by *E. coli, Klebsiella* spp., and MSSA and polymicrobial infections caused by aerobic and anaerobic organisms (in combination with metronidazole)
- Central nervous system infections including meningitis, caused by *H. influenzae* and *N. meningitidis, P. aeruginosa,* and *S. pneumoniae* (cefotaxime or ceftriaxone preferred for *S. pneumoniae*)

Non-FDA Approved Uses

Shunt Infections

- Diabetic foot infection (in combination with clindamycin)

FORMS

Brand name (mfr)	Forms	Cost*
Fortaz (GlaxoSmithKline and generic manufacturer)	IV or IM vial 500 mg; IV or IM vial 6 g	$7.41; $54.14
Tazicef (Hospira)	IV or IM vial 1 g; IV or IM vial 2 g; IV or IM vial 6 g	$9.05; $19.97; $54.14
*Prices represents Average Wholesale Price (AWP).		

USUAL ADULT DOSING

- Mild to moderate infections: 1 g IV q8–12h.
- Uncomplicated UTI: 500 mg IV q12h.
- Complicated UTI: 500 mg IV q8h–q12h.
- Severe infections or meningitis: 2 g IV q8 (8 g/day max).
- Bone and joint infections: 2 g IV q12h.
- *P. aeruginosa* pneumonia in CF pts: 2 g IV q6h to q8h.

Renal Dosing

Dosing for GFR 50–80: Usual dose.

Dosing for GFR 10–50: GFR >30–50 mL/min: 1 g q12h (2 g q12h for CNS or severe infections); GFR 10–29 mL/min: 1 g q24h (2 g q24 for CNS or severe infections).

Dosing for GFR <10: 0.5 g q24–48h (1 g q24h for CNS or severe infections).

Dosing in hemodialysis: 1 g loading, 1 g post-dialysis.

Dosing in peritoneal dialysis: 0.5–1.0 g loading, 250 mg per each 2 liter of dialysate exchange per day.

Dosing in hemofiltration: CVVH: 1–2 g q12h. CVVHD with flow rate 1.5–2.5 L/hr: 1–2 g q12h (2 g q12h for severe and CNS infections). CVVHD with flow rate 1 L/hr: 1–2 g q24h (2 g q24h for severe and CNS infections).

Adverse Drug Reactions

General

- Generally well tolerated

Occasional

- Phlebitis at infusion sites
- Allergic reactions (cross-reaction in PCN-allergic pts lower compared to 1st and 2nd generation cephalosporin)
- Diarrhea and *C. difficile* colitis
- Eosinophilia
- Positive Coombs' test

Rare

- Anaphylaxis
- Hemolytic anemia
- CNS: convulsions (high dose with renal failure), confusion, disorientation, and hallucinations
- Drug fever
- Neutropenia and thrombocytopenia
- Hepatitis
- Interstitial nephritis

Drug Interactions

Probenecid: increased in ceftazidime serum concentration due to inhibition of tubular secretion by probenecid. No dose adjustment needed; co-administer with caution in renal insufficiency.

Spectrum—See Appendix II, p. 792

Resistance

- MIC breakpoint for Enterobacteriaceae and Gram-negative non-lactose fermenters including *P. aeruginosa* is 8 mcg/mL.

Pharmacology

Mechanism

Cephalosporins like all beta-lactam antibiotics inhibit mucopeptide synthesis in the bacterial cell wall, this results in the formation of defective cell walls and osmotically unstable organisms susceptible to cell lysis.

Pharmacokinetic Parameters

- **Absorption** —
- **Cmax** 60 mcg/mL after 1 g IV dose administration.
- **Distribution** Widely distributed to tissues and fluids, including pleural fluid, synovial fluid, and bone. With inflamed meninges therapeutic concentrations attained. Good penetration into intracranial abscesses.
- **Protein binding** <10%
- **Metabolism/Excretion** Not metabolized. 80–90% of dose excreted unchanged in urine by glomerular filtration within 24 hrs.
- **T1/2** 1.8 hrs

Dosing for Decreased Hepatic Function

No data. Usual dose likely.

Pregnancy Risk

B: Cephalosporins are usually considered safe to use during pregnancy.

ANTIBACTERIAL DRUGS

Breast Feeding Compatibility

Excreted in breast milk at low concentrations. The American Academy of Pediatrics classifies cephalosporin antibiotics as compatible with breast feeding.

COMMENTS

Parenteral 3rd generation cephalosporin with good *P. aeruginosa* activity but resistance rates are up 20–25%. Acinetobacter is showing increasing resistance to ceftazidime (60–70% resistant). Cefepime is comparable to ceftazidime against GNB including *P. aeruginosa* but has better activity vs Gram-positive cocci.

SELECTED REFERENCES

American Thoracic Society, Infectious Diseases Society of America. Guidelines for the management of adults with hospital-acquired, ventilator-associated, and healthcare-associated pneumonia. *Am J Respir Crit Care Med*, 2005; Vol. 171; pp. 388–416.

Gaynes R, Edwards JR, National Nosocomial Infections Surveillance System. Overview of nosocomial infections caused by Gram-negative bacilli. *Clin Infect Dis*, 2005; Vol. 41; pp. 848–54.

CEFTRIAXONE

Paul A. Pham, PharmD and John G. Bartlett, MD

INDICATIONS

FDA

- Lower respiratory tract infections
- Acute otitis media
- Skin and skin-structure infections
- Urinary tract infections
- Uncomplicated gonorrhea
- Pelvic inflammatory disease
- Septicemia
- Bone and joint infections
- Intra-abdominal infections
- Meningitis and surgical prophylaxis

Non-FDA Approved Uses

- Brain abscess (with metronidazole)
- Appendicitis (with metronidazole)
- Peritonitis: spontaneous bacterial and secondary
- Endocarditis
- Diabetic foot infections (with metronidazole or clindamycin)
- Lyme disease: late Lyme arthritis and neuroborreliosis
- Meningococcal meningitis prophylaxis: 125 mg × 1 (<15 yrs); 250 mg × 1 (>15 yrs). Due to reports of fluoroquinolone resistance, rifampin, ceftriaxone, and azithromycin is recommended in selected counties in North Dakota and Minnesota (MMWR 2008; 57:173–175).
- Neurosyphilis
- Disseminated GC

FORMS

Brand name (mfr)	Forms	Cost*
Rocephin (Roche and generic manufacturers)	IV vial 250 mg; IV vial 500 mg IV vial 1 g; IV vial 2 g; IV vial 10 g; IV bag 1 g/50 mL IV bag 2 g/50 mL	$3.00; $2.68 $4.60; $9.14; $53.50; $6.96 $15.00

*Prices represents Average Wholesale Price (AWP).

USUAL ADULT DOSING

Use for meningitis treatment.

- Most infections: 1–2 g IM or IV q24h (up to 4 g max per day).
- Meningitis: 2 g IV q12h.
- Uncomplicated GC: 250 mg IM × 1.

- Surgical prophylaxis: 1 g IV within 1 hr before surgery.
- Obese pts: consider 2 g IV q12h.

RENAL DOSING

Dosing for GFR 50–80: Usual dose.
Dosing for GFR 10–50: Usual dose.
Dosing for GFR <10: Usual dose.
Dosing in hemodialysis: 1–2 g IV q24h (No extra doses needed post dialysis).
Dosing in peritoneal dialysis: Usual regimen.
Dosing in hemofiltration: Usual dose.

ADVERSE DRUG REACTIONS

General

- Generally well tolerated

Occasional

- Pseudocholelithiasis with sludge in gallbladder by ultrasound
- Minimal phlebitis at infusion sites
- Allergic reactions (eosinophilia): cross-allergy to PCN lower than 1st generation cephalosporins
- Diarrhea and *C.difficile* colitis
- Positive Coombs' test

Rare

- CNS: convulsions (high dose with renal failure); confusion, disorientation, and hallucinations
- Drug fever
- Neutropenia and thrombocytopenia
- Hepatitis
- Anaphylaxis reaction
- Hemolytic anemia
- Cholecystitis
- Interstitial nephritis

DRUG INTERACTIONS

- Calcium-ceftriaxone precipitates in the lungs and kidneys in both term and premature neonates (with calcium solution co-administration)
- Calcium containing solutions: ceftriaxone should not be mixed or administered simultaneously or within 48 hrs with calcium-containing solutions or products, even via different infusion lines. Consider using cefotaxime with calcium-containing solution co-administration.
- Probenecid: increase in cephalosporin serum concentration due to inhibition of tubular secretion by probenecid.
- Warfarin: anticoagulation effect may be enhanced.

SPECTRUM—See Appendix II, p. 792

RESISTANCE

- MIC breakpoint for *Enterobacteriaceae* and other Gram-negative *non-*Enterobacteriaceae: ≤8 mcg/mL (sensitive); 16–32 mcg/mL (intermediate); ≥64 mcg/mL (resistant).
- MIC breakpoint for *S. aureus:* ≤8 mcg/mL (sensitive); 16–32 mcg/mL (intermediate); ≥64 mcg/mL (resistant).
- MIC breakpoint for *S. viridans:* ≤1 mcg/mL (sensitive); 2 mcg/mL (intermediate); ≥4 mcg/mL (resistant).
- MIC breakpoint for *S. pneumoniae:* ≤0.5 mcg/mL (meningitis) and ≤1 mcg/mL (non-meningitis).
- MIC breakpoint for beta-hemolytic *Streptococcus* spp.: ≤0.5 mcg/mL.

PHARMACOLOGY

Mechanism

Cephalosporins like all beta-lactam antibiotics inhibit mucopeptide synthesis in the bacterial cell wall, this results in the formation of defective cell walls and osmotically unstable organisms susceptible to cell lysis.

Pharmacokinetic Parameters

- **Cmax** 150 mcg/mL after 1 g IV dose administration.
- **Distribution** Widely distributed to tissues and fluids, including pleural fluid, synovial fluid, and bone. With inflamed meninges therapeutic concentration can be attained with large doses.

ANTIBACTERIAL DRUGS

- **Protein binding** 85–95%; dose of 2 g IV q24h gives better tissue level than 1 g IV q12h because due to decrease in protein binding with larger single dose.
- **Metabolism/Excretion** 33–67% excreted as unchanged drug in urine by glomerular filtration. Remainder is excreted in feces by biliary route.
- **T1/2** 8 hrs.

Dosing for Decreased Hepatic Function
Maximum daily dose is 2 g with severe renal and hepatic impairment.

Pregnancy Risk
B: Cephalosporins are usually considered safe to use during pregnancy.

Breast Feeding Compatibility
Excreted in breast milk at low concentrations. The American Academy of Pediatrics classifies cephalosporin antibiotics as compatible with breast feeding.

COMMENTS
Parenteral 3rd generation cephalosporin w/ convenient once a day dosing often used for out-patient IV therapy. Cefotaxime is clinically equivalent, but given q6h. Excreted via biliary and urinary tracts. May cause biliary sludging and cholecystitis. Cefotaxime and ceftriaxone are the preferred cephalosporins for serious pneumococcal infections (meningitis and pneumonia), but 1.6 to 5+% of strains are resistant.

SELECTED REFERENCES

Doern GV, Richter SS, Miller A, et al. Antimicrobial resistance among *Streptococcus pneumoniae* in the United States: have we begun to turn the corner on resistance to certain antimicrobial classes? *Clin Infect Dis*, 2005; Vol. 41; pp. 139–48.

Fallon BA, Keilp JG, Corbera KM, et al. A randomized, placebo-controlled trial of repeated IV antibiotic therapy for Lyme encephalopathy. *Neurology*, 2008; Vol. 70; pp. 992–1003.

CEFUROXIME

Paul A. Pham, PharmD and John G. Bartlett, MD

INDICATIONS

FDA
- Uncomplicated urinary tract infections caused by *E. coli* or *K. pneumoniae*. (PO and IV)
- Uncomplicated skin and skin-structure infections caused by *S. aureus* or *S. pyogenes* (PO and IV) *E. coli*, *Klebsiella* spp., and *Enterobacter* spp. (IV)
- Uncomplicated urethral and endocervical gonorrhea and ano-rectal gonorrhea (females) caused by *N. gonorrhoeae* (oral and IV)
- Upper respiratory tract infections including acute otitis media, acute maxillary sinusitis, acute exacerbation of chronic bronchitis, and secondary infections of acute bronchitis (PO)
- Early Lyme disease (erythema migrans) caused by *B. burgdorferi* (PO)
- Lower respiratory tract infections including community-acquired pneumonia (CAP, IV)
- Septicemia caused by *S. aureus, S. pneumoniae, E. coli, H. influenzae, Klebsiella* spp. (IV only)
- Meningitis *S. pneumoniae, H. influenzae, N. meningitidis,* and *S. aureus* (MSSA) (IV only). Author's comment: nafcillin preferred for MSSA meningitis.
- Bone and joint infections caused by MSSA (IV)

Non-FDA Approved Uses
- Late Lyme arthritis
- CAP (oral cefuroxime)

FORMS

Brand name (mfr)	Forms	Cost*
Ceftin (GlaxoSmithKline and generic manufacturers)	PO tab 250 mg; PO tab 500 mg PO suspension 125 mg/5 mL; PO suspension 250 mg/5 mL	$4.38; $7.88 $68.51 per 100 mL; $116.61 per 100 mL

Brand name (mfr)	Forms	Cost*
Zinacef (GlaxoSmithKline and generic manufacturers)	IV vial 750 mg; IV vial 1.5 g; IV vial 7.5 g	$3.75; $7.38; $30.00

*Prices represents Average Wholesale Price (AWP).

USUAL ADULT DOSING

- **Parenteral dosing** (mild to moderate infections): 0.75 g IM or IV q8h.
- Bone/joint and severe infections: 1.5 g IV q8h or 1.5 g IV q6h.
- **Oral dosing:** 250–500 mg PO twice daily.
- CAP: treatment should be for a minimum of 5 days and pts should be afebrile for 48–72 hrs.
- Uncomplicated GC: 1000 mg × 1 (but cefixime preferred) **or** 1.5 g IM plus probenecid 1 g × 1 (ceftriaxone preferred).
- Surgical prophylaxis: 1.5 g IV × 1.
- Obese pts: consider 1.5 g IV q6h.

RENAL DOSING

Dosing for GFR 50–80: Usual dose.
Dosing for GFR 10–50: 0.75 g–1.5 g IV q8–12h; no dosage change for oral administration.
Dosing for GFR <10: 0.75 g IV q24h; 250 mg PO q24h.
Dosing in hemodialysis: 750 mg q24h (dose post-HD on HD day).
Dosing in peritoneal dialysis: 750 mg q24h.
Dosing in hemofiltration: No data. Consider 1.5 g IV q12h.

ADVERSE DRUG REACTIONS

Occasional

- Phlebitis at infusion sites
- Allergic reactions
- Diarrhea and *C. difficile* colitis
- Eosinophilia
- Positive Coombs' test

Rare

- Drug fever
- CNS: convulsions (high dose with renal failure), confusion, disorientation, and hallucinations
- Neutropenia and thrombocytopenia
- Hepatitis
- Interstitial nephritis
- Anaphylaxis reaction
- Hemolytic anemia

DRUG INTERACTIONS

Probenecid: increased cefuroxime serum concentration due to inhibition of tubular secretion by probenecid (no dose adjustment needed).

SPECTRUM—See Appendix II, p. 792

RESISTANCE

- MIC breakpoint for *S. pneumoniae:* 0.5 mcg/mL (IV) and 1 mcg/mL (oral).

PHARMACOLOGY

Mechanism

Cephalosporins like all beta-lactam antibiotics inhibit mucopeptide synthesis in the bacterial cell wall; this results in the formation of defective cell walls and osmotically unstable organisms susceptible to cell lysis.

Pharmacokinetic Parameters

- **Absorption** 52% oral absorption.
- **Cmax** 100 mcg/mL after 1.5 g IV dose administration; 4 mcg/mL after 250 mg oral dose administration.

ANTIBACTERIAL DRUGS

- **Distribution** Widely distributed to tissues and fluids, including pleural fluid, synovial fluid, and bone. With inflamed meninges therapeutic concentration can be attained with large doses but generally not used as first line agent.
- **Protein binding** 30–50%
- **Metabolism/Excretion** Not metabolized. 90–100% excreted primarily unchanged in the urine by glomerular filtration and tubular secretion within 24 hrs.
- **T1/2** 1.5 hrs.

Dosing for Decreased Hepatic Function
No data. Usual dose likely.

Pregnancy Risk
B: Cephalosporins are usually considered safe to use during pregnancy.

Breast Feeding Compatibility
Excreted in breast milk at low concentrations. The American Academy of Pediatrics classifies cephalosporin antibiotics as compatible with breast feeding.

COMMENTS
2nd generation oral and parenteral cephalosporin with convenient twice a day dosing schedule. One of the IDSA-ATS recommended 2nd generation cephalosporin for the treatment of CAP caused by PCN-susceptible *S. pneumoniae*.

SELECTED REFERENCES
Mandell LA, Wunderink RG, Anzueto A, et al. Infectious Diseases Society of America/American Thoracic Society consensus guidelines on the management of community-acquired pneumonia in adults. *Clin Infect Dis*, 2007; Vol. 44 Suppl 2; pp. S27–72.

Scott LJ, Ormrod D, Goa KL. Cefuroxime axetil: an updated review of its use in the management of bacterial infections. *Drugs*, 2001; Vol. 61; pp. 1455–500.

CEPHALEXIN

Paul A. Pham, PharmD and John G. Bartlett, MD

INDICATIONS
FDA
- Respiratory tract infections *S. pneumoniae* and *S. pyogenes* (author's comment: generally not recommended)
- Otitis media caused by *S. pneumoniae, H. influenzae*, MSSA, *S. pyogenes,* and *M. catarrhalis*
- Skin and skin-structure infections caused by *S. pyogenes* and *S. aureus* (MSSA)
- Osteomyelitis: MSSA and/or *P. mirabilis* (author's comment: not a first-line agent)
- Urinary tract infections including acute prostatitis caused by *E. coli, P. mirabilis*, and *K. pneumoniae* (author's comment: not a first-line agent)

Non-FDA Approved Uses
- Furuncle/carbuncle (MSSA)
- Impetigo
- Cellulitis/erysipelas
- Folliculitis (MSSA)
- Bacterial cystitis, acute, uncomplicated
- Mastitis (MSSA)

FORMS

Brand name (mfr)	Forms	Cost*
Panixine Disperdose (Ranbaxy)	PO tab 250 mg; PO tab 500 mg	$1.14; $2.25
Keflex (Advantus Pharm)	PO cap 250 mg; PO cap 500 mg; PO cap 750 mg PO susp 125 mg/5 mL; PO susp 250 mg/5 mL	$0.69; $1.21; $3.12 $8.93 per 100 mL; $18.90 per 100 mL
*Prices represents Average Wholesale Price (AWP).		

USUAL ADULT DOSING

* Mild skin infections (streptococcal pharyngitis and uncomplicated cystitis): consider 500 mg PO q12h.
* Mild to moderate infections: 250–500 mg PO q6h.
* Severe infections: consider an IV cephalosporin.

RENAL DOSING

Dosing for GFR 50–80: Usual dose.

Dosing for GFR 10–50: 0.25 g–1.0 g q8–12h.

Dosing for GFR <10: 0.25 g–1 g q24–48h.

Dosing in hemodialysis: 0.25 g–1 g q24h plus 0.25–1.0 g post-dialysis.

Dosing in peritoneal dialysis: 250 mg three times a day.

Dosing in hemofiltration: No data. Consider 1 g q12h.

ADVERSE DRUG REACTIONS

Common

* Generally well tolerated

Occasional

* Allergic reactions (eosinophilia)
* Diarrhea and *C. difficile* colitis
* Positive Coombs' test (without hemolytic anemia)

Rare

* Drug fever
* Neutropenia and thrombocytopenia
* Hepatitis
* Anaphylaxis reaction
* CNS: convulsions (high dose with renal failure), confusion, disorientation, and hallucinations.
* Hemolytic anemia (theoretical, case reports with ceftriaxone, cefotetan, cefoxitin, cefamandole, ceftazidime, and cefalothin)

DRUG INTERACTIONS

Probenecid: increase in cephalosporin serum concentration due to inhibition of tubular secretion by probenecid. No dose adjustment needed, but close monitoring recommended in ESRD.

SPECTRUM—See Appendix II, p. 792

PHARMACOLOGY

Mechanism

Cephalosporins like all beta-lactam antibiotics inhibit mucopeptide synthesis in the bacterial cell wall, this results in the formation of defective cell walls and osmotically unstable organisms susceptible to cell lysis.

Pharmacokinetic Parameters

* **Absorption** 90% absorbed
* **Cmax** 18–38 mcg/mL after 500 mg PO dose administration
* **Distribution** Widely distributed to tissues and fluids, including pleural fluid, synovial fluid, and bone. High concentration in purulent sputum of inflamed bronchi. Low CNS penetration.
* **Protein binding** 5–15%
* **Metabolism/Excretion** Mainly excreted unchanged in urine from glomerular filtration and tubular secretion. Small amount of biliary excretion.
* **T1/2** 1.0 hr.

Dosing for Decreased Hepatic Function

Usual dose.

Pregnancy Risk

B: Cephalosporins are usually considered safe to use during pregnancy.

Breast Feeding Compatibility

Excreted in breast milk at low concentrations. The American Academy of Pediatrics classifies cephalosporin antibiotics as compatible with breast feeding.

COMMENTS

Well absorbed 1st generation cephalosporin with good Gram-positive coverage and a low price but q6–8h dosing may decrease pt compliance. With the increasing prevalence of community-acquired MRSA soft tissue infections, use of cephalexin for moderate or serious infections should be guided by sensitivity data.

ANTIBACTERIAL DRUGS

SELECTED REFERENCES

Blaser MJ, Klaus BD, Jacobson JA, et al. Comparison of cefadroxil and cephalexin in the treatment of community-acquired pneumonia. *Antimicrob Agents Chemother*, 1983; Vol. 24; pp. 163–7.

Stevens DL, Bisno AL, Chambers HF, et al. Practice guidelines for the diagnosis and management of skin and soft-tissue infections. *Clin Infect Dis*, 2005; Vol. 41; pp. 1373–406.

CHLORAMPHENICOL

Paul A. Pham, PharmD and John G. Bartlett, MD

INDICATIONS

FDA

- Note: use only in those serious infections for which less potentially dangerous drugs are ineffective or contraindicated.
- Acute infections caused by *Salmonella typhi*
- Serious infections caused by *Salmonella* species, *H. influenzae,* specially meningeal infections, Rickettsia, Lymphogranuloma-psittacosis Chlamydia group, various Gram-negative bacteria causing bacteremia and meningitis.
- Part of a cystic fibrosis regimen when other agents are ineffective or contraindicated.
- Ocular infections (ophthalmic drops and ointments)

Non-FDA Approved Uses

- Lung abscess
- Gas gangrene (in PCN allergic pts)
- Brain abscess
- Paratyphoid fever
- Q fever (*Coxiella burnetii*)
- Rocky mountain spotted fever and other endemic (murine or scrub) typhus infections caused by Rickettsia species
- Ehrlichiosis
- Meningitis in PCN-allergic pts

FORMS

Brand name (mfr)	Forms	Cost*
Chloromycetin (Monarch)	IV vial 1000 mg	$29.94
Chloramphenicol (Various non-U.S. manufacturer)	PO capsule 250 mg Ophthalmic ophthalmic solution 0.5% Ophthalmic ophthalmic ointment 1%	n/a n/a n/a

*Prices represents Average Wholesale Price (AWP).

USUAL ADULT DOSING

- 50 mg/kg IV in 4 divided doses (up to 100 mg/kg/day).
- 250–500 mg PO q6h (usual dose is 500 mg PO q6h (oral formulation unavailable in U.S.).
- *S. typhi*: Administer for 8 to 10 days after the pts has become afebrile to decrease relapse rate.

RENAL DOSING

Dosing for GFR 50–80: Usual dose.
Dosing for GFR 10–50: Usual dose.
Dosing for GFR <10: Usual dose. Monitor serum concentrations.
Dosing in hemodialysis: Usual dose + 500 mg, dose post-dialysis. Monitor serum concentrations.
Dosing in peritoneal dialysis: Usual regimen.
Dosing in hemofiltration: Limited data; may be removed. Monitor serum concentrations.

ADVERSE DRUG REACTIONS

Occasional

- GI intolerance with oral administration.
- Bone marrow suppression (more likely with >4 g per day or with serum level >25 mcg/mL).

Rare
- Fatal aplastic anemia (not dose related). Occurs at a rate of 1 per 40,000
- "Gray baby syndrome" with cyanosis and circulatory collapse
- Optic neuritis
- Peripheral neuropathy
- Fever
- Allergic reactions
- *C. difficile* colitis

DRUG INTERACTIONS
- HIV protease inhibitors (e.g., atazanavir, indinavir): may increase chloramphenicol serum concentrations. Use with close monitoring for bone marrow suppression.
- Phenobarbital: may decrease chloramphenicol serum concentrations.
- Rifampin: may decrease serum concentration of chloramphenicol.
- Sulfonylureas (chlorpropamide, tolbutamide): chloramphenicol may inhibit hepatic metabolism of some sulfonylureas resulting in prolongation of half-life and resultant hypoglycemia.
- Vitamin B_{12}: hematologic effects of Vit B_{12} in pts with pernicious anemia may be decreased.
- Warfarin: may increase anticoagulant effect of warfarin. Monitor INR closely with co-administration.

SPECTRUM—See Appendix II, p. 804

PHARMACOLOGY
Mechanism
Chloramphenicol inhibits protein synthesis by binding to 50S ribosomal subunits, preventing binding of amino acyl t-RNA and inhibiting polypeptide synthesis.
- **Absorption** 80% absorbed.
- **Cmax** 11–18 mcg/mL after 1 g PO dose administration.
- **Distribution** Widely distributed into most body tissues and fluids including liver, kidney, saliva, ascitic fluid, pleural fluid, synovial fluid, and aqueous and vitreous humor. Good CNS penetration with inflamed meninges.
- **Protein binding** 60%.
- **Metabolism/Excretion** Metabolized in the liver by glucuronyl transferase. Metabolite and 30% of unchanged drug excreted in urine by glomerular filtration.
- **T1/2** 1.5–3.5 hrs.

Dosing for Decreased Hepatic Function
Use with caution with renal and/or hepatic failure; monitor serum levels to achieve levels between 5–20 mcg/mL.

Pregnancy Risk
C: A collaborative perinatal project monitored 98 exposures during the first trimester, 348 exposures anytime during pregnancy found no evidence of relationship with chloramphenicol and malformation. Although apparently nontoxic to the fetus, chloramphenicol should not be used near term due to the potential of "gray baby syndrome."

Breast Feeding Compatibility
Excreted in breast milk. The American Academy of Pediatrics classifies chloramphenicol as an agent whose effect on the nursing infant as unknown but may be of concern because of the potential of idiosyncratic bone marrow suppression.

COMMENTS
Oral and parenteral broad spectrum drug that is infrequently used in the U.S. due to rare idiosyncratic toxicity of aplastic anemia (1:40,000, more commonly associated with oral administration) and the availability of alternative agents. May be used as a second line agent (with vancomycin) for the empiric treatment of bacterial meningitis in PCN-allergic pts. Oral formulation unavailable in U.S.

SELECTED REFERENCES
Lennard ES, Minshew BH, Dellinger EP, et al. Stratified outcome comparison of clindamycin-gentamicin vs chloramphenicol-gentamicin for treatment of intra-abdominal sepsis. *Arch Surg*, 1985; Vol. 120; pp. 889–98.

Peltola H, Anttila M, Renkonen OV. Randomised comparison of chloramphenicol, ampicillin, cefotaxime, and ceftriaxone for childhood bacterial meningitis. Finnish Study Group. *Lancet*, 1989; Vol. 1; pp. 1281–7.

ANTIBACTERIAL DRUGS

CIPROFLOXACIN

Paul A. Pham, PharmD and John G. Bartlett, MD

INDICATIONS

FDA

- Uncomplicated UTI (Cipro XR and ciprofloxacin), complicated UTI (ciprofloxin)
- Post-exposure prophylaxis for inhalation anthrax. CDC recommends as first line agent + 1–2 additional agent(s) with *in vitro* activity (for inhalation anthrax, see "biodefense-anthrax" module)
- Complicated intra-abdominal infections (in combination with metronidazole)
- Infectious diarrhea
- Endocervical and urethral infections caused *N. gonorrhoeae* (note: high resistance rates reported in Hawaii and California)
- Empiric therapy for neutropenic fever (in combination with piperacillin); typhoid fever
- Nosocomial pneumonia
- Prostatitis
- Acute sinusitis
- Skin and soft tissue infections; bone and joint infections; bacterial conjunctivitis (opthalmic ointment); bacterial conjunctivitis and corneal ulcers (ophthalmic solution); Acute otitis externa (otic suspension)

Non-FDA Approved Uses

- MTB, MAI and other MOTT infections (2nd or 3rd line)
- Empiric therapy for neutropenic fever (in combination amoxicillin-clavulanate) in low-risk pts (defined as neutropenia expected to be present for no more than 10 days during CA chemotherapy).

FORMS

Brand name (mfr)	Forms	Cost*
Cipro (Bayer and various generic manufacturers)	Oral Tablet 250 mg; 500 mg; 750 mg IV Vial 200 mg; IV Vial 400 mg Oral Tablet 100 mg (6 pack) Oral XR tablet 500 mg; 1000 mg;	$5.49; $6.42; $6.73 $15.00; $30.00 $22.60 per pack $10.90; $12.40
Ciprodex (Alcon Labs)	Otic Suspension Cipro 0.3%/ Dexa 0.1% (7.5 mL)	$98.38
Cipro HC Otic (Alcon Labs)	Otic Suspension Cipro 0.2%/ HC 1% (10 mL)	$98.38
Ciloxan (Alcon Labs)	Topical Ophthalmic gtt 0.3% (2.5 mL; 5 mL; 10 mL) Topical Ophthalmic oint 0.3% (3.5 g)	$57.13 per 5 mL $67.38
*Prices represents Average Wholesale Price (AWP).		

USUAL ADULT DOSING

- Uncomplicated UTI: 250 mg PO twice daily or cipro XR 500 mg once daily PO × 3 days.
- Complicated UTI: 500 mg PO twice daily × 7–10 days.
- Nosocomial pneumonia (*P. aeruginosa*): 400 mg IV q8h, then 750 mg PO twice daily × 10–14 days.
- Salmonellosis: 500–750 mg PO twice daily or 400 mg IV twice daily × 7–14 days for mild disease (note: treat for 4–6 wks in HIV-infected pts w/ CD4 <200 and/or bacteremia).
- Traveler's diarrhea: 500 mg PO twice daily × 3 days.
- MTB/MAI and other MOTT: 750 mg PO twice daily.
- Acute otitis externa: 4 drops (cipro/dexamethasone) into the affected ear twice daily × 7 days.
- Bacterial conjunctivitis: 1–2 ophthalmic drops to the affected eye's conjunctival sac q2 hrs while awake × 2 days, then 1–2 drops q4h while awake × 5 days.

- Meningococcal meningitis prophylaxis in adults: 500 mg × 1. Due to reports of fluoroquinolone resistance, rifampin, ceftriaxone, and azithromycin is recommended in selected counties in North Dakota and Minnesota (*MMWR* 2008;57:173).
- Anthrax: see specific module.
- Obese pts: use 400 mg IV q8h.

RENAL DOSING
Dosing for GFR 50–80: Usual dose.
Dosing for GFR 10–50: GFR >30 mL/min: 400 mg IV q12h (250 mg–500 mg PO q12h). GFR <30 mL/min: 400 mg IV q24h (250 mg–500 mg PO q12h).
Dosing for GFR <10: 400 mg IV q24h (250 mg–500 mg PO q12h).
Dosing in hemodialysis: 200 mg–400 mg IV q24h (250 mg–500 mg PO q24h). Give post-HD on days of dialysis.
Dosing in peritoneal dialysis: 200 mg–400 mg IV q24h (250 mg–500 mg PO q24h).
Dosing in hemofiltration: CVVH: 200 mg IV q12h. CVVHD: 400 mg q12h.

ADVERSE DRUG REACTIONS
- Generally well tolerated.

Occasional
- GI intolerance: nausea and diarrhea
- CNS: headache, malaise, insomnia, restlessness, and dizziness
- Candida vaginitis
- *C. difficile*–associated colitis

Rare
- Tendon rupture (increased incidence especially seen in older pts over age 60, concurrent use of corticosteroids, kidney, heart, and lung transplant recipients)
- Photosensitivity /phototoxicity reaction (can be severe)
- Allergic reactions
- QTc prolongation
- Transaminases elevation and rare cases of hepatic failure
- Peripheral neuropathy
- Crystalluria
- Seizure
- Severe allergic reactions (TEN, Stevens-Johnsons syndrome, allergic pneumonitis, hepatitis, and bone marrow suppression)
- Interstitial nephritis

DRUG INTERACTIONS—See Appendix III, p. 808, for table of drug-to-drug interactions.
- Milk or dairy products: decreased GI absorption of ciprofloxacin by 36–47%. Administer ciprofloxacin 2 hrs before dairy products.

SPECTRUM—See Appendix II, p. 798
RESISTANCE
- *Pseudomonas aeruginosa, Acinetobacter* spp., *Enterobacteriaceae* spp., and other non-*Enterobacteriaceae* spp. breakpoints: ≤1 mcg/mL (sensitive); 2 mcg/mL (intermediate); ≥4 mcg/mL (resistant).
- *Staphylococcus* spp. and *Enterococcus* spp. breakpoints: ≤1 mcg/mL (sensitive); 2 mcg/mL (intermediate); ≥4 mcg/mL (resistant).

PHARMACOLOGY
Mechanism
Fluoroquinolones inhibits DNA topoisomerases (DNA gyrase and topoisomerase 4) by binding to DNA-enzyme complexes, thereby interfering with bacterial DNA replication and some aspects of transcription, repair, recombination, and transposition.

Pharmacokinetic Parameters
- **Absorption** 50–85% absorbed. Not significantly affected by food.
- **Cmax** 2.5–4.3 mcg/mL after 750 mg PO dose administration and 4.6 mcg/mL after 400 mg IV dose administration.
- **Distribution** Fluoroquinolones are widely distributed to most body fluids and tissues. High concentrations are attained in the kidneys, gallbladder, GYN tissues, liver, lung, prostatic tissue, phagocytic cells, urine, sputum, and bile. Skin, fat, muscle, bone, and cartilage. CNS

ANTIBACTERIAL DRUGS

penetration: 11–67% (use higher dose for CNS infections 400 mg IV q8h). Increased Vd and decreased tissue penetration in obese pts.

- **Protein binding** 13–43%
- **Metabolism/Excretion** 10–15% of dose is metabolized to desethylene, sulfo, oxo, N-formyl active metabolite. Metabolite and 15–50% of unchanged drug is excreted in urine by glomerular filtration and tubular secretion. 20–40% of dose excreted in feces mainly by biliary excretion.
- **T1/2** 4 hrs.

Dosing for Decreased Hepatic Function

No data. Usual dose likely.

Pregnancy Risk

C: In a prospective follow-up study conducted by the European Network of Teratology Information Services (ENTIS), 666 cases of fluoroquinolone exposure (the majority of the exposures were during the first trimester) showed a congenital malformation rate of 4.8%. From previous epidemiologic data, the 4.8% did not exceed the background rate. Animal data demonstrated arthropathy in immature animals with erosions in joint cartilage. Because of the animal data, and the availability of alternative antimicrobial agents, the use of fluoroquinolones during pregnancy is considered contraindicated due to concerns with arthropathy.

Breast Feeding Compatibility

Fluoroquinolones are not recommended during breast feeding due to the potential for arthropathy (based on animal data).

COMMENTS

Oral and parenteral fluoroquinolone with best clinical and *in vitro* data for activity against *P. aeruginosa*, but resistance rates have increased over the yrs. Experience is favorable and extensive for nosocomial pneumonia, osteomyelitis, neutropenic fever, travelers diarrhea, chronic prostatitis, and UTIs. Other fluoroquinolones (e.g., levofloxacin and moxifloxacin) are preferred for infections due to *S. pneumoniae*. Ciprofloxacin may be used as a 3rd or 4th line agent for MDR TB and MAC infections in HIV-infected pts. Like other fluoroquinolones, ciprofloxacin may result in false positive opiate screen (*JAMA* 2001;286:3115–9). No longer recommended for the gonococcus due to raising rates of FQ resistance.

SELECTED REFERENCES

Henry DC, Bettis RB, Riffer E, et al. Comparison of once daily extended-release ciprofloxacin and conventional twice daily ciprofloxacin for the treatment of uncomplicated urinary tract infection in women. *Clin Ther*, 2002; Vol. 24; pp. 2088–104.

Ho PL, Que TL, Chiu SS, et al. Fluoroquinolone and other antimicrobial resistance in invasive pneumococci, Hong Kong, 1995–2001. *Emerg Infect Dis*, 2004; Vol. 10; pp. 1250–7.

CLARITHROMYCIN

Paul A. Pham, PharmD and John G. Bartlett, MD

INDICATIONS

FDA

- Pharyngitis and tonsillitis
- Acute maxillary sinusitis (Biaxin and Biaxin XL)
- Acute bacterial exacerbation of chronic bronchitis (Biaxin and Biaxin XL)
- Community acquired pneumonia (Biaxin and Biaxin XL)
- Acute otitis media
- Uncomplicated skin and skin structure infections
- Treatment of disseminated mycobacterial infections due to *Mycobacterium avium*
- Prophylaxis of *Mycobacterium avium*
- Treatment of active duodenal ulcer associated with *H. pylori* infection (in combination with omeprazole or ranitidine bismuth citrate)

Non-FDA Approved Uses

- Bartonella

FORMS

Brand name (mfr)	Forms	Cost*
Biaxin (Abbott)	Oral tablet 250 mg; oral tablet 500 mg Oral suspension 125 mg/5 mL (50 mL and 100 mL bottle); Oral suspension 250 mg/5 mL (50 mL and 100 mL bottle)	$6.19; $6.19 $50.70 (100 mL bottle); $96.64 (100 mL bottle)
Biaxin XL (Abbott)	Oral XL tablet 500 mg	$6.62
Clarithromycin (Generic manufacturers)	Oral tablet 250 mg; oral tablet 500 mg Oral suspension 125 mg/5 mL (50 mL and 100 mL bottle); oral suspension 250 mg/5 mL (50 mL and 100 mL bottle)	$5.86; $5.86 $43.02 (100 mL bottle); $81.99 (100 mL bottle)

*Prices represents Average Wholesale Price (AWP).

USUAL ADULT DOSING
- Community acquired pneumonia, pharyngitis, tonsillitis, otitis media, and uncomplicated soft tissue infections: 250–500 mg PO twice daily or 1000 mg XL PO once daily × 7 days.
- Infections due to *H. influenzae* and *H. parainfluenzae:* 500 mg PO twice daily × 7–14 days.
- Acute bacterial sinusitis: 500 mg PO twice daily (immediate release formulation) or 1000 mg PO once daily w/ food (XL formulation) × 7–14 days.
- Acute exacerbation of chronic bronchitis: 500 mg PO twice daily (immediate release formulation) or 1000 mg PO once daily w/ food (XL formulation) × 7 days.
- MAC treatment: 500 mg PO twice daily or 1000 mg XL PO once daily (in combination with ethambutol) × 1 yr and treat until immune reconstitution (CD4 >100 × 6 mos).
- MAC prophylaxis: 500 mg PO twice daily (azithromycin 1200 mg q wk preferred).
- Peptic ulcer disease due to *H. pylori*: 500 mg PO (in combination with PPI and amoxicillin) twice daily × 10–14 days.

RENAL DOSING
Dosing for GFR 50–80: Usual dose.
Dosing for GFR 10–50: 50% of dose (500 mg once daily) with Cr clearance <30 mL/min, especially important with HIV protease inhibitor co-administration.
Dosing for GFR <10: 250 mg–500 mg q24h.
Dosing in hemodialysis: 500 mg q24h, on days of dialysis dose post-dialysis.
Dosing in peritoneal dialysis: No data. Consider 250–500 mg PO q24h.
Dosing in hemofiltration: No data. Consider 500 mg PO q24h.

ADVERSE DRUG REACTIONS
Occasional
- GI intolerance (diarrhea, nausea, vomiting)
- Metallic taste
- Transaminase elevations

Rare
- Headache
- Reversible hearing loss and tinnitus
- *C. difficile* colitis
- Rash

DRUG INTERACTIONS—See Appendix III, p. 809, for table of drug-to-drug interactions.
- Clarithromycin is a substrate and inhibitor of CYP3A4. May increase CYP3A4 substrate drugs. Inhibitors of CYP3A4 may increase clarithromycin serum concentrations. Inducers of CYP3A4 substrates may decrease clarithromycin serum concentrations.

SPECTRUM—See Appendix II, p. 800
RESISTANCE
- *S. pneumoniae* macrolide resistance ~26% but clinical significance unclear (especially with intermediate resistance); treatment failures not consistently reported.
- Use of clarithromycin monotherapy for MAC infections is associated with developing high rates of resistance. Combination therapy (usually with ethambutol +/– rifabutin) recommended. Drug sensitivity testing may help guide therapy but clinical significance is unclear.

ANTIBACTERIAL DRUGS

521

PHARMACOLOGY

Mechanism

Macrolides inhibit protein synthesis by binding to 50S ribosomal subunits, inhibiting transloca-tion of peptidase chain, and inhibiting polypeptide synthesis. Clarithromycin is methylated at position 6 of the lactone ring; this minimizes acid-catalyzed degradation of clarithromycin.

Pharmacokinetic Parameters

- **Absorption** 55% absorbed.
- **Cmax** 2–3 mcg/mL after 500 mg PO dose administration.
- **Distribution** Clarithromycin and 14-hydroxyclarithromycin has high intracellular concentration, resulting in higher tissue concentration than serum concentration. Poor CNS penetration.
- **Protein binding** 42–72%.
- **Metabolism/Excretion** Clarithromycin undergo extensive first-pass metabolism to the active 14-hydroxy metabolite. Both active metabolite and unchanged drug is excreted in urine (38%) and feces (40%).
- **T1/2** 5–7 hrs.

Dosing for Decreased Hepatic Function

No dose adjustment needed. Dosage adjustment with concomitant renal dysfunction (*Chu J Clin Pharmacol* 1993;33:480).

Pregnancy Risk

C: Studies in monkeys show growth retardation. The teratogen information service in Philadel-phia reported the outcome of 34 1st or 2nd trimester exposure were similar to those expected in nonexposed population.

Breast Feeding Compatibility

Excreted into breast milk. The American Academy of Pediatrics consider erythromycin compat-ible with breast feeding. Risk to clarithromycin exposure is probably minimal.

COMMENTS

Oral macrolide with debated *in vitro* activity vs. *H. influenzae*. However, clinical trials showed elim-ination of this pathogen support the contention that it has *in vivo* activity against *H. influenzae*. An important component of treatment of *H. pylori*, *M. avium* complex, and other MOTT infections. The XL formulation has comparable efficacy and toxicity to immediate release formulation, but is more expensive than generic clarithromycin.

SELECTED REFERENCES

Benson CA, Williams PL, Currier JS, et al. A prospective, randomized trial examining the efficacy and safety of clarithro-mycin in combination with ethambutol, rifabutin, or both for the treatment of disseminated *Mycobacterium avium* complex disease in persons with acquired immunodeficiency syndrome. *Clin Infect Dis*, 2003; Vol. 37; pp. 1234–43.

Hoban DJ and Zhanel GG. Clinical implications of macrolide resistance in community-acquired respiratory tract infec-tions. *Expert Rev Anti Infect Ther*, 2006; Vol. 4; pp. 973–80.

CLINDAMYCIN

Paul A. Pham, PharmD and John G. Bartlett, MD

INDICATIONS

FDA

- Skin and soft tissue infections caused by streptococci, staphylococci, and anaerobes
- Pelvic infections (endometritis, nongonococcal tubo-ovarian abscess, pelvic cellulitis, and postsurgical vaginal cuff infections)
- Intra-abdominal infections such as peritonitis and intra-abdominal abscess caused by anaerobes (note: IDSA no longer recommends clindamycin due to increased *B. fragilis* resistance rate)
- *Streptococcus pneumoniae* (empyema, pneumonitis, and lung abscess)
- Septicemia (no longer recommended)
- Acne vulgaris (topical gel)
- Bacterial vaginosis in non-pregnant women (vaginal ovules)

Non-FDA Approved Uses

- Treatment of PCP in combination with primaquine
- Treatment of CNS toxoplasmosis in combination with pyrimethamine and leucovorin

- CA-MRSA soft tissue infections.
- CA-MRSA pneumonia (may be considered in combination with vancomycin to decrease toxin production in severe cases)
- Actinomycosis
- Osteomyelitis
- Acute bacterial sinusitis

FORMS

Brand name (mfr)	Forms	Cost*
Cleocin (Pfizer and other generic manufacturers)	Oral capsule 150 mg; Oral capsule 300 mg	$1.20; $3.76
Cleocin phosphate (Pfizer)	IV vial 300 mg; 600 mg; 900 mg	$5.06; $9.16; $13.28
Cleocin pediatric solution (Pfizer)	Oral solution 75 mg/5 mL	$61.10 (100 mL)
Cleocin vaginal suppository (Pfizer)	Vaginal ovule suppository 100 mg	$23.51
Cleocin T (Pfizer)	Topical gel 1% (30 g; 60 g) Topical lotion 1% (60 mL)	$62.76; $113.03 $87.33

*Prices represents Average Wholesale Price (AWP).

USUAL ADULT DOSING

- Soft tissue infection: 300–450 mg PO q6h or 600 mg IV q8h × 14 days then reassess.
- Pelvic inflammatory disease: 900 mg IV q8h (in combination with gentamicin) × 14 days.
- Osteomyelitis: 600 mg IV q8h × 6–8 wks then reassess.
- Acute bacterial sinusitis: 300 mg PO q6h × 2–3 wks.
- Bacterial vaginosis: 100 mg vaginal suppository qhs × 3–7 days.
- Acne: 1–2 topical applications daily.
- Actinomycosis: 600 mg IV q8h × 2–6 wks, then clindamycin 300 mg PO q6h × 6–12 mos.
- PCP: clindamycin 600 mg IV q6h–q8h or 300 mg–450 mg PO q6h–8h + primaquine 15–30 mg (base) PO once daily +/– prednisone (recommended for $P_aO_2 < 70$) × 21 days.
- CNS toxoplasmosis: clindamycin 600 mg IV q6h or clindamycin 450 mg–600 mg PO q6h + pyrimethamine 200 mg PO loading dose, then 50–75 mg PO q24hd + leucovorin 10–20 mg q24hd until immune reconstitution (CD4 >200 on stable HAART for 6–12 mos).
- Cleocin caps should be taken with a full glass of water to avoid esophageal irritation.

RENAL DOSING

Dosing for GFR 50–80: Usual dose.
Dosing for GFR 10–50: Usual dose.
Dosing for GFR <10: Usual dose.
Dosing in hemodialysis: Usual regimen.
Dosing in peritoneal dialysis: Usual regimen.
Dosing in hemofiltration: Usual dose.

ADVERSE DRUG REACTIONS

Common

- Diarrhea (not due to *C.difficile* in 10–30%)
- GI intolerance: nausea, vomiting, and anorexia

Occasional

- Generalized morbilliform rash
- *C. difficile* colitis in 6% of pts

Rare

- Stevens-Johnson syndrome
- Allergic-type reactions (including bronchial asthma) in pts who have aspirin hyper-sensitivity (from tartrazine found in the 75 and 150 mg caps)

ANTIBACTERIAL DRUGS

ANTIBACTERIAL

Drug Interactions
- Erythromycin: *in vitro* antagonism. Clinical significance unclear. Avoid co-administration.
- Kaolin-pectin: decreases clindamycin absorption.
- Loperamide and diphenoxylate/atropine: may increase risk of diarrhea and *C. difficile*-associated colitis. Avoid use with clindamycin.
- Nondepolarizing muscle relaxant (pancuronium, tubocurarine): lincosamides may enhances the action of nondepolarizing muscle relaxants. Use with caution in pts receiving such agents.

Spectrum—See Appendix II, p. 800
Resistance
- MIC breakpoint of 0.5 mcg/mL for *Staphylococci*.

Pharmacology
Mechanism
Inhibits protein synthesis by binding to 50S ribosomal subunits, interfering with transpeptidation and early chain termination.

Pharmacokinetic Parameters
- **Absorption** 90% absorbed.
- **Cmax** 10 mcg/mL after 600 mg IV and 2.5 mcg/mL after 150 mg IV and PO dose administration, respectively.
- **Distribution** Distributed to many body tissues and fluids including ascites fluid, pleural fluid, synovial fluid, bone, bile, and saliva. Poor CNS penetration.
- **Protein binding** 85–94%.
- **Metabolism/Excretion** Metabolized to sulfoxide and N-dimethyl metabolites. Only 10% is excreted in urine within 24 hrs. Majority excreted as inactive metabolite in feces and bile.
- **T1/2** 2.4 hrs.

Dosing for Decreased Hepatic Function
Dose reduction recommended for severe hepatic failure.

Pregnancy Risk
B: In a surveillance study of Michigan Medicaid recipients, 647 exposures to clindamycin during the 1st trimester resulted in 4.8% birth defects. These data do not support an association between clindamycin and congenital effects.

Breast Feeding Compatibility
Excreted into breast milk. The American Academy of Pediatrics considers clindamycin to be compatible with breast feeding.

Comments
Oral and parenteral lincomycins have good activity vs. anaerobes; increasing resistance with *B. fragilis* makes metronidazole a more reliable agent for intrabdominal infections. On a per pt basis, clindamycin is the antimicrobial most likely to cause *C. difficile* colitis, but many more pts get diarrhea (antibiotic-related) without *C. difficile* colitis. Prescribe with caution in individuals with h/o colitis. Four times a day dosing may limit pt adherence. A first-line oral treatment option for CA-MRSA soft tissue infection due to good tissue penetration (and a theoretical benefit of toxin inhibition), but should not be used with bacteremia.

Selected References
Smego RA, Nagar S, Maloba B, et al. A meta-analysis of salvage therapy for *Pneumocystis carinii pneumonia*. *Arch Intern Med*, 2001; Vol. 161; pp. 1529–33.
Snydman DR, Jacobus NV, McDermott LA, et al. National survey on the susceptibility of *Bacteroides Fragilis* Group: report and analysis of trends for 1997–2000. *Clin Infect Dis*, 2002; Vol. 35; pp. S126–34.

COLISTIMETHATE (COLISTIN)

Paul A. Pham, PharmD and John G. Bartlett, MD

Indications
FDA
- Enteritis (caused by *E. coli*)
- External auditory canal infections (in combination with neomycin and hydrocortisone)
- Mastoid infections (in combination with neomycin and hydrocortisone)
- Shigella gastroenteritis

- Acute or chronic infections due to sensitive strains of *Pseudomonas aeruginosa*; cystic fibrosis; disease due to Gram-negative bacteria, Enterobacter aerogenes, *E. coli, Klebsiella pneumoniae*

Non-FDA Approved Uses

- Infections caused by multi-drug resistant *Acinetobacter baumannii, Klebsiella pneumoniae*, and *Pseudomonas aeruginosa.*

FORMS

Brand name (mfr)	Forms	Cost*
Coly-Mycin M (Monarch)	IV vial 150 mg	$57.00
Coly-Mycin S Otic (JHP Pharmaceuticals, LLC)	Otic drops 5 mL	$47.28
*Prices represents Average Wholesale Price (AWP).		

USUAL ADULT DOSING

- Severe infections caused by MDR Gram-negative organisms: 2.5–5 mg/kg/day IV divided q8–12h (5 mg/kg/day divided q12h for severe infections).
- Inhalation: 75 mg in 3 mL NS via nebulizer twice daily. Note: ask pharmacy to reconstitute drug shortly prior to inhalation, since otherwise prodrug colistimethate may convert to biologically active colistin which if given significantly by aerosol route may lead to ARDS.
- Intraventricular or intrathecal colistin: 5 mg q12h, up to 10 mg q12h (Falagas EM et al. *Int. J. Antimicrobial Agents* 2007; Guardado AR et al. *JAC* 2008).
- Unit conversion: colistin sulfate (used for MIC testing) 1 mg = 30,000 units. For colistin methanesulfonate (aka CMS, colistimethate, sulphomethate) 2.5 mg CMS = 30,000 units.
- PK modeling suggest the need for a loading dose in ICU pts (5–7.5 mg/kg). Without loading dose, therapeutic concentrations reached at 24 hrs (MIC = 1) and 60 hrs (MIC = 2)
- Otic preparation: 1–2 drops q8–6h to affected ear.

RENAL DOSING

Dosing for GFR 50–80: 5 mg/kg/day IV divided in 2 doses.

Dosing for GFR 10–50: GFR 20–50 mL/min: 2.5–3.8 mg/kg/day divided in 2 doses. GFR 5–20 mL/min: 2.5 mg/kg q24h.

Dosing for GFR <10: 1.5 mg/kg/day (approx 30% of daily dose) q24h.

Dosing in hemodialysis: 1.5 mg/kg/day (approx 30% of daily dose) q24h. Conflicting data on drug removal during HD. On days of HD, dose post-HD.

Dosing in peritoneal dialysis: 1.5 mg/kg/day (approx 30% of daily dose) q24h. No supplement dose required, not removed in PD.

Dosing in hemofiltration: Limited data. CVVH: 2.5 mg/kg q48h. CVVHD with 1 L/hr dialysis flow rate: 2.5 mg/kg q24h (2.5 mg/kg q12h can be considered in severe infections); CVVHD with >1 L/hr dialysis flow rate: 2.5 mg/kg q12h.

ADVERSE DRUG REACTIONS

General

- Topical form well tolerated
- Systemic administration may result in effects listed below but may be less nephrotoxic or neurotoxic than older literature suggests

Common

- Reversible dose dependent nephrotoxicity in up to 20% of pts
- Phlebitis at infusion site

Occasional

- Neurotoxicity: circumoral and peripheral paresthesia, dizziness, vertigo, ataxia, blurred vision, slurred speech with IV use
- Inhaled colistimethate: possible bronchospasm, ARDS (especially if drug reconstituted and not given quickly leading to administration of colistin rather than prodrug (see McCoy ref)

Rare

- Respiratory depression
- Allergic reactions

ANTIBACTERIAL DRUGS

DRUG INTERACTIONS

- Aminoglycosides: may increase risk of neuromuscular blockade.
- Nephrotoxic drugs (e.g., amphotericin B, aminoglycosides, cidofovir, foscarnet): may increase risk of nephrotoxicity. Avoid co-administration.
- Non-depolarizing muscle relaxants (atracurium, vecuronium, pancuronium, tubocurarine): neuromuscular blockade may be enhanced with IM or IV use.

SPECTRUM—See Appendix II, p. 804

RESISTANCE

- *Proteus* spp., *Providencia* spp., *Burkholderia* spp., and *Serratia marcescens* are generally resistant. *B. fragilis* are resistant, but colistin may have limited activity against *Prevotella* and *Fusobacterium* spp. No activity against Gram-positive bacteria.
- MIC break point for *P. aeruginosa* and non-*Enterobacteriaceae*: ≤2 mcg/mL (sensitive); 4 mcg/mL (intermediate resistance); ≥8 mcg/mL (resistant). MIC break point for *Acinetobacter* spp.: ≤2 mcg/mL (sensitive); ≥4 mcg/mL (resistant).

PHARMACOLOGY

Mechanism

Colistimethate is hydrolysed to colistin, colistin acts like a cationic detergent binding to the lipids of bacterial cytoplasmic membranes and causing damage that results in alteration of the osmotic barrier and leakage of essential intracellular metabolites.

Pharmacokinetic Parameters

- Absorption —
- Cmax 5–7.5 mcg/mL after 500 mg IM dose administration.
- Distribution Widely distributed into body tissue, low level is attained in synovial, pleural, and pericardial fluid. ~25% CNS penetration w/ meningeal inflammation (consider intraventricular or intrathecal administration but only 5% without inflammation (*AAC* 2009;53;4907).
- Protein binding 50%.
- Metabolism/Excretion Hydrolyzed to colistin and other metabolite. Both colistimethate and metabolite is excreted unchanged in the urine vial glomerular filtration.
- T1/2 1.5–8 hrs. ICU pts: 7.4–14 hrs.

Dosing for Decreased Hepatic Function

No data. Usual dose likely.

Pregnancy Risk

C: No reports linking colistimethate with congenital defects have been located, but adverse events observed in animal studies.

Breast Feeding Compatibility

Colistimethate is excreted in breast milk. Milk:plasma ratio is 0.17.

COMMENTS

Parenteral and topical polymyxin rarely used as first line therapy due to historical reports of nephrotoxicity and neurotoxicity; however, modern studies report less significant rates of side effects (e.g., *CID* 2003;36:1111, *J Infect* 2008;56:432). Inhaled use with resistant *Pseudomonas aeruginosa* or other Gram-negative MDR infections seen in cystic fibrosis pts, or nosocomial pneumonia. Delivery of aerosolized colistin not standardized. Active against virtually all *P. aeruginosa* and *Acinetobacter* strains but *Proteus* spp. are usually resistant and may cause superinfection. An acceptable second line agent for VAP.

SELECTED REFERENCES

Garnacho-Montero J, Ortiz-Leyba C, Jiménez-Jiménez FJ, et al. Treatment of multidrug-resistant Acinetobacter baumannii ventilator-associated pneumonia (VAP) with intravenous colistin: a comparison with imipenem-susceptible VAP. *Clin Infect Dis*, 2003; Vol. 36; pp. 1111–8.

Jensen T, Pedersen SS, Garne S, et al. Colistin inhalation therapy in cystic fibrosis pts with chronic Pseudomonas aeruginosa lung infection. *J Antimicrob Chemother*, 1987; Vol. 19; pp. 831–8.

Li J, Nation RL, Milne RW, et al. Evaluation of colistin as an agent against multi-resistant Gram-negative bacteria. *Int J Antimicrob Agents*, 2005; Vol. 25; pp. 11–25.

McCoy KS. Compounded colistimethate as possible cause of fatal acute respiratory distress syndrome. *N Engl J Med*, 2007; Vol. 357; pp. 2310–1.

Reina R, Estenssoro E, Saenz G, et al. Safety and efficacy of colistin in Acinetobacter and Pseudomonas infections: a prospective cohort study. *Intensive Care Med*, 2005; Vol. 31(8); pp. 1058–65.

DAPTOMYCIN

Paul A. Pham, PharmD and John G. Bartlett, MD

INDICATIONS
FDA
- Treatment of complicated skin and skin structure infections (caused by susceptible strains of Gram-positive microorganisms including MSSA and MRSA).
- *S. aureus* bacteremia, including those with right-sided endocarditis, caused by MSSA and MRSA.

Non-FDA Approved Uses
- Splenic abscess
- Surgical wound infections
- Hepatic abscess
- Osteomyelitis, acute
- Osteomyelitis, chronic
- Diabetic foot infection
- Septic arthritis, community-acquired

FORMS

Brand name (mfr)	Forms	Cost*
Cubicin (Cubist)	IV vial 500 mg	$248.34
*Prices represents Average Wholesale Price (AWP).		

USUAL ADULT DOSING
Soft tissue infection: 4 mg/kg IV qday. Bacteremia and endocarditis: 6 mg/kg IV qday. May consider higher doses (up to 10 mg/kg/day) for severe infections with close monitoring for myopathy.

RENAL DOSING
Dosing for GFR 50–80: Soft tissue infection: 4 mg/kg IV q24h. Bacteremia and endocarditis: 6–10 mg/kg IV q24h.
Dosing for GFR 10–50: CrCL >30 mL/min: 4 mg/kg IV q24h. IE: 6 mg/kg IV q24h. CrCL <30 mL/min: 4mg/kg IV q48h. IE: 6–10 mg/kg IV q48h.
Dosing for GFR <10: Soft tissue infection: 4 mg/kg IV q48h. IE: 6–10 mg/kg IV q48h.
Dosing in hemodialysis: 4 mg/kg IV q48h. Bacteremia and IE: 6–10 mg/kg IV q48h (minimal removal with HD, 15% removal following 4 hrs of HD).
Dosing in peritoneal dialysis: 4 mg/kg IV q48h. Bacteremia and IE: 6–10 mg/kg IV q48h (minimal removal with PD, 11% removal following 48 hrs of PD).
Dosing in hemofiltration: Limited data: consider 4 mg/kg IV q48h. Bacteremia and IE: 6–10 mg/kg IV q48h.

ADVERSE DRUG REACTIONS
General
- Generally well tolerated.
- 2-mercaptobenzothiazole (MBT) impurity has been isolated from reconstituted daptomycin stored in with ReadyMED elastomeric infusion pumps manufactured by Cardinal Health. MBT has been associated with dermal sensitization and increased risk of certain tumors (in rodent studies with chronic administration). No impurity has been isolated in daptomycin vials.

Occasional
- LFTs, alkaline phosphatase, and LDH elevation.
- Dose dependent CPK elevation (reversible) with or without myopathy. Higher incidence of myopathy has been reported with 4 mg/kg q12h dosing.

Rare
- Neuropathy
- Jaundice
- *C. difficile* associated colitis

ANTIBACTERIAL DRUGS

ANTIBACTERIAL

Drug Interactions
Daptomycin is not an inhibitor or inducer of human cytochrome P450 isoform.
- Pharmacokinetic and pharmacodynamic interaction studies involving aztreonam, tobramycin, warfarin (single dose study), simvastatin, and probenecid did not result in interactions.
- Statins: discontinue statin is recommended during daptomycin therapy.

Spectrum—See Appendix II, p. 804

Resistance
- In pts with persistent or relapsing bacteremia, 9/20 (45%) of daptomycin treated pts developed an increasing MIC of greater than 1 mcg/mL during treatment. Of these, eight pts had clinical failure.
- MIC breakpoint of 1 mcg/mL for *staphylococci* and 4 mcg/mL for *enterococci*.

Pharmacology

Mechanism
Daptomycin binds to bacterial membranes and causes rapid depolarization of membrane potential, which results in inhibition of protein, DNA, and RNA synthesis. This leads to rapid cell death.

Pharmacokinetic Parameters
- **Absorption** Poor oral absorption in animal studies.
- **Cmax** 58 mcg/mL, AUC: 494 mcg hr/mL.
- **Distribution** Vd = 0.096 L/kg; no CNS penetration (animal data); poor bone penetration in animal data (clinical significance unknown) [AAC 1989;33:689].
- **Protein binding** 92%.
- **Metabolism/Excretion** Primarily excreted as unchanged drug in the kidney (78%) with little metabolism to inactive metabolites.
- **T1/2** 8.1 hrs.

Dosing for Decreased Hepatic Function
4 mg/kg IV q24h (with moderate Child-Pugh Class B).

Pregnancy Risk
B: Animal data using 3–6 times the human dose did not result in teratogenicity. No human data.

Breast Feeding Compatibility
No data.

Comments
Daptomycin is active against virtually all Gram-positive organism including *S. aureus* (including MRSA) and *E. faecalis/E. faecium* including VRE (but MIC higher compared to *S. aureus*). Poor outcome has been described when daptomycin was used to treat VRE endocarditis (Pharmacotherapy 2006;26:347). Daptomycin should not be used for pneumonia due to high failure rates (drug binds to surfactant). Recently completed RCT of 235 pts with *S. aureus* bacteremia and endocarditis showed daptomycin to be non-inferior to vancomycin or semi-synthetic PCN.

Selected References
Fowler VG, Boucher HW, Corey GR, et al. Daptomycin versus standard therapy for bacteremia and endocarditis caused by Staphylococcus aureus. *N Engl J Med*, 2006; Vol. 355; pp. 653–65.
Pertel PE, Bernardo P, Fogarty C, et al. Effects of prior effective therapy on the efficacy of daptomycin and ceftriaxone for the treatment of community-acquired pneumonia. *Clin Infect Dis*, 2008; Vol. 46; pp. 1142–51.

DICLOXACILLIN

Paul A. Pham, PharmD and John G. Bartlett, MD

Indications

FDA
- Respiratory tract infections (pharyngitis and pneumonia)
- Staphylococcal infections (MSSA)
- Streptococcal infections
- Skin and soft tissue infections

Non-FDA Approved Uses
- Furuncle/carbuncle
- Impetigo
- Cellulitis/erysipelas

- Folliculitis
- Hidradenitis supparativa

FORMS

Brand name (mfr)	Forms	Cost*
Dynapen; Dycill; Pathocil (Various generic manufacturers)	PO cap 250 mg; PO cap 500 mg PO susp 62.5 mg/5 mL	$0.66; $1.20 $0.50 per 5 mL
*Prices represents Average Wholesale Price (AWP).		

USUAL ADULT DOSING

- Mild infections: 125 mg PO q6h.
- Moderate to severe infections: 250–500 mg PO q6h (parenteral therapy for severe infections recommended).

RENAL DOSING

Dosing for GFR 50–80: Usual dose.
Dosing for GFR 10–50: Usual dose.
Dosing for GFR <10: Usual dose.
Dosing in hemodialysis: Usual regimen.
Dosing in peritoneal dialysis: Usual regimen.
Dosing in hemofiltration: No data. Usual dose likely.

ADVERSE DRUG REACTIONS

Common

- Hypersensitivity reactions and rash

Occasional

- Drug fever
- Coombs' test positive without hemolytic anemia
- LFT elevations
- GI intolerance and diarrhea
- Herxheimer reaction (with treatment of spirochetal infections)
- *C. difficile*–associated colitis

Rare

- Anaphylaxis
- Hemolytic anemia
- Thrombocytopenia
- Leukopenia
- Interstitial nephritis

DRUG INTERACTIONS

Tetracyclines: *in vitro* antagonism when co-administered. Bactericidal effect of penicillins may be diminished *in vivo*. Avoid co-administration.

SPECTRUM—See Appendix II, p. 795

PHARMACOLOGY

Mechanism

Beta-lactam antibiotics inhibit mucopeptide synthesis in the bacterial cell wall, this results in the formation of defective cell walls and osmotically unstable organisms susceptible to cell lysis.

Pharmacokinetic Parameters

- **Absorption** 35% absorbed; with blood level 2 times greater than cloxacillin.
- **Cmax** 7–18 mcg/mL after 500 mg PO dose administration.
- **Distribution** Distributed to blister fluid, urine, peritoneal fluid, pleural fluid, middle ear fluid, intestinal mucosa, bone, gallbladder, lung, female reproductive tissue, bile, and inflamed meninges.
- **Protein binding** 95–98%
- **Metabolism/Excretion** Hepatic metabolism accounts for less than 30% of administered dose. Both unchanged drug and metabolites are excreted via glomerular filtration and tubular secretion. 10% Biliary excretion.
- **T1/2** 0.6–0.8 hr.

ANTIBACTERIAL DRUGS

Dosing for Decreased Hepatic Function
No data. Usual dose likely (less than 30% hepatic metabolism).

Pregnancy Risk
B: Several collaborative perinatal project reports involving over 12,000 exposures to penicillin derivatives during the first trimester indicated no association between penicillin derivative drugs and birth defects.

Breast Feeding Compatibility
Excreted in breast milk in low concentration. No adverse effects have been reported.

COMMENTS
Oral anti-staphylococcal penicillin with better bioavailability compared to cloxacillin. Four times a day administration may decrease adherence for some pts.

SELECTED REFERENCES
Marcy SM, Klein JO. The isoxazolyl penicillins: oxacillin, cloxacillin, and dicloxacillin. *Med Clin North Am*, 1970; Vol. 54; pp. 1127–43.

Stevens DL, Smith LG, Bruss JB, et al. Randomized comparison of linezolid (PNU-100766) versus oxacillin-dicloxacillin for treatment of complicated skin and soft tissue infections. *Antimicrob Agents Chemother*, 2000; Vol. 44; pp. 3408–13.

DORIPENEM

Paul A. Pham, PharmD

INDICATIONS
FDA
- Complicated intra-abdominal infection
- Complicated UTI

Non-FDA Approved Uses
- Skin and soft tissue infections (not due to MRSA)
- Nosocomial pneumonia including ventilator-associated pneumonia

FORMS

Brand name (mfr)	Forms	Cost*
Doribax (JOM Pharmaceutical)	IV vial 500 mg	$47.91
*Prices represents Average Wholesale Price (AWP).		

USUAL ADULT DOSING
- 500 mg IV q8h (infuse over 1 hr)
- To optimize PK/PD, infuse over 4 hrs

RENAL DOSING
Dosing for GFR 50–80: 500 mg IV q8h.
Dosing for GFR 10–50: 30–50 mL/min: 250 mg IV q8h; 10–30 mL/min: 250 mg IV q12h.
Dosing for GFR <10: No data; dose reduction needed.
Dosing in hemodialysis: No dosing data, but haemodialyzed.
Dosing in peritoneal dialysis: No data.
Dosing in hemofiltration: CVVHD: no data, but haemodialyzed.

ADVERSE DRUG REACTIONS
General
- Well tolerated
- ADRs comparable to levofloxacin and meropenem in clinical trials

Occasional
- Nausea
- Diarrhea
- Headache
- Phlebitis
- Hypersensitivity reaction, especially with history of PCN allergy
- *C. difficile*–associated colitis

Rare

- Anaphylaxis reaction
- Interstitial pneumonitis (described with inhaled doripenem)
- Stevens Johnson Syndrome, toxic epidermal necrolysis
- Seizure: in contrast to imipenem, doripenem did not cause EEG changes and seizures in animal studies (Horiuchi M, et al. *Toxicology* 2006;222:114–24). However, in a clinical trial seizures were reported in 1.1% and 3.8% of doripenem and imipenem treated pts, respectively.

DRUG INTERACTIONS

- *In vitro* doripenem is not an inducer or inhibitor of CYP450 isoenzymes.
- Probenecid: doripenem serum concentrations may be increased with probenecid co-administration.
- Valproic acid: may decrease valproic acid serum concentrations. Monitor valproic acid serum concentrations closely with co-administration.

RESISTANCE

- *S. maltophilia, S. aureus* (MRSA), and *E. faecium* are generally resistant.
- Doripenem exhibited the greatest ability to prevent the emergence of the carbapenem-resistant mutant *in vitro* (Sakyo S et al. *J Antibiot* (Tokyo) 2006;59:220–8).
- CLSI breakpoint not yet established.

PHARMACOLOGY

Mechanism

Doripenem inhibits cell wall biosynthesis by binding to several penicillin-binding proteins (PBP 2, 3, and 4).

Pharmacokinetic Parameters

- **Cmax** After 500 mg IV infusion: Cmax = 23 mcg/mL; AUC = 36.3 mcg hr/mL.
- **Distribution** Vd = 16.8 L (8–55 L); high retroperitoneal fluid, bile and urine concentrations. Limited gall bladder penetration.
- **Protein binding** 8%.
- **Metabolism/Excretion** Approximately 18% converted to an inactive ring-opened metabolite via dehydropeptidase-I. Active drug and metabolites are excreted primarily in the urine via glomerular filtration and active tubular secretion.
- **T1/2** 1 hr.

Dosing for Decreased Hepatic Function

No data, usual dose likely.

Pregnancy Risk

B: No human data. Not teratogenic in animal studies.

Breast Feeding Compatibility

No data; likely to be secreted in breast milk.

COMMENTS

Doripenem is a novel 1-beta-methylcarbapenem antibiotic with similar spectrum of activity to imipenem/cilastin and meropenem. Doripenem is active against all anaerobes and most GNB, including *P. aeruginosa*, inducible chromosomal beta-lactamases, and ESBL-producing organisms. The benefit of a lower a MIC to *P. aeruginosa* and a lower likelihood of resistance development observed *in vitro* remains to be evaluated in clinical studies.

SELECTED REFERENCES

Chastre J, Wunderink R, Prokocimer P. et al. Efficacy and safety of intravenous infusion of doripenem versus imipenem in ventilator-associated pneumonia: A multicenter, randomized study. *Critical Care Medicine*, 2008; Vol. 36; pp. 1089–1096.

FDA. *FDA approved labeling*, 2007.

DOXYCYCLINE

Paul A. Pham, PharmD and John G. Bartlett, MD

INDICATIONS

FDA

- Anthrax due to *Bacillus anthracis*, including inhalation anthrax (post-exposure). CDC recommends as first line agent + 1–2 additional agents with *in vitro* activity (for inhalation anthrax, see "biodefense-anthrax")

ANTIBACTERIAL DRUGS

- Granuloma inguinale caused by *Calymmatobacterium granulomatis*
- If PCN allergic: uncomplicated gonorrhea caused by *Neisseria gonorrhoeae*; syphilis caused by *Treponema pallidum*; yaws caused by *Treponema pertenue*; listeriosis due to *Listeria monocytogenes*; Vincent's infection caused by *Fusobacterium fusiforme*; Actinomycosis caused by *Actinomyces israelli*; infections caused by Clostridial species
- Psittacosis caused by *Chlamydia psittaci*
- Relapsing fever caused by *Borrelia recurrentis*
- *Mycoplasma pneumoniae*
- Rocky mountain spotted fever, typhus, Q fever, rickettsialpox, and tick fevers cased by Rickettsial species.
- Uncomplicated urethral, endocervical, or rectal infections caused by *Chlamydia trachomatis*; nongonococcal urethritis caused by *Ureaplasma urealyticum*; lymphogranuloma venereum caused by *Chlamydia* spp.
- Trachoma, inclusion conjunctivitis cause *by C. trachomatis*.
- Gram-negative infections caused by: *H. ducreyi, Y. pestis, F. tularensis, V. cholerae, C. fetus, Brucella* spp. *B. bacilliformis, C. granulomatis*.

Non-FDA Approved Uses
- Lyme disease
- Malaria prophylaxis

FORMS

Brand name (mfr)	Forms	Cost*
Vibramycin (Pfizer)	Oral suspension 25 mg/5 mL Oral capsule 100 mg	$321.76 per 16 oz $1.70; $26.35 per 2 oz
Doxycycline; Monodox; Adoxa (Generic manufacturers (Imiren, Watson/Schein and others))	Oral capsule 50 mg; 100 mg IV vial 100 mg Oral tablet 50 mg; 75 mg; 100 mg	$1.00 $14.75 $1.15
Periostat Collagenex Pharmaceutical and generic manufacturer (Mutual pharmaceutical)	Oral 20 mg caps	$1.32
Doryx DR (Warner Chilcott Labs)	Oral delayed release pellets 75 mg; 100 mg; 150 mg	$7.91; $9.32 $14.75
*Prices represents Average Wholesale Price (AWP).		

USUAL ADULT DOSING
- Respiratory tract infections (community-acquired pneumonia, otitis, sinusitis): 100 mg PO twice daily w/ food × 7–14 days.
- *C. trachomatis* (alternative to azithromycin): 100 mg PO twice daily w/ food × 7 days.
- Uncomplicated non-GC infections (urethral, endocervical, or rectal): 100 mg PO twice daily × 7 days.
- Bacillary angiomatosis: 100 mg twice daily w/ food × >3 mos; consider lifelong rx to prevent relapse in pts not on ART with immune reconstitution.

ADVERSE DRUG REACTIONS
General
- Stains and deforms teeth in children up to 8 yrs old
Occasional
- GI intolerance (dose related)
- Photosensitivity
Rare
- Candida overgrowth (vaginitis and esophagitis)
- Worsening azotemia in pts with renal failure

- Rash
- "Black tongue" syndrome; benign fungus infection that is generally reversible upon drug discontinuation
- Esophageal ulceration
- Elevated liver function tests
- Jarisch-Herxheimer reaction
- *C. difficile* -associated colitis (less likely compared to cephalosporins, carbapenems, and fluoroquinolones)

RESISTANCE

- *S. pneumoniae:* 12 and 27% resistance in bloodstream infection and pneumonia, respectively. Cross-resistance with PCN-resistant *S. pneumoniae* with only 60% susceptible.
- Many strains of CA-MRSA are sensitive doxycycline, but minocycline has better *in vitro* activity and demonstrated efficacy *in vivo*.
- MIC breakpoint for Enterobacteriaceae, *Staphylococcus* spp., and *Enterococcus* spp.: ≤4 mcg/mL (sensitive); 8 mcg/mL (intermediate); ≥16 mcg/mL (resistant).
- Isolates that are susceptible tetracycline are also considered susceptible to doxycycline and minocycline. However, tetracycline-intermediate or -resistant isolates may be susceptible to doxycycline or minocycline.

DRUG INTERACTIONS—See Appendix III, p. 812, for table of drug-to-drug interactions.
SPECTRUM—See Appendix II, p. 802

PHARMACOLOGY
Mechanism
Inhibit protein synthesis by mainly binding to 30S ribosomal subunit and blocking binding of aminoacyl transfer-RNA.

Pharmacokinetic Parameters
- **Absorption** 90% absorbed.
- **Cmax** 1.5–2.1 mcg/mL.
- **Distribution** Widely distributed into body tissues and fluids including pleural fluid, bronchial secretions, sputum, ascitic fluid, synovial fluid, aqueous and vitreous humor, and prostatic fluid. Better CSF penetration compared to tetracycline (26% of serum levels).
- **Protein binding** 25–91%.
- **Metabolism/Excretion** Excreted mainly by nonrenal routes. Possible liver metabolism and intestinal inactivation. 20–26% excreted in the urine, 20–40% excreted in the feces.
- **T1/2** 18 hrs.

Dosing for GFR 50–80: Usual dose.
Dosing for GFR 10–50: Usual dose.
Dosing for GFR <10: Usual dose.
Dosing in hemodialysis: Usual dose.
Dosing in peritoneal dialysis: Usual dose.
Dosing in hemofiltration: Usual dose.

Dosing for Decreased Hepatic Function
No data

Pregnancy Risk
D: Contraindicated in pregnancy due to retardation of skeletal development and bone growth; enamel hypoplasia and discoloration of teeth of fetus. Maternal liver toxicity have also been reported.

Breast Feeding Compatibility
Excreted in breast milk at very low concentrations. There is theoretical possibility of dental staining and inhibition of bone growth, but infants exposed to tetracyclines have serum levels less than 0.05 mcg/mL.

COMMENTS
Preferred tetracycline derivative due to more convenient twice daily dosing regimen and no food-drug interaction. Recommended tetracycline derivative in pts with renal failure. Agents of choice for rickettsial and vibrio infections. Minocycline is preferred by some for the treatment of mild to moderate soft tissue infections caused by CA-MRSA, but note that activity of tetracyclines against Streptococcus spp. is limited.

ANTIBACTERIAL DRUGS

SELECTED REFERENCES

Cunha BA. Methicillin-resistant Staphylococcus aureus: clinical manifestations and antimicrobial therapy. *Clin Microbiol Infect*, 2005; Vol. 11. Suppl 4; pp. 33–42.

Jones RN, Sader HS, Fritsche TR. Doxycycline use for community-acquired pneumonia: contemporary *in vitro* spectrum of activity against Streptococcus pneumoniae (1999–2002). *Diagn Microbiol Infect Dis*, 2004; Vol. 49; pp. 147–9.

ERTAPENEM

Paul A. Pham, PharmD and John G. Bartlett, MD

INDICATIONS
FDA
- (1) Complicated intra-abdominal infections. (2) Community-acquired pneumonia (CAP). (3) Complicated urinary tract infections.
- (4) Complicated Skin and Skin Structure Infections, including diabetic foot infections without osteomyelitis.
- (5) Elective colorectal surgical prophylaxis.
- (6) Acute pelvic infections (postpartum endomyometritis, septic abortion, and post surgical gynecologic infections).
- Ertapenem is now FDA indicated in pediatrics (3 mos–17 yo) for the above indications.

Non-FDA Approved Uses
- Mild-moderate intra-abdominal infections (cholecystitis, cholangitis, diverticulitis, splenic and hepatic abscess, peritonitis) not requiring drainage or surgery.

FORMS

Brand name (mfr)	Forms	Cost*
Invanz (Merck)	IV vial 500 mg; 1000 mg	$34.14 (500 mg); $68.58 (1000 mg)

*Prices represents Average Wholesale Price (AWP).

USUAL ADULT DOSING
- CAP, complicated UTI, complicated soft tissue infection, and intra-abdominal infection: 1 g IV or IM q24h × 10–14 days.
- For obese pts: 1 g q24h inadequate (*AAC* 2006;50:1222). Consider higher dose or use alternative antibiotic.

RENAL DOSING
Dosing for GFR 50–80: Usual dose.
Dosing for GFR 10–50: Usual dose.
Dosing for GFR <10: <30 mL/min: 500 mg q24h.
Dosing in hemodialysis: 500 mg q24h. Dose post-HD on days of HD. If daily dose given 6 hrs within HD (supplement with 150 mg post-HD).
Dosing in peritoneal dialysis: No data.
Dosing in hemofiltration: CVVH or CVVHD: no data. Ertapenem is not recommended for severe infections. Consider meropenem 1–2 g IV q12h.

ADVERSE DRUG REACTIONS
General
- Generally well tolerated

Occasional
- Diarrhea
- *C. difficile* colitis
- Minimal phlebitis
- Headache
- Nausea and vomiting
- ALT elevation

Rare
- Seizures (reported in 0.5% of pts; pts with renal insufficiency and/or CNS disorder are at increased risk)

DRUG INTERACTIONS

Does not interact with cytochrome p450 isoform (1A2, 2C9, 2C19, 2D6, 2E1, and 3A4) or P-glycoprotein.

- Probenecid: increases ertapenem AUC by 25%.
- Valproic acid: may decrease valproic acid serum concentrations. Monitor serum concentrations closely with co-administration.
- Not compatible with dextrose (do not co-infuse with dextrose or other medications).

SPECTRUM—See Appendix II, p. 789

RESISTANCE

- Cross-resistance to ertapenem seen in imipenem-1 metallo-beta-lactamase and SME-1 carbapenemase producing organisms [*AAC* 2001;45(10):2831–7].
- MIC breakpoint for Enterobacteriaceae: ≤2 mcg/mL (sensitive); 4 mcg/mL (intermediate); ≥8 mcg/mL (resistant).
- No CLSI MIC breakpoints exist for Gram-negative non-lactose fermenters.

PHARMACOLOGY

Mechanism

A carbapenem antibiotic, inhibits mucopeptide synthesis in the bacterial cell wall, this results in the formation of defective cell walls and osmotically unstable organisms susceptible to cell lysis.

Pharmacokinetic Parameters

- **Absorption** 90% after IM administration
- **Cmax** 155 mcg/mL. Cmin: 1 mcg/mL at 24 hrs (after 1 g IV).
- **Distribution** Well distributed, Vd = 8.2 L/kg. Inadequate data on CNS penetration. 13%–19% bone penetration and 41% synovial fluid penetration (Boselli E et al. *JAC* 2007; 60:893).
- **Protein binding** 85–95%.
- **Metabolism/Excretion** Hydrolyzing of beta-lactam ring. Metabolite and parent drug are renally excreted.
- **T1/2** 4 hrs.

Dosing for Decreased Hepatic Function

1 g q24h (usual dose).

Pregnancy Risk

B: not teratogenic in animal studies. No human data.

Breast Feeding Compatibility

Excreted in breast milk. Use only when clearly indicated.

COMMENTS

Ertapenem has a spectrum of activity that includes all anaerobes and many Gram-negative bacilli with the exception of *P. aeruginosa* and Acinetobacter. Risk of seizure is reported at 0.5% in clinical trials. T½ of 4–5 hrs suggests caution in using q24h dosing for severely ill pts (e.g., bacteremia and/or ICU pts). Although ertapenem is active against many ESBL-producing organisms, there are limited clinical data for the treatment of severe pneumonia or soft tissue infections caused by these organisms. May be used as a convenient once-a-day outpatient IV antibiotic for mild to moderate infections.

SELECTED REFERENCES

Goff DA, Mangino JE. Ertapenem: no effect on aerobic Gram-negative susceptibilities to imipenem. *J Infect*, 2008; Vol. 57; pp. 123–7.

Itani KM, Wilson SE, Awad SS, et al. Ertapenem versus cefotetan prophylaxis in elective colorectal surgery. *N Engl J Med*, 2006; Vol. 355; pp. 2640–51.

ERYTHROMYCIN

Paul A. Pham, PharmD and John G. Bartlett, MD

INDICATIONS

FDA

- Preoperative bowel preparation (with neomycin)
- Syphilis caused by *Treponema pallidum* (in pts allergic to the penicillins, but azithromycin preferred)
- Acute exacerbations of chronic bronchitis and sinusitis
- Acute otitis media and pharyngitis
- Diphtheria infections due to *Corynebacterium diphtheriae*, as an adjunct to antitoxin

- Intestinal amebiasis caused by *Entamoeba histolytica*
- Conjunctivitis in the newborn caused by *Chlamydia trachomatis*
- Legionnaires' disease
- Pertussis
- Rheumatic fever prophylaxis, also upper respiratory tract infections caused by *Streptococcus pyogenes, Streptococcus pneumoniae, Haemophilus influenzae* (when used concomitantly with adequate sulfonamide dosage), lower respiratory tract infections caused by *Streptococcus pyogenes* or *pneumoniae,* listeriosis, skin and soft tissue infections, respiratory tract infections caused by *Mycoplasma pneumoniae,* erythrasma, acute inflammatory pelvic disease, uncomplicated urethral, endocervical, or rectal infections caused by *Chlamydia trachomatis.*

FORMS

Brand name (mfr)	Forms	Cost*
PCE Dispertab (Abbott)	PO tab, EC 333 mg; PO tab, EC 500 mg PO cap 250 mg	$1.90; $2.50 $0.27
Eryc (Abbott)	PO cap, EC 250 mg	$0.27
Eryped (Abbott)	PO susp 200 mg/5 mL; PO susp 400 mg/5 mL	$0.41 per 5 mL; $0.65 per 5 mL
Erythrocin Lactobionate (Hospira)	IV vial 500 mg	$123 per vial
Erythromycin stearate (Abbott, Nycomed U.S.)	PO tab 250 mg; PO tab 500 mg Ophthalmic ointment 5 mg/g	$0.74; $0.28 $1.53 per g

*Prices represents Average Wholesale Price (AWP).

USUAL ADULT DOSING
- Erythromycin base 250–500 mg PO q6–8h.
- Erythromycin estolate 250–500 mg PO q6h.
- Erythromycin ethylsuccinate 400–800 mg PO q6h or 0.5–1 g IV q6h.
- Bowel prep: 1 g PO 1 pm, 2 pm and 11 pm prior to surgery (plus neomycin).

RENAL DOSING
Dosing for GFR 50–80: Usual dose.
Dosing for GFR 10–50: Usual dose.
Dosing for GFR <10: Usual dose.
Dosing in hemodialysis: Usual regimen.
Dosing in peritoneal dialysis: Usual regimen.
Dosing in hemofiltration: No data. Usual dose likely.

ADVERSE DRUG REACTIONS
Common
- GI intolerance (oral-dose related), diarrhea
- Phlebitis with IV administration

Occasional
- Stomatitis
- Cholestatic hepatitis (1:1000 especially with estolate salt formulation-reversible)
- Generalized rash
- Prolonged QTc (especially with high dose IV)
- LFTs elevation
- Rash
- Reversible ototoxicity (especially with high dose IV)

Rare
- *C. difficile* colitis
- Torsades de pointes (especially in women)
- Hypothermia
- Exacerbation of symptoms of myasthenia gravis and new onset of symptoms of myasthenic syndrome have been reported.

DRUG INTERACTIONS—See Appendix III, p. 813, for table of drug-to-drug interactions.
Substrate of CYP3A4 and potent inhibitor CYP3A4 and CYP1A2.

SPECTRUM—See Appendix II, p. 800

PHARMACOLOGY
Mechanism
Macrolides inhibit protein synthesis by binding to 50S ribosomal subunits, inhibiting translocation of peptidase chain and inhibiting polypeptide synthesis.

Pharmacokinetic Parameters
- **Absorption** 20–50% absorbed.
- **Cmax** 0.1–2 mcg/mL after 500 mg (erythromycin base, stearate, ethyl succinate) PO dose administration. 2 mcg/mL after 500 mg (erythromycin estolate) PO dose administration. 3–4 mcg/mL after 500 mg IV dose administration.
- **Distribution** Widely distributed into most body tissue and fluids. Poor CNS penetration (only 2–13% of serum level).
- **Protein binding** 70–90%.
- **Metabolism/Excretion** Partially metabolized to N-demethylation metabolite. Excreted primarily in feces as unchanged drug and metabolite via biliary excretion. Only small amount excreted in urine.
- **T1/2** 1.4–2.0 hrs.

Dosing for Decreased Hepatic Function
No data. May require dose adjustment with severe hepatic insufficiency.

Pregnancy Risk
B: In a surveillance study of Michigan Medicaid recipient, 6,972 pts were exposed to erythromycin during the first trimester, resulted in a 4.6% birth defect. This data does not support an association erythromycin and congenital malformation. The CDC recommends the use of erythromycin for the treatment of chlamydia in pregnancy.

Breast Feeding Compatibility
Erythromycin is excreted into breast milk. The American Academy of Pediatrics considers erythromycin compatible with breast feeding.

COMMENTS
Oral and parenteral macrolide that often causes GI distress especially with oral administration. It has decreasing activity against *S. pneumoniae* and it has multiple drug interactions with drug metabolized by cytochrome P450. Highest risk for QTc prolongation among antimicrobials (especially with high dose erythromycin). Therapeutically equivalent and better tolerated macrolides such as azithromycin and clarithromycin are preferred.

SELECTED REFERENCES
Iannini PB. Cardiotoxicity of macrolides, ketolides and fluoroquinolones that prolong the QTc interval. *Expert Opin Drug Saf*, 2002; Vol. 1; pp. 121–8.

Ray WA, Murray KT, Meredith S, et al. Oral erythromycin and the risk of sudden death from cardiac causes. *N Engl J Med*, 2004; Vol. 351; pp. 1089–96.

FOSFOMYCIN

Paul A. Pham, PharmD and John G. Bartlett, MD

INDICATIONS
FDA
- Treatment of uncomplicated urinary tract infections due to *E. coli* and *E. faecalis*.

Non-FDA Approved Uses
- Treatment of complicated UTI w/o bacteremia

FORMS

Brand name (mfr)	Forms	Cost*
Monurol (Forest)	PO pds 3 g	$46.25 per packet (3 g)

*Prices represents Average Wholesale Price (AWP).

USUAL ADULT DOSING
- Uncomplicated UTI: 3 g sachet PO × 1 dose with or without food.
- Complicated UTI: 3 g sachet PO every 2–3 days (up to 21 days) on an empty stomach preferred.
- Mix powder in 120 mL of cool water until it dissolves.

RENAL DOSING
Dosing for GFR 50–80: Usual dose.
Dosing for GFR 10–50: No data, consider dose adjustment. 3 g × 1 (uncomplicated UTI). Consider 3 g every 3 days for complicated UTI.
Dosing for GFR <10: No data, prolonged half-life consider dose adjustment or avoid due to decrease urinary excretion.
Dosing in hemodialysis: Redose after dialysis, due to removal during HD.
Dosing in peritoneal dialysis: 1 g q36 hrs.
Dosing in hemofiltration: CVVH: 77% removal during CVVH

ADVERSE DRUG REACTIONS
Occasional
- GI intolerance: diarrhea (10%), nausea, and dyspepsia
- Headache and dizziness
- Vaginitis
- Asthenia

Rare
- *C. difficile* colitis

DRUG INTERACTIONS
Antacids (calcium carbonate): reduction of fosfomycin absorption. Food decreases absorption of fosfomycin.

SPECTRUM—See Appendix II, p. 804

PHARMACOLOGY
Mechanism
Fosfomycin interferes with bacterial wall synthesis by inhibiting the enzyme enolpyruvyl transferase (this enzyme catalyzes the formation of uridine diphosphate N-acetylmuramic acid, which is the first step of bacterial cell wall synthesis).

Pharmacokinetic Parameters
- **Absorption** 30% absorbed with food; 37% absorbed without food.
- **Cmax** 64–128 mcg/mL; 3000 mcg/mL with a 3-g oral dose achieved in the urine.
- **Distribution** Distributed into bladder wall, kidneys, prostate, and seminal vesicles.
- **Protein binding** No protein binding.
- **Metabolism/Excretion** Converted to free acid fosfomycin. Excreted primarily in the urine. 18% excreted in the feces.
- **T1/2** 5.7 hrs.

Dosing for Decreased Hepatic Function
No data, usual dose likely.

Pregnancy Risk
B: Animal data shows no teratogenic effects. Several published reports studied the efficacy and safety of oral fosfomycin in all stages of pregnancy. In these studies fosfomycin did not cause harm to the fetus.

Breast Feeding Compatibility
No data, but expect excretion into breast milk due to low molecular weight of fosfomycin.

COMMENTS

Oral agent FDA approved only for uncomplicated UTI. Broad spectrum of activity includes all common uropathogenic bacteria. Single dose therapy (3 g) was equivalent to 7-day course of norfloxacin in randomized, blinded study. May be used for VRE in UTIs if renal function is good. Due to limited systemic absorption, fosfomycin should not be used for severe pyelonephritis and urosepsis.

SELECTED REFERENCES

Bayrak O, Cimentepe E, Inegöl I, et al. Is single-dose fosfomycin trometamol a good alternative for asymptomatic bacteriuria in the second trimester of pregnancy? *Int Urogynecol J Pelvic Floor Dysfunct*, 2007; Vol. 18; pp. 525–529.

Minassian MA, Lewis DA, Chattopadhyay D, et al. A comparison between single-dose fosfomycin trometamol (Monuril) and a 5-day course of trimethoprim in the treatment of uncomplicated lower urinary tract infection in women. *Int J Antimicrob Agents*, 1998; Vol. 10; pp. 39–47.

GENTAMICIN

Paul A. Pham, PharmD and John G. Bartlett, MD

INDICATIONS

FDA

- Serious infections caused by susceptible strains of organism. With the exception of uncomplicated UTI, aminoglycosides are generally used in combination.
- Bacterial septicemia, including neonatal sepsis
- Skin, bone, and soft tissue infections (including burns)
- Meningitis (poor penetration)
- Urinary tract
- Respiratory tract (poor penetration)
- Gastrointestinal tract (including peritonitis)
- Inflammatory ocular conditions that are steroid-responsive (opthalmic ointment and suspension)

Non-FDA Approved Uses

- Pneumonia, hospital-acquired (in combination with a beta-lactam, beta-lactam/beta-lactamase inhibitor, or a 3rd/4th generation cephalosporin)
- Intra-abdominal infection (in combination with an agent with Gram-positive and anaerobe coverage)
- Enterococcal endocarditis (in combination with ampicillin)
- Pelvic Inflammatory Disease (PID) (in combination with clindamycin)
- Pseudomonad infections (in combination with a beta-lactam, beta-lactam/beta-lactamase inhibitor, or a 3rd/4th generation cephalosporin)
- Brucella Species

FORMS

Brand name (mfr)	Forms	Cost*
Gentamicin (Various generic manufacturers)	IV vial 10 mg/mL (2 mL);	$5.00 per vial;
	IV vial 40 mg/mL (2 mL)	$0.90 per vial
	Topical cre 0.1% (15 g);	$360;
	Topical cre 0.1% (30 g)	$4.90
	Topical oint 0.1% (15 g);	$3.60;
	Topical oint 0.1% (30 g)	$4.90
	Topical oph gtt 3 mg/mL (5 mL);	$8.17;
	Topical oph gtt 3 mg/mL (15 mL);	$10.78;
	Topical oph gtt 0.3% (5 mL);	$9.54;
	Topical oph oint 0.3% (3.5 g)	$19.67

*Prices represents Average Wholesale Price (AWP).

USUAL ADULT DOSING

- **Once daily dosing:** 5–7 mg/kg IV. Therapeutic drug monitoring generally not recommended. Consider trough in pts at risk for nephrotoxicity (ICU pts, elderly, and concomitant nephrotoxin). Target trough <1 mcg/mL. Don't use once daily dosing in pts w/ unstable renal fxn, CrCl <60 mL/min, endocarditis, meningitis, or increased Vd (pregnancy, ascites, edema).

- **Traditional dosing (mild-moderate infections):** 2 mg/kg load, then 1.7–2 mg/kg IV q8h (goal peak >6 mcg/mL and trough <2 mcg/mL).
- **Traditional dosing (severe infections, e.g., Pseudomonas, pneumonia):** 3 mg/kg load, then 2 mg/kg IV q8h (goal peak >8 mcg/mL and trough <2 mcg/mL).
- Synergy w/ beta-lactams for gram-positive infections: 1 mg/kg IV q8h (goal peak 3–5 mcg/mL). 3 mg/kg once daily synergy dosing may be considered for *S. bovis* or viridans streptococci (MIC <0.5 mcg/mL only).
- Consider a higher loading dose and obtain a peak and trough after first dose in severe infections (+/– diffuse edema, ascites, shock, burns, CF, and pregnancy) in order to calculate pt-specific pharmacokinetic dose. Doses need to be adjusted based on changing renal function and/or volume status.
- Trough should be obtained (generally after 3rd dose) immediately before next dose.
- Peak should be obtained 30 mins after the end of a 30 mins infusion (generally after 3rd dose).
- For obese pts: use calculated lean body weight **plus** 40% of excess fat (Dosing Body Weight (DBW) = Ideal Body Weight (IBW) + 0.4 (actual body weight-IBW).
- IBW = 50 kg (for males) or 45.5 kg (for females) plus (2.3 × inches over 5 ft).
- Intraventricular or intrathecal administration: preservative free gentamicin 5 mg q24h (range 4–10 mg).

RENAL DOSING

Dosing for GFR 50–80: Standard loading dose for all levels of renal function. GRF >70 mL/min: Use standard dose. GFR 50–69 mL/min: calculated GFR × 0.045 = "mg/kg" q12h (Ex. for GFR 56 mL/min: 56 × 0.045 = "2.5" mg/kg q12h. Monitor peak and trough.

Dosing for GFR 10–50: Standard loading dose for all levels of renal function. GFR 40–49 mL/min: calculated GFR × 0.045 = "mg/kg" q12h (Ex. for GFR 45 mL/min: 45 × 0.045 = "2" mg/kg q12h). GFR 20–39: calculated GFR × 0.09 = "mg/kg" q24h. Monitor peak and trough.

Dosing for GFR <10: Standard loading dose for all levels of renal function. GFR <20 mL/min: 2–2.5 mg/kg × 1, then redose when level <2 mcg/mL. Monitor peak and trough.

Dosing in hemodialysis: Standard loading dose, then 1.7–2 mg/kg post-HD (treatment doses) or 1.0 mg/kg post-HD (for synergy). Peak (measure 2 hrs-post dose, target 7–10 mcg/mL) and trough (before next HD session, depending on residual renal function, expect 3–5 mcg/mL.)

Dosing in peritoneal dialysis: 2–4 mg per liter of dialysate exchange per day. Aminoglycosides given for prolonged periods to pts receiving continuous peritoneal dialysis have been associated with high rates of ototoxicity.

Dosing in hemofiltration: CVVH or CVVHD: loading dose 3 mg/kg, then 2 mg/kg q24–48 (measure peak 2 hrs-post dose, target 7–10 mcg/mL). Check a 24-hrs concentration (redose <2 mcg/mL).

ADVERSE DRUG REACTIONS

Common

- Renal failure (usually reversible). Risk factors: older pts, preexisting renal and hepatic disease, volume depletion, traditional Q8h dosing, large doses, concomitant nephrotoxic drug (including vancomycin), and length of therapy (most important). Controversial but trough may be associated with nephrotoxicity.

Occasional

- Irreversible vestibular toxicity (4–6%). Most pts compensate with visual and proprioceptive cues. Monitor for nausea, vomiting, nystagmus, and vertigo (exacerbated in the dark).
- Irreversible cochlear toxicity (3–14%). Risk factors: repeated exposure (cumulative dose and duration of therapy), genetic predisposition, renal impairment, specific aminoglycoside (neomycin > streptomycin >gentamicin > tobramycin > amikacin >netilmicin), elderly, age, bacteremia, hypovolemia, degree of temp elevation, and liver dysfunction (*JID* 1984:149:23–30). 62% of hearing lost were at frequency above 9 kHz (high pitch) at a mean of 9 days of therapy (*JID* 1992;165:1026–1032).

- Genetic predisposition in some cases vestibular and cochlear toxicity. Check family hx for aminoglycoside ototoxicity.
- Monitor for ototoxicity in any pts receiving >3 days of aminoglycoside. Vestibular toxicity monitoring: check baseline visual acuity using a Snellen pocket card. After 3 days of aminoglycoside, have pts shake head (side to side) while reading a line. Early sign of ototoxicity if pts loses 2 lines of visual acuity. Check Romberg sign. Cochlear toxicity monitoring: audiology test.

Rare
- Neuromuscular blockade (esp with myasthenia or Parkinsons and rapid infusion of large aminoglycoside doses)
- Allergic reaction (secondary to sulfites in some formulations)

DRUG INTERACTIONS
- Cephalothin: increased risk of nephrotoxicity.
- Loop diuretics (bumetanide, furosemide, ethacrynic acid, torsemide): cochlear toxicity (esp. w/ ethacrynic acid). Avoid co-administration.
- Nondepolarizing muscle relaxants (atracurium, pancuronium, tubocurarine, gallamine triethiodide): possible enhanced action of nondepolarizing muscle relaxant resulting in possible respiratory depression.
- Other nephrotoxic agents (e.g., amphotericin B, foscarnet, cidofovir, and IV contrast dyes): additive nephrotoxicity. Avoid co-administration.
- Penicillins: *in vitro* inactivation. Do not mix or run in the same tubing.
- Vancomycin: increased risk of nephrotoxicity.

SPECTRUM—See Appendix II, p. 795

RESISTANCE
- MIC breakpoint for Enterobacteriaceae and Gram-negative non-lactose fermenters including *P. aeruginosa* is 4 mcg/mL.
- *Enterococci* synergy with ampicillin if MIC <500 mcg/mL. If >500 mcg/mL to gentamicin, test for streptomycin sensitivity.

Pharmacology
Mechanism
Aminoglycosides inhibit protein synthesis by irreversibly binding to 30S ribosomal subunit.

Pharmacokinetic Parameters
- **Absorption** Aminoglycosides are rapidly absorbed after IM administration. Intrapleural and intraperitoneal administration results in rapid absorption. Poor absorption with oral administration.
- **Cmax** 6 mcg/mL after 1.5 mg/kg IV dose administration. In addition to the dose, Cmax will be affected by the volume of distribution.
- **Distribution** 0.2–0.4 L/kg (may be higher in pregnancy, ascites, edema, sepsis, and burn pts); Distributed in extracellular fluid, abscesses, ascitic fluid, pericardial fluid, pleural fluid, synovial fluid, lymphatic fluid, and peritoneal fluid. Not well distributed into bile, aqueous humor, bronchial secretions, abscess, sputum, and CSF.
- **Protein Binding** 0–10%
- **Metabolism/Excretion** Aminoglycosides are not metabolized in the liver, they are excreted unchanged in the urine.
- **T1/2** 2–4 hrs (Note: cystic fibrosis pts may have shorter half life of 1–2 hrs; burn and febrile pts may have increase clearance of aminoglycosides).

Dosing for Decreased Hepatic Function
No dose adjustment, but may increase risk of nephrotoxicity and ototoxicity. Use with close monitoring.

Pregnancy Risk
D: Animal studies show dose related nephrotoxicity. Reports of intra-amniotic instillations of gentamicin in pts (n=11) did not result in harm to the newborn. Ototoxicity has not been reported with in utero exposure, however eighth cranial nerve toxicity in the fetus is well known with exposure to other aminoglycosides (kanamycin and streptomycin) and can potentially occur with gentamicin.

Breast Feeding Compatibility
Excreted in low concentration in breast milk.

ANTIBACTERIAL DRUGS

COMMENTS

Enterococcal endocarditis and tularemia may be among the few infections in which gentamicin have a clearly defined role. Gentamicin appears more nephrotoxic but less ototoxic than tobramycin. Monitor renal function and watch for ototoxicity (auditory and vestibular). Don't use once daily dosing in pts w/ unstable renal fxn, CrCl <60 mL/min, endocarditis, meningitis, or increased Vd (e.g., pregnancy, ascites, edema).

SELECTED REFERENCES

American Thoracic Society, Infectious Diseases Society of America. Guidelines for the management of adults with hospital-acquired, ventilator-associated, and healthcare-associated pneumonia. *Am J Respir Crit Care Med*, 2005; Vol. 171; pp. 388–416.

Olaison L, Schadewitz K, Swedish Society of Infectious Diseases Quality Assurance Study Group for Endocarditis. Enterococcal endocarditis in Sweden, 1995–1999: can shorter therapy with aminoglycosides be used? *Clin Infect Dis*, 2002; Vol. 34; pp. 159–66.

IMIPENEM/CILASTATIN

Paul A. Pham, PharmD and John G. Bartlett, MD

INDICATIONS

FDA

- Bacterial endocarditis (caused by MSSA)
- Septicemia
- Skin/soft tissue infections (not MRSA)
- Lower respiratory tract infections (e.g., nosocomial pneumonia)
- Gynecologic infections
- Intra-abdominal infections
- Polymicrobial infections
- Uncomplicated and complicated urinary tract infections (pyelonephritis)

Non-FDA Approved Uses

- Gas gangrene
- Diabetic foot infection
- Bone/joint infections

FORMS

Brand name (mfr)	Forms	Cost*
Primaxin (Merck)	IV vial 250 mg; IV vial 500 mg	$21.68 per vial; $40.80 per vial
*Prices represents Average Wholesale Price (AWP).		

USUAL ADULT DOSING

- UTI: 250–500 mg IV q6h.
- Mild to moderate infections: 500 mg IV q6–8h.
- Severe or pseudomonal infections: 1 g IV q6–8h.
- Obese pts: consider 1 g IV q6h, but no clinical data.

RENAL DOSING

Dosing for GFR 50–80: GFR >70 mL/min: 0.5 g q6–8h (moderate infection) or 1 g q6–8h (severe infection).

Dosing for GFR 10–50: GFR 41–70 mL/min: 0.5 g q8h (moderate infection) or 0.5 g q6h (severe infection). GFR 21–40 mL/min: 0.25 g q6h (moderate infection) or 0.5 g q8h (severe infection). Consider using meropenem.

Dosing for GFR <10: GFR <20 mL/min: 0.25 g q12h (moderate infection) or 0.5 g q12h (severe infection). Consider using meropenem.

Dosing in hemodialysis: 0.25 g IV q12h with 0.25 g post dialysis on dialysis days. Consider meropenem.

Dosing in peritoneal dialysis: 0.25 g IV q12h. Consider meropenem.

Dosing in hemofiltration: CVVH: 250 mg IV q6h, CVVHD with dialysis flow rate <1.5L/hr: 500 mg IV q12h; CVVHD with dialysis flow rate 2 L/hr: 500 mg IV q8h. Consider meropenem.

ADVERSE DRUG REACTIONS

Occasional

- Phlebitis at infusion sites
- Allergic reactions (cross-allergy with PCN may be >50%, but clinically significant allergy may be much lower (see Romano reference)
- GI intolerance (nausea, vomiting, and diarrhea)
- LFTs elevation
- Eosinophilia
- Seizures (seen more in the elderly, pts w/ history of seizures, higher doses, and renal insufficiency)
- Drug fever

Rare

- Transient hypotension w/ infusion
- Myoclonus
- *C. difficile* colitis
- Bone marrow suppression
- Anaphylaxis

DRUG INTERACTIONS

- Probenecid: increases imipenem/cilastin concentrations. Avoid or use with caution in pts with renal failure or history of seizure disorders.
- Valproic acid: may decrease valproic acid serum concentrations. Monitor serum concentrations closely with co-administration.

SPECTRUM—See Appendix II, p. 789

RESISTANCE

- MRSA, *S. maltophilia*, *Burkholderia cepacia*, and *E. faecium* are generally resistant to Imipenem/cilastin.
- MIC breakpoint for Enterobacteriaceae: ≤4 mcg/mL (sensitive); 8 mcg/mL (intermediate); ≥16 mcg/mL (resistant).
- MIC breakpoint for Gram-negative non-lactose fermenters including *P. aeruginosa* and *Acinetobacter* spp.: ≤4 mcg/mL (sensitive); 8 mcg/mL (intermediate); ≥16 mcg/mL (resistant).

PHARMACOLOGY

Mechanism

A carbapenem antibiotic, inhibits mucopeptide synthesis in the bacterial cell wall, this results in the formation of defective cell walls and osmotically unstable organisms susceptible to cell lysis. Cilastatin is an inhibitor of dehydropeptidase I. Dehydropeptidase is present on the brush border of proximal renal tubular cells and inactivates imipenem by hydrolyzing the beta-lactam ring.

Pharmacokinetic Parameters

- **Absorption** —
- **Cmax** 40 mcg/mL after 500 mg IV dose administration
- **Distribution** Distributed in high concentration in pleural fluid, interstitial fluid, peritoneal fluid, pancreatic tissue, and reproductive organs. Also distributed in sputum, bile, aqueous humor, bone, and CSF in low concentration.
- **Protein Binding** 15–25%.
- **Metabolism/Excretion** 70–76% excreted in urine within 10 hrs via glomerular filtration and tubular secretion. Unknown nonrenal excretion mechanism accounts for the other 20–25%. Only 1–2% excreted via the bile in the feces.
- **T1/2** 1.0 hr.

Dosing for Decreased Hepatic Function

No data. Usual dose likely.

Pregnancy Risk

C: Animal studies (monkeys) shows increase in embryogenic loss and intolerance to mother. No data in humans.

Breast Feeding Compatibility
Excreted in breast milk.

COMMENTS
Parenteral carbapenem with very broad spectrum of activity that includes all anaerobes and most GNB, including *P. aeruginosa*, inducible chromosomal beta-lactamases, and ESBL-producing organisms but not MRSA, VRE, or *S. maltophilia*. The frequency of seizures range from 0.2% in pts without CNS or renal disease who were given the proper dose to 33% in those with CNS disease and renal insufficiency who were given a higher than recommended doses.

SELECTED REFERENCES
American Thoracic Society, Infectious Diseases Society of America. Guidelines for the management of adults with hospital-acquired, ventilator-associated, and healthcare-associated pneumonia. *Am J Respir Crit Care Med*, 2005; Vol. 171; pp. 388–416.

Romano A, Gueant-Rodrigues R, Gaeta F, et al. Imipenem in pts with immediate hypersensitivity to penicillins *NEJM*, 2006; Vol. 354; p. 26.

LEVOFLOXACIN

Paul A. Pham, PharmD and John G. Bartlett, MD

INDICATIONS
FDA
* Acute bacterial exacerbations of chronic bronchitis (ABECB); Acute bacterial sinusitis
* Community-acquired pneumonia (including those due to PCN-resistant *S. pneumoniae*) and nosocomial pneumonia
* Inhalational Anthrax (post-exposure)
* Uncomplicated and complicated skin and soft tissue infections (not MRSA)
* Uncomplicated and complicated urinary tract infections
* Bacterial conjunctivitis (Quixin 0.5% opthalmic drops); Treatment of corneal ulcer (1.5% ophthalmic solution)
* Chronic bacterial prostatitis

FORMS

Brand name (mfr)	Forms	Cost*
Levaquin (JOM)	Oral tablet 250 mg;	$13.35;
	Oral tablet 500 mg;	$15.30;
	Oral tablet 750 mg	$28.65
	IV vial 500 mg;	$45.65;
	IV vial 750 mg	$60.59
Quixin (JOM)	Topical ophthalmic gtt (5 mL) 0.5%	$73.50
Iquix (JOM)	Topical opthalmic gtt (5 mL) 1.5%	$73.50
*Prices represents Average Wholesale Price (AWP).		

USUAL ADULT DOSING
* Community acquired pneumonia: 500 mg IV or PO q24h × 7–14 days.
* Community acquired pneumonia: 750 mg IV or PO q24h × 5 days.
* Complicated skin and skin structure infections: 750 mg IV/PO q24h × 7–14 days.
* Nosocomial pneumonia: 750 mg IV/PO q24h × 7–14 days.
* ABECB: 500 mg PO q24h × 7 days.
* Acute bacterial sinusitis: 500 mg PO q24h × 7–14 days.
* UTI (uncomplicated): 250 mg PO q24h × 3 days,
* UTI (complicated): 250 mg PO q24h × 10 days.
* Chronic prostatitis: 500 mg PO q24h × 28 days.
* Anthrax: see anthrax modules.

- Bacterial conjunctivitis: 0.5% ophthalmic solution: 1–2 gtts into affected eye q2hrs (up to 8 times/day) × 2 days, then q4hrs while awake (up to 4 times/day) × 5 days.
- Corneal ulceration: day 1–2 (1.5%), gtt in the affected eye(s) every 30 mins to 2 hrs while awake and 4 and 6 hrs at night × 3 days, then 1 to 2 gtts in the affected eye(s) every 1 to 4 hrs while awake until completion.
- Obese pts: 750 mg IV or PO q24h.

RENAL DOSING

Dosing for GFR 50–80: 500–750 mg q24h.

Dosing for GFR 10–50: GFR 20–49 mL/min: 500–750 mg × 1, then 250 mg q24h or 750 mg q48h. GFR 10–19 mL/min: 500–750 mg × 1, then 250–500 mg q48h.

Dosing for GFR <10: 500–750 mg, then 250–500 mg q48h.

Dosing in hemodialysis: 500–750 mg, then 250–500 mg q48h.

Dosing in peritoneal dialysis: 500–750 mg, then 250–500 mg q48h.

Dosing in hemofiltration: CVVHD: 500–750 mg, then 250 mg q24h or 500 mg q48h.

ADVERSE DRUG REACTIONS

General

- Generally well tolerated

Occasional

- GI: diarrhea
- CNS: headache, malaise, insomnia, restlessness, dizziness
- Allergic reactions
- Photosensitivity/phototoxicity (can be severe)
- *C. difficile* colitis (a major agent of the NAP–1 strain of *C. difficile*)

Rare

- Peripheral neuropathy
- Increased hepatic enzymes
- QTc prolongation (elderly pts may be more susceptible)
- Tendon rupture (increased incidence seen in older pts with concurrent use of corticosteroids)
- Seizure
- Severe allergic reactions (TEN, Stevens-Johnsons syndrome, allergic pneumonitis, hepatitis, and bone marrow suppression)
- Interstitial nephritis
- Hepatitis (including severe, generally occurred within 14 days of initiation of therapy and most cases occurred within 6 days).

DRUG INTERACTIONS

- Divalent or trivalent cations (i.e., antacids, sucralfate, buffered ddI, vitamins, and minerals): interferes with levofloxacin absorption. Do not co-administer or administer levofloxacin 2 hrs before cation.
- Avoid concurrent use with other drugs that prolong the QT interval including class Ia or class III antiarrhythmic agents, in pts with hypokalemia, significant bradycardia, or cardiomyopathy.
- No significant interaction with HIV-protease inhibitor (nelfinavir) and non-nucleoside reverse transcriptase (nevirapine).
- NSAIDs: may increase risk of CNS side effects (clinical significance unknown).
- Sevelamer may decrease levofloxacin absorption. Avoid co-administration or give levofloxacin 2 hrs before sevelamer.
- Warfarin: may increase INR with co-administration. Monitor closely.

SPECTRUM—See Appendix II, p. 798

RESISTANCE

- PCN- resistant *S. pneumoniae* to levofloxacin is low (<3%) but with increasing use resistance is a concern.
- *Pseudomonas aeruginosa*, *Acinetobacter* spp., *Enterobacteriaceae* spp., and other *non-Enterobacteriaceae* spp. breakpoints: ≤2 mcg/mL (sensitive); 4 mcg/mL (intermediate); ≥8 mcg/mL (resistant).
- *Staphylococcus* spp. breakpoints: ≤1 mcg/mL (sensitive); 2 mcg/mL (intermediate); ≥4 mcg/mL (resistant).
- *S. pneumoniae* and *Enterococcus* spp. breakpoints: ≤2 mcg/mL (sensitive); 4 mcg/mL (intermediate); ≥8 mcg/mL (resistant).

ANTIBACTERIAL DRUGS

Mechanism

Fluoroquinolones inhibit DNA topoisomerases (DNA gyrase and topoisomerase 4) by binding to DNA-enzyme complexes, thereby interfering with bacterial DNA replication and some aspects of transcription, repair, recombination, and transposition.

Pharmacokinetic Parameters

- **Absorption** 98% absorbed. Can be administered without regard to food.
- **Cmax** 6.2 mcg/mL after 500 mg IV dose administration and 5.7 mcg/mL after 500 mg oral dose administration.
- **Distribution** Mean Vd 74–112 L. Widely distributed in kidneys, gallbladder, GYN tissues, liver, lung, prostatic tissue, phagocytic cells, urine, sputum, blister fluid, lungs, and bile. 30–50% of serum attained in CSF with inflamed meninges.
- **Protein binding** 24–38%.
- **Metabolism/Excretion** Minimal hepatic metabolism. 87% of dose excreted unchanged in the urine within 48 hrs via glomerular filtration and tubular secretion.
- **T1/2** 7 hrs.

Dosing for Decreased Hepatic Function

Usual dose likely.

Pregnancy Risk

C: In a prospective follow-up study conducted by the European Network of Teratology Information Services (ENTIS), 666 cases of fluoroquinolone exposure (the majority of the exposures were during the first trimester) showed a congenital malformation rate of 4.8%. From previous epidemiologic data, the 4.8% did not exceed the background rate. Animal data demonstrated arthropathy in immature animals with erosions in joint cartilage. Because of the animal data, and the availability of alternative antimicrobial agents, the use of fluoroquinolones during pregnancy is considered contraindicated.

Breast Feeding Compatibility

Fluoroquinolones are not recommended during breast feeding due to the potential for arthropathy (based on animal data).

COMMENTS

Levofloxacin is the L-isomer of ofloxacin with good *in vitro* and clinical experience against *S. pneumoniae* and atypical agents of pneumonia. Used primarily for lower respiratory tract infections and FDA approved for PCN-resistant *S. pneumoniae* and nosocomial pneumonia. Comparable to moxifloxacin for the treatment of community acquired pneumonia.

BASIS FOR RECOMMENDATIONS

Mandell LA, Wunderink RG, Anzueto A, et al. Infectious Diseases Society of America/American Thoracic Society consensus guidelines on the management of community-acquired pneumonia in adults. *Clin Infect Dis*, 2007; Vol. 44 Suppl 2; pp. S27–72.

Comments: The IDSA guidelines recommend a respiratory fluoroquinolone (i.e., levofloxacin, moxifloxacin, or gemifloxacin) for outpatient treatment of CAP in pts with comorbidities or in pts requiring hospital admissions (non-ICU). In ICU pts with CAP, cefotaxime or ceftriaxone should be used in combination with a respiratory fluoroquinolone.

SELECTED REFERENCES

Ho PL, Que TL, Chiu SS, et al. Fluoroquinolone and other antimicrobial resistance in invasive pneumococci, Hong Kong, 1995–2001. *Emerg Infect Dis*, 2004; Vol. 10; pp. 1250–7.

West M, Boulanger BR, Fogarty C, et al. Levofloxacin compared with imipenem/cilastatin followed by ciprofloxacin in adult pts with nosocomial pneumonia: a multicenter, prospective, randomized, open-label study. *Clin Ther*, 2003; Vol. 25; pp. 485–506.

LINEZOLID

Paul A. Pham, PharmD and John G. Bartlett, MD

INDICATIONS

FDA

- Pneumonia, hospital-acquired caused by MRSA, MSSA, and *S. pneumoniae*. Generally reserved for MRSA.
- Community acquired pneumonia caused by *S. pneumoniae* and MSSA. Not a preferred agent for CAP except for severe cases caused by MRSA.

- Infections due to vancomycin-resistant *Enterococcus faecium* (VRE), with or without concurrent bacteremia
- Complicated and uncomplicated skin and skin structure infection including diabetic foot ulcers (without osteomyelitis)

Non-FDA Approved Uses
- Vascular catheter associated sepsis (generally not recommended)
- Surgical wound infections
- Furuncle/carbuncle
- Cellulitis/erysipelas
- Osteomyelitis, acute (2nd line agent)
- Osteomyelitis, chronic (2nd line agent)
- Septic arthritis, community-acquired (limited data)
- Hardware associated septic arthritis (limited data)

FORMS

Brand name (mfr)	Forms	Cost*
Zyvox (Pfizer)	PO tab 600 mg PO susp 100 mg/5 mL IV soln 600 mg/300 mL	$86.90 $434.50 per 150 mL $111.35

*Prices represents Average Wholesale Price (AWP).

USUAL ADULT DOSING
- 600 mg IV or PO twice daily.
- Lower doses (400 mg PO twice daily) may be considered for uncomplicated soft tissue infection.
- Obese pts: consider linezolid 600 mg q8h for severe infections.

RENAL DOSING
Dosing for GFR 50–80: 600 mg twice daily.
Dosing for GFR 10–50: 600 mg twice daily.
Dosing for GFR <10: 600 mg twice daily.
Dosing in hemodialysis: 600 mg twice daily (give dose post-hemodialysis on days of dialysis).
Dosing in peritoneal dialysis: No data. Consider 600 mg twice daily.
Dosing in hemofiltration: Limited data. 600 mg twice daily.

ADVERSE DRUG REACTIONS
Occasional
- Reversible bone marrow suppression (thrombocytopenia and anemia) especially with >2 wks of treatment. Neutropenia has also been reported. In an open label study, thrombocytopenia and anemia occured in 4.7 % and 5.8 % of pts after a median treatment duration of 7–8 wks (*Eur J Clin Microbiol Infect Dis*. 2007;26:353).
- GI intolerance (nausea, vomiting, diarrhea)
- Headache

Rare
- Serotonin syndrome reported with SSRI co-administration
- Lactic acidosis
- *C. difficile*
- Optic neuritis or peripheral neuropathy (especially with long-term administration)
- Drug fever
- Rash
- Dizziness

DRUG INTERACTIONS
Linezolid is a reversible, nonselective inhibitor of monoamine oxidase. Tyramine rich foods, adrenergic and SSRI drugs should be avoided due to the potential interactions resulting in restlessness, myoclonus, mental status changes. It is recommended to discontinue SSRI or adrenergic agents 14 days before initiating linezolid. No interactions w/ CYP3A4.
- Buspirone: avoid coadministration.
- Meperidine: avoid coadministration.
- Serotonin 5-HT1 receptor agonists (triptans): avoid co-administration.

ANTIBACTERIAL DRUGS

- SSRIs (e.g., fluoxetine): avoid coadministration. (see Taylor et al.)
- Tricyclic antidepressants (e.g., nortryptyline, amitriptyline): avoid co-administration.

SPECTRUM—See Appendix II, p. 804

RESISTANCE

- MRSA and VRE resistance and emergence of resistance to linezolid have been reported [Potoski et al. *Emerg Infect Dis* Vol. 8, No. 12 December 2002. Birmingham et al *CID* 2003;36:159]
- MIC breakpoints of 4 mcg/mL for staphylococci and 2 mcg/mL for enterococci

PHARMACOLOGY

Mechanism

Linezolid inhibits the first step of protein synthesis by binding to f-met-t-RNA-mRNA-30s ribosome subunit.

Pharmacokinetic Parameters

- **Absorption** 100% absorbed (may be administered without regard to meals).
- **Cmax** 12.7 mcg/mL after a single dose of 600 mg administered orally.
- **Distribution** Volume of distribution of 50 L, widely distributed. Good CNS penetration (animal data). In osteomyelitis, inferior to cefazolin in an animal model (AAC 2000;44:3438), but achieves therapeutic bone concentrations (6–9 mcg/mL) (JAC 2002;50:73); however, bone marrow suppression may limit treatment duration >2 wks.
- **Protein binding** Low protein binding of 31%.
- **Metabolism/Excretion** Metabolized in the liver by oxidation with approximately 30% renal excretion and 70% non-renal excretion.
- **T1/2** 4.2–5.4 hrs.

Dosing for Decreased Hepatic Function

No dose adjustment needed.

Pregnancy Risk

C: Not teratogenic in animal studies.

Breast Feeding Compatibility

Excreted in breast milk (concentration similar to maternal plasma).

COMMENTS

Linezolid is active against nearly all antibiotic resistant Gram-positive bacteria and has a good short-term side effect profile. A retrospective study showed a significantly better survival and clinical cure rates compared to vancomycin in pts with nosocomial pneumonia due to MRSA, prospective confirmation of these results is needed. Linezolid may be considered for MRSA infections with documented vancomycin failure or intolerance. Since only minimal data to support the use of linezolid in MRSA endocarditis (Birmingham et al. *CID* 2003;36:159. Stevens et al. *CID* 2002;34:1481. Howden et al. *CID* 2004;38:521–8), daptomycin is preferred in cases of vancomycin failure or resistance. Susceptibility testing to linezolid should be performed for all MRSA and VRE isolates.

SELECTED REFERENCES

Adembri C, Fallani S, Cassetta MI, et al. Linezolid pharmacokinetic/pharmacodynamic profile in critically ill septic pts: intermittent versus continuous infusion. *Int J. Antimicrob Agents*, 2008; Vol. 31; pp. 122.

Taylor JJ, Wilson JW, Estes LL. Linezolid and serotonergic drug interactions: a retrospective survey. *Clin Infect Dis*, 2006; Vol. 43; pp. 180–7.

MEROPENEM

Paul A. Pham, PharmD and John G. Bartlett, MD

INDICATIONS

FDA

- Intra-abdominal infections (appendicitis and peritonitis) caused by viridans group streptococci, *E. coli, K. pneumoniae, P. aeruginosa, B. fragilis, B. thetaiotaomicron,* and *Peptostreptococcus* species.
- Meningitis (children 3 mos of age and older.) caused by *S. pneumoniae, H. influenzae,* and *N. meningitidis.*
- Complicated skin and soft tissue infections caused by *S. aureus* (MSSA only), *S. pyogenes, S. agalactiae,* viridans group streptococci, *E. faecalis* (not VRE), *P. aeruginosa, E. coli, P. mirabilis, B. fragilis,* and *Peptostreptococcus* species.

Non-FDA Approved Uses
- Brain abscess
- Shunt infections
- Other intra-abdominal infections (cholecystitis, cholangitis, diverticulitis, splenic abscess, hepatic abscess)

FORMS

Brand name (mfr)	Forms	Cost*
Merrem (Astra Zeneca)	IV vial 500 mg; IV vial 1000 mg	$38.39; $76.78
*Prices represents Average Wholesale Price (AWP).		

USUAL ADULT DOSING
- Mild to moderate infections: 1 g IV q8h.
- Severe and CNS infections: 2 g IV q8h.
- To enhance PK/PD parameters, some experts recommend extended infusion (over 4 hrs) for severe infections and/or treatment of intermediately-resistant organisms (in combination with an aminoglycoside).
- Obese pts: 2 g IV q8h (limited data).

RENAL DOSING

Dosing for GFR 50–80: Usual dose.

Dosing for GFR 10–50: GFR 26–50 mL/min: 1 g IV q12h (mild to moderate infections) or 1 g IV q8h (severe or CNS infections). GFR 10–25 mL/min: 0.5 g IV q12h (mild to moderate infections) or 1 g IV q12h (severe of CNS infections).

Dosing for GFR <10: GFR 0.5 g q24h (mild to moderate infections) or 1 g q24h (severe or CNS infections).

Dosing in hemodialysis: 0.5–1.0 g q24h. On days of HD, dose after dialysis.

Dosing in peritoneal dialysis: 0.5 g IV q24h.

Dosing in hemofiltration: CVVH: 1 g IV q12h to q8h, CVVHD: 1–2 g IV q12h; 2 g IV q12h for severe or CNS infections.

ADVERSE DRUG REACTIONS

Occasional
- Allergic reactions (skin test cross-reaction w/ PCN may be up to 50%, but clinically significant cross allergy reported to be much lower; see Romano ref)
- GI intolerance (nausea, vomiting, and diarrhea)

Rare
- Seizure (decreased incidence of seizures in animal studies compared to imipenem)
- *C. difficile* colitis
- Thrombocytopenia
- Anaphylaxis
- Drug fever

DRUG INTERACTIONS
- Probenecid: may increase meropenem serum concentrations. Avoid or use with caution in renal failure.
- Valproic acid: may decrease valproic acid serum concentrations. Monitor serum concentrations closely with co-administration.

SPECTRUM—See Appendix II, p. 789

RESISTANCE
- MRSA, *S. maltophilia*, *B. cepacia*, and *E. faecium* are generally resistant to meropenem.
- MIC breakpoint for *Enterobacteriaceae:* ≤4 mcg/mL (sensitive); 8 mcg/mL (intermediate); ≤16 mcg/mL (resistant).
- MIC breakpoint for Gram-negative non-lactose fermenters including *P. aeruginosa* and *Acinetobacter* spp.: ≤4 mcg/mL (sensitive); 8 mcg/mL (intermediate); ≥16 mcg/mL (resistant).

PHARMACOLOGY

Mechanism

A carbapenem antibiotic that inhibits mucopeptide synthesis in the bacterial cell wall, this results in the formation of defective cell walls and osmotically unstable organism which leads to cell lysis.

ANTIBACTERIAL DRUGS

Pharmacokinetic Parameters
- **Cmax** 26 mcg/mL after 500 mg IV dose administration.
- **Distribution** Well distributed into most body tissues and fluid including pancreatic tissue and CSF.
- **Protein binding** 2%.
- **Metabolism/Excretion** Primarily excreted unchanged via glomerular filtration and tubular secretion.
- **T1/2** 1.0 hrs.

Dosing for Decreased Hepatic Function
No data, usual dose likely.

Pregnancy Risk
B: Animal data shows no risk. No data in humans. Carbapenem antibiotic is considered safest to use during perinatal period (i.e., 28 wks gestation or later) and most likely meropenem can be classified this way. The fetal risk of use before this period is unknown.

Breast Feeding Compatibility
No data available.

Comments
Similar spectrum of activity to imipenem that includes *P. aeruginosa*, inducible chromosomal beta-lactamases, and ESBL producing organisms with comparable efficacy for intra-abdominal and soft tissue infections. May have an advantage over imipenem for the treatment of meningitis where up to 6 g per day has been used with minimal seizure complications. More expensive compared to imipenem.

Selected References
American Thoracic Society, Infectious Diseases Society of America. Guidelines for the management of adults with hospital-acquired, ventilator-associated, and healthcare-associated pneumonia. *Am J Respir Crit Care Med*, 2005; Vol. 171; pp. 388–416.

Romano A, Viola M, Guéant-Rodriguez RM, et al. Brief communication: tolerability of meropenem in pts with IgE-mediated hypersensitivity to penicillins. *Ann Intern Med*, 2007; Vol. 146; pp. 266–9.

METHENAMINE HIPPURATE

Paul A. Pham, PharmD and John G. Bartlett, MD

Indications

FDA
- Prophylactic or suppressive treatment of frequently recurring urinary tract infections. Use after eradication of the infection by other appropriate antibiotic.
- Chronic urinary tract infections.

Non-FDA Approved Uses
- Uncomplicated urinary tract infections.
- Bacteriuria

Forms

Brand name (mfr)	Forms	Cost*
Hiprex (Sanofi-Aventis)	Oral tablet 1000 mg	$2.06
Urex (Rising)	Oral tablet 1000 mg	$1.79
*Prices represents Average Wholesale Price (AWP).		

Usual Adult Dosing
Methenamine hippurate 1 g PO twice daily.

Renal Dosing
Dosing for GFR 50–80: Usual dose.
Dosing for GFR 10–50: Avoid use due to inadequate urine concentration and toxic serum level.
Dosing for GFR <10: Avoid use due to inadequate urine concentration and toxic serum level.
Dosing in hemodialysis: Avoid use due to inadequate urine concentration and toxic serum level.
Dosing in peritoneal dialysis: Avoid use due to inadequate urine concentration and toxic serum level.
Dosing in hemofiltration: No data. Avoid use.

ADVERSE DRUG REACTIONS
Occasional
- Nausea and dyspepsia
- Rash

Rare
- Crystalluria (with large doses)
- LFT elevation

DRUG INTERACTIONS
Urinary alkalinizers (sodium bicarbonate, sodium acetate, sodium lactate, sodium citrate) increases urine pH and may decrease hydrolysis of methenamine in urine to formaldehyde and ammonia, resulting in decreased efficacy. Avoid urinary alkalinizers.

RESISTANCE
Enterobacter aerogenes

PHARMACOLOGY
Mechanism
Methenamine is hydrolyzed by acid (mandelate acid or hippurate acid) to formaldehyde and ammonia. Formaldehyde is responsible for the antiseptic and antibacterial activity of methenamine.

Pharmacokinetic Parameters
- **Absorption** Rapidly absorbed.
- **Cmax** Inactive in blood and serum. Urinary formaldehyde of 18–60 mcg/mL after 1 g administration.
- **Distribution** Distributed to body tissues and fluids, but not hydrolyzed to formaldehyde and ammonia systemically (due to pH higher than 6.8).
- **Metabolism/Excretion** Excreted unchanged in urine via glomerular filtration and tubular secretion. Hydrolyzed in the urine to formaldehyde and ammonia.
- **T1/2** 4.3 hrs.

Dosing for Decreased Hepatic Function
No data. Usual dose likely.

Pregnancy Risk
C: In a surveillance study of Michigan Medicaid recipients reported 209 exposures to methenamine during the first trimester. The 3.8% birth defects reported did not support an association between methenamine and congenital defects.

Breast Feeding Compatibility
Methenamine is excreted in breast milk.

COMMENTS
Oral urinary antiseptic used for the prevention or treatment of uncomplicated urinary tract infections, but cotrimoxazole is the agent of choice.

SELECTED REFERENCES
Cronberg S, Welin CO, Henriksson L, et al. Prevention of recurrent acute cystitis by methenamine hippurate: double blind controlled crossover long term study. *Br Med J (Clin Res Ed)*, 1987; Vol. 294; pp. 1507–8.

Lee B, Bhuta T, Craig J, et al. Methenamine hippurate for preventing urinary tract infections. *Cochrane Database Syst Rev*, 2002; Vol. CD003265.

METRONIDAZOLE

Paul A. Pham, PharmD and John G. Bartlett, MD

INDICATIONS
FDA
- Anaerobic infections: intra-abdominal infections, skin, and skin structure infections, bone and joint infections
- Bacterial septicemia; endocarditis (caused by *Bacteroides* spp.)
- Gynecologic infections (endometritis, endomyometritis, tubo-ovarian abscess, and postsurgical vaginal cuff infection)
- Lower respiratory tract infections (in combination with another agent with activity against microaerophilic Streptococcus)

ANTIBACTERIAL DRUGS

- Adjunct treatment for gastritis and duodenal ulcer associated with *Helicobacter pylori*
- CNS infections (meningitis and brain abscess)
- Treatment of acute intestinal amebiasis and amoebic liver abscess
- Treatment of symptomatic and asymptomatic trichomoniasis
- Bacterial vaginosis (vaginal gel)
- Acne rosacea (topical gel)

Non-FDA Approved Uses
- Colitis, antibiotic-associated (*C. difficile*)
- Treatment of giardiasis and dracunculiasis
- Periodontal disease
- Elective colorectal surgery (classified as contaminated or potentially contaminated)
- Prophylaxis for elective colon surgery (with agent for coliforms)

FORMS

Brand name (mfr)	Forms	Cost*
Flagyl (Pfizer and generic manufacturers)	Oral tablet 250 mg; Oral tablet 500 mg Oral cap 375 mg IV minibag 500 mg	$0.16; $0.70 $4.08 $3.11
Metrocream; Metrolotion (Galderma)	Topical cream 0.75% (45 g) Topical gel 0.75% (70 g)	$70.35 $37.50
MetroGel (*Vaginal*)(Prasco)	Topical gel 0.75% (70 g)	$33.71
MetroGel (Galderma; Taro)	Topical gel 0.75% (1.5 oz); Topical gel 1% (60 g)	$71.15; $153.94
Flagyl ER (Pfizer)	Oral extended release tab 750 mg	$12.11
*Prices represents Average Wholesale Price (AWP).		

USUAL ADULT DOSING
- Susceptible anaerobic infections: 250–500 mg PO q8h or 500 mg IV q6h (manufacturer's recommendation) or consider 0.5–1 g PO or IV q12h (based on PK data).
- *C. difficile* colitis: 500 mg PO q8h or 250 mg PO four times a day × 10–14 days.
- Bacterial vaginosis: 500 mg twice daily PO × 7 days or *Flagyl ER* 750 mg PO once daily × 7 days.
- Trichomoniasis: single 2 g × 1 dose or 500 mg PO twice daily × 7 days (alternative).
- Amebiasis: 750 mg PO q8h × 5–10 days.
- Giardiasis: 250 mg PO q8h × 5–10 days.

RENAL DOSING
Dosing for GFR 50–80: Usual dose.
Dosing for GFR 10–50: Usual dose.
Dosing for GFR <10: Usual dose.
Dosing in hemodialysis: Usual regimen.
Dosing in peritoneal dialysis: Usual regimen.
Dosing in hemofiltration: No data. Usual dose likely.

ADVERSE DRUG REACTIONS
Common
- GI intolerance
- Metallic taste
- Headache
- Dark urine (harmless)

Occasional
- Peripheral neuropathy (with prolonged use, usually reversible)
- Phlebitis at injection sites

- Disulfiram-like reaction with alcohol
- Insomnia
- Stomatitis

Rare

- Seizures

DRUG INTERACTIONS

- Barbiturates: may decrease metronidazole levels.
- Disulfiram: contraindicated.
- Ethanol: nausea, vomiting, headache, abdominal cramps, and flushing. Acute of psychosis or confusional state may also occur (avoid co-administration). Alcohol should be avoided and disulfiram should be discontinued 2 wks prior to use of metronidazole.
- Lithium: lithium levels may be increased.
- Lopinavir liquid: disulfiram-like reaction (avoid co-administration).
- Phenytoin: phenytoin levels may be increased.
- Ritonavir liquid: due to the alcohol content in the RTV liquid formulation, a disulfiram-like reaction may occur (avoid co-administration).
- Tipranavir capsule: disulfiram-like reaction (avoid co-administration).
- Warfarin: INR may be increased.

SPECTRUM—See Appendix II, p. 804

PHARMACOLOGY

Mechanism

Exact mechanism not fully elucidated, but reduction of metronidazole may lead to a polar metabolite that disrupts DNA and inhibits nucleic acid synthesis.

Pharmacokinetic Parameters

- **Absorption** 90% absorbed with oral administration (IV only if oral administration is contraindicated).
- **Cmax** 20–25 mcg/mL after 500 mg PO or IV dose administration.
- **Distribution** Distributed to saliva, bile, seminal fluid, bone, liver, and liver abscesses, lungs, vaginal secretions. Good CSF penetration (30–100% of serum levels attained in the CSF).
- **Protein binding** 20%.
- **Metabolism/Excretion** Hepatic hydroxylation, oxidation and glucuronide conjugation to an active metabolite (2-hydroxy metronidazole) accounts for 30–60% of administered dose. 77% of the dose excreted in urine and 14% in feces as unchanged drug and metabolites within 5 days.
- **T1/2** 6–14 hrs.

Dosing for Decreased Hepatic Function

Decreased dose in severe hepatic impairment.

Pregnancy Risk

B: Animal (rodents) data show risk of carcinogenicity. The use of metronidazole in pregnancy is controversial, reports in humans have arrived at conflicting data (but most studies show no risk). The manufacturer and CDC consider metronidazole to be contraindicated in the first trimester.

Breast Feeding Compatibility

Excreted in breast milk. American Academy of Pediatrics recommends using metronidazole with caution, discontinuation of breast feeding for 12–24 hrs recommended to allow excretion of the drug.

COMMENTS

Metronidazole is the gold standard anti-anaerobic agent. Active against virtually all anaerobes with exception of actinomyces, *Propionibacterium acnes*, and *Lactobacillus* spp. Additional antibiotic coverage needed for combined aerobes/anaerobes infections (metronidazole only active against anaerobes). First line agent for giardiasis, trichomoniasis, and amebiasis. Oral vancomycin and metronidazole are equivalent in the treatment of MILD (but not severe) *C. difficile*—associated colitis with comparable rates of response and relapse.

SELECTED REFERENCES

Bartlett JG. Narrative review: the new epidemic of *Clostridium difficile*-associated enteric disease. *Ann Intern Med*, 2006; Vol. 145; pp. 758–64.

Chaudhry R, Mathur P, Dhawan B, et al. Emergence of metronidazole-resistant *Bacteroides fragilis*, India. *Emerg Infect Dis*, 2001; Vol. 7; pp. 485–6.

ANTIBACTERIAL DRUGS

MINOCYCLINE

Paul A. Pham, PharmD and John G. Bartlett, MD

INDICATIONS
FDA

- Pneumonia due to *Mycoplasma pneumoniae.*
- Granuloma inguinale caused by *Calymmatobacterium granulomatis.*
- Lymphogranuloma venereum caused by chlamydia species.
- Psittacosis caused by *Chlamydia psittaci.*
- Rocky Mountain spotted fever, typhus fever and the rickettsial typhus group, Q fever, rickettsialpox and other tick fevers caused by Rickettsiae.
- Relapsing fever due to *Borrelia recurrentis.*
- Chancroid caused by *Haemophilus ducreyi.*
- Cholera caused by *Vibrio cholerae* (resistance reported).
- Nongonococcal urethritis (caused by Ureaplasma urealyticum or Chlamydia trachomatis)
- Yaws caused by *T. pertenue.* Plague due to *Yersinia pestis.* Tularemia due to *Francisella tularensis.* Campylobacter fetus infections caused by *Campylobacter fetus.* Brucellosis due to *Brucella* species (in conjunction with streptomycin). Bartonellosis due to *Bartonella bacilliformis.* Granuloma inguinale caused by *Calymmatobacterium granulomatis,* mild-moderate acne vulgaris (age >12, minocycline ER only).

Non-FDA Approved Uses

- Hardware-associated septic arthritis
- Acne vulgaris (adjunctive treatment)
- Typhus infections

FORMS

Brand name (mfr)	Forms	Cost*
Minocin (Triax)	PO cap 50 mg; 100 mg	$0.57; $1.15
Dynacin and generic (Medicis Dermatologics and generic)	PO cap 50 mg; 75 mg; 100 mg PO tab 50 mg; 75 mg; 100 mg	$1.68; $1.98; $6.02 $6.93; $10.17; $12.15
Solodyn ER (Medicis Dermatologics)	Oral ER tab 45 mg; 90 mg; 135 mg	$19.35
*Prices represents Average Wholesale Price (AWP).		

USUAL ADULT DOSING

100 mg PO twice daily.

- Acne vulgaris: minocycline ER (age >12) dosed at approximately 1 mg/kg/day PO.

RENAL DOSING

Dosing for GFR 50–80: Usual dose.

Dosing for GFR 10–50: Usual dose, some recommend increasing the dosing interval. Doxycycline is preferred.

Dosing for GFR <10: Usual dose though some recommend increasing the dosing interval. Doxycycline is preferred.

Dosing in hemodialysis: Usual dose. No supplementation recommended. Doxycycline is preferred.

Dosing in peritoneal dialysis: Usual dose. Doxycycline is preferred.

Dosing in hemofiltration: No data. Usual dose likely. Doxycycline is preferred.

ADVERSE DRUG REACTIONS
Common

- Vertigo and ataxia

- GI intolerance (dose related), nausea and vomiting
- Stains and deforms teeth in children <8 yrs

Occasional
- Worsening azotemia (increased in pts with renal failure). Doxycycline preferred in pts with renal insufficiency.
- Hepatotoxicity (dose related, especially pregnant women, renal insufficiency, and with the use of expired medication).
- Esophageal ulcerations.
- Candidiasis (thrush and vaginitis)
- Photosensitivity.
- Skin hyperpigmentation (blue-black) reported with long-term treatment.

Rare
- Allergic reactions
- Visual disturbances
- Aggravation of myasthenia gravis (reversed with calcium)
- *C. difficile* colitis (less likely compared to cephalosporins, carbapenems, and fluoroquinolones)
- Hemolytic anemia
- Benign intracranial hypertension, papilledema
- Fanconi syndrome (with outdated drugs)
- Hypersensitivity reactions (anaphylaxis, angioneurotic edema, urticaria, rash, and pruritus)
- Stevens Johnson syndrome and erythema multiforme have been reported
- Lupus-like syndrome manifested by arthralgia, myalgia

RESISTANCE
- MIC breakpoint for *Enterobacteriaceae, Staphylococcus* spp., and *Enterococcus* spp.: <4 mcg/mL (sensitive); 8 mcg/mL (intermediate); >16 mcg/mL (resistant).
- Isolates that are susceptible tetracycline are also considered susceptible to doxycycline and minocycline. However, tetracycline-intermediate or -resistant isolates may be susceptible to doxycycline or minocycline.

DRUG INTERACTIONS—See Appendix III, p. 824, for table of drug-to-drug interactions.
SPECTRUM—See Appendix II, p. 802

PHARMACOLOGY
Mechanism
Tetracyclines inhibit protein synthesis by mainly binding to 30S ribosomal subunit and blocking binding of aminoacyl transfer-RNA.

Pharmacokinetic Parameters
- **Absorption** 90% absorbed.
- **Cmax** 4.2 mcg/mL after 200 mg IV dose administration. 2–3.5 mcg/mL after 200 mg PO dose administration.
- **Distribution** Widely distributed into body tissues and fluids including pleural fluid, bronchial secretions, sputum, ascitic fluid, synovial fluid, aqueous and vitreous humor, and prostatic fluid.
- **Protein binding** 55–88%.
- **Metabolism/Excretion** Possible liver metabolism. 4–19% excreted in the urine, 20–34% excreted in the feces.
- **T1/2** 16 hrs.

Dosing for Decreased Hepatic Function
No accumulation. Usual dose.

Pregnancy Risk
D: Tetracyclines are contraindicated in pregnancy due to retardation of skeletal development and bone growth; enamel hypoplasia and discoloration of teeth of fetus. Maternal liver toxicity have also been reported.

Breast Feeding Compatibility
Tetracyclines are excreted in breast milk at very low concentrations. There is theoretical possibility of dental staining and inhibition of bone growth, but infants exposed to tetracyclines have blood levels less than 0.05 mcg/mL.

ANTIBACTERIAL DRUGS

COMMENTS

Oral tetracycline that may be used in place of doxycycline, but dizziness may be very bothersome in some pts. Absorption is not significantly affected by food. Most active tetracycline against staphylococci (including CA-MRSA), but activity against *Streptococcus* spp. is limited. May be useful with rifampin in an attempt to provide chronic suppressive treatment of infected bone and joint prosthesis.

SELECTED REFERENCES

Barnes EV, Dooley DP, Hepburn MJ, et al. Outcomes of community-acquired, methicillin-resistant *Staphylococcus aureus*, soft tissue infections treated with antibiotics other than vancomycin. *Mil Med*, 2006; Vol. 171; pp. 504–7.

Keeney RE, Seamans ML, Russo RM, et al. The comparative efficacy of minocycline and penicillin-V in *Staphylococcus aureus* skin and soft tissue infections. *Cutis*, 1979; Vol. 23; pp. 711–8.

MOXIFLOXACIN

Paul A. Pham, PharmD and John G. Bartlett, MD

INDICATIONS

FDA

- Acute exacerbations of chronic bronchitis. Acute bacterial sinusitis.
- Community-acquired pneumonia (including those caused by multi-drug resistant).
- Uncomplicated skin and skin structure infections (oral, not MRSA). Complicated skin and skin structure infections, including diabetic foot infections (oral and IV, not MRSA).
- Complicated intra-abdominal infections, including polymicrobial infections such as abscesses. Author's opinion: due to the potential resistance of *B. fragilis*, use in mild to moderate intra-abdominal infections only. Consider the addition of metronidazole for severe infections.
- Bacterial conjunctivitis (ophthalmic drops).

Non-FDA Approved Uses

- Treatment of MTB (in combination)
- Treatment of MAI (in combination)

FORMS

Brand name (mfr)	Forms	Cost*
Avelox (Schering-Plough [Bayer])	Oral tablet 400 mg	$13.38
	IV piggyback 400 mg	$43.75
Vigamox (Alcon)	Ophthalmic gtts 0.5% (3 mL)	$69.44
*Prices represents Average Wholesale Price (AWP).		

USUAL ADULT DOSING

- Community-acquired pneumonia: 400 mg IV or PO once daily × 7–14 days.
- Uncomplicated skin and skin structure infections (not MRSA): 400 mg IV or PO once daily × 7 days. Complicated skin and skin structure infections: 400 mg IV once daily × 7–21 days.
- Acute sinusitis: 400 mg PO once daily × 5–10 days.
- Acute exacerbations of chronic bronchitis: 400 mg PO once daily × 5 days.
- Mild to moderate intra-abdominal infections, including polymicrobial infections: 400 mg IV or PO once daily × 5–21 days. Consider the addition of metronidazole for severe intra-abdominal infections.
- Bacterial conjunctivitis: 1 ophthalmic drop to affected eye(s) q8h × 7 days.
- Obese pts: no data, consider 600 mg once daily (based on PK of dose-ranging studies).

RENAL DOSING

Dosing for GFR 50–80: Usual dose.
Dosing for GFR 10–50: Usual dose.
Dosing for GFR <10: Usual dose.
Dosing in hemodialysis: No data, usual dose likely.
Dosing in peritoneal dialysis: No data, usual dose.
Dosing in hemofiltration: No data, usual dose.

ADVERSE DRUG REACTIONS
Occasional
- Generally well tolerated GI intolerance: diarrhea
- CNS: headache, malaise, insomnia, restlessness, dizziness. Use with caution in pts with CNS disorders, especially elderly
- Increased transaminases
- Photosensitivity/phototoxicity reactions (can be severe)
- *C. difficile* colitis

Rare
- Allergic reactions.
- QTc prolongation.
- Tendon rupture. FQ class effect. Increased incidence especially seen in older pts over age 60, concurrent use of corticosteroids, kidney, heart, and lung transplant recipients. D/C if pt experiences pain or tendon rupture.
- Peripheral neuropathy.
- Seizure.
- Severe allergic reactions (TEN, Stevens-Johnsons syndrome, allergic pneumonitis, hepatitis, and bone marrow suppression).
- Interstitial nephritis.

DRUG INTERACTIONS
- Any divalent and trivalent cations (i.e., antacid, multiple vitamin, zinc, calcium, iron, sucralfate, buffered ddI, etc.): significant decrease in moxifloxacin serum levels. Avoid co-administration or moxifloxacin should be taken 4 hrs before or 8 hrs after divalent/trivalent cations administration.
- Class IA (e.g., quinidine, procainamide) or Class III (e.g., amiodarone, sotalol) antiarrhythmic agents: avoid in pts with known prolongation of the QT interval and pts with uncorrected hypokalemia due to the potential for additive QTc prolongation. Other drugs that have the potential for causing QTc prolongation should be used with caution.
- Sevelamer-may decrease moxifloxacin absorption. Avoid co-administration or give moxifloxacin 2 hrs before sevelamer.

SPECTRUM—See Appendix II, p. 798
RESISTANCE
- *S. pneumoniae* resistance to newer fluoroquinolones remains very low (*Clin Microbiol Infect.* 2004;10:645–51) but drug resistant *S. pneumoniae* (DRSP) can be a concern.
- *S. pneumoniae* breakpoints: ≤ 1 mcg/mL (sensitive); 2 mcg/mL (intermediate); ≥ 4 mcg/mL (resistant).
- *Staphylococcus* spp. breakpoints: ≤ 0.5 mcg/mL (sensitive); 1 mcg/mL (intermediate); ≥ 2 mcg/mL (resistant).

PHARMACOLOGY
Mechanism
Inhibits DNA topoisomerases (DNA gyrase and topoisomerase 4) by binding to DNA-enzyme complexes, thereby interfering with bacterial DNA replication and some aspects of transcription, repair, recombination, and transposition.

Pharmacokinetic Parameters
- **Absorption** 90%; may be taken with or without meals.
- **Cmax** 4.5 mcg/mL; AUC 48 mcg/mL hr with 400 mg qd at steady-state.
- **Distribution** Vd2.7–3.5 L/kg; widely distributed.
- **Protein binding** 48%.
- **Metabolism/Excretion** Metabolized in the liver to an inactive metabolite. CYP450 enzymes are not involved in moxifloxacin metabolism, and are not affected by moxifloxacin.
- **T1/2** 13 hrs.

Dosing for Decreased Hepatic Function
No data.

Pregnancy Risk
C: No data for moxifloxacin. In a prospective follow-up study conducted by the European Network of Teratology Information Services (ENTIS), 666 cases of fluoroquinolone exposure (the majority of the exposures were during the first trimester) showed a congenital malformation rate of 4.8%.

ANTIBACTERIAL DRUGS

557

From previous epidemiologic data, the 4.8% did not exceed the background rate. Animal data demonstrated arthropathy in immature animals with erosions in joint cartilage. Because of the animal data, and the availability of alternative antimicrobial agents, the use of fluoroquinolones during pregnancy is considered contraindicated.

Breast Feeding Compatibility

No data. Fluoroquinolones are not recommended during breast feeding due to the potential for arthropathy.

COMMENTS

Oral and parenteral fluoroquinolone with spectrum of activity similar to levofloxacin (this include enhanced activity against *S. pneumoniae*). Best anaerobic and mycobacteria activity among quinolones. Activity against pseudomonas is poor compared to ciprofloxacin and levofloxacin. Lower urinary drug concentrations means this fluoroquinolone should not be used for complicated UTI's. May result in false positive opiate screening test (*JAMA*. 2001;286:3115–3119).

BASIS FOR RECOMMENDATIONS

Mandell LA, Wunderink RG, Anzueto A, et al. Infectious Diseases Society of America/American Thoracic Society consensus guidelines on the management of community-acquired pneumonia in adults. *Clin Infect Dis*, 2007; Vol. 44 Suppl 2; pp. S27–72.

Comments: The IDSA guidelines recommend a respiratory fluoroquinolone (i.e., levofloxacin, moxifloxacin, or gemifloxacin) for outpatient treatment of CAP in pts with comorbidities or in pts requiring hospital admissions (non-ICU). In ICU pts with CAP, cefotaxime or ceftriaxone should be used in combination with a respiratory fluoroquinolone.

SELECTED REFERENCES

Ho PL, Que TL, Chiu SS, et al. Fluoroquinolone and other antimicrobial resistance in invasive pneumococci, Hong Kong, 1995–2001. *Emerg Infect Dis*, 2004; Vol. 10; pp. 1250–7.

Malangoni MA, Song J, Herrington J, et al. Randomized controlled trial of moxifloxacin compared with piperacillin-tazobactam and amoxicillin-clavulanate for the treatment of complicated intra-abdominal infections. *Ann Surg*, 2006; Vol. 244; pp. 204–11.

MUPIROCIN

Paul A. Pham, PharmD and John G. Bartlett, MD

INDICATIONS

FDA

- Eradication of nasal colonization with methicillin-resistant *S. aureus* (nasal ointment)
- Treatment of secondarily infected traumatic skin lesions due to susceptible strains of *S. aureus* and Streptococcus pyogenes
- Impetigo due to *S. pyogenes* or *S. aureus*

FORMS

Brand name (mfr)	Forms	Cost*
Bactroban (GlaxoSmithKline)	Topical cream 2% (15 g; 30 g) Topical nasal oint 2% (1 g) Topical oint 2% (22 g)	$3.54 per g $9.95 per g $42.90 per 22 g tube
Mupirocin (Various generic manufacturers)	Topical ointment 2% (22 g)	$26 per tube
*Prices represents Average Wholesale Price (AWP).		

USUAL ADULT DOSING

- Staphylococcal nasal colonization: topical apply (1/2 nasal oint tube each nares or ointment applied to each nares) twice daily × 5 days.
- Skin infections: apply small amount three times daily to affected areas for 3–5 days. If unimproved, have condition re-evaluated.
- Ointment contains polyethylene glycol which may be absorbed from non-intact skin, care should be used if potential to absorb large quantities is possible, especially if there is evidence of moderate or severe renal impairment.

RENAL DOSING
Dosing for GFR 50–80: Usual dose.
Dosing for GFR 10–50: Usual dose.
Dosing for GFR <10: Usual dose.
Dosing in hemodialysis: Usual dose.
Dosing in peritoneal dialysis: Usual dose.
Dosing in hemofiltration: Usual dose.

ADVERSE DRUG REACTIONS
Occasional
* Local site reaction: burning, stinging (irritation of mucous membrane), pain, pruritus, and rash.

DRUG INTERACTIONS
None.

PHARMACOLOGY
Mechanism
Mupirocin binds to bacterial isoleucine-tRNA ligase (isoleucyl-tRNA synthase) and prevents translation of bacterial ribosomal RNA by interfering with incorporation of isoleucine into polypeptide chain.

Pharmacokinetic Parameters
* **Absorption** No systemic absorption following topical treatment.
* **Protein binding** >97%.
* **T1/2** 0.4–0.8 hr (in a study using IV).

Dosing for Decreased Hepatic Function
Usual dose.

Pregnancy Risk
Animal data show no risk. No human data available.

Breast Feeding Compatibility
No data available.

COMMENTS
Topical agent that may be used for temporarily eradication of *S. aureus* (including MRSA) nasal carriage. Approximately 30% recolonization within 4 wks after completion of mupirocin treatment.

SELECTED REFERENCES
Kluytmans JA, Wertheim HF. Nasal carriage of *Staphylococcus aureus* and prevention of nosocomial infections. *Infection*, 2005; Vol. 33; pp. 3–8.

Mupirocin Study Group. Nasal mupirocin prevents *Staphylococcus aureus* exit-site infection during peritoneal dialysis. Mupirocin Study Group. *J Am Soc Nephrol*, 1996; Vol. 7; pp. 2403–8.

NAFCILLIN

Paul A. Pham, PharmD and John G. Bartlett, MD

INDICATIONS
FDA
* Staphylococcal infections (not MRSA)

Non-FDA Approved Uses
* Parotitis (MSSA)
* Brain abscess (MSSA)
* Empyema (MSSA)
* Pyomyositis (MSSA)
* Osteomyelitis, acute (MSSA)
* Osteomyelitis, chronic (MSSA)
* Diabetic foot infection (mild-moderate infections)
* Septic arthritis, community-acquired (MSSA)
* Hardware associated septic arthritis (2 nd line treatment of MSSE; consider adding rifampin)
* Endocarditis (MSSA)
* Meningitis (MSSA)

ANTIBACTERIAL DRUGS

- Septicemia (MSSA)
- Skin and soft tissue infections (MSSA, strep species)

FORMS

Brand name (mfr)	Forms	Cost*
Nafcillin (Various generic manufacturers)	IV vial 1 g; IV vial 2 g; IV vial 10 g	$11.34; $13.78; $107.78
*Prices represents Average Wholesale Price (AWP).		

USUAL ADULT DOSING

- Streptococcal or MSSA native valve endocarditis, bacteremia: 2 g IV q4h (+/– aminoglycoside).
- Soft tissue infections: 1–2 g IV q4–6h.
- For obese pts: 2 g IV q4h or 3 g IV q6h.

RENAL DOSING

Dosing for GFR 50–80: Usual dose.
Dosing for GFR 10–50: Usual dose.
Dosing for GFR <10: Usual dose.
Dosing in hemodialysis: Usual dose, no supplement doses needed.
Dosing in peritoneal dialysis: Usual dose.
Dosing in hemofiltration: No data. Usual dose likely.

ADVERSE DRUG REACTIONS
Common
- Phlebitis at IV sites

Occasional
- Neutropenia
- Hypersensitivity reactions
- Rash (in up to 10%)
- Coombs' test positive without hemolytic anemia
- Sterile abscesses if given IM
- Tissue necrosis with extravasation
- Jarisch-Herxheimer reaction (with treatment of syphilis or other spirochetal infections)
- Interstitial nephritis
- *C. difficile*–associated colitis

Rare
- Hepatitis
- Hemolytic anemia
- Thrombocytopenia
- Leukopenia

DRUG INTERACTIONS
- Tetracyclines: *in vitro* antagonism, may decrease efficacy of nafcillin *in vivo*. Avoid co-administration.
- Warfarin: may significantly decrease warfarin effect (decrease PT INR). Monitor INR closely with co-administration.

SPECTRUM—See Appendix II, p. 795
RESISTANCE
- MIC breakpoint is 2 mcg/mL for *S. aureus* and 0.25 mcg/mL for *S. epidermidis*. Heteroresistance reported with *S. epidermidis* (use with caution).

PHARMACOLOGY
Mechanism
Beta-lactam antibiotics inhibit mucopeptide synthesis in the bacterial cell wall; this results in the formation of defective cell walls and osmotically unstable organisms susceptible to cell lysis.

Pharmacokinetic Parameters
- **Cmax** 40–57 mcg/mL after 500 mg IV dose administration.
- **Distribution** Distributed to blister fluid, urine, peritoneal fluid, pleural fluid, middle ear fluid, intestinal mucosa, bone, gallbladder, lung, female reproductive tissue, bile, and inflamed meninges.

- **Protein binding** 90%.
- **Metabolism/Excretion** Hepatic metabolism accounts for 60% of administered dose. Both unchanged drug and metabolites are excreted via glomerular filtration and tubular secretion. Biliary excretion also occurs accounting for the high biliary concentration.
- **T1/2** 0.5 hrs.

Dosing for Decreased Hepatic Function
Dose decrease needed only for combined severe hepatic and renal impairment.

Pregnancy Risk
B: Several collaborative perinatal project reports involving over 12,000 exposures to penicillin derivatives during the first trimester indicated no association between penicillin derivative drugs and birth defects.

Breast Feeding Compatibility
Excreted in breast milk in low concentration. No adverse effects have been reported.

COMMENTS
Parenteral anti-staphylococcal penicillin that is therapeutically equivalent to oxacillin. Incidence of hepatitis and rash appears to be lower with nafcillin than oxacillin, and may be used in pts developing oxacillin-induced hepatitis but may be associated with more neutropenia.

BASIS FOR RECOMMENDATIONS
ACC/AHA 2006 guidelines for the management of pts with valvular heart disease: a report of the American College of Cardiology/American Heart Association Task Force on Practice Guidelines (writing committee to revise the 1998 Guidelines for the Management of Pts With Valvular Heart Disease): developed in collaboration with the Society of Cardiovascular Anesthesiologists: endorsed by the Society for Cardiovascular Angiography and Interventions and the Society of Thoracic Surgeons. *Circulation*, 2006; Vol. 114(5); pp. e84–231.

Comments: Endocarditis guidelines. Nafcillin or oxacillin (2 g IV q4h) +/– gentamicin is recommended for MSSA native valve endocarditis.

SELECTED REFERENCES
Maraqa NF, Gomez MM, Rathore MH, et al. Higher occurrence of hepatotoxicity and rash in pts treated with oxacillin, compared with those treated with nafcillin and other commonly used antimicrobials. *Clin Infect Dis*, 2002; Vol. 34; pp. 50–4.

NEOMYCIN

Paul A. Pham, PharmD and John G. Bartlett, MD

INDICATIONS
FDA
- Bladder irrigation
- Bowel preparation (w/ erythromycin for elective colon surgery)
- Minor dermal infection (prophylaxis)
- Ocular infections (keratoconjunctivitis, keratitis, conjunctivitis, blepharoconjunctivitis, blepharitis, used as ophthalmic solution and suspension)
- Portal-systemic encephalopathy

FORMS

Brand name (mfr)	Forms	Cost*
Neomycin (Various)	PO tab 500 mg	$1.25
Neo-Rx Powder (X-Gen)	PO powder 100 g	$0.20 (per 1 g)
Cortisporin (Monarch)	Topical ointment 1% (0.5 oz)	$70.28
Neomycin + polymyxin (Bausch and Lomb (and generic manufacturers))	Opthalmic Drops 10 mL	$30.03
Coly-Mycin S Otic (Generic Manufacturer)	Otic Drops Susp 1% (10 mL)	$30.80
*Prices represents Average Wholesale Price (AWP).		

ANTIBACTERIAL DRUGS

561

USUAL ADULT DOSING
- Bowel Prep: neomycin 1 g oral at 19 hrs, 18 hrs, and 9 hrs before the start of surgery (plus erythromycin).
- Hepatic encephalopathy: 1–4 g PO three times a day (generally 4–12 g per day).
- Superficial ocular infections: 1–2 drops (ophthalmic) in the affected eye q3–4 hrs.
- Otitis externa: 4 drops (otic susp) in the affected ear q6–8h.

RENAL DOSING
Dosing for GFR 50–80: Usual dose.
Dosing for GFR 10–50: 1–4 g q12–18 hrs with long-term therapy.
Dosing for GFR <10: 1–4 g q18–24 hrs with long-term therapy.
Dosing in hemodialysis: No data, may require adjustment with long-term therapy.
Dosing in peritoneal dialysis: No data, may require adjustment with long-term therapy.
Dosing in hemofiltration: No data, may require adjustment with long-term therapy.

ADVERSE REACTION
Rare
- Renal failure.
- Vestibular and auditory damage may occur through systemic accumulation of oral doses in pts with decrease GFR.

DRUG INTERACTIONS
- Digoxin: may increase serum digoxin level due to the alteration of microbial gut flora by oral neomycin. Monitor for digoxin toxicity and serum concentrations. Dose of digoxin may need to be decreased.
- Loop diuretics (bumetanide, furosemide, ethacrynic acid, torsemide): may increase risk of ototoxicity, but less of an issue with oral administration in pts with normal renal function.
- Nephrotoxic agents (e.g., amphotericin B, foscarnet, cidofovir): may increase risk of nephrotoxicity, but less of an issue with oral administration in pts with normal renal function.

PHARMACOLOGY
Mechanism
Aminoglycosides inhibit protein synthesis by irreversibly binding to 30S ribosomal subunit.
Pharmacokinetic Parameters
- **Absorption** Poor absorption following oral administration.
- **Distribution** 0.2–0.4 L/kg; not adequately absorbed for systemic therapeutic level.
- **Metabolism/Excretion** Aminoglycosides are not metabolized in the liver, they are excreted unchanged in the urine.
- **T1/2** 2–3 hrs.
Pregnancy Risk
C: Ototoxicity has not been reported with *in utero* exposure, however eighth cranial nerve toxicity in the fetus is well known with exposure to other aminoglycosides (kanamycin and streptomycin) and can potentially occur with neomycin. In a report of 30 exposures in the first trimester to neomycin found no association between neomycin and congenital defects.
Breast Feeding Compatibility
No data available.

COMMENTS
Cochlear toxicity precludes parenteral use. Main use is for treatment of hepatic encephalopathy and with erythromycin as a bowel prep in pts undergoing elective colon surgery, although this latter use has been losing favor. Though usually used only in a topical applications, systemic effects may occur when used in large volumes.

SELECTED REFERENCES
Shah VH, Kamath P. Management of portal hypertension. *Postgrad Med*, 2006; Vol. 119; pp. 14–8.

Song F, Glenny AM. Antimicrobial prophylaxis in colorectal surgery: a systematic review of randomized controlled trials. *Br J Surg*, 1998; Vol. 85; pp. 1232–41.

NITROFURANTOIN

Paul A. Pham, PharmD and John G. Bartlett, MD

INDICATIONS

FDA

- Treatment of uncomplicated urinary tract infection

Non-FDA Approved Uses

- Urinary tract infection, recurrent [women]
- Urinary tract infections in pregnancy
- Prophylaxis of UTI

FORMS

Brand name (mfr)	Forms	Cost*
Macrodantin (Procter and Gamble and generic)	PO cap 25 mg; PO cap 50 mg; PO cap 100 mg	$1.13; $0.37; $0.59
Macrobid (Proctor and Gamble and generic)	PO cap 100 mg	$2.36
Furadantin (Sciele)	PO susp 25 mg/5 mL	$6.63 per 5 mL
*Prices represents Average Wholesale Price (AWP).		

USUAL ADULT DOSING

- Uncomplicated UTI (in pts with normal renal function): 50–100 mg PO q6h or nitrofurantoin monohydrate/macrocrystals (Macrobid) 100 mg PO twice daily.
- Agent not appropriate for short course (3 days) UTI therapy. Dose duration should be 7 days minimum.
- UTI suppression: 50–100 mg PO once daily.

RENAL DOSING

Dosing for GFR 50–80: Usual dose.

Dosing for GFR 10–50: Avoid due to inadequate urinary level and potential for toxic serum level.

Dosing for GFR <10: Avoid due to inadequate urinary level and potential for toxic serum level.

Dosing in hemodialysis: Avoid due to inadequate urinary level and potential for toxic serum level.

Dosing in peritoneal dialysis: Avoid due to inadequate urinary level and potential for toxic serum level.

Dosing in hemofiltration: Avoid.

ADVERSE DRUG REACTIONS

Common

- GI intolerance (macrocrystalline formulation better tolerated)

Occasional

- Hypersensitivity reactions with acute pulmonary symptoms: fever, cough, dyspnea w/ infiltrate and eosinophilia. Occurs within hrs-wks of dose.
- Lupus-like reaction
- Rash

Rare

- Methemoglobinemia and hemolytic anemia (with G6PD deficiency)
- Hepatitis +/– cholestatic jaundice
- Peripheral neuropathy
- Pancreatitis
- Pulmonary fibrosis with long-term use
- Lactic acidosis
- Trigeminal neuralgia
- Parotitis

ANTIBACTERIAL DRUGS

- Avoid long term co-administration with drugs associated peripheral neuropathy (e.g., metronidazole, stavudine, didanosine, linezolid).
- Norfloxacin: may be antagonistic, avoid concurrent administration.

PHARMACOLOGY

Mechanism

Nitrofurantoin is reduced by flavoproteins (bacterial enzyme) to active intermediates that may inactivate or damage ribosomal proteins and other macromolecules including DNA and RNA.

Pharmacokinetic Parameters

- **Absorption** Rapidly and completely absorbed (administer with food, increase bioavailability by 40%).
- **Cmax** 50–150 mcg in urine after 100 mg oral dose administration.
- **Distribution** Distributed in urine and kidneys in high concentrations, while serum concentration are very low.
- **Protein binding** 20–60%.
- **Metabolism/Excretion** 66% rapidly metabolized mainly in liver. Between 20–44% excreted unchanged in urine via glomerular filtration and tubular secretion.
- **T1/2** 0.4 hrs.

Dosing for Decreased Hepatic Function

No data.

Pregnancy Risk

B: In a surveillance study of Michigan Medicaid recipients, 1,292 exposures to nitrofurantoin resulted in 4.0% birth defects. This data did not support an association between nitrofurantoin and congenital defects.

Breast Feeding Compatibility

Excreted in breast milk. Theoretical chance of hemolytic anemia in G6PD deficiency. The American Academy of Pediatrics considers nitrofurantoin compatible with breast feeding.

COMMENTS

Antiseptic for uncomplicated UTI's. Caution when used in G6PD deficient pts. Avoid in pts w/ CrCl <40 mL/min since efficacy is decreased and side effects increased. Associated with acute allergic pneumonitis w/ short-term treatment; interstitial fibrosis w/ long-term use has been reported. Since *E. coli* resistance remains low, nitrofurantoin is a good alternative to fluoroquinolones in the treatment of uncomplicated UTI.

SELECTED REFERENCES

Iravani A, Klimberg I, Briefer C, et al. A trial comparing low-dose, short-course ciprofloxacin and standard 7 days therapy with co-trimoxazole or nitrofurantoin in the treatment of uncomplicated urinary tract infection. *J Antimicrob Chemother*, 1999; Vol. 43 Suppl A; pp. 67–75.

Kahlmeter G. Prevalence and antimicrobial susceptibility of pathogens in uncomplicated cystitis in Europe. The ECO. SENS study. *Int J Antimicrob Agents*, 2003; Vol. 22 Suppl 2; pp. 49–52.

NORFLOXACIN

Paul A. Pham, PharmD and John G. Bartlett, MD

INDICATIONS

FDA

- Uncomplicated endocervical and urethral gonorrhea
- Prostatitis due to *E. coli*
- Uncomplicated and complicated urinary tract infections
- Uncomplicated urinary tract infections (including cystitis) due to *Enterococcus faecalis, Escherichia coli, Klebsiella pneumoniae, Proteus mirabilis, Pseudomonas aeruginosa, Staphylococcus epidermidis, Staphylococcus saprophyticus, Citrobacter freundii, Enterobacter aerogenes, Enterobacter cloacae, Proteus vulgaris, Staphylococcus aureus,* or *Streptococcus agalactiae.*
- Complicated urinary tract infections due to *Enterococcus faecalis, Escherichia coli, Klebsiella pneumoniae, Proteus mirabilis, Pseudomonas aeruginosa,* or *Serratia marcescens.*

Non-FDA Approved Uses
- Spontaneous bacterial peritonitis prophylaxis
- Antibiotic prophylaxis in afebrile neutropenic pts with hematological malignancies

FORMS

Brand name (mfr)	Forms	Cost*
Noroxin (Merck)	PO tab 400 mg	$4.27

*Prices represents Average Wholesale Price (AWP).

USUAL ADULT DOSING
- UTI: 400 mg PO twice daily.
- Uncomplicated GC: 800 mg × 1.
- SBP prophylaxis: 400 mg PO once daily.
- Prostatitis: 400 mg PO twice daily.
- Prophylaxis in neutropenic pts: 400 mg PO twice daily.

RENAL DOSING
Dosing for GFR 50–80: Usual dose.
Dosing for GFR 10–50: 400 mg q12h–q24h.
Dosing for GFR <10: 400 mg once daily.
Dosing in hemodialysis: not removed in hemodialysis, dose 400 mg once daily.
Dosing in peritoneal dialysis: 400 mg once daily.
Dosing in hemofiltration: No data. Consider 400 mg q12h–24h.

ADVERSE DRUG REACTIONS
General
- Generally well tolerated

Occasional
- GI intolerance: diarrhea, dyspepsia and flatulence
- CNS: headache, malaise, insomnia, restlessness, dizziness
- Photosensitivity
- *C. difficile* colitis

Rare
- Increased LFTs
- QTc prolongation
- Seizure
- Tendon rupture (increased incidence especially seen in older pts over age 60, concurrent use of corticosteroids, kidney, heart, and lung transplant recipients)

DRUG INTERACTIONS
- Antiarrhythmics (with QT prolongation: avoid concurrent use with other drugs that prolong the QT interval including class Ia or class III antiarrhythmic agents, in pts with hypokalemia, significant bradycardia, or cardiomyopathy.
- Divalent or trivalent cations (i.e., antacids, sucralfate, buffered ddI, vitamins, and minerals): interferes with norfloxacin absorption. Do not co-administer or administer norfloxacin 2 hrs before cation.
- Nitrofurantoin: may be antagonistic, avoid concurrent administration.
- Warfarin: may increase INR with co-administration. Monitor closely.

SPECTRUM—See Appendix II, p. 804
PHARMACOLOGY
Mechanism
Fluoroquinolones inhibits DNA topoisomerases (DNA gyrase and topoisomerase 4) by binding to DNA-enzyme complexes, thereby interfering with bacterial DNA replication and some aspects of transcription, repair, recombination, and transposition.
Pharmacokinetic Parameters
- **Absorption** 30–40% absorbed.
- **Cmax** 1.4–1.8 mcg/mL after 400 mg PO dose administration.

ANTIBACTERIAL DRUGS

- **Distribution** Distributed in renal parenchyma, gallbladder, liver, prostatic tissue, testicle, seminal fluid, sputum, maxillary sinus mucosa, tonsils, blister fluid, uterus, fallopian tube, cervical and vaginal tissue, and high concentration in bile.
- **Protein binding** 10–15%.
- **Metabolism/Excretion** Hepatic metabolism to some active metabolites. Unchanged drug and metabolites are excreted in urine via glomerular filtration and tubular secretion. 30% excreted in feces via biliary route or unabsorbed drug.
- **T1/2** 4 hrs.

Dosing for Decreased Hepatic Function
Usual dose. Serum level unchanged in hepatic insufficiency.

Pregnancy Risk
C: In a prospective follow-up study conducted by the European Network of Teratology Information Services (ENTIS), 666 cases of fluoroquinolone exposure (the majority of the exposures were during the first trimester) showed a congenital malformation rate of 4.8%. From previous epidemiologic data, the 4.8% did not exceed the background rate. Animal data demonstrated arthropathy in immature animals with erosions in joint cartilage. Because of the animal data, and the availability of alternative antimicrobial agents, the use of fluoroquinolones during pregnancy is considered contraindicated.

Breast Feeding Compatibility
Fluoroquinolones are not recommended during breast feeding due to the potential for arthropathy (based on animal data).

COMMENTS

- Oral fluoroquinolone that is not well absorbed compared to most agents in this class. Main uses are as prophylaxis for spontaneous bacterial peritonitis (SBP) and prophylaxis of fever in neutropenic pts.

SELECTED REFERENCES

Gafter-Gvili A, Fraser A, Paul M, et al. Meta-analysis: antibiotic prophylaxis reduces mortality in neutropenic pts. *Ann Intern Med*, 2005; Vol. 142; pp. 979–95.

Grangé JD, Roulot D, Pelletier G, et al. Norfloxacin primary prophylaxis of bacterial infections in cirrhotic pts with ascites: a double-blind randomized trial. *J Hepatol*, 1998; Vol. 29; pp. 430–6.

OFLOXACIN

Paul A. Pham, PharmD and John G. Bartlett, MD

INDICATIONS

FDA

- Acute exacerbation of chronic bronchitis (AECB) and community-acquired pneumonia (CAP)
- Pelvic Inflammatory Disease (PID). Endocervical and urethral gonorrhea (note: high resistance rates in U.S. and world-wide, no longer recommended) and chlamydia infections. Nongonococcal urethritis and cervicitis due to *C. trachomatis*.
- Uncomplicated and complicated UTI.
- Prostatitis due to *E. coli*.
- Skin and soft tissue infections.
- Otitis externa, chronic suppurative otitis media, otitis media (otic solution).
- Conjunctivitis, keratitis, and corneal ulcers (ophthalmic solution).

Non-FDA Approved Uses

- Peritonitis, spontaneous bacterial and secondary
- Proctitis [sexually transmitted]
- Sexually-associated reactive arthritis (SARA)

FORMS

Brand name (mfr)	Forms	Cost*
Floxin (Ortho-McNeil and generic manufacturer)	PO tab 200 mg; PO tab 300 mg; PO tab 400 mg	$4.79; $5.70; $6.01

Brand name (mfr)	Forms	Cost*
Ocuflox (Allergan; Bausch and Lomb)	Ophthalmic gtt 0.3% (5 mL); Ophthalmic gtt 0.3% (10 mL)	$54.65; $83.30
Floxin (Falcon)	Otic gtt 0.3%(10 mL); Otic gtt 0.3% (5 mL)	$127.00; $82.50

*Prices represents Average Wholesale Price (AWP).

USUAL ADULT DOSING

- CAP, soft tissue infection and AECB: 400 mg PO twice daily.
- Uncomplicated UTI: 200 mg PO twice daily × 3–7 days.
- Non GC cervicitis/urethritis: 300 mg twice daily × 7 days.
- Conjunctivitis, keratitis: 1–2 ophthalmic drops q2–4hrs × 2 days then q6h for a total of 7–10 days.
- Corneal ulcer: 1–2 ophthalmic drops every 30 minutes while awake × 2 days, then hourly while awake during days 3–9, then four times daily (consult ophthalmology).
- Otitis externa: 10 drops (otic solution) into affected ear(s) once daily × 7 days.

RENAL DOSING

Dosing for GFR 50–80: Usual dose.
Dosing for GFR 10–50: 200–400 mg q24h.
Dosing for GFR <10: 100–200 mg q24h.
Dosing in hemodialysis: 200 mg, then 100 mg q24h.
Dosing in peritoneal dialysis: 100–200 mg q24h.
Dosing in hemofiltration: No data. Consider 400 mg q24h.

ADVERSE DRUG REACTIONS

General
- Generally well tolerated

Occasional
- GI: diarrhea
- CNS: headache, malaise, insomnia, restlessness, dizziness
- Allergic reactions: rash, hives
- *C. difficile* colitis
- Photosensitivity /phototoxicity (can be severe)

Rare
- Tendon rupture (increased incidence seen in older pts with concurrent use of corticosteroids)
- Increased LFTs
- Peripheral neuropathy
- QTc prolongation
- Seizure
- Severe allergic reactions (TEN, Stevens-Johnsons syndrome, allergic pneumonitis, hepatitis, and bone marrow suppression)
- Interstitial nephritis
- *C. difficile* colitis

DRUG INTERACTIONS

- Antiarrhythmic agents (prolong the QT interval including class Ia or class III): avoid especially in pts with hypokalemia, significant bradycardia, or cardiomyopathy.
- Divalent or trivalent cations (e.g., antacids, sucralfate, buffered ddI, vitamins, and minerals): interferes with ofloxacin absorption. Do not co-administer or give ofloxacin 2 hrs before cations.
- NSAIDS: may increase risk of CNS side effects (clinical significance unknown). Monitor closely.
- Procainamide: procainamide levels may be increased. Monitor closely with co-administration.
- Warfarin: may increase INR with co-administration. Monitor closely.

ANTIBACTERIAL DRUGS

PHARMACOLOGY

Mechanism

Fluoroquinolones inhibits DNA topoisomerases (DNA gyrase and topoisomerase 4) by binding to DNA–enzyme complexes, thereby interfering with bacterial DNA replication and some aspects of transcription, repair, recombination, and transposition.

Pharmacokinetic Parameters

- **Absorption** 98% absorbed.
- **Cmax** 4.6 mcg/mL after 400 mg PO dose administration. 5.2–7.2 mcg/mL after 400 mg IV dose administration.
- **Distribution** Fluoroquinolones are widely distributed to most body fluids and tissues; high concentrations are attained in the kidneys, gallbladder, GYN tissues, liver, lung, prostatic tissue, phagocytic cells, urine, sputum, and bile.
- **Protein binding** 98%.
- **Metabolism/Excretion** <10% hepatic metabolism. 68–90% excreted unchanged in urine. 4–8% excreted in feces.
- **T1/2** 7.0 hrs.

Dosing for Decreased Hepatic Function

No data. Usual dose likely.

Pregnancy Risk

C: In a prospective follow-up study conducted by the European Network of Teratology Information Services (ENTIS), 666 cases of fluoroquinolone exposure (the majority of the exposures were during the first trimester) showed a congenital malformation rate of 4.8%. From previous epidemiologic data, the 4.8% did not exceed the background rate. Animal data demonstrated arthropathy in immature animals with erosions in joint cartilage. Because of the animal data, and the availability of alternative antimicrobial agents, the use of fluoroquinolones during pregnancy is considered contraindicated.

Breast Feeding Compatibility

Fluoroquinolone are not recommended during breast feeding due to the potential for arthropathy (based on animal data).

COMMENTS

Oral FQ that has been largely supplanted by levofloxacin, its more active L-isomer. IV formulation is no longer available. Ofloxacin ophthalmic drops is equivalent to ciprofloxacin ophthalmic drops in the treatment of corneal ulcer. Ofloxacin is preferred over cipro due to a 20% incidence crystalline precipitate in the epithelial defect seen with ciprofloxacin drops.

SELECTED REFERENCES

Adachi JA, Ostrosky-Zeichner L, DuPont HL, et al. Empirical antimicrobial therapy for traveler's diarrhea. *Clin Infect Dis*, 2000; Vol. 31; pp. 1079–83.

Nouira S, Marghli S, Belghith M, et al. Once daily oral ofloxacin in chronic obstructive pulmonary disease exacerbation requiring mechanical ventilation: a randomised placebo-controlled trial. *Lancet*, 2001; Vol. 358; pp. 2020–5.

OXACILLIN

Paul A. Pham, PharmD and John G. Bartlett, MD

INDICATIONS

FDA

- Staphylococcal infections (MSSA)

Non-FDA Approved Uses

- Parotitis (MSSA)
- Empyema (MSSA)
- Vascular Graft Infections (2nd line treatment for MSSE; consider adding rifampin)
- Hepatic Abscess (MSSA)
- Pyomyositis (MSSA)
- Diabetic Foot Infection (mild-moderate infections)
- Septic Arthritis, Community-Acquired (MSSA)
- Hardware Associated Septic Arthritis (2nd line treatment for MSSE; consider adding rifampin)

- Endocarditis (MSSA)
- Treatment of bacterial septicemia (MSSA)
- Skin and soft tissue infections (MSSA)

FORMS

Brand name (mfr)	Forms	Cost*
Oxacillin (Various)	IV vial 1 g; IV vial 2 g; IV vial 10 g	$11.34; $22.00; $107.70
*Prices represents Average Wholesale Price (AWP).		

USUAL ADULT DOSING
- Cellulitis and other soft tissue infections: 1–2 g IV q4–6 hrs.
- MSSA native valve endocarditis: 2 g IV q4h (+/– aminoglycoside).
- For obese pts: 2 g IV q4h

RENAL DOSING
Dosing for GFR 50–80: Usual dose.
Dosing for GFR 10–50: Usual dose.
Dosing for GFR <10: Usual dose.
Dosing in hemodialysis: Usual regimen.
Dosing in peritoneal dialysis: Usual regimen.
Dosing in hemofiltration: No data. Usual regimen likely.

ADVERSE DRUG REACTIONS
Common
- Rash (in up to 32%)
- Hepatitis (in up to 22%)
- Phlebitis at infusion sites

Occasional
- *C. difficile*–associated colitis
- Coombs' test positive without hemolytic anemia
- Drug fever
- Jarisch-Herxheimer reaction (with treatment of syphilis or other spirochetal infections)

Rare
- Anaphylaxis, the frequency of anaphylaxis reaction is reported at 0.004–0.015% of PCN courses
- Hemolytic anemia
- Thrombocytopenia
- Leukopenia
- Interstitial nephritis

DRUG INTERACTIONS
Tetracyclines: *in vitro* antagonism; avoid co-administration. Bactericidal effect of penicillins may be diminished *in vivo*. In 2 studies involving a total of 79 pts with pneumococcal meningitis treated with either penicillin plus tetracyclines or penicillin monotherapy resulted in a higher mortality rate (79–85%) in the combination therapy compared to penicillin monotherapy (30–33%) [*Arch Intern Med* 1951;88:489, *Ann Intern Med* 1961;55:545]. However there was not a difference in mortality between penicillin monotherapy and penicillin plus tetracycline in the treatment of pneumococcal pneumonia [*Arch Intern Med* 1953;91:197].

SPECTRUM—See Appendix II, p. 795
RESISTANCE
- MIC breakpoint is 2 mcg/mL for *S. aureus* and 0.25 mcg/mL for *S. epidermidis*. Heteroresistance reported with *S. epidermidis* (use with caution).

PHARMACOLOGY
Mechanism
Beta-lactam antibiotics inhibit mucopeptide synthesis in the bacterial cell wall, this results in the formation of defective cell walls and osmotically unstable organisms susceptible to cell lysis.

ANTIBACTERIAL DRUGS

Pharmacokinetic Parameters

- **Absorption** 30% absorbed.
- **Cmax** 40–57 mcg/mL after 500 mg IV dose administration.
- **Distribution** Distributed to blister fluid, urine, peritoneal fluid, pleural fluid, middle ear fluid, intestinal mucosa, bone, gallbladder, lung, female reproductive tissue, bile, and inflamed meninges.
- **Protein binding** 90%.
- **Metabolism/Excretion** Hepatic metabolism accounts for 49% of administered dose. Both unchanged drug and metabolites are excreted via glomerular filtration and tubular secretion. 10% biliary excretion.
- **T1/2** 0.5 hrs.

Dosing for Decreased Hepatic Function

Use with caution. Consider using nafcillin.

Pregnancy Risk

B: Several collaborative perinatal project reports involving over 12,000 exposures to penicillin derivatives during the first trimester indicated no association between penicillin derivative drugs and birth defects.

Breast Feeding Compatibility

Excreted in breast milk in low concentration. No adverse effects have been reported.

COMMENTS

Anti-staphylococcal penicillin equivalent to nafcillin but more likely to cause reversible hepatitis and rash.

SELECTED REFERENCES

American College of Cardiology/American Heart Association Task Force on Practice Guidelines, Society of Cardiovascular Anesthesiologists, Society for Cardiovascular Angiography and Interventions, et al. ACC/AHA 2006 guidelines for the management of pts with valvular heart disease: a report of the American College of Cardiology/American Heart Association Task Force on Practice Guidelines (writing committee to revise the 1998 Guidelines for the Management of Pts With Valvular Heart Disease): developed in collaboration with the Society of Cardiovascular Anesthesiologists: endorsed by the Society for Cardiovascular Angiography and Interventions and the Society of Thoracic Surgeons. *Circulation*, 2006; Vol. 114; pp. e84–231.

Maraqa NF, Gomez MM, Rathore MH, et al. Higher occurrence of hepatotoxicity and rash in pts treated with oxacillin, compared with those treated with nafcillin and other commonly used antimicrobials. *Clin Infect Dis*, 2002; Vol. 34; pp. 50–4.

PENICILLIN

Paul A. Pham, PharmD and John G. Bartlett, MD

INDICATIONS

FDA

- Endocarditis.
- Skin and soft tissue infection (erysipelas, erysipeloid).
- Rat-bite fever.
- Syphilis.
- Vincent's infection fusospirochetosis (Vincent's gingivitis and pharyngitis).
- PCN procaine: anthrax due to *Bacillus anthracis*, including inhalation anthrax (post-exposure). However, CDC does not recommend as first line agent due to beta-lactamase production (see "biodefense-anthrax").
- Actinomycosis.
- Empyema.
- Pasteurella infections.
- Pneumonia, upper respiratory tract infection, Otitis media, venereal infections (penicillin G benzathine suspension), rheumatic fever prophylaxis, chorea prophylaxis, upper bacterial respiratory infection, syphilis and neurosyphilis, glomerulonephritis prophylaxis, prophylaxis for rheumatic fever, rheumatic heart disease, rheumatic chorea.

Non-FDA Approved Uses

- Brain abscess
- Lung abscess

- Endocarditis (*S. viridans*)
- Necrotizing fasciitis (*S. pyogenes*)
- Gas gangrene
- Lyme arthritis
- Neisseria meningitidis
- Neurosyphilis (*Treponema pallidum*)

FORMS

Brand name (mfr)	Forms	Cost*
Penicillin V Potassium (Various)	PO tab 250 mg; PO tab 500 mg PO susp 125 mg/5 mL; PO susp 250 mg/5 mL	$0.24; $0.40 $0.13 per 5 mL; $0.11 per 5 mL
Penicillin G potassium (Sandoz and various generic manufacturers)	IV vial 1 MU; IV vial 3 MU; IV vial 2 MU; IV vial 5 MU	$12.70; $13.70; $13.20; $6-$42.00
Bicillin L-A (Monarch)	IM syringe 0.6 MU/mL; IM syringe 1.2 MMU/2 mL; IM syringe 2.4 MMU/4 mL	$31.40 per mL; $53.30 per 2 mL; $110 per 4 mL
Bicillin C-R (King)	IM syringe 0.30 MU–0.30 U/mL	$16.40 per mL
Bicillin C-R 900/300 (Monarch)	IM syringe 0.9 MU-0.30 MU/2 mL; IM syringe 1.2 MMU/2 mL	$44.74; $42.99
Penicillin G sodium (Sandoz and various generic manufacturers)	IV vial 5 million units	$47.91

*Prices represents Average Wholesale Price (AWP).

USUAL ADULT DOSING
- **Parenteral:** Aqueous PCN G: 2–4 million units IV q4h.
- Infective endocarditis (IE): 4 million units IV q4h (see resistance section for duration of treatment).
- Skin and soft tissue infections, due to susceptible streptococci (rarely used): PCN benzathine/procaine (Bicillin C-R) 2.4 million units IM × 1.
- **Oral:** PCN VK: 250–500 mg PO q6h (amoxicillin generally preferred due to better bioavailability). Twice daily administration may be considered for streptococcal tonsillopharyngitis.
- **Syphilis**, including primary, secondary, and latent syphilis: PCN benzathine (Bicillin L-A) 2.4 million units × 1 dose. Note: not be be confused with Bicillin C-R.
- Late (latent) syphilis: PCN benzathine (Bicillin L-A) 2.4 million units × 3 doses at 7-day intervals. Note: not be be confused with Bicillin C-R.
- Neurosyphilis or ocular syphilis: Aqueous PCN G 3–4 million units IV q4h × 14 days. Alternative: Procaine PCN 2.4 million units q24h plus probenecid 500 mg PO q6h × 14 days.
- **Note:** Benzathine PCN (Bicillin L-A, use for syphilis) and benzathine/procaine PCN (Bicillin C-R use for skin/soft tissue infection) are **not** interchangeable.

RENAL DOSING
Dosing for GFR 50–80: Usual dose.
Dosing for GFR 10–50: Neurosyphilis, endocarditis or serious infections: 2–3 million units IV q4h. Mild-moderate infections: 1–1.5 million units IV q4h.
Dosing for GFR <10: Neurosyphilis, endocarditis or serious infections: 2 million units IV q4–6h. Mild-moderate infections: 1 million units IV q6h. No dose adjustment needed for oral PCN.
Dosing in hemodialysis: Neurosyphilis, endocarditis or serious infections: 2 million units IV q4–6h, dose post-HD on days of dialysis or supplement with 500,000 units post-dialysis. Mild-moderate infections: 1 million units IV q6h.

ANTIBACTERIAL DRUGS

Dosing in peritoneal dialysis: Neurosyphilis, endocarditis or serious infections: 2 million units IV q4–6h. Mild-moderate infections: 1 million units IV q6h.

Dosing in hemofiltration: No data. CVVH: consider 2–3 million units q6h for serious infections. CVVHD: consider 3 million units IV q4h for serious infections. 1.5 million units IV q6h for mild-moderate infections.

ADVERSE DRUG REACTIONS

Occasional

- Hypersensitivity reaction without anaphylaxis. The most common reaction is idiopathic with a maculopapular or morbilliform rash that occurs in 1–4% of penicillin recipients and 5.2–9.5% of ampicillin recipients (*Lancet* 1969;2:969; *JAMA* 1976;235:918).
- GI intolerance (with oral administration).
- Drug fever.
- Coombs' test positive without hemolytic anemia.
- Phlebitis at infusion sites and sterile abscesses at IM sites.
- Jarisch-Herxheimer reaction (with treatment of syphilis or other spirochetal infections).
- *C. difficile*—associated colitis.

Rare

- Anaphylaxis: the frequency of anaphylaxis reaction is reported at 0.004–0.015% of PCN courses
- Hemolytic anemia
- Thrombocytopenia
- Leukopenia
- Interstitial nephritis
- Hepatitis
- Seizure (higher doses in pts with renal failure)

DRUG INTERACTIONS

- Probenecid: increased PCN serum concentration (beneficial if high serum level needed). Avoid co-administration in renal failure.
- Tetracyclines: antagonism, avoid co-administration. Bactericidal effect of penicillins may be diminished *in vivo*. In 2 studies involving a total of 79 pts with pneumococcal meningitis treated with either penicillin plus tetracyclines or penicillin monotherapy resulted in a higher mortality rate (79–85%) in the combination therapy compared to penicillin monotherapy (30–33%) [*Arch Intern Med* 1951:88:489; *Ann Intern Med* 1961; 55:545]. However there was not a difference in mortality between penicillin monotherapy and penicillin plus tetracycline in the treatment of pneumococcal pneumonia [*Arch Intern Med* 1953;91:197].

SPECTRUM—See Appendix II, p. 795

RESISTANCE

S. pneumoniae: PCN resistance rate was 10.3% (using resistance break point 2 mcg/mL), but only 1.2% (using an MICs of 8 mcg/mL for IV PCN for non-meningeal involvement, MMWR 2008;57:1353) Without meningeal involvement, *S. pneumoniae* with MIC of 2 mcg/mL or lower can be treated with high dose PCN or amoxicillin (3–4 g/day; *CID* 2005;41:139–48).

- *S. pneumoniae* break points (non-meningeal, oral therapy PCN): ≤0.06 mcg/mL (sensitive); 0.12–1.0 mcg/mL (intermediate); ≥2 mcg/mL (resistant).
- *S. pneumoniae* break points (non-meningeal, parenteral therapy PCN): ≤2 mcg/mL (sensitive); 4 mcg/mL (intermediate); ≥8 mcg/mL (resistant).
- *S. pneumoniae* break points (meningeal isolates, PCN): ≤0.06 mcg/mL (sensitive); ≥0.12 mcg/mL (resistant).
- IE caused by Viridans Group Streptococci and *S. bovis* with MIC ≤0.12 mcg/mL: PCN monotherapy × 4 wks **or** PCN + gentamicin × 2 wks (short course in uncomplicated cases only).
- IE caused by Viridans Group Streptococci and *S. bovis* with MIC >0.12 mcg/mL to 0.5 mcg/mL: PCN × 4 wks + gentamicin × 2 wks.
- IE caused by Viridans Group Streptococci and *S. bovis* with MIC >0.5 mcg/mL: PCN + gentamicin × 4–6 wks.

PHARMACOLOGY

Mechanism

Beta-lactam antibiotics inhibit mucopeptide synthesis in the bacterial cell wall, this results in the formation of defective cell walls and osmotically unstable organisms susceptible to cell lysis.

Pharmacokinetic Parameters

- **Absorption** 15%.
- **Cmax** 5–6 mcg/mL after 500 mg PO dose administered. 0.15 mcg/mL after 1.2 million units benzathine pen G IM dose administered. 20 mcg/mL after administration of 12 mU per day.
- **Distribution** Distributed to blister fluid, urine, peritoneal fluid, pleural fluid, middle ear fluid, intestinal mucosa, bone, gallbladder, lung, female reproductive tissue, bile, and inflamed meninges.
- **Protein binding** 65%.
- **Metabolism/Excretion** Hepatic metabolism accounts for less than 30% of administered dose. Both unchanged drug and metabolites are excreted via glomerular filtration and tubular secretion. Biliary excretion also occurs accounting for the high biliary concentration.
- **T1/2** 0.5 hr.

Dosing for Decreased Hepatic Function

Dose decrease needed only for severe hepatic and renal impairment.

Pregnancy Risk

B: several collaborative perinatal project reports involving over 12,000 exposure to penicillin derivatives during the first trimester indicated no association between penicillin derivative drugs and birth defects.

Breast Feeding Compatibility

Excreted in breast milk in low concentration. No adverse effects have been reported.

COMMENTS

PCN is the gold standard for treating Group A strep infections and syphilis. Generic substitution of PCN G benzathine injection is not recommended.

- Penicillin skin test: This is useful only for Type I penicillin allergy. The testing requires both major determinants (commercially available as PrePen) and minor determinants (not commercially available in the U.S.). The use of major determinants alone will detect 75–95% of potentially positive reactions; testing with both major and minor determinants will identify 99% (*NEJM* 1971;285:22). A previous study showed that 80–90% of persons reporting penicillin allergy will have negative tests. The pts who need beta-lactams with a history of penicillin allergy with Type I reactions should have skin testing, and negative results when using both major and minor determinants will assure tolerance without sequelae in over 98%. Frequency of allergic reactions with cephalosporin administration to pts with a positive skin test was 5.6% and for those with a history of penicillin allergy plus a negative test, it was 1.7% (*Allergy Clin N Am* 1991;11:611).

SELECTED REFERENCES

Adam D, Scholz H, Helmerking M. Short-course antibiotic treatment of 4782 culture-proven cases of group A streptococcal tonsillopharyngitis and incidence of poststreptococcal sequelae. *J Infect Dis*, 2000; Vol. 182; pp. 509–16.

Centers for Disease Control and Prevention (CDC). Inadvertent use of Bicillin C-R to treat syphilis infection—Los Angeles, California, 1999–2004. *MMWR Morb Mortal Wkly Rep*, 2005; Vol. 54; pp. 217–9.

PIPERACILLIN

Paul A. Pham, PharmD and John G. Bartlett, MD

INDICATIONS

FDA

- Bone and joint infections
- Gonococcal infections
- Gynecologic infections
- Intra-abdominal infections
- Lower respiratory tract infections
- Septicemia
- Skin and skin structure infections

- Surgical prophylaxis (intra-abdominal procedure, vaginal hysterectomy, abdominal hysterectomy, c-section)
- Urinary tract infections

FORMS

Brand name (mfr)	Forms	Cost*
Piperacillin (Various generic manufacturers)	IV vial 3 g; IV vial 4 g; IV vial 40 g; IV vial 2 g	$13.05; $17.40; $161.25; $8.70
*Prices represents Average Wholesale Price (AWP).		

USUAL ADULT DOSING

- Moderate to severe infections: 3 g IV q4–6h (up to 24 g a day).
- Pneumonia and pseudomonal infections: 3 g IV q4h or 4 g IV q6h.

RENAL DOSING

Dosing for GFR 50–80: GFR >40 mL/min: 3 g q6h. Use 3 g q4h or 4 g q6h for severe infections or Pseudomonas.

Dosing for GFR 10–50: GFR 20–40 mL/min: 2 g q6h. For severe infection or Pseudomonas 4 g q8h.

Dosing for GFR <10: GFR: <20 mL/min: 2 g q8h or 3 g q12h. Use 4 g q12h for severe infections or Pseudomonas.

Dosing in hemodialysis: 2 g q8h plus 1 g post-dialysis. For severe infections 3 g q8h plus 1 g post dialysis.

Dosing in peritoneal dialysis: 2 g q8h. For severe infection 3 g q8h.

Dosing in hemofiltration: CVVH: 2 g q6h. CVVHD: 2–3 g q6h; severe infections: 3 g IV q6–8h.

ADVERSE DRUG REACTIONS

General

- Generally well tolerated

Occasional

- GI intolerance
- Phlebitis at infusion sites
- Jarisch–Herxheimer reaction (with syphilis or other spirochetal infections)
- *C. difficile* colitis
- LFTs elevations with rare cases of clinical hepatitis
- Hypersensitivity reactions
- Rash

Rare

- Drug fever
- Coombs' test positive w/ hemolytic anemia
- Interstitial nephritis
- Neutropenia and thrombocytopenia
- Abnormal platelet aggregation with bleeding diathesis
- CNS: seizures and twitching (with high doses in pts with renal failure)
- Hepatitis
- Anaphylaxis

DRUG INTERACTIONS

- Methotrexate: serum concentrations may be increased. Monitor with methotrexate-induced toxicity.
- Probenecid: may prolong piperacillin half-life. May be result in significant accumulation in renal failure.
- Tetracyclines: *in vitro* antagonism when co-administered. Bactericidal effect of penicillins may be diminished *in vivo*. Management recommendation: avoid concurrent administration. In two studies involving a total of 79 pts with pneumococcal meningitis treated with either penicillin plus tetracyclines or penicillin monotherapy resulted in a higher mortality rate (79–85%) in the combination therapy compared to penicillin monotherapy (30–33%) [*Arch Intern Med* 1951;88:489, *Ann Intern Med* 1961;55:545]. However there was not a difference in mortality between penicillin monotherapy and penicillin plus tetracycline in the treatment of pneumococcal pneumonia [*Arch Intern Med* 1953;91:197].

RESISTANCE
- MIC breakpoint for Enterobacteriaceae and Gram-negative non-lactose fermenters is 16 mcg/mL (except *P. aeruginosa*).
- Current MIC breakpoint for *P. aeruginosa* is 64 mcg/mL (in part due to historical use of piperacillin always combined with an aminoglycoside), but pharmacokinetics of piperacillin are suboptimal for strains with MIC of 32 and 64 mcg/mL. Avoid piperacillin in these cases or use in combination with an aminoglycoside.

PHARMACOLOGY
Mechanism
Beta-lactam antibiotics inhibit mucopeptide synthesis in the bacterial cell wall, this results in the formation of defective cell walls and osmotically unstable organisms susceptible to cell lysis.

Pharmacokinetic Parameters
- **Cmax** 400 mcg/mL after 4 g IV dose administration.
- **Distribution** 0.23 L/kg; Distributed to blister fluid, urine, peritoneal fluid, pleural fluid, middle ear fluid, intestinal mucosa, bone, gallbladder, lung, female reproductive tissue, bile. Moderate CNS penetration with inflamed meninges, may not be effective for *P. aeruginosa*.
- **Protein binding** 16–45%.
- **Metabolism/Excretion** Hepatic metabolism accounts for less than 30% of administered dose. Both unchanged drug and metabolites are excreted via glomerular filtration and tubular secretion. Biliary excretion also occurs accounting for the high biliary concentration.
- **T1/2** 1.0 hr.

Dosing for Decreased Hepatic Function
Limited metabolism. Consider standard dose.

Pregnancy Risk
B: Several collaborative perinatal project reports involving over 12,000 exposure to penicillin derivatives during the first trimester indicated no association between penicillin derivative drugs and birth defects.

Breast Feeding Compatibility
Excreted in breast milk in low concentration. No adverse effects have been reported.

COMMENTS
Parenteral anti-pseudomonal penicillin with superior enterococcal coverage compared to ticarcillin. Due to the high prevalence of plasmid-mediated beta-lactamases produced by Gram-negative bacteria, piperacillin without tazobactam is not recommended empirically for nosocomial infections. If sensitive to piperacillin, may be preferred over piperacillin-tazobactam for *P. aeruginosa* as the tazobactam does not add activity against pseudomonas.

SELECTED REFERENCES
Combes A, Luyt CE, Fagon JY, et al. Impact of piperacillin resistance on the outcome of Pseudomonas ventilator-associated pneumonia. *Intensive Care Med*, 2006; Vol. 32; pp. 1970–8.

Mattoes HM, Capitano B, Kim MK, et al. Comparative pharmacokinetic and pharmacodynamic profile of piperacillin/tazobactam 3.375 G Q4H and 4.5 G Q6H. *Chemotherapy*, 2002; Vol. 48; pp. 59–63.

PIPERACILLIN + TAZOBACTAM

Paul A. Pham, PharmD and John G. Bartlett, MD

INDICATIONS
FDA
- Gynecologic infections (pelvic inflammatory disease, post-partum endometritis)
- Intra-abdominal infections (peritonitis, appendicitis, cholecystitis, cholangitis, diverticulitis)
- Skin and skin structure infections (including diabetic foot infections)
- Community-acquired pneumonia
- Nosocomial pneumonia

Non-FDA Approved Uses
- Lung abscess
- Empyema
- Ventilator-associated pneumonia

ANTIBACTERIAL DRUGS

Brand name (mfr)	Forms	Cost*
Zosyn (Wyeth)	IV vial 2 g–0.25 g;	$14.50;
	IV vial 3 g–0.375 g;	$21.75;
	IV vial 4 g–0.5 g;	$27.55;
	IV vial 36 g–4.5 g	$261.03
*Prices represents Average Wholesale Price (AWP).		

USUAL ADULT DOSING

- 3.375 g IV q6h.
- Nosocomial pneumonia, pseudomonal infection or severe infection: 3.375 g q4h or 4.5 g q6h IV.

RENAL DOSING

Dosing for GFR 50–80: GFR >40 mL/min:3.375 g q6h (4.5 g q6h for severe infections or Pseudomonas).

Dosing for GFR 10–50: GFR 20–40 mL/min:2.25 g q6h, for severe infections or Pseudomonas, dose 4.5 g q8h.

Dosing for GFR <10: GFR <20 mL/min: 2.25 g q8h or 3.375 g q12h. For severe infections or Pseudomonas, dose 4.5 g q12h.

Dosing in hemodialysis: 2.25 g q8–12h plus 0.75 g post-dialysis. For severe infections or Pseudomonas, 2.25 g IV q8h plus 0.75 g post dialysis.

Dosing in peritoneal dialysis: 2.25 g q8–12h. For severe infection or Pseudomonas 2.25 g q8h.

Dosing in hemofiltration: CVVH: 2.25 g q6h. CVVHD: 2.25–3.375 IV g q6h; severe infections: 3.375 g IV q6–8h.

ADVERSE DRUG REACTIONS

General

- Generally well tolerated

Occasional

- GI intolerance
- Phlebitis at infusion sites
- Jarisch–Herxheimer reaction (with syphilis or other spirochetal infections)
- *C. difficile* colitis
- LFTs elevations with rare cases of hepatitis
- Hypersensitivity reactions
- Rash

Rare

- Drug fever
- Coombs' test positive w/ hemolytic anemia
- Interstitial nephritis
- Leukopenia and thrombocytopenia
- Abnormal platelet aggregation with bleeding diathesis
- CNS: seizures and twitching (with high doses in pts with renal failure)
- Hepatitis
- Anaphylaxis

DRUG INTERACTIONS

- Methotrexate serum concentrations may be increased. Monitor with methotrexate induced toxicity.
- Probenecid may prolong piperacillin half-life. May be result in significant accumulation in renal failure.
- Tetracyclines: *in vitro* antagonism when co-administered. Bactericidal effect of penicillins may be diminished *in vivo*. Management recommendation: avoid concurrent administration. In two studies involving a total of 79 pts with pneumococcal meningitis treated with either penicillin plus tetracyclines or penicillin monotherapy resulted in a higher mortality rate (79–85%) in the combination therapy compared to penicillin monotherapy (30–33%) [*Arch Intern Med* 1951:88:489, *Ann Intern Med* 1961;55:545]. However, there was not

a difference in mortality between penicillin monotherapy and penicillin plus tetracycline in the treatment of pneumococcal pneumonia [*Arch Intern Med* 1953;91:197].

SPECTRUM—See Appendix II, p. 795

RESISTANCE

- MIC breakpoint for Enterobacteriaceae and Gram-negative non-lactose fermenters is 16/4 mcg/mL (except *P. aeruginosa*).
- Current MIC breakpoint for *P. aeruginosa* is 64/4 mcg/mL, but higher mortality was associated with infections due to *P. aeruginosa* with MIC of 32 and 64 mcg/mL. Avoid piperacillin + tazobactam in these cases or use in combination with an aminoglycoside [*CID* 2008; 46:862–7].

PHARMACOLOGY

Mechanism

Beta-lactam antibiotics inhibit mucopeptide synthesis in the bacterial cell wall, this results in the formation of defective cell walls and osmotically unstable organisms susceptible to cell lysis. Tazobactam acts as a beta-lactamase inhibitor and inactivates both plasmid and chromosome-mediated beta-lactamases.

Pharmacokinetic Parameters

- Absorption —
- **Cmax** 209 mcg/mL after 3.375 g IV dose administration.
- **Distribution** 0.23 L/kg; distributed to blister fluid, urine, peritoneal fluid, pleural fluid, middle ear fluid, intestinal mucosa, bone, gallbladder, lung, female reproductive tissue, bile. Moderate CNS penetration with inflamed meninges, may not be effective for *P. aeruginosa*.
- **Protein binding** 16–45%.
- **Metabolism/Excretion** Hepatic metabolism accounts for less than 30% of administered dose. Both unchanged drug and metabolites are excreted via glomerular filtration and tubular secretion. Biliary excretion also occurs accounting for the high biliary concentration.
- **T1/2** 1.0 hr.

Dosing for Decreased Hepatic Function

Limited metabolism. Consider standard dose.

Pregnancy Risk

B: Animal data shows no risk. Human data lacking.

Breast Feeding Compatibility

Piperacillin is excreted in breast milk in low concentration. Tazobactam excretion is not known.

COMMENTS

Parenteral beta-lactam/beta-lactamase inhibitor with broad-spectrum activity that includes most *P. aeruginosa* strains, *Enterobacteriaceae*, Enterococci and all anaerobes. More frequent dosing interval (3.375 g IV q4h) or higher doses (4.5 g IV q6h) are recommended for serious pseudomonal pulmonary infections. Higher mortality was associated with infections due to *P. aeruginosa* isolates with MICs of 32 and 64 mcg/mL. Avoid piperacillin + tazobactam in these cases or use in combination with an aminoglycoside. Use galactomannan antigen assay when using piperacillin/tazobactam may result in false-positive results, although this is less so with current, refined formulations of the drug. Of note, *P. aeruginosa* infections can be treated with piperacillin alone, as tazobactam component does not add in this circumstance since resistance in PSA is not typically beta-lactamase driven.

SELECTED REFERENCES

American Thoracic Society, Infectious Diseases Society of America. Guidelines for the management of adults with hospital-acquired, ventilator-associated, and healthcare-associated pneumonia. *Am J Respir Crit Care Med*, 2005; Vol. 171; pp. 388–416.

Re'a-Neto A, Niederman M, Lobo SM, et al. Efficacy and safety of doripenem versus piperacillin/tazobactam in nosocomial pneumonia: a randomized, open-label, multicenter study. *Curr Med Res Opin*, 2008; Vol. 24; pp. 2113–26.

POLYMYXIN B

Paul A. Pham, PharmD and John G. Bartlett, MD

INDICATIONS

FDA

- Serious infections caused by *P. aeruginosa, H. influenzae, E. coli, A. aerogenes,* and *K. pneumoniae* when alternative agents are contraindicated.

- Ocular infections with or without steroids (e.g., bacterial conjunctivitis and blepharoconjunctivitis, ophthalmic drops).
- Meningitis (intrathecal route).

Non-FDA Approved Uses
- Prophylaxis of superficial skin infections (topical)
- Irrigation of urinary bladder (adjunctive treatment)

FORMS

Brand name (mfr)	Forms	Cost*
Polymyxin B (Bedford)	IV vial 500,000 U	$13.65
Polytrim (Allergan)	Ophthalmic gtts 0.1%(10 mL)	$34.55

*Prices represents Average Wholesale Price (AWP).

USUAL ADULT DOSING
- **Systemic:** 0.75–1.25 mg/kg (7500–12,500 U/kg)IV q12h.
- **Topical application:** (dermatologic or ophthalmic) instill 1 drop to the affected eye or skin q3h hrs (max of 6 doses/day) × 7–10 days.
- **Intrathecal:** 5 mg (50,000 units) once daily intrathecally for 3 to 4 days, then 50,000 units once every other day.
- Note 1 mg = 10,000 U.

RENAL DOSING
Dosing for GFR 50–80: For CrCL 50–80 mL/min: 2.5 mg/kg (day 1), then 1–1.5 mg/kg/day. Avoid if possible w/ impaired renal function.
Dosing for GFR 10–50: For CrCL 30–50 mL/min: 2.5 mg/kg (day 1), then 1–1.5 mg/kg/day. For CrCL <30 mL/min: 2.5 mg/kg (day 1), then 1–1.5 mg/kg every 2–3 days. Avoid if possible.
Dosing for GFR <10: For CrCL <30 mL/min: 2.5 mg/kg (day 1), then 1–1.5 mg/kg every 2–3 days.
Dosing in hemodialysis: Little data, some removal. 2.5 mg/kg (day 1), then 1 mg/kg every 5–7 days. Dose post-HD.
Dosing in peritoneal dialysis: Little data, some removal. 2.5 mg/kg (day 1), then 1 mg/kg every 5–7 days.
Dosing in hemofiltration: Limited data. CVVHD: 2.5 mg/kg (day 1), then 1 mg/kg on day 4 and day 8, then 0.8 mg/kg/day. Consider higher doses in critically ill pts.

ADVERSE DRUG REACTIONS
General
- Topical administration generally well tolerated

Common
- Nephrotoxicity (systemic)
- Neurotoxicity (systemic use: circumoral and peripheral paresthesia, dizziness, vertigo, ataxia, blurred vision, slurred speech)
- Severe pain at injection sites with IM administration (generally not recommended)

Rare
- Neuromuscular blockade

DRUG INTERACTIONS
Non-depolarizing muscle relaxant effect may be increased with systemic use of polymyxin. Avoid co-administration. If concurrent administration is needed, titrate the non-depolarizing muscle relaxant slowly and monitor neuromuscular function closely.

RESISTANCE
- Not active against Proteus, Serratia, Providencia, Burkholderia, Gram-negative cocci, all Gram-positives, or anaerobes.

PHARMACOLOGY
Mechanism
Polymyxin B acts like a cationic detergent that binds to the lipids of the bacterial cytoplasmic membrane and damage that results in alteration of osmotic barrier of the membrane and causes leakage of essential intracellular metabolites and nucleosides.

Pharmacokinetic Parameters
- **Absorption** Negligible.
- **Cmax** 1–8 mcg/mL after 30,000 u/kg IV dose administration.
- **Distribution** Little data, poor CNS penetration.
- **Protein binding** Low.
- **Metabolism/Excretion** No data.
- **T1/2** 4.3–6.0 hrs.

Dosing for Decreased Hepatic Function
No data.

Pregnancy Risk
B: A report of 7 exposures during the first trimester found no association with congenital defects.

Breast Feeding Compatibility
No data available.

COMMENTS
Agent in the polymyxin class thus active against *Pseudomonas aeruginosa* and other Gram-negative bacilli. Rarely used systemically due to renal toxicity (among other) and limited clinical data, but may be a last resort for resistant pseudomonal infections (1 mg = 10,000 U). Spectrum of activity similar to colistin and includes *P. aeruginosa*, *A. baumannii*, MDR Gram-negative, carbapenemase-producing *Enterobacteriaceae*. Has also been used intrathecally and by inhalation. Polymyxin E (colistin, colistimethate) is used more commonly.

SELECTED REFERENCES
Arnold TM, Forrest GN, Messmer KJ. Polymyxin antibiotics for Gram-negative infections. *Am J Health Syst Pharm*, 2007; Vol. 64; pp. 819–26.

Robert PY, Adenis JP. Comparative review of topical ophthalmic antibacterial preparations. *Drugs*, 2001; Vol. 61; pp. 175–85.

QUINUPRISTIN + DALFOPRISTIN

Paul A. Pham, PharmD and John G. Bartlett, MD

INDICATIONS
FDA
- Treatment of pts with serious or life-threatening infections associated with vancomycin-resistant *Enterococcus faecium* (VREF) bacteremia.
- Complicated skin and skin structure infections caused by *Staphylococcus aureus* (MSSA) or *Streptococcus pyogenes*.

Non-FDA Approved Uses
- Endocarditis (generally not recommended due to poor clearance of bacteremia)

FORMS

Brand name (mfr)	Forms	Cost*
Synercid (Monarch Pharmaceuticals)	IV vial 500 mg	$182.61

*Prices represents Average Wholesale Price (AWP).

USUAL ADULT DOSING
- Complicated skin and skin structure infections: 7.5 mg/kg IV 12 hrs.
- VRE (*E. faecium*) infection: 7.5 mg/kg IV q8h.
- Note: drug is ineffective versus *E. faecalis*.
- Infuse by central venous catheter.

RENAL DOSING
Dosing for GFR 50–80: Usual dose. No significant change in pharmacokinetic parameters.
Dosing for GFR 10–50: Usual dose. No significant change in pharmacokinetic parameters.
Dosing for GFR <10: No data. Usual dose likely.
Dosing in hemodialysis: No data.
Dosing in peritoneal dialysis: No data.
Dosing in hemodialysis: No data.

ANTIBACTERIAL DRUGS

ADVERSE DRUG REACTIONS
Common
- Dose-dependent infusion-related reaction at injection site (10% w/ 5 mg/kg, 68% w/ 10–15 mg/kg) such as pain, itching, burning
- Arthralgia/myalgia (15%)
- Asymptomatic hyperbilirubinemia (up to 25%)

Occasional
- Thrombophlebitis (5%)
- LFT elevations
- Nausea
- Headache

Rare
- *C. difficile*—associated colitis

DRUG INTERACTIONS
- CYP3A4 substrates (e.g., fentanyl, dofetilide, quinidine, irinotecan, tacrolimus, sirolimus, cyclosporine, clarithromycin, midazolam, triazolam, dihydropyridine calcium channel blockers (felodipine, amlodipine, nifedipine), ergotamine, amiodarone, simvastatin, and lovastatin): may increase serum concentrations of CYP3A4 substrates. Use with close monitoring.

SPECTRUM—See Appendix II, p. 804

RESISTANCE
- MIC breakpoint of 1 mcg/mL for *staphylococci* and *enterococci.*

PHARMACOLOGY
Mechanism
Each agent binds at a different site of bacterial 50S ribosomal subunit, resulting in interruption of protein synthesis.

Pharmacokinetic Parameters
- **Cmax** 5 mcg/mL after 7.5 mg/kg IV dose administration.
- **Distribution** Good tissue penetration. Good blister fluid penetration.
- **Protein binding** 50–56%.
- **Metabolism/Excretion** Extensively metabolized to RP 12536 (pristinamycin IIA derivative, active metabolite) and other active and non-active metabolite. Excreted primarily in the feces and less than 20% in the urine.
- **T1/2** 1.5 hrs.

Dosing for Decreased Hepatic Function
No data.

Pregnancy Risk
No data—does manufacturer currently does not recommend the use in pregnancy.

Breast Feeding Compatibility
No data.

COMMENTS
Parenteral agent with activity against most Gram-positive cocci including penicillin-resistant *S. pneumoniae*, vancomycin -intermediately-resistant *S. aureus*, *S. epidermidis,* and vancomycin-resistant *E. faecium*. It does not have activity against *E. faecalis*. Expensive at approximately $300–450.00 per day. May cause disabling myalgia that precludes continued use. Must be infused by central venous line.

SELECTED REFERENCES
Raad I, Hachem R, Hanna H, et al. Prospective, randomized study comparing quinupristin-dalfopristin with linezolid in the treatment of vancomycin-resistant Enterococcus faecium infections. *J Antimicrob Chemother*, 2004; Vol. 53; pp. 646–9.

Simonsen GS, Bergh K, Bevanger L, et al. Susceptibility to quinupristin-dalfopristin and linezolid in 839 clinical isolates of Gram-positive cocci from Norway. *Scand J Infect Dis*, 2004; Vol. 36; pp. 254–8.

RETAPAMULIN

Paul A. Pham, PharmD

INDICATIONS

FDA

• Indicated for the topical treatment of impetigo due to *S. aureus* (MSSA) or *S. pyogenes* in pts >9 mos old.

Non-FDA Approved Uses

• *In vitro* activity against MRSA, but no clinical data.

FORMS

Brand name (mfr)	Forms	Cost*
Altabax (GlaxoSmithKline)	Topical ointment 1% (5, 10, 15 g tubes)	$42.85 (5 g); $72.61(10 g); $88.78 (15 g)

*Prices represents Average Wholesale Price (AWP).

USUAL ADULT DOSING

• Apply to affected area (up to 100 cm²) twice daily × 5 days.

RENAL DOSING

Dosing for GFR 50–80: Usual dose.
Dosing for GFR 10–50: Usual dose.
Dosing for GFR <10: Usual dose.
Dosing in hemodialysis: Usual dose.
Dosing in peritoneal dialysis: Usual dose.
Dosing in hemofiltration: Usual dose.

ADVERSE DRUG REACTIONS

General

• Generally well tolerated

Occasional

• Application site pruritus and eczema

DRUG INTERACTIONS

• Ketoconazole and other CYP3A4 inhibitors (e.g., HIV-protease inhibitor and macrolides): may increase retapamulin serum concentrations, but unlikely to be clinically significant due to limited systemic absorption after topical administration.

RESISTANCE

• No resistance observed in early clinical trials, but *in vitro*, mutations in ribosomal protein L3 or efflux pump can lead to retapamulin resistance.

PHARMACOLOGY

Mechanism

Selective inhibition of 50S subunit of the bacterial ribosome.

Pharmacokinetic Parameters

• **Absorption** Limited systemic absorption. Only 11% of the treated pts had measurable concentration of 0.8 ng/mL.
• **Protein binding** 94%
• **Metabolism/Excretion** Metabolized via CYP3A4.
• **T1/2** —

Dosing for Decreased Hepatic Function

Limited systemic absorption. Usual dose likely.

Pregnancy Risk

B: Not teratogenic in animal studies. No human data.

Breast Feeding Compatibility

No data.

COMMENTS

Similar to mupirocin, retapamulin is effective in the treatment of impetigo. Retapamulin has the advantage of twice daily dosing vs. three times per day dosing with mupirocin; however, it is more

ANTIBACTERIAL DRUGS

expensive compared to mupirocin ($88 vs. $40 per 15 g tube). Unlike mupirocin, the intranasal administration of retapamulin is currently not recommended due to the lack of clinical data.

SELECTED REFERENCES

Free A, Roth E, Dalessandro M, et al. Retapamulin ointment twice daily for 5 days vs oral cephalexin twice daily for 10 days for empiric treatment of secondarily infected traumatic lesions of the skin. *Skinmed*, 2006; Vol. 5; pp. 224–32.

RIFAMPIN

Paul A. Pham, PharmD and John G. Bartlett, MD

INDICATIONS

FDA
- Treatment of active TB.
- Treatment of asymptomatic carriers of *Neisseria meningitidis* to eliminate meningococci from the nasopharynx.

Non-FDA Approved Uses
- Treatment of latent TB (2nd line agent)

FORMS

Brand name (mfr)	Forms	Cost*
Rifadin (Sanofi-Aventis U.S. and generic manufacturers)	Oral capsule 150 mg; 300 mg IV vial 600 mg	$2.27; $3.22 $124.28
Rifamate (Sanofi-Aventis U.S.)	Oral capsule 300 mg RIF/150 mg INH	$3.71
Rifater (Sanofi-Aventis U.S.)	Oral capsule 120 mg RIF/50 mg INH/300 mg PZA	$2.75
*Prices represents Average Wholesale Price (AWP).		

USUAL ADULT DOSING
- TB treatment (in combination with other anti-TB drugs): 10 mg/kg/day (max 600 mg PO [usual adult dose] or IV once daily). DOT: 600 mg 2–3×/wk. HIV-infected pts with CD4 <100 should received DOT 3×/wk (and not 2×/wk since they are more prone to rifamycin resistance).
- *Rifamate*: 2 caps (600 mg RIF/300 mg INH) once daily, 1 hr before or 2 hrs after meals.
- *Rifater*: ≥44 kg—4 tabs daily; 45–54 kg—5 tabs once daily; ≥55 kg—6 tabs once daily, administered 1 hr before or 2 hrs after meals.
- Treatment of latent TB: 10 mg/kg (max 600 mg) once daily for 4 mos (alternative to INH in pts intolerant of INH or exposed to INH-resistant TB).
- Meningococcal prophylaxis: 600 mg q12h × 2 days. Due to reports of fluoroquinolone resistance, rifampin is recommended in selected counties in North Dakota and Minnesota (*MMWR* 2008; 57:173).
- Prosthetic valve endocarditis: 300 mg three times daily (in combination with other drugs).
- Drug should never be used as monotherapy due to quick emergence of resistance.
- Obese pts: use 900–1200 mg/day in 2 divided doses.

RENAL DOSING
Dosing for GFR 50–80: Usual dose.
Dosing for GFR 10–50: Usual dose.
Dosing for GFR <10: Usual dose. Some recommend a 50% decrease in dose.
Dosing in hemodialysis: 300–600 mg once daily.
Dosing in peritoneal dialysis: 300–600 mg once daily.
Dosing in hemofiltration: No data. Usual dose likely.

ADVERSE DRUG REACTIONS

Common
- Orange discoloration of urine, tears, sweat

Occasional
- Hepatitis (2.7% w/ other TB drugs) with cholestatic changes in first mo; jaundice
- GI intolerance
- Flu-like syndrome (0.4–0.7% when taking RIF 2 ×/wks): symptoms include fever and chills, headache, dizziness, bone pain, abdominal pain, and generalized pruritus

Rare
- Hypersensitivity (0.07–0.3%)
- Thrombocytopenia and hemolytic anemia
- Headache and dizziness

SPECTRUM—See Appendix II, p. 804

RESISTANCE
- XDR TB: resistant to at least the first-line anti-TB drugs isoniazid and rifampin, as well as any fluoroquinolone and at least one of three second-line injectable TB drugs.
- MIC breakpoints for Staphylococcus spp.: ≤1 mcg/mL (sensitive); 2 mcg/mL (intermediate); ≥4 mcg/mL (resistant).

DRUG INTERACTIONS

PHARMACOLOGY

Mechanism

Inhibits initiation of chain formation for RNA synthesis by inhibiting DNA-dependent RNA polymerase.

Pharmacokinetic Parameters
- **Absorption** Well absorbed.
- **Cmax** 7–9 mcg/mL after 600 mg PO. 17.5 mcg/mL after 600 mg IV.
- **Distribution** Widely distributed into most tissue and fluids including liver, lungs, bile, pleural fluid, prostate, seminal fluid, bone and saliva. With inflamed meninges therapeutic CSF concentration attained.
- **Protein Binding** 75%.
- **Metabolism/Excretion** Hepatic metabolism to active deacetylated metabolite. Potent CYP3A4 inducer and prone to multiple drug interactions. Both unchanged drug and active metabolite primarily excreted via biliary excretion. Unchanged drug undergo enterohepatic circulation. 3–30% excreted in urine as metabolite and unchanged drug.
- **T1/2** 2–5 hrs.

Dosing for Decreased Hepatic Function

Clearance may be impaired. Should be given with close monitoring.

Pregnancy Risk

C: Considered safe in pregnancy. Animal data show congenital malformations: cleft palate, spina bifida, embryotoxicity. Administration in last wks of pregnancy may cause postnatal hemorrhage. Several reviews concluded that RIF is not proven teratogen and recommended use of RIF with INH and EMB if necessary.

Breast Feeding Compatibility

Excreted in breast milk. American Academy of Pediatrics considers RIF compatible with breast feeding.

COMMENTS

Oral and parenteral rifamycin used for treatment of active and latent TB, treatment and prophylaxis of MOTT, meningococcal prophylaxis, and occasional adjunctive therapy for infections involving *S. aureus*. Significant reduction of CYP3A4 substrate drugs serum level (i.e., HIV protease inhibitors, azole antifungal, and many other drugs). Although data are limited, rifampin biofilm penetration may make this agent an ideal candidate (in combination with other antibiotics) for treating infections associated with prosthetic devices.

SELECTED REFERENCES

Boulle A, Van Cutsem G, Cohen K, et al. Outcomes of nevirapine- and efavirenz-based antiretroviral therapy when coadministered with rifampicin-based antitubercular therapy. *JAMA*, 2008; Vol. 300; pp. 530–9.

Centers for Disease Control and Prevention (CDC). Managing Drug Interactions in the Treatment of HIV-Related Tuberculosis. http://www.cdc.gov/tb/TB_HIV_Drugs/default.htm, 2008.

ANTIBACTERIAL DRUGS

RIFAXIMIN

Paul A. Pham, PharmD and John G. Bartlett, MD

INDICATIONS

FDA

- Treatment of traveler's diarrhea due to noninvasive *E. coli*

Non-FDA Approved Uses

- *C. difficile*-associated diarrhea; relapsing disease after prolonged course of oral vancomycin
- Hepatic encephalopathy
- Small bowel bacterial overgrowth
- Irritable bowel syndrome

FORMS

Brand name (mfr)	Forms	Cost*
Xifaxan (Salix)	PO tab 200 mg	$5.71
*Prices represents Average Wholesale Price (AWP).		

USUAL ADULT DOSING

- Traveler's diarrhea: 200 mg PO three times daily with or without food × 3 days.
- *C. difficile*–associated diarrhea: 400 mg PO twice daily or 200 mg PO q8h × 14 days.
- Hepatic encephalopathy: 400 mg PO three times daily × 5–10 days.
- Small intestinal bacterial overgrowth: 400 mg PO three times daily × 7 days.

RENAL DOSING

Dosing for GFR 50–80: Usual dose.
Dosing for GFR 10–50: Usual dose likely.
Dosing for GFR <10: Usual dose likely.
Dosing in hemodialysis: Usual dose likely.
Dosing in peritoneal dialysis: Usual dose likely.
Dosing in hemofiltration: Usual dose likely.

ADVERSE DRUG REACTIONS

General

- Generally well tolerated

Occasional

- GI: flatulence, nausea, and vomiting, but comparable to placebo in trials

Rare

- Rash

DRUG INTERACTIONS

In vitro rifaximin is an inducer of CYP3A4, however since it is not systemically absorbed, interaction with drug substrate of CYP3A4 is unlikely.

- Ethinyl estradiol/norgestimate: no significant interaction.
- Midazolam: no significant interaction.

PHARMACOLOGY

Mechanism

- Rifaximin is a structural analog of rifampin, it acts by inhibiting RNA synthesis by binding to beta-subunit of bacterial DNA-dependent RNA polymerase.

Pharmacokinetic Parameters

- **Absorption** Not absorbed. Estimated 0.4% absorption.
- **Metabolism/Excretion** Not metabolized with 97% excretion in the feces.
- **T1/2** n/a.

Dosing for Decreased Hepatic Function

Usual dose.

Pregnancy Risk

C: No human data. Risk likely to be low since rifaximin is not systemically absorbed. Rifaximin was teratogenic in rats at doses 2 to 33-fold higher than human doses.

Breast Feeding Compatibility

No data.

COMMENTS

Rifaximin is effective and well tolerated in the treatment of uncomplicated traveler's diarrhea caused by *E. coli*. Rifaximin is not effective in diarrhea caused by invasive *C. jejuni* and has not been well studied in diarrhea caused by *Shigella* spp or *Salmonella* spp. Since rifaximin is not systemically absorbed, it should not be used in complicated cases of traveler's diarrhea. Rifamixin appears effective in the treatment of *C. difficile* associated diarrhea, but is much more expensive compared to metronidazole. Resistance is a major concern and use is limited after multiple relapses treated with a prolonged course of vancomycin ("the rifaximin chaser").

SELECTED REFERENCES

DuPont HL, Jiang ZD, Okhuysen PC, et al. A randomized, double-blind, placebo-controlled trial of rifaximin to prevent traveler's diarrhea. *Ann Intern Med*, 2005; Vol. 142; pp. 805–12.

Johnson S, Schriever C, Galang M, et al. Interruption of recurrent Clostridium difficile-associated diarrhea episodes by serial therapy with vancomycin and rifaximin. *Clin Infect Dis*, 2007; Vol. 44; pp. 846–8.

STREPTOMYCIN

Paul A. Pham, PharmD and John G. Bartlett, MD

INDICATIONS

FDA

* *Mycobacterium tuberculosis* (2nd line)
* *Yersinia pestis* (plague)
* *Francisella tularensis* (tularemia)
* Brucella infection
* *Klebsiella granulomatis* (Donovanosis, granuloma inguinale)
* *Haemophilus ducreyi* (chancroid); *Haemophilus influenzae*
* Urinary tract infections (not a first-line agent)
* Endocarditis caused by *Streptococcus viridans* (used in combination with PCN), *Enterococcus faecalis* (use with ampicillin)
* Gram-negative bacillary bacteremia (concomitantly with another antibacterial agent) (11)
  K. pneumoniae pneumonia

FORMS

Brand name (mfr)	Forms	Cost*
Streptomycin (X-Gen)	IM vial 1 g	$14.65

*Prices represents Average Wholesale Price (AWP).

USUAL ADULT DOSING

* TB: 15 mg/kg/days (max 1 g) IM once daily.
* TB DOT regimen: 25–30 mg/kg IM 2–3 ×/wk.
* Enterococcal endocarditis (synergy with ampicillin if resistant to gentamicin and sensitive to streptomycin): 7.5 mg/kg IM q12h (max dose per day is 2 g with a target peak 1 hr after IM dose of 20 mcg/mL and trough <10 mcg/mL).

RENAL DOSING

Dosing for GFR 50–80: TB: 15 mg/kg q24–72h (monitor serum concentrations; target trough <10 mcg/mL); Synergy for enterococcal endocarditis: 7.5 mg/kg q12–24h (monitor serum concentrations; target trough <10 mcg/mL).

Dosing for GFR 10–50: TB: 15 mg/kg q72–96h (monitor serum concentrations; target trough <10 mcg/mL). Synergy for enterococcal endocarditis: 7.5 mg/kg q24–72h (monitor serum concentrations; target trough <10 mcg/mL).

Dosing for GFR <10: TB and synergy for Enterococcal endocarditis: 7.5 mg/kg q72–96h (monitor serum concentrations; target trough <10 mcg/mL).

Dosing in hemodialysis: TB: 12–15 mg/kg 2–3 ×/wk (monitor serum concentrations; target trough <10 mcg/mL). Synergy for enterococcal endocarditis: 7.5 mg/kg q96h (monitor serum concentrations; target trough <10 mcg/mL).

ANTIBACTERIAL DRUGS

Dosing in peritoneal dialysis: 20–40 mg/Liter of dialysate per day (monitor serum concentrations closely; target trough <10 mcg/mL).

Dosing in hemofiltration: 15 mg/kg q24 to 72h (dose adjust based on serum concentrations; target trough <10 mcg/mL).

ADVERSE DRUG REACTIONS

Occasional

- Renal failure.
- Otological/vestibular damage. The most ototoxic of all aminoglycosides. Peak should not exceed 20–25 mcg/mL.

Rare

- Optic nerve dysfunction
- Peripheral neuritis
- Arachnoiditis
- Neuromuscular blockade
- Encephalopathy

DRUG INTERACTIONS

- Non-depolarizing muscle relaxants (e.g., atracurium, pancuronium, tubocurarine, gallamine triethiodide): may increase risk of neuromuscular blockade with large doses. Use with close monitoring.
- Loop diuretic (especially w/ ethacrynic acid): additive ototoxicity. Avoid co-administration with streptomycin.
- Nephrotoxic agents (e.g., cidofovir, foscarnet, pentamidine, ampho B): may increase risk of nephrotoxicity. Avoid co-administration with streptomycin.

SPECTRUM—See Appendix II, p. 797

Resistance

- *Enterococci* synergy with ampicillin if MIC <1000 mcg/mL.

PHARMACOLOGY

Mechanism

Aminoglycosides inhibit protein synthesis by irreversibly binding to 30S ribosomal subunit.

Pharmacokinetic Parameters

- **Absorption** Aminoglycosides are rapidly absorbed after IM administration. Intrapleural and intraperitoneal administration results in rapid absorption. Poor absorption with oral administration.
- **Cmax** 25–50 mcg/mL after 1 g IM dose administration.
- **Distribution** 0.2–0.4 L/kg; distributed in extracellular fluid, abscesses, ascitic fluid, pericardial fluid, pleural fluid, synovial fluid, lymphatic fluid and peritoneal fluid. Not well distributed into bile, aqueous humor, bronchial secretions, sputum, and CSF.
- **Protein binding** 0–10%.
- **Metabolism/Excretion** Aminoglycosides are not metabolized in the liver, they are excreted unchanged in the urine.
- **T1/2** 2–4 hrs (Note: cystic fibrosis pts may have shorter half life of 1–2 hrs; burn and febrile pts may have increased clearance of aminoglycosides).

Dosing for Decreased Hepatic Function

Usual dose, but monitor for hepato-renal syndrome in ESLD.

Pregnancy Risk

Strictly contraindicated in pregnancy. D: Eighth cranial nerve damage has been reported following *in utero* exposure to streptomycin.

Breast Feeding Compatibility

Excreted in breast milk. The American Academy of Pediatrics considers streptomycin compatible with breast feeding.

COMMENTS

Parenteral aminoglycoside with the most ototoxicity potential. Use is generally limited to treatment of multiple-drug resistant tuberculosis (MDRTB), but high rates of streptomycin resistance has been described in high-incidence countries. Also used for unusual infections: plague, tularemia and brucellosis. May be synergistic with ampicillin in cases of gentamicin resistant enterococcus endocarditis.

SELECTED REFERENCES

Ariza J, Gudiol F, Pallares R, et al. Treatment of human brucellosis with doxycycline plus rifampin or doxycycline plus streptomycin. A randomized, double-blind study. *Ann Intern Med*, 1992; Vol. 117; pp. 25–30.

Enderlin G, Morales L, Jacobs RF, et al. Streptomycin and alternative agents for the treatment of tularemia: review of the literature. *Clin Infect Dis*, 1994; Vol. 19; pp. 42–7.

SULFADIAZINE

Paul A. Pham, PharmD and John G. Bartlett, MD

INDICATIONS

FDA

- CNS and ocular toxoplasmosis (in combination with pyrimethamine); nocardiosis.
- Malaria due to chloroquine-resistant *P. falciparum* (in combination with quinine and pyrimethamine).
- UTI (also FDA indicated for pyelonephritis, but generally reserved for uncomplicated UTI), trimethoprim-sulfamethoxazole preferred.
- FDA indicated, but not generally recommended: chancroid, trachoma, inclusion conjunctivitis.
- FDA indicated, but not generally recommended: prophylaxis of meningococcal meningitis when sulfonamide-sensitive group A strains are known to prevail, meningococcal meningitis, acute otitis media due to *Haemophilus influenzae* (in combination with PCN), prophylaxis against recurrences of rheumatic fever (alternative to penicillin), *H. influenzae* meningitis (in combination with streptomycin).

FORMS

Brand name (mfr)	Forms	Cost*
Sulfadiazine (Eon Labs)	Oral tab 500 mg	$2.08 per 500 mg tab
*Prices represents Average Wholesale Price (AWP).		

USUAL ADULT DOSING

- CNS and ocular toxoplasmosis (induction phase): sulfadiazine 1–1.5 g PO q6h (+ leucovorin 10–20 mg PO once daily and pyrimethamine 100–200 mg PO loading dose, then 50–100 mg PO once daily × 6 wks).
- CNS and ocular toxoplasmosis (maintenance phase): sulfadiazine 500 mg PO q6h (+ leucovorin 10–20 mg PO once daily and pyrimethamine 25–50 mg PO once daily) until immune reconstitution (CD4 >200 × 6 mos and on stable HAART).
- Ocular toxoplasmosis: sulfadiazine 1 g q6h (+ leucovorin 15 mg PO once daily and pyrimethamine 100 mg PO × 1, then 50 mg PO once daily) × 4 wks. Additional treatment if pt has dense vitreous floaters, active retinal inflammation, or both (*Am J Ophthalmol*. 2002;134(1):34–40).
- Nocardia: 1.5 g PO q6h × ≥6 mos [SMX/TMP preferred (*CID* 1996;22(6):891–903)]. Target serum level: 100–150 g/mL (2 hrs after dose).
- Uncomplicated UTI: 500 mg PO q6h (SMX-TMP preferred).
- Malaria (in combination with quinine and pyrimethamine): 500–1000 mg PO q6h.
- Consider therapeutic drug monitoring for serious infections. Target 120 to 150 mcg/mL. Levels >200 mcg/mL associated with increased rates of adverse drug reactions.

RENAL DOSING

Dosing for GFR 50–80: 0.5–1.5 g PO q6h.

Dosing for GFR 10–50: 0.5–1.5 g PO q8–12h (approx. half dose).

Dosing for GFR <10: 0.5–1.5 g PO q12h–24h (approx. 1/3 dose).

Dosing in hemodialysis: No data, consider 0.5–1.5 g PO q12–24h, dose post-HD.

Dosing in peritoneal dialysis: No data, consider 0.5–1.5 g PO q12–24h.

Dosing in hemofiltration: No data, consider 0.5–1.5 g PO q8h–12h.

ANTIBACTERIAL DRUGS

ADVERSE DRUG REACTIONS

Common

- GI intolerance with nausea and vomiting
- Rash and pruritus

Occasional

- Bone marrow suppression (anemia, thrombocytopenia, leukopenia).
- Serum sickness and drug fever.
- Crystalluria with azotemia, urolithiasis, oliguria. May be prevented by adequate hydration (daily urinary output >1500 mL) and alkalinizing urine to pH >7.15.
- Photosensitivity.
- Hepatitis.

Rare

- TEN and Stevens-Johnson syndrome
- Encephalopathy
- Pancreatitis

DRUG INTERACTIONS

- Cyclosporine: may decrease cyclosporine serum levels. Monitor levels closely; may require dose increase.
- Para-aminobenzoic acid (PABA) and derivatives (such as benzocaine, procaine, tetracaine): theoretical antagonism. Avoid co-administration.
- Phenytoin: may increase phenytoin serum levels. Monitor free phenytoin levels with co-administration.
- Porfimer: may increase the risk of photosensitivity reaction. Avoid co-administration.
- Sulfonylurea: may increase hypoglycemia. Monitor closely with co-administration.
- Warfarin: may increase INR. Monitor closely.

PHARMACOLOGY

Mechanism

Structural analog of p-aminobenzoic acid (PABA); competitively inhibits dihydrofolic acid synthesis, which is necessary for conversion of PABA to folic acid.

Pharmacokinetic Parameters

- **Absorption** Well absorbed.
- **Cmax** 100–150 mcg/mL.
- **Distribution** 0.29 L/kg, 40–60% CSN penetration.
- **Protein binding** 38–48%.
- **Metabolism/Excretion** Metabolized extensively in liver to acetylated metabolite. 30–44% excretion of unchanged drug in urine, while 15–40% excreted as acetylated metabolite. Renal excretion dependent on urinary pH.
- **T1/2** 7–17 hrs of parent compound.

Dosing for Decreased Hepatic Function

No data. consider 0.5–1.0 g PO q6h.

Pregnancy Risk

C: contraindicated near term due to potential for kernicterus in newborn.

Breast Feeding Compatibility

Excreted in breast milk. Breast feeding generally not recommended with sulfonamide co-administration.

COMMENTS

Agent of choice for toxoplasmosis (with pyrimethamine) due to superior CNS penetration and extensive clinical data. Higher incidence of crystalluria compared to other sulfonamides. This regimen also provides PCP prophylaxis.

SELECTED REFERENCES

Dannemann B, McCutchan JA, Israelski D, et al. Treatment of toxoplasmic encephalitis in pts with AIDS. A randomized trial comparing pyrimethamine plus clindamycin to pyrimethamine plus sulfadiazine. The California Collaborative Treatment Group. *Ann Intern Med*, 1992; Vol. 116; pp. 33–43.

Katlama C, De Wit S, O'Doherty E, et al. Pyrimethamine-clindamycin vs. pyrimethamine-sulfadiazine as acute and long-term therapy for toxoplasmic encephalitis in pts with AIDS. *Clin Infect Dis*, 1996; Vol. 22; pp. 268–75.

SULFAMETHOXAZOLE

Paul A. Pham, PharmD and John G. Bartlett, MD

INDICATIONS
FDA
- Urinary tract infections (as TMP/SMX)
- Acute otitis media (TMP/SMX)
- Acute exacerbations of chronic bronchitis in adults (TMP/SMX)
- Traveler's diarrhea in adults (TMP/SMX)
- Prophylaxis and treatment of PCP pneumonia (TMP/SMX) and shigellosis (TMP/SMX)

USUAL ADULT DOSING
- Available in U.S. only in combination w/ trimethoprim (e.g., Bactrim or Septra formulations).
- Traveler's diarrhea: TMP-SMX DS PO twice daily.
- PCP: TMP-SMX DS or SS qday (prophylaxis); 25 mg/kg IV q8h (SMX component, treatment).

RENAL DOSING
Dosing for GFR 50–80: 1 g q12h.
Dosing for GFR 10–50: 1 g q18h.
Dosing for GFR <10: 1 g q24h.
Dosing in hemodialysis: 1 g q24h on days on dialysis dose post dialysis.
Dosing in peritoneal dialysis: 1 g q24h.
Dosing in hemofiltration: No data.

ADVERSE DRUG REACTIONS
Common
- Allergic reactions (rash, pruritus +/– fever)

Occasional
- GI intolerance
- Photosensitivity
- Hepatitis (especially with high doses)
- Bone marrow suppression (especially with high doses)
- Hemolytic anemia with G6PD deficiency
- Crystalluria (with high doses and dehydration)

Rare
- Stevens-Johnson syndrome, toxic epidermal necrolysis (TEN)
- Periarteritis nodosum
- Serum sickness
- Aseptic meningitis

DRUG INTERACTIONS
- Cyclosporine: may decreased cyclosporine metabolism. Monitor cyclosporine serum levels with co-administration.
- Para-aminobenzoic acid (PABA) derivatives (such as benzocaine, procaine, tetracaine): possible antagonism of antimicrobial effect of sulfonamide. Avoid concurrent administration.
- Phenytoin: may increase free phenytoin serum concentrations. Monitor free phenytoin serum concentration with co-administration.
- Porfimer: may increase risk of photosensitivity reaction. Counsel pts on avoidance of sunlight for 30 days after the last porfimer dose.
- Sulfonylureas: may increase hypoglycemic effects of sulfonylureas. Monitor blood sugar closely with co-administration.
- Warfarin: may increase anticoagulant effect. Monitor INR closely with co-administration.

PHARMACOLOGY
Mechanism
Sulfonamides are structural analogs of p-aminobenzoic acid (PABA), it competitively inhibits dihydrofolic acid synthesis which is necessary for the conversion of PABA to folic acid.

Pharmacokinetic Parameters
- **Absorption** Rapid and well absorbed.
- **Distribution** Good CSF penetration (80% of serum concentration attained in the CSF), may not be bacteriocidal against coliforms.

ANTIBACTERIAL DRUGS

- **Protein binding** 90%.
- **Metabolism/Excretion** Less than 5% liver metabolism. Primarily excreted in the urine.
- **T1/2** 1.5 hrs.

Dosing for Decreased Hepatic Function
Use with caution.

Pregnancy Risk
C: animal data show cleft palate and bone abnormalities with high doses. Extensive use in human without complication except 1 case of agranulocytosis. Due to the potential of kernicterus in the newborn sulfa drugs should be avoided near term/third trimester.

Breast Feeding Compatibility
Excreted in breast milk. The American Academy of Pediatrics considers sulfapyridine, sulfisoxazole, and sulfamethoxazole compatible with breast feeding. Avoid in hyperbilirubinemia and in G6PD deficiency.

COMMENTS
Oral and parenteral sulfonamide now only available in U.S. as a combination with trimethoprim.

SELECTED REFERENCES
Smith L. Evaluation of a new sulfonamide, sulfamethoxazole (gantanol). *JAMA*, 1964; Vol. 187; pp. 142.

TELAVANCIN

Paul A. Pham, PharmD

INDICATIONS

FDA
- Complicated skin and skin structure infections caused by susceptible Gram-positive bacteria (MSSA, MRSA, *S. pyogenes*, *S. agalactiae*, *S. anginosus* group, or vancomycin sensitive *E. faecalis*).

Non-FDA Approved Uses
- HAP and VAP (in combination with Gram-negative coverage).

FORMS

Brand name (mfr)	Forms	Cost*
Vibativ telavancin (Astellas Pharma U.S.)	IV vial 250 mg; IV vial 750 mg	tba; tba
*Prices represents Average Wholesale Price (AWP).		

USUAL ADULT DOSING
- Soft tissue infections: 10 mg/kg IV once daily (infuse over 1 hr) × 7–14 days.
- HAP and VAP: 10 mg/kg IV once daily (infuse over 1 hr).

RENAL DOSING
Dosing for GFR 50–80: 10 mg/kg IV q24hrs.
Dosing for GFR 10–50: CrCL 50–30 mL/min: 7.5 mg/kg IV q24hrs; CrCL <30 mL/min to 10 mL/min: 10 mg/kg q48hrs. Note: decreased efficacy (75% vs. 63%) reported with CrCL <50 mL/min (use with caution)
Dosing for GFR <10: Dose reduction likely, but insufficient clinical data for dose recommendation. Note: decreased efficacy (75% vs. 63%) reported with CrCL <50 mL/min (use with caution).
Dosing in hemodialysis: Limited data. Approximately 6% removal with HD. $T_{1/2}$ increased to 19.7 +/– 5 hrs in pts on HD.
Dosing in peritoneal dialysis: No data.
Dosing in hemofiltration: Limited data. CVVHD: using a polysulfone hemofilter (1 L/hr flow rate) drug clearance of 7.1 +/– 2.35 mL/min (approx. 50% that in healthy individuals), [Churchwell MD et al. *ECC Microbiology and ID*, 2006].

ADVERSE DRUG REACTIONS
GENERAL
- Generally well tolerated, but incidence of mild taste disturbance, nausea, vomiting, and renal dysfunction were reported more commonly in telavancin-treated pts compared to common vancomycin-treatment pts.
- Taste disturbance (33%)
- Nausea (27%) and vomiting (14%)
- Insomnia

Occasional
- Red-man Syndrome (flushing of the upper body, urticaria, pruritus, or rash) with rapid infusion (<1 hr)
- Headache and dizziness
- Foamy urine (13%)
- Diarrhea
- Mean corrected QTc F prolongation increase of 4 msec
- Nephrotoxicity (Scr >1.5 mg/dL in 6% vs. 2% in vancomycin-treated pts)

Rare
- C. difficile associated diarrhea
- Significant QTc prolongation >60 msec observed in 1.5% in telavancin-treated group compared to 0.6% in the vancomycin-treated group.

DRUG INTERACTIONS
Telavancin is not a substrate or inhibitor of CYP450 isoenzymes. Significant drug-drug interactions involving phase 1 oxidation unlikely.
- Avoid co-administration with drugs associated with QTc prolongation (e.g., moxifloxacin, clarithromycin, pimozide, etc.)
- No significant drug-drug interactions observed with midazolam, aztreonam, and piperacillin/tazobactam (J Clin Pharmacol. 2009;49:816).
- The combination of telavancin with amikacin, aztreonam, cefepime, ceftriaxone, ciprofloxacin, gentamicin, imipenem, meropenem, oxacillin, piperacillin/tazobactam, rifampin, and TMP/SMX is not antagonistic in vitro.

RESISTANCE
- No CLSI breakpoint, but FDA approved break points are: <1 mcg/mL for vancomycin-sensitive E. faecalis , MSSA, and MRSA. For S. pyogenes, S. agalactiae, S. anginosus group MIC breakpoint is <0.12 mcg/mL.
- VRE strains with high vancomycin MIC will be cross-resistant to telavancin, but telavancin retains activity against some Van B (vancomycin-resistant, teicoplanin-susceptible) strains (AAC 2008;52:2383).
- The telavancin MIC range of 60 CA-MRSA isolates was 0.25–1 mcg/mL (JAC 2007; 60:406).
- Telavancin is active against 26 VISA strains in vitro, but evolution of resistance can occur (AAC 2009; 53:4217).

PHARMACOLOGY
Mechanism
Telavancin is a semisynthetic, lipoglycopeptide antibiotic. Similar to vancomycin, telavancin inhibits bacterial cell wall synthesis by interfering cross-linking and polymerization of peptidoglycan. In addition, telavancin depolarizes the bacterial membrane and disrupts barrier function.

PHARMACOKINETIC PARAMETERS
Absorption n/a

Cmax =108 ± 26 mcg/mL; AUC=780 +/− 125 mcg/mL after 10 mg/kg at steady state. Telavancin displays concentration-dependent bactericidal effects with 4–6 hrs post-antibiotic effect. Pharmacodynamic parameters associated with rapid MRSA cidal activity: free telavancin AUC/MIC of 50–100.

Distribution Vd=0.133 L/kg. Blister fluid fluid penetration of ~40%. Good lung penetration (epithelial lining fluid is 73% of plasma) [AAC 2008; 52: 2300].

Protein binding 90%

ANTIBACTERIAL DRUGS

Metabolism/Excretion Telavancin is primarily eliminated by the kidney with 76% of the administered dose recovered from urine.
T1/2 8.0 ± 1.5 hrs.
Dosing for Decreased Hepatic Function
Moderate hepatic impairment (Child-Pugh B): usual dose. Severe hepatic impairment: no data, but usual dose likely.
Pregnancy Risk
C: Based on animal data, telavancin may cause fetal harm. Avoid administration in pregnancy. Women of childbearing potential should have a serum pregnancy test. Pregnancy registry (1-888-658-4228)
Breast Feeding Compatibility
No data.
COMMENTS
Telavancin is non-inferior to vancomycin for the treatment of complicated soft tissue infections and nosocomial pneumonia caused by susceptible Gram-positive organisms. The spectrum of activity of telavancin is similar to vancomycin, but it may be active against some VRE strains (Van B). The clinical significance of a lower telavancin MRSA MIC and better pulmonary penetration compared to vancomycin remains to be determined.
SELECTED REFERENCES

Stryjewski ME, Graham DR, Wilson SE, et al. Telavancin versus vancomycin for the treatment of complicated skin and skin-structure infections caused by Gram-positive organisms. *Clin Infect Dis,* 2008; Vol. 46; p. 1683.

Rubinstein E, Corey GR, Stryjewski ME, et al. Telavancin for Treatment of Hospital-Acquired Pneumonia (HAP) Caused by MRSA and MSSA: the ATTAIN studies. *48th Interscience Conference on Antimicrobial Agents and Chemotherapy,* 2008, Vol. abstract K-530.

TELITHROMYCIN

Paul A. Pham, PharmD and John G. Bartlett, MD

INDICATIONS
FDA
* Mild to moderate severe community-acquired pneumonia due to *S. pneumoniae* (including multi-drug resistant isolates), *H. influenzae, M. catarrhalis, C. pneumoniae,* or *M. pneumoniae.*
Non-FDA Approved Uses
* Sinusitis, acute (FDA indication withdrawn due to a low benefit vs. risk ratio)
* Chronic bronchitis, acute exacerbations (FDA indication withdrawn due to a low benefit vs. risk ratio)
FORMS

Brand name (mfr)	Forms	Cost*
Ketek (Sanofi-Aventis)	PO tab 400 mg	$6.00
*Prices represents Average Wholesale Price (AWP).		

USUAL ADULT DOSING
Community acquired pneumonia: 800 mg PO once daily with or without food × 7–1 0 days.
RENAL DOSING
Dosing for GFR 50–80: Usual dose.
Dosing for GFR 10–50: Usual dose.
Dosing for GFR <10: AUC increased by 1.9× in severe renal insufficiency. Consider dose reduction in pts with concurrent hepatic failure.
Dosing in hemodialysis: Usual dose (800 mg PO once daily, limited data).
Dosing in peritoneal dialysis: No data (consider 800 mg PO once daily).
Dosing in hemofiltration: No data. Usual dose likely.
ADVERSE DRUG REACTIONS
Common
* Nausea/diarrhea (7–10%)

Occasional
- Headache, dizziness
- Vomiting
- LFT elevation/hepatitis
- Reversible blurring, difficulty focusing, and diplopia observed in 1.1% of pts (females <40 yrs at increased risk)

Rare
- QTc prolongation
- Severe hepatitis w/ fatalities reported
- Loss of consciousness

DRUG INTERACTIONS—See Appendix III, p. 835, for table of drug-to-drug interactions.
Telithromycin is a substrate and an inhibitor of CYP3A4. Use with caution with CYP3A4 substrates, inducers, and inhibitors.

SPECTRUM—See Appendix II, p. 595

PHARMACOLOGY

Mechanism
Similar to that of macrolides, ketolides dually binds to 50S-ribosomal subunit (domains II and V) with inhibition of bacterial protein synthesis. Due to its binding at domain II, telithromycin retains activity against Gram-positive cocci in the presence of resistance mediated by methylases that alter the domain V binding site of this antibiotic.

Pharmacokinetic Parameters
- **Absorption** Bioavailability: 57%.
- **Cmax** 2–2.9 mcg/mL (1 hr after 800-mg dose administration; Cmin: 0.07–0.2 mcg/mL.
- **Distribution** Vd: large volume of distribution of 2.9 L/kg with telithromycin tissue level (i.e., bronchial mucosa, epithelial lining fluid, and alveolar macrophages) exceeding plasma level by 2 to 8-fold.
- **Protein binding** 60% to 70%.
- **Metabolism/Excretion** 70% of total dose is metabolized via CYP450 3A4 and non-CYP450 route, metabolites and unchanged drugs are excreted in the urine (13%) and feces (7%).
- **T1/2** 10 hrs.

Dosing for Decreased Hepatic Function
Use with caution. (Child Pugh Class A, B and C) standard dose: 800 mg PO once daily

Pregnancy Risk
C: No treatment related malformation seen in animal studies. No human data.

Breast Feeding Compatibility
No data.

COMMENTS
No longer FDA indicated for AECB or acute bacterial sinusitis due to reported rare but very serious and sometimes lethal cases of hepatoxicity. May be considered an alternative to fluoroquinolones (levofloxacin, moxifloxacin) in the treatment of moderate to severe CAP involving penicillin-resistant *S. pneumoniae*. Disadvantages: available only in oral formulation, relatively high rate of GI intolerance, reversible visual disturbance, loss of consciousness, and some incidence of apparently drug-related severe hepatitis. Many drug interactions with CYP3A4 substrate. Contraindicated in pts with myasthenia gravis.

SELECTED REFERENCES
Clay KD, Hanson JS, Pope SD, et al. Brief communication: severe hepatotoxicity of telithromycin: three case reports and literature review. *Ann Intern Med*, 2006; Vol. 144; pp. 415–20.

Ross DB. The FDA and the case of Ketek. *N Engl J Med*, 2007; Vol. 356; pp. 1601–4.

TETRACYCLINE

Paul A. Pham, PharmD and John G. Bartlett, MD

INDICATIONS

FDA
- Alternative in PCN-allergic pts: syphilis, yaws, Vincent's infections, and infections caused by *N. gonorrhoeae*, *B. anthracis*, *L. monocytogenes*, *Actinomyces* sp., and *Clostridium* sp.

ANTIBACTERIAL DRUGS

- URI and lower respiratory tract infections; skin and soft tissue infections; Granuloma inguinale; psittacosis caused by *Chlamydia psittaci*.
- Typhus infections, Rocky Mountain Spotted Fever, rickettsial infections, and Q fever.
- Infections caused by *Chlamydia trachomatis*.
- Urinary tract infections.
- Infections caused by *Borrelia* sp., *Bartonella bacilliformis*, *H. ducreyi*, *F. tularensis*, *Y. pestis*, *V. cholerae*, *Brucella* sp., *C. fetus*.
- Adjunctive to intestinal amebiasis cause by *E. histolytica*.
- Infections caused by susceptible strains of *E. coli*, *Enterobacter aerogenes*, *Shigella* sp., *Acinetobacter* sp. *Klebsiella* sp., *Bacteroides* sp.

Non-FDA Approved Uses

- *H. pylori*-related peptic ulcer disease (in combination with bismuth subsalicylate and metronidazole).
- Gingivitis/periodontitis.
- Acne vulgaris.

FORMS

Brand name (mfr)	Forms	Cost*
Sumycin (Par)	PO cap 250 mg; PO cap 500 mg PO susp 125 mg/5 mL (16 oz)	$0.08; $0.17; $75.00
Tetracycline (Various)	PO cap 250 mg; PO cap 500 mg	$0.09; $0.20
*Prices represents Average Wholesale Price (AWP).		

USUAL ADULT DOSING

250–500 mg PO four times a day on an empty stomach.

RENAL DOSING

Dosing for GFR 50–80: Usual dose.
Dosing for GFR 10–50: Avoid tetracycline, use doxycycline.
Dosing for GFR <10: Avoid tetracycline, use doxycycline.
Dosing in hemodialysis: Avoid tetracycline, use doxycycline.
Dosing in peritoneal dialysis: Avoid tetracycline, use doxycycline.
Dosing in hemofiltration: Avoid tetracycline, use doxycycline.

ADVERSE DRUG REACTIONS

Common

- GI upset and diarrhea
- Stains and deforms teeth in children <8 yrs
- Severe phlebitis with IV infusion (no longer available in the U.S.)

Occasional

- Hepatotoxicity (dose related, especially seen in pregnant women, pts w/ renal insufficiency, and with the use of expired medication).
- Worsening azotemia (increased in pts with renal failure). Doxycycline preferred in pts with renal insufficiency.
- Esophageal ulcerations.
- Candidiasis (thrush and vaginitis).
- Photosensitivity.

Rare

- Allergic reactions
- Visual disturbances
- Aggravation of myasthenia gravis (reversed with calcium)
- *C. difficile* colitis (less likely compared to cephalosporins, carbapenems, and fluoroquinolones)
- Hemolytic anemia
- Benign intracranial hypertension, papilledema
- Fanconi syndrome (with outdated drugs)

DRUG INTERACTIONS—See Appendix III, p. 839, for table of drug-to-drug interactions.
SPECTRUM—See Appendix II, p. 802

RESISTANCE
- MIC breakpoint for Enterobacteriaceae, *Staphylococcus* spp., and *Enterococcus* spp.: ≤4 mcg/mL (sensitive); 8 mcg/mL (intermediate); ≥16 mcg/mL (resistant).
- Isolates that are susceptible tetracycline are also considered susceptible to doxycycline and minocycline. However, tetracycline-intermediate or -resistant isolates may be susceptible to doxycycline or minocycline.

PHARMACOLOGY
Mechanism
Tetracyclines inhibit protein synthesis by mainly binding to 30S ribosomal subunit and blocking binding of aminoacyl transfer-RNA.

Pharmacokinetic Parameters
- **Absorption** 60–80% absorbed. Administer on empty stomach.
- **Cmax** 1.5–2.2 mcg/mL after 250 mg PO dose administration.
- **Distribution** Widely distributed into body tissues and fluids including pleural fluid, bronchial secretions, sputum, ascitic fluid, synovial fluid, aqueous and vitreous humor, and prostatic fluid. Poor CNS penetration.
- **Protein binding** 20–67%.
- **Metabolism/Excretion** Excreted unchanged mainly by glomerular filtration; also excreted into GI tract via bile and nonbiliary route.
- **T1/2** 6–11 hrs.

Dosing for Decreased Hepatic Function
Avoid with severe hepatic dysfunction.

Pregnancy Risk
D: Tetracyclines are contraindicated in pregnancy due to retardation of skeletal development and bone growth; enamel hypoplasia and discoloration of teeth of fetus. Maternal liver toxicity have also been reported.

Breast Feeding Compatibility
Tetracyclines are excreted in breast milk at very low concentrations. There is theoretical possibility of dental staining and inhibition of bone growth, but infants exposed to tetracyclines have blood levels less than 0.05 mcg/mL.

COMMENTS
Oral tetracycline has broad activity, but doxycycline is usually preferred due to twice a day dosing convenience without regard to meals. Tetracycline has role for the treatment of susceptible organisms causing UTIs since it achieves good urinary levels compared to the hepatically metabolized doxycycline, minocycline, and tigecycline.

SELECTED REFERENCES
Ariza J, Gudiol F, Pallarés R, et al. Comparative trial of rifampin-doxycycline versus tetracycline-streptomycin in the therapy of human brucellosis. *Antimicrob Agents Chemother*, 1985; Vol. 28; pp. 548–51.

TICARCILLIN + CLAVULANIC ACID

Paul A. Pham, PharmD and John G. Bartlett, MD

INDICATIONS
FDA
- Bone and joint infections
- Intra-abdominal infections (appendicitis, cholecystitis, cholangitis, diverticulitis)
- Lower respiratory tract infections
- Obstetric/gynecologic infections
- Septicemia
- Skin and soft-tissue infections
- Urinary tract infections

Non-FDA Approved Uses
- Pneumonia, hospital-acquired
- Empyema
- Diabetic foot infection

ANTIBACTERIAL DRUGS

Brand name (mfr)	Forms	Cost*
Timentin (GlaxoSmithKline)	IV minibag 3.1 g/100 mL IV vial 3.1 g	$19.25 $16.66

*Prices represents Average Wholesale Price (AWP).

USUAL ADULT DOSING

3.1 g IV q4–6h (up to 24 g per day). Pulmonary, pseudomonal and serious infections: 3.1 g IV q4h.

RENAL DOSING

Dosing for GFR 50–80: GFR >60 mL/min: 3.1 g IV q4–6h (up to 24 g per day). Pulmonary, Pseudomonad, and serious infections: 3.1 g IV q4h.

Dosing for GFR 10–50: <30 mL/min: 2 g q8h, if 30–60 mL/min: 2 g q4h.

Dosing for GFR <10: 2 g q12h.

Dosing in hemodialysis: 2 g q12h plus 3.1 g post-dialysis.

Dosing in peritoneal dialysis: 3.1 g q12h.

Dosing in hemofiltration: CVVH: 2 g q6–8h; CVVHD: 3.1 g q6h

ADVERSE DRUG REACTIONS

General
- Generally well tolerated

Occasional
- Hypersensitivity reactions
- Rash
- GI intolerance
- Phlebitis at infusion sites
- Jarisch-Herxheimer reaction (with syphilis or other spirochetal infections)
- *C. difficile* colitis
- LFTs elevations, rare cases of clinical hepatitis

Rare
- Drug fever
- Coombs' test positive w/ hemolytic anemia
- Interstitial nephritis
- Leukopenia and thrombocytopenia
- Abnormal platelet aggregation with bleeding diathesis (especially with higher dose in renal failure)
- CNS-seizures and twitching (with high doses in pts with renal failure)
- Hepatitis
- Anaphylaxis

DRUG INTERACTIONS
- Oral contraceptives: may decrease the efficacy of oral contraceptives with co-administration. Consider an additional barrier form of contraception.
- Probenecid: may prolong piperacillin levels. May be result in significant accumulation in renal failure.
- Tetracyclines: *in vitro* antagonism when co-administered. Bactericidal effect of penicillins may be diminished *in vivo*. Management recommendation: avoid concurrent administration. In 2 studies involving a total of 79 pts with pneumococcal meningitis treated with either penicillin plus tetracyclines or penicillin monotherapy resulted in a higher mortality rate (79–85 %) in the combination therapy compared to penicillin monotherapy (30–33%) [*Arch Intern Med* 1951;88:489, *Ann Intern Med* 1961;55:545]. However, there was not a difference in mortality between penicillin monotherapy and penicillin plus tetracycline in the treatment of pneumococcal pneumonia [*Arch Intern Med* 1953;91:197].

SPECTRUM—See Appendix II, p. 795

PHARMACOLOGY

Mechanism

Beta-lactam antibiotics inhibit mucopeptide synthesis in the bacterial cell wall, this result in the formation of defective cell walls and osmotically unstable organism which leads to cell lysis. Clavulanate inhibits plasmid-mediated beta-lactamases.

Pharmacokinetic Parameters

- **Absorption** —
- **Cmax** 324 mcg/mL after 3.1 g IV dose administration.
- **Distribution** 0.16 L/kg; Distributed to blister fluid, urine, peritoneal and pleural fluid, middle ear fluid, intestinal mucosa, bone, gallbladder, lung, female reproductive tissue, bile. Moderate CNS penetration w/ inflamed meninges, may not be effective for *P. aeruginosa*.
- **Protein binding** 35–45%.
- **Metabolism/Excretion** Hepatic metabolism accounts for less than 15% of administered dose. Both unchanged drug and metabolites are excreted via glomerular filtration and tubular secretion. Biliary excretion also occurs accounting for the high biliary concentration.
- **T1/2** 1.2 hrs.

Dosing for Decreased Hepatic Function

For pts with hepatic dysfunction and creatinine clearance <10 mL/min: 2 g IV/day in 1 or 2 doses, but consider 2 g q12h for serious infections.

Pregnancy Risk

B: In surveillance study of Michigan Medicaid recipients, 556 newborns was exposed to clavulanate/penicillins during the first trimester, there was no association between birth defects and clavulanate/penicillins.

Breast Feeding Compatibility

Excreted in breast milk. Clinical significance unknown.

COMMENTS

Parenteral beta-lactam-beta-lactamase inhibitor with spectrum similar to that of piperacillin/tazobactam but with less activity against *P. aeruginosa*, enterococcus, and *S. pneumoniae*. Contains 4.75 meq of sodium per Gram of ticarcillin. More frequent dosing interval (every 4 hrs) recommended for serious pseudomonal infections.

SELECTED REFERENCES

Dougherty SH, Sirinek KR, Schauer PR, et al. Ticarcillin/clavulanate compared with clindamycin/gentamicin (with or without ampicillin) for the treatment of intra-abdominal infections in pediatric and adult pts. *Am Surg*, 1995; Vol. 61; pp. 297–303.

Yellin AE, Johnson J, Higareda I, et al. Ertapenem or ticarcillin/clavulanate for the treatment of intra-abdominal infections or acute pelvic infections in pediatric pts. *Am J Surg*, 2007; Vol. 194; pp. 367–74.

TIGECYCLINE

Paul A. Pham, PharmD and John G. Bartlett, MD

INDICATIONS

FDA

- Complicated skin and skin structure infections (including those caused by MRSA and vancomycin-susceptible *E. faecalis*).
- Complicated intra-abdominal infections (as a single agent).
- Community-acquired bacterial pneumonia caused by *S. pneumoniae* (PCN-susceptible isolates), *H. influenzae* (beta-lactamase negative isolates), and *Legionella pneumophila*. Author's comment: not a first-line agent and rarely used for CAP.

Non-FDA Approved Uses

- Infections at multiple anatomical sites involving resistance Gram-negative bacilli such as Acinetobacter and KPC producing Enterobacteraceae.

FORMS

Brand name (mfr)	Forms	Cost*
Tygacil (Wyeth)	IV vial 50 mg/5 mL	$72.23
*Prices represents Average Wholesale Price (AWP).		

USUAL ADULT DOSING

100 mg IV × 1 (load), then 50 mg IV q12h × 5–14 days.

ANTIBACTERIAL DRUGS

RENAL DOSING

Dosing for GFR 50–80: Usual dose.
Dosing for GFR 10–50: Usual dose.
Dosing for GFR <10: Usual dose.
Dosing in hemodialysis: Not removed with HD. No dose adjustment needed.
Dosing in peritoneal dialysis: No data, usual dose likely.
Dosing in hemofiltration: No data, usual dose likely.

ADVERSE DRUG REACTIONS

Common

- Nausea and vomiting in 20–30%

Occasional

- Hyperbilirubinemia (2.3%)
- BUN increase (2.1%)

Rare

- *C. difficile* colitis (less likely compared to cephalosporins, carbapenems, and fluoroquinolones)
- Due to structural similarity, tetracycline-style photosensitivity may occur

DRUG INTERACTIONS

Does not interact with cytochrome p450 isoform (1A2, 2C8, 2C9, 2C19, 2D6, and 3A4) therefore drug-drug interaction with CYP450 is unlikely.

- Digoxin: no interaction.
- Warfarin: tigecycline increased warfarin-R AUC by 40% but did not affect INR.

PHARMACOLOGY

Pharmacokinetic Parameters

- **Cmax** 0.87 mcg/mL; AUC = 4.7 mcg/mL hr.
- **Distribution** Widely distributed. Vd = 500 to 700 L. Concentrated in epithelial lining fluid (1.32-fold higher than serum), alveolar macrophages (78-fold higher than serum), gallbladder (23-fold), and colon (2.6-fold). After a single dose administration, 31–58% of serum concentration is achieved in the synovial fluid, 35–41% of serum concentration is achieved in the bone, and 11% of serum concentration is achieved in the CSF.
- **Protein binding** 71–89%.
- **Metabolism/Excretion** Not extensively metabolized with 59% of the dose excreted in the biliary/feces, and 33% is excreted in the urine.
- **T1/2** 42 hrs at steady state.

Dosing for Decreased Hepatic Function

100 mg IV × 1, then 25 mg IV q12h (for Child Pugh C).

Pregnancy Risk

D: No human data. Avoid in pregnancy. Reduction in fetal weight and increased incidence of minor skeletal anomalies in rats and rabbits studies.

Breast Feeding Compatibility

Excreted in breast milk but tigecycline has limited oral bioavailability. Use only when clearly indicated.

COMMENTS

Tigecycline has a spectrum of activity that includes anaerobes, many Gram-positive cocci and Gram-negative bacilli w/ the exception of Pseudomonas, Proteus, and Providencia. Tigecycline is effective in the treatment of intra-abdominal infections, PNA, and complicated soft-tissue infections with a more convenient twice-a-day dosing compared to imipenem/cilastin and piperacillin/tazobactam. Main use is for treating multiply resistant GNB. A low achievable serum concentration may make treatment of bacteremia problematic (especially when treating organisms with a higher susceptibility break point of 2–4 mcg/mL). Nausea and vomiting may occur in up to a third of pts.

SELECTED REFERENCES

Babinchak T, Ellis-Grosse E, Dartois N, et al. The efficacy and safety of tigecycline for the treatment of complicated intra-abdominal infections: analysis of pooled clinical trial data. *Clin Infect Dis.* 2005; Vol. *41 Suppl 5;* pp. S354–67.

Ellis-Grosse EJ, Babinchak T, Dartois N, et al. The efficacy and safety of tigecycline in the treatment of skin and skin-structure infections: results of 2 double-blind phase 3 comparison studies with vancomycin-aztreonam. *Clin Infect Dis.* 2005; Vol. *41 Suppl 5;* pp. S341–53.

TOBRAMYCIN

Paul A. Pham, PharmD and John G. Bartlett, MD

INDICATIONS

FDA

- With the exception of uncomplicated UTI, aminoglycosides are generally used in combination.
- Septicemia, including serious central-nervous-system infections (use in combination)
- Lower respiratory tract infections (use in combination)
- Complicated urinary tract infections
- Intra-abdominal infections, including peritonitis (use in combination)
- Skin, bone, and skin structure infections (use in combination)
- Management of cystic fibrosis, with *P. aeruginosa* (as TOBI inhalation)
- Treatment of ocular infections (uncomplicated conjunctivitis-ophthalmic solution)

Non-FDA Approved Uses

- Pneumonia, Hospital-Acquired (in combination with a beta-lactam, beta-lactam/beta-lactamase inhibitor, or a 3rd/4th generation cephalosporin)
- Pseudomonal infections (in combination with a beta-lactam, beta-lactam/beta-lactamase inhibitor, carbapenem or a 3rd/4th generation cephalosporin)

FORMS

Brand name (mfr)	Forms	Cost*
Tobramycin (various generic manufacturers)	IV vial 10 mg/mL (2 mL); IV vial 40 mg/mL (30 mL) Opth soln drops 0.3% IV vial 1.2 g	$3.68 per vial; $37.50 per vial $14.25 (5 mL) $88.56
Tobi (Novartis)	Inhalation ampule 300 mg/5 mL	$76.58 per ampule.
Tobradex (ALCON LABORATORIES, Bausch and Lomb)	Opth suspension drops 0.3%/0.1%; Opth suspension drops 0.3%/0.5% Opth ointment ointment 0.3%/0.1%	$89.38 (5 mL); $178.75 (10 mL) $18.43; $70.44 (3.5 g)
*Prices represents Average Wholesale Price (AWP).		

USUAL ADULT DOSING

- **Once daily dosing:** 5–7 mg/kg IV. Therapeutic drug monitoring generally not recommended. Consider trough in pts at risk for nephrotoxicity (ICU pts, elderly, and concomitant nephrotoxin). Target trough <1 mcg/mL. Don't use once daily dosing in pts w/ unstable renal function, CrCl <60 mL/min, endocarditis, meningitis, or increased Vd (pregnancy, ascites, edema).
- **Traditional dosing mild-moderate infections:** 2 mg/kg load, then 1.7–2 mg/kg IV q8h (goal peak >6 mcg/mL and trough <2 mcg/mL).
- **Traditional dosing severe infections (Pseudomonas, pneumonia):** 3 mg/kg load, then 2 mg/kg IV q8h (goal peak >8 mcg/mL and trough <2 mcg/mL).
- Consider a higher loading dose and obtain a peak and trough after first dose in severe infections (+/– diffuse edema, ascites, shock, burns, CF, and pregnancy) in order to calculate pt-specific pharmacokinetic dose. Doses need to be adjusted based on changing renal function and/or volume status.
- Trough to be obtained (generally after 3rd dose) immediately before next dose.
- Peak to be obtained 30 mins after the end of a 30 mins infusion (generally after 3rd dose).
- For obese pts: use calculated lean body weight plus 40% of excess fat (i.e., Dosing Body Weight (DBW) = Ideal Body Weight (IBW) + 0.4 (actual body weight-IBW).
- IBW = 50 kg (for males) **or** 45.5 kg (for females) **plus** (2.3 × inches over 5 ft).
- Tobramycin by aerosol (nebs): 80–300 mg q12–24h.
- Intraventricular or intrathecal administration: use preservative free tobramycin 5 mg q24h (range 4–10 mg).

ANTIBACTERIAL DRUGS

Renal Dosing

Dosing for GFR 50–80: Standard loading dose for all levels of renal function. GRF >70 mL/min: use standard dose. GFR 50–69 mL/min: calculated GFR × 0.045 = mg/kg q12h (ex. for GFR 56 mL/min: 56 × 0.045 = 2.5 mg/kg q12h). Monitor peak and trough.

Dosing for GFR 10–50: Standard loading dose for all levels of renal function. GFR 40–49 mL/min: calculated GFR × 0.045 = mg/kg q12h (ex. for GFR 45 mL/min: 45 × 0.045 = 2 mg/kg q12h). GFR 20–39: calculated GFR × 0.09 = mg/kg q24h.

Dosing for GFR <10: Standard loading dose for all levels of renal function. GFR <20 mL/min: 2–2.5 mg/kg × 1, then redose when level <2 mcg/mL.

Dosing in hemodialysis: Standard loading dose, then 1.7–2 mg/kg post-HD. Peak (measure 2 hrs-post dose, target 7–10 mcg/mL) and trough (before next HD session, depending on residual renal function, expect 3–5 mcg/mL.)

Dosing in peritoneal dialysis: 2–4 mg/L of dialysate exchange per day. Aminoglycosides given for prolonged periods to pts receiving continuous peritoneal dialysis have been associated with high rates of ototoxicity.

Dosing in hemofiltration: CVVH or CVVHD: loading dose 3 mg/kg, then 2 mg/kg q24–48 (measure peak 2 hrs-post dose, target 7–10 mcg/mL). Check a 24-hr concentration (redose <2 mcg/mL).

Adverse Drug Reactions

Common

- Renal failure (usually reversible), risk factors: older pts, preexisting renal and hepatic disease, volume depletion, traditional Q8h dosing, large doses, concomitant nephrotoxic drug (including vancomycin), and length of therapy (most important). Controversial but trough may be associated with nephrotoxicity.

Occasional

- Irreversible vestibular toxicity (4–6%). Most pt compensate with visual and proprioceptive cues. Monitor for nausea, vomiting, nystagmus, and vertigo (exacerbated in the dark).
- Irreversible cochlear toxicity (3–14%). Risk factors: repeated exposure (cumulative dose and duration of therapy), genetic predisposition, renal impairment, specific aminoglycoside (neomycin > streptomycin > gentamicin > tobramycin > amikacin > netilmicin), elderly, age, bacteremia, hypovolemia, degree of temp elevation and liver dysfunction (*JID* 1984:149:23–30). 62% of hearing lost were at frequency above 9 kHz (high pitch) at a mean of 9 days of therapy (*JID* 1992;165:1026–1032).
- Genetic predisposition in some cases vestibular and cochlear toxicity. Check family hx for aminoglycoside ototoxicity.
- Monitor for ototoxicity in any pts receiving >3 days of aminoglycoside. Vestibular toxicity monitoring: Check baseline visual acuity using a Snellen pocket card. After 3 days of aminoglycoside, have pt shake head (side to side) while reading a line. Early sign of ototoxicity if pt loses 2 lines of visual acuity. Check Romberg sign. Cochlear toxicity monitoring: audiology test.

Rare

- Neuromuscular blockade (esp with myasthenia or Parkinsons and rapid infusion of large aminoglycoside doses).
- Allergic reaction (secondary to sulfites in some formulation).

Drug Interactions

- Cephalothin: increased risk of nephrotoxicity.
- Loop diuretics (bumetanide, furosemide, ethacrynic acid, torsemide): cochlear toxicity (esp. w/ ethacrynic acid). Avoid co-administration.
- Nondepolarizing muscle relaxants (atracurium, pancuronium, tubocurarine, gallamine triethiodide): possible enhanced action of nondepolarizing muscle relaxant resulting in possible respiratory depression.
- Nephrotoxic agents (e.g., amphotericin B, foscarnet, cidofovir, and contrast agents): additive nephrotoxicity. Avoid co-administration.
- Penicillins: *in vitro* inactivation. Do not mix or run in the same tubing.
- Vancomycin: increased risk of nephrotoxicity.

Spectrum—See Appendix II, p. 797

Resistance

- MIC breakpoint for *Enterobacteriaceae* and other Gram-negative non-lactose fermenters including *P. aeruginosa* is 4 mcg/mL.

Pharmacology

Mechanism

Aminoglycosides inhibit protein synthesis by irreversibly binding to 30S ribosomal subunit.

Pharmacokinetic Parameters

- **Absorption** Aminoglycosides are rapidly absorbed after IM administration. Intrapleural and intraperitoneal administration results in rapid absorption. Poor absorption with oral administration.
- **Cmax** 6 mcg/mL after 1.5 mg/kg IV dose administration. In addition to the dose, Cmax will be affected by the volume of distribution.
- **Distribution** 0.2–0.4 L/kg (may be higher in pregnancy, ascites, edema, sepsis, and burn pts); Distributed in extracellular fluid, abscesses, ascitic fluid, pericardial fluid, pleural fluid, synovial fluid, lymphatic fluid, and peritoneal fluid. Not well distributed into bile, aqueous humor, bronchial secretions, abscess, sputum, and CSF.
- **Protein binding** 0–10%.
- **Metabolism/Excretion** Aminoglycosides are not metabolized in the liver, they are excreted unchanged in the urine.
- **T1/2** 2–4 hrs (Note: cystic fibrosis pts may have shorter half life of 1–2 hrs; burn and febrile pts may have increased clearance of aminoglycosides).

Dosing for Decreased Hepatic Function

No dose adjustment, but may increase risk of nephrotoxicity and ototoxicity. Use with close monitoring.

Pregnancy Risk

D: Animal studies did not demonstrate teratogenicity. Case reports exist of irreversible bilateral congenital deafness in children whose mothers received streptomycin. Can potentially occur with tobramycin.

Breast Feeding Compatibility

Only trace amount of tobramycin was found in some nursing infants. Due to the poor absorption of aminoglycoside the systemic toxicity should not occur, but alteration in normal bowel flora may occur in nursing infants.

Comments

Parenteral aminoglycoside with slightly better anti-pseudomonal activity compared to gentamicin. May also be less nephrotoxic, but may be more ototoxic compared to gentamicin. Once daily dosing should not be used in pts w/ unstable renal function, cr clearance <60 mL/min, endocarditis, meningitis, and any pts with increased vol (pregnancy, burn, ascites, edema, shock). Aminoglycoside monotherapy for systemic pseudomonal infections associated with worsened outcomes.

Selected References

American Thoracic Society, Infectious Diseases Society of America. Guidelines for the management of adults with hospital-acquired, ventilator-associated, and healthcare-associated pneumonia. *Am J Respir Crit Care Med*, 2005; Vol. 171; pp. 388–416.

Wiesemann HG, Steinkamp G, Ratjen F, et al. Placebo-controlled, double-blind, randomized study of aerosolized tobramycin for early treatment of *Pseudomonas aeruginosa* colonization in cystic fibrosis. *Pediatr Pulmonol*, 1998; Vol. 25; pp. 88–92.

TRIMETHOPRIM

Paul A. Pham, PharmD and John G. Bartlett, MD

Indications

FDA

- Urinary tract infections (uncomplicated) caused by *E. coli, P. mirabilis, K. pneumoniae, Enterobacter* species, and *S. saprophyticus*

Non-FDA Approved Uses

- *Pneumocystis jiroveci* pneumonia (in combination with dapsone)
- *Campylobacter jejuni*

ANTIBACTERIAL DRUGS

FORMS

Brand name (mfr)	Forms	Cost*
Proloprim (Various generic manufacturers)	PO tab 100 mg	$0.69
Primsol (FSC Laboratories)	PO sol 50 mg/5mL (473 mL)	$156.25
*Prices represents Average Wholesale Price (AWP).		

USUAL ADULT DOSING
- Uncomplicated UTI: 200 mg PO daily in 1–2 doses (note: TMP/SMX preferred for this indication, but TMP alone used if sulfa intolerant)
- Mild-moderate PCP: TMP 5 mg/kg PO q8h + dapsone 100 mg PO once daily

RENAL DOSING
Dosing for GFR 50–80: Usual dose.
Dosing for GFR 10–50: UTI: 100 mg q24h. PCP: 5 mg/kg q8–12h.
Dosing for GFR <10: Manufacturer recommends avoiding, but for PCP: 5–7.5 mg/kg/day (1/2–1/3 standard dose) in combination with dapsone.
Dosing in hemodialysis: PCP: 5–7.5 mg/kg/day. On days of HD, dose 5 mg/kg post dialysis in combination with dapsone.
Dosing in peritoneal dialysis: PD does not efficiently remove TMP. UTI: 100–200 mg q48h. PCP: no data, consider 5–7.5 mg/kg/day.
Dosing in hemofiltration: No data. See TMP/SMX.

ADVERSE DRUG REACTIONS
Common
- GI upset (dose related)

Occasional
- Megaloblastic anemia
- Neutropenia
- Thrombocytopenia
- Reversible hyperkalemia (with high dose trimethoprim)
- Liver enzyme elevation
- Pancytopenia
- Rash and pruritis

Rare
- Erythema multiforme, Stevens-Johnson syndrome and TEN (unclear association)

DRUG INTERACTIONS
- Dapsone: increased serum level of both dapsone (40%) and trimethoprim (48%). This interaction may be beneficial in the treatment of *Pneumocystis carinii* pneumonia. No dose adjustment needed.
- Methotrexate: plasma concentration of methotrexate may be increased due to decreased renal clearance. Monitor for pancytopenia with co-administration. Dose of methotrexate may need to be decreased.
- Phenytoin: phenytoin concentration may be increased due to trimethoprim Inhibition of hepatic metabolism. Management recommendation: monitor for phenytoin toxicity (drowsiness, nystagmus, dysarthria and tremor) and serum levels. Dose may need to be adjusted.
- Procainamide: elevated procainamide and N-acetylprocainamide (NAPA) serum level secondary to competitive inhibition of renal tubular secretion between trimethoprim and procainamide. Monitor serum level of procainamide and N-acetylprocainamide in addition to monitoring EKG for QTc prolongation and arrythmia.

PHARMACOLOGY
Mechanism
Trimethoprim binds to dihydrofolate reductase, therefore inhibiting the reduction of dihydrofolic acid to tetrahydrofolic acid (folinic acid).

Pharmacokinetic Parameters
- **Absorption** Complete absorption.
- **Cmax** 2 mcg/mL after 200 mg PO dose administration.
- **Distribution** Widely distributed into tissues and fluid including aqueous humor, middle ear, saliva, lung tissue, sputum, seminal fluid, prostatic fluid, bile, bone. 13–44% of serum concentration attained in CSF.
- **Protein binding** 45%.
- **Metabolism/Excretion** Metabolized to oxide and hydroxylated metabolite. Unchanged drug and metabolite are excreted in the urine. Small amount of drug is excreted in feces via biliary elimination.
- **T1/2** 8–10 hrs.

Dosing for Decreased Hepatic Function
No data. See TMP/SMX.

Pregnancy Risk
C: Animal data show teratogenicity as 40 times the human dose. Should be avoided in the first 3 mos of pregnancy during the formation of vital organs. This agent should only be used in pregnancy if the potential benefits outweigh the risk. If used, it should be administered with a supplemental multivitamin containing folic acid.

Breast Feeding Compatibility
Excreted in breast milk. The American Academy of Pediatrics considers trimethoprim compatible with breast feeding.

Comments
Generally used in combination with sulfamethoxazole. Only acceptable indication for monotherapy is acute uncomplicated UTI. TMP/dapsone is an alternative to TMP/SMX in the treatment of mild to moderately severe PCP, but should not be used with severe disease.

Selected References
Safrin S, Finkelstein DM, Feinberg J, et al. Comparison of 3 regimens for treatment of mild to moderate Pneumocystis carinii pneumonia in pts with AIDS. A double-blind, randomized, trial of oral trimethoprim-sulfamethoxazole, dapsone-trimethoprim, and clindamycin-primaquine. ACTG 108 Study Group. *Ann Intern Med*, 1996; Vol. 124; pp. 792–802.

TRIMETHOPRIM + SULFAMETHOXAZOLE

Paul A. Pham, PharmD and John G. Bartlett, MD

Indications

FDA
- Acute exacerbation of acute bronchitis
- Otitis media
- *Pneumocystis jiroveci* pneumonia prophylaxis
- *Pneumocystis jiroveci* pneumonia treatment
- Traveler's diarrhea; Shigellosis
- Urinary tract infections

Non-FDA Approved Uses
- Nocardia infections
- Toxoplasmosis treatment and prophylaxis
- Bacterial cystitis prophylaxis
- Isospora infections
- Salmonella infections
- MSSA and community acquired MRSA soft tissue infections
- Legionella (2nd line)
- Listeria treatment (2nd line for PCN allergic pts)

ANTIBACTERIAL DRUGS

FORMS

Brand name (mfr)	Forms	Cost*
Bactrim and Septra and Sulfatrim (Generic manufacturers)	Oral tablet 400 mg/80 mg (SS); Oral tablet 800 mg/160 mg (DS) IV vial 80 mg/16 mg per mL (30 mL) Oral suspension 200–40 mg/5 mL (480 mL bottle)	$0.67; $0.91 $11.44 /30 mL $57.95/480 mL bottle

*Prices represents Average Wholesale Price (AWP).

USUAL ADULT DOSING

- PCP treatment: 5 mg/kg (TMP component) IV or PO q8h × 21 days (usually 5–6 DS/day but must dose based upon TMP component).
- PCP prophylaxis: 1 DS or 1SS PO once daily or 1 DS 3 ×/wk (alternative).
- Toxoplasmosis prophylaxis: 1 DS PO once daily.
- Toxoplasmosis treatment: 5 mg/kg (TMP component) PO or IV q12h × 6 wks, then 1/2 dose for maintenance (sulfadiazine + pyrimethamine preferred).
- UTI: 1 DS PO twice daily × 3–14 days, (3 days recommended for uncomplicated cystitis in women).
- Traveler's diarrhea (*Salmonella, Shigella, E. coli,* and *Cyclospora*): 1DS PO twice daily × 5–7 days.
- Skin and soft tissue infections: 1–2 DS PO q12h.
- Nocardia: 2–3 DS PO twice daily × >6 mos.
- Isospora: 1 DS PO twice daily × 7–10 days, then 1DS 3 ×/wk.
- Gradual dose escalation over 6 days may improves long term tolerance of TMP/SMX compared to direct rechallenge, but dosing may be impractical for some pts. Start with 12.5% of SS TMP/SMX (10 mg TMP component), then increase by 12.5%/days until target dose of 1SS TMP/SMX on day 6 (*J Infect Dis*. 2001;184:992–7).
- Obese pts: consider using ABW for severe infections, but no data to support this.

RENAL DOSING

Dosing for GFR 50–80: Usual dose.
Dosing for GFR 10–50: GFR 10–30 mL/min: 5 mg/kg IV q12h; oral 50% of dose.
Dosing for GFR <10: Manufacturer recommends avoiding. For severe PCP or serious infections, the author recommend 5–7.5 mg/kg/day in 2–3 divided doses (1/2–1/3 standard dose) for GFR <10 mL/min.
Dosing in hemodialysis: Dialyzed, consider 5–7.5 mg/kg/day in 2–3 divided doses (dose post-HD on days of dialysis). PCP prophylaxis: consider 1SS PO every day.
Dosing in peritoneal dialysis: Not dialyzed out. PCP prophylaxis: consider 1 DS PO q48h. PCP treatment: consider 5 mg/kg/day.
Dosing in hemofiltration: CVVH: no data. CVVHD: limited data. Consider 5 mg/kg IV q8–12h.

ADVERSE DRUG REACTIONS

- Generally well tolerated in the immunocompetent host. HIV-infected pts are at increased risk for developing SMX-TMP-associated ADRs.

Common

- GI intolerance with nausea and vomiting (in 20–50% receiving high dose >15 mg/kg)
- Rash and pruritus (usually 7–14 days after starting SMX/TMP)
- Continue treatment if symptoms not disabling
- Pseudo elevation in serum creatinine (an average increase of 18%) [Kainer et al. *Chemotherapy*. 1981;27:229–32]

Occasional

- Reversible hyperkalemia (with higher TMP doses +/– chronic renal insufficiency)
- Bone marrow suppression (anemia with folate deficiency, thrombocytopenia, and leukopenia; more common with higher doses)
- Serum sickness and drug fever
- Hepatitis (may be cholestatic)
- Photosensitivity

- Methemoglobinemia (with severe G6PD deficiency). African American pts with mild to moderate G6PD deficiency can tolerate TMP-SMX.

Rare

- Crystalluria with azotemia, urolithiasis, and oliguria (more common with sulfadiazine)
- Stevens-Johnson syndrome or toxic epidermal necrolysis (TEN)
- Aseptic meningitis
- Pancreatitis
- Neurologic toxicity (tremor, ataxia, apathy, and ankle clonus)
- Interstitial nephritis

DRUG INTERACTIONS—See Appendix III, p. 841, for table of drug-to-drug interactions.

SPECTRUM—See Appendix II, p. 802

RESISTANCE

- *E. coli:* (urine isolates) certain regions in U.S. and world-wide >20% resistance.
- *S. pneumoniae:* 15–30% resistance rate.
- *P. jiroveci:* increasing rates of mutations in the dihydropteroate synthase (DHPS) gene of *P. jiroveci* associated with resistance to sulfonamide and dapsone but not clinically significant since clinical outcome was not worse with DHPS mutation in a prospective trial (*Lancet.* 2001;358:545–9).
- CA-MRSA: low incidence of resistance.
- TMP/SMX MIC breakpoint for Enterobacteriaceae and Gram-negative non-Enterobacteriaceae: ≤2/38 mcg/mL (sensitive); ≥4/76 mcg/mL (resistant).
- TMP/SMX MIC breakpoint for *Staphylococcus* spp.: ≤2/38 mcg/mL (sensitive); ≥4/76 mcg/mL (resistant).
- TMP/SMX MIC breakpoint for *S. maltophilia:* ≤2/38 mcg/mL (sensitive); ≥4/76 mcg/mL (resistant).

PHARMACOLOGY

Mechanism

TMP act synergistically with SMX by interfering with folic acid production. TMP binds to dihydrofolate reductase inhibiting the reduction of dihydrofolic acid to tetrahydrofolic acid (folinic acid). Sulfonamides are structural analog of p-aminobenzoic acid (PABA), it competitively inhibits dihydrofolic acid synthesis which is necessary for the conversion of PABA to folic acid.

Pharmacokinetic Parameters

- **Absorption** 90–100% absorption.
- **Cmax** 3.4 mcg/mL TMP after 160 (TMP component) IV dose administration, steady-tate peak concentration is 9 mcg/mL with 160 mg IV q8h administration.
- **Distribution** TMP: 2.0 L/kg; SMX: 360 mL/kg. Good CSF penetration.
- **Protein binding** SMZ (70%). TMP (44% to 62%).
- **Metabolism/Excretion** Extensive liver metabolism of SMZ to n-acetyl and n-glucuronidate metabolite. 10–30% of SMZ and 50–70% of TMP excreted in urine.
- **T1/2** 11 hrs (TMP), 9 hrs (SMX).

Dosing for Decreased Hepatic Function

No data. Consider usual dose with close monitoring.

Pregnancy Risk

C: In a surveillance study of Michigan Medicaid recipients, 2296 exposures to SMX/TMP in the first trimester resulted in 5.5% birth defect. This incident is suggestive of an association between the drug and congenital defects (cardiovascular); however, other factors such as mother's disease, concurrent drug used and chance, may be involved. Contraindicated near term/late third trimester.

Breast Feeding Compatibility

Excreted in breast milk at low concentrations. The American Academy of Pediatrics considers trimethoprim-sulfamethoxazole to be compatible.

COMMENTS

First line agent for PCP prophylaxis and treatment. Active against other pathogens (*T. gondii, Listeria, Legionella,* 70% of *S. pneumoniae,* many *S. aureus* including CA-MRSA, and) which may protect pts against CAP and soft tissue infections. A good first line agent for CA-MRSA soft tissue infection. Although it is generally well tolerated in the immunocompetent host, there is a higher incidence of intolerance requiring discontinuation in HIV-infected pts.

ANTIBACTERIAL DRUGS

BASIS FOR RECOMMENDATIONS
National Institutes of Health (NIH), the Centers for Disease Control and Prevention (CDC), and the HIV Medicine Association of the Infectious Diseases Society of America (HIVMA/IDSA). Guidelines for Prevention and Treatment of Opportunistic Infections in HIV-Infected Adults and Adolescents, 2008; Vol. 58; pp. 1–207.

SELECTED REFERENCES
Green H, Paul M, Vidal L, et al. Prophylaxis of Pneumocystis pneumonia in immunocompromised non-HIV-infected pts: systematic review and meta-analysis of randomized controlled trials. *Mayo Clin Proc.*, 2007; Vol. 82; pp. 1052–9.

Safrin S, Finkelstein DM, Feinberg J, et al. Comparison of three regimens for treatment of mild to moderate *Pneumocystis carinii* pneumonia in pts with AIDS. A double-blind, randomized, trial of oral trimethoprim-sulfamethoxazole, dapsone-trimethoprim, and clindamycin-primaquine. ACTG 108 Study Group. *Ann Intern Med*, 1996; Vol. 124; pp. 792–802.

VANCOMYCIN

Paul A. Pham, PharmD and John G. Bartlett, MD

INDICATIONS
FDA
- Bone and joint infections
- Pneumonia
- Septicemia
- Endocarditis treatment and prophylaxis (in PCN allergic pts)
- Oral vancomycin: antibiotic-associated pseudomembranous colitis caused by *C. difficile* and enterocolitis caused by *S. aureus* (including MRSA)

Non-FDA Approved Uses
- Hardware-associated infections

FORMS

Brand name (mfr)	Forms	Cost*
Vancocin, Lyphocin (Generic manufacturers, Eli Lilly, Fujisawa, Schein, and others)	IV vial 500 mg; 1000 mg	$4.70; $9.65
Vancocin Pulvule (Viropharma)	Oral pulvule 125 mg; 250 mg	$17.70; $35.66

*Prices represents Average Wholesale Price (AWP).

USUAL ADULT DOSING
- **Systemic infections** caused by MRSA and other resistant Gram-positive organisms: MIC ≤ 1: 15 mg/kg IV q12h (up to 20 mg/kg q8h dose based on actual body weight). Loading dose of 25–30 mg/kg × 1 can be considered in critically ill pts. Consider 22.5 mg/kg IV q12h for CNS infections.
- Consider an alternative agent in the treatment of MRSA with an MIC ≥ 2 (especially when treating pneumonia and meningitis).
- Target trough concentrations: 15–20 mcg/mL (endocarditis, osteomyelitis, pneumonia, and CNS); 20 mcg/mL recommended by some for CNS infections. Trough 10–15 mcg/mL likely to be adequate in pts with mild infections due to MRSA w/ low MIC.
- *C. difficile* colitis: 125 mg PO q6h × 7–10 days. Higher doses 250–500 mg PO q6h (+/– IV metronidazole) may be given in the setting of ileus or severe disease.
- Oral preparation is not systemically absorbed and is ineffective for any infections other than *C. difficile* colitis and *S. aureus* enterocolitis. The parenteral formulation is not effective for treatment of staphylococcal enterocolitis and pseudomembranous colitis caused by *C. difficile*.
- **Staphylococcal enterocolitis:** 500–2000 mg PO per day in 3–4 divided doses × 7–10 days.
- IV vancomycin can be given orally for *C. difficile* colitis to decrease cost ($5 vs. $80 per day).
- Intraventricular or intrathecal dose: vancomycin 20 mg q24h (up to 30 mg). Use preservative-free vancomycin 1 g vial for reconstitution.

RENAL DOSING

Dosing for GFR 50–80: GFR >60 ml/min: 15 mg/kg IV q12 (monitor serum concentrations, target Cmin: 10–20 mcg/ml).

Dosing for GFR 10–50: GFR 30–59 ml/min: 15 mg/kg q24h. GFR 15–29 ml/min: 15 mg/kg IV q48h (monitor serum concentrations, target Cmin:10–20 mcg/ml).

Dosing for GFR <10: 15 mg/kg IV, then redose based on serum concentrations, redose with Cmin <10–20 mcg/ml

Dosing in hemodialysis: 15 mg/kg, then redose based on on serum concentrations, redose with Cmin <10–20 mcg/ml) IV. Generally twice a week administration required, but more frequent dosing with residual renal function.

Dosing in peritoneal dialysis: 0.5–1.0 g IV/wk (monitor serum concentrations, redose when Cmin <10–20 mcg/ml). More frequent dosing with residual renal function.

Dosing in hemofiltration: CVVH 15 mg/kg q48h. CVVHD: 15 mg/kg IV q24h (monitor serum concentrations, redose when Cmin <10–20 mcg/ml).

ADVERSE DRUG REACTIONS

General

• Generally well tolerated.

Occasional

• Red man syndrome: flushing over chest/face +/– hypotension & pruritis (infusion over >60 min may reverse or prevent; pretreatment w/ antihistamine may alleviate symptoms). Red man syndrome should not be construed as a true allergy.

• Phlebitis

• Renal function impairment (most often in combination with aminoglycosides). Uncommon with modern formulations of drug, but rates up to 1.4%–5% have been reported.

Rare

• Neutropenia

• Eosinophilia

• Drug fever

• Allergic reactions w/ rash

• Tissue irritation

• Ototoxicity

• Thrombocytopenia

DRUG INTERACTIONS

• Non-depolarizing muscle relaxants (succinylcholine, atracurium, vecuronium, pancuronium, tubocurarine): case reports of enhanced neuromuscular blockade. Monitor closely with co-administration.

• Cholestyramine: binds to oral vancomycin. **Do not co-administer**; consider oral metronidazole with cholestyramine co-administration.

• Aminoglycoside: Higher incidence of nephrotoxicity associated with vancomycin and aminoglycoside co-administration.

SPECTRUM—See Appendix II, p. 804

RESISTANCE

• Vancomycin resistant *S. aureus* (VRSA): MIC = 16 mcg/mL (7 isolates reported to date).

• Vancomycin intermediate resistant *S. aureus* (VISA): MIC range 4–8 mcg/mL.

• Heteroresistant *S. aureus* (hetero VISA): MIC = 4 mcg/mL (but contain subpopulation of organisms that have MICs of 4–8 mcg/mL).

• Vancomycin sensitive *S. aureus*: MIC = 2 mcg/mL or lower (former breakpoint was 4 mcg/mL).

• *Enterococci* MIC breakpoint: 4 mcg/mL.

PHARMACOLOGY

Mechanism

Inhibits bacterial cell wall biosynthesis by binding to D-alanyl-D-alanine precursor thereby blocking peptidoglycan polymerization.

Pharmacokinetic Parameters

• **Absorption** Oral vancomycin is not absorbed in the GI tract (therefore should not be given for systemic infections).

• **Cmax** 20–50 mcg/ml and Cmin 10 mcg/ml after 1 g IV dose administration.

ANTIBACTERIAL DRUGS

- **Distribution** Following parenteral administration, widely distributed in body tissue and fluids. Good level attained in pericardial, pleural, ascitic, and synovial fluid. Low concentration attained in CSF with inflamed meninges (1–53% of serum concentration attained with high dose with inflamed meninges).
- **Protein binding** 50–60%.
- **Metabolism/Excretion** Excreted unchanged in the urine by primarily by glomerular filtration.
- **T1/2** 4–6 hrs.

Dosing for Decreased Hepatic Function
Usual dose.

Pregnancy Risk
C: The manufacturer has received reports on the use of vancomycin in pregnancy without adverse fetal effects.

Breast Feeding Compatibility
Excreted in breast milk.

COMMENTS
Vancomycin is appropriate in the following conditions: 1) For treatment of serious infections caused by beta-lactam resistant Gram-positive microorganisms, 2) Treatment of infections caused by Gram-positive microorganisms in pts who have serious allergies to beta-lactam antimicrobials, 3) When antibiotic-associated colitis fails to respond to metronidazole therapy or is moderate to severe and potentially life-threatening, 4) Prophylaxis, as recommended by the American Heart Association, for endocarditis following certain procedures in pts at high risk for endocarditis, 5) Prophylaxis for major surgical procedures involving implantation of prosthetic materials or devices (e.g., cardiac and vascular procedures and total hip replacement) at institutions that have a high rate of infections caused by MRSA or methicillin-resistant *S. epidermidis*. A single dose of vancomycin administered immediately before surgery is sufficient unless the procedure lasts greater than 6 hrs, in which case the dose should be repeated. Prophylaxis should be discontinued after a maximum of 2 doses.

SELECTED REFERENCES
Hidayat LK, Hsu DI, Quist R, et al. High-dose vancomycin therapy for methicillin-resistant Staphylococcus aureus infections: efficacy and toxicity. *Arch Intern Med*, 2006; Vol. 166; pp. 2138–44.

Zar FA, Bakkanagari SR, Moorthi KM, et al. A comparison of vancomycin and metronidazole for the treatment of Clostridium difficile-associated diarrhea, stratified by disease severity. *Clin Infect Dis*, 2007; Vol. 45; p. 302.

Antifungal

AMPHOTERICIN B

Paul A. Pham, PharmD and John G. Bartlett, MD

INDICATIONS

FDA

- Aspergillosis
- Blastomycosis
- Disseminated candidiasis
- Leishmaniasis
- Cryptococcosis
- Histoplasmosis
- Cryptococcal meningitis (treatment and suppression)
- Meningitis caused by organisms such as *Coccidioides immitis*, *Candida* spp, *Sporothrix schenckii*, and *aspergillus* spp
- Coccidioidomycosis
- Disseminated sporotrichosis

FORMS

Brand name (mfr)	Forms	Cost*
Fungizone (Sandoz and generic manufacturers)	IV vial 50 mg	$24.50/50 mg vial
*Prices represents Average Wholesale Price (AWP).		

USUAL ADULT DOSING

Dosing range: 0.3–1.5 mg/kg/day IV (infuse over 2–4 hrs). Oral form no longer commercially available.

- Aspergillosis, invasive pulmonary or extrapulmonary: 1.0–1.5 mg/kg once daily (voriconazole preferred; if unable to tolerate voriconazole, lipid amphotericin preferred over ampho B).
- Blastomycosis, severe pulmonary or disseminated: 0.7–1.0 mg/kg once daily (total amphotericin B dose of 2.0–2.5 g).
- Candida esophagitis: 0.3–0.7 mg/kg IV q24h (in azole-resistant esophagitis).
- Candidemia or disseminated deep organ infection: 0.7–1.0 mg/kg. Add flucytosine 100 mg/kg/day in 4 divided doses in endocarditis. Consider adding flucytosine in meningitis and endophthalmitis.
- Coccidioidomycosis, severe pulmonary or progressive: 0.5–0.7 mg/kg/day (total amphotericin B dose of 7–20 mg/kg). With meningitis, fluconazole preferred, but intrathecal amphotericin can be used for fluconazole failures.
- Cryptococcal meningitis: 0.7 mg/kg IV q24h + flucytosine 25 mg/kg PO q6h × 2 wks, then fluconazole 400 mg PO q24h × 8 wks. Maintenance therapy with fluconazole 200 mg PO q24h.
- Histoplasmosis, disseminated: 0.7–1.0 mg/kg/day until stable, then switch to itraconazole. With meningitis, a total dose of 35 mg/kg is recommended. Consider intrathecal amphotericin for failure or relapse.
- Zygomycosis (*Rhizopus* spp., *Mucor* spp., *Absidia* spp.): 1.0–1.5 mg/kg/day (total dose of 30–40 mg/kg). Posaconazole and lipid amphotericin formulations are preferred.
- Obese pts: use actual body weight.

RENAL DOSING

Dosing for GFR 50–80: Usual dose.
Dosing for GFR 10–50: Usual dose.
Dosing for GFR <10: Consider alternative lipid formulation.
Dosing in hemodialysis: Usual dose, no supplement needed post HD.
Dosing in peritoneal dialysis: Usual dose.
Dosing in hemofiltration: No data. Usual dose likely.

ANTIFUNGAL DRUGS

ADVERSE DRUG REACTIONS
Common

- Nephrotoxicity: can occur with or without nephrocalcinosis. Reduced with adequate hydration, salt loading (500 cc NS pre and post amphotericin B infusion), and avoidance of concurrent nephrotoxic agents.
- Renal tubular acidosis.
- Electrolyte abnormalities: hypokalemia, hypomagnesemia, and hypocalcemia.
- Fever and chills: can be managed with meperidine or hydrocortisone 10–50 mg added to infusion. Alternatively, could premedicate with meperidine or ibuprofen.
- Anemia (normocytic normochromic).
- Phlebitis (improved with the addition of 1000 U heparin to infusion).

Occasional

- Hypotension
- Nausea and vomiting
- Metallic taste
- Headache

DRUG INTERACTIONS

- Digoxin: may increase digitalis toxicity secondary to hypokalemia (consider potassium supplementation).
- Diuretics and corticosteroids: may result in additive hypokalemia.
- Nephrotoxic agents (e.g., foscarnet, cidofovir, aminoglycosides, and cyclosporine): may result in additive nephrotoxicity.

RESISTANCE

- Some species of *Fusarium oxysporum* and *F. solani* and most species of *Pseudallescheria boydii* are resistant.
- *Candida lusitaniae.*

PHARMACOLOGY
Mechanism

Binds to ergosterol and disrupts fungal cell membrane resulting in leakage of intracellular contents.

Pharmacokinetic Parameters

- **Absorption** Not absorbed from the GI tract.
- **Cmax** 0.5–3.5 mcg/mL after 0.4–0.7 mg/kg IV dose administration.
- **Distribution** Vd = 4 L/Kg. Widely distributed in body tissue and fluids such as inflamed pleura, peritoneum, synovium, aqueous humor, vitreous humor, and pericardial fluid. Poor CNS penetration (only 3% of serum concentration is attained in the CSF) but effective in the treatment of cryptococcal meningitis.
- **Protein binding** 90%.
- **Metabolism/Excretion** Metabolism not fully understood. Undergoes slow renal excretion.
- **T1/2** 24 hrs (up to 15 days).

Dosing for Decreased Hepatic Function

No data.

Pregnancy Risk

B-A: Collaborative Perinatal Project identified 9 1st trimester exposure to amphotericin, found no adverse fetal effect. Animal studies demonstrated amphotericin to be harmless in pregnancy.

Breast Feeding Compatibility

No data available.

COMMENTS

Use is complicated by high rate of infusion and dose dependent related reactions such as anemia, electrolyte imbalance and renal failure. A switch to the lipid formulation (liposomal amphotericin) is generally recommended in pts at risk for renal failure or when serum creatinine is elevated to an arbitrary threshold (>2.5 used at Hopkins). Infusion-related side effects is higher than *Ambisome* and *Abelcet* but lower than *Amphotec*. When indicated, agents such as caspofungin or lipid amphotericin may also be considered for candidemia.

SELECTED REFERENCES

Pappas PG, Rex JH, Sobel JD, et al. Guidelines for treatment of candidiasis. *Clinical Infectious Diseases*, 2004; Vol. 38; pp. 161–189.

Walsh TJ, Anaissie EJ, Denning DW, et al. Treatment of aspergillosis: clinical practice guidelines of the Infectious Diseases Society of America. *Clinical Infectious Diseases*, 2008; Vol. 46; pp. 327–60.

AMPHOTERICIN B CHOLESTERYL SULFATE COMPLEX (ABCD)

Paul A. Pham, PharmD and John G. Bartlett, MD

INDICATIONS

FDA

- Invasive aspergillosis in pts who are refractory to or intolerant of amphotericin B deoxycholate therapy

FORMS

Brand name (mfr)	Forms	Cost*
Amphotec (Three River Pharmaceutical)	IV vial 50 mg	$93.00
*Prices represents Average Wholesale Price (AWP).		

USUAL ADULT DOSING

- 3–4 mg/kg/day (may be increased up to 7.5 mg/kg).
- Invasive aspergillosis: 6 mg/kg/day (voriconazole usual first-line therapy; if unable to tolerate voriconazole, Ambisome or Abelcet is preferred).
- For obese pts: use ideal body weight (limited data).

RENAL DOSING

Dosing for GFR 50–80: Usual dose.
Dosing for GFR 10–50: Usual dose. Monitor closely for worsening renal function.
Dosing for GFR <10: Usual dose.
Dosing in hemodialysis: Not removed in dialysis, no supplement needed post HD. Usual dose.
Dosing in peritoneal dialysis: Usual dose.
Dosing in hemofiltration: Standard dose.

ADVERSE DRUG REACTIONS

Common

- Infusion reactions: fever (27%), chills (53%), phlebitis, pain at infusion site.
- Infusion related reactions were the highest in amphotec treated pts compared to all amphotericin products, including regular amphotericin.
- Infusion reactions lower with premedication (hydrocortisone, NSAID, ASA, APAP, meperidine).

Occasional

- Creatinine elevation (>2 × baseline) observed in up to 25% on ABCD
- Anemia
- Electrolyte wasting: hypokalemia, hypomagnesemia, and hypocalcemia
- Nausea, vomiting, diarrhea, abdominal pain
- Metallic taste
- Headache and insomnia
- Hypotension
- Transaminase elevations
- Increased in bilirubin (>1.5 × baseline)

Rare

- Rash and pruritis

DRUG INTERACTIONS

- Digoxin: potential increase in digitalis toxicity secondary to amphotericin-induced potassium depletion. Monitor potassium closely with co-administration.
- Diuretics: may result in additive hypokalemia. Monitor potassium closely with co-administration.
- Nephrotoxic agents (aminoglycosides, cidofovir, foscarnet, pentamidine): may result in additive nephrotoxicity. Avoid co-administration or use with close monitoring.

ANTIFUNGAL DRUGS

- Pentamidine: potential for additive hypocalcemia and/or nephrotoxicity. Avoid co-administration or use with close monitoring.
- Skeletal muscle relaxants: may enhance curariform effect of skeletal muscle relaxants (e.g., tubocurarine) due to hypokalemia. Monitor potassium closely with co-administration.

PHARMACOLOGY

Mechanism

Amphotericin binds to ergosterol in fungal cell membrane, resulting in the disruption of the cell membrane. As a result, the cell membrane is no longer able to function as a selective barrier and leakage of intracellular contents occurs. The lipid formulations are designed to reduce binding of amphotericin to mammalian cell membranes, therefore reducing toxicities.

Pharmacokinetic Parameters

- **Absorption** Not absorbed from the GI tract.
- **Cmax** 2–9 mcg/mL after 4 mg/kg IV dose administration.
- **Distribution** Attains lower serum concentration but has greater volume of distribution (vd = 4L/kg) compared to conventional amphotericin. Increased uptake by the liver and spleen and decreased kidney concentration. Poor fat distribution (animal data).
- **Protein binding** No data.
- **Metabolism/Excretion** No data.
- **T1/2** 25 hrs.

Dosing for Decreased Hepatic Function

No data. Usual dose likely in mild and moderate hepatic insufficiency.

Pregnancy Risk

B: There is limited data on the use of Amphotericin B cholesteryl sulfate complex in pregnancy therefore the use should be limited to pts where the benefit outweighs the risk.

Breast Feeding Compatibility

No data available.

COMMENTS

Parenteral lipid amphotericin that is the least expensive of all lipid formulations but also associated with the highest infusion-related side effects compared to standard amphotericin B and other lipid amphotericin formulations. Ambisome and Abelcet are generally preferred over Amphotec for most indications.

SELECTED REFERENCES

Bowden R, Chandrasekar P, White MH, et al. A double-blind, randomized, controlled trial of amphotericin B colloidal dispersion versus amphotericin B for treatment of invasive aspergillosis in immunocompromised pts. *Clin Infect Dis*, 2002; Vol. 35; pp. 359–66.

Walsh TJ, Anaissie EJ, Denning DW, et al. Treatment of aspergillosis: clinical practice guidelines of the Infectious Diseases Society of America. *Clin Infect Dis*, 2008; Vol. 46; pp. 327–60.

AMPHOTERICIN B LIPID COMPLEX (ABLC)

Paul A. Pham, PharmD and John G. Bartlett, MD

INDICATIONS

FDA

- Aspergillosis infections in pts who are refractory to or intolerant of conventional amphotericin B therapy.

Non-FDA Approved Uses

- Studied in pts with aspergillosis, candidiasis, zygomycosis, cryptococcosis, and fusariosis.

FORMS

Brand name (mfr)	Forms	Cost*
Abelcet (Enzon)	IV vial 100 mg (5 mg/mL 20 mL)	$240 per vial
*Prices represents Average Wholesale Price (AWP).		

USUAL ADULT DOSING

- 5 mg/kg/day IV
- For obese pts: consider ideal body weight (limited data)

RENAL DOSING

Dosing for GFR 50–80: Usual dose.
Dosing for GFR 10–50: Usual dose.
Dosing for GFR <10: Usual dose.
Dosing in hemodialysis: Not removed in dialysis, no supplement needed post HD. Usual dose.
Dosing in peritoneal dialysis: Usual dose.
Dosing in hemodialysis: No data.

ADVERSE DRUG REACTIONS

Common

- Infusion reactions: fever, chills, phlebitis, pain at infusion site.
- Infusion related reactions were higher compared to ambisome but lower compared to amphotericin B.
- Infusion reactions lower with premedication (hydrocortisone, NSAID, ASA, APAP, meperidine).

Occasional

- Creatinine elevation (>2 × baseline) observed in up to 8% (with low dose Abelcet)
- Anemia
- Electrolyte wasting: hypokalemia, hypomagnesemia, and hypocalcemia
- Nausea, vomiting, diarrhea, abdominal pain
- Metallic taste
- Headache and insomnia
- Hypotension
- Transaminases elevation
- Increased in bilirubin (>1.5 × baseline)

Rare

- Rash and pruritis

DRUG INTERACTIONS

- Digoxin: potential increase in digitalis toxicity secondary to amphotericin-induced potassium depletion. Monitor potassium closely with co-administration.
- Diuretics: may result in additive hypokalemia. Monitor potassium closely with co-administration.
- Nephrotoxic agents (aminoglycosides, cidofovir, foscarnet, pentamidine): may result in additive nephrotoxicity. Avoid co-administration or use with close monitoring.
- Pentamidine: potential for additive hypocalcemia and/or nephrotoxicity. Avoid co-administration or use with close monitoring.
- Skeletal muscle relaxants: may enhance curariform effect of skeletal muscle relaxants (e.g., tubocurarine) due to hypokalemia. Monitor potassium closely with co-administration.

PHARMACOLOGY

Mechanism

Amphotericin binds to ergosterol in fungal cell membrane, resulting in the disruption of the cell membrane. As a result the cell membrane is no longer able to function as a selective barrier and leakage of intracellular contents occurs. The lipid formulations are designed to reduce binding of amphotericin to mammalian cell membranes, therefore reducing toxicities.

Pharmacokinetic Parameters

- **Absorption** Not absorbed from the GI tract.
- **Cmax** 0.9–2.5 mcg/mL after 5 mg/kg IV dose administration.
- **Distribution** Attains lower serum concentration but has greater volume of distribution compared to conventional amphotericin. Increased uptake by the liver and spleen and decreased kidney concentration. Poor fat distribution (animal data).
- **Protein binding** No data.
- **Metabolism/Excretion** Slow renal excretion. Approximately 0.9% of dose excreted in the first day.
- **T1/2** 7.2 days.

ANTIFUNGAL DRUGS

Dosing for Decreased Hepatic Function
No data.

Pregnancy Risk
B: There is limited data on the use of Amphotericin B lipid complex in pregnancy therefore the use should be limited to pts where the benefit outweighs the risk.

Breast Feeding Compatibility
No data available.

COMMENTS
Abelcet has comparable cost to Amphotec but generally better tolerated with less infusion related reactions. Compared to Ambisome, Abelcet has a lower cost, but resulted in a higher incidence of nephrotoxicity and infusion related side effects.

SELECTED REFERENCES
Fleming RV, Kantarjian HM, Husni R, et al. Comparison of amphotericin B lipid complex (ABLC) vs. ambisome in the treatment of suspected or documented fungal infections in pts with leukemia. *Leuk Lymphoma*, 2001; Vol. 40; pp. 511–20.

Walsh TJ, Anaissie EJ, Denning DW, et al. Treatment of aspergillosis: clinical practice guidelines of the Infectious Diseases Society of America. *Clin Infect Dis*, 2008; Vol. 46; pp. 327–60.

AMPHOTERICIN B LIPOSOMAL

Paul A. Pham, PharmD and John G. Bartlett, MD

INDICATIONS
FDA
- Aspergillosis (in pts refractory to or intolerant of amphotericin B deoxycholate)
- Candidiasis (in pts refractory to or intolerant of amphotericin B deoxycholate)
- Cryptococcosis (in pts refractory to or intolerant of amphotericin B deoxycholate)
- Empiric therapy for presumed fungal infection in pts with febrile neutropenia
- Visceral leishmaniasis (high relapse rate in immunocompromised pts with response rate of only 12%)

Non-FDA Approved Uses
- Zygomycetes and other invasive molds

FORMS

Brand name (mfr)	Forms	Cost*
AmBisome (Astellas)	IV vial 50 mg	$196 per vial
*Prices represents Average Wholesale Price (AWP).		

USUAL ADULT DOSING
- Empiric treatment of fever in neutropenic pts not responding to antibiotic: 3 mg/kg/day IV. Higher doses (5 mg/kg/day) may be considered in pts with neutropenia >10 days, evidence of fungal infection, and/or clinically unstable.
- Cryptococcal meningitis (alternative to amphotericin B deoxycholate): 4 mg/kg IV once daily.
- Candidemia: 5 mg/kg IV once daily. Lower dose (3 mg/kg/day) may be considered in clinically stable pts.
- Invasive aspergillosis: 5 mg/kg IV once daily.
- Zygomycoses: higher doses (up to 10–15 mg/kg IV q24h) have been employed in refractory zygomycosis infections though little data supports this dosing. Posaconazole may be considered in refractory cases.
- For obese pts: consider ideal body weight (limited data)

RENAL DOSING
Dosing for GFR 50–80: Usual dose.
Dosing for GFR 10–50: Usual dose.
Dosing for GFR <10: Usual dose.
Dosing in hemodialysis: Limited data. No change in PK parameters. Usual dose likely.
Dosing in peritoneal dialysis: No data.
Dosing in hemofiltration: Limited data. No change in PK parameters. Usual dose likely.

ADVERSE DRUG REACTIONS
Common
- Infusion reactions: fever (8%), chills (18%), phlebitis, pain at infusion site
- Infusion related reactions were lower compared to other amphotericin products
- Infusion reactions lower with premedication (hydrocortisone, NSAID, ASA, APAP, meperidine)

Occasional
- Creatinine elevation (>2 × baseline) observed in up to 19% on Ambisome
- Anemia
- Electrolyte wasting: hypokalemia, hypomagnesemia, and hypocalcemia
- Nausea, vomiting, diarrhea, abdominal pain
- Metallic taste
- Headache and insomnia
- Hypotension
- Transaminases elevation (>2 × ULN with cumulative dose of >2000 mg)
- Increased in bilirubin (>1.5 × baseline)

Rare
- Rash and pruritis

DRUG INTERACTIONS
- Digoxin: potential increase in digitalis toxicity secondary to amphotericin-induced potassium depletion. Monitor potassium closely with co-administration.
- Diuretics: may result in additive hypokalemia. Monitor potassium closely with co-administration.
- Nephrotoxic agents (aminoglycosides, cidofovir, foscarnet, pentamidine): may result in additive nephrotoxicity. Avoid co-administration or use with close monitoring.
- Pentamidine: potential for additive hypocalcemia and/or nephrotoxicity. Avoid co-administration or use with close monitoring.
- Skeletal muscle relaxants: may enhance curariform effect of skeletal muscle relaxants (e.g., tubocurarine) due to hypokalemia. Monitor potassium closely with co-administration.

PHARMACOLOGY
Mechanism
Amphotericin binds to ergosterol in fungal cell membrane, resulting in the disruption of the cell membrane. As a result the cell membrane is no longer able to function as a selective barrier and leakage of intracellular contents occurs. The lipid formulations are designed to reduce binding of amphotericin to mammalian cell membranes, therefore reducing toxicities.

Pharmacokinetic Parameters
- **Absorption** Not absorbed from the GI tract.
- **Cmax** 13–49 mcg/mL after 2.5 mg/kg IV dose administration.
- **Distribution** Attains lower serum concentration but has greater volume of distribution compared to conventional amphotericin. Increased uptake by the liver and spleen and decreased kidney concentration. Poor fat distribution (animal data).
- **Protein binding** No data.
- **Metabolism/Excretion** No data.
- **T1/2** 100–153 hrs.

Dosing for Decreased Hepatic Function
No data. Usual dose likely.

Pregnancy Risk
B: There is limited data on the use of Amphotericin B liposomal complex in pregnancy therefore the use should be limited to pts where the benefit outweighs the risk.

Breast Feeding Compatibility
No data available.

COMMENTS
The only truly liposomal amphotericin that is also the most expensive of the lipid formulations (but cost will vary between institutions). Compared to Abelcet, Ambisome resulted in less nephrotoxicity and fewer infusion related side effects. No difference in efficacy compared to conventional amphoB, w/ the possible exception of disseminated histoplasmosis in AIDS pts, but generally preferred due to reduced toxicity (main concern is cost).

ANTIFUNGAL DRUGS

SELECTED REFERENCES

Cornely OA, Maertens J, Bresnik M, et al. Liposomal amphotericin B as initial therapy for invasive mold infection: a randomized trial comparing a high-loading dose regimen with standard dosing (AmBiLoad trial). *Clin Infect Dis*, 2007; Vol. 44(10); pp. 1289–97.

Walsh TJ, Anaissie EJ, Denning DW, et al. Treatment of Aspergillosis: Clinical Practice Guidelines of the Infectious Diseases Society of America. *Clin Infect Dis*, 2008; Vol. 46; p. 327.

ANIDULAFUNGIN

Paul A. Pham, PharmD and John G. Bartlett, MD

INDICATIONS

FDA

- Candidemia and other candida infections (intra-abdominal abscess, peritonitis). Not studied in endocarditis, osteomyelitis, and meningitis (poor CNS penetration).
- Esophageal candidiasis.

Non-FDA Approved Uses

- Aspergillosis (with or without voriconazole), no data.

FORMS

Brand name (mfr)	Forms	Cost*
Eraxis (Pfizer)	IV Vial 50 mg; IV Vial 100 mg	$112.50; $225.00
*Prices represents Average Wholesale Price (AWP).		

USUAL ADULT DOSING

- Candidemia: 200 mg IV × 1 (dL), then 100 mg IV q24h × 14 days from last positive culture.
- Esophageal candidiasis: 100 mg IV × 1 (dL), then 50 mg IV q24h × 7–14 days following resolution of symptoms.
- Infusion rate should not exceed 1.1 mg/min.

RENAL DOSING

Dosing for GFR 50–80: Usual dose.

Dosing for GFR 10–50: Usual dose.

Dosing for GFR <10: Usual dose.

Dosing in hemodialysis: Usual dose. Not dialyzable, thus no supplemental doses needed post dialysis.

Dosing in peritoneal dialysis: No data, usual dose likely.

Dosing in hemofiltration: No data, usual dose likely.

ADVERSE DRUG REACTIONS

General

- Well tolerated with ADRs comparable to fluconazole.

Occasional

- Histamine-mediated symptoms may including rash, urticaria, flushing, pruritus, dyspnea, and hypotension. This is infrequent if IV rate <1.1 mg/min.
- Phlebitis
- Fever
- Diarrhea
- Hypokalemia
- LFT elevation

DRUG INTERACTIONS

Not a substrate, inducer, or inhibitor of CYP450 isoenzymes.

- No significant drug-drug interactions with voriconazole, tacrolimus, ambisome, and rifampin.
- Cyclosporin: anidulafungin AUC increased by 22% with cyclosporine co-administration (use standard dose). Unlike caspofungin, no significant increase in LFTs observed.

RESISTANCE

- *In vitro* development of resistance appears difficult to produce.
- *C. neoformans* has intrinsic resistance to echinocandins such as anidulafungin.

PHARMACOLOGY
Mechanism
Anidulafungin is a non-competitive inhibitor of Beta (1,3) beta-D-glucan synthase, a critical enzyme responsible for polysaccharide formation in the fungal cell wall.

Pharmacokinetic Parameters
- **Cmax** 8.6 mcg/mL; AUC: 111.8 mcg/mL hr (200 mg load, then 100 mg every day at steady state).
- **Distribution** Vd = 30–50 L. Poor CNS penetration.
- **Protein binding** 84%.
- **Metabolism/Excretion** No hepatic metabolism observed. Undergoes slow chemical degradation that is eliminated in the feces (30% over 9 days).
- **T1/2** 52 hrs.

Dosing for Decreased Hepatic Function
For Child-Pugh class A, B, or C: usual dose.

Pregnancy Risk
C: No human data. Animal studies: skeletal changes in rat fetuses and reduced fetal weight in rabbit fetuses.

Breast Feeding Compatibility
Excreted in breast milk. Use with caution.

COMMENTS
Anidulafungin is an echinocandin antifungal with a similar spectrum to caspofungin and micafungin that includes all Candida species and Aspergillus spp. Randomized clinical trials are limited to esophageal candidiasis (would reserve for azole-refractory cases) and candidemia (non-neutropenic w/ APACHE II score <20). Prospective comparison to other echinocandin or amphotericin products has not been performed, but it is recommended by the IDSA for the treatment of candidemia in non-neutropenic and neutropenic pts (AIII recommendation). Anidulafungin has not been evaluated in invasive aspergillosis. Cost (AWP) is lower than caspofungin, but purchased price is often comparable.

SELECTED REFERENCES
Pappas PG, Kauffman CA, Andes D, et al. Clinical practice guidelines for the management of candidiasis: 2009 update by the Infectious Diseases Society of America. *Clin Infect Dis*, 2009; Vol. 48(5); pp. 503–35.

Reboli AC, Rotstein C, Pappas PG, et al. Anidulafungin versus fluconazole for invasive candidiasis. *N Engl J Med*, 2007; Vol. 356(24); pp. 2472–82.

CASPOFUNGIN ACETATE

Paul A. Pham, PharmD and John G. Bartlett, MD

INDICATIONS
FDA
- Treatment of invasive aspergillosis in pts who are refractory or intolerant to other anti-fungal therapy.
- Candidemia and the following candida infections: intra-abdominal abscesses, peritonitis and pleural space infections. Not well studied in endocarditis, osteomyelitis, and meningitis (low CNS penetration) due to Candida.
- Esophageal candidiasis (authors' opinion: would reserve caspofungin for azole-resistant cases).
- Empiric treatment of presumed fungal infections in febrile neutropenic pts.

FORMS

Brand name (mfr)	Forms	Cost*
Cancidas (Merck)	IV vial 50 mg; IV vial 70 mg	$422.14; $438.60
*Prices represents Average Wholesale Price (AWP).		

ANTIFUNGAL DRUGS

USUAL ADULT DOSING

- 70 mg IV load on day 1, then 50 mg IV q24h (infuse over 1 hr).
- Dosing for Child-Pugh score of 7–9: after initial 70 mg load on day 1, decrease daily dose to 35 mg q24h. Use with caution with Child-Pugh score >9.
- Obese pts: 70 mg IV q24h.
- Co-administration of caspofungin and CYP enzyme inducer: 70 mg IV q24h (see drug-drug interaction section below).

RENAL DOSING

Dosing for GFR 50–80: Usual dose.

Dosing for GFR 10–50: Usual dose.

Dosing for GFR <10: Usual dose.

Dosing in hemodialysis: Not dialyzable, thus no supplemental doses needed post dialysis. Usual dose.

Dosing in peritoneal dialysis: No data, usual dose likely.

Dosing in hemofiltration: No data, usual dose likely.

ADVERSE DRUG REACTIONS

General

- Generally well tolerated

Occasional

- Histamine-mediated symptoms including rash, facial swelling, pruritus and sensation of warmth (infusion rate related, consider antihistamine)
- LFT/bilirubin elevation (monitor at baseline and every 1–2 wks thereafter)
- Elevated alkaline phosphatase

Rare

- Fever
- Phlebitis
- Nausea/vomiting
- Headache
- Eosinophilia
- Proteinuria
- Hypokalemia

DRUG INTERACTIONS

Caspofungin did not induce or inhibited the cytochrome P450 system, but a poor substrate of CYP450 enzymes. Caspofungin PK parameters are not altered by itraconazole, amphotericin B, mycophenolate, nelfinavir, or tacrolimus. Itraconazole, amphotericin B, and the active metabolite of mycophenolate are not affected by caspofungin co-administration.

- Carbamezapine: may decrease caspofungin concentrations, monitor for clinical response. Increase caspofungin dose to 70 mg once-daily **or** consider anidulafungin or micafungin.
- Cyclosporin: increased caspofungin AUC by 35%. Co-administration not recommended, close monitoring of liver enzyme recommended with co-administration.
- Dexamethasone: may decrease caspofungin concentrations, monitor for clinical response. Increase caspofungin dose to 70 mg once-daily **or** consider anidulafungin or micafungin.
- Efavirenz: may decrease caspofungin concentrations, monitor for clinical response. Increase caspofungin dose to 70 mg once-daily **or** consider anidulafungin or micafungin.
- Etravirine: may decrease caspofungin concentrations, monitor for clinical response. Increase caspofungin dose to 70 mg once-daily **or** consider anidulafungin or micafungin.
- Nevirapine: may decrease caspofungin concentrations, monitor for clinical response. Increase caspofungin dose to 70 mg once-daily **or** consider anidulafungin or micafungin.
- Phenobarbital: may decrease caspofungin concentrations, monitor for clinical response. Increase caspofungin dose to 70 mg once-daily **or** consider anidulafungin or micafungin.
- Phenytoin: may decrease caspofungin concentrations, monitor for clinical response. Increase caspofungin dose to 70 mg once-daily.
- Rifabutin: may decrease caspofungin concentrations, monitor for clinical response. Increase caspofungin dose to 70 mg once-daily **or** consider anidulafungin or micafungin.
- Rifampin: decreased caspofungin AUC by 30%. Increase dose to 70 mg q24h with co-administration **or** consider anidulafungin or micafungin.

- Rifapentine: may decrease caspofungin concentrations, monitor for clinical response. Increase caspofungin dose to 70 mg once-daily **or** consider anidulafungin or micafungin.
- Tacrolimus: AUC decreased by 20% with caspofungin, monitor tacrolimus serum concentration closely with co-administration.

RESISTANCE
- *C. neoformans* has intrinsic resistance to caspofungin.
- Similar to other echinocandins, caspofungin is not active against *zygomycetes*, Trichosporon spp. and *Fusarium* spp.

PHARMACOLOGY
Mechanism
Beta (1,3)-D-glucan, an integral component of fungal cell wall, is inhibited by caspofungin.

Pharmacokinetic Parameters
- **Cmax** = 9.39 mcg/mL; Cmin = 2.01 mcg/mL.
- **Distribution** Well distributed into tissues by 36–48 hrs. Poor penetration into CNS and urinary tract.
- **Protein binding** 97%.
- **Metabolism/Excretion** Metabolized by N-acetylation and hydrolysis. Spontaneous chemical degradation. 35% and 41% of metabolites are excreted in the feces and urine respectively. Only 1.4% of unchanged drug is excreted in the urine.
- **T1/2** Half-life (beta-phase) of 9–11 hrs.

Dosing for Decreased Hepatic Function
For Child-Pugh score of 7–9, after initial 70 mg load on day 1, decrease daily dose to 35 mg q24h.

Pregnancy Risk
C: No human data. Animal data with exposure similar to a 70 mg-dose in human resulted in incomplete ossification of skull, torso, cervical ribs and talus/calcaneus. Amphotericin B is preferred.

Breast Feeding Compatibility
No data.

COMMENTS
Caspofungin offers clinicians an alternative to voriconazole and liposomal amphotericin for the treatment of invasive aspergillosis that is refractory or intolerant to first line therapy. It has established efficacy for the treatment of azole-resistant candidal esophagitis and invasive candidiasis. It is second line (oral) azoles for most candida infections, but has reliable activity against azole-resistant *C. albicans*, *C. glabrata*, *C. tropicalis*, and *C. krusei* which makes it the preferred agent for the empiric treatment of invasive candidiasis. Compared to micafungin and anidulafungin, caspofungin has the highest price (AWP), but the purchased prices are often comparable.

SELECTED REFERENCES
Caillot D, Thiébaut A, Herbrecht R, et al. Liposomal amphotericin B in combination with caspofungin for invasive aspergillosis in pts with hematologic malignancies: a randomized pilot study (Combistrat trial). *Cancer*, 2007; Vol. 110; pp. 2740–6.

Pappas PG, Kauffman CA, Andes D, et al. Clinical practice guidelines for the management of candidiasis: 2009 update by the Infectious Diseases Society of America. *Clin Infect Dis*, 2009; Vol. 48(5); pp. 503–35.

CLOTRIMAZOLE

Paul A. Pham, PharmD and John G. Bartlett, MD

INDICATIONS
FDA
- Oral candidiasis (thrush)
- Vaginal candidiasis
- Dermatomycoses

ANTIFUNGAL DRUGS

Brand name (mfr)	Forms	Cost*
Mycelex (Generic manufacturers)	Oral troche 10 mg	$1.60
Alpharma; Ivax (Generic manufacturers)	Vaginal cream 1% (45 g) Vaginal tablet 200 mg (3); Vaginal tablet 500 mg (1) Topical cream (1%) 15 g and 30 g tube Topical solution/lotion (1%) 10 mL and 30 mL	$12.00 $9.00; $13.88 $8.29/15 g $6.00/10 mL
*Prices represents Average Wholesale Price (AWP).		

USUAL ADULT DOSING
- Thrush: 10 mg troche 5 × /day (dissolve in mouth).
- Candida vaginitis: 100 mg intravaginal tab twice daily × 3 days (preferred) or 100 mg daily × 7 days or 500 mg × 1.
- Cutaneous candidiasis: apply cream, solution, or lotion to affected areas twice daily × 2–8 wks.

RENAL DOSING
Dosing for GFR 50–80: Usual dose.
Dosing for GFR 10–50: Usual dose.
Dosing for GFR <10: Usual dose.
Dosing in hemodialysis: Usual dose.
Dosing in peritoneal dialysis: Usual dose.
Dosing in hemofiltration: Usual dose.

ADVERSE DRUG REACTIONS
General
- Generally well tolerated.

Occasional
- Burning, itching, erythema (intravaginal and topical administration).
- Nausea and vomiting (lozenge).

Rare
- Elevated transaminases.

DRUG INTERACTIONS
No known drug interactions.

PHARMACOLOGY
Mechanism
Alteration of cell membrane permeability by binding with phospholipids resulting in cellular destruction.

Pharmacokinetic Parameters
- **Absorption** Very small amount absorbed systemically after intravaginal administration. Systemic absorption after lozenge administration has not been determined.
- **Distribution** Attains therapeutic concentration in saliva for up to 3 hrs after lozenge dissolution.

Dosing for Decreased Hepatic Function
Usual dose, monitor LFTs.

Pregnancy Risk
C: Teratogenic in animal studies at high doses. No human data available with lozenge. No adverse effect seen with intravaginal administration during the 2nd and 3rd trimester.

Breast Feeding Compatibility
No data.

COMMENTS
Slightly less effective (measured as disease free period post-therapy) than fluconazole for oropharyngeal candidiasis but preferred as 1st line due to the concern over azole-resistant candidiasis with long-term use of fluconazole.

SELECTED REFERENCES

Mikamo H, Kawazoe K, Sato Y, et al. Comparative study on the effectiveness of antifungal agents in different regimens against vaginal candidiasis. *Chemotherapy*, 1998; Vol. 44; pp. 364–8.

Pons V, Greenspan D, Debruin M. Therapy for oropharyngeal candidiasis in HIV-infected pts: a randomized, prospective multicenter study of oral fluconazole versus clotrimazole troches. The Multicenter Study Group. *J Acquir Immune Defic Syndr*, 1993; Vol. 6; pp. 1311–6.

FLUCONAZOLE

Paul A. Pham, PharmD and John G. Bartlett, MD

INDICATIONS

FDA

- Candidiasis prophylaxis (pts undergoing bone marrow transplant who receive cytotoxic chemotherapy and/or radiation therapy)
- Treatment of oropharyngeal and esophageal candidiasis
- Disseminated candidiasis (including peritonitis, pneumonia, and UTIs)
- Chronic mucocutaneous candidiasis
- Vulvovaginal candidiasis
- Disseminated cryptococcosis
- Treatment and suppression of cryptococcal meningitis

Non-FDA Approved Uses

- Coccidioidomycosis (itraconazole is alternative)
- Pityriasis versicolor
- Histoplasmosis (mild–moderate disease, itraconazole preferred)
- Candidal infections prophylaxis in critically ill surgical pts

FORMS

Brand name (mfr)	Forms	Cost*
Diflucan (Pfizer and generic manufacturers)	PO tablet 50 mg;	$5.77;
	PO tablet 100 mg;	$9.07;
	PO tablet 150 mg;	$14.42;
	PO tablet 200 mg	$14.80
	PO suspension 10 mg/mL;	$35–$44 per 35 mL bottle;
	PO suspension 40 mg/mL	$130–$160 per 35 mL bottle
	IV piggyback 200 mg;	$107.00;
	IV piggyback 400 mg	$186

*Prices represents Average Wholesale Price (AWP).

USUAL ADULT DOSING

- Non-meningeal cryptococcosis: 400 mg PO once daily.
- Cryptococcal meningitis, induction phase: 800–1200 mg PO/IV once daily × 10–12 wks + flucytosine 100 mg/kg/day × 6 wks (amphotericin B IV × 2 wks is preferred regimen).
- Cryptococcal meningitis, consolidation phase: 400 mg PO once daily × 8 wks.
- Cryptococcal meningitis, maintenance phase: 200 mg PO once daily (until CD4 >200 × >6 mos).
- Vaginal candidiasis: 150 mg PO × 1. Multiple recurrences: fluconazole 150 mg PO once per wk (topical azoles alternative).
- Esophageal candidiasis: 200 mg PO once daily × 14–21 days (or IV up to 800 mg/day). Use chronic maintenance therapy (same dose) for recurrent esophagitis.
- Oropharyngeal candidiasis (thrush): 100–200 mg PO once daily × 7–14 days (topical therapy with clotrimazole preferred to avoid azole resistance).

ANTIFUNGAL DRUGS

- Coccidioidomycosis, meningitis: 400–800 mg IV or PO. Non-meningeal (diffuse pulmonary or disseminated): fluconazole 400–800 mg PO once daily, (amB preferred) maintenance: 400 mg PO once daily.
- Candidal infections prophylaxis in critically ill surgical pts: 400 mg PO once daily.
- Candidemia: 800 mg × 1, the 400 mg once daily (must know sensitivity before use in severely ill). Empiric use of echinocandins or lipid amphotericin is preferred in severely ill pts.

RENAL DOSING

Dosing for GFR 50–80: Usual dose: 200–1200 mg once daily (see indication).

Dosing for GFR 10–50: 50% of dose.

Dosing for GFR <10: 25%–50% of dose.

Dosing in hemodialysis: 200–400 mg post-HD.

Dosing in peritoneal dialysis: 25–50% of dose once daily.

Dosing in hemofiltration: CVVH: 200–400 mg once daily. CVVHD: 400–800 mg once daily.

ADVERSE DRUG REACTIONS

General

- Generally well tolerated

Occasional

- GI intolerance w/ bloating, nausea, vomiting, pain, anorexia
- Reversible alopecia (with >400 mg/day)
- Transaminase elevations

Rare

- Hepatitis (fatal hepatotoxicity in pts with serious underlying medical conditions; monitor LFTs)
- Dizziness
- Headache
- Hypokalemia

DRUG INTERACTIONS—See Appendix III, p. 819, for table of drug-to-drug interactions.

RESISTANCE

- Up to 30–40% of *C. glabrata* are fluconazole-resistant. *C. albicans* resistance associated with long term exposure. *C. krusei* and *C. lusitaniae* are resistant.

PHARMACOLOGY

Mechanism

Triazoles alter fungal cell membrane function by inhibiting C-14 alpha anosterol demethylase, thereby interfering with ergosterol synthesis, which results in increased cell permeability and leakage of essential elements.

Pharmacokinetic Parameters

- **Absorption** >90% absorbed independent of gastric acidity.
- **Cmax** 6.72 mcg/mL after 400 mg PO dose administration. 3.9–5 mcg/mL after 6 days of 100 mg IV administration.
- **Distribution** Widely distributed throughout body tissues and fluids such as kidney, skin, saliva, sputum, nail, blister fluid, prostate. Good CSF penetration (50–94% of plasma serum concentration attained in the CSF).
- **Protein binding** 11–12%.
- **Metabolism/Excretion** Partial metabolism. Both metabolite (11%) and unchanged drug (60–80%) excreted in urine.
- **T1/2** 30 hrs.

Dosing for Decreased Hepatic Function

Use with caution.

Pregnancy Risk

C: Teratogenic in animal studies. Case reports of craniofacial, limb, and cardiac defects have been reported in 3 infants with 1st trimester exposure to high dose fluconazole. The risk of low dose intermittent use has not been fully evaluated but appears to be low.

Breast Feeding Compatibility

Fluconazole excreted into breast milk at high concentration (up to 83% of plasma concentration). Since no drug-induced toxicity encountered in infants during therapy with fluconazole, likelihood of toxicity during breast feeding is low.

COMMENTS

Oral and parenteral azole with best oral bioavailability in its class, independent of stomach pH. Use of fluconazole for treatment or suppression of thrush not recommended due to risk of azole-resistance; topical therapy (e.g., clotrimazole) preferred. Itraconazole has better *in vitro* activity against *C occidioides immitis*, however due to better CNS penetration, fluconazole is recommended for meningitis. Due to increasing rates of *C. glabrata* resistance, fluconazole should not be used to empirically treat candidemia in severely ill pts (echinocandins and lipid amphotericin are preferred).

BASIS FOR RECOMMENDATIONS

NIH, CDC, and HIVMA/IDSA. Guidelines for Prevention and Treatment of Opportunistic Infections in HIV-Infected Adults and Adolescents. *http://aidsinfo.nih.gov/*

Comments: Treatment guidelines recommend fluconazole for the treatment of initial episodes of oropharyngeal candidiasis Secondary prophylaxis for recurrent oropharyngeal or vulvovaginal candidiasis is generally not recommended because of the potential for resistant candidiasis. However, if recurrences are frequent or mucocutaneous candidiasis is severe, oral fluconazole can be used for either oropharyngeal or vulvovaginal. In addition, it is prudent to institute secondary prophylaxis in pts with fluconazole-refractory oropharyngeal or esophageal candidiasis who have responded to echinocandins, voriconazole, or posaconazole therapy because of high relapse rate until ART produces immune reconstitution.

SELECTED REFERENCES

Pappas PG, Rex JH, Sobel JD, et al. Guidelines for Treatment of Candidiasis. *Clinical Infectious Diseases*, 2004; Vol. 38; pp. 161–189.

Pelz RK, Hendrix CW, Swoboda SM, et al. Double-blind placebo-controlled trial of fluconazole to prevent candidal infections in critically ill surgical pts. *Ann Surg*, 2001; Vol. 233; pp. 542–548.

FLUCYTOSINE

Paul A. Pham, PharmD and John G. Bartlett, MD

INDICATIONS

FDA

- Cryptococcal and *Candida* endocarditis (in addition to amphotericin B).
- Cryptococcal meningitis (in addition to amphotericin B).
- Cryptococcal and *Candida* pneumonia (in addition to amphotericin B).
- Cryptococcal and *Candida* septicemia (in addition to amphotericin B).
- Cryptococcal and *Candida* urinary tract infections (in addition to amphotericin B).

FORMS

Brand name (mfr)	Forms	Cost*
Ancobon (ICN Pharmaceuticals)	Oral capsule 250 mg; Oral capsule 500 mg	$5.29; $10.52
*Prices represents Average Wholesale Price (AWP).		

USUAL ADULT DOSING

- 25 mg/kg PO q6h.
- Therapeutic drug monitoring recommended with renal insufficiency.
- Goal peak of 50–100 mcg/mL 2 hrs post-dose at steady-state.
- Obese pts: use IBW (follow serum concentrations to guide dose adjustment).

RENAL DOSING

Dosing for GFR 50–80: 25 mg/kg q6h.

Dosing for GFR 10–50: 25 mg/kg q12–24h (monitor CBC and serum levels with appropriate dose adjustments).

Dosing for GFR <10: 25 mg/kg q24–48h (monitor CBC serum levels closely with appropriate dose adjustments).

Dosing in hemodialysis: 25 mg/kg q24–48h. Dose post-dialysis on days of dialysis (monitor CBC and serum levels w/ appropriate dose adjustment).

Dosing in peritoneal dialysis: 0.5–1.0 g q24h (monitor CBC and serum levels w/ appropriate dose adjustments).

ANTIFUNGAL DRUGS

Dosing in hemofiltration: CVVH and CVVHD: no data. Consider 25 mg/kg q24 for dialysis rate of 1 L/hr and 25 mg/kg q12h for dialysis rate > or = 1.5 L/hr (monitor CBC and serum levels with appropriate dose adjustments).

ADVERSE DRUG REACTIONS

Occasional

- GI intolerance: diarrhea, dyspepsia, and abdominal pain
- Marrow suppression w/ leukopenia or thrombocytopenia (with concentrations >100 mcg/mL)
- Headache
- Taste perversion
- Pruritis

Rare

- Confusion
- Rash
- Hepatitis
- Peripheral neuropathy
- Enterocolitis
- Photosensitivity

DRUG INTERACTIONS

- Cytarabine: antagonism (avoid co-administration).
- Drugs that cause bone marrow suppression (e.g., AZT, ganciclovir, and interferon): increased bone marrow suppression.

PHARMACOLOGY

Mechanism

Flucytosine interferes with protein synthesis by incorporation into fungal RNA after being converted to 5-FU intracellularly.

Pharmacokinetic Parameters

- **Absorption** 75–90%.
- **Cmax** 30–40 mcg/mL after 2 g PO.
- **Distribution** Widely distributed into body tissues and fluids such as liver, kidney, spleen, heart, aqueous humor, and bronchial secretion. Good CNS penetration (60–100% of serum concentration attained in the CSF).
- **Protein binding** 2–4%.
- **Metabolism/Excretion** Minimal metabolism; principally excreted unchanged in the urine. Unabsorbed drug excreted in feces.
- **T1/2** 2.5–6 hrs.

Dosing for Decreased Hepatic Function

No data. Usual dose likely.

Pregnancy Risk

C: Teratogenicity reported in animal studies. 3 case reports of 2nd and 3rd exposure found no defects in infants.

Breast Feeding Compatibility

No data. Breast feeding during flucytosine therapy not recommended.

COMMENTS

May be used with amphotericin for treatment of cryptococcal meningitis, resulting in more rapid CSF sterilization, but clinical outcome similar with or without flucytosine. Should be used if tolerated, but can treat with amphotericin B alone if toxicity develops. Goal: peak of 50–100 mcg/mL 2 hrs post-dose at steady-state. Close monitoring of renal function and serum level critical to prevent bone marrow suppression. 5-FC may be considered in combination with amphotericin (and surgery) in the treatment of candidal endocarditis. Flucytosine should never be used alone due to the rapid development of resistance, with perhaps the sole exception of candidal UTI.

SELECTED REFERENCES

Saag MS, Cloud GA, Graybill JR, et al. A comparison of itraconazole versus fluconazole as maintenance therapy for AIDS-associated cryptococcal meningitis. National Institute of Allergy and Infectious Diseases Mycoses Study Group. *Clin Infect Dis*, 1999; Vol. 28; pp. 291–6.

van der Horst CM, Saag MS, Cloud GA, et al. Treatment of cryptococcal meningitis associated with the acquired immunodeficiency syndrome. National Institute of Allergy and Infectious Diseases Mycoses Study Group and AIDS Clinical Trials Group. *N Engl J Med*, 1997; Vol. 337; pp. 15–21.

GRISEOFULVIN

Paul A. Pham, PharmD and John G. Bartlett, MD

INDICATIONS
FDA
- Dermatomycosis
- Tinea capitis, T. corporis, T. pedis, T. unguium, T. cruris, and T. barbae

Non-FDA Approved Uses
- Tinea corporis/Tinea cruris
- Tinea pedis
- Tinea capitis/Tinea Barbae
- Onychomycosis

FORMS

Brand name (mfr)	Forms	Cost*
Gris-PEG (Generic manufacturers)	PO tab 125 mg; PO tab 250 mg	$1.98; $2.62
Grifulvin V (Generic manufacturers)	PO tab 500 mg PO susp 125 mg/5 mL (4 oz)	$3.98 $75.78
*Prices represents Average Wholesale Price (AWP).		

USUAL ADULT DOSING
- Tineas: 500–1000 mg (griseofulvin micronized) once daily or 375–750 mg (griseofulvin ultramicronized) once daily × 4–6 wks.
- Tinea unguium should be treated for at least 4 mos.

RENAL DOSING
Dosing for GFR 50–80: Usual dose.
Dosing for GFR 10–50: Usual dose.
Dosing for GFR <10: Usual dose.
Dosing in hemodialysis: No data. Usual dose likely.
Dosing in peritoneal dialysis: No data. Usual dose likely.
Dosing in hemofiltration: No data. Usual dose likely.

ADVERSE DRUG REACTIONS
Common
- GI: nausea, vomiting, diarrhea, flatulence, and heartburn
- Headache

Occasional
- Angular stomatitis
- Disulfiram-like reaction
- Photosensitivity
- Glossodynia
- Thirst
- Black-furred tongue

Rare
- Porphyria
- Hypersensitivity reactions (drug eruption, Erythema multiforme, TEN and Stevens-Johnson syndrome)
- CNS: irritability, confusion, impaired co-ordination, burry vision, and vertigo
- Peripheral neuritis and paresthesias after prolonged therapy
- Interstitial nephritis
- Albuminuria
- Leukopenia and neutropenia
- Hepatitis
- Myositis

ANTIFUNGAL DRUGS

DRUG INTERACTIONS
- Barbiturates: may decrease griseofulvin concentrations. Monitor for therapeutic response; consider an alternative antifungal.
- Cyclosporin: may decrease serum concentrations. Monitor cyclosporin serum concentrations closely with co-administration.
- Oral contraceptives: may decrease oral contraceptive efficacy. Consider an additional barrier form of contraception.
- Warfarin: may decrease anticoagulation effect. Monitor INR closely with co-administration.

PHARMACOLOGY
Mechanism
Griseofulvin binds to the keratin precursor cells which becomes highly resistant to fungal invasion.
Pharmacokinetic Parameters
- **Absorption** Slow but complete absorption but may vary between pts (best when administered after meals).
- **Cmax** 0.8 mcg/mL after 500 mg dose.
- **Distribution** Well distributed into stratum corneum.
- **Metabolism/Excretion** Extensive liver metabolism to 6-demethylgriseofulvin metabolite. High hepatobiliary clearance with minimal renal excretion.
- **T1/2** 9–22 hrs.
Dosing for Decreased Hepatic Function
May need dose reduction.
Pregnancy Risk
C: Not recommended due to possible association with hypoplastic heart failure, conjoined twins, abortion, and cleft palate.
Breast Feeding Compatibility
No data.

COMMENTS
Griseofulvin is an older antifungal agent that has been shown to be equivalent to azoles in the treatment of dermatomycosis caused by *Microsporum*, *Epidermophyton* and *Trichophyton* spp. (but not active against *C. albicans*).

SELECTED REFERENCES
Faergemann J, Mörk NJ, Haglund A, et al. A multicentre (double-blind) comparative study to assess the safety and efficacy of fluconazole and griseofulvin in the treatment of tinea corporis and tinea cruris. *Br J Dermatol*, 1997; Vol. 136; pp. 575–7.

Wingfield AB, Fernandez-Obregon AC, Wignall FS, et al. Treatment of tinea imbricata: a randomized clinical trial using griseofulvin, terbinafine, itraconazole and fluconazole. *Br J Dermatol*, 2004; Vol. 150; pp. 119–26.

ITRACONAZOLE

Paul A. Pham, PharmD and John G. Bartlett, MD

INDICATIONS
FDA
- Aspergillosis treatment in pts intolerant of or refractory to amphotericin B therapy
- Pulmonary and extrapulmonary blastomycosis in immunocompromised and non immunocompromised pts
- Oropharyngeal and esophageal candidiasis (oral liquid)
- Histoplasmosis, including chronic cavitary pulmonary disease and disseminated non-meningeal histoplasmosis
- Neutropenic fever in pts with a suspected fungal infection (oral liquid). Onychomycosis (oral capsule)
Non-FDA Approved Uses
- Coccidioidomycosis
- Cryptococcosis (fluconazole preferred)
- Penicilliosis
- Sporotrichosis
- *Candida vaginitis*
- Fluconazole-resistant esophageal candidiasis

FORMS

Brand name (mfr)	Forms	Cost*
Sporanox (Ortho Biotech Products and generic manufacturers)	Oral capsule 100 mg Oral solution 10 mg/mL (150 mL) IV vial 10 mg/mL (250 mg)	$9.30 $180.40 (150 mL) IV formulation no longer available in the U.S.
*Prices represents Average Wholesale Price (AWP).		

USUAL ADULT DOSING

- Aspergillosis: 200 mg twice-daily. Voriconazole is the preferred azole for invasive aspergillosis. Allergic bronchopulmonary aspergillosis: itraconazole 200 mg twice daily × 16 wks.
- Blastomycosis: 200 mg once or twice daily. Itraconazole is the preferred azole for non-meningeal cases, but fluconazole preferred for meningeal cases. With initial therapy with amphotericin B recommended.
- *Candida esophagitis*: 200 mg liquid swish and swallow once daily × 14 days (fluconazole or posaconazole preferred).
- *Candida* vaginitis: 200 mg once daily × 3 days or 200 mg q12h × 1 day (fluconazole preferred).
- Histoplasmosis: 200 mg q8h × 3 days (loading dose) then 200 mg PO twice daily. Preferred azole but amphotericin B is indicated for initial treatment of severe disseminated disease.
- Onychomycosis: pulse therapy with 200 mg twice daily × 1 wk per mo × 2 mos (fingernails). For toenails treat with 200 mg once daily × 3 mos. Note: treatment not recommended in pts with CHF.
- Coccidioidomycosis: 200–400 mg PO twice daily (acute treatment of non-meningeal coccidioidomycosis) then maintenance with 200 mg PO twice daily. Preferred azole for non-meningeal coccidioidomycosis (fluconazole is preferred for meningeal cases).
- Cryptococcal meningitis: 200 mg once daily maintenance (after 2 wks of amphotericin B then 400 mg/day × 8 wks in pts who can not tolerate fluconazole).
- Non-meningeal cryptococcosis: 200 mg twice daily × 8 wks then 200 mg once daily maintenance (fluconazole preferred).
- Penicilliosis: 200 mg PO twice daily (+ amphotericin B 0.7 mg/kg × 1–2 wks) then 200 mg PO twice-daily maintenance (preferred azole).
- Sporotrichosis: 200 mg twice daily × 3–6 mos Preferred azole for lymphocutaneous cases. Amphotericin B preferred for disseminated cases.
- Neutropenic fever in pts with suspected fungal infection: no longer generally used for acute treatment of suspected invasive fungal infections (IFI), but still employed by some institutions for prophylaxis of IFI, 200 mg twice daily. (lipid amphotericin, and caspofungin are preferred).
- **Administration notes:** take capsule with food and acidic beverage (Coca-cola), absorption dependent on acidity. Avoid PPIs and H2 blockers that reduce gastric acidity.
- Liquid preparation with superior bioavailability, take on empty stomach (food decreases absorption of liquid by 30%).
- Most studies have been performed with capsule formulation but liquid should be considered if desired serum levels are not achieved.
- Target serum concentration (Cmax at steady-state): >1 mcg/mL 2 hrs post-dose after 5 days of therapy.
- Loading doses: 200 mg caps q8h × 3 days and monitoring of serum concentrations is recommended for all serious systemic infections.
- Dose conversion from capsule to liquid: 200 mg capsule = 100 mg liquid (variable serum concentrations therefore serum concentration monitoring is recommended).

RENAL DOSING

Dosing for GFR 50–80: Usual dose.
Dosing for GFR 10–50: Usual dose.
Dosing for GFR <10: Usual dose, some recommend decrease dose by 50%.
Dosing in hemodialysis: 100 mg q12–24h.

ANTIFUNGAL DRUGS

Dosing in peritoneal dialysis: 100 mg q12–24h.
Dosing in hemofiltration: No data.

ADVERSE DRUG REACTIONS

Common
- GI intolerance (nausea and vomiting)

Occasional
- Headache
- Rash
- Increased transaminases

Rare
- Hypokalemia
- Cardiotoxicity with negative inotropic effect
- Severe hepatitis
- Neuropathy
- Adrenal insufficiency (generally with long-term use of high dose itraconazole)
- Impotency
- Gynecomastia
- Leg edema associated with high dose (>600 mg/day)

DRUG INTERACTIONS—See Appendix III, p. 820, for table of drug-to-drug interactions.

PHARMACOLOGY

Mechanism

Triazoles alter fungal cell membrane function by inhibiting C-14 alpha anosterol demethylase, thereby interfering with ergosterol synthesis which results in increased cell permeability and leakage of essential elements.

Pharmacokinetic Parameters
- **Absorption** Variable and dependent on gastric acidity (decreased absorption with achlorhydria; common in AIDS); increased absorption with solution (administer on empty stomach); capsule (administer with food).
- **Cmax** 2 mcg/mL steady-state concentration after 200 mg PO twice daily dose administration. Range of .5–1.1 mcg/mL after single dose 100 mg dose administration.
- **Distribution** Good tissue penetration including (skin, liver, bone, adipose tissue, endometrium cervical mucus). Good nail and bronchial fluid distribution. Negligible CSF penetration, however treatment has been successfully reported for cryptococcal and coccidioidal meningitis.
- **Protein binding** 90–99%.
- **Metabolism/Excretion** Extensive liver metabolism to active (hydroxyitraconazole) and inactive metabolite. 55% biliary excretion and 35% renal excretion of both active and inactive metabolites.
- **T1/2** 56–64 hrs.

Dosing for Decreased Hepatic Function

Use with caution. Usual dose likely based on a small study. Consider monitoring serum levels.

Pregnancy Risk

C: Teratogenic in animal studies. Generally not recommended in pregnancy but some studies have found it to be safe (*Am J Obstet Gynecol.* 2000;183:617–20).

Breast Feeding Compatibility

High breast milk excretion (up to 177% of plasma concentration). Because the safety of itraconazole has not been evaluated, the use of itraconazole during breast feeding should be avoided.

COMMENTS

Absorption of capsules is pH dependent therefore H-2 blockers, PPIs, and antacid co-administration should be avoided. Improved absorption is achieved with acidic gastric environment (Coca-cola). Liquid formulation may be preferred due to better absorption but most studies have been performed with the capsule formulation. Itraconazole is a CYP3A4 substrate and inhibitor with potential for many drug-drug interactions. Parenteral formulation no longer available in the U.S.

SELECTED REFERENCES

Pappas PG, Rex JH, Sobel JD, et al. Guidelines for treatment of candidiasis. *Clin Infect Dis*, 2004; Vol. 38; pp. 161–89.

Walsh TJ, Anaissie EJ, Denning DW, et al. Treatment of aspergillosis: clinical practice guidelines of the Infectious Diseases Society of America. *Clin Infect Dis*, 2008; Vol. 46; pp. 327–60.

KETOCONAZOLE

Paul A. Pham, PharmD and John G. Bartlett, MD

INDICATIONS
FDA
- Treatment of severe recalcitrant cutaneous dermatophyte infections (tinea corporis and tinea cruris) unresponsive to topical therapy or oral griseofulvin.
- Treatment of candidiasis, mucocutaneous candidiasis (esophagitis, oral thrush) and candiduria.
- Treatment of blastomycosis, coccidioidomycosis, histoplasmosis, chromomycosis, and paracoccidioidomycosis.

FORMS

Brand name (mfr)	Forms	Cost*
Nizoral (Janssen and generics manufacturer)	Oral tablet 200 mg	$4.74(brand); $3.03(generic)
Nizoral shampoo (McNeil and generic manufacturers)	Topical shampoo 2% (120 mL)	$27.75
Nizoral cream (Generic manufacturers)	Topical cream 2% (15 g)	$16.45
*Prices represents Average Wholesale Price (AWP).		

USUAL ADULT DOSING
- Thrush: 200 mg PO q12–24h × 7–10 days (topical therapy with clotrimazole preferred).
- *Candida* esophagitis: 200–400 mg PO twice daily (fluconazole preferred) × 2–3 wks.
- *Candida* vaginitis: 200–400 mg/day × 7 days or 400 mg/day × 3 days.
- Non-meningeal blastomycosis: 400–800 mg/day >6 mos (itraconazole preferred).
- Non-meningeal coccidioidomycosis: 400 mg/day >1 yr (itraconazole or fluconazole preferred).
- Histoplasmosis: not generally recommended (itraconazole preferred).
- Chromomycosis: not generally recommended (itraconazole preferred).
- Tinea: 200 mg PO once daily × 2–4 wks.
- Absorption dependent on gastric acidity, which decreases with age, acid-suppression therapy and advanced HIV disease. Administer with acidic drinks (orange juice, colas, etc).

RENAL DOSING
Dosing for GFR 50–80: Usual dose.
Dosing for GFR 10–50: Usual dose.
Dosing for GFR <10: Usual dose.
Dosing in hemodialysis: Not removed in HD, usual dose.
Dosing in peritoneal dialysis: Not removed in peritoneal dialysis, usual dose.
Dosing in hemofiltration: No data, usual dose likely.

ADVERSE DRUG REACTIONS
Common
- GI upset and abdominal pain
- Transient transaminitis

Occasional
- Decreased steroid and testosterone synthesis generally seen with prolong use of higher doses, >600 mg/day. Impotence, gynecomastia, oligospermia, reduced libido, and menstrual abnormalities secondary to decreased steroid synthesis.
- CNS: headache, somnolence, dizziness, photophobia.
- Hepatitis (more common compared to other azoles).
- Asthenia.

Rare
- Hepatic necrosis
- Bone marrow suppression
- Hallucination
- Hypothyroidism

ANTIFUNGAL DRUGS

DRUG INTERACTIONS—See Appendix III, p. 822, for table of drug-to-drug interactions.
Substrate and potent inhibitor of CYP3A4. Many potential drug interactions.
- **Contraindicated** (Do not co-administer):
- terfenadine
- astemizole
- cisapride
- pimozide
- midazolam
- triazolam
- quinidine

PHARMACOLOGY
Mechanism
Imidazoles alter fungal cell membrane function by interfering with ergosterol synthesis, which results in increased cell permeability and leakage of essential elements.

Pharmacokinetic Parameters
- **Absorption** Variable absorption. Dependent on gastric acidity; decreased absorption with achlorhydria (common in AIDS).
- **Cmax** 4.2 mcg/mL after 200 mg dose oral administration.
- **Distribution** High concentration attained in liver, pituitary, adrenals. Lung, kidney, bladder, bone marrow, myocardium, and various glandular tissue distribution also noted. Low and unpredictable CSF concentration.
- **Protein binding** 84–99%.
- **Metabolism/Excretion** Partially metabolized. Primarily excreted as unchanged drug and metabolite in feces via biliary excretion. Only a small amount excreted in urine.
- **T1/2** 8 hrs.

Dosing for Decreased Hepatic Function
Use with caution or avoid.

Pregnancy Risk
C: Teratogenic in animal studies. In surveillance study of Michigan Medicaid recipients, no birth defects found in 20 newborns exposed to oral ketoconazole during the 1st trimester. Since this study, FDA has received 6 reports of limb defects.

Breast Feeding Compatibility
Breast milk excretion likely. Effect on the fetus unknown.

COMMENTS
Oral azole with pH-dependent absorption. Improved absorption achieved with an acidic gastric environment; avoid proton-pump inhibitor, H_2 blocker, and antacid coadministration. Somewhat cheaper than fluconazole, but fluconazole preferred for treatment of *Candida* esophagitis due to more predictable absorption, better efficacy, and fewer drug-drug interactions.

SELECTED REFERENCES
de Repentigny L, Ratelle J. Comparison of itraconazole and ketoconazole in HIV-positive pts with oropharyngeal or esophageal candidiasis. Human Immunodeficiency Virus Itraconazole Ketoconazole Project Group. *Chemotherapy*, 1997; Vol. 42; pp. 374–83.

Pappas PG, Rex JH, Sobel JD, et al. Guidelines for treatment of candidiasis. *Clin Infect Dis*, 2004; Vol. 38; pp. 161–89.

MICAFUNGIN

Paul A. Pham, PharmD and John G. Bartlett, MD

INDICATIONS
FDA
- Prophylaxis of candida infections in hematopoietic stem cell transplant pts (HSCT)
- Esophageal candidiasis (author's opinion: would reserve micafungin for azole-resistant cases)
- Treatment of pts with candidemia, acute disseminated candidiasis, candida peritonitis, and abscesses

Non-FDA Approved Uses
- Invasive aspergillosis (known data limited to open-label studies.)

FORMS

Brand name (mfr)	Forms	Cost*
Mycamine (Astellas Pharma)	IV vial 50 mg; IV vial 100 mg	$116.88; $233.75

*Prices represents Average Wholesale Price (AWP).

USUAL ADULT DOSING
- Esophageal candidiasis: 150 mg IV once daily.
- Invasive candidiasis: 100–150 mg IV once daily (150 mg for severe infections).
- Candida prophylaxis in HSCT: 50 mg IV once daily.

RENAL DOSING
Dosing for GFR 50–80: Usual dose.
Dosing for GFR 10–50: Usual dose.
Dosing for GFR <10: Usual dose.
Dosing in hemodialysis: Usual dose. Not dialyzable, thus no supplemental doses needed post dialysis.
Dosing in peritoneal dialysis: No data, usual dose likely.
Dosing in hemofiltration: No data, usual dose likely.

ADVERSE DRUG REACTIONS
General
- Well tolerated with ADR profile comparable to caspofungin and fluconazole.
- Compared to liposomal amphotericin B, micafungin is associated with less fever, chills, back pain, and renal failure.

Occasional
- Histamine-mediated symptoms including rash, facial swelling, pruritus, and vasodilation
- Local phlebitis
- Fever, chills
- LFT elevations
- Diarrhea, nausea, vomiting
- Hypokalemia
- Thrombocytopenia
- Headache

Rare
- Anaphylaxis
- Hemolytic anemia

DRUG INTERACTIONS
No significant drug-drug interactions with mycophenolate, cyclosporine, tacrolimus, predniso-lone, fluconazole, voriconazole, amphotericin B, ritonavir, and rifampin.
- Itraconazole: AUC increased 11% with micafungin co-administration.
- Nifedipine: AUC increased by 18% with micafungin co-administration.
- Sirolimus: AUC increased by 21% with micafungin co-administration. Monitor sirolimus serum concentrations with co-administrations.

RESISTANCE
- *C. neoformans:* intrinsically resistant to echinocandins such as micafungin.

PHARMACOLOGY
Mechanism
Lipopeptide. Beta (1,3) beta-D-glucan is an integral component of fungal cell wall, is inhibited by micafungin.

Pharmacokinetic Parameters
- **Cmax** 16.4 mcg/mL; AUC: 167 mcg/mL hr (150 mg once-daily at steady state).
- **Distribution** Vd = 0.39 +/− 0.11 L/kg. Limited CNS and bone penetration.
- **Protein binding** >99%.
- **Metabolism/Excretion** Metabolized to methoxyl and hydroxyl-metabolite that is primarily excreted in the feces.
- **T1/2** 13–17 hrs.

ANTIFUNGAL DRUGS

Dosing for Decreased Hepatic Function
For Child-Pugh score of 7–9: no dose adjustment needed. No data for severe hepatic dysfunction.
Pregnancy Risk
C: No human data. Visceral abnormalities and abortion with high dose in animal studies.
Breast Feeding Compatibility
Excreted in breast milk. Use with caution.

COMMENTS
Micafungin is an echinocandin antifungal with similar spectrum of activity to caspofungin and anidulafungin which includes most all *Candida* spp. and *Aspergillus* spp. Clinical data established for the treatment of esophageal candidiasis, candida prophylaxis in hematopoietic stem cell transplant pts, and invasive candidiasis. Cost (AWP) is much lower than caspofungin, but purchased prices are often comparable.

SELECTED REFERENCES
Pappas PG, Kauffman CA, Andes D, et al. Clinical practice guidelines for the management of candidiasis: 2009 update by the Infectious Diseases Society of America. *Clin Infect Dis*, 2009; Vol. 48(5); pp. 503–35.

Pappas PG, Rotstein CM, Betts RF, et al. Micafungin versus caspofungin for treatment of candidemia and other forms of invasive candidiasis. *Clin Infect Dis*, 2007; Vol. 45(7); pp. 833–93.

NYSTATIN

Paul A. Pham, PharmD and John G. Bartlett, MD

INDICATIONS
FDA
• Oropharyngeal candidiasis
• Vulvovaginal candidiasis
• Cutaneous candidiasis
FORMS

Brand name (mfr)	Forms	Cost*
Nystatin (Generic manufacturers (Paddock, Teva and others))	Oral tablet 500,000 U Vaginal tablet 100,000 U	$0.68 $0.47
Mycostatin (Generic manufacturers (Apothecon, Bristol-Myers Squibb, and others))	Oral suspension 100,000 U/mL (60 mL or 480 mL) Topical powder 100,000 U/g Topical cream or ointment 100,000 U/g (15 g, 30 g)	$1.66 per 5 mL $5.50 $4.25 (15 g) $6.50 (30 g)
*Prices represents Average Wholesale Price (AWP).		

USUAL ADULT DOSING
• Thrush: 500,000 to 1,000,000 Units (1–2 tabs or 5–10 mL) in mouth 3–5 × day. Put ½ of suspension in left side of mouth, hold as long as possible before swallowing. Repeat for right side of mouth.
• Vaginitis: 1 vaginal tablet (100,000 units) daily for 2 wks.
• Topical candidiases: Apply cream or ointment to affected areas twice daily.

RENAL DOSING
Dosing for GFR 50–80: Usual dose
Dosing for GFR 10–50: Usual dose
Dosing for GFR <10: Usual dose
Dosing in hemodialysis: Usual dose
Dosing in peritoneal dialysis: Usual dose
Dosing in hemofiltration: Usual dose

ADVERSE DRUG REACTIONS
Common
- Oral preparations: bad taste.

Occasional
- Oral preparations: GI distress including nausea, vomiting and diarrhea.
- Topical preparations: skin irritation.

DRUG INTERACTIONS
None

PHARMACOLOGY
Mechanism
Binds to sterols in the fungal cell membrane resulting in loss of function.

Pharmacokinetic Parameters
- **Absorption** No systemic absorption.
- **Cmax** Minimal absorption. Salivary concentration 1000 u/mL 1 hr post-dose.
- **Distribution** Concentrated in saliva.
- **Metabolism/Excretion** Not metabolized.
- **T1/2** 4 hrs.

Dosing for Decreased Hepatic Function
Usual dose.

Pregnancy Risk
B: No fetal harm has been reported.

Breast Feeding Compatibility
Compatible with breastfeeding.

COMMENTS
Causes GI side effects and may not be as effective as clotrimazole since the bitter taste prevents pts from keeping it in their mouth for prolong periods of time. Poor adherence due to frequent administration (suspension). Efficacy dependent on contact time with mucosa. Clotrimazole lozenges preferred by most pts. In contrast to topical clotrimazole, topical nystatin not effective for *Tinea corporis*.

BASIS FOR RECOMMENDATIONS
National Institutes of Health (NIH), the Centers for Disease Control and Prevention (CDC), and the HIV Medicine Association of the Infectious Diseases Society of America (HIVMA/IDSA). Guidelines for Prevention and Treatment of Opportunistic Infections in HIV-Infected Adults and Adolescents. *http://AIDSinfo.nih.gov/*, 2008.

Comments: Initial episodes of oropharyngeal candidiasis can be treated with topical therapy, such as clotrimazole troches or nystatin suspension.

SELECTED REFERENCES
Pappas PG, Rex JH, Sobel JD, et al. Guidelines for treatment of candidiasis. *Clin Infect Dis*, 2004; Vol. 38; pp. 161–89.

Pons V, Greenspan D, Lozada-Nur F, et al. Oropharyngeal candidiasis in pts with AIDS: randomized comparison of fluconazole versus nystatin oral suspensions. *Clin Infect Dis*, 1997; Vol. 24; pp. 1204–7.

PENTAMIDINE

Paul A. Pham, PharmD and John G. Bartlett, MD

INDICATIONS
FDA
- Treatment and prophylaxis of PCP.

FORMS

Brand name (mfr)	Forms	Cost*
Pentam 300 (Generic manufacturers)	IV vial 300 mg	$98.75
NebuPent (Generic manufacturers)	Inhalation powder 300 mg	$98.75
*Prices represents Average Wholesale Price (AWP).		

ANTIFUNGAL DRUGS

USUAL ADULT DOSING

- PCP treatment: 4 mg/kg IV once daily over 1 hr × 21 days (TMP-SMX or clindamycin/primaquine preferred).
- PCP prophylaxis: 300 mg aerosolized pentamidine (AP) q mo (TMP-SMX or dapsone preferred). 300 mg diluted in 6 mL sterile water delivered at 6 L/min by a Respigard II nebulizer.
- Aerosolized pentamidine should not be used for PCP treatment.

RENAL DOSING

Dosing for GFR 50–80: Usual dosing.
Dosing for GFR 10–50: 4 mg/kg q24–36h.
Dosing for GFR <10: Consider dose adjustment to 4 mg/kg q48h.
Dosing in hemodialysis: Nonsignificant increase in elimination half-life during hemodialysis. No dosage adjustment needed.
Dosing in peritoneal dialysis: No data, no supplemental dose needed.
Dosing in hemofiltration: No data.

ADVERSE DRUG REACTIONS

Common

- Nephrotoxicity (25–50%): usually reversible with discontinuation but may progress to ARF.
- Hypoglycemia: most commonly seen after 5–7 days but can occur at anytime, including after therapy have been stopped (treat with IV glucose and/or diazoxide).
- Hyperglycemia and insulin-dependent diabetes mellitus.
- GI intolerance: anorexia, abdominal pain, dysgeusia, nausea, and vomiting.
- Phlebitis at IV infusion site.
- Cough and wheezing with AP: consider pretreatment with inhaled beta-2 agonist.

Occasional

- Hypotension: avoid by giving IV over 60 min in supine position with hydration to reduce risk.
- Marrow suppression: leukopenia and thrombocytopenia.
- Electrolyte abnormalities: hypocalcemia, hypomagnesemia, and hypokalemia; laboratory monitoring recommended.

Rare

- Pancreatitis
- Torsade de pointes
- Fever
- Rash, including TEN
- Dizziness and confusion
- Hepatitis
- Laryngitis, chest pain, and dyspnea with aerosolized pentamidine

DRUG INTERACTIONS

- Amphotericin B and foscarnet: may increase risk of severe hypocalcemia.
- ddI: may increase risk of pancreatitis.
- Nephrotoxic agents (aminoglycoside, foscarnet, cidofovir, amphotericin B): may increase risk of nephrotoxicity.

PHARMACOLOGY

Mechanism

Exact mechanism of action of pentamidine not fully elucidated but may involve interference with incorporation of nucleotides into RNA and DNA and inhibition of oxidative phosphorylation and biosynthesis of DNA, RNA, protein, and phospholipid.

Pharmacokinetic Parameters

- **Absorption** N/A
- **Cmax** 0.5–3.4 mcg/mL after 4 mg/kg IV dose administration.
- **Distribution** High concentration attained in liver, kidney, adrenal glands, and spleen. Slow CNS penetration, only detected 30 days after the start of therapy. Lung concentration also attained.
- **Protein binding** 69%.

- **Metabolism/Excretion** Unknown metabolism. 4–17% excreted in the urine, due to the long terminal half life excretion can last up to 8 wks following last dose.
- **T1/2** 7 hrs (terminal half life up to 4 wks).

Dosing for Decreased Hepatic Function

No data. Usual dose likely.

Pregnancy Risk

C: Both manufacturer and CDC advices against the use of pentamidine in pregnancy. Spontaneous abortion reported, however causal relationship has not been established.

Breast Feeding Compatibility

No data.

COMMENTS

Parenteral agent used for treatment of severe PCP in pts intolerant or unresponsive to TMP/SMX or clindamycin/primaquine. Aerosolized pentamidine used for PCP prophylaxis in pts intolerant of TMP/SMX or dapsone. Parenteral: toxicities such as hypotension, hypoglycemia, and renal failure limit its use. Close monitoring of vital signs and blood sugar with infusion recommended. Avoid concurrent administration of nephrotoxic drugs due to additive nephrotoxicity. Unclear whether aerosolized pentamidine may increase risk of extrapulmonary infection and pneumothorax. Risk of TB transmission to health care workers during aerosolized pentamidine administration: do not use if suspicion of active TB.

BASIS FOR RECOMMENDATIONS

National Institutes of Health (NIH), the Centers for Disease Control and Prevention (CDC), and the HIV Medicine Association of the Infectious Diseases Society of America (HIVMA/IDSA). Guidelines for Prevention and Treatment of Opportunistic Infections in HIV-Infected Adults and Adolescents. *http://AIDSinfo.nih.gov*, 2008.

Comments: Current OI treatment guidelines. Alternative therapeutic regimens for pts with moderate-to-severe PCP include clindamycin-primaquine or intravenous pentamidine, but IV pentamidine is generally the drug of second choice for severe disease.

SELECTED REFERENCES

Bozzette SA, Finkelstein DM, Spector SA, et al. A randomized trial of three antipneumocystis agents in pts with advanced human immunodeficiency virus infection. NIAID AIDS Clinical Trials Group. *N Engl J Med*, 1995; Vol. 332; pp. 693–9.

Klein NC, Duncanson FP, Lenox TH, et al. Trimethoprim-sulfamethoxazole versus pentamidine for Pneumocystis carinii pneumonia in AIDS pts: results of a large prospective randomized treatment trial. *AIDS*, 1992; Vol. 6; pp. 301–5.

POSACONAZOLE

Paul A. Pham, PharmD and John G. Bartlett, MD

INDICATIONS

FDA

- Prophylaxis of invasive aspergillus and disseminated candidiasis in severely immunocompromised hosts, such as hemapoietic stem cell transplant recipients with graft vs. host (GVH) disease or those with hematologic malignancies with prolonged neutropenia from chemotherapy.
- Treatment of oropharyngeal candidiasis, including itraconazole and/or fluconazole refractory cases.

Non-FDA Approved Uses

- Treatment of invasive fungal infections due to *Aspergillus* spp., *Candida* spp., and zygomycoses (e.g., Rhizomucor, Cunninghamella, *Absidia* species).

FORMS

Brand name (mfr)	Forms	Cost*
Noxafil (Schering Corporation)	Oral Suspension 40 mg/mL (105 mL)	$650.40 per 105 mL bottle
*Prices represents Average Wholesale Price (AWP).		

ANTIFUNGAL DRUGS

USUAL ADULT DOSING

- Administration of oral drug with a full meal or liquid nutritional supplement significantly increases drug levels. Food is critical for absorption.
- Prophylaxis of invasive fungal infections: 200 mg (5 mL) PO q8h.
- Treatment of invasive fungal infections: 200 mg PO q6h or 400 mg PO q12h.
- Oropharyngeal candidiasis: 100 mg q12h × 2 (loading dose on day 1), then 100 mg q24h × 13 days. Generally not recommended due to high cost and the availability of alternatives (including topical clotrimazole).
- Oropharyngeal and esophageal candidiasis refractory to itraconazole and/or fluconazole: 400 mg q12h (duration of therapy based on clinical response).

RENAL DOSING

Dosing for GFR 50–80: Standard dose

Dosing for GFR 10–50: Use standard dose. Due to a large pharmacokinetic variability (CV = 96%), closer monitoring for breakthrough infection is recommended with CrCL <20 mL/min.

Dosing for GFR <10: Use standard dose. Due to a large pharmacokinetic variability (CV = 96%), closer monitoring for breakthrough infection is recommended with CrCL <20 mL/min.

Dosing in hemodialysis: No data. Standard dose likely. Dose post-HD on days of HD.

Dosing in peritoneal dialysis: No data. Standard dose likely.

Dosing in hemofiltration: No data. Standard dose likely.

ADVERSE DRUG REACTIONS

General

- Generally well tolerated with comparable side effect profile to fluconazole.

Occasional

- Nausea, vomiting, diarrhea, abdominal pain.
- Increased liver enzymes.
- Hyperbilirubinemia.

Rare

- Adrenal insufficiency.
- Hypersensitivity reaction.
- QTc prolongation (clinical significance unknown)

DRUG INTERACTIONS—See Appendix III, p. 827, for table of drug-to-drug interactions.

Posaconazole is metabolized via UDP glucuronidation (phase II enzymes). It is a substrate of P-gp efflux and an inhibitor of CYP3A4. As a result, CYP3A4 substrate may be increased. Posaconazole serum concentrations may be decreased with the co-administration of UDP glucuronidation or P-gp inducers.

PHARMACOLOGY

Mechanism

Mechanism of action: posaconazole is a triazole antifungal that inhibits fungal ergosterol synthesis.

Pharmacokinetic Parameters

- **Absorption** Well absorbed when administered with food or a nutritional supplement (e.g., Boost Plus). The mean AUC and Cmax of posaconazole were approximately 3–4 × higher with food. Acidic beverage increases posaconazole AUC 70%.
- **Cmax** Mean average concentration after 200 mg PO three times a day with food at steady state: 583–1103 g/mL with a relative large CV% of 65–67%.
- **Distribution** Widely distributed with a Vd of 1774L.
- **Protein binding** >98%.
- **Metabolism/Excretion** Primarily metabolized in the liver, where it undergoes glucuronidation and is transformed into biologically inactive metabolites. Posaconazole is predominantly eliminated in the feces (71%). Renal clearance is a minor elimination pathway (13%).
- **T1/2** 35 hrs (steady-state attained at 7–10 days). Although the half-life would suggest less frequent dosing, more frequent dosing results in better bioavailability.

Dosing for Decreased Hepatic Function

Limited data, consider standard dose. Use with caution.

Pregnancy Risk
C: No human data. Posaconazole has been shown to cause skeletal malformations in rats, but not in rabbits, given 3–5 × human exposure.
Breast Feeding Compatibility
No human data. Posaconazole is excreted in milk of lactating rats.
COMMENTS
Posaconazole is active against all *Candida* spp. (including many azole-resistant *Candida* spp, but cross-resistance reported) and *Aspergillus* spp. (including *A. terreus*). Although *Fusarium* spp. are generally resistant *in vitro*, clinical successes have been reported. The high pharmacokinetic variability (dependent on fatty food administration), the lack of IV formulation and the 1 wk lag time to reach steady-state may limit the use of posaconazole in severe invasive fungal infections. Nevertheless, activities against certain *Zygomycetes* spp. and good efficacy in preliminary open-label observational studies are encouraging. Prospective, randomized studies are needed to better define the role of posaconazole in invasive fungal infections.
BASIS FOR RECOMMENDATIONS
FDA labeling.
Comments: The FDA approval of posaconazole was based on 2 prophylaxis studies comparing posaconazole to fluconazole (or itraconazole) in hematopoeitic stem cell transplant recipients with Graft vs. Host Disease (study 1) and hematologic malignancies with prolonged neutropenia from chemotherapy (study 2). In stem cell recipient, clinical failure rate of posaconazole (33%) was similar to fluconazole (37%). In hematologic malignancies with prolonged neutropenia pts, clinical failure rate (27% vs. 42%) and mortality (14% vs, 21%) were lower in posaconazole treated pts compared fluconazole or itraconazole treated pts. The difference was attributed to fewer breakthrough infections caused by Aspergillus spp. in posaconazole treated pts.

SELECTED REFERENCES
Greenberg RN, Mullane K, van Burik JA, et al. Posaconazole as salvage therapy for zygomycosis. *Antimicrob Agents Chemother*, 2006; Vol. 50; pp. 126–33.

SATURATED SOLUTION OF POTASSIUM IODIDE (SSKI)

Paul A. Pham, PharmD and John G. Bartlett, MD

INDICATIONS
FDA Indications
- Hyperthyroidism
- Post radiation exposure to prevent radiation-induced thyroid neoplasm
Non-FDA Approved Uses
- Cutaneous sporotrichosis
FORMS

Brand name (mfr)	Forms	Cost*
SSKI (Upsher-Smith)	Oral oral solution 1 g/mL (1 oz and 8 oz)	$12.10 (1 oz) and $56.31 (8 oz)
*Prices represents Average Wholesale Price (AWP).		

USUAL ADULT DOSING
For cutaneous/lymphocutaneous sporotrichosis (second line to itraconazole): 5–10 drops PO q8h initially, then advance to 40–50 drops q8h as tolerated (24–40 drops in pediatrics) × 6–24 wks until skin lesion resolution.
RENAL DOSING
Dosing for GFR 50–80: Usual dose.
Dosing for GFR 10–50: Usual dose likely.
Dosing for GFR *<10:* Usual dose likely.
Dosing in hemodialysis: No data.
Dosing in peritoneal dialysis: No data.
Dosing in hemofiltration: No data.

ANTIFUNGAL DRUGS

ADVERSE DRUG REACTIONS
Common
- Bad taste
Occasional
- GI: nausea, diarrhea, and anorexia
- Parotid or lacrimal gland enlargement (side effects are dose dependent and may resolve with lower doses)
Rare
- Hypersensitivity reaction
- Hypothyroidism
- Thyroid adenoma

DRUG INTERACTIONS
- Lithium: may result in additive hypothyroidism. Monitor for sign and symptoms of hypothyroidism.
- Warfarin: may decrease anticoagulation efficacy. Monitor INR closely with co-administration.

PHARMACOLOGY
Pharmacokinetic Parameters
- **Absorption** Well absorbed after oral administration.
Dosing for Decreased Hepatic Function
No data.
Pregnancy Risk
D: May cause hypothyroidism and goiter in the fetus with prolong use (>10 days). The American Academy of Pediatrics considers iodide preparation contraindicated in pregnancy.
Breast Feeding Compatibility
Excreted in breast milk, but no problems or alterations in thyroid test were noted in these breast-fed infants. The American Academy of Pediatrics considers iodide compatible with breast feeding.

COMMENTS
Saturated solution potassium iodide (SSKI) is an effective agent for cutaneous sporotrichosis. Itraconazole has been shown to be effective and most authorities prefer itraconazole as first line therapy. SSKI is not effective in extracutaneous sporotrichosis.

SELECTED REFERENCES
Kauffman CA, Hajjeh R, Chapman SW. Practice guidelines for the management of pts with sporotrichosis. For the Mycoses Study Group. Infectious Diseases Society of America. *Clin Infect Dis*, 2000; Vol. 30; pp. 684–7.

Tripathy S, Vijayashree J, Mishra M, et al. Rhinofacial zygomycosis successfully treated with oral saturated solution of potassium iodide: a case report. *J Eur Acad Dermatol Venereol*, 2007; Vol. 21; pp. 117–9.

TERBINAFINE

Paul A. Pham, PharmD and John G. Bartlett, MD

INDICATIONS
FDA
- Onychomycosis
- *Tinea capitis*
- *Tinea corporis*
- *Tinea cruris*
- *Tinea pedis*
Non-FDA Approved Uses
- *Tinea versicolor*
- *Tinea barbae*

FORMS

Brand name (mfr)	Forms	Cost*
Lamisil (Novartis)	Topical spray 1% (30 mL) PO tab 250 mg Topical cream 1% (12 g); Topical cream 1% (24 gg) PO granules 125 mg; PO granules 187.5 mg	$8.15 $15.97 $8.15; $12.23 $8.78; $13.14
Terbinafine (Generic manufacturers)	PO tab 250 mg	$0.62

*Prices represents Average Wholesale Price (AWP).

USUAL ADULT DOSING
- Onychomycosis: 250 mg PO once daily (6 wks in fingernail infections and 12 wks in toenail infections).
- **Note**: pretreatment liver function testing (AST/ALT) recommended for long-term therapy for all pts. Use of drug not recommended for pts with chronic or active liver disease.
- Tinea cruris or tinea corporis: terbinafine 1% cream or spray applied once daily to affected area × 1 wk.
- Terbinafine 250 mg PO once daily × 1 wk can be used for tinea corporis, tinea cruris, and cutaneous candidiasis (azole preferred), but topical therapy is preferred.

RENAL DOSING
Dosing for GFR 50–80: 250 mg once daily.
Dosing for GFR 10–50: No data, avoid.
Dosing for GFR <10: No data, avoid.
Dosing in hemodialysis: No data, avoid.
Dosing in peritoneal dialysis: No data, avoid.
Dosing in hemofiltration: No data, avoid.

ADVERSE DRUG REACTIONS
Occasional
- GI intolerance: diarrhea, dyspepsia and abdominal pain
- Rash and pruritis
- Taste perversion

Rare
- Severe hepatitis (FDA black box warning)
- Erythema multiforme and Stevens-Johnson syndrome
- Cholestatic hepatitis
- CNS: headache, lethargy, and sedation

DRUG INTERACTIONS
- Cimetidine: may increase terbinafine serum concentration. Consider an alternative H-2 blocker (e.g., ranitidine or famotidine) with terbinafine co-administration.
- Cyclosporine: may decrease cyclosporine serum concentrations. Monitor cyclosporine serum concentration closely with co-administration.
- Ethanol: potential additive hepatoxicity. Avoid concurrent use.
- Hepatotoxic drugs (e.g., HIV-protease inhibitors, nevirapine, INH, telithromycin...): potential additive hepatotoxicity. Avoid concurrent administration; monitor liver enzymes closely.
- Rifampin: rifampin significantly decreased terbinafine serum concentrations. Monitor for terbinafine therapeutic response.

PHARMACOLOGY
Mechanism
Exact mechanism not understood but may interfere with sterol synthesis.

ANTIFUNGAL DRUGS

Pharmacokinetic Parameters

- **Absorption** 80%.
- **Cmax** 0.8–1.5 mg/mL serum concentration after 250 mg PO dose administration. 250–550 ng/mL nail concentration after 250 mg once daily administration 3–18 wks after start of therapy.
- **Distribution** Highly distributed in the stratum corneum, dermis, epidermis and nails. High concentration in adipose tissue.
- **Protein binding** 99%.
- **Metabolism/Excretion** Extensively metabolized in the liver. 70% of the dose undergo renal clearance with the remainder recovered in the feces.
- **T1/2** 22–26 hrs.

Dosing for Decreased Hepatic Function

Not recommended.

Pregnancy Risk

B: Animal studies have shown adverse effect but no human data available.

Breast Feeding Compatibility

Considered unsafe during breastfeeding; not recommended by the manufacturer.

COMMENTS

Terbinafine is superior to pulse dose itraconazole in the management of onychomycosis. Monitoring of liver enzymes recommended with long-term therapy if abnormal LFT's or liver disease is preexisting. Generics now available.

SELECTED REFERENCES

Gupta AK, Ryder JE, Lynch LE, et al. The use of terbinafine in the treatment of onychomycosis in adults and special populations: a review of the evidence. *J Drugs Dermatol*, 2005; Vol. 4; pp. 302–8.

Sigurgeirsson B, Olafsson JH, Steinsson JB, et al. Long-term effectiveness of treatment with terbinafine vs itraconazole in onychomycosis: a 5-yrs blinded prospective follow-up study. *Arch Dermatol*, 2002; Vol. 138; pp. 353–7.

VORICONAZOLE

Paul A. Pham, PharmD and John G. Bartlett, MD

INDICATIONS

FDA

- Invasive aspergillosis.
- *P. boydii* (*S. apiospermum*) and *Fusarium* spp. (including *F. solani*) infections in persons intolerant of, or refractory to, other therapy.
- Esophageal candidiasis.
- Treatment of candidemia in non-neutropenic pts.

FORMS

Brand name (mfr)	Forms	Cost*
VFEND (Pfizer)	Oral tablet 50 mg; 200 mg	$12.09; $48.38
	IV vial 200 mg/20 mL	$142.36
	Oral suspension 45 g per bottle (40 mg/mL)	$830.59/45 g bottle
*Prices represents Average Wholesale Price (AWP).		

USUAL ADULT DOSING

- Invasive aspergillosis (IV): 6 mg/kg IV q12h × 2 doses (load), then 4 mg/kg IV q12h infused over 1–2 hrs.
- Invasive aspergillosis (PO): 200 mg PO q12h (for pts >40 kg, but 300 mg PO q12h should be used for severe disease). For pts <40 kg: 100 mg PO q12h, may be increased to 150 mg PO q12h for severe disease.
- Candidemia in non-neutropenic pts: 6 mg/kg IV q12h × 2 then 3 mg/kg q12h.
- Candida esophagitis (may be active against fluconazole resistant esophagitis): 200 mg PO q12h (>40 kg) or 100 mg PO q12h (<40 kg) × 14 days or 7 days after symptoms resolution.

- Administer oral doses on an empty stomach, avoid high fat food.
- Consider therapeutic drug monitoring in severe disease, target Cmin >2.05 mcg/mL (*AAC* 2006; 50:1570–1572.)
- Although not robustly prospectively studied, voriconazole trough concentrations <1 mg/L associated with higher rates of failure in treatment of aspergillus, while troughs >5.5 mg/L associated with development of encephalopathy.

RENAL DOSING

Dosing for GFR 50–80: Standard dose.

Dosing for GFR 10–50: Standard dosing of oral voriconazole. IV voriconazole is not recommended due to potential for toxicity of the sulfobutylether—cyclodextrin (SBECD) vehicle, but have been used in severe infections.

Dosing for GFR <10: Standard dosing of oral voriconazole. IV voriconazole is not recommended due to potential for toxicity of the sulfobutylether—cyclodextrin (SBECD) vehicle, but have been used in severe infections.

Dosing in hemodialysis: Voriconazole is dialyzed. Standard dosing of oral voriconazole (dose after HD). IV voriconazole is not recommended, but have been used in severe infections.

Dosing in peritoneal dialysis: No data. Standard oral dose likely. IV voriconazole is not recommended.

Dosing in hemofiltration: CVVHDF: usual dose recommended (*JAC* 2007; 60:1085–90.)

ADVERSE DRUG REACTIONS
Common

- Visual disturbances ("abnormal vision" described as blurriness, color changes, and enhanced vision) seen in 20.6% of pts but less than <1% required discontinuation. Duration of abnormality usually less than 30 minutes, typically starting 30 minutes after dosing.

Occasional

- Increased transaminases (13%) and alkaline phosphatase. Discontinuance required in 4–8%
- Rash (6%)
- Hallucination (4.3%)
- Nausea and vomiting
- Increase in total bilirubin
- Encephalopathy (associated with trough >5.5 mcg/mL)

RESISTANCE

- Isolates with low level resistance to fluconazole and/or itraconazole exhibit 15% cross-resistance to voriconazole. However, high level resistance to fluconazole results in 50% cross-resistance to voriconazole.
- No reliable activity against members of the zygomycetes family, e.g., mucor, rhizopus. 83% and 60% *in vitro* resistance seen with *Fusarium* and *Rhizopus*, respectively (Diekema D.J. et al. *J Clin Microbiol* 2003; 41: 3623). Case reports of clinical success with *Fusarium* spp.

DRUG INTERACTIONS—See Appendix III, p. 843, for table of drug-to-drug interactions.
PHARMACOLOGY
Mechanism

Voriconazole is a triazole antifungal that inhibits fungal ergosterol biosynthesis.

Pharmacokinetic Parameters

- **Absorption** 96% (CV13%) absorbed on an empty stomach (1 hr before or 2 hrs after meals). Absorption is independent of gastric pH but is reduced by 24% with high fat meals.
- **Cmax** 2.51–4.6 mcg/mL.
- **Distribution** Widely distributed with a Vd of 4.6 L/kg. CSF: serum ratio of 0.5:1 [animal data]. CNS tissue:serum ratio of 2:1 [animal data].
- **Protein binding** 58% (low).
- **Metabolism/Excretion** Metabolized by CYP2C19/CYP2C9/CYP3A4 (based on *in vitro* data) to inactive metabolite (N-oxide voriconazole) that is excreted in the urine. Less than 2% of unchanged drug excreted in the urine.
- **T1/2** Dose dependent terminal half-life.

Dosing for Decreased Hepatic Function

Mild to moderate hepatic insufficiency (Child-Pugh Class A and B): 6 mg/kg q12h × 2 doses (load), then 2 mg/kg IV q12h. Monitor serum concentrations.

ANTIFUNGAL DRUGS

Pregnancy Risk

D: Avoid in pregnancy. No human data, but teratogenic in animal studies.

Breast Feeding Compatibility

No data. Not recommended.

COMMENTS

Voriconazole is active against *P. boydii*, *Fusarium* spp., *Candia* spp. (including *C. glabrata* and *C. krusei*), and aspergillosis. In the treatment of aspergillosis, voriconazole resulted in better clinical response at 12 wks compared to amphotericin. Generally well tolerated with reversible visual disturbances (blurriness, color changes, and enhanced vision) reported in 20.6% of pts. May be considered for the treatment of fluconazole resistant esophagitis but similar to itraconazole, up to 50% cross-resistance to other azoles has been reported.

BASIS FOR RECOMMENDATIONS

National Institutes of Health (NIH), the Centers for Disease Control and Prevention (CDC), and the HIV Medicine Association of the Infectious Diseases Society of America (HIVMA/IDSA). Guidelines for Prevention and Treatment of Opportunistic Infections in HIV-Infected Adults and Adolescents. *http://AIDSinfo.nih.gov*, 2008.

Comments: Voriconazole, posaconazole, amphotericin, anidulafungin, caspofungin, and micafungin can be considered in fluconazole- and itraconazole-refractory esophageal candidiasis.

SELECTED REFERENCES

Herbrecht R, Denning DW, Patterson TF, et al. Voriconazole versus amphotericin B for primary therapy of invasive aspergillosis. *N Engl J Med*, 2002; Vol. 347; pp. 408–15.

Pascual A, Calandra T, Bolay S, et al. Voriconazole therapeutic drug monitoring in pts with invasive mycoses improves efficacy and safety outcomes. *Clin Infect Dis*, 2008; Vol. 46; pp. 201–11.

Antimycobacterial

CAPREOMYCIN

Paul A. Pham, PharmD and John G. Bartlett, MD

INDICATIONS

FDA

- Pulmonary tuberculosis caused by *Mycobacterium tuberculosis* after failure w/ of primary medications (isoniazid, rifampin, pyrazinamide, aminosalicylic acid, ethambutol, and/or streptomycin)

FORMS

Brand name (mfr)	Forms	Cost*
Capastat (Lilly)	IV vial 1000 mg/10 mL	$26.60
*Prices represents Average Wholesale Price (AWP).		

ADULT DOSING

15–30 mg/kg/day (max: 1 G/day) IM or IV once daily or 2–3×/wk.

RENAL DOSING

Dosing for GFR 50–80: Usual dose.
Dosing for GFR 10–50: 7.5 mg/kg q1–2 days.
Dosing for GFR <10: 7.5 mg/kg 2 ×/wk.
Dosing in hemodialysis: 12–15 mg/kg 2–3×/wk.
Dosing in peritoneal dialysis: No additional doses needed after peritoneal dialysis.
Dosing in hemofiltration: No data.

ADVERSE DRUG REACTIONS

Common

- Nephrotoxicity (20–36%): tubular dysfunction, azotemia, proteinuria

Occasional

- Ototoxicity in 11% of pts (vestibular>auditory), monitor vestibular function before and during treatment
- Electrolyte abnormalities
- Pain, induration and sterile abscesses at injection sites (for IM administration)

Rare

- Allergic reactions
- Leukopenia or leukocytosis
- Neuromuscular blockade with large IV doses (reversed with neostigmine)
- Hepatitis

DRUG INTERACTIONS

Non-depolarizing muscle relaxants (atracurium, vecuronium, pancuronium, tubocurarine): neuromuscular blockade may be enhanced. Use with caution.

PHARMACOLOGY

Mechanism

Exact mechanism of action unknown but inhibits protein synthesis through ribosomal binding.

Pharmacokinetic Parameters

- **Absorption** Not absorbed in GI tract; IM absorption.
- **Cmax** No data.
- **Distribution** No data on tissue distribution. Highly concentrated in urine.
- **Protein Binding** No data.
- **Metabolism/Excretion** 50–60% excreted via glomerular filtration. Small amount of biliary excretion.
- **T1/2** 3–6 hrs.

Dosing for Decreased Hepatic Function

Usual dose.

ANTIMYCOBACTERIAL DRUGS

643

Pregnancy Risk

C: Animal studies show teratogenic effect ("wavy ribs" when given 3.5 times the human dose). Avoid in pregnancy.

Breast Feeding Compatibility

No data available.

COMMENTS

Parenteral aminoglycoside that is a second line TB agent for MDR-TB and XDR-TB (especially useful when there is streptomycin resistance). Vertigo, tinnitus and hearing loss has occurred in approximately 11% of pts. Use with caution in pts with impaired renal function. Tubular dysfunction and tubular necrosis has been reported in up to 36% of pts treated with capreomycin.

SELECTED REFERENCES

Chan ED, Laurel V, Strand MJ, et al. Treatment and outcome analysis of 205 pts with multidrug-resistant tuberculosis. *Am J Respir Crit Care Med*, 2004; Vol. 169; pp. 1103–9.

Mitnick CD, Shin SS, Seung KJ, et al. Comprehensive treatment of extensively drug-resistant tuberculosis. *NEJM*, 2008; Vol. 359; pp. 563–74.

CYCLOSERINE

Paul A. Pham, PharmD and John G. Bartlett, MD

INDICATIONS

FDA

- Second line tuberculosis treatment [combine w/ other antitubercular agents for failure of primary medications (e.g., pyrazinamide, isoniazid, rifampin, ethambutol +/– streptomycin)].
- Second line in the treatment of acute urinary tract infection treatment caused by *Enterobacter* spp. and *Escherichia coli* (generally not recommended).

FORMS

Brand name (mfr)	Forms	Cost*
Seromycin (The Chao Center)	PO cap 250 mg	$6.25
*Prices represents Average Wholesale Price (AWP).		

USUAL ADULT DOSING

- TB: 10–15 mg/kg/day (maximum daily dose 1000 mg, but hard to tolerate), usual dose is 500–750 mg per day given in two divided doses.
- Dose should be guided by serum concentration monitoring (1–2 hrs goal peak): 20–35 mg/ml.
- Seizures may be prevented with large doses of pyridoxine 100 mg PO q8h.

RENAL DOSING

Dosing for GFR 50–80: Usual dose (monitor cycloserine levels).

Dosing for GFR 10–50: Not recommended, due to accumulation.

Dosing for GFR <10: Not recommended unless pt is receiving HD.

Dosing in hemodialysis: 250 mg once daily or 500 mg 3×/wk. Monitor cycloserine serum concentrations.

Dosing in peritoneal dialysis: No data, no supplementation required. Monitor cycloserine serum concentrations.

Dosing in hemofiltration: No data. Monitor cycloserine serum concentrations.

ADVERSE DRUG REACTIONS

Common

- CNS: anxiety, confusion, somnolence, disorientation, headache, hallucinations, tremor, hyperreflexia, depression (with suicidal ideation), psychotic disturbances
- CNS toxicity associated with peak serum concentration greater than 30 mcg/mL

Occasional

- Increased CSF protein and pressure (dose related and reversible)
- Seizure (dose dependent, 3% with 500 mg/day and 8% with 1000 mg/day). Seizures may be prevented with large doses of pyridoxine 100 mg q8h

Rare
- Peripheral neuropathy
- Drug fever
- Rash
- Heart failure

DRUG INTERACTIONS
- Ethionamide: may increase risk of neurotoxicity. Monitor closely with co-administration.
- Isoniazid: may increase risk of peripheral neuropathy. Monitor closely with co-administration.
- Phenytoin: may increase phenytoin serum concentrations. May require phenytoin dose adjustments.

PHARMACOLOGY

Mechanism

Cycloserine inhibits cell wall synthesis in susceptible organisms by competing with d-alanine during peptidoglycan synthesis.

Pharmacokinetic Parameters
- **Absorption** 70–90% absorbed.
- **Cmax** 10 mcg/ml after 250 mg PO dose administration.
- **Distribution** Widely distributed into body tissue and fluids such as lung, bile, ascitic fluid, pleural fluid, synovial fluid, lymph, sputum. Good CSF penetration (80–100% of serum concentration attained in the CSF, higher level with inflamed meninges).
- **Protein binding** No data.
- **Metabolism/Excretion** 60–70% excreted unchanged in the urine via glomerular filtration. Small amount excreted in feces. Small amount metabolized.
- **T1/2** 10 hrs.

Dosing for Decreased Hepatic Function

No data. Usual dose likely.

Pregnancy Risk

C: The CDC does not recommend the use of cycloserine in pregnancy.

Breast Feeding Compatibility

No data.

COMMENTS

Second line agent for TB due to propensity for CNS side effects (e.g., somnolence; headache; tremor; dysarthria; vertigo; confusion and seizures) that tend to occur more frequently during the first 2 wks of therapy. Use with caution in pts with a psychiatric history due to reports of acute psychosis and paranoia. May be considered on a temporary basis in pts with acute hepatitis. Contraindicated in pts with a history of seizures. Generally reserved for MDRTB and XDRTB. Target peak concentration of 20–35 mg/l are often useful in determining the optimum dose for a given pt.

SELECTED REFERENCES

Chan ED, Laurel V, Strand MJ, et al. Treatment and outcome analysis of 205 pts with multidrug-resistant tuberculosis. *Am J Respir Crit Care Med,* 2004; Vol. 169; pp. 1103–9.

Mitnick CD, Shin SS, Seung KJ, et al. Comprehensive treatment of extensively drug-resistant tuberculosis. *NEJM,* 2008; Vol. 359; p. 563.

ETHAMBUTOL

Paul A. Pham, PharmD and John G. Bartlett, MD

INDICATIONS

FDA
- Treatment of all forms of TB in combination with other antituberculous drugs.

Non-FDA Approved Uses
- Treatment of *Mycobacterium avium* complex (MAC) infection (in combination with a macrolide).
- Treatment of *Mycobacterium kansasii* infection (in combination with INH and rifampin).

ANTIMYCOBACTERIAL DRUGS

ANTIMYCOBACTERIAL

FORMS

Brand name (mfr)	Forms	Cost*
Myambutol (Elan)	Oral tablet 100 mg; Oral tablet 400 mg	$0.59; $1.78

*Prices represents Average Wholesale Price (AWP).

USUAL ADULT DOSING
- TB: 15–20 mg/kg (max 2 g) once daily (plus INH, PZA, Rifamycin).
- DOT regimens: 50 mg/kg 2×/wk (max 4 g) or 25–30 mg/kg 3×/wk (max 2 g).
- MAC: 15 mg/kg/day (plus macrolide with or without rifabutin).
- *M. kansasii*: 15 mg/kg/day (max 2.5 g/day) (plus INH and Rifampin)

RENAL DOSING
Dosing for GFR 50–80: 15 mg/kg/ q24h (consider dose reduction with clearance, 70 mL/min).
Dosing for GFR 10–50: 15 mg/kg/ q24–36h. Monitor closely for visual acuity.
Dosing for GFR <10: 15 mg/kg/ q48h. Monitor closely for visual acuity.
Dosing in hemodialysis: 15–20 mg/kg post-HD 3×/wk.
Dosing in peritoneal dialysis: 15 mg/kg/q48 hrs.
Dosing in hemofiltration: No data. Consider dose reduction.

ADVERSE DRUG REACTIONS
Occasional
- Optic neuritis: decreased acuity, reduced color discrimination, constricted fields, and scotomata (infrequent with 15 mg/kg/day; increased risk w/ 25 mg/kg/day). Pts receiving 25 mg/kg/day should have baseline visual and color perception screening; repeated visual screening monthly. Ocular manifestation reversible with discontinuation, but irreversible blindness has been described.
- GI intolerance: anorexia, nausea, vomiting, and abdominal pain.

Rare
- Peripheral neuropathy.
- Hypersensitivity reaction.
- Confusion and dizziness.
- Acute gout.
- Hematologic: leukopenia, thrombocytopenia, eosinophilia, neutropenia, and lymphadenopathy.
- Dermatologic: rash, pruritus, dermatitis, and exfoliative dermatitis.
- Interstitial nephritis.

DRUG INTERACTIONS
- Ethionamide: may increase adverse effects of EMB.

PHARMACOLOGY
Mechanism
Mechanism of action not fully elucidated, but it appears to suppress multiplication by interfering with RNA synthesis.

Pharmacokinetic Parameters
- **Absorption** 75–80% absorbed.
- **Cmax** 2–5 mcg/mL after 25 mg/kg PO.
- **Distribution** Widely distributed to most tissues and fluids, attaining high concentrations in kidneys, lungs, saliva, and erythrocyte. Poor CSF concentration (therapeutic levels usually not attained). Penetrates CSF with inflammation and is indicated as part of a four drug regimen, but the added benefit of ethambutol has not been fully evaluated in TB meningitis.
- **Protein Binding** 22%.
- **Metabolism/Excretion** Partially metabolized in the liver. Both unchanged drug and metabolite are excreted in the urine. Unabsorbed drug excreted unchanged in the feces.
- **T1/2** 3–4 hrs.

Dosing for Decreased Hepatic Function
No data.

Pregnancy Risk
B: No congenital defects have been reported. CDC considers EMB safe in pregnancy
Breast Feeding Compatibility
Excreted in breast milk. American Academy of Pediatrics considers EMB compatible with breast feeding.

COMMENTS
First line agent in combination for treatment of MTB, MAC, *M. kansasii*. Monitor visual acuity in pts receiving higher doses (25 mg/kg/day).

SELECTED REFERENCES
American Thoracic Society, CDC, Infectious Diseases Society of America. Treatment of tuberculosis. *MMWR Recomm Rep*, 2003; Vol. 52; pp. 1–77.

Ward TT, Rimland D, Kauffman C, et al. Randomized, open-label trial of azithromycin plus ethambutol vs. clarithromycin plus ethambutol as therapy for Mycobacterium avium complex bacteremia in pts with human immunodeficiency virus infection. Veterans Affairs HIV Research Consortium. *Clin Infect Dis*, 1998; Vol. 27; pp. 1278–85.

ISONIAZID

Paul A. Pham, PharmD and John G. Bartlett, MD

INDICATIONS
FDA
• Treatment and prevention of TB (in combination).
Non-FDA Approved Uses
• Treatment of *M. kansasii* (in combination with EMB and RIF).

FORMS

Brand name (mfr)	Forms	Cost*
Isoniazid (Generic manufacturers [Barr, Eon and others])	Oral tablet 100 mg 300 mg Oral syrup 50 mg/5 mL (16oz)	$0.09, $0.34 $58.00
Nydrazid (Geneva)	IM vial 100 mg/mL (10 mL)	$24.90
Rifamate (Aventis)	Oral capsule INH 150 mg/RIF 300 mg	$3.71
Rifater (Aventis)	Oral capsule INH 50 mg/RIF 120 mg/pyrazinamide (PZA) 30 mg	$2.32
*Prices represents Average Wholesale Price (AWP).		

USUAL ADULT DOSING
• Treatment of latent TB (prophylaxis): INH 5 mg/kg (max 300 mg) PO daily × 9 mos or DOT: 15 mg/kg (max 900 mg) 2×/wk × 9 mos.
• Active TB treatment (with other anti-TB agents): 5 mg/kg (max 300 mg) PO daily × 6–9 mos or directly observed therapy (DOT): 15 mg/kg (max 900 mg) 2–3×/wk × 6–9 mos.
• Active TB treatment duration: 6 mos for most forms except severe cavitary pulmonary (9 mos), bone/joint (9 mos +), miliary (9 mos), CNS (9–12 mos).
• Coadminister with pyridoxine 50 mg/day or 100 mg 2×/wk to prevent neuropathy.
• DOT preferred for active TB in all pts.
• Obtain CBC and LFTs at baseline and periodically throughout course of therapy. Monitor monthly for hepatitis sx; consider monthly LFTs in pts with other risks for hepatotoxicity.
• Administer 1 hr before or 2 hrs after meals.
• Treatment of *M. kansasii*: isoniazid 300 mg daily plus pyridoxine 50 mg daily (in combination with ethambutol and rifampin +/– clarithromycin).

RENAL DOSING
Dosing for GFR 50–80: Usual dose.
Dosing for GFR 10–50: Usual dose.
Dosing for GFR <10: If slow acetylator use 150 mg PO once daily.

ANTIMYCOBACTERIAL DRUGS

Dosing in hemodialysis: 5 mg/kg/day dose post-dialysis on days of HD (50% of dose if slow acetylator).

Dosing in peritoneal dialysis: 5 mg/kg/day dose post-dialysis exchange (50% of dose if slow acetylator).

Dosing in hemofiltration: No data.

ADVERSE DRUG REACTIONS

Common

- Increased transaminases: increased ALT in 10–20% (d/c if LFTs >5× ULN).

Occasional

- GI intolerance (diarrhea with liquid INH, crushed tabs typically better tolerated in infants/children).

Rare

- Clinical hepatitis in 0.6% and fatal hepatitis in 0.02% (risk increased with age, alcohol, prior liver disease, concurrent RIF, and pregnancy). May occur even after mos on treatment. In most cases, enzyme levels return to normal with discontinuation of therapy. Recommend monthly clinical and lab monitoring. Instruct pts to report sxs of hepatitis. Discontinue if sxs or signs of hepatic damage. Consider non/less hepatotoxic alternatives. Reinstitute only after symptoms and lab abnormalities resolved. Restart with gradual dose escalation. Withdraw with any indication of recurrent liver damage.
- Peripheral neuropathy and optic neuropathy (dose-related and generally prevented by pyridoxine co-administration).
- Hypersensitivity reaction (rash, exfoliative dermatitis, urticaria, and edema).
- Fever.
- CNS toxicity: psychosis.
- Arthralgia.
- Bone marrow suppression.

DRUG INTERACTIONS

- Antacids: may decrease INH absorption (avoid co-administration).
- Benzodiazepines (e.g., diazepam, triazolam, midazolam): may increase benzodiazepine serum levels. Consider using oxazepam or lorazepam with INH co-administration.
- Carbamazepine: may increase carbamazepine levels. Monitor closely.
- Cycloserine: may increase central nervous system adverse effects. Monitor closely and discontinue if severe.
- Enflurane: in rapid acetylators of INH, high output renal failure may occur. Monitor closely.
- Ethanol: May increase risk of hepatotoxicity. Avoid.
- Ethionamide: may increase INH serum level. Monitor for toxicity (peripheral neuritis and hepatotoxicity) with co-administration.
- Ketoconazole: may decrease ketoconazole levels (based on case reports, clinical significance unknown).
- Phenytoin: may increase phenytoin levels. Monitor closely.
- Prednisone and prednisolone: may decrease INH serum levels. Monitor INH for therapeutic efficacy.
- Rifampin: possible additive hepatotoxicity due to production of secondary pathway metabolite of INH (hydrazine and isonicotinic acid). Clinical significance unknown.
- Theophylline: serum level may be increased. Monitor theophylline serum concentrations, dose may need to be decreased.
- Tyramine rich foods (wine, cheese, etc.): may develop monoamine poisoning (avoid tyramine rich foods).
- Warfarin: may increase INR, monitor closely.

PHARMACOLOGY

Mechanism

Inhibits mycolic acid synthesis which results in loss of acid-fastness and disruption of bacterial cell wall. May interfere with metabolism of bacterial proteins, nucleic acid, lipids and carbohydrate.

Pharmacokinetic Parameters

- **Absorption** 90%; readily absorbed.
- **Cmax** 3–7 mcg/ml after 300 mg PO.

- **Distribution** 0.57–0.76 L/kg; widely distributed in all fluid and tissue, pleural and ascitic fluid, skin, sputum, saliva, lungs, muscle and caseous tissue. Good CSF penetration (20–90% of serum levels attained in the CSF); therapeutic level attained in CSF.
- **Protein Binding** 0–10%.
- **Metabolism/Excretion** Hepatic acetylation via N-acetyl transferase (rate of acetylation is genetically determined). 75–95% excreted by the kidney mainly as inactive metabolite (90% as metabolite in fast acetylator, 63% as metabolite in slow acetylator). Approximately 50% of whites and AA are slow acetylators. Rate of acetylation not affect efficacy of standard daily or DOT regimens.
- **T1/2** 0.5–4 hrs.

Dosing for Decreased Hepatic Function

Use with caution in hepatic impairment. Use is contraindicated if acute liver disease or history of INH-associated hepatitis.

Pregnancy Risk

C: Animal studies show embryocidal effect, but not teratogenic. Retrospective analysis of more than 4900 exposures to INH did not result in an increased rate of fetal malformation. Pregnant women with active TB should be treated immediately. The American Academy of Pediatrics recommends that pregnant women with + PPD should receive INH if HIV +, have recent contact or X-ray showing old TB; begin after 1st trimester if possible. Treatment of latent TB should be deferred in pts with acute hepatic diseases.

Breast Feeding Compatibility

Excreted in breast milk at levels insufficient for tx of active or latent TB. The American Academy of Pediatrics considers INH compatible with breast feeding.

COMMENTS

First line agent for treatment and prophylaxis of TB. Because of high prevalence of INH resistance, treatment with RIF-containing regimen should be strongly considered in the treatment of latent TB for immigrants from Vietnam, Haiti, and the Philippines [*NEJM* 2002;347:1850].

SELECTED REFERENCES

American Thoracic Society. Targeted tuberculin testing and treatment of latent tuberculosis infection. This official statement of the American Thoracic Society was adopted by the ATS Board of Directors, July 1999. This is a Joint Statement of the American Thoracic Society (ATS) and the Centers for Disease Control and Prevention (CDC). This statement was endorsed by the Council of the Infectious Diseases Society of America. (IDSA), September 1999, and the sections of this statement. *Am J Respir Crit Care Med*, 2000; Vol. 161; pp. S221–47.

Blumberg HM, Burman WJ, Chaisson RE, et al. American Thoracic Society/Centers for Disease Control and Prevention/Infectious Diseases Society of America: treatment of tuberculosis. *Am J Respir Crit Care Med*, 2003; Vol. 167; pp. 603–62.

PYRAZINAMIDE

Paul A. Pham, PharmD and John G. Bartlett, MD

INDICATIONS

FDA

- TB (active, latent) treatment (in combination with other antituberculous drugs).

FORMS

Brand name (mfr)	Forms	Cost*
Pyrazinamide (Several generic manufacturers [Stada, UD, and others])	Oral tablet 500 mg	$1.19
Rifater (Aventis)	Oral capsule PZA 300 mg/ INH 50 mg / RIF 120 mg	$1.92
*Prices represents Average Wholesale Price (AWP).		

USUAL ADULT DOSING

- Active TB (induction phase): 20–25 mg/kg (max 2 g) once daily in combination with rifampin (RIF), ethambutol (EMB), and isoniazid (INH) × 8 wks.

- DOT active TB treatment (in combination with RIF + EMB + INH): 40–55 kg: 1500 mg 3×/wk or 2000 mg 2×/wk; 56–75 kg: 2500 3×/wk or 3000 mg 2×/wk; 76–90 kg: 3000 mg 3×/wk or 4000 mg 2×/wk. Max dose: 2000 mg/day; 3000 mg 3×/wk; 4000 mg 2×/wk.
- Pts with CD4 <100 should receive once daily or 3×/wk therapy for active TB.
- PZA + RIF × 2 mos for treatment of latent TB no longer recommended by the CDC due to hepatotoxicity in HIV and non-HIV infected pts; however, a subsequent analysis showed no deaths or serious reactions among the 792 HIV-infected pts who took RIF/PZA; the rate of AST >250 U/l at 2 mos was 2.1% (*CID* 2004; 39: 561).
- Treatment with *Rifat*er: wt. <65 kg 1 tab/10 kg/day; > 65 kg 6 tabs/day.

RENAL DOSING
Dosing for GFR 50–80: Usual dose.
Dosing for GFR 10–50: Usual dose.
Dosing for GFR <10: 12–20 mg/kg/day. Risk of hyperuricemia may be increased.
Dosing in hemodialysis: Usual dose post-HD on days of HD. Risk of hyperuricemia may be increased.
Dosing in peritoneal dialysis: No data. Avoid if possible.
Dosing in hemofiltration: No data.

ADVERSE DRUG REACTIONS
For Rifater ADRs see also INH and RIF
Common
- Non-gouty polyarthralgia (up to 40%, treat with ASA)
- Asymptomatic hyperuricemia
Occasional
- Dose related hepatitis (1% at 25 mg/kg, but up to 15% with >3 g/day). Monitor for sxs suggestive of hepatitis at baseline and 2, 4, 6, and 8 wks. Bilirubin, AST and ALT at baseline and 2, 4 and 6 wks. Discontinue if LFTs >5 × ULN asymptomatic pt or at any level above the normal range in symptomatic pt. Risk increased with alcohol consumption.
- GI intolerance.
Rare
- Gout (treat w/ allopurinol and probenecid). Discontinue and do not restart if hyperuricemia accompanied by acute gouty arthritis.

DRUG INTERACTIONS
For *Rifater* Drug Interactions see also INH and RIF.
- Ethionamide: may increase risk of hepatotoxicity.

RESISTANCE
- XDR TB: resistant to at least the first-line anti-TB drugs isoniazid and rifampin, as well as any fluoroquinolone and at least one of three second-line injectable TB drugs.

PHARMACOLOGY
Mechanism
Converted to pyrazinoic acid (in susceptible strains). Pyrazinoic acid may lower pH of local environment below that necessary for growth of *M. tuberculosis;* also may have direct antimycobacterial activity though unknown mechanism.
Pharmacokinetic Parameters
- **Absorption** Near complete absorption.
- **Cmax** 30–50 mcg/ml after 20–25 mg/kg oral dose.
- **Distribution** Widely distributed into body tissues and fluids. Good levels in liver and lungs. Good CNS penetration, with therapeutic levels attained (85–100% of serum levels).
- **Protein Binding** 17%.
- **Metabolism/Excretion** Metabolized in liver to pyrazoic acid (active metabolite). Both metabolite and small amount of unchanged drug are excreted in urine.
- **T1/2** 9.5 hrs.
Dosing for Decreased Hepatic Function
Consider withholding. Consult with a TB expert.
Pregnancy Risk
C: No animal data available. No human data available. For active TB tx during pregnancy, CDC guidelines for U.S. are INH + RIF + EMB (without PZA, due to insufficient safety data) for 2 mos

then INH + RIF for additional 7 mos (9 mos total). Worldwide, the W.H.O. recommends PZA for routine use in pregnant women with active TB.

Breast Feeding Compatibility

Excreted in breast milk.

Comments

1st line agent in combination with other antituberculous drugs for TB treatment. Monitor LFTs closely with RIF co-administration; use with caution in pts with gout due to potential for PZA-induced hyperuricemia.

Selected References

Blumberg HM, Burman WJ, Chaisson RE, et al. American Thoracic Society/Centers for Disease Control and Prevention/Infectious Diseases Society of America: treatment of tuberculosis. *Am J Respir Crit Care Med*, 2003; Vol. 167; pp. 603–62.

Centers for Disease Control and Prevention (CDC). Emergence of mycobacterium tuberculosis with extensive resistance to second-line drugs—worldwide, 2000–2004. *MMWR*, 2007; Vol. 55; pp. 301–305.

RIFABUTIN

Paul Pham, PharmD and John G. Bartlett, MD

Indications

FDA

- Prophylaxis of *Mycobacterium avium* complex (MAC) in pts with AIDS.

Non-FDA Approved Uses

- Treatment of disseminated MAC in pts with AIDS (in combination with macrolide plus ethambutol).
- Treatment of TB in pts with AIDS who are taking PIs or NNRTIs.
- Treatment of latent TB in pts intolerant to INH. Rifabutin × 4 mos can be considered.

Forms

Brand name (mfr)	Forms	Cost*
Mycobutin (Pfizer)	Oral capsule 150 mg	$12.18
*Prices represents Average Wholesale Price (AWP).		

Usual Adult Dosing

- MAC prophylaxis: 300 mg PO once daily (azithromycin preferred).
- MAC treatment: 5 mg/kg (300 mg) PO once daily combined with ethambutol and clarithromycin or azithromycin.
- With HIV protease inhibitors (PIs), HIV non-nucleoside reverse transcriptase inhibitors, integrase inhibitors, and CCR5 blockers: see drug-drug interaction section for dose recommendations.

Renal Dosing

Dosing for GFR 50–80: Usual dose.

Dosing for GFR 10–50: 50% of dose once daily with CrCL <30 ml/min.

Dosing for GFR <10: 50% of dose once daily.

Dosing in hemodialysis: No data, no supplementation needed.

Dosing in peritoneal dialysis: No data.

Dosing in hemofiltration: No data.

Adverse Drug Reactions

Common

- Orange discoloration of urine, tears, and sweat

Occasional

- Uveitis: seen with high doses, dose-related (≥600 mg/day or concurrent use with CYP3A4 inhibitors such as fluconazole, clarithromycin or most PIs). Discontinue immediately and consult an ophthalmologist.

Rare

- Neutropenia
- Hepatotoxicity (<1%)
- Pseudo jaundice (w/ normal bilirubin)

ANTIMYCOBACTERIAL DRUGS

DRUG INTERACTIONS—See Appendix III, p. 830, for table of drug-to-drug interactions.
Pharmacology
Mechanism
Inhibits initiation of chain formation for RNA synthesis by inhibiting DNA-dependent RNA polymerase.
Pharmacokinetic Parameters
- **Absorption** 20%.
- **Cmax** 375 ng/ml after 300 mg.
- **Distribution** Widely distributed with high intracellular uptake due to high lipophilicity. 50% of serum concentration penetrates into CSF; penetrates inflamed meninges.
- **Protein Binding** 85%.
- **Metabolism/Excretion** Extensive hepatic metabolism via CYP3A4 (25–O-desacetyl and 31–hydroxy most predominant metabolite; activity equivalent to rifabutin). CYP3A4 inducer, although effect less pronounced than rifampin. Metabolites excreted in urine. 30% of drug also excreted in feces. Small amount of drug excreted unchanged in urine and bile.
- **T1/2** 2–4 hrs.
Dosing for Decreased Hepatic Function
Dose reduction may be necessary with severe liver dysfunction. Use with caution.
Pregnancy Risk
B: Animal data show skeletal abnormalities. No human data available.
Breast Feeding Compatibility
No data available.

COMMENTS
Addition of rifabutin to clarithromycin + ethambutol in treatment of disseminated MAC has been debated. Fear of drug interactions should not deter clinicians, since rifabutin may have survival benefit in addition to protecting against macrolide resistance. The addition of rifabutin should be considered in pts with advanced immunosuppression, high mycobacterial burden, or in the absence of effective ART. Good alternative to rifampin for treatment of active and latent TB when needed for concurrent use with highly active antiretroviral therapy (HAART).

BASIS FOR RECOMMENDATIONS
Department of Health and Human Services Centers for Disease Control and Prevention. Managing Drug Interactions in the Treatment of HIV-Related Tuberculosis, 2007.
Comments: Recommendations on the management of drug interactions between rifamycin and ARVs.

SELECTED REFERENCES
Benson CA, Williams PL, Currier JS, et al. A prospective, randomized trial examining the efficacy and safety of clarithromycin in combination with ethambutol, rifabutin, or both for the treatment of disseminated Mycobacterium avium complex disease in persons with acquired immunodeficiency syndrome. *Clin Infect Dis*, 2003; Vol. 37; pp. 1234–43.
Di Mario F, Cavallaro LG, Scarpignato C. 'Rescue' therapies for the management of Helicobacter pylori infection. *Dig Dis*, 2006; Vol. 24; pp. 113–30.

RIFAMPIN see p. 582 in Antibacterial Section

RIFAPENTINE

Paul A. Pham, PharmD and John G. Bartlett, MD

INDICATIONS
FDA
- Tuberculosis (in combination with other anti-tubercular drugs).

FORMS

Brand name (mfr)	Forms	Cost*
Priftin (Aventis)	PO cap 150 mg	$3.63
*Prices represents Average Wholesale Price (AWP).		

USUAL ADULT DOSING
- Induction phase: 600 mg PO twice weekly for two mos (in combination with INH, PZA and ethambutol in immunocompetent pts).
- Continuation phase: 10 mg/kg (600 mg) PO q wk (w/ INH as part of the continuation phase in HIV-negative pts only) or 600 mg PO 2 ×/wk.

RENAL DOSING
Dosing for GFR 50–80: Usual dose.
Dosing for GFR 10–50: Usual dose likely (only 17% excreted via kidneys).
Dosing for GFR <10: Usual dose likely (only 17% excreted via kidneys).
Dosing in hemodialysis: Usual dose, not removed in HD.
Dosing in peritoneal dialysis: No data; usual dose likely.
Dosing in hemofiltration: No data; usual dose likely.

ADVERSE DRUG REACTIONS
Common
- Orange discoloration of urine, tears (contact lens), sweat

Occasional
- Hepatitis
- Flu-like syndrome
- GI intolerance

Rare
- Hypersensitivity
- Thrombocytopenia and hemolytic anemia
- Headache and dizziness

DRUG INTERACTIONS — See Appendix III, p. 833, for table of drug-to-drug interactions.
Substrate and potent inducer of CYP3A4. Inducer of CYP 2B6, 2C8, 2C9, 2C19, and 2D6, and glucuronosyltransferase. May significantly decrease serum concentrations of CYP 3A4, 2B6, 2C8, 2C9, 2C19, and 2D6 substrates. Inducers of CYP3A4 may decrease rifapentine drug concentrations. Inhibitors of CYP3A4 may increase rifapentine drug concentrations.

PHARMACOLOGY
Mechanism
Rifapentine inhibits initiation of chain formation for RNA synthesis by inhibiting DNA-dependent RNA polymerase.

Pharmacokinetic Parameters
- **Absorption** Well absorbed.
- **Cmax** Mean AUC of 325 mcg-hr/ml after 600 mg dose.
- **Distribution** Widely distributed. CNS penetration: no data.
- **Protein Binding** 93–97%.
- **Metabolism/Excretion** Hepatic metabolism to active deacetylated metabolite. 70% excreted via biliary excretion. 17% excreted in the urine. Autoinduction at steady-state.
- **T1/2** 16–19 hrs.

Dosing for Decreased Hepatic Function
No data.

Pregnancy Risk
C: Animal data demonstrated teratogenicity. No adequate data is available in humans. Administration in last wks of pregnancy may cause postnatal hemorrhage. Most experts feel that rifamycins have not proven teratogenic and recommend use of the drug with INH and ethambutol if necessary.

Breast Feeding Compatibility
No data.

COMMENTS
Oral rifamycin with a prolonged half-life. May be used once weekly w/ INH in the continuation phase treatment in HIV-negative pts with noncavitary, drug-susceptible pulmonary TB who have negative sputum smears at completion of the initial phase of treatment. Once weekly dosing should not be used in HIV-infected pts due to a high relapse rate and the development of rifamycin resistance. Short course (3 mos) INH + rifapentine is under investigation for latent TB.

ANTIMYCOBACTERIAL DRUGS

SELECTED REFERENCES

Benator D, Bhattacharya M, Bozeman L, et al. Rifapentine and isoniazid once a wk versus rifampicin and isoniazid twice a wk for treatment of drug-susceptible pulmonary tuberculosis in HIV-negative pts: a randomised clinical trial. *Lancet*, 2002; Vol. 360; pp. 528–34.

Vernon A, Burman W, Benator D, et al. Acquired rifamycin monoresistance in pts with HIV-related tuberculosis treated with once-weekly rifapentine and isoniazid. *Lancet*, 1999; Vol. 353; pp. 1843–47.

STREPTOMYCIN see p. 585 in Antibacterial Section

Antiparasitic

ALBENDAZOLE

Paul A. Pham, PharmD and John G. Bartlett, MD

INDICATIONS

FDA

- Neurocysticercosis caused by *Taenia solium*.
- Hydatid disease caused by *Echinococcus granulosis*.

Non-FDA Approved Uses

- Microsporidiosis
- Trichuris

FORMS

Brand name (mfr)	Forms	Cost*
Albenza (GlaxoSmithKline)	Oral tablet 200 mg	$1.65
Eskazole; Zentel (non-U.S. brands) (non-U.S. manufacturer)	Oral tablet 200 mg	n/a
*Prices represents Average Wholesale Price (AWP).		

USUAL ADULT DOSING

- Hydatid (echinococcal) disease: 400 mg PO twice daily with meals × 28 days followed by a 14-day drug-free interval for a total of 3 cycles. Note: when medically feasible, surgery is considered the treatment of choice.
- Neurocysticercosis: 400 mg PO twice daily with meals for 8 to 30 days with corticosteroid during the first wk of treatment in order to prevent cerebral hypertensive episodes.
- Hookworm: 400 mg PO × single dose.
- Microsporidiosis: 400 mg PO twice daily with meals (AIDS: treat until CD4 count >200).
- Toxocariasis: 400 mg PO twice daily with meals × 5 days.

RENAL DOSING

Dosing for GFR 50–80: Usual dose.
Dosing for GFR 10–50: Usual dose.
Dosing for GFR <10: Usual dose.
Dosing in hemodialysis: Not removed in hemodialysis. Use usual dose.
Dosing in peritoneal dialysis: No data.
Dosing in hemofiltration: No data. Usual dose likely.

ADVERSE DRUG REACTIONS

General

- Generally well tolerated

Occasional

- Reversible hepatoxicity (monitor LFTs q2wks)
- GI intolerance: nausea, vomiting, diarrhea and abdominal pain

Rare

- Bone marrow suppression (e.g., pancytopenia, aplastic anemia, agranulocytosis, and leukopenia), especially in pts with liver disease, including echinococcosis.
- Dizziness and headache.
- Hypersensitivity reaction.
- Alopecia.

DRUG INTERACTIONS

- Dexamethasone: some case reports describe trough concentration of albendazole increased up to 56%. Monitor for albendazole toxicity; dose may need to be decreased.

ANTIPARASITIC DRUGS

- Praziquantel: some case reports show mean plasma concentration of albendazole increased up to 50%. Monitor adverse events of albendazole. Dose of albendazole may need to be decreased.

PHARMACOLOGY
Mechanism
Albendazole causes degenerative alterations in the tegument and intestinal cells of the parasite by inhibiting its polymerization into microtubules; this results in the inability to uptake glucose by the larva and adult stage.

Pharmacokinetic Parameters
- **Absorption** Poor and erratic absorption (enhanced 5-fold with fatty food).
- **Cmax** 1.3 mcg/mL after 400 mg PO dose administration.
- **Distribution** Distributed in bile, hydatid cyst and CSF.
- **Protein binding** 70%.
- **Metabolism/Excretion** Hepatic metabolism to active sulfoxide metabolite then excreted by enterohepatic circulation. Metabolites excreted in urine. Only a small amount is found in the feces.
- **T1/2** 8–9 hrs.

Dosing for Decreased Hepatic Function
No data.

Pregnancy Risk
C: Teratogenicity demonstrated in laboratory animals. Avoid in first trimester of pregnancy.

Breast Feeding Compatibility
Unknown.

COMMENTS
Well-tolerated oral, broad-spectrum anti-helminthic. An effective agent against microsporidiosis involving *Encephalitozoon intestinalis*. Unfortunately, 80% of microsporidiosis in AIDS are caused by *Enterocytozoon bieneusi*, which has poor response to albendazole. Albendazole (400 mg × 1) resulted in higher cure rate compared to mebendazole in the treatment of *Ascaris*, hookworm, and *Trichuris*. In the treatment of Hydatid disease, surgery is considered the treatment of choice since clinical cure is achieved in only ~30% of pts with medical therapy alone.

SELECTED REFERENCES
Kelly P, Lungu F, Keane E, et al. Albendazole chemotherapy for treatment of diarrhoea in pts with AIDS in Zambia: a randomised double blind controlled trial. *BMJ*, 1996; Vol. 312; pp. 1187–91.

Molina JM, Chastang C, Goguel J, et al. Albendazole for treatment and prophylaxis of microsporidiosis due to *Encephalitozoon intestinalis* in pts with AIDS: a randomized double-blind controlled trial. *J Infect Dis*, 1998; Vol. 177; pp. 1373–7.

ARTESUNATE

Paul A. Pham, PharmD

INDICATIONS
FDA
- Not FDA approved, but now available for emergency use in the United States (contact CDC) for severe falciparum malaria.

Non-FDA Approved Uses
- Mild to moderate malaria falciparum.

FORMS

Brand name (mfr)	Forms	Cost*
Artesunate (Available through a treatment IND in the U.S. [call the CDC: 1-770-488-7788])	IM or IV Ampules 60 mg (anhydrous artesunic acid)	n/a
*Prices represents Average Wholesale Price (AWP).		

USUAL ADULT DOSING

- U.S. treatment IND (CDC): 4 equal doses of artesunate 2.4 mg/kg each over a 3-day period followed by oral treatment with atovaquone-proguanil, doxycycline, clindamycin, or mefloquine (to avoid emergence of resistance).
- WHO recommendations: IV artesunate 2.4 mg/kg IV or IM given on admission (time = 0), then 12 hrs and 24 hrs, then once a day in low transmission area or outside the malaria endemic area.
- Ongoing phase II trial for the treatment of severe malaria: artesunate 2.4 mg/kg/dose IV over 3 days with dosings at 0, 12, 24, 48 and 72 hrs. For quinine-resistant *P. falciparum*, combine with tetracycline or mefloquine.

RENAL DOSING

Dosing for GFR 50–80: Usual dose.
Dosing for GFR 10–50: Usual dose.
Dosing for GFR <10: Usual dose.
Dosing in hemodialysis: Usual dose.
Dosing in peritoneal dialysis: No data. Usual dose likely.
Dosing in hemofiltration: No data. Usual dose likely.

ADVERSE DRUG REACTIONS

General

- Generally well tolerated

Occasional

- Bradycardia
- Dizziness
- Nausea and vomiting

Rare

- Cerebellar dysfunction (ataxic gait, slurred speech)
- Hypersensitivity reactions
- Seizure

DRUG INTERACTIONS

No known drug interactions. However, artesunate is a substrate of CYP3A4.

- Clarithromycin, erythromycin, and telithromycin: may increase artesunate serum concentrations.
- CYP3A4 inducers (e.g., rifampin, rifapentine, rifabutin, phenytoin, carbamazepine, phenobarbital): may decrease artesunate serum concentrations. Avoid co-administration if possible. Monitor closely for therapeutic efficacy; artesunate dose may need to be increased with co-administration.
- Ketoconazole, fluconazole, itraconazole, voriconazole, and posaconazole: may increase artesunate serum concentrations.
- Protease-inhibitors, HIV: may increase artesunate serum concentrations.

RESISTANCE

- The genetic events conferring to for artemisinin resistance are uncommon. These genetic events may result in moderate changes in drug susceptibility, such that the drug still remains effective (e.g., as in the 108AsnDHFR mutation for pyrimethamine resistance) or, less commonly, very large reductions in susceptibility such that achievable concentrations of the drug are completely ineffective (e.g., as the cytochrome B mutations giving rise to atovaquone resistance).

PHARMACOLOGY

Mechanism

Derivative of artemisinin (other antimalarial members of this group include artemether, arteether and dihydroartemisinin), from the sweet wormwood plant. Antimalarial activity dependent on endoperoxide (radical) interaction with intraparasitic heme, which is lethal through the accumulation of non-polymerizable redox-active heme adducts.

Pharmacokinetic Parameters

- **Absorption** Rapidly absorbed after IM administration.
- **Cmax** Artesunate/dihydroartemisinin: 16 mcg/mL / 2.7 mcg/mL following 120 mg IV administration.

- **Distribution** *In vitro* data: significant dihydroartemisinin accumulation in *Plasmodium falciparum*-infected erythrocytes (erythrocyte/plasma ratio, 300)—Vd = 0.2 to 1.5 L/kg.
- **Protein binding** High.
- **Metabolism/Excretion** Rapidly converted to dihydroartemisinin (active metabolite) with extensive hydrolysis via plasma and tissue cholinesterases.
- **T1/2** Dihydroartemisinin $t_{1/2}$ = 45 min, but following IM administration elimination $t_{1/2}$ phase is prolonged because of continued absorption.

Dosing for Decreased Hepatic Function
Usual dose.

Pregnancy Risk
No evidence of physical or neurological abnormalities during development observed with first trimester exposure in small studies (n = 44 in SE Asia, n = 80 in Africa). WHO recommends artesunate as a first line agent in second and third trimesters, while in first trimester, until more evidence becomes available, both artesunate and quinine may be considered.

Breast Feeding Compatibility
No significant physical or neurological abnormalities during development observed with breast-feeding.

COMMENTS
IV artesunate provides U.S. clinicians an alternative to IV quinidine (in case of unavailability or failure/intolerance/contraindication of quinidine) for the treatment of severe malaria falciparum.

- Eligibility criteria for IV artesunate under CDC's IND protocol: (1) severe malaria falciparum, (2) high-density parasitemia (>5%), (3) unable to take oral medications, (4) acute respiratory distress syndrome or severe anemia. In addition, for these pts, one of the following must be true: (1) artesunate is available more rapidly than quinidine (if the drugs are equally available, attending clinicians will decide which drug to use in consultation with CDC), (2) the pt has experienced quinidine failure or intolerance, or (3) use of quinidine is contraindicated.
- In a small randomized trial, IV artesunate resulted in a higher survival rate compared to IV quinine.
- Based on the level of resistance in Africa, artemisinin-based combination therapy (artemether-lumefantrine and artesunate + amodiaquine) is currently the WHO recommended treatment of choice for the treatment of uncomplicated falciparum malaria.

BASIS FOR RECOMMENDATIONS
WHO. Guidelines for treatment of malaria. *www.who.int/malaria/docs/TreatmentGuidelines2006.pdf*.
Comments: WHO malaria treatment guidelines.

SELECTED REFERENCES
Newton P, Angus BJ, Chierkul W, et al. Randomised comparison of intravenous artesunate or quinine in the treatment of severe falciparum malaria. *Clin Infect Dis*, 2003; Vol. 37; pp. 7–16.

ATOVAQUONE

Paul A. Pham, PharmD and John G. Bartlett, MD

INDICATIONS
FDA
- Atovaquone in combination with proguanil indicated for the prevention and treatment of malaria due to *Plasmodium falciparum* (including chloroquine-resistant strains) in adults and pediatric pts weighing 5–11 kg.
- Prevention of *Pneumocystis jiroveci* pneumonia in pts who are intolerant to TMP-SMX.
- Oral treatment of mild-to-moderate *Pneumocystis jiroveci* pneumonia (2nd or 3rd line).

Non-FDA Approved Uses
- Toxoplasmosis treatment alone (limited data with atovaquone 750 mg four times a day).
- Toxoplasmosis treatment in combination with pyrimethamine or sulfadiazine.
- Babesiosis.

FORMS

Brand name (mfr)	Forms	Cost*
Mepron (GlaxoSmithKline)	Oral Suspension 750 mg/5 mL (210 mL)	$941.96 per 210 mL (21-day supply)
Malarone (GlaxoSmithKline)	Oral Tablet 250 g/100 mg; Oral Tablet 62.5 mg/25 mg	$6.81; $2.51
*Prices represents Average Wholesale Price (AWP).		

USUAL ADULT DOSING
- Treatment of mild-to-moderate PCP (A-a O_2 gradient <35 mmHg and PAO2 >60 mmHg): 750 mg (5 mL) PO twice daily × 21 days with food.
- PCP prophylaxis: 750 mg PO twice daily or 1500 mg PO once daily with food.
- *P. falciparum* treatment: Malarone 4 tabs/day (1000 mg/400 mg) × 3 days with food.
- Malaria prophylaxis: Malarone 1 tab (250 mg/100 mg) once daily with food (beginning 1–2 days before and ending 1 wk after travel).
- Toxoplasmosis (alternative to pyrimethamine + sulfadiazine or clindamycin): atovaquone 1500 mg PO twice daily with food combined with pyrimethamine 200 mg × 1, then followed by 75 mg/day.
- Babesiosis: 750 mg PO q12 hrs plus azithromycin (500 × day 1, then 250 mg q24h) × 7–10 days.

RENAL DOSING
Dosing for GFR 50–80: Usual dose.
Dosing for GFR 10–50: Usual dose.
Dosing for GFR <10: Usual dose.
Dosing in hemodialysis: Usual dose.
Dosing in peritoneal dialysis: Usual dose.
Dosing in hemofiltration: No data.

ADVERSE DRUG REACTIONS
General
- Up to 7–9% discontinued due to side effects (rash accounts for 4% of discontinuances).
Common
- Rash (20%).
- GI intolerance and diarrhea (20%).
Rare
- Stevens-Johnson syndrome reported with Malarone (CID 2003;37E5–7).
- Headache.
- Fever.
- Insomnia.
- LFTs elevation and severe hepatitis (atovaquone/proguanil prophylactic use). A single case of hepatic failure requiring liver transplantation has been reported.

DRUG INTERACTIONS
- Atovaquone serum levels increased by 70% with food and up to 6-fold with fatty meal.
- AZT: AZT AUC increased by 31% with concomitant atovaquone. Clinical significance unknown. Monitor for AZT associated anemia.
- Rifabutin: decreases atovaquone AUC by 34%.
- Rifampin: decreases atovaquone AUC by 50%. Avoid co-administration.
- Tetracycline: decreases atovaquone AUC by 40%. Avoid co-administration.

RESISTANCE
Pneumocystis jiroveci, *Plasmodium falciparum* (when atovaquone combined with proguanil), and *Toxoplasma gondii*.

PHARMACOLOGY
Mechanism
Not well understood but may inhibit mitochondrial electron-transport chain of *Plasmodium falciparum*.

ANTIPARASITIC DRUGS

Pharmacokinetic Parameters
- **Absorption** 47% (liquid formulation) with meals. Significant individual variation in absorption.
- **Cmax** 24 mcg/mL (suspension).
- **Distribution** Poor CSF penetration (<1%); Vd = 0.6 L/kg.
- **Protein binding** >99.9%.
- **Metabolism/Excretion** Excreted in the feces; 0.6% renal excretion.
- **T1/2** 2.2–2.9 days.

Dosing for Decreased Hepatic Function
No data.

Dosing Pregnancy Risk
C: Not teratogenic in animal studies; no studies in humans.

Breast Feeding Compatibility
No human data, breast milk excretion in animal studies.

COMMENTS
Pro: equivalent to dapsone for PCP prophylaxis. Combination drug malarone is effective and well tolerated compared to weekly mefloquine for malaria prophylaxis.
Con: high cost, GI intolerance, and needs to be administered with a fatty meal. Inferior to TMP/SMX for the treatment of PCP.

SELECTED REFERENCES
Chirgwin K, Hafner R, Leport C, et al. Randomized phase II trial of atovaquone with pyrimethamine or sulfadiazine for treatment of toxoplasmic encephalitis in pts with acquired immunodeficiency syndrome: ACTG 237/ANRS 039 Study. AIDS Clinical Trials Group 237/Agence Nationale de Recherche sur le SIDA, Essai 039. *Clin Infect Dis*, 2002; Vol. 34; pp. 1243–50.

Krause PJ, Lepore T, Sikand VK, et al. Atovaquone and azithromycin for the treatment of babesiosis. *N Engl J Med*, 2000; Vol. 343; pp. 1454–8.

ATOVAQUONE + PROGUANIL

Paul A. Pham, PharmD and Joseph Vinetz, MD

INDICATIONS

FDA
- *P. falciparum* malaria prophylaxis and treatment

Non-FDA Approved Uses
- *Plasmodium vivax*

FORMS

Brand name (mfr)	Forms	Cost*
Malarone (Glaxo Smithkline)	PO tab 62.5 mg/25 mg PO tab 250 mg/100 mg	$2.26 $6.12
*Prices represents Average Wholesale Price (AWP).		

USUAL ADULT DOSING
- Treatment of malaria: atovaquone 1000 mg/proguanil 400 mg (4 tabs, single dose) PO daily × 3 days.
- Prevention of malaria: atovaquone 250 mg/proguanil 100 mg (1 tab) once daily beginning 1–2 days before travel and continuing for 1 wk after leaving endemic area.

RENAL DOSING
Dosing for GFR 50–80: Usual dose.
Dosing for GFR 10–50: No data.
Dosing for GFR <10: No data, may need to be decreased.
Dosing in hemodialysis: No data, unlikely to be removed.
Dosing in peritoneal dialysis: No data, unlikely to be removed.
Dosing in hemofiltration: No data.

ADVERSE DRUG REACTIONS
General
- Malarone side effect profile comparable to the placebo in studies.

Occasional
- GI: abdominal pain, nausea, vomiting, diarrhea, anorexia
- Headache, asthenia, dizziness (generally with treatment doses)
- Reversible elevation of LFTs

Rare
- Stevens-Johnson syndrome

DRUG INTERACTIONS
- Atazanavir/ritonavir: compared to historical control, atovaquone and proguanil AUC decreased by 33% and 74%, respectively with ATV/r co-administration. Consider alternative or increasing atovaquone + proguanil with ATV/r co-administration.
- Efavirenz: compared to historical control, atovaquone and proguanil AUC decreased by 69% and 58%, respectively with EFV co-administration. Consider alternative or increasing atovaquone + proguanil with EFV co-administration.
- Lopinavir/ritonavir: compared to historical control, atovaquone and proguanil AUC decreased by 65% and 68%, respectively with LPV/r co-administration. Consider alternative or increasing atovaquone + proguanil with LPV/r co-administration.
- Metoclopramide: may decrease atovaquone serum concentration. Avoid co-administration.
- Proguanil component: no known drug interactions. Potential for drug interactions with substrates, inhibitors and inducers at CYP2C19.
- Rifampin: atovaquone decreased 50%. Avoid co-administration.
- Rifabutin: decreases atovaquone 34%. Avoid co-administration.
- Tetracycline: atovaquone decreased 40%. Use an alternative tetracycline.

PHARMACOLOGY
Mechanism
Atovaquone is a selective inhibitor of parasite mitochondrial electron transport. Proguanil active metabolite (cycloguanil) is a dihydrofolate reductase inhibitor that disrupts deoxythymidylate synthesis. Treatment failure associated with point mutation in cytochrome b.

Pharmacokinetic Parameters
- **Absorption** Atovaquone: only 23% (best when taken with fatty food). Proguanil: well absorbed with or without food.
- **Distribution** Proguanil is widely distributed into erythrocytes.
- **Protein binding** Atovaquone: >99% protein bound. Proguanil: 75% protein bound.
- **Metabolism/Excretion** Atovaquone: limited metabolism with 94% of administered drug is excreted unchanged in the feces. Proguanil: metabolized via CYP2C19 to an active metabolite with 40–60% excreted in the urine.
- **T1/2** Atovaquone: 2–3 days. Proguanil: 12–21 hrs.

Dosing for Decreased Hepatic Function
No data: may need to be decreased with severe hepatic dysfunction.

Pregnancy Risk
C: Atovaquone not teratogenic in rat studies. Maternal and fetal toxicities (decreased fetal weight, early fetal resorption and post-implantation fetal loss) reported in rabbits. No human data. Proguanil: not teratogenic in rat studies. In a study of 200 pregnant Nigerian women in the first two trimesters, proguanil 100 mg/day resulted in reduction of parasitemia from 35% to 2%, reduction of anemia from 18% to 3% and increases in mean birth weights by 132 g [*Lancet* 1990; 335(8680):45].

Breast Feeding Compatibility
No data.

COMMENTS
Malarone offers a well-tolerated alternative to mefloquine for the treatment and prevention of chloroquine-resistant *P. falciparum*. Disadvantages of Malarone include a higher price and the need for daily administration.

ANTIPARASITIC DRUGS

SELECTED REFERENCES

Borrmann S, Faucher JF, Bagaphou T, et al. Atovaquone and proguanil versus amodiaquine for the treatment of *Plasmodium falciparum* malaria in African infants and young children. *Clin Infect Dis*, 2003; Vol. 37; pp. 1441–7.

Camus D, Djossou F, Schilthuis HJ, et al. Atovaquone-proguanil versus chloroquine-proguanil for malaria prophylaxis in nonimmune pediatric travelers: results of an international, randomized, open-label study. *Clin Infect Dis*, 2004; Vol. 38; pp. 1716–23.

CHLOROQUINE

Paul A. Pham, PharmD and John G. Bartlett, MD

INDICATIONS

FDA

- Malaria prophylaxis and treatment (caused by *P. vivax, P. malariae, P. ovale*, and chloroquine-susceptible strains of *P. falciparum*)
- Amoebic liver abscess

FORMS

Brand name (mfr)	Forms	Cost*
Aralen phosphate (Various generic manufacturers)	PO tab 250 mg; PO tab 500 mg	$2.47; $5.42
*Prices represents Average Wholesale Price (AWP).		

USUAL ADULT DOSING

P. vivax, P. ovale, P. malariae, and chloroquine-sensitive *P. falciparum*: chloroquine phosphate 1 g salt (600 mg base) once, then 500 mg salt (300 mg base) 6 hr later, then 500 mg at 24 hrs and 48 hrs. Chloroquine HCL 160–200 mg (base) IM or IV q6h (IV n/a in U.S.).

RENAL DOSING

Dosing for GFR 50–80: Usual dose.
Dosing for GFR 10–50: Usual dose.
Dosing for GFR <10: 150–300 mg PO once daily.
Dosing in hemodialysis: No data.
Dosing in peritoneal dialysis: No data.
Dosing in hemofiltration: No data.

ADVERSE DRUG REACTIONS

Occasional

- Visual disturbances
- Hemolysis with G6PD deficiency
- GI intolerance
- Pruritus
- Weight loss
- Alopecia

Rare

- CNS: headache, confusion, dizziness, and psychosis
- Peripheral neuropathy
- Extraocular muscle palsies
- QTc prolongation

DRUG INTERACTIONS

- Aluminum and magnesium salts: decrease absorption of chloroquine. Administer chloroquine 2–4 hrs before antacid.
- Cimetidine: may increase chloroquine serum concentrations. Monitor for toxicity.
- Any drugs that can prolong QTc (macrolides, antipsychotics, tricyclic antidepressants, amiodarone, fluoroquinolones, methadone . . .): may result in additive QTc prolongation with chloroquine co-administration. Avoid co-administration.

PHARMACOLOGY

Mechanism

The exact mechanism of action of chloroquine is not fully understood but may be related to ability of chloroquine to bind to DNA and alter its properties or to interfere with the parasite's ability to metabolize and utilize erythrocyte hemoglobin.

Pharmacokinetic Parameters

- **Absorption** 89%.
- **Cmax** 26 mg of chloroquine base in 4 divided dose over 72 hrs resulted in levels above 1 mmol/L (note that mean toxic dose is 4.7 mg/dL).
- **Distribution** Widely distributed in body tissues such as eyes, heart, kidney, liver and lungs. High levels attained in erythrocytes.
- **Protein binding** 50–65%.
- **Metabolism/Excretion** Hepatic metabolism to desethyl metabolite. 47% of unchanged drug and 7–12% of metabolite are excreted unchanged in the urine.
- **T1/2** 4 days to 1 mo.

Dosing for Decreased Hepatic Function

30–50% decrease in dose is recommended.

Pregnancy Risk

C: Embryotoxic and teratogenic in animals studies. In a report of 169 infants exposed to in utero to 300 mg of chloroquine weekly throughout pregnancy did not result in increase teratogenicity. Chloroquine is the antimalarial prophylaxis considered probably safe in pregnancy, there is no other antimalarial prophylaxis with enough data in pregnancy, therefore pregnant women should be strongly discouraged to travel in a chloroquine-resistant malarial region.

Breast Feeding Compatibility

2.8% of dose is excreted in breast milk. The American Academy of Pediatrics considers chloroquine to be compatible with breast feeding.

COMMENTS

Oral antimalarial agent. Effective as malaria prophylaxis in Mexico and Central America above the Panama Canal. Some chloroquine resistance in the Middle East. Substantial resistance in continental South America. Mefloquine or Malarone recommended for travel to areas with chloroquine-resistant *P. falciparum*.

SELECTED REFERENCES

Baird JK. Effectiveness of antimalarial drugs. *N Engl J Med*, 2005; Vol. 352; pp. 1565–77.

Laufer MK, Thesing PC, Eddington ND, et al. Return of chloroquine antimalarial efficacy in Malawi. *N Engl J Med*, 2006; Vol. 355; pp. 1959–66.

DAPSONE

Paul A. Pham, PharmD and John G. Bartlett, MD

INDICATIONS

FDA

- Leprosy
- Dermatitis herpetiformis
- Acne vulgaris (dapsone 5% gel)

Non-FDA Approved Uses

- PCP prophylaxis
- Treatment of mild to moderately severe PCP (with trimethoprim)
- Toxoplasmosis prophylaxis (with pyrimethamine and leucovorin)

FORMS

Brand name (mfr)	Forms	Cost*
Dapsone (Generic manufacturers)	Oral tablet 25 mg Oral tablet 100 mg	$0.20 $0.21
Aczone (QLT)	Topical gel 5% (30 g)	tba
*Prices represents Average Wholesale Price (AWP).		

ANTIPARASITIC DRUGS

USUAL ADULT DOSING
- PCP prophylaxis: 100 mg PO daily.
- Treatment of mild to moderately severe PCP: dapsone 100 mg PO daily + trimethoprim 5 mg/kg q8h × 21 days.
- PCP and toxoplasmosis prophylaxis: dapsone 50 mg PO daily + pyrimethamine 50 mg PO qwk + leucovorin 25 mg PO qwk **or** dapsone 200 mg PO qwk + pyrimethamine 75 mg PO qwk + leucovorin 25 mg q wk.
- Multibacillary leprosy: dapsone 100 mg daily in combination with rifampicin 600 mg once a mo plus clofazimine 300 mg once a mo and 50 mg daily. Duration = 12 mos.
- Paucibacillary leprosy: dapsone 100 mg daily in combination with rifampicin: 600 mg once a mo. Duration = 6 mos.
- Acne: dapsone 5% topical gel, applied pea-sized amount to affected skin twice daily. G-6-PD level assessment recommended prior to use.

RENAL DOSING
Dosing for GFR 50–80: Usual dose.
Dosing for GFR 10–50: Usual dose.
Dosing for GFR <10: No data, metabolite excreted renally, may need adjustment.
Dosing in hemodialysis: No data.
Dosing in peritoneal dialysis: No data.
Dosing in hemofiltration: No data.

ADVERSE DRUG REACTIONS
Common
- Nausea and anorexia
- Hemolytic anemia with G6PD deficiency

Occasional
- Blood dyscrasias (methemoglobinemia and sulfhemoglobinemia with or without G6-PD deficiency)
- Hepatitis
- Rash
- Pruritus
- Dose dependent hemolytic anemia without G6PD deficiency

Rare
- Sulfone syndrome: fever, malaise, exfoliative dermatitis, hepatic necrosis, lymphadenopathy, and hemolytic anemia w/ methemoglobinemia
- Nephrotic syndrome
- Neutropenia
- Blurred vision
- Photosensitivity
- Tinnitus
- Insomnia
- Irritability
- Headache

DRUG INTERACTIONS—See Appendix III, p. 813, for table of drug-to-drug interactions.

PHARMACOLOGY
Mechanism
Mechanism of action has not been fully elucidated, but most likely involves inhibition of dihydropteroate synthase, to disrupt folate synthesis.

Pharmacokinetic Parameters
- **Absorption** Complete absorption (except with achlorhydria).
- **Cmax** 3.1–3.3 mcg/mL after 100 mg PO dose administration.
- **Distribution** Widely distributed in body tissue including skin, muscle, kidneys, liver, and sputum.
- **Protein binding** 50–90%.
- **Metabolism/Excretion** Enterohepatic circulation. Hepatic metabolism to monoacetyl and diacetyl metabolite. Both unchanged drug (20%) and metabolite (70–85%) are excreted in urine.
- **T1/2** 30 hrs.

Pregnancy Risk
C: No adverse effect reported with the use of dapsone in pts with Hansen's disease (leprosy).
Breast Feeding Compatibility
Excreted in breast milk. The American Academy of Pediatrics considers dapsone compatible with breast feeding.

Comments
Oral agent used for treatment and prevention of PCP. Dapsone in combination with rifampin and clofazimine is the WHO recommended treatment regimen for multibacillary leprosy. Strong oxidizing agent, G6-PD deficiency screening is recommended (especially in high-risk pts including African American men and Mediterranean descendent males). Contraindicated use with the Mediterranean but not the African variant of G6-PD deficiency. In addition to hemolytic anemia, may cause methemoglobinemia and bone marrow suppression.

Selected References
Benson CA, Kaplan JE, Masur HM, et al. Treating Opportunistic Infections Among HIV-Infected Adults and Adolescents. *MMWR*, 2004; Vol. 53; pp. (RR15); 1–112.

National Institutes of Health (NIH), the Centers for Disease Control and Prevention (CDC), and the HIV Medicine Association of the Infectious Diseases Society of America (HIVMA/IDSA). Guidelines for Prevention and Treatment of Opportunistic Infections in HIV-Infected Adults and Adolescents. *http://AIDSinfo.nih.gov*, 2008.

IVERMECTIN

Paul A. Pham, PharmD and John G. Bartlett, MD

Indications
FDA
- Onchocerciasis (river blindness)
- Strongyloidiasis (GI tract)

Non-FDA Approved Uses
- *Sarcoptes scabiei var. hominis* (Scabies)
- Lymphatic Filaria
- Strongyloides stercoralis
- Loa Loa
- Cutaneous Larva Migrans

Forms

Brand name (mfr)	Forms	Cost*
Stromectol (Merck)	PO tab 3mg	$5.44
*Prices represents Average Wholesale Price (AWP).		

Usual Adult Dosing
- Strongyloidiasis: 200 mcg/kg × 1 (70 kg: 15 mg or 2.5 × 6 mg tabs).
- Onchocerciasis: 150 mcg/kg × 1.
- Cutaneous Larva Migrans: 200 mcg/kg × 1 (retreatment may be needed).
- Filariasis: 150 μg/kg × 1 (retreatment often needed).
- Scabies (severe crusted scabies in immunodeficient pts): ivermectin in 2 doses (of 200 micrograms/kg) separated by 2 wks.

Renal Dosing
Dosing for GFR 50–80: Usual dose.
Dosing for GFR 10–50: Usual dose.
Dosing for GFR <10: Usual dose.
Dosing in hemodialysis: No data; usual dose likely.
Dosing in peritoneal dialysis: No data; usual dose likely.
Dosing in hemofiltration: No data; usual dose likely.

Adverse Drug Reactions
General
- Generally very well tolerated.

ANTIPARASITIC DRUGS

Occasional

- Mazzotti reaction in onchocerciasis with hypotension, fever, pruritis, bone and joint pain (mild in 10–15% in first time users but can be severe in 5%).

DRUG INTERACTIONS

None reported, but CYP 3A4 substrate *in vitro*.

PHARMACOLOGY

Mechanism

The exact mechanism of action of ivermectin has not been fully elucidated, but it appears that it act as an agonist of the neurotransmitter GABA, thereby disrupting GABA-mediated central nervous system neurosynaptic transmission which result in paralysis of the parasite's CNS and death of the parasite.

Pharmacokinetic Parameters

- **Absorption** Well absorbed, administer on an empty stomach.
- **Cmax** 46 ng/mL after 12 mg PO dose administration.
- **Distribution** Animal studies demonstrated high fat and liver distribution.
- **Protein binding** 93%.
- **Metabolism/Excretion** In animal studies demonstrated Principal excreted in the feces, with less than 2% found in the urine.
- **T1/2** 22–28 hrs.

Dosing for Decreased Hepatic Function

No data; usual dose likely.

Pregnancy Risk

Animal data show risk of teratogenicity. In 203 exposures to ivermectin (85% during the first trimester) found that there was no association with congenital malformation.

Breast Feeding Compatibility

Excreted in breast milk.

COMMENTS

Well-tolerated oral agent that is the preferred treatment for onchocerciasis, strongyloidiasis, cutaneous larva migrans and may be helpful with severe scabies. Ivermectin is a second line to diethyl-carbamazine in the treatment of filariasis. When using ivermectin to treat onchocerciasis in a Loa loa-endemic area, it is recommended to screen for loiasis in order to prevent serious or even fatal encephalopathy.

SELECTED REFERENCES

Bouchaud O, Houze S, Schiemann R, et al. Cutaneous larva migrans in travelers: a prospective study, with assessment of therapy with ivermectin. *Clinical Infectious Diseases*, 2000; Vol. 31; pp. 493–498.

Stolk WA, VAN Oortmarssen GJ, Pani SP, et al. Effects of ivermectin and diethylcarbamazine on microfilariae and overall microfilaria production in bancroftian filariasis. *Am J Trop Med Hyg*, 2005; Vol. 75; pp. 881–7.

MEBENDAZOLE

Paul A. Pham, PharmD and John G. Bartlett, MD

INDICATIONS

FDA

- Enterobiasis (pinworm)
- Hookworm
- Ascariasis (roundworm)
- Trichuriasis (whipworm)

Non-FDA Approved Uses

- Echinococcus (second line)

FORMS

Brand name (mfr)	Forms	Cost*
Vermox (Generic)	PO chew tab 100 mg	$5.25
*Prices represents Average Wholesale Price (AWP).		

USUAL ADULT DOSING

- Roundworm (ascaris): 100–200 mg PO twice daily × 5 days or 500 mg PO × 1.
- Hookworm: 100 mg PO twice daily × 3 days or 500 mg PO × 1.
- Pinworm: 100 mg PO × 1 (may be repeated if infection persists for 3 wks).
- Echinococcus: 40–50 mg/kg/day in 3 divided doses.

RENAL DOSING

Dosing for GFR 50–80: Usual dose.

Dosing for GFR 10–50: Usual dose.

Dosing for GFR <10: Usual dose.

Dosing in hemodialysis: Drug concentration not affected by dialysis; use usual dose.

Dosing in peritoneal dialysis: No data.

Dosing in hemofiltration: No data.

ADVERSE DRUG REACTIONS

Occasional

- Diarrhea
- Abdominal pain

Rare

- Leukopenia
- Agranulocytosis
- Hepatitis

DRUG INTERACTIONS

Carbamazepine: may decrease mebendazole serum levels. Consider valproic acid with co-administration.

PHARMACOLOGY

Mechanism

Mebendazole binds to beta-tubulin, prevents microtubule assembly, and inhibits glucose uptake; this ultimately results in immobilization and death of worm or clearance by peristalsis.

Pharmacokinetic Parameters

- **Absorption** 5–10% absorbed (absorption may be increase if administered with fatty food).
- **Cmax** 0.3 mcg/mL peak concentration after 100 mg PO twice daily for 3 days.
- **Distribution** Distributed to cyst fluid, liver, omental fat, pelvic, pulmonary and hepatic cyst.
- **Protein binding** 90–95%.
- **Metabolism/Excretion** Hepatic metabolism to inactive amino, hydroxy, and hydroxyamino metabolites. Metabolite and unchanged drug are excreted primarily in the feces. Only 2–5% excreted in urine as unchanged or as metabolite.
- **T1/2** 2.5–5.5 hrs (prolonged to 35 hrs in hepatic impairment).

Dosing for Decreased Hepatic Function

No data.

Pregnancy Risk

C: Embryotoxic and teratogenic in animal studies. One manufacturer reported 170 first trimester exposures which resulted in no identifiable teratogenic risk. In a Michigan Medicaid recipient surveillance study, 64 first trimester exposures did not result in a significant increase in teratogenicity risk.

Breast Feeding Compatibility

Amount excreted in breast milk unknown.

COMMENTS

Well-tolerated oral agent with broad-spectrum antihelmintic. Mean cure rates are >95% for pinworm, roundworm, and hookworm infections, and 35–68% for whipworm infection.

SELECTED REFERENCES

Legesse M, Erko B, Medhin G. Efficacy of albendazole and mebendazole in the treatment of Ascaris and Trichuris infections. *Ethiop Med J*, 2002; Vol. 40; pp. 335–43.

ANTIPARASITIC DRUGS

MEFLOQUINE

Paul A. Pham, PharmD and John G. Bartlett, MD

INDICATIONS

FDA

- Treatment of mild to moderate acute malaria (*P. falciparum* and *P. vivax*) caused by chloroquine-resistant, chloroquine-susceptible, and multiple drug-resistant (including sulfadoxine and pyrimethamine-resistant) strains.
- Malaria (*P. falciparum* and *P. vivax*) prophylaxis including prophylaxis of chloroquine-resistant strains of *P. falciparum*.

FORMS

Brand name (mfr)	Forms	Cost*
Lariam (Roche)	Oral tablet 250 mg	$12.93
Mefloquine (Generic)	Oral tablet 250 mg	$10.59

*Prices represents Average Wholesale Price (AWP).

USUAL ADULT DOSING

- Uncomplicated malaria treatment: 1250 mg PO × 1 **or** 750 mg once then 500 mg 12 hrs later.
- Malaria prophylaxis: 250 mg PO once a wk (malaria prophylaxis), start 1 wk prior to departure to an endemic area and continue for 4 wks after leaving endemic area.
- Note: In the treatment of *P. vivax*, mefloquine does not eliminate exoerythrocytic (hepatic phase) parasites; to prevent relapse, pts should subsequently be treated with primaquine.

RENAL DOSING

Dosing for GFR 50–80: Usual dose.
Dosing for GFR 10–50: Usual dose.
Dosing for GFR <10: Usual dose.
Dosing in hemodialysis: Usual dose, not removed in dialysis.
Dosing in peritoneal dialysis: No data, not removed in peritoneal dialysis.
Dosing in hemofiltration: No data, usual dose likely.

ADVERSE DRUG REACTIONS

Common

- CNS: vertigo; light-headedness, nightmares, headache, decreased fine motor function
- GI: nausea and diarrhea
- Visual disturbances (dose-related)

Occasional

- CNS: psychosis, panic attacks, seizures, disorientation (dose-related rare at prophylaxis dose)
- Extrasystole
- Sinus bradycardia

Rare

- Suicidal thoughts
- Dyspnea secondary to pneumonitis (of possible allergic etiology)

DRUG INTERACTIONS

- Avoid coadministration w/ any drugs that may prolong QTc (e.g., fluoroquinolones, antiarrhythmics (procainamide, sotalol, amiodarone), clarithromycin, and erythromycin...).
- Beta-blockers, quinine, and quinidine: may result in additive depression of cardiac conduction. Avoid co-administration.
- Gold compounds: potential additive effect for blood dyscrasias. Avoid co-administration.
- Ketoconazole (and other inhibitors of CYP3A4 such as macrolides, HIV-protease inhibitors...): mefloquine serum concentrations increased by 79%. Avoid co-administration due to the potential for QTc prolongation.
- Rifampin (and other inducers of CYP3A4 such as phenobarbital, phenytoin, carbamazepine.): mefloquine serum concentrations decreased by 68%. Use with caution or avoid co-administration.

- *P. falciparum* from Thailand or other parts of Southeast Asia may be resistant to mefloquine.

PHARMACOLOGY

Mechanism

The exact mechanism of action of mefloquine is not fully understood but may be related to interference with the parasite's ability to metabolize and utilize erythrocyte hemoglobin.

Pharmacokinetic Parameters
- **Absorption** 85% absorbed; slow absorption (absorption may be increase if administered with food).
- **Cmax** 540–1240 ng/mL after 1 g PO dose administration.
- **Distribution** Widely distributed in tissues. High concentration in erythrocytes. Good CSF penetration.
- **Protein binding** 98–99%.
- **Metabolism/Excretion** Hepatic metabolized to carboxylic acid metabolite. Primarily excreted in feces by biliary excretion. Only 5% of dose excreted in urine.
- **T1/2** 20 days.

Dosing for Decreased Hepatic Function

No data.

Pregnancy Risk

C: Embryotoxic and teratogenic in animal studies. CDC accepts mefloquine as safe and effective in second and third trimester; advises contraception during prophylaxis and for 2 mos after. A double-blind, placebo-controlled trial involving 360 pregnant pts (2nd trimester) found the incidence of stillbirth similar between mefloquine and placebo [*Ann Trop Med Parasitol*. 1998 Sep;92(6):643-53].

Breast Feeding Compatibility

Excreted in small concentration in breast milk. Long term effects of mefloquine exposure via breast milk have not been studied.

COMMENTS

Oral antimalarial that is commonly used for prophylaxis where chloroquine-resistance is found. May cause vivid dreams, acute psychosis and seizures, therefore contraindicated in pts with psychiatric illness and epilepsy. Has generally fallen out of favor in the U.S. for prophylaxis in travelers due to concerns about CNS side-effects with malarone now the favored drug.

SELECTED REFERENCES

Chen LH, Wilson ME, Schlagenhauf P. Controversies and misconceptions in malaria chemoprophylaxis for travelers. *JAMA*, 2007; Vol. 297; pp. 2251–63.

Griffith KS, Lewis LS, Mali S, et al. Treatment of malaria in the United States: a systematic review. *JAMA*, 2007; Vol. 297; pp. 2264–77.

NITAZOXANIDE

Paul A. Pham, PharmD and John G. Bartlett, MD

INDICATIONS

FDA
- Diarrhea caused by Cryptosporidia and Giardia in immunocompetent children (1 yr of age or older).
- Cryptosporidiosis in immunocompetent adults.

Non-FDA Approved Uses
- Cryptosporidiosis in HIV-infected pts.
- Entamoeba histolytica.

FORMS

Brand name (mfr)	Forms	Cost*
Alinia (Romark)	PO susp 100 mg/5 mL (60 mL)	$90.75
	PO tab 500 mg	$22.43
*Prices represents Average Wholesale Price (AWP).		

ANTIPARASITIC DRUGS

669

Usual Adult Dosing
- Immunocompetent adult: 500 mg PO q6–12h × 3 days.
- Immunocompetent child 4–11 y: 200 mg PO q12h × 3 days.
- Immunocompetent child 1–3 y: 100 mg PO q12h × 3 days.
- Most experts would treat for 4–6 wks in immunocompromised pts.

Renal Dosing
Dosing for GFR 50–80: No data; usual dose likely.
Dosing for GFR 10–50: No data; usual dose likely.
Dosing for GFR <10: No data; usual dose likely.
Dosing hemodialysis: No data.
Dosing in peritoneal dialysis: No data.
Dosing in hemofiltration: No data.

Adverse Drug Reactions
General
- Generally well tolerated with ADR comparable to placebo.

Occasional
- GI: abdominal pain (food improves GI tolerance)
- Headache
- Nausea

Rare
- Hypotension with tachycardia

Drug Interactions
No data.

Pharmacology
Mechanism
The antiprotozoal activity of nitazoxanide is believed to be due to interference with the pyruvate: ferredoxin oxidoreductase (PFOR) enzyme-dependent electron transfer reaction, which is essential to anaerobic energy metabolism.

Pharmacokinetic Parameters
- **Absorption** No data.
- **Protein binding** 98%.
- **Metabolism/Excretion** Metabolized in gut wall and liver with extensive biliary excretion. Minimal renal excretion (less 10%).
- **T1/2** 1.0–1.6 hrs.

Dosing for Decreased Hepatic Function
No data.

Pregnancy Risk
No data.

Breast Feeding Compatibility
No data.

Comments
Nitazoxanide is effective in the treatment of diarrhea caused by *Cryptosporidium parvum* in immunocompetent host (adult and children). Its efficacy in immunocompromised pts (e.g., HIV) has been disappointing. Avoid use in pts with hypersensitivity to aspirin or salicylates due to structural similarities. Some have used for *C. difficile* diarrhea, although large trials are lacking.

Selected References
Anderson VR, Curran MP. Nitazoxanide: a review of its use in the treatment of gastrointestinal infections. *Drugs*, 2007; Vol. 67; pp. 1947–67.

Musher DM, Logan N, Hamill RJ, et al. Nitazoxanide for the treatment of Clostridium difficile colitis. *Clin Infect Dis*, 2006; Vol. 43; pp. 421–7.

PRIMAQUINE

Paul A. Pham, PharmD and John G. Bartlett, MD

INDICATIONS

FDA

- Malaria prevention of relapses (radical cure) caused by *Plasmodium vivax* and *P. ovale*. Also effective against gametocytes of *P. falciparum*.

Non-FDA Approved Uses

- Treatment of PCP (in combination with clindamycin).

FORMS

Brand name (mfr)	Forms	Cost*
Primaquine (Sanofi-Aventis U.S.)	Oral tablet 26.3 mg (15 mg base)	$1.33

*Prices represents Average Wholesale Price (AWP).

USUAL ADULT DOSING

- Treatment of PCP: 15–30 mg (base) PO once daily with food (in combination with clindamycin).
- Eradication of dormant liver forms of *P. vivax* and *P. ovale*: 30 mg (base) once daily × 2 wks.

RENAL DOSING

Dosing for GFR 50–80: Usual dose.

Dosing for GFR 10–50: Usual dose.

Dosing for GFR <10: Usual dose.

Dosing in hemodialysis: No data, dose post-HD.

Dosing in peritoneal dialysis: No data.

Dosing in hemofiltration: No data.

ADVERSE DRUG REACTIONS

Occasional

- Hemolytic anemia (in pts with G6-PD deficiency). Screen for G6-PD deficiency (African American men and Mediterranean descendent males).
- Methemoglobinemia.
- Neutropenia and leukopenia (incidence may be higher with primaquine 30 mg).
- GI intolerance: abdominal pain, nausea, and vomiting.

Rare

- Blurred vision
- Headache
- Pruritis

DRUG INTERACTIONS

Bone marrow suppressive drugs (e.g., AZT, ganciclovir, pyrimethamine, flucytosine): potential for additive bone marrow suppression with co-administration.

PHARMACOLOGY

Mechanism

Exact mechanism of action not fully elucidated, but appears to interfere with pyrimidine synthesis and mitochondrial electron transport chain.

Pharmacokinetic Parameters

- **Absorption** Well absorbed.
- **Cmax** 104 ng/mL steady-state concentration after 30 mg PO.
- **Distribution** Lack of data, however appears to be widely distributed.
- **Protein binding** No data.
- **Metabolism/Excretion** Hepatic metabolism to carboxy metabolite. Both metabolite and a small amount of unchanged drug are excreted unchanged in urine.
- **T1/2** 5.8 hrs.

Pregnancy Risk

C: No studies available. Theoretical concern is hemolytic anemia in G6-PD deficient fetus.

Breast Feeding Compatibility

No data available.

ANTIPARASITIC DRUGS

COMMENTS

Primaquine in combination with clindamycin is a good second line treatment for mild, moderate, and severe *P. carinii* in pts intolerant of TMP/SMX. Prior screening for G6-PD deficiency recommended to prevent hemolytic anemia.

BASIS FOR RECOMMENDATIONS

National Institutes of Health (NIH), the Centers for Disease Control and Prevention (CDC), and the HIV Medicine Association of the Infectious Diseases Society of America (HIVMA/IDSA). Guidelines for Prevention and Treatment of Opportunistic Infections in HIV-Infected Adults and Adolescents. *http://AIDSinfo.nih.gov*, 2008.

Comments: Although primaquine/clindamycin efficacy data are not as robust as data supporting IV pentamidine for the treatment of severe PCP, the OI treatment guidelines recommend that primaquine/clindamycin **or** IV pentamidine be considered as alternative therapeutic regimens to TMP/SMX for pts with moderate-to-severe PCP.

SELECTED REFERENCES

Baird JK, Hoffman SL. Primaquine therapy for malaria. *Clin Infect Dis*, 2004; Vol. 39; pp. 1336–45.

Rowland M, Durrani N. Randomized controlled trials of 5- and 14-days primaquine therapy against relapses of vivax malaria in an Afghan refugee settlement in Pakistan. *Trans R Soc Trop Med Hyg*, 2000; Vol. 93; pp. 641–3.

PYRIMETHAMINE

Paul A. Pham, PharmD and John G. Bartlett, MD

INDICATIONS

FDA

- Malaria (acute) in combination with sulfadoxine and quinine in the treatment of chloroquine-resistant *Plasmodium falciparum* malaria. Resistance prevalent worldwide; not recommended as a prophylactic agent for travelers to most areas.
- Toxoplasmosis (in combination with sulfadiazine **or** clindamycin plus leucovorin).

FORMS

Brand name (mfr)	Forms	Cost*
Daraprim (GlaxoSmithKline)	Oral tablet 25 mg	$0.58
Fansidar (Roche)	Oral tablet Pyrimethamine 25 mg + sulfadoxine 500 mg	$3.92
*Prices represents Average Wholesale Price (AWP).		

USUAL ADULT DOSING

- CNS toxoplasmosis, induction therapy: 200 mg × 1, then 50–75 mg once daily (+ folinic acid 10–20 mg/day + sulfadiazine 1.5 g q6h or clindamycin 600 mg IV q6h) × ≥6 wks.
- CNS toxoplasmosis, maintenance therapy: 25–50 mg (+ folinic acid 15 mg + sulfadiazine 0.5–1 g q6h or clindamycin 300–450 mg q6h) until immune reconstitution (CD4 >200 × 6 mos, induction therapy completed, and asymptomatic). Reintroduced maintenance therapy if CD4+ count decreases to <200 cells/mL.
- Toxoplasmosis prophylaxis: 50 mg/wk (+ folinic acid 25 mg/wk + dapsone 50–100 mg daily + leucovorin 25 mg/wk **or** atovaquone 1500 mg/day +/– pyrimethamine 25 mg/day + leucovorin 10 mg/day). Note: TMP/SMX 1DS daily preferred. Toxoplasmosis primary prophylaxis should be discontinued in pts who have responded to ART with an increase in CD4 + counts to >200 cells/mL for >3 mos, but should be reintroduced if the CD4 + count decreases to <100–200 cells/mL.
- Acute malaria, acute: Fansidar 2 to 3 tabs (pyrimethamine 50–75 mg/sulfadoxine 1000–1500 mg) as a single dose. May also be used in sequence with quinine where Fansidar 3 tabs is given on the last day of quinine therapy.
- Malaria prophylaxis (generally not recommended due to a high incidence of rash): Fansidar 1 tab (pyrimethamine 25 mg/sulfadoxine 500 mg) q wk or **or** 2 tabs every other wk; start 1 to 2 days before arrival in endemic area and continue during stay and for 4 to 6 wk after leaving endemic area.

RENAL DOSING

Dosing for GFR 50–80: Usual dose.

Dosing for GFR 10–50: Usual dose.

Dosing for GFR <10: Usual dose.

Dosing in hemodialysis: No data, usual dose likely (dose post-HD on days of HD).

Dosing in peritoneal dialysis: 47% removed after PD.

Dosing in hemofiltration: No data. Usual dose likely.

ADVERSE DRUG REACTIONS

Occasional

- Reversible pancytopenia (megaloblastic anemia, leucopenia, agranulocytosis, and thrombocytopenia) secondary to depletion of folic acid stores. Generally prevented with co-administration of leucovorin. Consider increasing leucovorin dose to 50–100 mg/day if hematologic toxicity observed.
- GI intolerance: abdominal pain and vomiting (improved by administration with meals).
- Headache, dizziness, and insomnia.
- With sulfonamide co-administration: rash, hepatitis.

Rare

- Neurologic: tremors, ataxia, and seizure.
- With sulfonamide co-administration: Stevens-Johnson syndrome, TEN, erythema multiforme and anaphylaxis can occur.

DRUG INTERACTIONS

- Lorazepam: may increase risk of hepatotoxicity (unclear association).
- TMP/SMX, dapsone, ganciclovir, AZT, and interferon: potential for additive bone marrow suppression.

PHARMACOLOGY

Mechanism

Binds to dihydrofolate reductase inhibiting the reduction of dihydrofolic to tetrahydrofolic acid (folinic acid).

Pharmacokinetic Parameters

- **Absorption** Well absorbed.
- **Cmax** 0.13–0.31 mcg/mL after 25 mg PO.
- **Distribution** Distributed into kidneys, lungs, liver and spleen. 13–26% of serum concentration penetrates the CSF.
- **Protein binding** 80–87%
- **Metabolism/Excretion** Hepatic metabolism. Both metabolite and 20–30% of unchanged drug excreted in the urine.
- **T1/2** 80–123 hrs (139 +/– 34 hr in pts with AIDS; *Antimicrob Agents Chemother* 1996;40:1360–5).

Pregnancy Risk

C: Teratogenic in animal studies. No adverse fetal effects reported in 2 reviews of treatment of toxoplasmosis in pregnancy. If pyrimethamine used during pregnancy, folinic acid 5 mg/day supplementation recommended, especially during 1st trimester, to prevent folate deficiency.

Breast Feeding Compatibility

Excreted in breast milk. The American Academy of Pediatrics considers pyrimethamine compatible with breast feeding.

COMMENTS

Treatment of choice (with sulfadiazine and leucovorin) for CNS toxoplasmosis. Fansidar (pyrimethamine/sulfadoxine) is not a first line agent for malaria prophylaxis due to high incidence of rash and the availability of better tolerated alternatives (e.g., atovaquone/proguanil, mefloquine, and doxycycline).

BASIS FOR RECOMMENDATIONS

National Institutes of Health (NIH), the Centers for Disease Control and Prevention (CDC), and the HIV Medicine Association of the Infectious Diseases Society of America (HIVMA/IDSA). Guidelines for Prevention and Treatment of Opportunistic Infections in HIV-Infected Adults and Adolescents. *http://AIDSinfo.nih.gov*, 2008.

Comments: The initial therapy of choice for CNS toxoplasmosis is pyrimethamine + sulfadiazine + leucovorin.

ANTIPARASITIC DRUGS

673

SELECTED REFERENCES

Chen LH, Wilson ME, Schlagenhauf P. Prevention of malaria in long-term travelers. *JAMA*, 2006; Vol. 296; pp. 2234–44.

Katlama C, De Wit S, O'Doherty E, et al. Pyrimethamine-clindamycin vs. pyrimethamine-sulfadiazine as acute and long-term therapy for toxoplasmic encephalitis in pts with AIDS. *Clin Infect Dis*, 1996; Vol. 22; pp. 268–75.

QUINIDINE

Joseph Vinetz, MD and Paul Pham, PharmD

INDICATIONS

FDA

- Serious *P. falciparum* malaria treatment
- [non-ID indications: atrial and ventricular arrhythmias]

FORMS

Brand name (mfr)	Forms	Cost*
Quinidine gluconate (Eli Lilly)	IV vial 800 mg/10 mL	$22.46
*Prices represents Average Wholesale Price (AWP).		

USUAL ADULT DOSING

Loading dose: 10 milligrams/kilogram over 1 to 2 hrs followed by a maintenance dose of 0.02 milligrams/kilogram/minute for up to 72 hrs or until parasitemia decreases to less than 1% or oral therapy can be started.

- Start doxycycline 100 mg PO/IV twice daily along with quinidine.
- If parasitemia >5–10%, consider exchange transfusion.
- Pts should be on cardiac telemetry with administration if available.

RENAL DOSING

Dosing for GFR 50–80: Usual dose.

Dosing for GFR 10–50: Usual dose.

Dosing for GFR <10: 75% of dose (levels may be higher with renal failure). Dose based on clinical response. Levels may be useful.

Dosing in hemodialysis: Removed with HD. Supplement with 100–200 mg post dialysis. Levels may be useful.

Dosing in peritoneal dialysis: No data: unlikely to be removed. Dose based on clinical response. Levels may be useful.

Dosing in hemofiltration: No data. Dose based on clinical response. Levels may be useful.

ADVERSE DRUG REACTIONS

Common

- EKG changes (e.g., prolongation of the QT interval and QRS widening), arrhythmias and hypotension with infusion (close cardiac monitoring in the ICU recommended)

Occasional

- Hemolytic anemia (with G6PD deficiency)
- Drug-induced SLE
- Hypoglycemia

Rare

- Thrombocytopenia
- Transaminase elevation
- Rash

DRUG INTERACTIONS

- Antiarrhythmic drugs that prolong QTc (e.g., erythromycin, clarithromycin, amiodarone, TCAs, fluoroquinolones): may increase the risk of QTc prolongation with co-administration. Avoid or use with close monitoring.
- CYP3A4 inhibitors (e.g., macrolides, azoles, HIV protease inhibitors and cimetidine): may increase quinidine serum concentrations. Monitor quinidine serum concentrations closely with co-administration.

- CYP3A4 inducers (e.g., rifamycin, nevirapine, efavirenz, phenobarbital, carbamazepine, phenytoin): may decrease quinidine serum concentrations. Monitor quinidine serum concentrations closely.
- Digoxin serum concentration may be significantly increased with co-administration. Digoxin dose may need to be decreased.

PHARMACOLOGY
Mechanism
Inhibit the heme polymerase activity responsible for polymerizing heme into malarial pigment and may also inhibit the aspartic and cysteine proteases that degrade hemoglobin and alkalinize the plasmodial food vacuole.

Pharmacokinetic Parameters
- **Absorption** 70–80% with oral formulation.
- **Distribution** Wide volume of distribution 2–3 L/kg. High levels in the liver.
- **Protein binding** 80–88%.
- **Metabolism/Excretion** 50% to 90% is metabolized in the liver by cytochrome P4503A4 to several different hydroxylated metabolites and excreted in the urine. 20–50% of unchanged drug excreted in the kidney.
- **T1/2** 6–8 hrs.

Dosing for Decreased Hepatic Function
May need to be decreased with severe hepatic dysfunction.

Pregnancy Risk
C: Untreated malaria in pregnancy is universally fatal. Treatment is recommended.

Breast Feeding Compatibility
Excreted in breast milk.

COMMENTS
IV quinidine (plus doxycycline) is the agent of choice for treatment of complicated *P. falciparum*. Close monitoring with telemetry recommended (QT prolongation, hypotension, and hypoglycemia).

SELECTED REFERENCES
Stauffer W, Fischer PR. Diagnosis and treatment of malaria in children. *Clin Infect Dis*, 2003; Vol. 37; pp. 1340–8.

QUININE

Paul A. Pham, PharmD and John G. Bartlett, MD

INDICATIONS
FDA
- Oral quinine is indicated for the treatment of uncomplicated malaria (concurrently with tetracycline, doxycycline, clindamycin, or pyrimethamine plus sulfadiazine, or pyrimethamine plus sulfadoxine in the treatment of chloroquine-resistant malaria caused by *Plasmodium falciparum*).
- IV quinine is not available in the U.S.

Non-FDA Approved Uses
- Babesia species

FORMS

Brand name (mfr)	Forms	Cost*
Qualaquin (AR Scientific Inc.)	Oral capsule 324 mg	$5.46
*Prices represents Average Wholesale Price (AWP).		

USUAL ADULT DOSING
- Uncomplicated malaria: quinine 650 mg q8h × 3–7 days plus doxycycline 100 mg twice daily × 7 days **or** clindamycin 450 mg q8h × 7 days **or** pyrimethamine/sulfadoxine 3 tabs on last day of quinine.
- Babesiosis: quinine 650 mg PO q8h × 7 days plus clindamycin 600 mg PO q8h × 7 days.

ANTIPARASITIC DRUGS

- Quinine dihydrochloride: typical parenteral dose for malaria, 600 mg IV q8h (IV not commercially available in the U.S.). Pts should be closely monitored re: ECG changes, and blood glucose levels.
- Monitor quinine blood levels in pts with renal or hepatic dysfunction, also when drug interactions suspected.

RENAL DOSING
Dosing for GFR 50–80: Usual dose.
Dosing for GFR 10–50: Usual dose.
Dosing for GFR <10: Usual dose, but some recommend increasing dosing interval to q24h. Therapeutic drug monitoring recommended.
Dosing in hemodialysis: Usual dose, days of dialysis dose post dialysis. Therapeutic drug monitoring recommended.
Dosing in peritoneal dialysis: 650 mg q24h. Therapeutic drug monitoring recommended.
Dosing in hemofiltration: CVVHD: limited data. Use standard dose with close monitoring (*CID* 2004;39:288–289). Therapeutic drug monitoring recommended.

ADVERSE DRUG REACTIONS
Occasional
- GI intolerance
- Cinchonism (tinnitus, headache, nausea, abdominal pain, visual disturbances)
- Hemolytic anemia (G6PD deficiency)

Rare
- Cardiac arrhythmia
- Hypoglycemia
- Hepatitis
- Thrombocytopenia
- Hypotension (with rapid IV infusion)

DRUG INTERACTIONS
- Protease inhibitors may increase serum quinine levels.
- Quinine serum level may be decreased by CYP3A4 inducers (rifampin, phenytoin, phenobarbital, NNRTIs...).

PHARMACOLOGY
Mechanism
The exact mechanism of action has not been fully elucidated, but the quinine appears to interfere with the function of plasmodial DNA.

Pharmacokinetic Parameters
- **Absorption** Complete absorption.
- **Cmax** 7 mcg/mL after chronic administration of 1 g PO per day.
- **Distribution** Widely distributed in body tissues. Only 2–7% of serum concentration penetrates the CNS.
- **Protein binding** 70–90%.
- **Metabolism/Excretion** Extensively metabolized to hydroxy metabolite. Metabolite is excreted in the urine. Less than 5% is excreted unchanged in the urine.
- **T1/2** 11–18 hrs.

Dosing for Decreased Hepatic Function
Usual dose with therapeutic drug monitoring.

Pregnancy Risk
X: Animal data show teratogenic effects. Human data reports stillbirths and congenital malformation with large doses used for attempted abortions. CDC recommends quinidine gluconate for the treatment of malaria.

Breast Feeding Compatibility
Excreted in breast milk. The American Academy of Pediatrics considers quinine compatible with breast feeding.

COMMENTS
IV quinine (not available in the U.S.) is the drug of choice for complicated *Plasmodium falciparum* malaria. Monitor quinine blood levels in pts with renal or hepatic dysfunction. For parenteral

therapy, IV quinidine may be substituted for quinine (see quinidine module). Oral quinine plus doxycycline or pyrimethamine/sulfadoxine is recommended for uncomplicated malaria.

SELECTED REFERENCES

Flanagan KL, Buckley-Sharp M, Doherty T, et al. Quinine levels revisited: the value of routine drug level monitoring for those on parenteral therapy. *Acta Trop*, 2006; Vol. 97; pp. 233–7.

Griffith KS, Lewis LS, Mali S, et al. Treatment of malaria in the United States: a systematic review. *JAMA*, 2007; Vol. 297; pp. 2264–77.

TINIDAZOLE

Paul A. Pham, PharmD and John G. Bartlett, MD

INDICATIONS
FDA
- Trichomoniasis
- Giardiasis (including ages >3 yrs)
- Intestinal and amoebic liver abscess caused by *E. histolytica* (including ages >3 yrs)
- Bacterial vaginosis

Non-FDA Approved Uses
- *C. difficile* colitis

FORMS

Brand name (mfr)	Forms	Cost*
Tindamax (Presutti)	PO tab 250 mg	$3.29
	PO tab 500 mg	$5.88

*Prices represents Average Wholesale Price (AWP).

USUAL ADULT DOSING
- **Adult dosing.**
- Trichomoniasis: 2 g PO × 1 with food.
- Giardiasis: 2 g PO × 1 with food.
- Intestinal amebiasis: 2 g PO once daily with food × 3 days.
- Liver amebiasis: 2 g PO once daily with food × 3–5 days.
- Bacterial vaginosis: 1 g PO once daily × 5 days or 2 g PO once daily × 2 days.
- **Pediatric dosing:** giardiasis and amebiasis for children >3 yrs: 50 mg/kg with food as a single dose.

RENAL DOSING
Dosing for GFR 50–80: Standard dose.
Dosing for GFR 10–50: Standard dose.
Dosing for GFR <10: Standard dose.
Dosing in hemodialysis: 43% removed with HD, supplement with 50% (1 g) post-HD.
Dosing in peritoneal dialysis: No data. Usual dose likely.
Dosing in hemofiltration: No data. Usual dose likely.

ADVERSE DRUG REACTIONS
General
- Generally well tolerated with occasional GI intolerance, but lower compared to metronidazole in clinical trials

Occasional
- GI: nausea (9%), vomiting (3%), metallic/bitter taste (10%), anorexia (4.5%)
- Candidiasis

Rare
- Seizure
- Peripheral neuropathy
- Leukopenia and neutropenia

ANTIPARASITIC DRUGS

DRUG INTERACTIONS—See Appendix III, p. 842, for table of drug-to-drug interactions.

PHARMACOLOGY

Mechanism

Tinidazole, a 5-nitroimidazole, is chemically related to metronidazole, it exerts antiprotozoal activity by formation of free nitro radical with subsequent cell destruction.

Pharmacokinetic Parameters

- **Absorption** Absorption: Tinidazole is rapidly and completely absorbed.
- **Cmax** 48 mcg/mL.
- **Distribution** Widely distributed (Vd = 50 L) to all tissue including CNS.
- **Metabolism/Excretion** Metabolized via CYP3A4, 2-hydroxymethyl metabolite and unchanged drug are excreted in the urine (20–25%) and feces (12%).
- **T1/2** 12–14 hrs.

Dosing for Decreased Hepatic Function

No data. Increased in serum level of tinidazole may occur; use standard dose with close monitoring.

Pregnancy Risk

C: No human data. Animal studies did not find any embryo-fetal toxicity or malformation.

Breast Feeding Compatibility

Excreted in breast milk. No safety data.

COMMENTS

Tinidazole can be used as an alternative to metronidazole but is more expensive. It may be preferred for the treatment of intestinal amoebiasis and giardiasis due to better GI tolerance and superior efficacy.

SELECTED REFERENCES

Anjaeyulu R, Gupte SA, Desai DB. Single-dose treatment of trichomonal vaginitis: a comparison of tinidazole and metronidazole. *J Int Med Res*, 1977; Vol. 5; pp. 438–41.

Livengood CH, Ferris DG, Wiesenfeld HC, et al. Effectiveness of two tinidazole regimens in treatment of bacterial vaginosis: a randomized controlled trial. *Obstet Gynecol*, 2007; Vol. 110; pp. 302–9.

Antiviral

ACYCLOVIR

Paul A. Pham, PharmD and John G. Bartlett, MD

INDICATIONS

FDA

- Treatment of initial episode of herpes genitalis in immunocompromised pts.
- Treatment of herpes simplex encephalitis in immunocompetent pts.
- Treatment of herpes zoster.
- Treatment of varicella in immunocompetent pts when started within 24 hrs of onset of typical chickenpox rash (American Academy of Pediatrics does not recommend its use for treatment of uncomplicated chickenpox in healthy children).

FORMS

Brand name (mfr)	Forms	Cost*
Zovirax (Generic Manufacturer)	Oral capsule 200 mg	$1.12
	Oral tablet 800 mg	$4.21
	IV vial 500 mg	$35
	Oral tablet 400 mg	$2.17
	Topical ointment 5%	$5.71
	Oral suspension 200 mg/5 mL	$138 per 480 5 mL
*Prices represents Average Wholesale Price (AWP).		

USUAL ADULT DOSING

Some expert recommends higher doses for immunocompromised pts. Valacyclovir or famciclovir generally preferred for oral administration due to better pharmacokinetic parameters and more convenient dosing.

- Mild HSV labialis (cold sore/fever blister): 400 mg PO three times a day × 7 days.
- Mild genital or perirectal HSV: 400 PO three times a day × 7 days.
- Severe genital or perirectal HSV: 5–10 mg/kg IV q8h × 7–14 days.
- HSV or VZV encephalitis:10 mg/kg IV q8h × 3 wks.
- Mild chickenpox: 800 mg PO 5×/day × 5 days.
- Severe chickenpox: 10 mg/kg IV q8h × 7–10 days.
- Severe dermatomal or visceral zoster: 10 mg/kg IV q8h until lesions resolved.
- VZV retinal necrosis: 10 mg/kg IV q8h plus IV foscarnet 90 mg/kg IV 12h.
- For obese pts: manufacturer recommends using IBW, but can consider [IBW + 0.4(TBW-IBW)] for severe CNS infections.

RENAL DOSING

Dosing for GFR of 50–80: 5–10 mg/kg IV q8h; 200–800 mg PO 5 × day.

Dosing for GFR of 10–50: GFR 25–50 mL/min: 5–10 mg/kg q12. GFR 10–24 mL/min: 5–10 mg/kg IV q24h; 200–800 mg PO q8h.

Dosing for GFR <10: 2.5–5 mg/kg IV q24h; 200–800 mg PO q12h.

Dosing in hemodialysis: 2.5–5 mg/kg IV q24h, dose after HD.

Dosing in peritoneal dialysis: 2.5–5 mg/kg IV q24h.

Dosing in hemofiltration: CAVH: 3.5 mg/kg/day. CVVHD: 5–10 mg/kg/day (10 mg/kg/day for zoster and CNS).

ADVERSE DRUG REACTIONS

General

- Generally very well tolerated.

Occasional

- Irritation and phlebitis at infusion site (IV preparation).
- Nausea and vomiting.
- Rash.

- Renal toxicity (especially crystallization w/ rapid IV infusion, underlying renal disease and nephrotoxic drugs co-administration). Incidence may be decreased with good hydration status.

Rare
- Dizziness
- CNS (especially with high dose in renal failure): agitation, encephalopathy, lethargy, tremor, transient hemiparesis, disorientation, seizures, hallucinations
- Anemia, neutropenia
- Transaminase elevations
- Pruritis
- Headache
- Hypotension

DRUG INTERACTIONS
- Theophylline: may increase theophylline plasma concentration.
- Meperidine: may increase normeperidine plasma concentration.
- Probenecid: increase in acyclovir levels due to competitive tubular secretion by probenecid; no dose adjustment usually needed.

RESISTANCE
- Development of resistance to acyclovir (HSV, VZV) generally only seen in severely immunocompromised hosts after long duration of acyclovir treatment.
- Cross-resistance with ganciclovir generally observed. Consider foscarnet or cidofovir.

PHARMACOLOGY
Mechanism
Converted by viral thymidine kinase to active acyclovir monophosphate; cellular enzyme catalase converts acyclovir monophosphate to acyclovir triphosphate, which competitively inhibits viral DNA polymerase.

Pharmacokinetic Parameters
- **Absorption** 10–30% bioavailability; decreased absorption with increased dose.
- **Cmax** 1.2 mcg/mL after 400 mg PO administration; 1.6 mcg/mL after 800 mg PO administration. 9.8 mcg/mL after 5 mg/kg IV administration; 22.9 mcg/mL after 10 mg/kg IV administration.
- **Distribution** High concentration found in kidneys, liver, and intestines. CNS penetration 50% of serum. Also distributed to lung, aqueous humor, tears, muscle, spleen, breast milk, uterine, vaginal mucosa, semen, and amniotic fluid.
- **Protein binding** 9–33%.
- **Metabolism/Excretion** Only 9–14% of dose metabolized to inactive metabolite. 45–79% excreted unchanged in the urine via glomerular filtration and tubular secretion.
- **T1/2** 2.5 hrs.

Dosing for Decreased Hepatic Function
No data. Dose reduction unlikely.

Pregnancy Risk
C: Not teratogen but potential to cause chromosomal damage at high dose. CDC recommends use of acyclovir for life threatening disease but does not advocate use for treatment or prophylaxis of genital herpes in pregnancy.

Breast Feeding Compatibility
Acyclovir is concentrated at high level in breast milk. Because acyclovir has been used in newborn to treat HSV infection without adverse events, the American Academy of Pediatrics considers acyclovir to be safe during breast feeding.

COMMENTS
Well tolerated oral and parenteral antiviral agent with activity against HSV and VZV. In immunocompromised pts, valacyclovir or famciclovir generally preferred over oral acyclovir due to better pharmacokinetic profiles and more convenient dosing. Topical use not effective. Monitor for crystalluria in pts receiving large IV doses with dehydration and/or renal insufficiency. Oral valacyclovir or famciclovir significantly reduced the duration of postherpetic neuralgia compared to oral acyclovir.

SELECTED REFERENCES
Conant MA, Schacker TW, Murphy RL, et al. Valaciclovir versus aciclovir for herpes simplex virus infection in HIV-infected individuals: two randomized trials. *Int J STD AIDS*, 2002; Vol. 13; pp. 12–21.

Spruance SL, Nett R, Marbury T, et al. Acyclovir cream for treatment of herpes simplex labialis: results of two random-ized, double-blind, vehicle-controlled, multicenter clinical trials. *Antimicrob Agents Chemother*, 2002; Vol. 46; pp. 2238–43.

ADEFOVIR

Paul A. Pham, PharmD and John G. Bartlett, MD

INDICATIONS
FDA
- Chronic hepatitis B (pts w/ clinical evidence of lamivudine-resistant HBV with either compensated or decompensated liver function)

FORMS

Brand name (mfr)	Forms	Cost*
Hepsera (Gilead)	PO tab 10 mg	$26.82

*Prices represents Average Wholesale Price (AWP).

USUAL ADULT DOSING
10 mg once daily (with or without food) × 48–92 wks.

RENAL DOSING
Dosing for GFR of 50–80: 10mg PO once daily.
Dosing for GFR of 10–50: GFR 20–49 mL/min:10mg q48h. GFR 10–19 mL/min: 10 mg every 72 hrs.
Dosing for GFR <10: No data.
Dosing in hemodialysis: 10 mg every 7 days following HD.
Dosing in peritoneal dialysis: No data.
Dosing in hemofiltration: CVVHD: no data, consider 10 mg every 48 hrs.

ADVERSE DRUG REACTIONS
General
- Generally well tolerated

Common
- Asthenia

Occasional
- Nephrotoxicity (w/ underlying renal insufficiency)
- Exacerbation of hepatitis (with discontinuation of therapy or development of HBV resistance)
- Abdominal pain, nausea, vomiting, diarrhea
- Cough
- Pruritus
- Headache

Rare
- Lactic acidosis, but less likely to occur compared to other NRTIs
- Fanconi syndrome (reported with large doses)

DRUG INTERACTIONS
Ibuprofen increases adefovir AUC by 23%. Drugs that inhibit tubular secretion (i.e., probenecid) may increase adefovir serum level.

RESISTANCE
- In a genotype analysis of an open-label pilot study evaluating the efficacy of adefovir (10 mg every day) in the treatment of lamivudine-resistance HBV infection, adefovir at a suboptimal concentration for (HIV-1) for 12 mos did not result in selection for either adefovir mutations at codons 65 and 70 or any other particular HIV-1 reverse transcriptase resistance in pts with uncontrolled HIV-1 replication [Delaugerre C et al. *AAC* 2002;46:1586]. Larger analysis that includes major and minor viral population with a longer follow-up should be performed before this cross-resistance issue can be settled.

ANTIVIRAL DRUGS

- Another concern regarding adefovir monotherapy for HBV is the potential for the development of adefovir resistant HBV. Thus far, adefovir resistant HBV has not been detected in approximately 78 wks of follow-up. However, longer follow-up is needed.
- Clinical trials of the various combinations involving interferon, lamivudine, and adefovir are underway, the hope is to prevent the evolution of resistant mutation and improve clinical outcome.

PHARMACOLOGY

Mechanism

Adefovir diphosphate inhibits HBV DNA polymerase which results in DNA chain termination after its incorporation into viral DNA.

Pharmacokinetic Parameters

- **Absorption** 59% (unaffected by food).
- **Cmax** 18.4 +/– 6.26 ng/mL.
- **Distribution** Vd = 393 +/– 75 mL/kg.
- **Protein binding** <4%.
- **Metabolism/Excretion** Adefovir dipivoxil is converted to adefovir which is excreted via glomerular filtration and active tubular secretion.
- **T1/2** serum: 1.6. Intracellular (diphosphate): 16 to 18 hrs.

Dosing for Decreased Hepatic Function

10 mg once daily.

Pregnancy Risk

C: Parenteral adefovir, when given at 20 mg/kg (systemic exposure 38 times human), resulted in embryotoxicity and fetal malformations. No human data.

Breast Feeding Compatibility

No data, not recommended.

COMMENTS

Adefovir is an effective treatment of chronic HBV infection, but entecavir, telbivudine, and tenofovir may be better choices due to higher potency. In HIV-co-infected pts, a concern w/ the use of low dose adefovir is the potential for the development of cross- resistance w/ nucleoside analogues and/or future activity of tenofovir. Preliminary data didn't show selection of adefovir mutations. Most HBV experts recommend the use of adefovir (tenofovir preferred) plus lamivudine for the treatment of HBV infection.

SELECTED REFERENCES

Peters MG, Andersen J, Lynch P, et al. Randomized controlled study of tenofovir and adefovir in chronic hepatitis B virus and HIV infection: ACTG A5127. *Hepatology*, 2006; Vol. 44; pp. 1110–6.

Sung JJ, Lai JY, Zeuzem S, et al. Lamivudine compared with lamivudine and adefovir dipivoxil for the treatment of HBeAg-positive chronic hepatitis B. *J Hepatol*, 2008; Vol. 48; pp. 728–35.

AMANTADINE

Paul A. Pham, PharmD and John G. Bartlett, MD

INDICATIONS

FDA

- Influenza A (prophylaxis and treatment: no longer recommended due to high incidence of resistant influenza strains, unless annual strain known to be susceptible)
- Parkinsonism

FORMS

Brand name (mfr)	Forms	Cost*
Symmetrel (Sandoz)	PO cap 100 mg	$0.73
	PO syrup 50 mg/5 mL (16 oz)	$72.75
*Prices represents Average Wholesale Price (AWP).		

USUAL ADULT DOSING
- Influenza treatment: 100 mg PO q12h (within 48 hrs of symptoms) × 5 days. Note: only use if circulating strains known to be susceptible to drug.
- Influenza prophylaxis: 100 mg PO q12h continued for at least 10 days after exposure or 2–4 wks after vaccination.
- 2009–2010 influenza season: pandemic H1N1 influenza A virus is expected to be the predominant circulating virus; amantadines are not recommended. Unknown if oseltamivir-resistant seasonal H1N1 virus seen in 2008–2009 season will circulate. See CDC website for any changed recommendations: Updated Interim Recommendations for the Use of Antiviral Medications in the Treatment and Prevention of Influenza for the 2009–2010 Season.

RENAL DOSING
Dosing for GFR 50–80: 100 mg q24–48hrs.
Dosing for GFR 10–50: 100 mg q48–72hrs.
Dosing for GFR <10: 100 mg q7d.
Dosing in hemodialysis: 100 mg q7d, no supplement needed post-dialysis.
Dosing in peritoneal dialysis: 100 mg q7d, no supplement needed post-dialysis.
Dosing in hemofiltration: No data.

ADVERSE DRUG REACTIONS
Common
- CNS: insomnia, lethargy, dizziness, inability to concentrate.

Occasional
- GI intolerance, esp. nausea
- Rash
- Depression
- Livedo reticularis

Rare
- CNS: tremor, confusion, psychosis, visual hallucination, paranoia, mania, seizure (esp. in elderly with renal failure and/or a seizure history)
- Heart failure, cardiac arrythmia (with high serum level)
- Eczematoid dermatitis and photosensitivity
- Oculogyric episodes (rotation of eyeball) and sudden loss of vision
- Orthostatic hypotension
- Peripheral edema
- Bone marrow suppression
- Urinary retention

DRUG INTERACTIONS
- Anticholinergic agents (e.g., tricyclic antidepressants, diphenhydramine): may increase the incidence of CNS side effects.
- Probenecid: may decrease renal clearance of amantadine, as a result, may enhance CNS side effects (confusion, tremors, seizures).
- Triamterene: may decrease renal clearance of amantadine, as a result, may enhance CNS side effects (confusion, tremors, seizures).
- Trimethoprim: may decrease renal clearance of amantadine, as a result, may enhance CNS side effects (confusion, tremors, seizures).

PHARMACOLOGY
Mechanism
Interferes with early step in influenza A replication (inhibits viral uncoating) inhibits ion channel function of M2 protein.

Pharmacokinetic Parameters
- **Absorption** Well absorbed.
- **Cmax** 0.3 mcg/mL after 2.5 mg/kg administration.
- **Distribution** animal data showed distribution in saliva, nasal secretion, lung tissues.
- **Protein binding** 60–67%.
- **Metabolism/Excretion** Excreted primarily unchanged in the urine.
- **T1/2** 24 hrs (range 9–37 hrs).

Dosing for Decreased Hepatic Function
100 mg q24h.

ANTIVIRAL DRUGS

Pregnancy Risk

C: Embryotoxic and teratogenic in animal studies. Of 51 exposures during the first trimester in a Michigan Medicaid surveillance study, the incidence of defects was 9.8%; though high, the numbers of exposures were too small to draw any conclusions.

Breast Feeding Compatibility

Excreted in low concentration in breast milk, potential for urinary retention, vomiting, and skin rash.

COMMENTS

Oral agent for prophylaxis and treatment of influenza A (but not active against influenza B). Amantadine prophylaxis is 70–90% effective in preventing influenza A if strains are susceptible, but offer only modest benefit in acute illness (1 day reduction in fever if given within 48 hrs of symptoms). CNS side effects may be bothersome, esp in elderly pts and in pts with renal impairment. Due to CNS toxicity, may prefer rimantadine or neuraminidase inhibitors which are more expensive. Can be used as an alternative to rimantidine in the treatment of influenza A (H1N1) resistant to oseltamivir.

BASIS FOR RECOMMENDATIONS

Fiore AE, Shay DK, Broder K, et al. Prevention and control of influenza: recommendations of the Advisory Committee on Immunization Practices (ACIP), 2008. *MMWR Recomm Rep*, 2008; Vol. 57; pp. 1–60.

Comments: Amantadine should not be used for the treatment or prevention of influenza A in the U.S. until evidence of susceptibility has been reestablished.

SELECTED REFERENCES

Bright RA, Shay DK, Shu B, et al. Adamantane resistance among influenza A viruses isolated early during the 2005–2006 influenza season in the United States. *JAMA*, 2006; Vol. 295; pp. 891–4.

T. O. Jefferson, et al. Cochrane Review. *The Cochrane Library, Oxford, February 1999 as reviewed in the ACP Journal Club*, 1999; Vol. 131; p. 68.

CIDOFOVIR

Paul A. Pham, PharmD and John G. Bartlett, MD

INDICATIONS

FDA

• Treatment of CMV retinitis in pts with AIDS.

Non-FDA Approved Uses

• Treatment of CMV colitis and pneumonitis (efficacy not established).
• Treatment of acyclovir-resistant HSV.
• Treatment of adenovirus infection in severely immune compromised.

FORMS

Brand name (mfr)	Forms	Cost*
Vistide (Gilead)	IV Vial 375 mg (75 mg/mL)	$888.00
*Prices represents Average Wholesale Price (AWP).		

USUAL ADULT DOSING

CMV retinitis: **induction:** 5 mg/kg IV over 1 hr qwk × 2, **maintenance:** 5 mg/kg IV over 1 hr q2 wks.

• Give probenecid 2 g given 3 hrs prior to cidofovir and 1 g given 2 and 8 hrs after infusion (blocks tubular secretion of cidofovir). Prehydrate with >1 L NS immediately before cidofovir infusion. Cidofovir is diluted in 100 mL 9% saline.
• Acyclovir-resistant HSV: cidofovir 1% gel to affected area once daily × 5 days (must be compounded by the pharmacy).

RENAL DOSING

Dosing for GFR of 50–80: 5 mg/kg.
Dosing for GFR of 10–50: Contraindicated for serum creat >1.5 mg/dL or creat clearance <55 mL/min.
Dosing for GFR <10: Contraindicated.

Dosing in hemodialysis: 52% +/– 11% cleared during high-flux hemodialysis. (*Clin Pharm Ther* 1999;65:21–8). Dose post-HD.

Dosing in peritoneal dialysis: Not significantly cleared.

Dosing in hemofiltration: No data.

ADVERSE DRUG REACTIONS

Common

- Dose-dependent **nephrotoxicity** in ~25% (proteinuria, azotemia, and proximal tubular dysfunction). Increased rate w/ other nephrotoxins, reduced w/ prehydration and probenecid. Monitor renal function 48 hrs prior to each dose.
- GI intolerance, rash, fever, and chills due to high dose probenecid (reduced by antiemetics, antihistamines, antipyretics, and food intake).
- Neutropenia (15%): monitor ANC.

Occasional

- Metabolic acidosis with Fanconi's syndrome: proteinuria, normoglycemic glycosuria, hypophosphatemia, and hypouricemia.

Rare

- Uveitis and ocular hypotony
- Asthenia

DRUG INTERACTIONS

Contraindicated with other nephrotoxic drugs: aminoglycosides, amphotericin B, foscarnet, NSAIDs, and pentamidine. One wk washout from nephrotoxic drugs recommended before cidofovir administration. Probenecid inhibits tubular secretion of acyclovir, beta-lactam antibiotics, AZT, and TDF; clinical significance unclear without prolonged co-administration.

PHARMACOLOGY

Mechanism

Cidofovir converted intracellularly by host enzymes to cidofovir diphosphate, which inhibits viral DNA polymerase.

Pharmacokinetic Parameters

- **Absorption** n/a
- **Cmax** 19.6 mcg/mL after 5 mg/kg administration.
- **Distribution** Undetectable CSF levels.
- **Protein binding** Low protein binding (0.5%).
- **Metabolism/Excretion** 80–100% of drug excreted unchanged in urine within 24 hrs.
- **T1/2** Active intracellular metabolite: 17–65 hrs.

Dosing for Decreased Hepatic Function

No data. Usual dose likely.

Pregnancy Risk

C: Carcinogenic, teratogenic and causes hypospermia in animal studies, no human data available.

Breast Feeding Compatibility

No data: avoid due to potential for severe toxicity.

COMMENTS

With the availability of ganciclovir ocular implant and oral valganciclovir, cidofovir now considered 2nd or 3rd line agent for treatment of CMV retinitis. Advantage of every other wk dosing and activity against ganciclovir-resistant CMV, but nephrotoxicity and probenecid side effects (chills, fever, headache, rash and nausea in 30–50% of pts) limit routine use. IV and/or topical cidofovir gel can be considered in acyclovir-resistant HSV. Occasionally used for adenovirus treatment in the severely immunosuppressed (see Neofytos ref).

SELECTED REFERENCES

Lalezari JP, Holland GN, Kramer F, et al. Randomized, controlled study of the safety and efficacy of intravenous cidofovir for the treatment of relapsing cytomegalovirus retinitis in pts with AIDS. *J Acquir Immune Defic Syndr Hum Retrovirol*, 1998; Vol. 17; pp. 339–44.

Neofytos D, Ojha A, Mookerjee B, et al. Treatment of adenovirus disease in stem cell transplant recipients with cidofovir. *Biol Blood Marrow Transplant*, 2007; Vol. 13; pp. 74–81.

ANTIVIRAL DRUGS

ENTECAVIR

Paul A. Pham, PharmD and John G. Bartlett, MD

INDICATIONS

FDA

- Treatment of chronic hepatitis B (HBV) infection in adult pts with evidence of active disease (active viral replication, elevated ALT or AST or histologic evidence of active disease)

FORMS

Brand name (mfr)	Forms	Cost*
Baraclude (Bristol-Myers Squibb)	Oral tablets 0.5 mg, 1mg Oral solution 0.05 mg/mL (210 mL)	$28.41 $596.70 /210 mL
*Prices represents Average Wholesale Price (AWP).		

USUAL ADULT DOSING

- For nucleoside-naive pts: 0.5 mg PO daily on an empty stomach (2hrs before or after food).
- For lamivudine (3TC) refractory pts: 1 mg PO daily on an empty stomach (2 hrs before or after food).

RENAL DOSING

Dosing for GFR 50–80: Usual dosing.

Dosing for GFR 10–50: CrCl 30–49 mL/min, NRTI naive: 0.25 mg daily; lamivudine (3TC)-resistant: 0.5 mg daily. CrCl 10–29 mL/min, NRTI naive: 0.15 mg daily; lamivudine (3TC)-res. 0.30 mg daily.

Dosing for GFR <10: Cr Clearance <10 mL/min: nucleoside naive: 0.05 mg daily; lamivudine (3TC)-refractory: 0.1 mg daily.

Dosing in hemodialysis: Nucleoside naive: 0.05 mg daily (dose post HD on days of dialysis); lamivudine (3TC)-refractory: 0.1 mg daily (dose post HD on days of dialysis).

Dosing in peritoneal dialysis: Nucleoside naive: 0.05 mg daily; lamivudine (3TC)-refractory: 0.1 mg daily.

Dosing in hemofiltration: No data. Consider 0.5–1.0 mg daily.

ADVERSE DRUG REACTIONS

Common

- Generally well tolerated with side effect profile comparable to lamivudine and placebo in clinical trials.

Rare

- Headache
- Fatigue
- Nausea, diarrhea
- Insomnia
- Low likelihood of lactic acidosis

DRUG INTERACTIONS

No drug interactions observed with the co-administration of entecavir and adefovir, tenofovir or lamivudine. *In vitro,* entecavir was not antagonistic with abacavir, didanosine, lamivudine, stavudine, tenofovir, or zidovudine.

RESISTANCE

- Lamivudine-resistant strains are 8–30-fold less sensitive to entecavir. Resistance to entecavir can emerge during treatment but is infrequent.
- HBV strains from pts who failed entecavir are resistant to lamivudine.
- In pts with lamivudine-refractory infections, emergence of entecavir resistance occurs in 7% of pts by wk 48.

PHARMACOLOGY

Mechanism

Entecavir is a guanosine nucleoside analogue that specifically inhibits the HBV polymerase. A 150 to 1300-fold higher entecavir concentration would be needed to inhibit human cellular DNA polymerase.

Pharmacokinetic Parameters
- **Absorption** Food decreases absorption by 18–20%.
- **Cmax** Cmin, and AUC: Cmax = 4.2 ng/mL (with 0.5 mg) and 8.2 ng/mL (with 1 mg); AUC decreased by 18–20% and Cmax decreased by 44–46% when taken with food.
- **Distribution** PK studies suggest it is widely distributed in tissues.
- **Protein binding** 13% (*in vitro*).
- **Metabolism/Excretion** Renal excretion via glomerular filtration and tubular secretion accounts for 63–73%.
- **T1/2** Serum: 128–149 hrs; intracellular: 15 hrs.

Dosing for Decreased Hepatic Function
Usual dose.

Pregnancy Risk
C: negative embryotoxicity and maternal toxicity in rat and rabbit studies at 28 and 212 times the levels achieved with the highest daily dose (1 mg/day). Rat and rabbit embryo and fetal toxicities seen at 3100 times the human drug levels. No studies in humans. Pregnancy registry for entecavir: 1-800-258-4263.

Breast Feeding Compatibility
No human data, breast milk excretion in animal studies. Breast feeding is not recommended.

COMMENTS
Entecavir is well tolerated and superior to lamivudine for treatment of HBV-infected pt who are treatment naive or lamivudine-resistant. Similar to adefovir and lamivudine, recent evidence suggests that entecavir has activity against HIV, therefore HIV cross-resistance has been reported when entecavir is used as monotherapy in co-infected pts. Although monotherapy entecavir is FDA approved for the treatment of chronic HBV, most ID experts recommend combination therapy.

SELECTED REFERENCES
Gish RG, Lok AS, Chang TT, et al. Entecavir therapy for up to 96 wks in pts with HBeAg-positive chronic hepatitis B. *Gastroenterology*, 2007; Vol. 133; pp. 1437–44.

Sherman M, Yurdaydin C, Sollano J, et al. Entecavir for treatment of lamivudine-refractory, HBeAg-positive chronic hepatitis B. *Gastroenterology*, 2006; Vol. 130; pp. 2039–49.

FAMCICLOVIR

Paul A. Pham, PharmD and John G. Bartlett, MD

INDICATIONS

FDA
- Recurrent genital herpes (suppression and treatment) in immunocompetent and HIV-infected pts.
- Treatment of herpes zoster.

FORMS

Brand name (mfr)	Forms	Cost*
Famvir (Norvartis Pharmaceuticals)	Oral tablet 125 mg Oral tablet 250 mg Oral tablet 500 mg	$5.57 $6.06 $12.17
Famciclovir (Teva, generic manufacturers)	Oral tablet 125 mg Oral tablet 250 mg Oral tablet 500 mg	$4.63 $5.03 $10.13
*Prices represents Average Wholesale Price (AWP).		

USUAL ADULT DOSING
- HSV (initial): 250 mg PO q8h or 500 mg PO twice daily × 7 days.
- Recurrent HSV (orolabial or genital herpes infection): 125 mg PO q8h or 250–500 mg PO twice daily × 7 days.
- Suppression of recurrent genital HSV: 250 mg twice daily (up to 1 yr).

ANTIVIRAL DRUGS

- Herpes zoster: 500 mg PO q8h × 7–10 days.
- Famciclovir is a prodrug of the antiviral agent penciclovir.

RENAL DOSING
Dosing for GFR 50–80: Usual dose with GFR >60 mL/min.
Dosing for GFR 10–50: GFR 40 to 59 mL/min: 500 mg q12h. GFR 20–39 mL/min: 125–250 mg q12 hrs.
Dosing for GFR <10: GFR <20 mL/min: 125–250 mg q24 hrs.
Dosing in hemodialysis: 125–250 mg q48h, dose after HD.
Dosing in peritoneal dialysis: No data.
Dosing in hemofiltration: No data.

ADVERSE DRUG REACTIONS
- Generally very well tolerated

Occasional
- Headache and dizziness
- GI intolerance: nausea and diarrhea

DRUG INTERACTIONS
Probenecid: may increase penciclovir concentrations.

PHARMACOLOGY
Mechanism
Converted to penciclovir, a guanosine analog transformed in HSV and VZV infected cells into triphosphate form which inhibits viral DNA polymerase.

Pharmacokinetic Parameters
- **Absorption** 77%.
- **Cmax** 3.3–4.2 mcg/mL after a single dose of 500 mg.
- **Distribution** Good tissue penetration with blood/plasma ratio of 1.
- **Protein binding** 20%.
- **Metabolism/Excretion** Deacetylated and then oxidized to penciclovir (active), less than 1.5% of total dose is metabolized to inactive metabolite. 60–65% of dose is excreted as penciclovir in the urine; 27% of dose excreted in feces.
- **T1/2** 2–3 hrs.

Dosing for Decreased Hepatic Function
No data. Usual dose likely.

Pregnancy Risk
B: Carcinogenic, but not embryotoxic or teratogenic in animal studies. No human data.

Breast Feeding Compatibility
No data, but due to the probable excretion into breast milk and the carcinogenicity potential in animal studies, not recommended when breastfeeding.

SELECTED REFERENCES
Aoki FY, Tyring S, Diaz-Mitoma F, et al. Single-day, patient-initiated famciclovir therapy for recurrent genital herpes: a randomized, double-blind, placebo-controlled trial. *Clin Infect Dis*, 2006; Vol. 42; pp. 8–13.

Romanowski B, Aoki FY, Martel AY, et al. Efficacy and safety of famciclovir for treating mucocutaneous herpes simplex infection in HIV-infected individuals. Collaborative Famciclovir HIV Study Group. *AIDS*, 2000; Vol. 14; pp. 1211–7.

FOSCARNET

Paul A. Pham, PharmD and John G. Bartlett, MD

INDICATIONS
FDA
- CMV retinitis in immunocompromised pts.
- Acyclovir-resistant mucocutaneous herpes simplex virus (HSV-1 and HSV-2) infections in immunocompromised pts.

Non-FDA Approved Uses
- Ganciclovir-resistant CMV retinitis.
- Extraocular CMV infection.

FORMS

Brand name (mfr)	Forms	Cost*
Foscavir (Astra Zeneca and generic manufacturer [Pharmaforce])	IV vial 24 mg/mL (250 mL, 500 mL)	$73 per 250 mL vial; $143.25 per 500 vial

*Prices represents Average Wholesale Price (AWP).

USUAL ADULT DOSING

- CMV retinitis: **induction** 90 mg/kg IV q12h × 14 days over 1 hr via infusion pump, **maintenance** 90–120 mg/kg IV once daily over 2 hrs via infusion pump (120 mg/kg IV once daily after reinduction for a relapse).
- Extraocular CMV disease (e.g., GI, neuro): 90 mg/kg IV q12 × 14–21 days. Role of maintenance dose unclear but most recommend maintenance dose with reoccurrences.
- Acyclovir-resistant HSV and VZV: 60 mg/kg IV q8h × 3 wks.
- Note: infuse foscarnet over 2 hrs with 500 cc NS pre- and post-hydration.
- **Dose adjustment in renal failure:** >1.4 mL/min/kg or >98 mL/min for a 70 kg pt: 90 mg/kg q12h (induction); 90 mg/kg once daily (maintenance).
- CrCl of 1.0–1.4 mL/min/kg: 70 mg/kg q12h (induction); 70 mg/kg once daily (maintenance).
- CrCl of 0.8–1.0 mL/min/kg: 50 mg/kg q12h (induction); 50 mg/kg once daily (maintenance).
- CrCl of 0.6–0.8 mL/min/kg: 80 mg/kg q24h (induction); 80 mg/kg every other day (maintenance).
- CrCl of 0.5–0.6 mL/min/kg: 60 mg/kg q24h (induction); 60 mg/kg every other day (maintenance).
- CrCl of 0.4–0.5 mL/min/kg: 50 mg/kg q24h (induction); 50 mg/kg every other day (maintenance).
- Administer by controlled IV infusion (24 mg/mL via central venous line or 12 mg/mL via peripheral vein). Solutions (with NL saline or 5% dextrose) should be used within 24 hrs of first entry into sealed foscarnet bottle. Do not co-administer with other drugs or supplements concurrently via the same catheter.
- CrCl of <0.4 mL/min/kg: not recommended.

RENAL DOSING

Dosing for GFR <10: Contraindicated for CrCl <20 mL/min (unless irreversible renal failure on HD).

Dosing in hemodialysis: 38% removal, 60 mg/kg post HD (consider monitoring serum levels: goal of 500–800 *mcgM*).

Dosing in peritoneal dialysis: Dose for GFR <10 mL/min.

Dosing in hemofiltration: No data.

ADVERSE DRUG REACTIONS

Common

- **Renal failure** (creat 2 mg/dL in up to 37% of pts); often reversible if discontinued early; hydrate adequately and monitor creat 2–3 ×/wk during induction and qwk during maintenance. Discontinue if creat >2.9 mg/dL.
- **Electrolyte imbalance** (hypocalcemia, hypophosphatemia, hypomagnesemia, and hypokalemia (8–15%)—monitor chem 2 ×/wk during induction and qwk during maintenance.

Occasional

- Paresthesias and seizures secondary to electrolyte imbalance.
- Penile ulcers.
- Nausea and vomiting.

Rare

- Fever
- Rash
- Bone marrow suppression
- LFTs elevation
- Headache

ANTIVIRAL DRUGS

- Pentamidine (IV): additive hypocalcemia and nephrotoxicity with co-administration.
- Amphotericin B, aminoglycoside, cidofovir and other nephrotoxic agents: additive nephrotoxicity with foscarnet co-administration. Avoid co-administration.
- Imipenem: possible increase in risk of seizure.

RESISTANCE
- CMV cross-resistance to foscarnet is rare.
- UL54 resistance mutation in the DNA polymerase gene (without UL97) is uncommon in ganciclovir treated pts but can confer foscarnet resistance (N495K) (*Antivir Ther.* 2006;11:537–40.)
- Foscarnet resistance mutations in the DNA polymerase gene include V787L and E756Q and is associated with retinitis progression (odds ratio, 14; P = .016) (*J Infect Dis.* 2003;187:777–84.)
- The incidence of foscarnet resistance after 6, 9, and 12 mos of therapy is 13%, 24%, and 37%, respectively.

PHARMACOLOGY
Mechanism
Pyrophosphate analog of phosphonoacetic acid that directly blocks pyrophosphate binding site of viral DNA polymerase, preventing cleavage of pyrophosphate from deoxynucleoside triphosphate and elongation of viral DNA chains. Unlike acyclovir and ganciclovir, foscarnet does not require thymidine kinase for activation.

Pharmacokinetic Parameters
- **Absorption** Poor absorption 12–22% (only given IV).
- **Cmax** 575 mcg/L after 57 mg/kg administration.
- **Distribution** 43% CNS penetration; sequestered in bone and cartilage.
- **Protein binding** 14–17%.
- **Metabolism/Excretion** Not metabolized; approximately 80–87% of drug excreted unchanged in the urine via glomerular filtration and tubular secretion.
- **T1/2** 3 hrs.

Dosing for Decreased Hepatic Function
No data. Usual dose likely.

Pregnancy Risk
C: Skeletal malformation or variation in animal studies. No human data available; however, some OB/GYN experts feel that foscarnet should be used as first line agent for sight-threatening CMV retinitis in pregnant women (due to high incidence of nephrotoxicity, antepartum testing of fetus and close monitoring of the amniotic fluid to observe for fetal nephrotoxicity recommended).

Breast Feeding Compatibility
No data: Most likely excreted in human milk; excreted in breast milk in animal studies. Due to the potential for severe adverse reaction to foscarnet mother should avoid foscarnet when breast feeding.

COMMENTS
Parenteral antiviral agent with activity against HSV, VZV, and CMV. Generally considered the second line to ganciclovir for CMV infections due to unfavorable side effect profile (nephrotoxicity and electrolyte imbalance). Close monitoring of electrolytes and renal function needed. Active against ganciclovir-resistant CMV and acyclovir-resistant HSV and VZV.

SELECTED REFERENCES
Jacobson MA, Wulfsohn M, Feinberg JE, et al. Phase II dose-ranging trial of foscarnet salvage therapy for cytomegalovirus retinitis in AIDS pts intolerant of or resistant to ganciclovir (ACTG protocol 093). AIDS Clinical Trials Group of the National Institute of Allergy and Infectious Diseases. *AIDS*, 1994; Vol. 8; pp. 451–9.

National Institutes of Health (NIH), the Centers for Disease Control and Prevention (CDC), and the HIV Medicine Association of the Infectious Diseases Society of America (HIVMA/IDSA). Guidelines for Prevention and Treatment of Opportunistic Infections in HIV-Infected Adults and Adolescents. *http://AIDSinfo.nih.gov*, 2008.

GANCICLOVIR

Paul A. Pham, PharmD and John G. Bartlett, MD

INDICATIONS

FDA

- Treatment of CMV retinitis (IV) in immunocompromised pts.
- Prophylaxis and prevention of CMV disease recurrence in pts with AIDS and solid organ transplant recipients (use for primary prophylaxis in HIV is FDA approved but not currently recommended).

FORMS

Brand name (mfr)	Forms	Cost*
Cytovene (Roche)	IV vial 500 mg	$66.80
Ganciclovir (generic) (Ranbaxy)	Oral capsule 250 mg; 500 mg	$4.72; $9.44
Vitrasert ocular implant (Bausch and Lomb)	Ocular implant 4.5 mg	$19,200.00/per implant
*Prices represents Average Wholesale Price (AWP).		

USUAL ADULT DOSING

- **CMV retinitis induction:** 5 mg/kg IV q12h × 2 wks (alternative is valganciclovir 900 mg PO twice daily × 3 wks)+ ganciclovir implant then maintenance valganciclovir.
- **CMV retinitis maintenance:** 5 mg/kg IV once daily until immune reconstitution (CD4 >150 for 3–6 mos with inactive disease and follow-up by ophthalmologist). Decision to stop ganciclovir maintenance should take into account anatomic location of the retinal lesions, vision in the contralateral eye, and the feasibility of regular ophthalmologic monitoring. IV reserved for pts unable to take oral medications or for seriously ill pts. For pts with small peripheral lesions, oral valganciclovir alone may be adequate.
- Preferred maintenance regimen is valganciclovir (900 mg PO once daily). Provides serum concentrations comparable to those achieved with IV ganciclovir.
- **Implant:** 4.5 mg ocular implant every 6–9 mos (+ oral valganciclovir). Ganciclovir implant provides longest time to relapse. Many ophthalmologists recommend initial intravitreous injection of ganciclovir ASAP, until the ganciclovir implant can be placed.
- **CMV encephalitis and CMV polyradiculitis:** 5 mg/kg IV q12h (consider combination therapy with foscarnet), then 5 mg/kg q24h until immune reconstitution.
- **CMV (GI):** 5 mg/kg q12h × 3–6 wks. The role of maintenance ganciclovir is unclear. In an open label study, after an initial response, the time to progression was not significantly different between recipients (16 wks) and non-recipient (13 wks) of maintenance therapy (Blanshard et al. *J Infect Dis*. 1995;172:622–8).
- **CMV pneumonitis prophylaxis in HSCT recipients:** Ganciclovir 5 mg/kg/dose intravenously every 12 hrs for 5 to 7 days (up to 14 days), followed by 5 mg/kg intravenously daily for 5 days/wk from engraftment until day 100 after HSCT or until antigenemia or PCR is negative.
- CMV disease in BMT: if antigenemia/positive PCR persists > 4 wks of ganciclovir IV or levels increase after 3 wks, assume resistance; discontinue ganciclovir, begin foscarnet.

RENAL DOSING

Dosing for GFR 50–80: Induction dose: CrCL >80 mL/min: 5 mg/kg IV q12h; 1000 mg PO three times daily. CrCL 50–79 mL/min: 2.5 mg/kg q12h or 500 mg PO three times daily.

Dosing for GFR 10–50: Induction dose: CrCL 25–49 mL/min: 2.5 mg/kg IV q24h or 1000 mg PO q24h. CrCL 10–25 mL/min: 1.25 mg/kg IV q24h or 500 mg PO q24h.

Dosing for GFR <10: Induction dose: 1.25 mg/kg IV three times per wk or 500 mg PO three times per wk.

Dosing in hemodialysis: 50% of dose removed after 4 hrs of HD. Induction dose: 1.25 mg/kg IV or 500 mg PO three times per wk given post HD.

Dosing in peritoneal dialysis: No data, likely to be removed.

ANTIVIRAL DRUGS

Dosing in hemofiltration: Removed in CVVHD. Limited data, consider 5 mg/kg q48h (induction) or 2.5 mg/kg q48h (maintenance)

ADVERSE DRUG REACTIONS

Common

- Neutropenia (reversible and responds to G-CSF).
- Reversible thrombocytopenia.
- Monitor CBC 2–3/wk and discontinue or add G-CSF if ANC <500. Discontinue for PLT <25,000.

Occasional

- Anemia
- Fever
- Rash
- Headache, seizures, confusion, change in mental status
- GI intolerance

Rare

- Coma
- Hepatoxicity

DRUG INTERACTIONS

- AZT: additive risk of neutropenia with co-administration.
- Didanosine (ddI): ddI AUC increased 111% with oral ganciclovir and 50–70% with IV ganciclovir. Avoid or use with close monitoring for ddI induced toxicity. Consider an alternative NRTI.
- Imipenem-cilastatin: potential for generalized seizures.
- Pyrimethamine, 5-FC, interferon: potential for additive bone marrow suppression.

RESISTANCE

- The detection of cytomegalovirus resistant (genotype UL97 in the protein kinase associated with ganciclovir resistance only) to ganciclovir was associated with a 4 to 6-fold increase in the odds of retinitis progression (*Am J Ophthalmol*. 2003;135:26–34).
- In high-risk solid-organ transplant recipients receiving valganciclovir, no resistance mutation (UL97) was detected after 100 days of therapy (*J Infect Dis*. 2004;189:1615–8).
- UL54 resistance mutation in the DNA polymerase gene (with or without UL97) is uncommon but can confer cidofovir cross-resistance (L545S) and possibly foscarnet resistance (N495K) (*Antivir Ther*. 2006;11:537–40. *J Med Virol*. 2005;77:425–9).

PHARMACOLOGY

Mechanism

Guanosine that requires TK (HSV/VZV) or protein kinase (CMV) as first step to convert to triphosphate, which inhibits viral DNA polymerase.

Pharmacokinetic Parameters

- **Absorption** 5% (fasting); 6–9% (with food).
- **Cmax** 9.5–11.6 mcg/mL after 5 mg/kg IV.
- **Distribution** 7–67% CNS penetration. Good intraocular penetration.
- **Protein binding** 1–2%, low protein binding.
- **Metabolism/Excretion** Not metabolized, 90–99% excreted unchanged in the urine.
- **T1/2** 2.5–4 hrs.

Dosing for Decreased Hepatic Function

No data: usual dose likely.

Pregnancy Risk

C: Teratogenic, carcinogenic, and embryogenic; growth retardation; aplastic organ and aspermatogenesis in animal studies. No human data, use only for life threatening CMV infection and warn pt of possible teratogenic effect.

Breast Feeding Compatibility

No data: due to the potential for serious toxicity, mother should avoid breast feeding.

COMMENTS

Agent of choice for CMV infection due to better side effect profile vs. foscarnet and cidofovir. Acyclovir-resistant HSV usually cross-resistant to ganciclovir. Oral ganciclovir replaced by valganciclovir for maintenance therapy of CMV retinitis due to poor absorption, high pill burden. Neutropenia (ANC < 500) or thrombocytopenia (<25,000) are contraindications to initial use.

BASIS FOR RECOMMENDATIONS

Recommendations of the National Institutes of Health (NIH), the Centers for Disease Control and Prevention (CDC), and the HIV Medicine Association of the Infectious Diseases Society of America (HIVMA/IDSA). Guidelines for Prevention and Treatment of Opportunistic Infections in HIV-Infected Adults and Adolescents. *http://AIDSinfo.nih.gov*, 2008.

Comments: Valganciclovir, IV ganciclovir, IV ganciclovir followed by valganciclovir, IV foscarnet, IV cidofovir, and ganciclovir intraocular implant + valganciclovir are all effective treatments for CMV retinitis.

SELECTED REFERENCES

Martin DF, Sierra-Madero J, Walmsley S, et al. A controlled trial of valganciclovir as induction therapy for cytomegalovirus retinitis. *N Engl J Med*, 2002; Vol. 346; pp. 1119–26.

Martin DF, Parks DJ, Mellow SD, et al. Treatment of cytomegalovirus retinitis with an intraocular sustained-release ganciclovir implant. A randomized controlled clinical trial. *Arch Ophthalmol*, 1994; Vol. 112; pp. 1531–9.

INTERFERON ALPHA

Paul A. Pham, PharmD and John G. Bartlett, MD

INDICATIONS

FDA

- Hepatitis C and AIDS-related KS (interferon [IFN] alpha 2a and IFN alpha 2b).
- CML and hairy cell leukemia (IFN alpha 2a).
- Hepatitis B (IFN alpha 2b).
- Condyloma acuminata, hairy cell leukemia, malignant melanoma, follicular lymphoma (IFN alpha 2b).
- Pegylated Interferon (Peg-Intron and Pegasys): Hepatitis C. Only Pegasys plus Copegus have the indication for HCV in HIV coinfected pts.

FORMS

Brand name (mfr)	Forms	Cost*
Intron A (Schering)	SC vial 10 million units	$174.71
	18 million units	$314.51
	25 million units	$505.74
	50 million units	$873.71 per vial
	SC pen injection kit 3 million units	$364.10
	5 million units	$606.88
	10 million units	$1048.45 (6 pen per kit)
	SC vial kit 10 million units	$1017.91 (6 vial per kit)
Roferon A (Roche3)	SC vial kit 3 million units	$50.94
	6 million units	$101.84
	9 million units/0.5 mL	$143.38/vial kit
Peg-Intron (Schering)	SC vial kit 50 mcg	$495
	80 mcg	$520
	120 mcg	$546
	150 mcg	$573 (4 vial per kit)
Pegasys (Roche)	SC vial 180 mcg/mL	$570.85
	SC vial kit 180 mcg/0.5 mL	$2283.40 per vial kit (4 vial per kit)

*Prices represents Average Wholesale Price (AWP).

USUAL ADULT DOSING

- HBV: 10 million units SQ or IM 3 ×/wk or 5 million units q24h × 16–24 wks (HBeAg+). Pts with negative HBeAg may require >12 mos treatment.
- KS: Intron A or Roferon A 30–36 million units 3–7 ×/wk until lesion resolution.
- Condylomata: Intron A 1 million units intralesional 3 ×/wk. 2–4 million units IM three times a wk for a total of 6 wks as also been effective, but associated with ADRs.
- HCV: 3 million units SQ or IM 3 ×/wk in combination w/ ribavirin × 48 wks (pegylated interferon preferred).

ANTIVIRAL DRUGS

- HCV: *Peg-Intron* 1.5 mcg/kg SC q wk + ribavirin 1000 mg (<75 kg) or 1200 mg (≥75 kg) × 48 wks. Dose reduction to 0.5 mcg/kg for ANC<750 or PLT <80 K;D/C if ANC<500 or PLT <50 K. Monotherapy with 1 mcg/kg q wk and lower ribavirin doses of 800 mg in combination with *Peg-Intron* is FDA indicated but not recommended.
- HCV (genotype I and 4): *Pegasys* 180 mcg SC q wk + ribavirin 1000 mg (<75 kg) or 1200 mg (≥75 kg) × 48 wks (may reduce ribavirin to 800 mg/day and shorten treatment duration to 24 wks for genotype 2 and 3). For ANC <750: dose reduce to *Pegasys* 135 mcg/wk. For PLT <50 K: dose *Pegasys* 90 mcg/wk. D/C if ANC <500 or Plt <25 K.

RENAL DOSING
Dosing for GFR 50–80: Usual dose.
Dosing for GFR 10–50: Limited data. Usual dose likely.
Dosing for GFR <10: Limited data. Usual dose likely.
Dosing in hemodialysis: Usual dose.
Dosing in peritoneal dialysis: No data. Usual dose likely.
Dosing in hemofiltration: No data. Usual dose likely.

ADVERSE DRUG REACTIONS
Most pts experience dose-related side effects (more common with >18 million units).

Common
- Flu-like syndrome (50–98%): fever, chills, fatigue, headache, arthralgias, usually within 6 hrs of administration, lasting 2–12 hrs. NSAIDs may alleviate sx.
- GI intolerance (20–65%): anorexia, abdominal pain, nausea, vomiting, diarrhea.
- Neuropsychiatric toxicity (20–50%): irritability, depression, confusion, anxiety.
- Hepatitis (dose related in up to 40% receiving high doses).
- Marrow suppression.
- Rash and alopecia (up to 25%).
- Proteinuria.
- Metallic taste.

Occasional
- Dyspnea and cough.
- Elevations of bilirubin and alkaline phosphatase.
- Insomnia.

Rare
- Suicidal ideation or behavior.
- Thyroiditis with hyperthyroidism or hypothyroidism.
- Retinopathy.
- Rash with rare cases of EM, Stevens Johnson Syndrome and TEN reported.
- Injection site necrosis.
- Myositis.
- ITP and TTP.

DRUG INTERACTIONS
- ACE inhibitors (captopril and enalapril): case reports of neutropenia and thrombocytopenia with coadministration. Monitor closely.
- AZT, ganciclovir, pyrimethamine, cancer chemotherapy, and 5FC: additive bone marrow suppression with INF coadministration. Monitor CBC closely.
- Phenobarbital: phenobarbital serum levels may be increased. Monitor levels closely.
- Theophylline: theophylline serum levels may be increased. Monitor levels closely.

PHARMACOLOGY
Mechanism
Glycoprotein cytokine (intracellular messenger) with complex immunomodulating, antineoplastic, and antiviral properties after binding new cellular RNA and effector proteins are synthesized, mediating antiviral effect.

Pharmacokinetic Parameters
- **Absorption** 80% absorption from SQ and IM site.
- **Cmax** Mean concentration levels at steady-state: Peg-IFN-a2a: 20,000 pg/mL > Peg-IFN-a2b: 1000 pg/mL hrs >> IFN-a: 100 pg/mL.
- **Distribution** No data.
- **Protein binding** No data.

- **Metabolism/Excretion** IFN: undergoes rapid proteolytic degradation during tubular reabsorption with only minor hepatic metabolism. Reabsorption of intact compound is minimal, and parent compound does not appear in urine. Peg-IFN: liver metabolism by non-specific proteases (no renal metabolism). Excreted primarily in the bile (with little renal clearance).
- **T1/2** Peg-IFN-a2a: 77 hrs > Peg-IFN-a2b: 40 hrs >> IFN-a: 2–5 hrs.

Dosing for Decreased Hepatic Function
Usual dose.

Pregnancy Risk
C: Abortifacient in animal studies at high doses. In case reports of maternal administration does not appear to pose significant risk to the fetus; however, due to antiproliferative activity of interferon, should be avoided during gestation.

Breast Feeding Compatibility
Avoid during breastfeeding.

COMMENTS
For parenteral treatment for hepatitis C (in combination with ribavirin), Peg-IFN now preferred due to superior efficacy and more convenient weekly dosing. *Pegasys* has more prolonged $T_{1/2}$ and reaches higher serum levels compared to *Peg-Intron*. Despite these differences, 2 products have comparable in efficacy. Pts with <2 log drop in HCV DNA after 12-wk treatment with Peg-IFN unlikely to achieve virological suppression. Consider D/C if HCV RNA detectable after 24 wks. Obtain CBC and chemistries (baseline, wk 2 and q6wks) and TSH (baseline and q12wks). Obtain EKG (baseline and PRN) for pts with cardiac disease and pregnancy test (4–6 wks) for women of childbearing potential. IFN may be more efficacious than 3TC for treatment of HBV, but side effect profile, including flu-like symptoms and depression, may complicate treatment. Uncontrolled psychiatric illness and decompensated liver disease are contraindications to interferon therapy. Lower rate of SVR for genotype 1 in HIV-coinfected pts compared to non-HIV infected pts with genotype 2 and 3. Rapid virological response (RVR) obtained at wk 4 of therapy is a very good positive predictive factor of sustained virologic response (PPV at 97%).

SELECTED REFERENCES
Abergel A, Hezode C, Leroy V, et al. Peginterferon alpha-2b plus ribavirin for treatment of chronic hepatitis C with severe fibrosis: a multicentre randomized controlled trial comparing two doses of peginterferon alpha-2b. *J Viral Hepat*, 2006; Vol. 13; pp. 811–20.

Payan C, Pivert A, Morand P, et al. Rapid and early virological response to chronic hepatitis C treatment with IFN alpha2b or PEG-IFN alpha2b plus ribavirin in HIV/HCV co-infected pts. *Gut*, 2007; Vol. 56; pp. 1111–6.

LAMIVUDINE

Paul A. Pham, PharmD and John G. Bartlett, MD

INDICATIONS

FDA
- Treatment of HIV infection in combination with other antiretrovirals.
- Treatment of HBV (*Epivir HB*).

Non-FDA Approved Uses
- Treatment of hepatitis in HIV-HBV co-infected pts.

FORMS

Brand name (mfr)	Forms	Cost*
Epivir (GlaxoSmithKline)	Oral tablet 150 mg; 300 mg	$7.08; $14.17
	Oral solution 10 mg/mL (240 mL)	$113.34
Epivir HB (for HBV infection) (GlaxoSmithKline)	Oral tablet 100 mg	$13.55
	Oral solution 5 mg/mL (240 mL)	$162.66
Combivir (GlaxoSmithKline)	Oral tablet 150 mg 3TC/300 mg AZT	$15.36

ANTIVIRAL DRUGS

Brand name (mfr)	Forms	Cost*
Trizivir (GlaxoSmithKline)	Oral tablet ABC 300 mg + AZT 300 mg + 3TC 150 mg	$24.87
Epzicom (GlaxoSmithKline)	Oral tablet ABC 600 mg + 3TC 300 mg	$33.20
Kivexa (brand name available in Europe) (GlaxoSmithKline)	Oral tablet ABC 600 mg + 3TC 300 mg	variable
*Prices represents Average Wholesale Price (AWP).		

USUAL ADULT DOSING
Pill burden: 1–2 tabs once daily (for HIV). HBV: 100 mg once daily.
- As *Epivir:* 3TC 300 mg PO once daily or 150 mg PO twice daily.
- As *Combivir* or *Trizivir:* 1 tab PO twice daily.
- As *Epzicom:* 1 tab PO once daily.

RENAL DOSING
Dosing for GFR 50–80: 300 mg once daily or 150 mg PO twice daily.
Dosing for GFR 10–50: Cr Clearance 30–49 mL/min: 150 mg PO once daily; Cr Clearance 15–29 mL/min: 150 mg × 1 then 100 mg once daily.
Dosing for GFR <10: 150 mg × 1 then 25–50 mg once daily.
Dosing in hemodialysis: 150 mg × 1, then 25–50 mg once daily (post HD).
Dosing in peritoneal dialysis: 150 mg × 1, then 25–50 mg once daily (limited data).
Dosing in hemofiltration: No data consider 150 mg PO once daily.

ADVERSE DRUG REACTIONS
One of the best tolerated NRTIs with side effect profile comparable to placebo in hepatitis trials.

Occasional
- Headache, nausea, diarrhea, abdominal pain, and insomnia (association unclear; may be due to co-administered ARVs).
- Hepatitis flare or fulminant hepatitis (in HBV co-infected pts if 3TC withdrawn or with development 3TC-resistant HBV)

Rare
- Lactic Acidosis: listed as NRTI class effect, but unlikely to be caused by 3TC. *In vitro*, 3TC, along with TDF, FTC, and ABC, are not associated with mitochondrial toxicity.
- Pancreatitis (reported in pediatric pts).

DRUG INTERACTIONS—See Appendix III, p. 826, for table of drug-to-drug interactions.
No pertinent drug interactions since it is not a substrate, inhibitor, or inducer of CYP450 isoforms.

RESISTANCE
- 184 V: selected by 3TC, resulting in high-level resistance to 3TC and FTC, slight decrease in susceptibility to ddI and ABC, and enhanced susceptibility to AZT, d4T, and TDF.
- TAMs (41 L, 210 W, 215 Y/F, 219 Q/E, 67 N, 70 R): resistance likely with multiple TAMs.
- T69 S: high-level resistance.
- Q151 M complex: high-level resistance.
- K65R: intermediate resistance.
- 44D and 119I: increase 3TC resistance in combination with TAMs.

PHARMACOLOGY
Mechanism
Intracellular phosphorylation to active lamivudine triphosphate, which competitively inhibits HIV DNA polymerase.

Pharmacokinetic Parameters
- **Absorption** 86%.
- **Cmax** = 3 mcg/mL; Intracellular carbovir triphosphate 100 FM/million cells.
- **Distribution** Widely distributed. Vd = 1.3 L/kg.
- **Protein binding** 36%.

- **Metabolism/Excretion** Renal excretion accounts for 71%.
- **T1/2** Serum: 5–7 hrs; Intracellular: 12 hrs.

Dosing for Decreased Hepatic Function
Usual dose.

Pregnancy Risk
C: Negative carcinogenicity and teratogenicity studies in rodents. Placental passage ratio of 1.0 (newborn:mother). Well tolerated in pregnant pts.

Breast Feeding Compatibility
No human data, breast milk excretion in animal studies. Breast feeding is not recommended in the U.S. in order to avoid post-natal transmission of HIV to the child, who may not yet be infected.

COMMENTS

- Pros: very well tolerated; active against HBV; convenient coformulations available; once daily dosing with low pill burden (1 tab once daily); resistance (184 V mutation) increases susceptibility to AZT, d4T, and TDF, and delays accumulation of TAMs; 3TC or FTC are essential components of all recommended initial regimens; coformulated with AZT (*Combivir*), ABC (*Epzicom*), and AZT + ABC (*Trizivir*). Decreased fitness with 184 V mutation, which may result in partial antiviral activity.
- Cons: high-level resistance with single point mutation (184 V); risk of hepatitis flare or fulminant hepatitis if 3TC withdrawn or if resistance develops in co-infected pts; high rate of HBV resistance with prolonged therapy if not used in combination with other anti-HBV agent (typically TDF); shorter intracellular half-life compared to FTC; more frequent emergence of 184 V with AZT/3TC than TDF/FTC in GS934 study.

SELECTED REFERENCES
Castagna A, Danise A, Menzo S, et al. Lamivudine monotherapy in HIV-1-infected pts harbouring a lamivudine-resistant virus: a randomized pilot study (E-184V study). *AIDS*, 2006; Vol. 20; pp. 795–803.

Fox Z, Dragsted UB, Gerstoft J, et al. A randomized trial to evaluate continuation versus discontinuation of lamivudine in individuals failing a lamivudine-containing regimen: the COLATE trial. *Antivir Ther*, 2006; Vol. 11; pp. 761.

OSELTAMIVIR

Paul A. Pham, PharmD and Johns G. Bartlett, MD

INDICATIONS

FDA

- Uncomplicated acute illness due to influenza A and B infection in adults who have been symptomatic for no more than 2 days.
- Prevention of influenza during an outbreak/epidemic for age >1 yr of age (82% effective).

Non-FDA Approved Uses

- Severe illness due to influenza A and B infection in immunocompromised and elderly pts who are hospitalized.

FORMS

Brand name (mfr)	Forms	Cost*
Tamiflu (Roche)	PO cap 75 mg	$10.17
	PO cap 30 mg	$10.17
	PO cap 45 mg	$10.17
	PO susp 12 mg/mL (25 mL)	$50.85
*Prices represents Average Wholesale Price (AWP).		

USUAL ADULT DOSING

- Influenza treatment (adults): 75 mg PO q12h × 5 days (must be started within 48 hrs of symptoms for documented efficacy, use after 48 hs now recommended for hospitalized pts or those with severe illness).

ANTIVIRAL DRUGS

- Influenza prophylaxis (adults): 75 mg PO once daily × at least 7 days following close contact or up to 6 wks during a community outbreak.
- Influenza treatment (children >1 yo): <15 kg = 30 mg q12h; 15–23 kg = 45 mg q12h; 23–40 kg = 60 mg q12h; >40 kg = 75 mg q12h.
- Influenza prophylaxis (children >1 yo): <15 kg = 30 mg q24h; 15–23 kg = 45 mg q24h; 23–40 kg = 60 mg q24h; >40 kg = 75 mg q24h.
- 2009–2010 season: pandemic H1N1 influenza A expected to be predominant isolate, or unknown influenza-type illness: use oseltamivir **or** inhaled zanamivir.
- 2009–2010 season, influenza B: oseltamivir monotherapy.
- Note: unknown if seasonal H1N1 influenza A with oseltamivir resistance will circulate in 2009–2010 season, see CDC site: Updated Interim Recommendations for the Use of Antiviral Medications in the Treatment and Prevention of Influenza for the 2009–2010 Season for latest recommendations.

Renal Dosing
Dosing for GFR 50–80: Usual dose.

Dosing for GFR 10–50: 10–30 mL/min: 75 mg q24h (treatment) or 75 mg every other day (prophylaxis).

Dosing for GFR <10: No data. Consider dose reduction.

Dosing in hemodialysis: Limited data Consider 30 mg post-HD every other HD session (*Nephrol Dial Transplant* 2006; 21: 2556).

Dosing in peritoneal dialysis: Limited data. Consider 30 mg once weekly (*Nephrol Dial Transplant* 2006; 21: 2556).

Dosing in hemofiltration: No data; Consider 75 mg q12h–24h.

Adverse Drug Reactions
Common
- GI: nausea, vomiting, and diarrhea in up to 10–20% of pts (generally resolves after several days; food may improve tolerance)

Rare
- Allergic reactions: rash, erythema multiforme, and Stevens Johnson syndrome
- Insomnia
- Confusion
- LFTs elevation
- Delirium with disturbed behavior, suicidal events, panic attacks, delusions, convulsions, depressed consciousness, and loss of consciousness (most of the reports were in children and came from Japan)

Drug Interactions
- No significant interaction between oseltamivir and warfarin, amoxicillin, acetaminophen, cimetidine, or antacids (magnesium and aluminum hydroxides and calcium carbonates).
- Probenecid: co-administration resulted in a 2.5-fold increase in oseltamivir. The clinical significance of this interaction is unknown but may allow dose reduction of oseltamivir to 75 mg q48h (prophylaxis) when in short supply.

Resistance
- Influenza A and B resistance reported in up to 5% in children.
- Influenza A (H1N1) viruses identified in the U.S. and elsewhere to be resistant to oseltamivir remain sensitive to zanamivir.
- 2008–2009 influenza season: Over 98% of seasonal flu (H1N1) strains were resistant to oseltamivir, but over 99% of 2009 pandemic influenza A (H1N1) were sensitive to oseltamivir.

Pharmacology
Mechanism
Inhibits influenza virus neuraminidase with the possible alteration of virus particle aggregation and release.

Pharmacokinetic Parameters
- **Absorption** 75% bioavailability.
- **Cmax** 348 mcg (of active drug) after 75 mg q12h multiple dosing.

- **Distribution** Widely distributed with a Vd of 23–26 L.
- **Protein binding** 42%.
- **Metabolism/Excretion** Extensive hepatic metabolism to the active carboxylate metabolite. Active metabolite excreted primarily in the urine with less than 20% eliminated in the feces.
- **T1/2** 6–10 hrs. Shelf life of 5 yrs.

Dosing for Decreased Hepatic Function
Usual dose recommended with moderate liver impairment (Snell et al. *Br J Clin Pharmacol.* 2005;59:598–601).

Pregnancy Risk
C: No data in human. Animal data using large dose resulted in maternal toxicity.

Breast Feeding Compatibility
No data.

COMMENTS
High rates of oseltamivir resistance among influenza A (H1N1) observed in 2008–2009, but appears lower for the 2009–2010 season (see CDC for updated resistance data), but >99% of pandemic ("swineflu") influenza A (H1N1) strains were sensitive. This drug works best if given within 48 hrs of on set of influenza symptoms, but the CDC urges initiating treatment for any pt sick enough to require hospitalization. Effective for prevention of influenza. More expensive compared to rimantadine or amantadine. GI side effects may be bothersome. Unlike rimantadine and amantadine, oseltamivir is active against influenza B and avian influenza (at least *in vitro*).

BASIS FOR RECOMMENDATIONS

Fiore AE, Shay DK, Broder K, et al. Prevention and control of influenza: recommendations of the Advisory Committee on Immunization Practices (ACIP), 2008. *MMWR Recomm Rep*, 2008; Vol. 57; pp. 1–60.

Comments: Oseltamivir or zanamivir continue to be the recommended agents for treatment and chemoprophylaxis of influenza in the U.S. Clinicians should check for up-to-date resistance rates (http://www.cdc.gov/flu/professionals/antivirals/index.htm).

Fiore AE, Shay DK, Haber P, et al. Prevention and control of influenza. Recommendations of the Advisory Committee on Immunization Practices (ACIP), 2007. *MMWR Recomm Rep*, 2007; Vol. 56; pp. 1–54.

Comments: Current guidelines from the ACIP.

SELECTED REFERENCES

McGeer A, Green KA, Plevneshi A, et al. Antiviral therapy and outcomes of influenza requiring hospitalization in Ontario, Canada. *Clin Infect Dis*, 2007; Vol. 45(12); pp. 1568–75.

PERAMIVIR

Paul A. Pham, PharmD

INDICATIONS

FDA
- Not FDA approved, but is available under an Emergency Use Authorization program during the 2009 H1N1 influenza season. http://emergency.cdc.gov/h1n1antivirals/3.asp

NON-FDA APPROVED USES
- Treatment of influenza for hospitalized adult and pediatric pts for whom therapy with an IV anti-influenza drug is needed. Peramivir can be considered for treatment failure occuring with use of currently approved anti-influenza drugs (e.g., oseltamivir and zanamivir) but cross-resistance possible and in pts who are unable to take oral or inhaled anti-viral therapy. Mandatory reporting of serious adverse events to FDA's MedWatch program required.

FORMS

Brand name (mfr)	Forms	Cost*
Peramivir (BioCryst Pharmaceuticals, Inc.)	IV vial 200 mg per 20 mL (10 mg per mL)	TBA
*Prices represents Average Wholesale Price (AWP).		

ANTIVIRAL DRUGS

USUAL ADULT DOSING
- 600 mg IV once daily × 5–10 days (infuse over 60 mins in 0.9% or 0.45% NaCL solution).
- No data, but longer treatment duration can be considered in critically ill pts, unresolved clinical influenza illness, or continued viral shedding.
- Peds: limited data with only case reports of 5 to 10 days treatment duration. See table under Other Information.

RENAL DOSING
Dosing for GFR 50–80: 600 mg IV once daily × 5–10 days.
Dosing for GFR 10–50: CrCl 31–49 mL/min = 150 mg once daily; CrCl 10–30 mL/min = 100 mg once daily.
Dosing for GFR <10: 100 mg × 1, then 15 mg once daily.
Dosing in hemodialysis: 100 mg × 1, then 100 mg post-HD (dose 2 hrs post-HD).
Dosing in peritoneal dialysis: No data.
Dosing in hemodialysis: CVVHD: No data. Significant removed likely.

ADVERSE DRUG REACTIONS
General
- Peramivir is generally well tolerated. No significant differences between Peramivir and placebo or oseltamivir were reported in phase 2/3 trials involving over 1800 pts.

Common
- GI: nausea, vomiting, and diarrhea (13% vs. 2% for oseltamivir treated pts)
- Neutropenia

OCCASIONAL
- Psychiatric: including depression, confusion, insomnia, delirium, restlessness, anxiety, nightmare, and alteration of mood reported in 11% (vs. 4% of oseltamivir treated pts)
- Hyperglycemia

Rare
- Based on data with other neuraminidase inhibitor, anaphylaxis, rash, neurologic and psychiatric behavioral symptoms are possible.
- Avoid use in oseltamivir or zanamivir allergic pts. Cross-allergic reaction between peramivir and oseltamivir or zanamivir is possible.

DRUG INTERACTIONS
- No known drug interaction.
- Probenecid may increase peramivir serum concentrations.

RESISTANCE
- Should not be used for treatment of 2009 H1N1 virus infection in pts with documented or highly suspected oseltamivir resistance (H275Y mutation), but as of September 5, 2009, resistance rates in isolates from treated and untreated pts has been <1% (source: http://www.cdc.gov/flu/weekly/index.htm#whomap)
- In pts with documented resistance (neuraminidase mutations E119D or R292K) or highly suspected zanamivir resistance, the activity of peramivir IV is unknown.

PHARMACOLOGY
Mechanism
Inhibits neuraminidase of influenza A and B
Dosing for Decreased Hepatic Function
Usual dose likely.
Pregnancy Risk
No data.
Breast Feeding Compatibility
No data.

COMMENTS
- To date, four clinical trials involving 1891 pts evaluated the safety and efficacy of peramivir. For uncomplicated influenza, peramivir appears to be similar to other neuraminidase inhibitor in alleviating symptoms by 1 day. Limited data are available in high-risk pts (e.g., diabetes, chronic respiratory disease, immunosuppressed).

- In a randomized trial, 42 pts received 300 mg IV or 600 mg IV for one to five days. Based on thirty seven evaluable pts, multiple dose treated group appears to have a shorter duration of symptoms (64 hrs vs 92 hrs), but further analysis of this study is needed.
  A randomized study in hospitalized pts with severe influenza compared lower peramivir dose (200 mg once daily and 400 mg once daily) to oral oseltamivir 75 mg twice daily × 5 days. No difference in time to clinical stability or time to hospital discharge between the three treatment groups was observed.

BASIS FOR RECOMMENDATIONS

FDA.http://www.fda.gov/downloads/Drugs/DrugSafety/PostmarketDrugSafetyInformationforPtsandProviders/UCM18 7811.pdf.

Comments: Fact Sheet for health care providers

OTHER INFORMATION

Pediatric Daily Dosage Recommendations*

Age	Dose (mg/kg)
Birth through 30 Days	6 mg/kg
31 Days through 90 Days	8 mg/kg
91 Days through 180 Days	10 mg/kg
181 Days through 5 Yrs	12 mg/kg
6 Yrs through 17 Yrs	10 mg/kg

*Maximum Daily Dose is 600 mg IV

Pediatric Impaired Renal Function Daily Dosage Recommendations

Age	CrCl (mL/min) 50–80 mL/min	31–49 mL/min	10–30 mL/min	<10 mL/min	HD#
Birth through 30 days	6 mg/kg once daily	1.5 mg/kg once daily	1 mg/kg once daily	1 mg/kg × 1 day, then 0.15 mg/kg once daily	1 mg/kg × 1, then post-HD
31 Days through 90 Days	8 mg/kg once daily	2 mg/kg once daily	1.3 mg/kg once daily 0.2 mg/kg once daily	1.3 mg/kg × 1 day, then 0.25 mg/kg once daily	1.3 mg/kg × 1, then post-HD
91 Days through 180 Days	10 mg/kg once daily	2.5 mg/kg once daily	1.6 mg/kg once daily	1.6 mg/kg × 1 day, then 0.25 mg/kg once daily	1.6 mg/kg × 1, then post-HD
181 Days through 5 Yrs	12 mg/kg once daily	3.0 mg/kg once daily	1.9 mg/kg once daily	1.9 mg/kg × 1 day, then 0.3 mg/kg once daily	1.9 mg/kg × 1, then post-HD
6 Yrs through 17 Yrs	10 mg/kg once daily	2.5 mg/kg once daily	1.6 mg/kg once daily	1.6 mg/kg × 1 day, then 0.25 mg/kg once daily	1.6 mg/kg × 1, then post-HD

Peramivir IV should be administered 2 hrs after hemodialysis is completed.

ANTIVIRAL DRUGS

RIBAVIRIN

Paul A. Pham, PharmD and John G. Bartlett, MD

INDICATIONS

FDA

- Hepatitis C (in combination with interferon alpha or peginterferon alpha)
- Respiratory syncytial virus (RSV) infection (including bronchiolitis and pneumonia)

Non-FDA Approved Uses

- Treatment of progressive vaccinia in combination with vaccinia immune globulin (VIG) [Kesson AM et al. *CID* 1997; 25:911].
- Treatment of hemorrhagic fever.

FORMS

Brand name (mfr)	Forms	Cost*
Virazole (Valeant Pharmaceutical)	Inhalation vial 6 g	$15,570 (per 4 vials)
Rebetol (Schering)	Oral capsule 200 mg Oral solution 40 mg/mL	$11.04 242.50 (4oz)
RibaPak (Three River Pharmaceutics)	Oral tab pak 800 mg Oral tab pak 1000 mg Oral tab pak 1200 mg	$17.35 $21.76 $26.13
Copegus (Roche)	Oral tablet 200 mg	$12.52
Ribavirin (Various generic manufacturers)	Oral capsule 200 mg	$9.93
*Prices represents Average Wholesale Price (AWP).		

USUAL ADULT DOSING

- Hepatitis C (genotype I): ribavirin 1200 mg/day (>75 kg) or 1000 mg/day (<75 kg) or 800 mg/day (<40 kg) × 48 wks + peginterferon. For Hep C (genotype II and III): RBV 800 mg/day + peginterferon × 24 wks.
- In pts without cardiovascular history:consider dose reduction to 600 mg/day with Hgb <10 g/dL or D/C with Hgb <8.5 g/dL. Consider erythropoietin.
- In pts with cardiovascular history: consider dose reduction to 600 mg/day with a Hgb drop > or = to 2 g/dL. If Hgb remains <12 g/dL over the next 4 wks after the reduction to 600 mg, ribavirin should be discontinued. Consider erythropoietin.
- Hemorrhagic fever (for contained casualty setting): 30 mg/kg IV (load), then 16 mg/kg (max 1000 mg) every 6 hrs × 4 days, followed by 8 mg/kg (max 500 mg) every 8h × 6 days.
- Hemorrhagic fever (for mass casualty setting): 2000 mg PO (load), then 1200 mg/day in two divided dose for >70 kg pt or 1000 mg/day in two divided dose for <70 kg pt × 10 days.
- To obtain IV ribavirin call Valeant Pharmaceutical (formerly known as ICN): 1-800-548-5100.

RENAL DOSING

Dosing for GFR 50–80: Usual dose.

Dosing for GFR 10–50: Not recommended per manufacturer due to the lack of data. Consider dose reduction with close monitoring.

Dosing for GFR <10: Not recommended per manufacturer due to the lack of data. Consider dose reduction with close monitoring.

Dosing in hemodialysis: Not recommended per manufacturer due to the lack of data. Consider dose reduction with close monitoring. Small amount removed in dialysis; dose post dialysis.

Dosing in peritoneal dialysis: No data. Not recommended.

Dosing in hemodialysis: No data. Not recommended.

ADVERSE DRUG REACTIONS

Common

- Hemolytic anemia (dose-related and reversible. Develops in 2–4 wks; avg drop 2.5–3 g Hb). Consider erythropoietin co-administration.

- Dry cough.
- Dyspnea.

Occasional

- Fatigue
- Dyspepsia (may respond to antacid)
- Headache
- Insomnia
- Bronchospasm (aerosolized ribavirin)
- Anorexia
- Nausea
- Gout

Rare

- Lactic acidosis (esp. when combined with ddI)

DRUG INTERACTIONS

- Abacavir: potential antagonism. Avoid co-administration.
- didanosine (ddI): increases intracellular concentrations of ddI; may increase risk of lactic acidosis and/or pancreatitis. Avoid co-administration.
- Zidovudine (AZT), dapsone, pyrimethamine, ganciclovir, ampho B: may increase risk of anemia. Monitor for anemia with co-administration; consider alternative NRTI or use with Procrit.

PHARMACOLOGY

Mechanism

Synthetic guanosine nucleoside analog that interferes with synthesis of guanosine triphosphate thereby inhibiting nucleic acid synthesis. May also inhibit some viral RNA polymerases.

Pharmacokinetic Parameters

- **Absorption** 64% (increased with high fat meal).
- **Cmax** 5.1 micromol/L (600 mg dose).
- **Distribution** Large volume of distribution (Vd: 802L). Concentrated in plasma, respiratory tract secretion and RBCs. CNS concentration found (up to 67%) after prolong administration.
- **Protein binding** No significant protein binding.
- **Metabolism/Excretion** Metabolized by phosphorylation and deribosylation. Metabolites excreted in urine.
- **T1/2** Inhalation-9.5 hrs; IV and oral-0.5–2 hrs; erythrocyte intracellular half-life 40 days.

Dosing for Decreased Hepatic Function

Usual dose.

Pregnancy Risk

X: Embryotoxic and teratogenic in all animal species. **Contraindicated in pregnant women and in male partners of pregnant women per manufacturer and CDC. Women of childbearing age must use effective form of contraception during treatment and 6-mos post-treatment.**

Breast Feeding Compatibility

No data

COMMENTS

Preferred agent for hepatitis C infection when combined with pegylated alpha interferon. Monitor closely for hemolytic anemia in the first few wks of therapy. In the management of hemolytic anemia, the addition of erythropoietin is preferred over decreasing ribavirin dose since sustained virologic response rate is higher with standard dose (1000–1200 mg). Contraindicated in pregnancy and co-administration with didanosine. Warn pts of the teratogenic effect of ribavirin and need for adequate forms of contraception. Avoid use with renal failure and/or hemoglobinopathies. SVR is lower in HIV-coinfected pts.

BASIS FOR RECOMMENDATIONS

Borio L; Inglesby T; Peters, C. J. et al. Hemorrhagic Fever Viruses as Biological Weapons. *JAMA*, 2002; Vol. 287; pp. 2391–2405.

Comments: Recommendations for the use of ribavirin in the treatment of hemorrhagic fever.

ANTIVIRAL DRUGS

SELECTED REFERENCES

Hadziyannis SJ, Sette H, Morgan TR, et al. Peginterferon-alpha2a and ribavirin combination therapy in chronic hepatitis C: a randomized study of treatment duration and ribavirin dose. *Ann Intern Med*, 2004; Vol. 140; pp. 346–55.

Payan C, Pivert A, Morand P, et al. Rapid and early virological response to chronic hepatitis C treatment with IFN alpha2b or PEG-IFN alpha2b plus ribavirin in HIV/HCV co-infected pts. *Gut*, 2007; Vol. 56; pp. 1111–6.

RIMANTADINE

Paul A. Pham, PharmD and John G. Bartlett, MD

INDICATIONS

FDA

- Influenza A (prophylaxis and treatment)

FORMS

Brand name (mfr)	Forms	Cost*
Flumadine (Generic manufacturers)	PO tab 100 mg PO syrup 50 mg/5 mL (8 oz)	$1.83 $55.79

*Prices represents Average Wholesale Price (AWP).

USUAL ADULT DOSING

- Prophylaxis: 100 mg PO twice daily.
- Treatment: 100 mg PO twice daily within 48 hrs of symptoms × 7 days.
- Consider dose reduction in severe hepatic dysfunction, renal failure and in the elderly.
- 2009–2010 influenza season: pandemic H1N1 influenza A virus is expected to be the predominant circulating virus; amantadines are not recommended. Unknown if oseltamivir-resistant seasonal H1N1 virus seen in 2008–2009 season will circulate. See CDC website for any changed recommendations: Updated Interim Recommendations for the Use of Antiviral Medications in the Treatment and Prevention of Influenza for the 2009–2010 Season.

RENAL DOSING

Dosing for GFR 50–80: 100 mg twice daily.
Dosing for GFR 10–50: 100 mg twice daily.
Dosing for GFR <10: 100 mg twice daily.
Dosing in hemodialysis: Not removed, dose at 100 mg once daily (not removed in HD).
Dosing in peritoneal dialysis: No data.
Dosing in hemofiltration: No data. Consider 100 mg once daily.

ADVERSE DRUG REACTIONS

Occasional

- GI intolerance
- CNS: light headedness, insomnia, reduced ability to concentrate, and nervousness (4–8%, about half the rate compared with amantadine, more likely with older pts and renal failure).

Rare

- Seizures (reported in pts with seizure disorder).
- Tremors.
- Cardiac arrhythmias have been reported with high drug plasma concentrations.

DRUG INTERACTIONS

None

PHARMACOLOGY

Mechanism

Interferes with early step in influenza A replication (inhibits viral uncoating) inhibits ion channel function of M2 protein.

Pharmacokinetic Parameters

- **Absorption** 96%.
- **Cmax** 0.25 mcg/mL in plasma; 0.42 mcg/mL in mucus.

- **Distribution** Large volume of distribution attaining high concentration in respiratory secretions.
- **Protein binding** 40%.
- **Metabolism/Excretion** Extensive liver metabolism. Metabolites exceed in urine. Less than 1% excreted as unchanged drug in the urine.
- **T1/2** 6 to 9 hrs.

Dosing for Decreased Hepatic Function
In severe hepatic insufficiency: 100 mg once daily.

Pregnancy Risk
C.

Breast Feeding Compatibility
No data.

COMMENTS
Oral agent for influenza A that is more expensive compared to amantadine, but CNS side effects are less bothersome. Less expensive than zanamivir or oseltamivir (see http://www.cdc.gov/flu/professionals/antivirals/index.htm for Interim recommendations that may change).

BASIS FOR RECOMMENDATIONS
Fiore AE, Shay DK, Broder K, et al. Prevention and control of influenza: recommendations of the Advisory Committee on Immunization Practices (ACIP), 2008. *MMWR Recomm Rep*, 2008; Vol. 57; pp. 1–60.
Comments: Rimantadine should not be used for the treatment or prevention of influenza A in the U.S. until evidence of susceptibility has been reestablished.

SELECTED REFERENCES
CDC; Antiviral medication for influenza; www.cdc.gov/flu/professionals/treatment/; accessed 2/20/09.
Jefferson TO, et al.

TCA (TRICHLOROACETIC ACID), BCA (BICHLOROACETIC ACID)

Paul A. Pham, PharmD and John G. Bartlett, MD

INDICATIONS
FDA
Non-FDA Approved Uses
- Human papillomavirus (HPV)

FORMS

Brand name (mfr)	Forms	Cost*
Trichloroacetic acid (Various generic manufacturers)	Topical solution 80% (15 mL); Topical crystal 4 oz	$51.25; $30.75

*Prices represents Average Wholesale Price (AWP).

USUAL ADULT DOSING
Apply small amount to warts and allow to dry. Repeat weekly if necessary (note: cryotherapy preferred).

RENAL DOSING
Dosing for GFR 50–80: Usual dose.
Dosing for GFR 10–50: Usual dose.
Dosing for GFR <10: Usual dose.
Dosing in hemodialysis: Usual dose.
Dosing in peritoneal dialysis: Usual dose.
Dosing in hemofiltration: Usual dose.

ADVERSE DRUG REACTIONS
General
- Irritation and erythema at the site of administration.

ANTIVIRAL DRUGS

DRUG INTERACTIONS
None known

PHARMACOLOGY

Mechanism
Caustic and astringent agent used as a quick escharotic for warts.

Pharmacokinetic Parameters
• Absorption —

Dosing for Decreased Hepatic Function
Usual dose.

Pregnancy Risk
No data, but considered by some to be safe in the pregnancy setting to treat warts.

Breast Feeding Compatibility
No data.

COMMENTS
Though not as effective as some strategies, TCA and BCA are best used on smaller areas of warts to avoid local reactions on normal skin. Efficacy at best ~60%, accounting for why cryotherapy often preferred.

SELECTED REFERENCES

Sherrard J, Riddell L. Comparison of the effectiveness of commonly used clinic-based treatments for external genital warts. *Int J STD AIDS*, 2007; Vol. 18; pp. 365–8.

Wiley DJ, Douglas J, Beutner K, et al. External genital warts: diagnosis, treatment, and prevention. *Clin Infect Dis*, 2002; Vol. 35; pp. S210–24.

TELBIVUDINE

Paul A. Pham, PharmD and Chloe Thio, MD

INDICATIONS

FDA
• Treatment of chronic hepatitis B (HBeAg-negative or -positive) with ongoing viral replication and evidence of transferase elevation or histologically active disease.

FORMS

Brand name (mfr)	Forms	Cost*
Tyzeka (Novartis)	Oral tablet 600 mg	$25.77 per tablet
*Prices represents Average Wholesale Price (AWP).		

USUAL ADULT DOSING
• 600 mg PO once daily with or without food.

RENAL DOSING
Dosing for GFR 50–80: GFR >50 mL/min: 600 mg once daily.
Dosing for GFR 10–50: GFR 30–49 mL/min: 600 mg every other day; GFR <30 mL/min (no HD): 600 mg q72h.
Dosing for GFR <10: GFR <30 mL/min (no HD): 600 mg q72h.
Dosing in hemodialysis: ESRD (HD): 600 mg q96h (on days of HD, dose post-HD).
Dosing in peritoneal dialysis: No data.
Dosing in hemofiltration: No data.

ADVERSE DRUG REACTIONS

General
• Generally well tolerated with adverse reactions comparable to lamivudine and adefovir.

Occasional
• Compared to lamivudine, CK elevation more common in telbivudine treated pts (9% vs 3%).
• Potential for acute exacerbations of hepatitis B with discontinuation.

Rare

- Although lactic acidosis and severe hepatomegaly with steatosis not reported with telbivudine, nucleoside analogs have potential for causing these potentially fatal adverse reactions.

DRUG INTERACTIONS

Not a substrate, inducer, or inhibitor of CYP450 isoenzymes.

- Interactions with PIs and NNRTI unlikely.
- No antagonism observed with other NRTIs *in vitro*. No significant interactions observed with lamivudine, adefovir, cyclosporine, and pegylated IFN-alfa.

RESISTANCE

- M204I genotypic substitution accounts for 74%–94% of observed mutations associated with resistance (*Gastro* 2006;130:A765; Standring, et al. *EASL* 2006). Additional reported mutations include L80I/V, A181T, L180M, L229W/V.
- In 2-yr follow-up, resistance developed in 8.6% and 21.6% of telbivudine-treated pts who were HBeAg– and HBeAg+, respectively. Although overall resistance rates were high, in subset of pts who successfully suppressed to undetectable at 24 wks, resistance rates were only 2–4%. Clinical implication of this finding unclear, but some experts advocate using monotherapy for 24 wks with "intensification" only if VL remains detectable. Efficacy of telbivudine against HBV harboring lamivudine and adefovir resistance remains to be determined. *In vitro*, telbivudine active against lamivudine-resistant virus with M204V mutation alone, but not against lamivudine-treated virus with L180M/M204V double mutation or M204I mutation. However, clinical relevance of these *in vitro* observations unclear.
- Adefovir-resistant HBV with A181V mutation associated with 3–5-fold reduction in susceptibility.

PHARMACOLOGY

Mechanism

Telbivudine, a synthetic thymidine analog, inhibits HBV DNA polymerase reverse transcriptase by competing with natural substrate thymidine 5'-triphosphate.

Pharmacokinetic Parameters

- **Absorption** Well absorbed
- **Cmax** 3.69, AUC 26.1 mcg hr/mL, and Cmin 0.2–0.3 mcg/mL after 600 mg once daily at steady-state
- **Distribution** Widely distributed
- **Protein binding** Low (3.3%)
- **Metabolism/Excretion** Not metabolized, and is primarily excreted via glomerular filtration
- **T1/2** Terminal half-life of 40–49 hrs.

Dosing for Decreased Hepatic Function

600 mg once daily.

Pregnancy Risk

B: Not teratogenic in animal studies. No human data.

Breast Feeding Compatibility

Excreted in breast milk (animal data).

COMMENTS

In treatment of chronic hepatitis B, telbivudine is more potent than lamivudine and adefovir. Active *in vitro* against lamivudine-resistant strains with M204V mutation, but due to similar resistance mutation, some experts do not recommend telbivudine for treatment of lamivudine-resistant HBV. Compared to lamivudine, resistance less likely and slower to develop. In addition, a unique mutation (M204I), may allow sequencing. In contrast to tenofovir, entecavir links, adefovir, lamivudine, and emtricitabine, telbivudine does not have HIV activity. Head-to-head comparison with more potent agents (e.g., entecavir), combination studies, and studies evaluating sequencing strategies needed to establish role of telbivudine. This drug inactive vs HIV and can therefore be used in pts with HBV + HIV co-infections when treatment vs HIV is not desired.

SELECTED REFERENCES

Chan HL, Heathcote EJ, Marcellin P, et al. Treatment of hepatitis B e antigen positive chronic hepatitis with telbivudine or adefovir: a randomized trial. *Ann Intern Med*, 2007; Vol. 147; pp. 745–54.

Lai CL, Gane E, Liaw YF, et al. Telbivudine versus lamivudine in pts with chronic hepatitis B. *N Engl J Med*, 2007; Vol. 357; pp. 2576–88.

ANTIVIRAL DRUGS

TENOFOVIR DF

Paul A. Pham, PharmD and John G. Bartlett, MD

INDICATIONS

FDA
- Treatment of HIV-infection in combination with other antiretroviral drugs.
- Treatment of HBV.

Non-FDA Approved Uses
- Treatment of hepatitis in HIV-HBV co-infected pts.

FORMS

Brand name (mfr)	Forms	Cost*
Viread (Gilead Sciences)	Oral tablet 300 mg	$23.00
Truvada (Gilead Sciences)	Oral tablet 300/200 mg	$35.00
Atripla (Bristol-Myers Squibb and Gilead)	Oral tablet EFV 600 mg + TDF 300 mg + FTC 200 mg	$55.10
*Prices represents Average Wholesale Price (AWP).		

USUAL ADULT DOSING

Pill burden: 1 tab per day.
- TDF: 1 tab once daily without regard to meals. Fatty meals improve absorption by 40% (clinical significance unknown but not thought to be significant).
- TDF/FTC (*Truvada*): 1 tab once daily without regard to meals.
- EFV/TDF/FTC (*Atripla*): 1 tab once daily. Evening dosing on an empty stomach recommended with initial therapy to decrease EFV-associated side effects.

RENAL DOSING

Dosing for GFR 50–80: Usual dose.

Dosing for GFR 10–50: 30–49 mL/min TDF 300 mg q48h or Truvada (TDF/FTC co-formulation) 1 tab q48h. <30 mL/min: TDF 300 mg q72–96h. Atripla (TDF/TDF/FTC co-formulation) not recommended with GFR <50 mL/min.

Dosing for GFR <10: TDF 300 mg q 7 days. Atripla (TDF/TDF/FTC co-formulation) not recommended with GFR <50 mL/min.

Dosing in hemodialysis: TDF 300 mg q 7 days following HD (may require more if more than three 4-hr HD session). Atripla (TDF/TDF/FTC co-formulation) not recommended with GFR <50 mL/min.

Dosing in peritoneal dialysis: No data. Consider dose reduction. Atripla (TDF/TDF/FTC co-formulation) not recommended with GFR <50 mL/min.

Dosing in hemofiltration: No data. Consider dose reduction.

ADVERSE DRUG REACTIONS

General
- Generally well tolerated. For *Atripla*, see EFV for EFV-associated side effects.

Occasional
- Flatulence, nausea, and vomiting. Asymptomatic elevation of CPK in 12%; transaminase elevation in 4–5%. Neutropenia in 3% and increased amylase in 9%.
- Pts with underlying renal insufficiency or other conditions predisposing to renal insufficiency may be at increased risk for nephrotoxicity.

Rare
- Case reports of nephrotoxicity with characteristic features of Fanconi syndrome (hypophosphatemia, hypouricemia, proteinuria, and normoglycemic glycosuria), especially in pts with prior history of Fanconi syndrome on adefovir.
- **Lactic acidosis and hepatic steatosis**: Causal relationship not established. *In vitro*, TDF is one of the NRTIs least associated with mitochondrial toxicity. In a clinical trial, d4T resulted in significantly more hyperlactemia (>2.2 mmol/L) compared to TDF (27% vs 4%, p <0.0001).

DRUG INTERACTIONS—See Appendix III, p. 840, for table of drug-to-drug interactions.
Low likelihood drug-drug interactions with PIs (with the exception of ATV and LPV) and NNRTIs, since TDF is not a substrate, inhibitor, or inducer of CYP 3A4.

RESISTANCE

- TAMs (41L, 210W, 215Y/F, 219Q/E, 67N, 70R): high-level resistance with 3 or more TAMs that include 41L and 210W.
- 65R: selected by TDF, causing intermediate tenofovir resistance, and intermediate resistance to ddI, 3TC, FTC, low-level resistance to ABC and possibly d4T. Susceptibility to AZT retained (may be hypersusceptible).
- 184V: increased susceptibility;may partially reverse 65R—or TAM-mediated resistance.
- T69 insertion: intermediate resistance in setting of multi-NRTI resistance.
- Q151M complex: tenofovir sensitivity retained.
- 74V: increased susceptibility to tenofovir (clinical significance unknown).

PHARMACOLOGY

Mechanism

TDF inhibits the activity of HIV reverse transcriptase by competing with the natural substrate deoxyadenosine 5'-triphosphate causing DNA chain termination.

Pharmacokinetic Parameters

- **Absorption** Oral absorption: 30% (fasting) and 40% with fatty meal.
- **Cmax** Mean Cmax = 296 +/− 90 ng/mL; AUC = 2287 +/− 685 ng h/mL.
- **Distribution** Vd = 1.2 +/− 4 L/kg.
- **Protein binding** <7.2%.
- **Metabolism/Excretion** Renal excretion by glomerular filtration and active tubular secretion by MRP4.
- **T1/2** Serum: 11–14 hrs; intracellular: 12–50 hrs.

Dosing for Decreased Hepatic Function

No data. Usual dose likely.

Pregnancy Risk

B: Gravid rhesus monkeys study showed normal fetal development, but reduction in body weight, insulin-like growth factor, and fetal bone porosity observed (*JAIDS* 2002; 29:207). Lower TDF exposure during third trimester than postpartum period. Because of lack of data on use in human pregnancy and concern regarding potential fetal bone effects, TDF should be used as component of a maternal ART regimen only after careful consideration of alternatives. Pregnancy Registry through July 2007 showed birth defects in 6/380 (1.6%) first trimester exposures; this is substantially lower than expected rate.

Breast Feeding Compatibility

Not recommended.

COMMENTS

- Pros: once daily administration; well tolerated with few short-term side effects and no clear mitochondrial or other long-term toxicity; few drug interactions; activity against some NRTI-resistant strains; longer intracellular half-life than most NRTIs; active against HBV. Coformulations available, including the only single-pill, once daily regimen.
- Cons: potential for nephrotoxicity; resistance with selection of K65R.

SELECTED REFERENCES

Arribas JR, Pozniak AL, Gallant JE, et al. Tenofovir DF, emtricitabine, and efavirenz compared with zidovudine, lamivudine, and efavirenz in treatment-naive pts. 144-Wk Analysis. *J Acquir Immune Defic Syndr*, 2008; Vol. 47; p. 75.

Jemsek J, Hutcherson P, Harper E. Poor virologic response and early emergence of resistance in treatment naive, HIV-infected pts receiving a once daily triple nucleoside regimen of ddI, 3TC, and TDF. *11th CROI*. San Francisco, California, 2004. Abstract 51, 2004.

ANTIVIRAL DRUGS

VALACYCLOVIR

Paul A. Pham, PharmD and John G. Bartlett, MD

INDICATIONS

FDA

- Treatment of initial episode of herpes genitalis in immunocompetent adults.
- Suppression of recurrent episodes of herpes genitalis in immunocompetent and HIV-infected adults.
- Treatment of recurrent episodes of herpes genitalis in immunocompetent adults.
- Treatment of herpes zoster in immunocompetent adults.
- Treatment of herpes labialis.

Non-FDA Approved Uses

- Treatment of initial episode and recurrent episodes of herpes genitalis in immunocompromised pts.
- Treatment of herpes zoster in immunocompromised pts.
- Treatment of perianal HSV and other forms of disseminated HSV.
- Prevention of CMV disease in solid organ transplant.

FORMS

Brand name (mfr)	Forms	Cost*
Valtrex (GlaxoSmithKline)	Oral tablet 500 mg; 1000 mg	$7.45; 13.29
*Prices represents Average Wholesale Price (AWP).		

Usual Adult Dosing

- Dermatomal zoster: 1 g PO q8h × 7–10 days.
- Treatment of first episode of genital HSV: 1 g PO twice daily × 7–10 days.
- Treatment of recurrent genital HSV: 500 mg PO twice daily (1 g PO twice daily if severe).
- Suppressive therapy for genital HSV: 500 mg PO twice daily.
- Herpes labialis: 2 g PO q12h × 1d.
- Treatment of adult varicella: consider 1 g PO twice daily within 24 hrs of rash onset (no data with valacyclovir but efficacy demonstrated with ACV [*Ann Intern Med*. 1992; 117(5):358–63]).

RENAL DOSING

Dosing for GFR 50–80: Usual dose.

Dosing for GFR 10–50: Cr clearance 30–49 mL/min: 1000 mg PO q12h. Cr clearance 10–29 mL/min: 1000 mg q24h.

Dosing for GFR <10: 500 mg PO q day.

Dosing in hemodialysis: 500 mg q day, 33% removed with HD. On days of dialysis dose after dialysis.

Dosing in peritoneal dialysis: 500 mg PO q24–48h, no supplemental dose needed (*Nephron*. 2002; 91:164).

Dosing in hemofiltration: Not effectively removed. Consider 500 mg PO q day.

ADVERSE DRUG REACTIONS

General

- Generally well tolerated

Occasional

- Nausea and vomiting
- Rash

Rare

- Agitation, dizziness, headache, confusion, hallucination, seizure
- Transaminase elevations
- Anemia, neutropenia
- Hypotension
- Thrombotic thrombocytopenic purpura/hemolytic uremic syndrome (TTP/HUS) reported in immunocompromised pts receiving valacyclovir 8 g/day

DRUG INTERACTIONS

Probenecid: may increase acyclovir levels. No dose adjustment needed.

PHARMACOLOGY

Mechanism

Cleaved by valine hydrolase into ACV. ACV converted by viral thymidine kinase (TK) to active ACV monophosphate; cellular enzyme catalase converts ACV monophosphate to ACV triphosphate, which competitively inhibits viral DNA polymerase.

Pharmacokinetic Parameters

- **Absorption** 54% (3–5-fold increase in bioavailability compared to oral ACV).
- **Cmax** 3.3–3.7 mcg/mL after 500 mg administration; AUC: 18–20 hr/mcg/mL. Cmax: 4.6–5.5 mcg/mL after 1 g oral administration.
- **Distribution** High concentration found in kidneys, liver, and intestines. CNS penetration 50% of serum. Also distributed to lung, aqueous humor, tears, muscle, spleen, breast milk, uterine, vaginal mucosa, semen, and amniotic fluid.
- **Protein binding** 14–18%.
- **Metabolism/Excretion** Rapidly converted to ACV via intestinal and hepatic first pass metabolism. ACV converted to inactive metabolites by alcohol and aldehyde dehydrogenase. 80–89% of ACV recovered in the urine unchanged.
- **T1/2** 2.5–3.3 hrs.

Dosing for Decreased Hepatic Function

No data. Dose reduction unlikely.

Pregnancy Risk

B: Not teratogenic in animal studies. No human data available but likely to be similar to ACV. Prophylaxis not recommended in pregnancy.

Breast Feeding Compatibility

No data: most likely distributed into breast milk as ACV. Not associated with any problems in the newborn.

COMMENTS

Pro-drug of ACV with better absorption, higher blood levels, and more convenient dosing vs. oral ACV. Alternatives are ACV and famciclovir. More effective at decreasing post-herpetic neuralgia than ACV in immunocompetent host.

SELECTED REFERENCES

Hodson EM, Barclay PG, Craig JC, et al. Antiviral medications for preventing cytomegalovirus disease in solid organ transplant recipients. *Cochrane Database Syst Rev*, 2005; Vol. 4; pp. CD003774.

MacDougall C, Guglielmo BJ. Pharmacokinetics of valaciclovir. *J Antimicrob Chemother*, 2004; Vol. 53; pp. 899–901.

VALGANCICLOVIR

Paul A. Pham, PharmD and John G. Bartlett, MD

INDICATIONS

FDA

- Treatment of CMV retinitis in pts with AIDS.
- Prevention of CMV disease in kidney, heart, and kidney-pancreas transplant pts at high risk for CMV disease (e.g., donor positive, recipient negative). Not indicated in liver transplant pts.

Non-FDA Approved Uses

- Prevention of disseminated CMV disease of the contralateral eye in pts treated with intraocular ganciclovir implant.

FORMS

Brand name (mfr)	Forms	Cost*
Valcyte (Roche)	Oral tablet 450 mg	$42.83
*Prices represents Average Wholesale Price (AWP).		

ANTIVIRAL DRUGS

Usual Adult Dosing

- CMV retinitis (induction): 900 mg PO q12h with food × 3 wks (plus ganciclovir implant).
- CMV retinitis (maintenance): 900 mg PO daily with food until immune reconstitution (CD4> 150 × 3–6 mos w/ ophthalmology consultation confirming quiescence).
- Gastrointestinal CMV disease: 900 mg q12h with food × 3–6 wks (consider maintenance therapy with severe disease and/or with relapse).
- Prevention of CMV disease in kidney, heart, and kidney-pancreas transplant pts at high risk for CMV disease (e.g., donor [+] CMV/recipient negative): 900 mg daily with food beginning within 10 days of transplantation and continuing through day 100 post-transplantation.
- Monitor CBC 2–3 ×/wk. Discontinue drug or add G-CSF if ANC <500. Discontinue if platelet count <25,000 or consider d/c if Hgb <8 g/dL.

RENAL DOSING

Dosing for GFR 50–80: >60 mL/min: 900 mg twice daily (induction); 900 mg q24h (maintenance).

Dosing for GFR 10–50: 40–59 mL/min: 450 mg twice daily (induction) then 450 mg q24h (maintenance). 25–39 mL/min: 450 mg q24h (induction) then 450 mg every other day (maintenance). 10–24 mL/min: 450 mg every other day (induction) then 450 mg biweekly (maintenance).

Dosing for GFR <10: Not recommended by manufacturer.

Dosing in hemodialysis: Not recommended by manufacturer (HD removes approx. 50% of GCV). Consider 900 mg q48h (induction) or 450 mg q48h (maintenance).

Dosing in peritoneal dialysis: No data.

Dosing in hemofiltration: No data. Consider 900 mg q48h (induction) or 450 mg q48h (maintenance).

ADVERSE DRUG REACTIONS

Common

- Neutropenia (reversible and responds to G-CSF). Reversible within 3–7 days of discontinuation or dose reduction.
- Reversible thrombocytopenia.
- Diarrhea and nausea.

Occasional

- Anemia
- Fever
- Rash
- Headache
- Confusion
- Mental status changes

Rare

- Hepatoxicity
- Seizures

DRUG INTERACTIONS

- Myelosuppressive drugs (e.g., AZT, interferon, 5-FC, pyrimethamine, etc.): may increase risk of hematologic toxicity. Monitor closely with co-administration. Consider alternative agents or support with GCSF.
- Didanosine (ddI): not studied with valganciclovir but ddI levels may be increased. PK study with ddI and ganciclovir (GCV) resulted in a 111% increase in ddI AUC. GCV AUC decreased by 21%. Monitor closely for ddI toxicity. Consider ddI dose reduction or use an alternative NRTI.
- Probenecid: may increase GCV serum levels. Monitor for GCV toxicity.
- Trimethoprim: may increase GCV serum levels. Monitor for GCV toxicity.

RESISTANCE

- The detection of cytomegalovirus resistant (genotype UL97 in the protein kinase associated with ganciclovir resistance only) to ganciclovir was associated with a 4- to 6-fold increase in the odds of retinitis progression (*Am J Ophthalmol.* 2003; 135:26–34)
- In high-risk solid-organ transplant recipients receiving valganciclovir, no resistance mutation (UL97) was detected after 100 days of therapy (*J Infect Dis.* 2004; 189:1615–8.)

- UL54 resistance mutation in the DNA polymerase gene (with or without UL97) is uncommon but can confer cidofovir cross-resistance (L545S) and possibly foscarnet resistance (N495K) (*Antivir Ther*. 2006; 11:537–40. *J Med Virol*. 2005; 77:425–9.)

PHARMACOLOGY

Mechanism

Prodrug of GCV with improved bioavailability. GCV is a synthetic analogue of 2-deoxyguanosine. Once phosphorylated, GCV triphosphate inhibits viral DNA synthesis.

Pharmacokinetic Parameters

- **Absorption** 60% (well absorbed, should be administered with food).
- **Cmax** 5.61 mcg/mL after 900 mg dose (with food). AUC = 29 mcg hr/mL after 900 mg dose (comparable to 5 mg/kg GCV IV).
- **Distribution** Vd = 0.7 L/kg.
- **Protein binding** 1–2%.
- **Metabolism/Excretion** Rapidly hydrolyzed to GCV, which is renally excreted via glomerular filtration and active tubular secretion.
- **T1/2** 4 hrs (serum), 18 hrs (intracellular).

Dosing for Decreased Hepatic Function

No data. Usual dose likely.

Pregnancy Risk

C: Teratogenic, carcinogenic, embryogenic, and causes aspermatogenesis; growth retardation; aplastic organ in animal studies. No human data, use only for life threatening CMV infection and warn pt of possible teratogenic effect. Effective form of contraception is recommended.

Breast Feeding Compatibility

No data. Due to potential for serious toxicity, mother should avoid breast feeding.

COMMENTS

Oral valganciclovir has 10-fold better absorption than oral GCV. AUC of oral valganciclovir 900 mg comparable to GCV 5 mg/kg IV. Oral valganciclovir equivalent to IV GCV for treatment of CMV retinitis in HIV+ pts and is preferred due to oral administration. Contraindicated by manufacturer in pts with severe neutropenia (ANC <500/dL), thrombocytopenia (<25,000/dL), severe anemia (Hgb <8 g/dL), and renal failure. Neutropenia and anemia generally responsive to G-CSF and erythropoietin.

BASIS FOR RECOMMENDATIONS

Recommendations of the National Institutes of Health (NIH), the Centers for Disease Control and Prevention (CDC), and the HIV Medicine Association of the Infectious Diseases Society of America (HIVMA/IDSA). Guidelines for Prevention and Treatment of Opportunistic Infections in HIV-Infected Adults and Adolescents *http://aidsinfo.nih.gov/*, 2008.

Comments: In pts tolerating PO intake, oral valganciclovir + ganciclovir implant is recommended for the treatment of CMV retinitis.

SELECTED REFERENCES

Khoury JA, Storch GA, Bohl DL, et al. Prophylactic versus preemptive oral valganciclovir for the management of cytomegalovirus infection in adult renal transplant recipients. *Am J Transplant*, 2006; Vol. 6; pp. 2134–43.

Lalezari J, Lindley J, Walmsley S, et al. A safety study of oral valganciclovir maintenance treatment of cytomegalovirus retinitis. *J Acquir Immune Defic Syndr*, 2002; Vol. 30; pp. 392–400.

ZANAMIVIR

Paul A. Pham, PharmD and John G. Bartlett, MD

INDICATIONS

FDA

- Indicated for treatment of uncomplicated acute illness due to influenza A and B infection (pts >7 yrs of age with <48 hr symptoms).
- Influenza prophylaxis in those 5 yrs of age or older.

Non-FDA Approved Uses

- Bronchitis, acute uncomplicated (due to influenza)
- Chronic bronchitis, acute exacerbations (due to influenza)
- Influenza, avian

ANTIVIRAL DRUGS

FORMS

Brand name (mfr)	Forms	Cost*
Relenza (GlaxoSmithKline)	Inhalation pow 5 mg	$16.80

*Prices represents Average Wholesale Price (AWP).

USUAL ADULT DOSING
- **Treatment:** two 5 mg inhalations twice a day × 5 days (must be administered within 2 days of symptom onset).
- **Prophylaxis:** one 5 mg inhalation q24h (84% effective).
- 2009–2010 influenza season: inhaled zanamivir can be used as an alternative to oseltamivir for any pandemic H1N1 influenza A or any influenza-type illness, if not otherwise contraindicated due to pre-existing respiratory diseases.
- For most current treatment recommendations visit CDC website: Updated Interim Recommendations for the Use of Antiviral Medications in the Treatment and Prevention of Influenza for the 2009–2010 Season.

RENAL DOSING
Dosing for GFR 50–80: Limited data, normal dose likely due to limited systemic absorption.
Dosing for GFR 10–50: Limited data, normal dose likely due to limited systemic absorption.
Dosing for GFR <10: Limited data, normal dose likely due to limited systemic absorption.
Dosing in hemodialysis: No data, normal dose likely due to limited systemic absorption.
Dosing in peritoneal dialysis: No data, normal dose likely.
Dosing in hemofiltration: No data, normal dose likely.

ADVERSE DRUG REACTIONS
General
- Bronchospasm may especially occur with use in pts with COPD or asthma. Avoidance or caution advised in this population with use.

Occasional
- Cough

Rare
- Headache
- Nausea, vomiting, diarrhea
- Dizziness
- Increase in liver function tests
- Allergic reactions
- Delirium and abnormal behavior (including suicide attempts) in pts receiving neuraminidase inhibitors, including zanamivir have been reported (mostly from Japan).

DRUG INTERACTIONS
No known drug interactions.

PHARMACOLOGY
Mechanism
Inhibits influenza virus neuraminidase with the possible alteration of virus particle aggregation and release.

Pharmacokinetic Parameters
- **Absorption** Poorly absorbed with only 4–17% systemic absorption.
- **Cmax** Wide variation in peak serum level of 17–142 ng/mL within 1–2 hrs after 10 mg dose.
- **Distribution** Pulmonary.
- **Protein binding** Less than 10%.
- **Metabolism/Excretion** Excreted unchanged in the urine.
- **T1/2** 2.5–5.1 hrs.

Dosing for Decreased Hepatic Function
No data, normal dose likely.

Pregnancy Risk
B: No malformation, maternal toxicity, or embryotoxicity were observed in animal studies. No data available in humans.

Breast Feeding Compatibility

No data in humans. Excreted in breast milk in animal data.

COMMENTS

Aerosolized anti-influenza agent w/ activity against influenza A and B. Influenza A (H1N1) resistant to oseltamivir remains sensitive to zanamivir. Requires manual dexterity for use. Avoid or use with caution in pts with COPD or asthma due to the risk of bronchospasm (have bronchodilator handy). IV formulation available from CDC for emergency use on compassionate basis.

BASIS FOR RECOMMENDATIONS

Fiore AE, Shay DK, Broder K, et al. Prevention and control of influenza: recommendations of the Advisory Committee on Immunization Practices (ACIP), 2008. *MMWR Recomm Rep*, 2008; Vol. 57; pp. 1–60.

Comments: Oseltamivir or zanamivir continue to be the recommended agents for treatment and chemoprophylaxis of influenza in the U.S. Clinicians should check for up-to-date resistance rates (http://www.cdc.gov/flu/professionals/antivirals/index.htm).

Lalezari J, Campion K, Keene O, et al. Zanamivir for the treatment of influenza A and B infection in high-risk pts: a pooled analysis of randomized controlled trials. *Arch Intern Med*, 2001; Vol. 161; pp. 212–7.

Comments: The authors reviewed the experience with zanamivir trials during the 1998–99 influenza season. Of a total of 2,751 participants, 321 were considered high-risk (COLD, cardiovascular disease, and age >65 yrs), and, of those, 151 were randomized to zanamivir. The results showed that zanamivir recipients in this subset had a median reduction in symptoms by 2.5 days (p = 0.015), a median time to return to normal daily activities of 3 days earlier (p = 0.02), and a 43% reduction in the incidence of complications requiring antibiotic use (p = 0.05).

SELECTED REFERENCES

Centers for Disease Control and Prevention (CDC). Oseltamivir-resistant novel influenza A (H1N1) virus infection in two immunosuppressed pts—Seattle, Washington, 2009. *MMWR Morb Mortal Wkly Rep*, 2009; Vol. 58; pp. 893–6.

Harper SA, Fukuda K, Uyeki TM et al. Prevention and control of influenza. Recommendations of the Advisory Committee on Immunization Practices (ACIP). *MMWR Recomm Rep*, 2005; Vol. 54; pp. 1–40.

Moscona A. Neuraminidase inhibitors for influenza. *N Engl J Med*, 2005; Vol. 353; pp. 1363–73.

ANTIVIRAL DRUGS

Biological

DROTRECOGIN ALPHA

Paul A. Pham, PharmD and John G. Bartlett, MD

INDICATIONS
FDA
- Drotrecogin is FDA indicated for the reduction of mortality in adult pts with severe sepsis (sepsis associated with acute organ dysfunction) who have a high risk of death (e.g., as determined by APACHE II score).
- Not indicated in the pediatric population. (Drotrecogin showed no improvement over placebo in the primary endpoint of "Composite Time to Complete Organ Failure Resolution" in a interim analysis of a RCT. Risk of bleed may be higher.)

FORMS

Brand name (mfr)	Forms	Cost*
Xigris (Eli Lilly)	IV vial 5 mg	$364
	IV vial 20 mg	$1456
*Prices represents Average Wholesale Price (AWP).		

USUAL ADULT DOSING
- Contraindications: active internal bleeding, recent hemorrhagic stroke (within 3 mos), recent intracranial or intraspinal surgery or severe head trauma, trauma with an increased risk of life-threatening bleed, presence of an epidural catheter, intracranial neoplasm or mass lesion or evidence of cerebral herniation.
- 24 mcg/kg/hr × 96 hrs, if infusion is interrupted drotrecogin should be restarted at 24 mcg/kg/hr (no bolus dose recommended).

RENAL DOSING
Dosing for GFR 50–80: Limited data. Usual dose: 24 mcg/kg/hr × 96 hrs.
Dosing for GFR 10–50: Limited data. Usual dose: 24 mcg/kg/hr × 96 hrs.
Dosing for GFR <10: Limited data. Usual dose: 24 mcg/kg/hr × 96 hrs.
Dosing in hemodialysis: Limited data. Usual dose: 24 mcg/kg/hr × 96 hrs.
Dosing in peritoneal dialysis: Limited data. Usual dose: 24 mcg/kg/hr × 96 hrs.
Dosing in hemodialysis: No data. Usual dose likely: 24 mcg/kg/hr × 96 hrs.

ADVERSE DRUG REACTIONS
General
- Bleeding reported in 25% of drotrecogin treated pts compared to 18% in placebo treated pts. Serious bleeding event reported in 3.5% of drotrecogin treated vs. 2% in placebo treated pts (P = 0.06). Intracranial hemorrhage reported in 0.2–2.5%.
- **WARNING:** The following conditions below may result in an increased risk of bleed that led to the exclusion from phase 3 trial. Careful considerations to bleeding risk must be given before the administration of drotrecogin:
- Platelet count <30,000 even if platelet count is increased after transfusion prothrombin time INR >3.0. Chronic severe hepatic disease
- Recent gastrointestinal bleeding (within 6 wks)
- Recent ischemic stroke (within 3 mos)
- Intracranial arteriovenous malformation or aneurysm
- Known bleeding diathesis

DRUG INTERACTIONS
- Avoid following drugs due to potential increased risk of bleed: thrombolytic therapy (within 3 days), warfarin (within 7 days), glycoprotein IIb/ IIIa inhibitors, aspirin (within 3 days), antithrombin III (within 12 hrs), LMW heparin (within 12 hrs), IV heparin.

PHARMACOLOGY
Mechanism
Sepsis syndrome results in thrombosis, impaired fibrinolysis, and induces an inflammatory response. Activated protein C exerts antithrombotic effect by inhibiting Factor Va and VIIIa, increases fibrinolysis, and invitro inhibits synthesis of tumor necrosis factor.

Pharmacokinetic Parameters
- **Absorption** —.
- **Cmax** Mean steady state concentration: 45 ng/mL.
- **Metabolism/Excretion** Drotrecogin is inactivated by endogenous protease inhibitors.
- **T1/2** Approx: 30 min.

Dosing for Decreased Hepatic Function
Limited data. Usual dose: 24 mcg/kg/hr × 96 hrs.

Pregnancy Risk
C: No data.

Breast Feeding Compatibility
No data.

COMMENTS
Due to the risk of severe bleed and lack of demonstrable benefit in pts with APACHE II score of <25 the recommended criteria for use are: (1) pts with severe sepsis as determined by an APACHE II score of >25 with a suspected or proven source of infection, with 3 or more signs of systemic inflammation (see Sepsis module); and (2) sepsis-induced organ dysfunction of >1 organ. The use of drotrecogin in pts at risk for bleed is a relative contraindication.

SELECTED REFERENCES
Abraham E, Laterre PF, Garg R, et al. Drotrecogin alfa (activated) for adults with severe sepsis and a low risk of death. *N Engl J Med*, 2005; Vol. 353; pp. 1332–41.

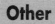

Other

LINDANE

Paul A. Pham, PharmD and John G. Bartlett, MD

INDICATIONS
FDA
- Treatment of Sarcoptes scabiei (scabies) in pts who are intolerant or have failed first-line therapy with safer agents (e.g., permethrin) for pediculosis or scabies.

NON-FDA Approved Uses
- Lice

FORMS

Brand name (mfr)	Forms	Cost*
Lindane (Generic)	Topical lotion 1% (60 mL)	$5.43
	Topical shampoo 1% (2oz)	$5.16

*Prices represents Average Wholesale Price (AWP).

USUAL ADULT DOSING
- Lice: apply 1 ounce of 1% shampoo to hair and scalp (for at least 4 min).
- Scabies: 1% topical cream apply from head to toe (leave in place for 6–12 hrs before rinsing). In epidemic setting or if live lice is still present after 2 wks, a second application is recommended.

RENAL DOSING
Dosing for GFR 50–80: Usual dose.
Dosing for GFR 10–50: No data, usual dose likely.

OTHER DRUGS

Dosing for GFR <10: No data, usual dose likely.
Dosing in hemodialysis: No data.
Dosing in peritoneal dialysis: No data.
Dosing in hemofiltration: No data.

ADVERSE DRUG REACTIONS

Common
- Pruritis

Occasional
- Neurotoxicity (more common in pts <50 kg, young children, and elderly pts): seizures, headache, lethargy, hallucinations, motor tics, paresthesias, myoclonic contractions.

Rare
- Death associated with seizures reported with repeated and prolong use.

DRUG INTERACTIONS
None known.

PHARMACOLOGY

Mechanism
A cyclic chlorinated hydrocarbon stimulates the nervous system of arthropods, resulting in seizures and death.

Pharmacokinetic Parameters
- **Absorption** 9% Systemic absorption after topical administration.
- **Cmax** 3–28 ng/ml after topical administration.
- **Distribution** Distributed in adipose tissue.
- **Metabolism/Excretion** Hepatic metabolism.
- **T1/2** 17.9–21.4 hrs.

Dosing for Decreased Hepatic Function
Avoid prolong exposure.

Pregnancy risk
B: No human data. Not teratogenic in animal studies. Due to the potential for neurotoxicity, permethrin is a safer alternative.

Breast Feeding Compatibility
No data. Due to the potential for neurotoxicity, permethrin is a safer alternative.

COMMENTS
Permethrin is the preferred agent for scabies due to comparable efficacy with lower risk of neurotoxicity compared to lindane [Schultz et al. Arch Dermatol 1990;126:167–70]. Contraindicated in neonates, in pts with seizure disorder, and Norwegian scabies. Avoid in pts <50 kg due to the increased risk of neurotoxicity.

SELECTED REFERENCES
Schultz MW, Gomez M, Hansen RC, et al. Comparative study of 5% permethrin cream and 1% lindane lotion for the treatment of scabies. *Arch Dermatol*, 1990; Vol. 126; pp. 167–70.

Singal A, Thami GP. Lindane neurotoxicity in childhood. *Am J Ther*, 2006; Vol. 13; pp. 277–80.

MALATHION

Paul A. Pham, PharmD and John G. Bartlett, MD

INDICATIONS

FDA
- Pediculus humanus capitis (head Lice), children >4 yrs of age

FORMS

Brand name (mfr)	Forms	Cost*
Ovide (Taro)	Topical lotion 0.5% packet	$133.73 per 2 oz
*Prices represents Average Wholesale Price (AWP).		

USUAL ADULT DOSING

Apply to dry hair in sufficient quantity to make wet, leave to dry off naturally, then rinse with shampoo 8–12 hrs later. Use fine-toothed comb to remove dead lice and eggs. May repeat in 1 wk if lice are still present. A randomized study suggests that a 20 minutes application of malathion is also effective.

RENAL DOSING

Dosing for GFR 50–80: Usual dose.

Dosing for GFR 10–50: Usual dose.

Dosing for GFR <10: No data. Usual dose likely.

Dosing in hemodialysis: No data. Usual dose likely.

Dosing in peritoneal dialysis: No data. Usual dose likely.

Dosing in hemofiltration: No data. Usual dose likely.

ADVERSE DRUG REACTIONS

Occasional

- Local skin irritation
- Caution: flammable lotion

Rare

- Recommended for topical application only. Fatal intentional ingestion has been reported (organophosphate poisoning management recommended with acute ingestion).

DRUG INTERACTIONS

None known

PHARMACOLOGY

Mechanism

Malathion is an organophosphate pesticide with anticholinesterase activity. Lice and nits are killed within 3 seconds by direct application of malathion.

Pharmacokinetic Parameters

- **Absorption** Less than 10% absorbed systemically with rapid metabolism and excretion.
- **Metabolism/Excretion** Rapid metabolism and excretion.
- **T1/2** n/a, if ingested half-life of 7.6 hrs.

Dosing for Decreased Hepatic Function

No data. Usual dose likely.

Pregnancy Risk

B: Not teratogenic in animal studies.

Breast Feeding Compatibility

No data.

COMMENTS

Malathion is safe and effective for the management of pediculosis capitis. Unlike lindane or permethrin, malathion needs to remain applied for 8–10 hrs, but a recent study found that an application time of 20 minutes was also effective.

SELECTED REFERENCES

Meinking TL, Vicaria M, Eyerdam DH, et al. Efficacy of a reduced application time of Ovide lotion (0.5% malathion) compared to Nix creme rinse (1% permethrin) for the treatment of head lice. *Pediatr Dermatol*, 2004; Vol. 21; pp. 670–4.

PERMETHRIN

Paul A. Pham, PharmD and John G. Bartlett, MD

INDICATIONS

FDA

- Pediculosis
- Scabies (*Sarcoptes scabiei var hominis*)

NON-FDA Approved Uses

- Lice

OTHER DRUGS

FORMS

Brand name (mfr)	Forms	Cost*
Elimite (Allergan)	Topical cream 5% (60 g)	$72.45
Permethrin (Alpharma and other generic manufactures)	Topical solution 1% (60 mL) Topical spray 0.5% (5 oz) Topical cream 5% (60 g)	$8.18 $5.12 $29.25
*Prices represents Average Wholesale Price (AWP).		

USUAL ADULT DOSING
- Pediculosis capitis: 1% cream rinse apply to hair and scalp for at least 10 min. Remove nits with nit comb; repeat application if live lice present 7 days after initial treatment.
- Scabies: 5% topical cream apply from head to toe; leave in place for 8–12 hrs before rinse. In epidemic setting or if live lice is present after 2 wks, a second application is recommended.

RENAL DOSING
Dosing for GFR 50–80: Usual dose.
Dosing for GFR 10–50: Usual dose.
Dosing for GFR <10: Usual dose.
Dosing in hemodialysis: Usual dose.
Dosing in peritoneal dialysis: Usual dose.
Dosing in hemofiltration: No data; usual dose likely.

ADVERSE DRUG REACTIONS
General
- Generally well tolerated
Common
- Pruritis
Occasional
- Burning and stinging

DRUG INTERACTIONS
None known

PHARMACOLOGY
Mechanism
Acts as a neurotoxin by depolarizing nerve cell membranes of parasites.
Pharmacokinetic Parameters
- **Absorption** Little to no systemic absorption
- **Metabolism/Excretion** Metabolized to inactive metabolite which is excreted in the urine
Dosing for Decreased Hepatic Function
No data; usual dose likely.
Pregnancy risk
B: No human data. Not teratogenic in animal studies. CDC considers permethrin the drug of choice in pregnancy.
Breast Feeding Compatibility
No human data; breast milk excretion in animal studies. CDC considers permethrin the drug of choice in breast feeding women.

COMMENTS
Permethrin is the preferred agent for scabies due to comparable efficacy with lower risk of neurotoxicity compared to lindane [Schultz et al. *Arch Dermatol* 1990;126:167–70].

SELECTED REFERENCES
Schultz MW, Gomez M, Hansen RC, et al. Comparative study of 5% permethrin cream and 1% lindane lotion for the treatment of scabies. *Arch Dermatol*, 1990; Vol. 126; pp. 167–70.

SECTION 5
VACCINES

ANTHRAX VACCINE

Paul A. Pham, PharmD and John G. Bartlett, MD

Vaccine Type

Anthrax Vaccine (AVA, BIOTHRAX), killed vaccine made from the cell-free filtrate of nonencapsulated, attenuated strain of *B. anthracis* culture that contains no dead or live bacteria (note: a live attenuated vaccine was manufactured in the former USSR, but no longer available).

Indications

ACIP Recommendations

- Routine vaccination with anthrax vaccine is indicated for persons engaged a) in work involving production quantities or concentrations of *B. anthracis* cultures and b) in activities with a high potential for aerosol production. Laboratory personnel using standard Biosafety Level 2 practices in the routine processing of clinical samples are not at increased risk for exposure to *B. anthracis* spores.
- Routine vaccination of veterinarians in the U.S. is not recommended because of the low incidence of animal cases. Vaccination may be considered in high-risk persons handling potentially infected animals in areas with a high incidence of anthrax cases.
- Routine vaccination is not recommended for bioterrorism preparedness (e.g., first responders, federal responders, medical practitioners, and private citizens), but The Working Group on Civilian Biodefense does recommend vaccination of exposed persons following a biological attack in conjunction with abx administration for 60 days following exposure.
- ACIP recommends that If antimicrobial prophylaxis is administered in combination with postexposure vaccination, it is prudent to continue antibiotics until 7–14 days after the third vaccine dose.

Other Information

- Post-exposure prophylaxis: AVA given as a sole agent was not effective in one primate study. AVA was effective if abx with activity against anthrax was given concurrently. The duration of postexposure antimicrobial prophylaxis should be 60 days if used alone for PEP of unvaccinated exposed persons.
- Department of Defense has mandated all U.S. military active- and reserve-duty personnel receive pre-exposure (vaccine) prophylaxis as an adjunct to prolonged postexposure antibiotic prophylaxis.
- Pre-exposure vaccination of some persons deemed to be in high-risk groups should also be considered.

Forms

Brand name (mfr)	Forms	Cost*
BioThrax (Bioport Corp, Lansing, Michigan)	SQ Vial 10 doses/vial	$900 per vial
*Prices represents Average Wholesale Price (AWP).		

Pathogen-Directed Protection

- *B. anthracis*

Dose/Administration

Primary Series

Dose (pre-exposure prophylaxis): 0.5 mL SQ × 6 doses (0, 2, and 4 wks followed by injections at 6, 12, and 18 mos). Six dose regimen used, because this regimen won FDA approval during registration trials in the 1950s (Brachman).

Booster

Revaccination: yearly booster dose (0.5 mL) required to maintain immunity.

ADVERSE DRUG REACTIONS

General
- No long-term sequelae reported
- Generally well tolerated

Common
- Injection site nodule: most frequently reported local reaction and more common in women for unexplained reasons (60% vs 30% in men).
- About 4% develop extensive erythema and swelling that may extend to the antecubital fossa—often misdiagnosed as bacterial cellulitis.

Occasional
- Headache (0.4%)
- Myalgia or arthralgia
- Headache
- Fatigue

Rare
- Anaphylaxis

VACCINE/DRUG INTERACTIONS
- No known drug interaction

CONTRAINDICATIONS
- History of an anaphylactic reaction to the vaccine. Previous anthrax infection (re: more severe adverse events among recipients with a vaccine history of anthrax).

IMMUNE RESPONSE
Relationship between immunity and quantitative antibody levels has not been evaluated. Onset of protection: antibody titer increased 3–4 × approximately 7 days after the second dose (3–4 wks from first dose), however clear minimum therapeutic antibody response has not been established, but appears to be sufficient to prevent development of disease once antibiotics were discontinued. An estimated 83% of human vaccinees develop a vaccine-induced immune response after 2 doses of the vaccine and >95% develop a four fold rise in antibody titer after 3 doses.

CLINICAL EFFICACY
- Effective in a placebo-controlled human trial against cutaneous anthrax. Primate models showed that antibiotic prevented inhalation anthrax, but were not protected from rechallenge.
- However, all animals given vaccine **plus** antibiotic were protected with re-challenge (Friedlander et al. *JID* 1993;167:1239).

OTHER INFORMATION
- Vaccine indicated only for risk of inhalation anthrax, but prevents cutaneous anthrax as well. Until ample reserve stockpiles of vaccine are available, reliance must be placed upon abx protection.
- The risk for persons who come in contact in the workplace with imported animal hides, furs, bone meal, wool, animal hair, or bristles has been reduced by changes in industry standards and import restrictions. Routine preexposure vaccination is recommended only for persons in this group for whom these standards and restrictions are insufficient to prevent exposure to anthrax spores.
- Safety in Pregnancy: Category D. Earlier unpublished study of infants born to women in the U.S. military service worldwide in 1998 and 1999 suggest that the vaccine may be linked with an increase in the number of birth defects. However, a published study found no effect on pregnancy or adverse birth outcomes in a cohort involving 4092 women [Wiesen AR et al. *JAMA* 2002;287:1556].
- Potentially exposed persons should be observed for signs of febrile illness.

BASIS FOR RECOMMENDATIONS
Advisory Committee on Immunization Practices. Use of anthrax vaccine in the United States. *MMWR Recomm Rep*, 2000; Vol. 49; pp. 1–20.
Comments: ACIP recommendations.

Centers for Disease Control and Prevention (CDC). Use of anthrax vaccine in response to terrorism: supplemental recommendations of the Advisory Committee on Immunization Practices. *MMWR Morb Mortal Wkly Rep*, 2002; Vol. 51; pp. 1024–6.
Comments: ACIP recommendations.

DIPHTHERIA VACCINE

John G. Bartlett, MD and Paul A. Pham, PharmD

VACCINE TYPE
Td, DT, DTP, and Tdap absorbed (diphtheria toxoid plus tetanus and/or pertussis).

INDICATIONS

ACIP Recommendations

- Tdap (single dose) as soon as 2 yrs after prior Td vaccination is recommended for a) postpartum women, b) close contacts of infants <12 mos (administer at least 2 wks before contact), and c) all healthcare workers with pt contacts.
- Tdap should replace Td for adults <65 yrs without prior Tdap dose. (This is a single one time dose of Adacel; otherwise subsequently use Td for boosting.)
- Adult with history of pertussis should receive Tdap.
- Pregnant women without Td for 10 yrs.
- Adults with uncertain histories of a complete primary vaccination series with tetanus and diphtheria toxoid-containing vaccines should begin or complete a primary vaccination series. (see "adult Td, primary series" under dosing recommendations).

Other Information

- Travelers: give if diphtheria acquisition risk high

FORMS

Brand name (mfr)	Forms	Cost*
ADACEL (Sanofi pasteur)	IM vial 2–2.5–5/.5 mL	$46.90
Infanrix (GlaxoSmithKline)	IM syringe 25–58–10 per .5 mL IM vial 25–58–10 per .5 mL	$26.24 $26.20
DECAVAC (sanofi pasteur)	IM syringe 5–2 LFU/0.5 IM vial 5–2 LFU	$23.55 $23.55
DT (sanofi pasteur)	IM vial 0.5 mL	$29.00
BOOSTRIX (GlaxoSmithKline)	IM syringe 2.5–8-5/.5 IM vial 2.5-8-5/.5	$45.31 $45.31
Pediarix (GlaxoSmithKline)	IM syringe 10–25–25 IM vial per .5 mL	$83.71 $83.71
DADPTACEL (Sanofi pasteur)	IM vial 2–2.5–5/.5	$46.23
TriHIBit for use as a booster only (Sanofi pasteur)	IM KIT 6.7–46–8.5	$52.86
Tripedia (Sanofi pasteur)	vial 6.7–46.8–5	$26.18
*Prices represents Average Wholesale Price (AWP).		

DOSE/ADMINISTRATION

Primary Series

ADACEL (adult Tdap): one dose (0.5 mL) IM. **DECAVAC** (adult Td): three 0.5 mL doses; 4 to 8 wks between the first and second dose, and 6 to 12 mos between the second and third dose. **INFANRIX** (pediatric Tdap): 0.5 mL IM (× 5 doses) 2, 4, and 6 mos of age, followed by 2 booster doses, administered at 15 to 20 mos of age and at 4 to 6 yrs of age. DT (pediatric DT): starting at 6 wks administer three doses of 0.5 mL IM 4 to 8 wks apart, then a another dose is given 6 to 12 mos after the third injection. **PEDIARIX** (pediatric Tdap + Inactivated Poliovirus Vaccine): 3 doses of 0.5 mL IM at 8-wk intervals starting at 2 mos of age. **DADPTACEL** (pediatric Tdap): 0.5 mL IM.

Booster

Booster is recommended every 10 yrs. Adult: ADACEL (× once only) or DECAVAC 0.5 mL IM q10 yrs. Pediatric: DT (for children between 4 and 6 yrs of age) 0.5 mL IM. Those who receive all four primary immunizing doses before their fourth birthday should receive a single dose of DT just before entering kindergarten or elementary school. This booster dose is not necessary if the fourth dose in the primary series was given after the fourth birthday. Thereafter, routine booster immunizations should be with tetanus and diphtheria toxoids adsorbed for adult use, at intervals of 10 yrs. Persons 7 yrs of age or older should not be immunized with DT (for pediatric use). **BOOSTRIX**: single 0.5 mL IM in individuals 10 through 18 yrs of age. TriHIBit (Tdap+Hib): 0.5 mL IM.

ADVERSE DRUG REACTIONS

General
• Generally well tolerated.

Common
• Pain and tenderness at injection site; rate increases with more doses.

Rare
• Anaphylaxis
• Encephalopathy
• Arthralgia
• Fever
• Guillain-Barre syndrome
• Arthus reaction (severe pain, swelling, induration, edema, hemorrhage, and occasional local necrosis)

VACCINE/DRUG INTERACTIONS
• The simultaneous administration of DT, MMR, OPV, or inactivated poliovirus vaccine (IPV), and Haemophilus b Conjugate Vaccine (HbCV) is acceptable.
• Immunosuppressive therapies, including irradiation, antimetabolites, alkylating agents, cytotoxic drugs, and corticosteroids (used in greater than physiologic doses), may reduce the immune response to vaccines.

CONTRAINDICATIONS
• History of anaphylaxis to vaccine components.
• Encephalopathy within 7 days of administration of pertussis vaccine should not receive Tdap.
• Use with caution with history of Guillain-Barre syndrome (within 6 wks after previous tetanus toxoid-containing vaccine), moderate or acute severe illness, unstable neurological conditions, and Arthus hypersensitivity reaction.

IMMUNE RESPONSE
Response usually good, but reduced in elderly. Anti-tetanus response: anti-tetanus levels >0.1 IU/mL achieved in nearly 100% and booster response was 90–93%. anti-diphtheria response: 99.9% had seroprotective anti-diphtheria levels >0.1 IU/mL and booster response was 91–96%. Anti-pertussis antigen response to pertussis antigens was 89% and booster response was 95%.

CLINICAL EFFICACY
• Vaccine is very effective.
• Diphtheria U.S. cases in 1999 – 0 cases.

OTHER INFORMATION
• Td preferred for adults (less local reactions) and during pregnancy
• DT: Pediatric preparation, contraindicated in persons >7 yrs.
• ADACEL contains the same tetanus toxoid, diphtheria toxoid, and 5 pertussis antigens as those in DAPTACEL (pediatric DTaP), but ADACEL is formulated with reduced quantities of diphtheria toxoid and detoxified pertussis toxin.

BASIS FOR RECOMMENDATIONS
Kretsinger K, Broder KR, Cortese MM, et al. Preventing tetanus, diphtheria, and pertussis among adults: use of tetanus toxoid, reduced diphtheria toxoid and acellular pertussis vaccine recommendations of the Advisory Committee on Immunization Practices (ACIP) and recommendation of ACIP, supported by the Healthcare Infection Control Practices Advisory Committee (HICPAC), for use of Tdap among health-care personnel. *MMWR Recomm Rep*, 2006; Vol. 55; pp. 1–37.
Comments: The ACIP recommendations for 2006 were changed to include Tdap as a one time single dose vaccine for persons <65 yrs.

ACIP. Recommended Adult immunization schedule. United States, October 2007. September 2008. *MMWR*, 2007; Vol. 56; p. 41.
Comments: ACIP recommended adult immunization.

HAEMOPHILUS INFLUENZAE (HIB) VACCINE

Paul A. Pham, PharmD and John G. Bartlett, MD

VACCINE TYPE
Haemophilus influenzae type b Conjugate Vaccine

INDICATIONS

ACIP Recommendations
• All children should be vaccinated, beginning routinely at 2 mos of age.

Other Information
• Recommended to be administered before splenectomy, 2 wks if possible.

FORMS

Brand name (mfr)	Forms	Cost*
Comvax (Merck)	IM vial 5–7.5–125 per 0.5 mL	$52.58 per vial
PedvaxHIB (Merck)	IM vial 7.5 mcg/0.5 mL	$27.53 per vial
*Prices represents Average Wholesale Price (AWP).		

PATHOGEN-DIRECTED PROTECTION
• *H. influenzae* type b

DOSE/ADMINISTRATION

Primary Series
Comvax: infants born to HBsAg negative mothers should be vaccinated with three 0.5 mL IM doses, ideally at 2, 4, and 12–15 mos of age. Infants born to HBsAg-positive mothers should receive Hepatitis B Immune Globulin and Hepatitis B Vaccine at birth and should complete the hepatitis B vaccination series. **PedvaxHIB:** Infants 2 to 14 mos of age should receive a 0.5 mL dose of vaccine ideally beginning at 2 mos of age followed by a 0.5 mL dose 2 mos later. When the primary two-dose regimen is completed before 12 mos of age, a booster dose is required.

Booster
Booster dose in infants completing the primary 2-dose regimen before 12 mos of age, a booster dose (0.5 mL) should be administered at 12 to 15 mos of age, but not earlier than 2 mos after the second dose.

ADVERSE DRUG REACTIONS

General
• Generally well tolerated with adverse reactions comparable to placebo

Occasional
• Fever (3%–4.3% after second dose)
• Injection site reaction (erythema in 0.7%–1.2%, swelling and induration in 0.9%–3.7% after the second dose)
• Irritability
• Drowsiness

Rare
• Allergic reaction

VACCINE/DRUG INTERACTIONS
• May be co-administered with DTP, DTaP, poliovirus vaccine live oral (OPV), MMR, hepatitis B vaccine, and inactivated poliovirus vaccine (IPV).
• Immunosuppressive therapies, including irradiation, antimetabolites, alkylating agents, cytotoxic drugs, and corticosteroids (used in greater than physiologic doses), may reduce the immune response to vaccines.

CONTRAINDICATIONS
• Hypersensitivity to components of the vaccine.

IMMUNE RESPONSE
An antibody serum level of >1.0 mcg/mL following vaccination corresponds with long-term protection against *H. influenzae* type b disease. ActHIB vaccine induced, on average anti-PRP levels >1.0 mcg/mL in 90% of infants after the primary series and in more than 98% of infants after a booster dose.

CLINICAL EFFICACY
- Efficacy of 93% reported in randomized placebo controlled trial. Observational studies reported an efficacy rate of up to 100%.

BASIS FOR RECOMMENDATIONS
No authors listed. Haemophilus b conjugate vaccines for prevention of Haemophilus influenzae type b disease among infants and children two mos of age and older. Recommendations of the immunization practices advisory committee (ACIP). *MMWR Recomm Rep*, 1991; Vol. 40; pp. 1–7.
Comments: ACIP recommendations.

HEPATITIS A VACCINE (HAV)

Paul A. Pham, PharmD and John G. Bartlett, MD

VACCINE TYPE
Killed, formalin inactivated vaccine

INDICATIONS

ACIP Recommendations
- Indicated for routine active immunization of persons aged >12 mos to protect against disease caused by hepatitis A virus.
- **High-risk pts** include: gay men, injection drug users, persons with clotting disorders, persons with chronic liver disease including HCV or chronic HBV, lab workers handling HAV, persons working with HAV or with nonhuman primates.
- **Travel**: travelers to countries with endemic HAV (see http://wwwn.cdc.gov/travel/contentDiseases.aspx). HAV vaccination not needed in northern and western Europe, New Zealand, Australia, Canada, and Japan.

FORMS

Brand name (mfr)	Forms	Cost*
Havrix (GlaxoSmithKline)	IM vial 1440 U/mL	$74.93
	IM vial 720 U/0.5 mL	$35.93
	IM syringe 1440 U/mL	$74.93
	IM syringe 720 U/0.5 mL	$35.93
VAQTA (Merck)	IM vial 50 U/mL	$74.80
	IM vial 25 U/0.5 mL	$37.78
Twinrix (HBV+HAV	IM vial 20 MCG-720 U	$106.18
vaccines) (GlaxoSmithKline)	IM syringe 20 MCG-720 U	$106.18
*Prices represents Average Wholesale Price (AWP).		

PATHOGEN-DIRECTED PROTECTION
- Hepatitis A virus

DOSE/ADMINISTRATION

Primary Series
Havrix 1440 ELISA units (1 mL) IM × 1 plus an additional dose at 6 to 12 mos is recommended for prolonged immunity. HAVRIX IM 720 units/0.5 mL × 1 (from 12 mos–18 yrs), then repeat × 1 6–12 mos later. Adults: VAQTA IM 50 units/1 mL × 1 plus an additional dose administered 6 to 18 mos later. Peds: VAQTA IM 25 units/0.5 mL × 1 (from 12 mos old through 18 yrs of age), then 25 units/0.5 mL × 16–18 mos later. Twinrix (combined HAV/HBV) 1 mL (720 units HAV vaccine/20 mcg HBV vaccine) IM at 0, 1, and 6 mos **or** alternate dosing schedule of at 0, 7, 21–30 days, followed by a dose at 12 mos. Injection should be given in the deltoid region. TWINRIX should not be administered in the gluteal region; such injections may result in a suboptimal response. Primary immunization for adults consists of 3 doses, given on a 0–, 1–, and 6-mo schedule. Twinrix is not approved for ≤18 yrs of age.

Booster
Duration of protection: 10 yrs minimum (no booster recommendations exist). Protective anti-HAV levels greater than 20 mIU/mL 8 yrs after initial dose.

ADVERSE DRUG REACTIONS

Common
- Local reactions in up to 56% (soreness, tenderness, and pain at immunization site).

Occasional
- Fever (4%)
- Headache (14%)
- Malaise (7%)
- Irritability, drowsiness, and loss of appetite in children

Rare
- Anaphylaxis
- Guillain-Barre syndrome (0.2 cases per 100,000 person-yrs. No higher than background incidence rates).

VACCINE/DRUG INTERACTIONS
- Immunosuppressant therapy may decrease response to vaccination.

CONTRAINDICATIONS
- Hypersensitivity to any component of the vaccine, including neomycin (contained in Twinrix and Havrix).

IMMUNE RESPONSE
80% seroconvert in 15 days, >96% at 30 days. With second dose nearly 100% respond. Anti-HAV levels greater than 10 to 20 mIU/mL have been protective.

CLINICAL EFFICACY
- In children, protection against clinical hepatitis A was 94% with HAVRIX and 100% with VAQTA.
- In adults, 97% who received one dose of VAQTA had anti-HAV levels greater than 10 mIU/mL.
- Onset of protection: 15–30 days.
- For adequate protection, Hepatitis A Vaccine must be administered 2 wks before expected exposure. For travelers expecting high-risk exposure within 2 wks, pooled immunoglobulin suggested instead.
- Not recommended for post exposure prophylaxis; if at least one dose of vaccine received >30 days prior to exposure, no immunoglobulin necessary.

OTHER INFORMATION
- See Hepatitis A pathogen module for details of HAV
- Pregnancy: Category C. No animal or human data. Use only if clearly indicated.
- Immunosuppressed pts may be unable to develop antibodies or may require additional boosters.

FOLLOW UP
- Long term immunity known for at least 8 yrs.
- No booster recommendations exist.

SELECTED REFERENCES

Advisory Committee on Immunization Practices (ACIP), Fiore AE, Wasley A, et al. Prevention of hepatitis A through active or passive immunization: recommendations of the Advisory Committee on Immunization Practices (ACIP). *MMWR Recomm Rep*, 2006; Vol. 55; pp. 1–23.

HEPATITIS B VACCINES (HBV)

Paul A. Pham, PharmD and John G. Bartlett, MD

VACCINE TYPE
Recombivax HB: recombinant vaccine produced by *Saccharomyces cerevisiae* (baker's yeast). **Engerix-B:** recombinant vaccine, also produced by *Saccharomyces cerevisiae*. **Twinrix:** bivalent vaccine providing protection against both hepatitis A and B: HAV (720 ELISA units/mL) and HBV(20 mcg HBsAg/mL).

INDICATIONS

ACIP Recommendations
- All infants and children by the age of 12 yrs.

- Persons w/ occupational risks (e.g., health care workers); persons w/ lifestyle risks (e.g., IVDU, hx of STDs, homosexual and bisexual men, and >1 sex partners in the past 6 mos), persons in correctional facilities.
- Hemodialysis, hemophiliac, chronic liver disease, and HIV-infected pts.
- Environmental risk factors: close contact of HBV carriers, sex partner of person with chronic HBV, clients and staff of institutions for those with developmental disabilities.
- HBV and pregnancy: (1) all pregnant women should be tested for HBsAg. (2) Infants born to HBsAg-positive mother, should receive HBIG (0.5 mL) IM ×1 and HB vaccine (0.5 mL) IM (w/in 12 hrs of delivery); the infant should complete the series with HB vaccine (0.5 mL) IM (5 mcg Recombivax or 10 mcg Engerix-B) at 1 and 6 mos. HBIG can be given up to 7 days of life. (3) If maternal HBsAg unknown, infant should receive HB vaccine w/in 12 hrs of delivery, and HBIG w/in 7 days if subsequent maternal HBsAg+. If infant preterm and <2000 g, HBIG should be given w/in 12 hrs due to lowered efficacy of HBV vaccine. (4) Routine HB vaccination for infants of HBsAg-negative mothers (HB vaccine (0.5 mL) IM × 3 (5 mcg Recombivax or 10 mcg Engerix-B) at 0, 1, and 6 mos).

Other Information

- Travellers: consider in those who plan to reside × 6 mos or longer in areas with prevalence of chronic HBV >2%, and who will have high risk contact with the local population (see http://wwwn.cdc.gov/travel/contentDiseases.aspx.htm).
- Post-exposure prophylaxis in occupational or non-occupational exposures

FORMS

Brand name (mfr)	Forms	Cost*
Engerix-B (GlaxoSmithKline)	IM vial 20 MCG/mL	$64.69
	IM vial 10 MCG/0.5 mL	$26.77
	IM syringe 20 MCG/mL	$64.69
	IM syringe 10 MCG/0.5 mL	$26.71
Recombivax HB (Merck)	IM vial 10 mcg/mL	$74.44 per vial
Comvax (Merck)	IM vial 5–7.5–125 per 0.5 mL	$53.32
Twinrix (GlaxoSmithKline)	IM syringe 20 MCG-720	$106.18
	IM vial 20 MCG-720	$106.18
*Prices represents Average Wholesale Price (AWP).		

PATHOGEN-DIRECTED PROTECTION

- Hepatitis B virus

DOSE/ADMINISTRATION

Primary Series

Recombivax HB (standard dose): 10 mcg/mL IM at 0, 1, and 6 mos. Recombivax HB (high dose): 40 mcg/mL IM at 0, 1, and 6 mos for pts on hemodialysis (and possibly other immunocompromised pts). **Engerix-B:** 20 mcg (1 mL) IM at 0, 1, and 6 mos (or 0, 1, 2, and 12 mos for more rapid induction of immunity). In HD pts double the dose (Engerix-B 2 doses of 20 mcg/mL). **Note:** if schedule is interrupted, may resume with good result providing that the second and third dose are separated by >2 mos. **Comvax:** infants born to HBsAg negative mothers should be vaccinated with three 0.5 mL doses IM of Comvax, ideally at 2, 4, and 12–15 mos of age. **Twinrix:** 1 mL (20 mcg-720 u) IM, given on a 0–, 1–, and 6–mo schedule **or** alternate dosing schedule at 0, 7, 21–30 days, followed by a dose at 12 mos.

Booster

Revaccination: controversial, since Ab levels do not measure immunologic memory; immunologic protection proven to last >12 yrs regardless of antibody levels. If done, response in 30–50% w/ 3 doses.

ADVERSE DRUG REACTIONS

General

- **No** role in the etiology or relapse of multiple sclerosis.

- Generally well tolerated. Among children receiving both hepatitis B vaccine and DTP, mild side effects have been observed no more frequently than among children receiving only DTP.

Common
- Injection site reaction (induration, pain, erythema) in 3%–29%

Occasional
- Fever >37.7°C (1–6%), but comparable to placebo

Rare
- Anaphylaxis
- No association with GBS

Vaccine/Drug Interactions
- No known drug interactions.
- Can be co-administered with DTP.

Contraindications
- Hypersensitivity to any component of the vaccine, including yeast.

Immune Response
Onset of protection: one mo after 3rd dose. Response: >95% for young and healthy adults. Response rate lower if >40 yrs (86%), certain HLA haplotypes, smoking history, obesity, diabetics (70–80%), HIV (18–72%) with lower response observed when CD4 <200, HD, renal and liver dz (60–70%).

Clinical Efficacy
- 80–95% for preventing HBV infection in gay men and virtually 100% if protective antibody response (>10 mIU/mL) is achieved.

Other Information
- Post-vaccination serologic testing recommended for pts w/ lower response rates (e.g., HIV pts) and whose subsequent management depends on this knowledge (e.g., health care workers and HD pts).
- Response defined as HBsAb level >10 mIU/mL, checked >1 mo after the 3rd dose.
- HBV deposited into fat rather than muscle results in lower seroconversion rates, so needle length is important.
- 60–90 Kg women and men: use 2.5 cm needle length. >90 Kg men and women: 3.8 cm needle length. <60 kg women: 1.6 cm needle length.
- Safety in pregnancy: Category C. Unless pt is at high risk for becoming infected during pregnancy, most experts recommend that HBV be deferred until after delivery.
- Double dose (40 mcg) more effective in HD and HIV-infected pts.

Basis for Recommendations
Mast EE, Margolis HS, Fiore AE, et al. A comprehensive immunization strategy to eliminate transmission of hepatitis B virus infection in the United States: recommendations of the Advisory Committee on Immunization Practices (ACIP) part 1: immunization of infants, children, and adolescents. *MMWR Recomm Rep*, 2005; Vol. 54; pp. 1–31.
Comments: ACIP recommendations.

HUMAN PAPILLOMA VIRUS (HPV) VACCINE

Paul A. Pham, PharmD and Khalil G. Ghanem, MD

Vaccine Type
Quadrivalent (types 6, 11, 16, 18) recombinant vaccine. Virus-like particle (VLP) does not contain genetic material—so non-infectious.

Indications

ACIP Recommendations
- The recommended age for vaccination of females is 11–12 yrs. Vaccine can be administered as young as age 9 yrs. Catch-up vaccination is recommended for females aged 13–26 yrs who have not been previously vaccinated.

Other Information
- FDA-approved indication: girls and women 9–26 yrs of age for prevention of cervical, vulvar (VIN), and vaginal (VaIN) neoplasia caused by HPV types 6, 11, 16, and 18.
- FDA approved for males 9–26 yrs to prevent genital warts caused by HPV 6 and 11.

FORMS

Brand name (mfr)	Forms	Cost*
Gardasil (Merck)	IM vial 20–40 ug/0.5 mL	$156.43
	IM syringe 20–40 ug/0.5 mL	$158.86

*Prices represents Average Wholesale Price (AWP).

PATHOGEN-DIRECTED PROTECTION
• HPV 6, 11, 16, and 18.

DOSE/ADMINISTRATION

Primary Series

Administer as 3 separate IM 0.5 mL inoculations at 0, 2, and, 6 mos. Give at deltoid or thigh sites. Minimum time between between 1st and 2nd dose is 4 wks. Minimum time between 2nd and 3rd doses is, 12 wks.

ADVERSE DRUG REACTIONS

General
• Serious adverse events were comparable between the vaccine and placebo groups.
• Generally well tolerated.

Common
• Mild to moderate injection site reactions—erythema (25%), pain (84%), and swelling (25%). These rates were only slightly higher than aluminum-containing placebo injection.

Occasional
• Pruritis (3%)
• Fever (10%)

Rare
• Syncope
• Headache (0.03%), gastroenteritis (0.03%), appendicitis (0.02%), and PID (0.02%). Unclear association with HPV vaccine

VACCINE/DRUG INTERACTIONS
• HPV vaccine may be co-administered with hepatitis B vaccine. No data on co-administration with other vaccines.
• Hormonal contraceptive did not affect HPV vaccine efficacy.
• Immunosuppressive therapies may decrease the efficacy of HPV vaccine.

CONTRAINDICATIONS
• Not recommended in pregnant pts. Pregnancy: Category B. Not teratogenetic in animal studies. In clinical studies, exposure in 1115 pregnant pts did not result in higher adverse reaction or teratogenicity compared to placebo. If inadvertent administration to a pregnant woman notify CDC (1-800-986-8999).
• Severe allergic reaction to yeast or other vaccine components.

IMMUNE RESPONSE

Response: 99.5% of girls and women were seropositive 1 mo post dose 3. Minimum anti-HPV 6, 11, 16, 18 antibody levels that protect against clinical disease have not been established.

CLINICAL EFFICACY
• HPV 6, 11, 16, and 18 seronegative pts: efficacy rate for prevention of CIN (any grade) or CIS was 95.2%.
• The efficacy rate was 100% for prevention of HPV 16- or 18-related CIN 2/3 or CIS.
• Not protective when given to pts who were already infected with one or more HPV types contained in the vaccine, but can be protective against the remaining vaccine HPV types.
• Response may be diminished in pts with immune deficiency (e.g., HIV) or those taking immunosuppressants.

OTHER INFORMATION
• By 50 yrs of age, at least 80% of women will have acquired genital HPV infection.
• Although up to 91% of HPV infections spontaneously clear within 2 yrs, certain HPV types (e.g., HPV 16 and 18) are more likely to persist and can significantly increase the risk of cervical cancer.

- HPV 16 and 18 account for 67.7% of all cervical cancers (Bosch FX, et al.).
- The quadrivalent HPV vaccine is effective in preventing cervical cancer and genital warts, as well as CIS, CIN 1–3, VIN 2/3, and VaIN 2/3 caused by HPV 6, 11, 16, and 18.
- May be administered to immunocompromised pts (including HIV-infected pts with CD4 count <200 cells/mL).

FOLLOW UP

- Vaccinated women must continue to undergo routine Papanicolaou (Pap) smear testing following a schedule identical to unvaccinated women.
- Vaccinated women should be advised to utilize barrier protection if sexually active.

BASIS FOR RECOMMENDATIONS

Markowitz LE, Dunne EF, Saraiya M, et al. Quadrivalent human papillomavirus vaccine: recommendations of the Advisory Committee on Immunization Practices (ACIP). *MMWR Recomm Rep*, 2007; Vol. 56; pp. 1–24.
Comments: ACIP recommendations.

SELECTED REFERENCES

Kim JJ, Goldie SJ. Health and economic implications of HPV vaccination in the United States. *N Engl J Med*, 2008; Vol. 359; pp. 821–32.
Villa LL, Costa RL, Petta CA, et al. Prophylactic quadrivalent human papillomavirus (types 6, 11, 16, and 18) L1 virus-like particle vaccine in young women: a randomised double-blind placebo-controlled multicentre phase II efficacy trial. *Lancet Oncol*, 2005; Vol. 6; pp. 271–8.

INFLUENZA VACCINE

John G. Bartlett, MD and Paul A. Pham, PharmD

Trivalent inactivated influenza purified split-virus preparation (TIV, IM preparation); live attenuated trivalent vaccine (LAIV, intranasal preparation); split-virus 2009 novel H1N1 influenza vaccine available as injection form as killed virus and as nasal spray as live attenuated virus. Note that there is a cross-protection between these vaccines.

INDICATIONS

ACIP Recommendations

- High risk: >50 yrs, residents of chronic care homes, chronic pulmonary/cardiac disease, chronic illness (diabetes; chronic lung, liver, heart, or renal disease; asthma; immunosuppression; sickle cell). Pregnancy: if during influenza season, give during 2nd/3rd trimesters.
- Transmission risk to high risk pts: medical personnel who serve high risk pts, household member of high risk pts.
- All persons, including school-aged children, who want to reduce the risk of becoming ill with influenza or of transmitting influenza to others should be vaccinated.
- "Consider" category: HIV, asplenia, anyone who wants it, or who provide essential services. Travellers: high risk pts to tropics (all yr), or to southern hemisphere in April-September. All children aged 5–18 yrs is now recommended beginning in September. All children aged 6 mos–4 yrs are priority targets, and older children with conditions that place them at increased risk for complications from influenza should continue.
- Priority groups to receive 2009 novel H1N1 vaccine: (1) pregnant women, (2) persons who live with or provide care for infants aged <6 mos (e.g., parents, siblings, and daycare providers), (3) health-care and emergency medical services personnel, (4) persons aged 6 mos–24 yrs, and (5) persons aged 25–64 yrs who have medical conditions that put them at higher risk for influenza-related complications.

Other Information

- FluMist: live attenuated virus; don't use if immunocompromised, pregnant, asthma, chronic lung disease, <2 yrs of age, or >49 yrs. No reports of transmission person-person.
- Either TIV or LAIV can be used when vaccinating healthy persons aged 2–49 yrs.

VACCINES

FORMS

Brand name (mfr)	Forms	Cost*
Fluvirin (McKesson Med Surgical)	IM vial 45MCG/.5 mL	$10.98
Flumist (Medimmune)	Intranasal syringe 1 dose	$22.74
Flulaval (indicated in adults only) (GSK)	IM vial 45 mcg/0.5 mL	tba
Afluria (CLS limited)	IM syringe 0.5 mL IM multidose vial 5 mL	tba tba
Influenza A (H1N1) Vaccine (Novartis Vaccines and Diagnostics Limited)	IM syringe 0.5 mL IM multidose vial 5 mL	tba tba
Influenza A (H1N1) 2009 Monovalent Vaccine (MedImmune, LLC)	Intranasal syringe 1 dose	tba
*Prices represents Average Wholesale Price (AWP).		

PATHOGEN-DIRECTED PROTECTION

- Influenza A and B
- The 2009–10 trivalent vaccine contains A/Brisbane/59/2007, IVR-148 (H1N1), A/Uruguay/716/2007, NYMC x-175C (H3N2) (an A/Brisbane/10/2007-like virus), and B/Brisbane/60/2008.
- Current novel H1N1 vaccine uses strain A/California 07/2009 (H1N1). Approx. 10 days to acquire immunologic protection with seroconversion in 76% and 66% in adults ages 18–49 and 50–64, respectively. Titers $>$ or $= 1:40$ was achieved in 100% and 94% of adults ages 18–49 and 50–64, respectively.

DOSE/ADMINISTRATION

Primary Series

Fluvirin (pediatric): not recommended if <4 yrs; 4–8 yrs: 0.5 mL × 1 dose (if previously unvaccinated give a second dose 1 mo later); <9 yrs vaccinated for the first time last season, but only received one dose: 2 doses of vaccine are required for protection, at least 4 wks apart; >8 yrs: 0.5 mL ×1. ACIP recommends FluZone 0.25 mL if aged 6–35 mos and 0.5 mL if aged $>$ or $= 3$ yrs. **FluLaval (adult):** 0.5 mL IM × 1 annually. **FluMist (LAIV):** for healthy children age 5–8 yrs not previously vaccinated: two 0.5 mL (0.25 mL/nostril) doses intranasally 6 wks apart before peak flu season (generally before December). For healthy children 5–8 yrs previously vaccinated, children 8–17 yrs, and adults (<49 yrs of age): 0.5 mL (0.25 mL/nostril) intranasally per season. **Novartis Influenza A (H1N1) vaccine:** Children 4 through 9 yrs: Two 0.5-mL intramuscular injections approx. 1 mo apart. **Sanofi Pasteur Influenza (H1N1) vaccine:** 6 through 35 mos of age: Two 0.25 mL doses approx. one mo apart; Children 3 yrs through 9 yrs of age: Two 0.5 mL doses approximately one mo apart. For Children 10–17 yrs and Adults: Sanofi Pasteur or Novartis Influenza A (H1N1) vaccine 0.5-mL IM ×1. Intranasal H1N1 live vaccine: 2–9 yrs: 2 doses (0.2 mL each, approximately 1 mo apart). >9 yrs and adults: 1 dose (0.2 mL).

Booster

Each season.

ADVERSE DRUG REACTIONS

General

- The new H1N1 vaccine is generally well tolerated. Mild to moderate local injection site reaction (46%) and headache (45%) were the most commonly reported ADR in the initial clinical trials.
- Intranasal H1N1 vaccine is not recommended in children <24 mos of age because of increased risk of hospitalization and wheezing.

Common
- Soreness at injection site (for TIV), usually >2 days in ~30%
- LAIV: runny nose/nasal congestion; incidence of headache, cough, and sore throat were comparable to placebo

Occasional
- Fever and malaise
- Wheezing with LAIV (especially in children 6–11 mos). Avoid Flumist in children aged <5 yrs with possible reactive airways disease (e.g., recurrent wheezing or a recent wheezing episode).

Rare
- Guillain-Barre syndrome (not associated with flu vaccine since 1993–94 season)
- Allergy: hives, angioedema, asthma

VACCINE/DRUG INTERACTIONS
- Immunosuppressive therapies (corticosteroids, alkylating drugs, antimetabolites, and radiation): do not co-administer. May increase risk of disseminated disease.
- May be co-administered with pneumococcal vaccine.
- Reports of the influenza vaccine inhibiting the clearance of warfarin, theophylline, phenytoin, although controlled studies have shown inconsistent results.
- Attenuated intranasal influenza vaccine should not be administered until 48 hrs after cessation of flumadine and flumadine should not be administered until two wks after the administration of live attenuated intranasal influenza vaccine.

CONTRAINDICATIONS
- IM vaccine (inactivated vaccine): allergy to eggs or prior severe allergic reaction, or fever >40C; no contraindication if only prior local reaction.
- Live attenuated vaccine: history of hypersensitivity to vaccine components, including eggs or egg products, children and adolescents (5–17 yrs of age) receiving aspirin, individuals who have a history of Guillain-Barre syndrome, and individuals with immune deficiency diseases.
- Children 6 to 12 mos may have a higher rate of wheezing and hospitalization with FluMist.

IMMUNE RESPONSE
6 mos–8 yrs: 86% had antibody response with 2 doses, but only 27% with one dose (The ACIP emphasized the importance of administering 2 doses of vaccine to all children aged 6 mos–8 yrs if they have not been vaccinated previously at any time with either live, attenuated influenza vaccine (doses separated by >6 wks) or trivalent inactivated influenza vaccine (doses separated by >4 wks).

CLINICAL EFFICACY
- Young adults or healthy elderly: ~70%. Elderly in nursing homes: 30–40%, but reduces influenza mortality by 80%. Vaccine efficacy depends on match of epidemic and vaccine strains-good in 14 of 16 past yrs.
- Vaccine efficacy may be decreased in elderly and immunosuppression.
- In young children (6 to 59 mos), intranasally administered live attenuated influenza vaccine was more effective than IM inactivated vaccine with 54.9% fewer cases of cultured-confirmed influenza.
- In adults, intranasally administered live attenuated vaccine resulted in a 40.9% reduction in febrile upper respiratory tract illnesses during a season with a poor match of epidemic and vaccine influenza strains (Nichol KL et al. *JAMA* 1999).

OTHER INFORMATION
- Estimated vaccination coverage remains <50% among certain groups for whom routine annual vaccination is recommended, including young children and adults with risk factors for influenza complications, health-care personnel (HCP), and pregnant women.
- Influenza—major infectious cause of death in U.S.; nearly all are elderly, in nursing homes, or have chronic diseases.
- Vaccine to healthy adults appears to generally reduce URI's and employee absenteeism; conflicting data on cost effectiveness. Health care workers—vaccination indicated to protect pts and infected health care workers; must avoid pt contact w/ FluMist × 7 days post-administration.
- LAIV must be kept frozen in the freezer. It may be thawed and kept in the refrigerator between 36–46°F for no more than 60 hrs.

- Children with reactive airways disease, persons with underlying medical conditions with higher risk for influenza complications, children aged 6–23 mos, and persons aged >49 yrs should receive not receive FluMist.
- Reported response rate with the new H1N1 vaccine: 96% in adults ages 16–64 and 56% >65 yrs (Sanofi-aventis vaccine). 80% and 60% in adults ages <65 and >65, respectively with the CSL Biotherapeutic's vaccine.
- Currently available H1N1 vaccine does not contain thimerosal.

BASIS FOR RECOMMENDATIONS

Use of influenza A (H1N1) 2009 monovalent vaccine. Recommendations of the Advisory Committee on Immunization Practices (ACIP), 2009. *MMWR*, 2009; Vol. 58;(Early Release) pp. 1–8.

Comments: ACIP H1N1 influenza vaccination recommendations.

SELECTED REFERENCES

Belshe RB, Edwards KM, Vesikari T, et al. Live attenuated versus inactivated influenza vaccine in infants and young children. *N Engl J Med*, 2007; Vol. 356; pp. 685–96.

Monto AS, Ohmit SE, Petrie JG, et al. Comparative efficacy of inactivated and live attenuated influenza vaccines. *N Engl J Med*, 2009; Vol. 361; pp. 1260–67.

JAPANESE ENCEPHALITIS VACCINE

Paul A. Pham, PharmD and John G. Bartlett, MD

VACCINE TYPE

Two types: (1) monovalent or polyvalent vaccines derived from infected mouse brain prepared by protamine precipitation of lipids followed by formalin viral inactivation (historical vaccine JE-VAX with supply expected to be exhausted by 2009), (2) new inactivated virus grown in Vero cells (Ixiaro).

INDICATIONS

ACIP Recommendations

- Individuals traveling to or residing (>1 mo) in areas where the mosquito-borne viral disease is endemic. (e.g., Far East and Southeast Asia; rice growing regions especially).
- Laboratory workers at risk for exposure to the Japanese encephalitis virus.
- Consider if travel <1 mo in epidemic area with extensive outdoor activities in rural area w/ rice paddies. Precaution should also be taken to reduce exposure to mosquitos.

FORMS

Brand name (mfr)	Forms	Cost*
JE-VAX (Sanofi pasteur)	SC vial 1 mL	N/A
Ixiaro (Intercell)	SC vial	TBA

*Prices represents Average Wholesale Price (AWP).

DOSE/ADMINISTRATION

Primary Series

Adults: 1 mL SC at days 0, 7, and 30. For 3 yrs of age and older: single dose is 1.0 mL of vaccine. For children 1 yr to 3 yrs of age: a single dose is 0.5 mL of vaccine.

Booster

Revaccination: booster dose of 1 mL may be administered every 2 yrs after the primary immunization series if pt is still at risk.

ADVERSE DRUG REACTIONS

Common

- Tenderness, redness, and swelling at the site of injection (20%).

Occasional

- Systemic side effects (fever, headache, malaise, rash, chills, dizziness, myalgia, nausea, and abdominal pain) (10%).

Rare

- Vaccine-related encephalitis, encephalopathy, or encephalomyelitis reported in 1–2.3 per million vaccinees (murine-derived vaccine).
- Generalized urticaria, EM, and angioedema (occur after a median of 12 hrs, and 3 hrs after the 1st and 2nd dose, respectively, but can occur within minutes to as long as 2 wks after vaccination).
- Hypotension
- Seizure

VACCINE/DRUG INTERACTIONS

- May be co-administered with DTP vaccine.

CONTRAINDICATIONS

- Hypersensitivity to thimerosal. Pts with a past history of **urticaria** are at increased risk of developing a severe allergic reaction to JE vaccine.
- Safety in Pregnancy: Category C. CDC does not recommend vaccination in pregnancy unless there is a very high risk of Japanese encephalitis transmission.
- Not recommended in persons <1 yr old.

IMMUNE RESPONSE

Onset of protection: effective titers of neutralizing antibodies reached within 60 days of immunization. Active immunity usually lasts for 6–24 mos. Response: based on animal studies, neutralizing antibody titer = or > 1:10 was protective. The new Japanese encephalitis vaccine (Ixiaro) immunogenicity was comparable to that of the older vaccine (JE-VAX).

CLINICAL EFFICACY

- Efficacy: 80–91% effective.

OTHER INFORMATION

- Crude estimate of acquiring Japanese B encephalitis among U.S. travelers ≤1 case per million annually.
- Japanese encephalitis has a mortality rate of approximately 25% and residual neuropsychiatric sequelae in 30% of survivors.
- Travel should not commence for at least 10 days after the last dose of vaccine, to allow adequate antibody formation and recognition of any delayed adverse reactions.
- Vaccinees should be observed for 30 mins after vaccination and warned about the possibility of delayed urticaria and angioedema of face and airways.
- New Ixiaro vero-based vaccine efficacy based on sero-responsiveness and safety appears comparable to JE-VAX with perhaps better local side effect profile.

BASIS FOR RECOMMENDATIONS

[No authors listed]. Inactivated Japanese encephalitis virus vaccine. Recommendations of the Advisory Committee on Immunization Practices (ACIP). *MMWR Recomm Rep*, 1993; Vol. 42; pp. 1–15.

Comments: ACIP recommendations.

SELECTED REFERENCES

Duggan ST, Plosker GL. Japanese encephalitis vaccine (inactivated, adsorbed) [Ixiaro]. *Drugs*, 2009; Vol. 69; pp. 115–22.

Tauber E, Kollaritsch H, Korinek M, et al. Safety and immunogenicity of a Vero-cell-derived, inactivated Japanese encephalitis vaccine: a non-inferiority, phase III, randomised controlled trial. *Lancet*, 2007; Vol. 370; pp. 1847–53.

MEASLES VACCINES

Paul A. Pham, PharmD

VACCINE TYPE

Live attenuated measles virus vaccine

INDICATIONS

ACIP Recommendations

- All adults and children should have routine vaccination at 12–15 mos (first MMR dose) and 4–6 yrs (second dose of MMR).
- All persons who work in health-care facilities must have an acceptable evidence of immunity.
- All adults born during or after 1957 should receive >1 dose of MMR unless they have a medical contraindication, documentation of >1 dose, history of measles based on health-care provider diagnosis, or laboratory evidence of immunity.

- Second dose of MMR is recommended for adults who (1) have been recently exposed to measles or are in an outbreak setting, (2) received killed measles vaccine or have been vaccinated with an unknown type of measles vaccine during 1963–1967, (3) are students in postsecondary educational institutions, (4) work in a health-care facility, or (5) plan to travel internationally.

Other Information

- Vaccination is recommended for susceptible international travelers leaving the U.S.
- Vaccination following exposure to natural measles may provide protection if the vaccine is given within 3 days of the exposure.
- High risk, susceptible individuals should receive measles immune globulin within 6 days of exposure. HIV infected children and adolescents receive IG regardless of immunization status.

FORMS

Brand name (mfr)	Forms	Cost*
ProQuad (Chiron)	SC vial 3–4.3–3	$160.38
M-M-R II (Merck)	SC vial 12500/0.5	$59.83
Attenuvax (Merck)	SC vial one vial	$21.30
*Prices represents Average Wholesale Price (AWP).		

PATHOGEN-DIRECTED PROTECTION

- Measles

DOSE/ADMINISTRATION

Primary Series

M-M-R II or ProQuad: 0.5-mL SC at 12–15 mos (revaccination with M-M-R II is recommended prior to elementary school entry). 2nd dose must be at least 4 wks after first dose. **Attenuvax (measles):** 0.5 mL SC for children 6–11 mos if needed for travel, but must be revaccinated with two doses of M-M-R. If not previously vaccinated, persons aged 7–18 yrs may receive 2 doses of MMR during any visit (with second dose at least 4 wks apart).

ADVERSE DRUG REACTIONS

Common

- Fevers (associated with the measles component of vaccine, occurs in ~5%)
- Transient rashes (5%)
- Urticaria or a wheal and flare at the injection site
- Pain at injection site

Occasional

- Transient lymphadenopathy
- Arthralgia and transient arthritis (associated with rubella components)

Rare

- Parotitis
- Anaphylaxis reaction
- Thrombocytopenia
- Febrile seizure (9 per 10,000 vaccinations among MMRV vaccine recipients vs. 4 per 10,000 vaccinations among MMR + varicella vaccine recipients; adjusted **or** of 2.3)
- Aseptic meningitis (associated with the Urabe strain mumps vaccine)
- Encephalitis
- Guillain-Barre Syndrome (but no increase incidence over background rates)

VACCINE/DRUG INTERACTIONS

- M-M-R II may be co-administered with varicella virus vaccine live and Haemophilus b conjugate vaccine using a separate injection sites and syringes.
- Although data are limited concerning the simultaneous administration of the entire recommended vaccine series (i.e., DTaP, IPV [or OPV], Hib with or without Hepatitis B vaccine, and varicella vaccine), data from numerous studies have indicated no interference between routinely recommended childhood vaccines (either live, attenuated, or killed).
- Avoid immune globulin administration within 3 mos of vaccination.

- Measles vaccine administration should be delayed for 3–12 mos after receiving immune globulin (source: AAP Red Book 2006).

CONTRAINDICATIONS

- Immunosuppressed pts (e.g., blood dyscrasias, leukemia, lymphomas, malignant neoplasms of bone or lymphatics, cellular immune deficiencies, hypogammaglobulinemia, dysgammaglobulinemia.
- Severe allergy to components of vaccine (including neomycin and gelatin).
- Severe febrile illness.
- Pregnancy (should be avoided for 30 days postvaccination).
- Use with caution in pts with a history seizure and severe thrombocytopenia.
- Eggs allergy is not a contraindication (risk of serious reaction to M-M-R is extremely low).
- May be administered in HIV pts if not severely immunosuppressed (CD4 % <15%), although there is the possibility of inadequate immune response.

IMMUNE RESPONSE

Immune response is measured by the presence of detectable antibody in the serum using the ELISA assay for measles. A protective antibody response to measles was seen with greater than 255 mIU/mL. In several randomized trials, children 12 to 23 mos of age received a single dose of ProQuad and achieved a response rates of the following: 97.4% for measles, 95.8% to 98.8% for mumps, 98.5% for rubella.

CLINICAL EFFICACY

- Since the introduction of MMR, the number of reported cases of measles, mumps, and congenital rubella syndrome have decreased by more than 99%.

OTHER INFORMATION

- Almost all recent cases of measles in the U.S. have been initiated as a consequence of an imported strain of virus carried by a susceptible traveler or immigrant (*MMWR*, 2008 / 57(29);796–799)

BASIS FOR RECOMMENDATIONS

ACIP. Recommended Adult immunization schedule—United States, October 2007–September 2008. *MMWR*, 2007; Vol. 56; p. 41.
Comments: ACIP recommended adult immunization.

Watson JC, Hadler SC, Dykewicz CA, et al. Measles, mumps, and rubella—vaccine use and strategies for elimination of measles, rubella, and congenital rubella syndrome and control of mumps: recommendations of the Advisory Committee on Immunization Practices (ACIP). *MMWR Recomm Rep*, 1998; Vol. 47; pp. 1–57.
Comments: ACIP recommendations

MENINGOCOCCAL VACCINES

Paul A. Pham, PharmD and John G. Bartlett, MD

VACCINE TYPE

Menactra (MCV4) is a conjugate vaccine. **Menomune** (MPSV4) is a meningococcal polysaccharide vaccine (Groups A, C, Y, and W-135 combined): older version, probably w/ less durable serologic response than newer conjugated version.

INDICATIONS

ACIP Recommendations

- ACIP Meningococcal vaccine recommendation for the general population: MCV4 (Menactra) at age 11–12 or at high school entry (approx. 15 yrs).
- High risk groups: Age 2–10: new recommendations from ACIP state that MCV4 is preferable to MPSV4. If previously received MPSV4 and remain at high risk, vaccinate with MCV4 at 3 yrs after receipt of MPSV4. If last received MPSV4 more than 3 yrs ago and remain at high risk, vaccinate with MCV4 as soon as possible. If lifelong high risk, subsequent doses of MCV4 likely will be needed. If history of Guillain-Barré syndrome (GBS), MPSV4 is an acceptable alternative. Providers may elect to vaccinate children aged 2–10 yrs infected with HIV; however efficacy of MCV4 among HIV-infected children is unknown.
- High risk groups: college freshmen living in dormitories, microbiologist with occupational exposure, military recruits, outbreak settings, terminal complement component deficiencies and asplenia.

- Travel: indicated if travel to epidemic area, most frequently sub-Saharan Africa during epidemics (Dec–June). Saudi Arabia requires certificate of vaccination for pilgrims to Mecca or Medina.
- Outbreaks of *N. meningitidis* serotype C disease; offer to college freshman living in dormitories.

Other Information

- Group B serotype is not covered by either commercially available vaccine.
- Routine vaccination of children 2–10 yrs is not recommended, but can be considered in high risk pts.

FORMS

Brand name (mfr)	Forms	Cost*
Menactra (Sanofi pasteur)	IM vial 4 MCG/0.5 mL	$117.15
Menomune-A/C/Y/W-135 (Sanofi pasteur)	IM vial 1 vial	$119.41
*Prices represents Average Wholesale Price (AWP).		

PATHOGEN-DIRECTED PROTECTION

- *N. meningitidis* (sero groups A, C, Y and W-135). Menactra has improved immune response (especially in adolescents), but still also does not cover serogroup B.

DOSE/ADMINISTRATION

Primary Series

Menomune (MPSV4): 0.5 mL SC × 1 (for age 2–10 high risk pts and ages >55). Menactra (MCV4): 0.5 mL IM ×1 (preferred for age 11–15+, but Menomune is acceptable alternative). ACIP recommends MCV4 in children aged 2–10 yrs at high risk for invasive meningococcal disease. Administer in the deltoid region. Menactra may be co-administered with Typhim Vi and Td vaccines.

Booster

Revaccination 2–3 yrs after initial immunization may be indicated for individuals at high-risk for infection especially if receiving MPSV4 vaccine, and children who were first vaccinated at less than 4 yrs.

ADVERSE DRUG REACTIONS

General

- Generally well tolerated.
- Incidence of mild to moderate pain, swelling, induration, and redness at injection site is higher with MCV4 (Menactra).

Occasional

- Erythema at the site of injection (4%)
- Irritability in young children (6%)
- Fatigue
- Headache
- Malaise
- Arthralgia

Rare

- Paresthesia
- Allergic reaction +/– anaphylaxis.
- Seizure
- Fever
- Five cases of Guillain-Barr Syndrome reported among MCV4 recipient (*MMWR* October 6, 2005 / 54(Dispatch);1–3). Evidence is insufficient to conclude that MCV4 causes GBS.
- Transverse myelitis

VACCINE/DRUG INTERACTIONS

- Immunosuppressive therapies, including irradiation, antimetabolites, alkylating agents, cytotoxic drugs, and corticosteroids (used in greater than physiologic doses), may reduce the immune response to vaccines.

CONTRAINDICATIONS
- Hypersensitivity to thimerosal.

IMMUNE RESPONSE
Seroconversion rates for these polysaccharides are >90%. Seroconversion of group A and C is lower in children <2–4 yrs of age.

CLINICAL EFFICACY
- Varies based on serogroup and pt population; 87% reduction of meningococcal meningitis from serogroup C in adult military recruits. Lower efficacy in children (<30% in children <4 yrs).

OTHER INFORMATION
- Menactra: $117/dose; Menomune: $119/dose
- Onset of protection: protective antibody levels at 7–10 days. Antibody level declines over 2–3 yr period.
- Menactra is a new meningococcal (Grps A, C, Y, and W-135) polysaccharide diphtheria toxoid conjugate vaccine, produces >4 × rise in titers in 82–97% of adolescents (11–18 yrs).
- Due to the poor immunogenicity in children <2 yrs old and lack vaccine to serogroup B, chemoprophylaxis (for *N. meningitidis*) is recommended in lieu of vaccine for prevention of secondary cases in daycare centers.
- Meningococcal B vaccine available, but not licensed in U.S., and not thought to be entirely effective.
- Meningococcal vaccine should not be administered concomitantly with whole-cell pertussis or whole-cell typhoid vaccines, but may be administered with other vaccines.
- Pregnancy: Category C. No teratogenicity or growth abnormalities were observed among the 34 infants born to mothers immunized while pregnant [Letson GW et al. *Pediatr Infect Dis J* 1998;17:261].

BASIS FOR RECOMMENDATIONS
Bilukha OO, Rosenstein N, National Center for Infectious Diseases, Centers for Disease Control and Prevention (CDC). Prevention and control of meningococcal disease. Recommendations of the Advisory Committee on Immunization Practices (ACIP). *MMWR Recomm Rep*, 2005; Vol. 54; pp. 1–21.
Comments: Recommendations on the prevention of Meningococcal disease of the Advisory Committee on Immunization Practices (ACIP).

Centers for Disease Control and Prevention (CDC). Report from the Advisory Committee on Immunization Practices (ACIP): decision not to recommend routine vaccination of all children aged 2–10 yrs with quadrivalent meningococcal conjugate vaccine (MCV4). *MMWR*, 2008; Vol. 57; pp. 462–465.
Comments: Routine vaccination of children 2–10 yrs is not recommended, but can be considered in high-risk pts.

Centers for Disease Control and Prevention (CDC). Recommendation from the Advisory Committee on Immunization Practices (ACIP) for use of quadrivalent meningococcal conjugate vaccine (MCV4) in children aged 2–10 yrs at increased risk for invasive meningococcal disease. *MMWR Morb Mortal Wkly Rep*, 2007; Vol. 56; pp. 1265–1266.
Comments: Updated recommendations on the prevention of meningococcal disease. MCV4 conjugate vaccine is preferred in children aged 2–10 yrs at risk for invasive meningococcal disease.

SELECTED REFERENCES
Centers for Disease Control and Prevention (CDC). Guillain-Barré syndrome among recipients of menactra meningococcal conjugate vaccine—United States, June-July 2005. *MMWR Morb Mortal Wkly Rep*, 2005; Vol. 54; pp. 1023–5.

MUMPS VACCINE

Paul A. Pham, PharmD

VACCINE TYPE
Live mumps virus vaccine

INDICATIONS
ACIP Recommendations
- All adults and children should have routine vaccination at 12–15 mos (first MMR dose) and 4–6 yrs (second dose of MMR) separated by at least 4 wks.
- All persons who work in health-care facilities must have an acceptable evidence of immunity.
- Adults born during or after 1957 should receive 1 dose of MMR unless they have a medical contraindication, history of mumps based on health-care provider diagnosis, or laboratory evidence of immunity.

• A second dose of MMR is recommended for adults who (1) are in an age group that is affected during a mumps outbreak; (2) are students in post secondary educational institutions; (3) work in a health-care facility; or (4) plan to travel internationally. For unvaccinated health-care workers born before 1957 who do not have other evidence of mumps immunity, consider administering 1 dose on a routine basis and strongly consider administering a second dose during an outbreak.

Other Information

• Vaccination is recommended for susceptible international travelers leaving the U.S.

FORMS

Brand name (mfr)	Forms	Cost*
M-M-R II (Merck)	SC vial 20000/0.5	$57.62
Mumpsvax (Merck)	SC vial 0.5 mL	$27.61
ProQuad (Chiron)	SC vial 3-4.3-3	$154.71
*Prices represents Average Wholesale Price (AWP).		

PATHOGEN-DIRECTED PROTECTION

• Mumps virus

DOSE/ADMINISTRATION

Primary Series

M-M-R II or ProQuad: 0.5-mL SC at 12–15 mos (revaccination with M-M-R II is recommended prior to elementary school entry). **Mumpsvax:** The dose for any age is 0.5 mL SC (note: the recommended age for primary vaccination is 12 to 15 mos and revaccination with M-M-R II is recommended prior to elementary school entry).

ADVERSE DRUG REACTIONS

Common

• Fevers (associated with the measles component in ~5%)
• Transient rashes (5%)
• Urticaria or a wheal and flare at the injection site
• Pain at injection site

Occasional

• Transient lymphadenopathy
• Arthralgia and transient arthritis (associated with rubella components)

Rare

• Parotitis
• Anaphylaxis reaction
• Thrombocytopenia
• Seizure
• Aseptic meningitis (associated with the Urabe strain mumps vaccine)
• Encephalitis
• Guillain-Barre Syndrome (but no increase incidence over background rates)

VACCINE/DRUG INTERACTIONS

• M-M-R II may be co-administered with varicella virus vaccine live and Haemophilus b conjugate vaccine using a separate injection sites and syringes.
• Although data are limited concerning the simultaneous administration of the entire recommended vaccine series (i.e., DTaP, IPV [or OPV], Hib with or without Hepatitis B vaccine, and varicella vaccine), data from numerous studies have indicated no interference between routinely recommended childhood vaccines (either live, attenuated, or killed).
• Avoid immune globulins within 3 mos of vaccination.
• Vaccination should be delayed 3–12 mos after receive immune globulins (Source: AAP Red Book 2006).

CONTRAINDICATIONS
- Immunosuppressed pts (i.e., blood dyscrasias, leukemia, lymphomas, malignant neoplasms of bone or lymphatics, cellular immune deficiencies, hypogammaglobulinemia, dysgammaglobulinemia.
- Severe allergy to components of vaccine (including neomycin and gelatin).
- Severe febrile illness.
- Pregnancy (should be avoided for 30 days post vaccination).
- Use with caution in pts with a history seizure and severe thrombocytopenia.
- Eggs allergy is not a contraindication (risk of serious reaction to M-M-R is extremely low); those w/ anaphylactic reaction may be at increased risk.
- May be administered in HIV if not severely immunosuppressed (CD4% <15%).

IMMUNE RESPONSE
Immune response is measured by the presence of detectable antibody in the serum using the ELISA assay for measles. A protective antibody response to mumps was seen with greater than 10 ELISA units/mL. In several randomized trials, children 12 to 23 mos of age received a single dose of Proquad and achieved a response rates of the following: 97.4% for measles, 95.8% to 98.8% for mumps, 98.5% for rubella.

CLINICAL EFFICACY
- Since the introduction of MMR, the number of reported cases of measles, mumps, and congenital rubella syndrome have decreased by more than 99%.

OTHER INFORMATION
- Recent mumps outbreak (2004–2005) in U.S. likely attributed to waning immunity in college age students, but not certain.
- Vaccine administration after exposure does not prevent disease, but can be given to protect against subsequent exposure.

BASIS FOR RECOMMENDATIONS
ACIP. Recommended Adult immunization schedule—United States, October 2007–September 2008. *MMWR*, 2007; Vol. 56; p. 41.
Comments: ACIP recommended adult vaccination.

Watson JC, Hadler SC, Dykewicz CA, et al. Measles, mumps, and rubella—vaccine use and strategies for elimination of measles, rubella, and congenital rubella syndrome and control of mumps: recommendations of the Advisory Committee on Immunization Practices (ACIP). *MMWR Recomm Rep*, 1998; Vol. 47; pp. 1–57.
Comments: ACIP recommendations.

PNEUMOCOCCAL VACCINES

Paul A. Pham, PharmD and John G. Bartlett, MD

VACCINE TYPE
Pneumovax: 23 valent polysaccharide vaccine w/ serotype antigens covering 87% bacteremic cases and most PCN-resistant serotypes. **Prevnar:** 7-valent conjugate vaccine (diphtheria CRM197 protein) covers serotypes 4, 9V, 14, 18C, 19F, 23F, and 6B.

INDICATIONS
ACIP Recommendations
- Adult recommendations—Age: >65 yrs.
- Chronic disease: pulmonary/cardiac disease, alcoholism, cirrhosis, diabetes, renal failure, nephrosis.
- Compromised host: HIV, asplenia/splenectomy, sickle-cell disease, lymphoma, leukemia, multiple myeloma, Hodgkins disease, organ or marrow transplant, iatrogenic immune suppression.
- Hospitalized pts w/ indications: considered ideal time to vaccinate.
- Specific populations: Native Americans, homeless, CSF leak, cochlear implants, Alaskan natives, residents of long-term care facilities.

Other Information
- HIV: best response w/ CD4 > 200.
- Travel: no indications.
- Pregnancy: not contraindicated.

- Pediatrics: Prevnar is recommended in all children aged 2–23 mos and for children aged 24–59 mos who are at increased risk for pneumococcal disease (e.g., children with sickle cell disease, human immunodeficiency virus infection, and other immunocompromising or chronic medical conditions). Consider Prevnar for all other children aged 24–59 mos, with priority given to a) children aged 24–35 mos, b) children who are of Alaska Native, American Indian, and African-American descent, and c) children who attend group day care centers.
- Catch-up immunization schedule: administer 1 dose of Prevnar to all healthy children aged 24–59 mos having any incomplete schedule.
- Catch-up immunization schedule in children with underlying medical conditions: administer 2 doses of Prevnar at least 8 wks apart if previously received less than 3 doses **or** 1 dose of Prevnar if previously received 3 doses.

FORMS

Brand name (mfr)	Forms	Cost*
Pneumovax 23 (Merck)	IM vial 25 MCG/0.5 mL	$46.29
Prevnar-7 (Wyeth)	IM vial 0.5 mL	$14.74
*Prices represents Average Wholesale Price (AWP).		

DOSE/ADMINISTRATION

Primary Series

Pneumovax: 0.5 mL IM. Best administered 2 wks before splenectomy or as long as possible before planned immunosuppression if possible. **Prevnar** (for pediatric use only): 3 doses of 0.5 mL IM each, at approximately 2-mos intervals (starting at 2 mos of age), followed by a fourth dose of 0.5 mL at 12–15 mos of age.

Booster

Revaccination, Pneumovax (at 5 yrs): if >5 yrs and immunosuppression, asplenia, turned >65 yrs, dialysis, CD4 increased from <200 to >200 (for HIV pts).

ADVERSE DRUG REACTIONS

General

- Revaccination (Pneumovax): local reaction increased 3.3×; severe reactions not increased.
- Prevnar is generally well tolerated in pediatrics with only occasional injection site reaction and fever.

Common

- Pain/erythema at injection site, rates ~50%.

Occasional

- Fever, myalgia, severe local reaction in <4%.

Rare

- Anaphylactoid reaction: 5 per/million

VACCINE/DRUG INTERACTIONS

- Influenza vaccine may be given together with Pneumovax; give at separate injection sites.
- Prevnar may be given together with DTaP.
- Immunosuppressive therapies, including irradiation, antimetabolites, alkylating agents, cytotoxic drugs, and corticosteroids (used in greater than physiologic doses), may reduce the immune response to vaccines.

CONTRAINDICATIONS

- Pneumovax for those <13 mos of age (reactions increased).
- Hypersensitivity to any component of (e.g., diphtheria toxoid in Prevnar)

IMMUNE RESPONSE

Most adults have 2× rise in type specific Ab at 2–3 wks; less if immunosuppressed.

CLINICAL EFFICACY

- Adults: best data show prevention of pneumococcal bacteremia, but not pneumonia.

OTHER INFORMATION

- Protection: starts within 2 wks; lasts >9 yrs; degree of protection—controversial.
- Highest priority: asplenia, CSF leak, renal failure; possibly those at high risk of bacteremia—e.g., smokers (author opinion).

- Benefit: good evidence Pneumovax reduces pneumococcal bacteremia.
- Inconsistent evidence that Pneumovax reduces pneumonia or pneumococcal infections.
- Protein conjugated vaccine (Prevnar) works well in pediatric populations, and this vaccine when given to children <2 yrs has great benefit in preventing invasive pneumococcal infections and in preventing inventing pneumococcal infections in adults, especially >65 yrs. This is presumed to be due to herd immunity. Problem with Prevnar-7, is the emergence of "replacement strains," especially serotype 19A that is not in Prevnar-7, is now a major cause of invasive pneumococcal infections and is relatively resistant to antibiotics. Prevnar-13 which includes serotype 19A, is being tested on adults.
- Inadequate current data to recommend protein conjugate vaccine (Prevnar) to adult pts.

BASIS FOR RECOMMENDATIONS

Modlin JF, et al. Preventing Pneumococcal Disease Among Infants and Young Children. *MMWR*, 2000; Vol. 49(RR09); pp. 1–38.
Comments: ACIP recommendations.

No authors listed. Prevention of pneumococcal disease: recommendations of the Advisory Committee on Immunization Practices (ACIP). *MMWR Recomm Rep*, 1997; Vol. 46; pp. 1–24.
Comments: Guidelines based on this document. Revaccination recommended for persons >65 yrs who were vaccinated when <65 and previously vaccinated persons who are immunocompromised.

SELECTED REFERENCES

Jefferson T, Demicheli V. Polysaccharide pneumococcal vaccines. *BMJ*, 2002; Vol. 325; pp. 292–3.

Kyaw MH, Lynfield R, Schaffner W, et al. Effect of introduction of the pneumococcal conjugate vaccine on drug-resistant Streptococcus pneumoniae. *N Engl J Med*, 2006; Vol. 354; pp. 1455–63.

Vila-Córcoles A, Ochoa-Gondar O, Hospital I, et al. Protective effects of the 23-valent pneumococcal polysaccharide vaccine in the elderly population: the EVAN-65 study. *Clin Infect Dis*, 2006; Vol. 43; pp. 860–8.

POLIO VACCINE

Paul A. Pham, PharmD

VACCINE TYPE

Inactivated poliovirus vaccine (IPV, routine use in U.S.). Oral polio vaccine (OPV, use in endemic regions only).

INDICATIONS

ACIP Recommendations

- Routine childhood polio vaccination in the United States. All children should receive 4 doses of IPV at ages 2, 4, 6–18 mos, and 4–6 yrs.
- Due to the risk of paralytic poliomyelitis, oral polio vaccine (OPV) is only recommended to eradicate polio from endemic countries.
- Unvaccinated adults at risk: travelers to endemic area, laboratory workers who handle polioviruses, health-care workers in close contact with pts who might be excreting wild polioviruses, and unvaccinated adults whose children will be receiving oral poliovirus vaccine.

Other Information

- If the poliovirus vaccination series was initiated with one or more doses of OPV, they should receive IPV to complete the series.
- Vaccine-derived polioviruses can produce outbreaks in areas with low rates of Sabin OPV coverage (MMWR 2009;58: 1002). OPV should be used in endemic regions only

FORMS

Brand name (mfr)	Generic	Mfg	Brand Forms	Cost*
IPOL	Polio (inactivated)	Sanofi Pasteur	IM or SCvial (multidose) 5 mL	$28.30 per dose
*Prices represents Average Wholesale Price (AWP).				

PATHOGEN-DIRECTED PROTECTION

- Poliovirus: type 1 (Mahoney), type 2 (MEF-1), and type 3 (Saukett).

DOSE/ADMINISTRATION

Primary Series

Peds: Three 0.5 mL IM or SC at ages 2, 4, and 6 to 18 mos (must be given at least 4 wks apart). The first immunization may be administered as early as 6 wks of age. **Adults at risk:** Two doses of IPV IM or SC at 4–8 wks intervals; a third dose should be administered 6–12 mos after the second.

Booster

Booster dose at 4 to 6 yrs unless 3rd dose received after 4th birthday

ADVERSE DRUG REACTIONS

General

- Generally well tolerated

Occasional

- Injection site tenderness
- Irritability and tiredness

Rare

- Vaccine-associated paralytic poliomyelitis (VAPP) associated with oral polio vaccine only (one case among 2.4 million vaccine recipient).

VACCINE/DRUG INTERACTIONS

- IPV may be co-administered with DTP, DTaP, Hib, HepB, varicella vaccine, and measles-mumps-rubella vaccine.
- No known drug interactions.

CONTRAINDICATIONS

- Severe allergic reaction to components of the vaccine including streptomycin, polymyxin B or neomycin.
- OPV should not be administered to immunosuppressed pts (IPV is recommended).

IMMUNE RESPONSE

IPV: 90% to 100% of children develop protective antibodies to all three types of poliovirus after 2 doses IPV, and 99%–100% develop protective antibodies after 3 doses. Immunosuppressed pts may have a decreased immune response. **OPV:** After 3 doses of OPV, >95% of recipients develop long-lasting. OPV consistently induces immunity of the gastrointestinal tract that provides a substantial degree of resistance to reinfection with poliovirus (including wild poliovirus). Both IPV and OPV induce immunity of the mucosa of the gastrointestinal tract, but the mucosal immunity induced by OPV is superior.

CLINICAL EFFICACY

- Effective in eradicating polio. One dose of IPV administered to persons during an outbreak of poliovirus type 1 in Senegal during 1986–1987 was 36% effective; the effectiveness of 2 doses was 89%.

BASIS FOR RECOMMENDATIONS

Modlin JF et al. Poliomyelitis Prevention in the United States. Updated Recommendations of the Advisory Committee on Immunization Practices (ACIP) *MMWR* 2000 49(RR05);1-22

Comments: ACIP recommendations.

RABIES VACCINES

Paul A. Pham, PharmD and John G. Bartlett, MD

VACCINE TYPE

Imovax rabies vaccine: human diploid cell (HDCV). **RabAvert rabies vaccine:** purified chick embryo (PCEC).

INDICATIONS

ACIP Recommendations

- Preexposure vaccination: should be offered to persons in high-risk groups, such as veterinarians, animal handlers, and certain laboratory workers. Vaccination can be consider for other persons whose activities bring them into frequent contact with rabies virus or potentially rabid bats, raccoons, skunks, cats, dogs, or other species at risk for having rabies. Preexposure prophylaxis eliminates the need for rabies immune globulin (RIG) and decreases the number of doses of vaccine needed, in addition, it protects persons whose postexposure therapy is delayed.

Other Information

- Major risk: bats in U.S. and Europe, dog bites in developing countries. Risk with bite from rabid dog and no prophylaxis: 36–57%.
- 32/35 rabies cases in U.S. 1958–2000 were bat associated, although 26/32 had no known prior hx of bat bite.
- Dog/cat bites (U.S.): quarantine × 10 days, if pet gets symptoms of rabies—start prophylaxis and necropsy animal. Escaped pet—consult health department but low risk in U.S.
- Skunks, raccoons, fox bite: consider rabid unless negative necropsy; consider immediate prophylaxis, but rare cause of human rabies.
- Livestock, rodents (gerbils, mice, rats, guinea pigs), rabbits, beavers, etc.—almost never cause rabies, but consult public health official.
- Combine vaccination with rabies immune globulin for severe exposures, obtain RIG: 800-822-2463 or 800-288-8370.

FORMS

Brand name (mfr)	Forms	Cost*
RabAvert (Chiron)	Intradermal KIT 2.5 UNIT 1 mL	$247.50

*Prices represents Average Wholesale Price (AWP).

PATHOGEN-DIRECTED PROTECTION

- Rabies virus

DOSE/ADMINISTRATION

Primary Series

Pre-exposure prophylaxis (primary vaccination in high risk groups): 1.0 mL IM injection on day 0 and one on day 7 and one either on day 21 or 28. **Post-exposure prophylaxis** (previously unvaccinated): **Imovax** rabies vaccine (HDCV) 1 mL IM in the deltoid day 0, 3, 7, and 14. **RabAvert** (PCEC) 1 mL intradermally day 0, 3, 7, and 14, intradermally. Post-exposure prophylaxis (previously vaccinated): two IM doses (1.0 mL each) of vaccine, one immediately and one 3 days later. If no prior vaccination and severe exposure: administer rabies immune globulin (RIG) 20 IU/kg at wound site and also IM in addition to vaccination (note: administer at distant site from vaccine administration site).

Booster

In high risk populations: booster doses of vaccine should be administered to maintain a serum titer corresponding to at least complete neutralization at a 1:5 serum dilution by the RFFIT. Monitor antibody levels q2yrs.

ADVERSE DRUG REACTIONS

Common

- Injection site reaction (e.g., erythema, induration, and pain)

Occasional

- Flu-like symptoms (e.g., fatigue, fever, headache, myalgia, dizziness, malaise, arthralgia)
- Lymphadenopathy

Rare

- Allergic reactions

VACCINE/DRUG INTERACTIONS

- Radiation, antimalarials, and immunosuppressive therapies (e.g., antimetabolites, alkylating agents, cytotoxic drugs, and corticosteroids (used in greater than physiologic doses): may reduce the immune response to vaccines.

Contraindications

- Hypersensitivity to any component of the vaccine (relative); however, benefit generally outweigh the risk for post-exposure prophylaxis.

IMMUNE RESPONSE

Response to vaccine: neutralizing Ab in 7–10 days, persists >2 yrs. At 1 yr 88–100% had protective levels of antibody. Intradermal produces a better antigenic response than intramuscular.

CLINICAL EFFICACY

- 100% effective when given pre-exposure.

OTHER INFORMATION
- Most important: immediate cleansing of wound with viricidal reduces risk by 50%. See rabies module for more detailed information.
- Wound: immediately clean with soap; irrigate with viricidal agent, e.g., povidone, iodine, etc.
- Main concern in U.S.: bats, many exposures unwittingly while asleep.
- Main concern with travelers: dog bite in endemic area (developing countries).
- Rabies prophylaxis guidelines: conservative, expensive ($1500), demanding (5 injections), and w/ side effects. Consider for occupational reasons (vets, animal handlers).
- Pregnancy or HIV: no differences, routine recommendations.
- HIV: vaccine response is poor with low CD4; double dose or use intradermal route.
- Recent studies have suggested that 4 immunizations are sufficient without the need for the prior recommended total of 5.

FOLLOW UP
- Antibody response, absence should guide reimmunization in at risk populations.

BASIS FOR RECOMMENDATIONS
[No authors listed]. Human rabies prevention—United States, 2008. Recommendations of the Advisory Committee on Immunization Practices (ACIP). *MMWR Recomm Rep*, 2008; Vol. 57; pp. RR–3.

Comments: In 2006, a total of 79 cases of rabies were reported in domestic animals in the U.S., but none were attributed to enzootic dog-to-dog transmission, and 3 human cases. Two of the human rabies cases were attributed to bat exposures and one case was associated with dog bite (where canine rabies is enzootic). None of the 2006 human rabies cases were from indigenous domestic animals.

SELECTED REFERENCES
CDC. Compendium of animal rabies prevention and control. *MMWR*, 2006; Vol. 55; pp. RR1–8.

Messenger SL, Smith JS, Rupprecht CE. Emerging epidemiology of bat-associated cryptic cases of rabies in humans in the United States. *Clin Infect Dis*, 2002; Vol. 35; pp. 738–47.

Morris J, Crowcroft NS. Pre-exposure rabies booster vaccinations: a literature review. *Dev Biol (Basel)*, 2006; Vol. 125; pp. 205–15.

Warrell MJ, Warrell DA. Rabies and other lyssavirus diseases. *Lancet*, 2004; Vol. 363; pp. 959–69.

Willoughby RE, Tieves KS, Hoffman GM, et al. Survival after treatment of rabies with induction of coma. *N Engl J Med*, 2005; Vol. 352; pp. 2508–14.

RUBELLA VACCINE

Paul A. Pham, PharmD

VACCINE TYPE
Live attenuated rubella virus vaccine

INDICATIONS
ACIP Recommendations
- All adults and children should have routine vaccination at 12–15 mos (first MMR dose) and 4–6 yrs (second dose of MMR) separated by at least 4 wks.
- All persons who work in health-care facilities must have an acceptable evidence of immunity.
- Administer 1 dose of MMR vaccine to women whose rubella vaccination history is unreliable or who lack laboratory evidence of immunity.

Other Information
- Vaccination is recommended for susceptible international travelers leaving the U.S.
- Vaccination following exposure to natural measles may provide protection if the vaccine is given within 3 days of the exposure.

FORMS

Brand name (mfr)	Forms	Cost*
ProQuad (Chiron)	SC vial 3–4.3–3	$154.71
M-M-R II (Merck)	SC vial 20000/0.5	$57.62
Meruvax II (Merck)	SC vial 0.5 mL	$23.75
*Prices represents Average Wholesale Price (AWP).		

PATHOGEN-DIRECTED PROTECTION
- Rubella

DOSE/ADMINISTRATION

Primary Series

M-M-R II or ProQuad: 0.5-mL SC at 12–15 mos (revaccination with M-M-R II is recommended prior to elementary school entry). **Meruvax:** 0.5 mL SC × 1 dose.

ADVERSE DRUG REACTIONS

Common
- Fevers (associated with the measles component in ~5%)
- Transient rashes (5%)
- Urticaria or a wheal and flare at the injection site

Occasional
- Transient lymphadenopathy
- Arthralgia and transient arthritis (associated with rubella components)

Rare
- Parotitis
- Anaphylaxis reaction
- Thrombocytopenia
- Seizure
- Aseptic meningitis (associated with the Urabe strain mumps vaccine)
- Encephalitis
- Guillain-Barre Syndrome (but no increase incidence over background rates)

VACCINE/DRUG INTERACTIONS
- M-M-R II may be co-administered with varicella virus vaccine live and Haemophilus b conjugate vaccine using a separate injection sites and syringes.
- Although data are limited concerning the simultaneous administration of the entire recommended vaccine series (i.e., DTaP, IPV [or OPV], Hib with or without Hepatitis B vaccine, and varicella vaccine), data from numerous studies have indicated no interference between routinely recommended childhood vaccines (either live, attenuated, or killed).
- Avoid immune globulins within 3 mos of vaccination.
- Vaccine should be delayed for at lease 3–12 mos after immune globulin (Source: AAP Red Book 2006)

CONTRAINDICATIONS
- Immunosuppressed pts (i.e., blood dyscrasias, leukemia, lymphomas, malignant neoplasms of bone or lymphatics, cellular immune deficiencies, hypogammaglobulinemia, dysgammaglobulinemia.
- Severe allergy to components of vaccine (including neomycin)
- Severe febrile illness
- Pregnancy (should be avoided for 30 days postvaccination)
- Use with caution in pts with a history seizure and severe thrombocytopenia
- Eggs allergy is not a contraindication (risk of serious reaction to M-M-R is extremely low).
- May be administered in HIV if not severely immunosuppressed (CD4% <15%).

IMMUNE RESPONSE

Immune response is measured by the presence of detectable antibody in the serum using the ELISA assay for measles. A protective antibody response to rubella was seen with greater than >10 IU rubella antibody/mL. In several randomized trials, children 12 to 23 mos of age received a single dose of Proquad and achieved a response rates of the following: 97.4% for measles, 95.8% to 98.8% for mumps, 98.5% for rubella.

CLINICAL EFFICACY
- Since the introduction of MMR, the number of reported cases of measles, mumps, and congenital rubella syndrome have decreased by more than 99%.

OTHER INFORMATION
- For women of childbearing age, regardless of birth year, routinely determine rubella immunity and counsel women regarding congenital rubella syndrome. Women who do not have evidence of immunity should receive MMR vaccine on completion of pregnancy and before discharge from the health-care facility.

Basis for Recommendations

ACIP. Recommended Adult immunization schedule—United States, October 2007–September 2008. *MMWR*, 2007; Vol. 56; p. 41.

Comments: ACIP recommendation.

Watson JC, Hadler SC, Dykewicz CA, et al. Measles, mumps, and rubella—vaccine use and strategies for elimination of measles, rubella, and congenital rubella syndrome and control of mumps: recommendations of the Advisory Committee on Immunization Practices (ACIP). *MMWR Recomm Rep*, 1998; Vol. 47; pp. 1–57.

Comments: ACIP recommendations.

TETANUS VACCINES

Paul A. Pham, PharmD and John G. Bartlett, MD

Vaccine Type

Td absorbed (tetanus + diphtheria toxoids). Tdap (Td + acellular pertussis vaccine). For other combinations see formulations.

Indications

ACIP Recommendations

- Tetanus prophylaxis in wound care: <3 prior doses, unknown vaccination, >10 yrs post Td or severe injury + >5 yrs post Td.
- Tdap (single dose) as soon as 2 yrs after prior Td vaccination is recommended for a) postpartum women, b) close contacts of infants <12 mos (administer at least 2 wks before contact), and c) all healthcare workers with pt contacts.
- Tdap should replace Td for adults <65 yrs without prior Tdap dose. (This is a single one time dose; otherwise subsequently use Td for boosting.). Adult with history of pertussis should receive Tdap.
- Adults with uncertain histories of a complete primary vaccination series with tetanus and diphtheria toxoid containing vaccines should begin or complete a primary vaccination series (see "adult Td, primary series" under dosing recommendations).
- Td routinely recommended in pregnant women if last tetanus toxoid vaccination was given >10 yrs earlier.

Forms

Brand name (mfr)	Forms	Cost*
ADACEL (Sanofi pasteur)	IM vial 2–2.5–5/.5 mL	$46.90
Infanrix (GlaxoSmithKline)	IM syringe 25–58–10 per .5 mL	$26.24
	IM vial 25–58–10 per .5 mL	$26.20
DECAVAC (Sanofi pasteur)	IM syringe 5–2 LFU/0.5	$23.55
	IM vial 5–2 LFU	$23.55
DT (Sanofi pasteur)	IM vial 0.5 mL	$29.00
Boostrix (GlaxoSmithKline)	IM syringe 2.5–8-5/.5	$45.31
Pediarix (GlaxoSmithKline)	IM syringe 10–25–25	$83.71
	IM vial 10–25–25 per .5 mL	$83.71
DADPTACEL (Sanofi pasteur)	IM vial 2–2.5–5/.5	$46.23
TriHIBit (Sanofi pasteur)	IM KIT 6.7–46–8.5	$52.86
Tripedia (Sanofi pasteur)	IM vial 6.7–46.8–5	$26.18
*Prices represents Average Wholesale Price (AWP).		

Pathogen-Directed Protection

- *Clostridium tetani*, Tetanus

DOSE/ADMINISTRATION
Primary Series

ADACEL (adult Tdap, booster): 1 dose (0.5 mL) IM. DECAVAC (adult Td, primary series): three 0.5 mL doses; 4 to 8 wks between the first and second dose, and 6 to 12 mos between the second and third dose. INFANRIX (pediatric Tdap): 0.5 mL IM ($\times$ 5 doses) 2, 4, and 6 mos of age, followed by 2 booster doses, administered at 15 to 20 mos of age and at 4 to 6 yrs of age. DT (pediatric DT): starting at 6 wks administer 3 doses of 0.5 mL IM 4 to 8 wk apart, then a another dose is given 6 to 12 mos after the third injection. Pediarix (pediatric Tdap + Inactivated Poliovirus Vaccine): 3 doses of 0.5 mL IM at 8-wk intervals starting at 2 mos of age. DAPTACEL (pediatric Tdap): 0.2 mL IM. Catch-up schedule for persons aged 7–18 yrs who received their first dose before age 12 mos should receive 4 doses, with at least 4 wks (not 8 wks) between doses 2 and 3.

Booster

Booster is recommended every 10 yrs. **Adult:** ADACEL (once if <65 yrs) or DECAVAC 0.5 mL IM q10 yrs. **Pediatric:** DT (for children between 4 and 6 yrs of age) 0.5 mL IM. Those who receive all four primary immunizing doses before their fourth birthday should receive a single dose of DT just before entering kindergarten or elementary school. This booster dose is not necessary if the fourth dose in the primary series was given after the fourth birthday. Thereafter, routine booster immunizations should be with tetanus and diphtheria toxoids adsorbed for adult use, at intervals of 10 yrs. Persons 7 yrs of age or older should not be immunized with DT (for pediatric use). BOOSTRIX: single 0.5 mL IM in individuals 10 through 18 yrs of age. TriHIBit (Tdap +Hib): 0.5 mL IM.

ADVERSE DRUG REACTIONS
General
- Generally well tolerated

Common
- Pain and tenderness at injection site; rate increases with more doses

Rare
- Anaphylaxis
- Encephalopathy
- Arthralgia
- Fever
- Guillain-Barre syndrome
- Arthus reaction (severe pain, swelling, induration, edema, hemorrhage, and occasional local necrosis)

VACCINE/DRUG INTERACTIONS
- The simultaneous administration of DT, MMR, OPV, or inactivated poliovirus vaccine (IPV), and Haemophilus b Conjugate Vaccine (HbCV) is acceptable.
- Immunosuppressive therapies, including irradiation, antimetabolites, alkylating agents, cytotoxic drugs, and corticosteroids (used in greater than physiologic doses), may reduce the immune response to vaccines.

CONTRAINDICATIONS
- History of anaphylaxis to vaccine components.
- Encephalopathy within 7 days of administration of pertussis vaccine.
- Use with caution with history of Guillain-Barre syndrome (within 6 wks after previous tetanus toxoid-containing vaccine), moderate or acute severe illness, unstable neurological conditions, and Arthus hypersensitivity reaction.

IMMUNE RESPONSE
Response usually good, but reduced in elderly. Antitetanus response: antitetanus levels >0.1 IU/mL achieved in nearly 100% and booster response was 90–93%. Antidiphtheria response: 99.9% had seroprotective antidiphtheria levels >0.1 IU/mL and booster response was 91–96%. Antipertussis antigen response to pertussis antigens was 89% and booster response was 95%.

CLINICAL EFFICACY
- Vaccine is very effective. Vaccine efficacy against confirmed pertussis was 92%. Tetanus: 1999, total U.S.—40 cases; diphtheria: 1999 total U.S.—0 cases.

OTHER INFORMATION
- Need: about 25% of U.S. adults >70 yrs to have protective tetanus ab titers.

VACCINES

- Most cases in U.S. occur in elderly population; presumed underimmunized, waning or no immunity.

FOLLOW UP
- Td preferred for adults (less local reactions) and during pregnancy. Adults should receive Tdap × 1 as primary series, booster or with wound management.
- Wounds, minor: <3 prior Td doses or unknown—give Td; >3 doses—Td if >10 yrs since last booster.
- Wounds, severe or contaminated: <3 prior Td doses, give Td + TIG; if >3 doses—give Td if >5 yrs since last Td booster.
- TIG: tetanus immune globulin, administer if <3 doses Td or unknown + contaminated wound (dirt, stool, saliva, soil), crush, burn or frostbite.
- DT: Pediatric preparation, contraindicated in persons >7 yrs.
- TIG: tetanus Immune globulin 500 units IM (prophylaxis), or 3,000–10,000 units (active tetanus).
- ADACEL contains the same tetanus toxoid, diphtheria toxoid, and five pertussis antigens as those in DAPTACEL (pediatric DTaP), but ADACEL is formulated with reduced quantities of diphtheria toxoid and detoxified pertussis toxin.

BASIS FOR RECOMMENDATIONS

ACIP. Recommended Adult immunization schedule. United States, October 2007. September 2008. *MMWR*, 2007; Vol. 56; p. 41.

Comments: ACIP recommended adult immunization.

Kretsinger K, Broder KR, Cortese MM, et al. Preventing tetanus, diphtheria, and pertussis among adults: use of tetanus toxoid, reduced diphtheria toxoid and acellular pertussis vaccine recommendations of the Advisory Committee on Immunization Practices (ACIP) and recommendation of ACIP, supported by the Healthcare Infection Control Practices Advisory Committee (HICPAC), for use of Tdap among health-care personnel. *MMWR Recomm Rep*, 2006; Vol. 55; pp. 1–37.

Comments: The ACIP recommendations for 2006 were changed to include Tdap as a one time single dose vaccine for persons <65 yrs.

SELECTED REFERENCES

Gergen PJ, McQuillan GM, Kiely M, et al. A population-based serologic survey of immunity to tetanus in the United States. *N Engl J Med*, 1995; Vol. 332; pp. 761–6.

TYPHOID VACCINES

Paul A. Pham, PharmD and John G. Bartlett, MD

VACCINE TYPE
Two forms: (1) live oral attenuated bacterial vaccine (Ty 21a, Vivotif), (2) polysaccharide IM vaccine (Typhim Vi).

INDICATIONS
ACIP Recommendations
- Prevention of *S. typhi* infection.
- Travelers to endemic areas; laboratory microbiologists with expected frequent contact with *Salmonella typhi*.
- Travel: rural areas of countries where typhoid fever is endemic (especially Peru, India, Pakistan, and Chile) or in areas with outbreaks.

Other Information
- Immunosuppression: Vivotif is a live bacterial vaccine; immunosuppressed pts should receive Typhim Vi (though response rates may be lower).

FORMS

Brand name (mfr)	Forms	Cost*
Typhim Vi (Sanofi pasteur)	IM vial 25 MCG/0.5 IM syringe 25 MCG/0.5	$56.94 $56.94
Vivotif berna (Berna Products)	Oral cap 1 cap	$12.06
*Prices represents Average Wholesale Price (AWP).		

PATHOGEN-DIRECTED PROTECTION
- *Salmonella typhi*

DOSE/ADMINISTRATION
Primary Series
Vivotif: 1 capsule every other day (1 hr before meals with cold or luke-warm drink) × 4 doses for children ages >6 and adults (starting at least 2 wks before travel). Do not take antimalarials or antibiotics for 2 wks as may decrease efficacy. **Typhim Vi:** 0.5 mL (25 mcg) IM in the deltoid or vastus lateralis × 1 (for children >2 yrs of age and adults).

Booster
Revaccination: recommended every 2 yrs for the Typhim Vi vaccine and every 5 yrs for the Vivotif oral vaccine in individuals with continued exposure risks to *Salmonella typhi*.

ADVERSE DRUG REACTIONS
General
- Ty21a (oral vaccine) produces fewer adverse reactions than the ViCPS (IM vaccine).
- Pts with hypersensitivity to parenteral vaccine may tolerate oral vaccine.
- Pregnancy: Category C for both oral and IM polysaccharide vaccine. No data. ACOG (Bulletin No. 160) recommends vaccination during pregnancy only for close continued exposure or travel to endemic areas.

Common
- Heat-phenol inactivated vaccine (no longer commercially available) had a high incidence of systemic side effects (fever, headache, and local pain at injection site). Current IM formulation (Typhim Vi) generally well tolerated.

Occasional
- Oral formulation: nausea, vomiting, and abdominal discomfort (comparable to placebo).
- IM formulation: erythema or induration greater than or equal to 1 cm (7% of vaccinees).

Rare
- Oral vaccine: fever, headache, and rash or urticaria, but comparable to placebo.
- IM formulation: fever (occurring in 0%–1% of vaccines) and headache (1.5%–3% of vaccines).

VACCINE/DRUG INTERACTIONS
- Antibiotics: may decrease the efficacy of oral Vivotif vaccine. Avoid co-administration within 2 wks
- Immunosuppressive therapies, including irradiation, antimetabolites, alkylating agents, cytotoxic drugs, and corticosteroids may reduce the immune response to vaccines and increase risk of infection by the live vaccine (oral TY21a vaccine).

CONTRAINDICATIONS
- Oral typhoid vaccine: acute febrile illness, respiratory or gastrointestinal illness, immunodeficiency states, concurrent antibiotic use (especially sulfa abx) may impair adequate immune response.

IMMUNE RESPONSE
Onset of protection: within 1 wk from the last dose.

CLINICAL EFFICACY
- Efficacy 67% in U.S. military recruits while in endemic areas if immunized w/ the enteric coated oral typhoid vaccine.
- Protective efficacy of 77.4% seen with polysaccharide IM vaccine.

OTHER INFORMATION
- Oral typhoid vaccine is preferred over the parenteral killed bacterial vaccine because of comparable efficacy, longer protection (5 yrs vs 2 yrs) [*Lancet* 1990;336:891].
- Many travel clinics suggest IM vaccine for simplicity, as many travelers do not complete appropriately four pill oral vaccine dosing.
- Oral vaccine heat intolerant, keep in cool location. Excessive heat (e.g., car trunk in the summer) may reduce potency of vaccine.

BASIS FOR RECOMMENDATIONS
Centers for Disease Control and Prevention. Typhoid immunization recommendations of the Advisory Committee on Immunization Practices (ACIP). *MMWR*, 1994; Vol. 43; pp. 1–7.
Comments: ACIP typhoid immunization recommendations.

VARICELLA VACCINE

Paul A. Pham, PharmD and John G. Bartlett, MD

VACCINE TYPE
Live attenuated virus vaccine

INDICATIONS

ACIP Recommendations
- Prevention of primary varicella, VZV, children 12–18 mos targeted for first dose.
- Routine vaccination of all healthy persons aged >13 yrs without evidence of immunity.

FORMS

Brand name (mfr)	Forms	Cost*
Varivax (Merck)	SC vial 0.5 mL	$96.70

*Prices represents Average Wholesale Price (AWP).

PATHOGEN-DIRECTED PROTECTION
- Varicella zoster virus
- This vaccine is not used for zoster prevention, but rather the zoster vaccine (Zostavax) which has ~14× more virus.

DOSE/ADMINISTRATION

Primary Series
Adult: 0.5 mL SC × 2, separated by 4–8 wks. Pediatric (ACIP recommendation): first dose (0.5 mL) of varicella vaccine at 12 to 18 mos of age and a second dose (0.5 mL) be given at 4 to 6 yrs of age. A second dose catch-up varicella vaccination is recommended for all children, adolescents, and adults who previously had received 1 dose.

Booster
Some recommend a booster dose at 9–10 yrs.

ADVERSE DRUG REACTIONS

Common
- Local reaction at injection site (30% in 0–2 days).

Occasional
- Fever >100°F (10%)
- Varicella-like rash at injection site (3%)
- Generalized varicella rash: occurs in 10% within 7–21 days (usually consists of <10 lesions and lasting >3 days and may be potential source of VZV transmission).

Rare
- Transmission of the vaccine strain reported in three cases out of 15 million vaccinees (*MMWR* 48(RR-6), 1999).

VACCINE/DRUG INTERACTIONS
- Immunosuppressants: may increase risk of severe vaccine-related infection.

CONTRAINDICATIONS
- Pregnancy or this possibility within 1 mo
- Immunosuppressed pts
- Active TB
- Persons who have received blood products within 6 mos
- Anaphylaxis to gelatin or neomycin

IMMUNE RESPONSE
Seroconversion rate in adults is 78% with one dose; 99% with two doses given 4–8 wks later. Protection at 7–10 yrs is 70–90% against infection and 95% against severe disease. 97% of infants and children 1–12 yrs of age develop detectable antibody titers after 1 dose. Vaccine-induced immunity is believed to be long-lasting.

CLINICAL EFFICACY
- Rate of zoster in vaccine recipients was 2.6/100,000 person-yr in vaccine recipients compared with 68/100,000 person-yr in a general population of persons age <20 yrs.
- Vaccine efficacy estimated 90% against VZV infection, and 95% against severe disease.

Other Information

- Vaccine must be stored frozen ≤5°C to maintain potency. Once reconstituted it must be used within 30 min.
- 90% current adults likely infected as children (pre-vaccine era) and therefore will not require varicella vaccine.
- 10% population over 15 yrs of age susceptible to infection. Adult clinical hx of chickenpox often unreliable; varicella serology may wane by adult yrs. If pt thought susceptible, check serology [if negative, immunize].
- Report involving an outbreak in a day-care center that showed the effectiveness of the vaccine was only 44 percent [Galil K, et al. *NEJM* 2002;347:1909].
- New ACIP (2007) also recommended prenatal assessment and postpartum vaccination; expanding the use of the varicella vaccine for HIV-infected children with age-specific CD4+ T lymphocyte percentages of 15%–24% and adolescents and adults with CD4+ T lymphocyte counts ≥200 cells/microL; and establishing middle school, high school, and college entry vaccination requirements.
- Evidence of immunity to varicella adults includes any of the following: (1) 2 doses of varicella vaccine at least 4 wks apart. (2) U.S. born before 1980 (note: pregnant pts, health-care personnel, and immunocompromised pts born before 1980 should have immunity confirmed by laboratory evidence of immunity). (3) history of varicella or Zoster confirmed by health-care provider. (4) laboratory evidence of immunity.

Basis for Recommendations

Marin M, Güris D, Chaves SS, et al. Prevention of varicella: recommendations of the Advisory Committee on Immunization Practices (ACIP). *MMWR Recomm Rep*, 2007; Vol. 56; pp. 1–40.

Comments: ACIP recommendations now endorse a two dose pediatric schedule because of high rates of breakthrough infection with the one dose strategy. Other new recommendations include guarded use in non-advanced HIV, college entrance verification of vaccination and routine immunization of all >13 yrs as well as catch-up vaccination for all individuals who only received one dose of the varicella vaccine.

Selected References

Chaves SS, Gargiullo P, Zhang JX, et al. Loss of vaccine-induced immunity to varicella over time. *N Engl J Med*, 2007; Vol. 356; pp. 1121–9.

YELLOW FEVER VACCINE

Paul A. Pham, PharmD and John G. Bartlett, MD

Vaccine Type

Live, attenuated virus preparation made from 17D yellow fever virus strain.

Indications

ACIP Recommendations

- Recommended with travel to endemic areas: tropical South America and most of Africa between 15° North and 15° South latitudes.
- Consider in children between 4–9 mos with exposure risk.
- Required vaccine for travel in some countries.

Forms

Brand name (mfr)	Forms	Cost*
YF-VAX (Sanofi-Pasteur (available only in U.S. only at designated yellow fever vaccination centers))	SC vial 0.5 mL	$62.00
*Prices represents Average Wholesale Price (AWP).		

Pathogen-Directed Protection

- Yellow fever virus

DOSE/ADMINISTRATION
Primary Series
Yellow fever vaccine: 0.5 milliliter SC × 1 (for adults and children >9 mos).

Booster
Revaccination: booster every 10 yrs if still at risk.

ADVERSE DRUG REACTIONS
General
- Pregnancy: Category C. Contraindicated unless exposure to YF can not be avoided. The yellow fever vaccine was not apparently harmful effects to the fetuses of 101 women who received YF vaccine.

Common
- Local reactions: including edema, hypersensitivity, pain or mass at the injection site.

Occasional
- Headache
- Myalgia
- Low-grade fevers

Rare
- Allergy with anaphylaxis in 1:116,000 (desensitization protocol available)
- Encephalitis
- Hepatitis
- ACIP has reported 7 cases of multiple organ failure in recipients of 17 D derived yellow fever vaccine; all became ill within 2–5 days of vaccination and six died (*MMWR* 2001;50–643)
- May cause severe encephalitis and hepatitis complications, especially with immunosuppression and age >65 yrs. Risk of vaccine often exceeds risk of travel

VACCINE/DRUG INTERACTIONS
- Immunosuppressive drugs: may increase risk of infectious complications.
- Yellow fever vaccine may be co-administered with the following vaccines without diminished efficacy: measles, smallpox, BCG, hepatitis A or hepatitis B vaccines, typhoid fever vaccine (Typhim Vi), and meningococcal vaccine(Menomune).

CONTRAINDICATIONS
- Known hypersensitivity to egg, chicken protein or gelatin.
- Infants less than 4 mos of age (increased risk of encephalitis).
- Pregnancy (relative): vaccination should be administered if travel to an endemic area is unavoidable and if an increased risk for exposure exists.
- Immunosuppression, including HIV with CD4 <200/mm^3 (since live virus vaccine).
- Age >65 is a relative contraindications.

IMMUNE RESPONSE
Immunity in more than 95% of recipients. Less immunogenic in pregnant women (39%), asymptomatic HIV-infected adults (77%), and HIV-infected infants (17%). Protection lasts 10 yrs in normal hosts.

CLINICAL EFFICACY
- Practically complete disappearance of yellow fever in French-speaking Africa following the launch of a mandatory vaccination campaign in 1941.
- Neutralizing antibodies developed in over 95% of pts.

OTHER INFORMATION
- Onset of protection: 10 days.
- If exposure cannot be avoided, vaccination should be offered to pregnant women and HIV-infected pts, in small studies no adverse events have been reported.

BASIS FOR RECOMMENDATIONS
Cetron MS, Marfin AA, Julian KG, et al. Yellow fever vaccine. Recommendations of the Advisory Committee on Immunization Practices (ACIP), 2002. *MMWR Recomm Rep*, 2002; Vol. 51; pp. 1–11; quiz CE1–4.
Comments: ACIP recommendations.

SELECTED REFERENCES
Chadwick DR, Geretti AM. Immunization of the HIV infected traveller. *AIDS*, 2007; Vol. 21; pp. 787–94.
Khromava AY, Eidex RB, Weld LH, et al. Yellow fever vaccine: an updated assessment of advanced age as a risk factor for serious adverse events. *Vaccine*, 2005; Vol. 23; pp. 3256–63.

ZOSTER VACCINE

Paul A. Pham, PharmD and John G. Bartlett, MD

VACCINE TYPE

Live attenuated virus vaccine. Modified version of existing Oka varicella vaccine, 14 × more potent.

INDICATIONS

ACIP Recommendations

• Indicated for prevention of herpes zoster (shingles) in pts 60 yrs of age and older.

Other Information

• Also reduces incidence of post-herpetic neuralgia.

FORMS

Brand name (mfr)	Forms	Cost*
Zostavax (Merck)	Subcutaneously vial 19400 U per .65 mL	$192.41
*Prices represents Average Wholesale Price (AWP).		

PATHOGEN-DIRECTED PROTECTION

• Varicella-zoster virus

DOSE/ADMINISTRATION

Primary Series

Administer the content of one vial (0.65 mL) subcutaneously in the deltoid region within 30 minutes of reconstitution. Note: Zostavax is stored frozen and should be reconstituted immediately upon removal from the freezer. The diluent should be stored separately at room temperature or in the refrigerator.

Booster

Efficacy has demonstrated through 4 yrs of follow-up. Unclear if a booster is needed after 4–5 yrs.

ADVERSE DRUG REACTIONS

General

• Generally well tolerated.
• In the overall study population, serious adverse events were comparable between the vaccinated and placebo groups.

Common

• Mild injection site reaction (erythema, pain/tenderness, and swelling) occurred in one third of vaccinated pts.

Occasional

• Pruritis (6.6%)
• Hematoma (1.4%)
• Warmth (1.5%)
• Headache (1.4%)

Rare

• Respiratory infection, fever, flu-like syndrome, diarrhea, rhinitis, skin disorder, respiratory disorder, and asthenia were uncommon—occurring in less than 2% of pts. Vaccinated pts had 0.1–0.3% higher rates of these adverse events compared to placebo.
• In the adverse event monitoring sub-study, cardiovascular events were 0.2% higher in the vaccinated group compared to placebo. The clinical significance of this difference is unclear.

VACCINE/DRUG INTERACTIONS

• Immunosuppressive therapy, including high-dose corticosteroids: contraindicated vaccine administration due to live virus and theoretical potential for zoster dissemination.

CONTRAINDICATIONS

• Immunosuppressed pts or pts on immunosuppressive therapy.
• Anaphylaxis to neomycin, gelatin or other component of the vaccine.
• Pts with active, untreated tuberculosis.
• Pregnancy or possibility of pregnancy within 1 mo.

VACCINES

IMMUNE RESPONSE

The specific antibody level that correlates with protection from zoster has not been established. VZV antibody levels 6 wks post vaccination increased 1.7-fold (95% CI: 1.6 to 1.8) compared to placebo.

CLINICAL EFFICACY

- Overall efficacy for the prevention of herpes zoster: 51%. Overall efficacy for the prevention of post-herpetic neuralgia: 39%.
- Subgroup efficacy prevention of zoster: 60–69 yrs old, 64%; 70–79 yrs old, 41%; >80 yrs old: 18% (not statistically significant).
- Prevention of postherpetic neuralgia in: 60–69 yrs old, not effective; 70–79 yrs old: 55%; >80 yrs old: 26% (not statistically significant).

OTHER INFORMATION

- In pts older than 80, the vaccine was less effective with only an 18% reduction in the incidence of herpes zoster at a cost of $191,000 per quality-adjusted life yr saved.
- Although transmission of the attenuated vaccine virus has not been reported, potential for transmission between vaccinees who develop a varicella-like rash and susceptible contacts is possible.
- Herpes zoster vaccine provides protection in half of all vaccinated pts and decreases the risk of a debilitating post herpetic neuralgia syndrome.
- Not to be confused with the varicella (Varivax) vaccine (aka chickenpox vaccine). **Not** interchangeable with varicella vaccine and should **not** be given to children.
- The zoster vaccine compared with the chickenpox vaccine contains more plaque-forming units (PFU) of Oka/Merck varicella virus (minimum of 19,400 PFU vs minimum of 1350 PFU).
- Vaccine must be stored frozen.
- Zoster vaccine is recommended for all persons aged >60 yrs, including persons who report a previous episode of zoster or who have chronic medical conditions. Can be given to individuals without moderate-to-high immunosuppression (e.g., <prednisone 20 mg daily dose).
- Pts do not need to be asked about their history of varicella (chickenpox). Serologic testing are not needed to determine varicella immunity.

FOLLOW UP

- Unclear if a booster is needed after 4–5 yrs.

BASIS FOR RECOMMENDATIONS

Advisory Committee on Immunization Practices (ACIP). Prevention of Herpes Zoster. *MMWR*, 2008; Vol. 57; pp. 1–30.

Comments: ACIP recommends Zoster vaccine in all persons aged >60 yrs who have no contraindications.

SELECTED REFERENCES

Oxman MN, Levin MJ, Johnson GR, et al. A vaccine to prevent herpes zoster and postherpetic neuralgia in older adults. *N Engl J Med*, 2005; Vol. 352; pp. 2271–84.

Rothberg MB, Virapongse A, Smith KJ. Cost-effectiveness of a vaccine to prevent herpes zoster and postherpetic neuralgia in older adults. *Clin Infect Dis*, 2007; Vol. 44; pp. 1280–8.

APPENDIX I
THERAPEUTIC TABLES FOR SPECIFIC DIAGNOSES AND PATHOGENS

TABLE 1. DEFINITIONS FOR THE DIAGNOSIS OF INFECTIVE ENDOCARDITIS ACCORDING TO THE DUKE CRITERIA*

Definite infective endocarditis

Pathologic criteria

- Micrgoorganisms: demonstrated by culture of histologic examination in a vegetation that has embolized, *or* in an intracardiac abscess, *or*
- Pathologic lesions: vegetation *or* intracardiac abscess present, confirmed by histological examination showing active endocarditis

Clinical criteria, using specific criteria listed in Table 2

2 major criteria, *or*

1 major and 3 minor criteria, *or*

5 minor criteria

Possible infective endocarditis

Findings consistent with infective endocarditis that fall short of "definite" but are not "rejected"

Rejected

Firm alternate diagnosis for manifestations of endocarditis, *or*

Resolution of manifestations of endocarditis, with antibiotic therapy for 4 days or less, *or*

No pathologic evidence of infective endocarditis at surgery or autopsy, after antibiotic therapy for 4 days or less

*See Table 2 for definitions of terminology.

Source: Durack DT, Lukes AS, Bright DK. New criteria for diagnosis of infective endocarditis: utilization of specific echocardiographic findings: Duke Endocarditis Service. *Am J Med.* 96:200–209, 1994. Reprinted with permission.

TABLE 2. DEFINITIONS OF TERMINOLOGY USED IN THE DUKE CRITERIA

Major Criteria

Positive blood culture for infective endocarditis

Typical microorganism for infective endocarditis from 2 separate blood cultures:

Viridans streptococci,* *Streptococcus bovis,* HACEK† group

OR

Community-acquired *Staphylococcus aureus* or enterococci, in the absence of a primary focus

OR

Persistently positive blood culture, defined as recovery of a microorganism conistent with infective endocarditis from:

1) Blood cultures drawn more than 12 hrs apart; *OR*
2) All of 3 or a majority of 4 or more separate blood cultures, with first and last drawn at least 1 hr apart

Evidence of endocardial involvement

Positive echocardiogram for infective endocarditis

1) Oscillating intracardiac mass, on valve or supporting structures, *OR* in the path of regurgitant jets, *OR* on implanted material in the absence of an alternative anatomic explanation, *OR*
2) Abscess, *OR*
3) New partial dehiscence of prosthetic valve

OR

New valvular regurgitation (increase or change in preexisting murmur not sufficient)

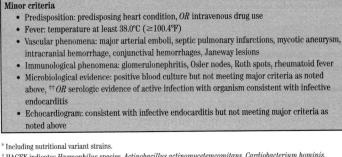

Minor criteria

- Predisposition: predisposing heart condition, *OR* intravenous drug use
- Fever: temperature at least 38.0°C (≥100.4°F)
- Vascular phenomena: major arterial emboli, septic pulmonary infarctions, mycotic aneurysm, intracranial hemorrhage, conjunctival hemorrhages, Janeway lesions
- Immunological phenomena: glomerulonephritis, Osler nodes, Roth spots, rheumatoid fever
- Microbiological evidence: positive blood culture but not meeting major criteria as noted above, †† *OR* serologic evidence of active infection with organism consistent with infective endocarditis
- Echocardiogram: consistent with infective endocarditis but not meeting major criteria as noted above

* Including nutritional variant strains.
† HACEK indicates *Haemophilus* species, *Actinobacillus actinomycetemcomitans, Cardiobacterium hominis, Eikenella* species, and *Kingella kingae.*
†† Excluding single positive cultures for coagulase-negative staphylococci and organisms that do not cause endocarditis.
Source: Durack DT, Lukes AS, Bright DK. New criteria for diagnosis of infective endocarditis: utilization of specific echocardiographic findings: Duke Endocarditis Service. *Am J Med.* 96:200–209, 1994. Reprinted with permission.

TABLE 3. MISCELLANEOUS CAUSES OF FEVER OF UNKNOWN ORIGIN (FUO)

Etiology	Clues to the Diagnosis
Common	
Drug fever*	Temperature–pulse dissociation, eosinophilia
Thromboembolism	Dyspnea, chest pain (blood-gas measurements may remain normal). Pt recovering from pelvic surgery or parturition at greatest risk.
Alcoholic liver disease	Hepatomegaly, increased serum aspartate aminotransferase levels
Factitious fever	Absence of diurnal temperature variation, discrepancy between concomitant oral and rectal temperature measurements
Cryptic hematoma	Recent history of blunt trauma or anticoagulant therapy
Rare	
Occult dental infection	Poor dentition, history of recent dental procedure
Familial Mediterranean Fever	Episodic fever with abdominal pain, serositis, skin rash, arthritis, family history
Idiopathic pericarditis	Chest pain, pleuritic quality
Subacute granulomatous thyroiditis	Neck pain, pharyngeal swelling
New Causes	
Kikuchi's disease	Histiocytic necrotizing adenitis, leucopenia, elevated serum transaminase levels, splenomegaly
Hypergammaglobulinemia IgD syndrome	Periodic and prolonged fevers, rash, large joint arthritis

TABLE 3. *(CONT.)*

'Drugs Commonly Implicated in Development of Fever		
Common	**Less Common**	**Rare**
Atropine	Allopurinol	Aminoglycosides
Amphotericin B	Azathionprine	Chloramphenicol
Asparaginase	Cimetidine	Clindamycin
Barbiturates	Hydralazine	Corticostreroids
Bleomycin	Imipenem	Macrolides
Cephalosporins	Iodides	Salicylates (therapeutic doses)
Interferon	Isoniazid	Tetracylines
Methyldopa	Metroclopramide	Vitamin preparation
Penicillins	Nifedipine	
Phenytoin	NSAIDs	
Procainamide	Rifampin	
Quinidine	Streptokinase	
Salicylates (including sulfa-containing laxatives)	Vancomycin	
Sulfanamides		

Source: Johnson DH, et al. *Infect Dis Clin North Am*. 1996 Mar;10(1):85–91.

TABLE 4. HISTORICAL CLUES IN FUO (FEVER OF UNKNOWN ORIGIN)

Exposure	Possible Diagnosis
Birds	Salmonellosis, psittacosis, tuberculosis
Cats	Cat scratch fever, Q fever, toxoplasmosis
Dogs	Leptospirosis
Cattle	Brucellosis, Q fever, leptospirosis
Rodents	Leptospirosis, relapsing fever
Ticks	Ehrlichiosis, Lyme disease
Travel	Malaria, tularemia, tuberculosis
Sexual	HIV, hepatitis, gonorrhea, syphilis
Spelunking	Relapsing fever
Dairy products	Salmonellosis, yersinial infection, brucellosis, Q Fever
Chicken, pork	Salmonellosis, yersinial infection
Shellfish	Salmonellosis

TABLE 5. PHYSICAL EXAMINATION FINDINGS IN FEVER OF UNKNOWN ORIGIN (FUO)

Evaluation	Finding	Possible Diagnosis
Vital signs	High fever with slow pulse	Typhoid fever, legionnaires' disease, brucellosis, factitious fever, drug fever
Head	Nasal discharge and sinus tenderness	Sinusitis
	Nodules or reduced pulsations in temporal artery	Temporal arteritis
	Oropharyngeal ulceration	Disseminated hisoplasmosis
	Tender tooth	Apical abscess
Thyroid*	Enlarged, tender	Thyroiditis
Ocular	Conjunctivitis	Fungal infection, tuberculosis
	Roth's spots	Subacute bacterial endocarditis, leukemia
	Icterus	Hepatitis, cholestasis
Lymphatic system	Abnormality or any nodes, including the epitrochlear and supraclavicular nodes	Infectious mononucleosis, other systemic infection, lymphoma
Heart	Murmur or changes in heart sounds	Endocarditis
Abdomen	Splenomegaly	Various viral and bacterial diseases, lymphoma, lymphoreticular neoplasm
	Hepatic enlargement or tenderness	Hepatic infection or intra-abdominal abscess
	Flank tenderness or swelling	Perinephric or intrarenal abscess
Anus and rectum*	Perirectal or prostatic tenderness or fluctuance	Abscess
Genitalia*	Epididymal nodule	Disseminated granulomatosis
	Testicular nodule	Periarteritis nodosa
	Cervical discharge and uterine tenderness	Pelvic inflammatory disease
Joints	Stiffness, swelling, redness	Rheumatic disease
Lower extremities	Deep venous tenderness, swelling	Thrombophlebitis
Skin and mucous membranes	Rash	Drug fever, viral infection
	Petechiae with vasculitis (palpable purpuric lesions)	Collagen vascular disease
	Purpura with petechiae	Meningococcal or gonococcal bacteremia
	Janeway's spots	Subacute bacterial endocarditis
	Osler's nodes	Subacute bacterial endocarditis

*Mackowiak PA, Durack DT: *Mandell, Douglas, and Bennett's Principles and Practice of Infectious Diseases, 5th ed.* Edited by Mandell GL, Bennett JE, Dolin R. Philadelphia: Churchill Livingstone; 2000:623–33.

TABLE 6. ROUTINE LABORATORY TESTS FOR FUO (FEVER OF UNKNOWN ORIGIN)

Test	Finding	Significance
Complete blood count (CBC) with differential	Leukocytosis, leucopenia, anemia, thrombocytopenia	Wide range of underlying diseases
Erythrocyte sedimentation rate (ESR)	Elevation	Infection or collagen vascular disease
Liver enzyme (transaminase and alkaline phosphatase) levels	Elevation	Hepatitis, hepatic abscess or tumor, cholestasis
Syphilis serology	Positive	Syphilis
HIV screen	Positive	HIV infection (requires confirmatory test)
Urinalysis with culture	Presence of pathogens	Urinary-tract infection
Blood culture	Presence of pathogens	Bacteremia, especially bacterial endocarditis
Stool examination	Parasites or ova	Parasitic infection
Tuberculin skin test	Positive	Tuberculosis
Chest film	Infiltrates	Tuberculosis or malignancy

TABLE 7. COMPARISON OF INFLUENZA DRUGS

	Amantadine*	Rimantadine*	Zanamivir (Relanza)	Oseltamivir (Tamiflu)
Year approved—FDA	1966	1993	1999	1999
Activity	A	A	A & B	A & B
FDA Approved				
Treatment	+	+	+	+
Prophylaxis	+	+	+	+
Efficacy for:				
Treatment	+	+	+	+
Studies in high-risk pts	+	−	−	+
Start Rx within	48 hrs	48 hrs	48 hrs	48 hrs
Reduction in Sx	1–1.5 days	1–1.5 days	1–1.5 days	1–1.5 days
Efficacy for Prevention	+	+	+	+
Treatment Duration	5 days	7 days	5 days	5 days
Dose–Treatment				
Age 14–64 yrs	100 mg BID	100 mg BID	10 mg BID	75 mg BID
Age >65 yrs	100 mg BID	100 mg BID	10 mg BID	75 mg BID
Renal failure	Adjust	Standard	10 mg BID	Adjust
Liver failure	Standard	Standard	No data	No data
Side Effects	CNS	CNS	Bronchospasm	GI
Cost AWP 5 days	$7	$18	$168	$101.70

*Not recommended for the 2009–2010 season.

FIGURE 8. IDENTIFYING PATIENTS IN RISK CLASS I IN THE DERIVATION OF THE PREDICTION RULE

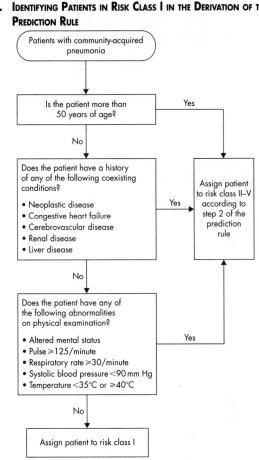

In step 1 of the prediction rule, the following were independently associated with mortality: an age of more than 50 yrs, 5 coexisting illnesses (neoplastic disease, congestive heart failure, cerebrovascular disease, renal disease, and liver disease), and five physical-examination findings (altered mental status; pulse, ≥125 per minute; respiratory rate, ≥30 per minute; systolic blood pressure, <90 mm Hg; and temperature, <35°C or ≥40°C). In the derivation cohort, 1372 pts (9.7%) with none of these 11 risk factors were assigned to risk class I. All 12,827 remaining pts were assigned to risk class II, III, IV, or V according to the sum of the points assigned in step 2 of the prediction rule (see Table 10).

Source: Fine MJ, Auble TE, Yealy DM, et al. *N Enlg J Med.* 1997;336(4):243–250. Copyright © 2004 Massachusetts Medical Society. All rights reserved. Reprinted with permission.

TABLE 9. POINT SCORING SYSTEM FOR STEP 2 OF THE PREDICTION RULE FOR ASSIGNMENT TO RISK CLASSES II, III, IV, AND V

Patient characteristics	Points assigned*
Demographic factors	
Age (1 point/yr)	
Men	Age (yr)
Women	Age (yr) -10
Nursing home resident	+10
Comorbid illnesses†	
Neoplastic disease	+30
Liver disease	+20
Congestive heart failure	+10
Cerebrovascular disease	+10
Renal disease	+10
Physical examination findings	
Altered mental status‡	+20
Respiratory rate ≥30 breaths/minute	+20
Systolic blood pressure <90 mm Hg	+20
Temperature <35°C or ≥40°C	+15
Pulse ≥125 beats/minute	+10
Laboratory findings	
PH <7.35	+30
Blood urea nitrogen >10.7 mmol/L	+20
Sodium <130 mEq/L	+20
Glucose >13.9 mmol/L	+10
Hematocrit <30%	+10
PO_2 <60 mm Hg (or SaO_2 <90%)§	+10
Pleural effusion	+10

*A total point score for a given patient is obtained by summing the patient's age in years (age –10 for women) and the points for each applicable characteristic. The points assigned to each predictor variable were based on coefficients obtained from the logistic-regression model used in step 2 of the prediction rule.

†Neoplastic disease is defined as any cancer except basal- or squamous-cell cancer of the skin that was active at the time of presentation or diagnosed within 1 year of presentation. Liver disease is defined as a clinical or histologic diagnosis of cirrhosis or another form of chronic liver disease, such as chronic active hepatitis. Congestive heart failure is defined as systolic or diastolic ventricular dysfunction documented by history, physical examination, and chest radiograph, echocardiogram, multiple gated acquisition scan, or left ventriculogram. Cerebrovascular disease is defined as a clinical diagnosis of stroke or transient ischemic attack or stroke documented by magnetic resonance imaging or computed tomography. Renal disease is defined as a history of chronic renal disease or abnormal blood urea nitrogen and creatinine concentrations documented in the medical record.

‡Altered mental status is defined as disorientation with respect to person, place, or time that is not known to be chronic, stupor, or coma.

§In the Pneumonia PORT cohort study, an oxygen saturation of <90% on pulse oximetry or intubation before admission was also considered abnormal.

Source: Fine MJ, Auble TE, Yealy DM, et al. *N Enlg J Med*. 1997;336(4):243–250. Copyright © 2004 Massachusetts Medical Society. All rights reserved. Reprinted with permission.

TABLE 10. COMPARISON OF RISK-CLASS–SPECIFIC MORTALITY RATES IN THE DERIVATION AND VALIDATION COHORTS*

Risk Class (no. of Points)†	MedisGroups Derivation Cohort		MedisGroups Validation Cohort		Pneumonia PORT Validation Cohort					
					INPATIENTS		OUTPATIENTS		ALL PATIENTS	
	no. of pts	% who died	no. of pts	% who died	no. of pts	% who died	no. of pts	% who died	no. of pts	% who died
I	1,372	0.4	3,034	0.1	185	0.5	587	0.0	772	0.1
II ($\leq$70)	2,412	0.7	5,778	0.6	233	0.9	244	0.4	477	0.6
III (71–90)	2,632	2.8	6,790	2.8	254	1.2	72	0.0	326	0.9
IV (91–130)	4,697	8.5	13,104	8.2	446	9.0	40	12.5	486	9.3
V (>130)	3,086	31.1	9,333	29.2	225	27.1	1	0.0	226	27.0
Total	14,199	10.2	38,039	10.6	1343	8.0	944	0.6	2287	5.2

*There were no statistically significant differences in overall mortality or mortality within risk class among pts in the MedisGroups derivation, MedisGroups validation, or overall Pneumonia PORT validation cohort. The P values for the comparisons of mortality across risk classes are as follows: class I, P= 0.22; class II, P= 0.67; class III, P= 0.12; class IV, P= 0.69; and class V, P= 0.09.
†Inclusion in risk class I was determined by the absence of all predictors identified in step 1 of the prediction rule. Inclusion in risk classes II, III, IV, and V was determined by a pt's total risk score, which was computed according to the scoring system shown in Table 8.

Source: Fine MJ, Auble TE, Yealy DM, et al. *N Engl J Med.* 1997;336(4):243–250. Copyright © 2004 Massachusetts Medical Society. All rights reserved. Reprinted with permission.

DIAGNOSES AND PATHOGENS

TABLE 11. DIAGNOSTIC CRITERIA FOR STAPHYLOCOCCAL TOXIC SHOCK SYNDROME

1. Temperature >38.8°C
2. Systolic blood pressure ≤90 mm Hg for adults, less than the 5th percentile for children, or >15 mm Hg orthostatic drop in diastolic blood pressure or orthostatic dizziness/syncope
3. Diffuse macular rash with subsequent desquamation
4. Three of the following organ systems involved:
   - *Liver:* bilirubin, AST, ALT more than twice the upper normal limit
   - *Blood:* platelets <100,000/mm^3
   - *Renal:* BUN or creatinine more than twice the upper normal limit or pyuria without urinary tract infection
   - *Mucous membranes:* hyperemia of the vagina, oropharynx, or conjunctivae
   - *Gastrointestinal:* diarrhea or vomiting
   - *Muscular:* myalgias or CPK more than twice the normal upper limit
   - *Central nervous system:* disorientation or lowered level of consciousness in the absence of hypotension, fever, or focal neurologic deficits
5. Negative serologies for measles, leptospirosis, and Rocky Mountain spotted fever. Blood or CSF cultures negative for organisms other than *Staphylococcus aureus*

AST = aspartate transaminase; ALT = alanine aminotransferase; BUN = blood urea nitrogen; CPK = creatine phosphokinase; CSF = cerebrospinal fluid.
Source: MMWR. 1980;29:229.

TABLE 12. DIAGNOSTIC CRITERIA FOR STREPTOCOCCAL TOXIC SHOCK SYNDROME

1. Isolation of group A streptococci:
   - From a sterile site for a *definite* case
   - From nonsterile site for a *probable* case
2. Clinical criteria—Hypotension *and* two of the following:
   - Renal dysfunction
   - Erythematous macular rash
   - Liver involvement
   - Soft-tissue necrosis

Source: JAMA. 1993;269:390.

FIGURE 13. NECROTIZING FASCIITIS TREATMENT ALGORITHM

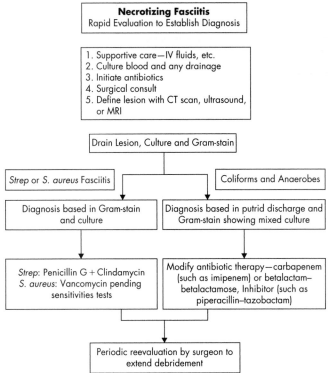

Necrotizing Fasciitis
Rapid Evaluation to Establish Diagnosis

1. Supportive care—IV fluids, etc.
2. Culture blood and any drainage
3. Initiate antibiotics
4. Surgical consult
5. Define lesion with CT scan, ultrasound, or MRI

Drain Lesion, Culture and Gram-stain

Strep or *S. aureus* Fasciitis

Coliforms and Anaerobes

Diagnosis based in Gram-stain and culture

Diagnosis based in putrid discharge and Gram-stain showing mixed culture

Strep: Penicillin G + Clindamycin
S. aureus: Vancomycin pending sensitivities tests

Modify antibiotic therapy—carbapenem (such as imipenem) or betalactam–betalactamose, Inhibitor (such as piperacillin–tazobactam)

Periodic reevaluation by surgeon to extend debridement

FIGURE 14.

Recommended Adult Immunization Schedule
UNITED STATES · 2010

Note: These recommendations *must* be read with the footnotes that follow containing number of doses, intervals between doses, and other important information.

Figure 1. Recommended adult immunization schedule, by vaccine and age group

VACCINE ▼ / AGE GROUP ▶	19–26 years	27–49 years	50–59 years	60–64 years	≥65 years
Tetanus, diphtheria, pertussis (Td/Tdap)[1,*]	Substitute 1-time dose of Tdap for Td booster; then boost with Td every 10 yrs				Td booster every 10 yrs
Human papillomavirus (HPV)[2,*]	3 doses (females)				
Varicella[3,*]	2 doses				
Zoster[4]				1 dose	
Measles, mumps, rubella (MMR)[5,*]	1 or 2 doses			1 dose	
Influenza[6,*]	1 dose annually				
Pneumococcal (polysaccharide)[7,8]	1 or 2 doses				1 dose
Hepatitis A[9,*]	2 doses				
Hepatitis B[10,*]	3 doses				
Meningococcal[11,*]	1 or more doses				

*Covered by the Vaccine Injury Compensation Program.

For all persons in this category who meet the age requirements and who lack evidence of immunity (e.g., lack documentation of vaccination or have no evidence of prior infection)	Recommended if some other risk factor is present (e.g., on the basis of medical, occupational, lifestyle, or other indications)	No recommendation

Report all clinically significant postvaccination reactions to the Vaccine Adverse Event Reporting System (VAERS). Reporting forms and instructions on filing a VAERS report are available at www.vaers.hhs.gov or by telephone, 800-822-7967.

Information on how to file a Vaccine Injury Compensation Program claim is available at www.hrsa.gov/vaccinecompensation or by telephone, 800-338-2382. To file a claim for vaccine injury, contact the U.S. Court of Federal Claims, 717 Madison Place, N.W., Washington, D.C. 20005; telephone, 202-357-6400.

Additional information about the vaccines in this schedule, extent of available data, and contraindications for vaccination is also available at www.cdc.gov/vaccines or from the CDC-INFO Contact Center at 800-CDC-INFO (800-232-4636) in English and Spanish, 24 hours a day, 7 days a week.

Use of trade names and commercial sources is for identification only and does not imply endorsement by the U.S. Department of Health and Human Services.

Figure 2. Vaccines that might be indicated for adults based on medical and other indications

VACCINE ▼ / INDICATION ▶	Pregnancy	Immuno-compromising conditions (excluding human immunodeficiency virus [HIV])[c,d,e,g]	HIV infection[c,d,e,g,n] CD4+ T lymphocyte count <200 cells/µL	HIV infection ≥200 cells/µL	Diabetes, heart disease, chronic lung disease, chronic alcoholism	Asplenia[d] (including elective splenectomy and persistent complement component deficiencies)	Chronic liver disease	Kidney failure, end-stage renal disease, receipt of hemodialysis	Health-care personnel
Tetanus, diphtheria, pertussis (Td/Tdap)[c,*]	Td	Substitute 1-time dose of Tdap for Td booster; then boost with Td every 10 yrs							
Human papillomavirus (HPV)[c,*]		3 doses for females through age 26 yrs							
Varicella[c,*]	Contraindicated			2 doses					
Zoster[*]	Contraindicated			1 dose					
Measles, mumps, rubella (MMR)[c,*]	Contraindicated			1 or 2 doses					
Influenza[c,*]	1 dose TIV annually								1 dose TIV or LAIV annually
Pneumococcal (polysaccharide)[c,d]				1 or 2 doses					
Hepatitis A[c,*]				2 doses					
Hepatitis B[c,*]				3 doses					
Meningococcal[c,d]				1 or more doses					

*Covered by the Vaccine Injury Compensation Program.

For all persons in this category who meet the age requirements and who lack evidence of immunity (e.g., lack documentation of vaccination or have no evidence of prior infection)

Recommended if some other risk factor is present (e.g., on the basis of medical, occupational, lifestyle, or other indications)

No recommendation

These schedules indicate the recommended age groups and medical indications for which administration of currently licensed vaccines is commonly indicated for adults ages 19 years and older, as of January 1, 2010. Licensed combination vaccines may be used whenever any components of the combination are indicated and when the vaccine's other components are not contraindicated. For detailed recommendations on all vaccines, including those used primarily for travelers or that are issued during the year, consult the manufacturers' package inserts and the complete statements from the Advisory Committee on Immunization Practices (www.cdc.gov/vaccines/pubs/acip-list.htm).

The recommendations in this schedule were approved by the Centers for Disease Control and Prevention's (CDC) Advisory Committee on Immunization Practices (ACIP), the American Academy of Family Physicians (AAFP), the American College of Physicians (ACP), the American College of Obstetricians and Gynecologists (ACOG), and the American College of Physicians (ACP).

DEPARTMENT OF HEALTH AND HUMAN SERVICES
CENTERS FOR DISEASE CONTROL AND PREVENTION — CDC

FIGURE 14. (CONT.)

Footnotes

Recommended Adult Immunization Schedule—UNITED STATES • 2010

For complete statements by the Advisory Committee on Immunization Practices (ACIP), visit www.cdc.gov/vaccines/pubs/ACIP-list.htm.

1. Tetanus, diphtheria, and acellular pertussis (Td/Tdap) vaccination

Tdap should replace a single dose of Td for adults aged 19 through 64 years who have not received a dose of Tdap previously.

Adults with uncertain or incomplete history of primary vaccination series with tetanus and diphtheria toxoid-containing vaccines should begin or complete a primary vaccination series. A primary series for adults is 3 doses of tetanus and diphtheria toxoid-containing vaccines; administer the first 2 doses at least 4 weeks apart and the third dose 6–12 months after the second; Tdap can substitute for any one of the doses of Td in the 3-dose primary series. The booster dose of tetanus and diphtheria toxoid-containing vaccine should be administered to adults who have completed a primary series and if the last vaccination was received ≥10 years previously. Tdap or Td vaccine may be used, as indicated.

If a woman is pregnant and received the last Td vaccination ≥10 years previously, administer Td during the second or third trimester. If the woman received the last Td vaccination <10 years previously, administer Tdap during the immediate postpartum period. A dose of Tdap is recommended for postpartum women, close contacts of infants aged <12 months, and all health-care personnel with direct patient contact if they have not previously received Tdap. An interval as short as 2 years from the last Td is suggested; shorter intervals can be used. Td may be deferred during pregnancy and Tdap substituted in the immediate postpartum period, or Tdap can be administered instead of Td to a pregnant woman.

Consult the ACIP statement for recommendations for giving Td as prophylaxis in wound management.

2. Human papillomavirus (HPV) vaccination

HPV vaccination is recommended at age 11 or 12 years with catch-up vaccination at ages 13 through 26 years.

Ideally, vaccine should be administered before potential exposure to HPV through sexual activity; however, females who are sexually active should still be vaccinated consistent with age-based recommendations. Sexually active females who have not been infected with any of the four HPV vaccine types (types 6, 11, 16, 18 all of which HPV4 prevents) or any of the two HPV vaccine types (types 16 and 18 both of which HPV2 prevents) receive the full benefit of the vaccination. Vaccination is less beneficial for females who have already been infected with one or more of the HPV vaccine types. HPV4 or HPV2 can be administered to persons with a history of genital warts, abnormal Papanicolaou test, or positive HPV DNA test, because these conditions are not evidence of prior infection with vaccine HPV types.

A complete series for either HPV4 or HPV2 consists of 3 doses. The second dose should be administered 1–2 months after the first dose; the third dose should be administered 6 months after the first dose.

HPV4 may be administered to males aged 9 through 26 years to reduce their likelihood of acquiring genital warts. HPV4 would be most effective when administered before exposure to HPV through sexual contact.

Although HPV vaccination is not specifically recommended for persons with the medical indications described in Figure 2, "Vaccines that might be indicated for adults based on medical and other indications," it may be administered to these persons because the HPV vaccine is not a live-virus vaccine. However, the immune response and vaccine efficacy might be less than that in persons with a history of genital warts, abnormal warts, abnormal Papanicolaou test, or positive HPV DNA test. However, the immune response and vaccine efficacy might be less in persons who do not have the medical indications described in Figure 2 than in persons with the medical indications described. Health-care personnel are not at increased risk because of occupational exposure, and should be vaccinated consistent with age-based recommendations.

3. Varicella vaccination

All adults without evidence of immunity to varicella should receive 2 doses of single-antigen varicella vaccine if not previously vaccinated or the second dose if they have received only 1 dose, unless they have a medical contraindication. Special consideration should be given to those who 1) have close contact with persons at high risk for severe disease (e.g., health-care personnel and family contacts of persons with immunocompromising conditions) or 2) are at high risk for exposure or transmission (e.g., teachers; child-care employees; residents and staff members of institutional settings, including correctional institutions; college students; military personnel; adolescents and adults living in households with children; nonpregnant women of childbearing age; and international travelers).

Evidence of immunity to varicella in adults includes any of the following: 1) documentation of 2 doses of varicella vaccine at least 4 weeks apart; 2) U.S.-born before 1980 (although for health-care personnel and pregnant women, birth before 1980 should not be considered evidence of immunity); 3) history of varicella based on diagnosis or verification of varicella by a health-care provider (for a patient reporting a history of or presenting with an atypical case, a mild case, or both, health-care providers should seek either an epidemiologic link with a typical varicella case or to a laboratory-confirmed case or evidence of laboratory confirmation, if it was performed at the time of acute disease); 4) history of herpes zoster based on diagnosis or verification of herpes zoster by a health-care provider; or 5) laboratory evidence of immunity or laboratory confirmation of disease.

Pregnant women should be assessed for evidence of varicella immunity. Women who do not have evidence of immunity should receive the first dose of varicella vaccine upon completion or termination of pregnancy and before discharge from the health-care facility. The second dose should be administered 4–8 weeks after the first dose.

4. Herpes zoster vaccination

A single dose of zoster vaccine is recommended for adults aged ≥60 years regardless of whether they report a prior episode of herpes zoster. Persons with chronic medical conditions may be vaccinated unless their condition constitutes a contraindication.

5. Measles, mumps, rubella (MMR) vaccination

Adults born before 1957 generally are considered immune to measles and mumps.

Measles component: Adults born during or after 1957 should receive 1 or more doses of MMR vaccine unless they have 1) a medical contraindication; 2) documentation of vaccination with 1 or more doses of MMR vaccine; 3) laboratory evidence of immunity; or 4) documentation of physician-diagnosed measles.

A second dose of MMR vaccine, administered 4 weeks after the first dose, is recommended for adults who 1) have been recently exposed to measles or are in an outbreak setting; 2) have been vaccinated previously with killed measles vaccine; 3) have been vaccinated with an unknown type of measles vaccine during 1963–1967; 4) are students in postsecondary educational institutions; 5) work in a health-care facility; or 6) plan to travel internationally.

Mumps component: Adults born during or after 1957 should receive 1 dose of MMR vaccine unless they have 1) a medical contraindication; 2) documentation of vaccination with 1 or more doses of MMR vaccine; 3) laboratory evidence of immunity; or 4) documentation of physician-diagnosed mumps.

A second dose of MMR vaccine, administered 4 weeks after the first dose, is recommended for adults who 1) live in a community experiencing a mumps outbreak and are in an affected age group; 2) are students in postsecondary educational institutions; 3) work in a health-care facility; or 4) plan to travel internationally.

Rubella component: 1 dose of MMR vaccine is recommended for women who do not have documentation of rubella vaccination, or who lack laboratory evidence of immunity. For women of childbearing age, regardless of birth year, rubella immunity should be determined and women should be counseled regarding congenital rubella syndrome. Women who do not have evidence of immunity should receive MMR vaccine upon completion or termination of pregnancy and before discharge from the health-care facility.

Health-care personnel born before 1957: For unvaccinated health-care personnel born before 1957 who lack laboratory evidence of measles, mumps, and/or rubella immunity or laboratory confirmation of disease, health-care facilities should consider vaccinating personnel with 2 doses of MMR vaccine at the appropriate interval (for measles and mumps) and 1 dose of MMR vaccine (for rubella), respectively.

During outbreaks, health-care facilities should recommend that unvaccinated health-care personnel born before 1957, who lack laboratory evidence of measles, mumps, and/or rubella immunity or laboratory confirmation of disease, receive 2 doses of MMR vaccine during an outbreak of measles or mumps, and 1 dose during an outbreak of rubella.

Complete information about evidence of immunity is available at www.cdc.gov/vaccines/recs/provisional/default.htm.

6. Seasonal Influenza vaccination

Vaccinate all persons aged ≥50 years and any younger persons who would like to decrease their risk of getting influenza. Vaccinate persons aged 19 through 49 years with any of the following indications.

Medical: Chronic disorders of the cardiovascular or pulmonary systems, including asthma; chronic metabolic diseases, including diabetes mellitus; renal or hepatic dysfunction, hemoglobinopathies, or immunocompromising conditions (including immunocompromising conditions caused by medications or HIV); cognitive, neurologic or neuromuscular disorders; and pregnancy during the influenza season. No data exist on the risk for severe or complicated influenza disease among persons with asplenia; however, influenza is a risk factor for secondary bacterial infections that can cause severe disease among persons with asplenia.

Occupational: All health-care personnel, including those employed by long-term care and assisted-living facilities; and caregivers of children aged <5 years.

Other: Residents of nursing homes and other long-term care and assisted-living facilities; persons likely to transmit influenza to persons at high risk (e.g., in-home household contacts and caregivers of children aged <5 years, persons aged ≥50 years, and persons of all ages with high-risk conditions).

Healthy, nonpregnant adults aged <50 years without high-risk medical conditions who are not contacts of severely immunocompromised persons in special-care units may receive either intranasally administered live, attenuated influenza vaccine (FluMist) or inactivated vaccine. Other persons should receive the inactivated vaccine.

7. Pneumococcal polysaccharide (PPSV) vaccination

Vaccinate all persons with the following indications.

Medical: Chronic lung disease (including asthma); chronic cardiovascular diseases; diabetes mellitus; chronic liver diseases, cirrhosis; chronic alcoholism; functional or anatomic asplenia (e.g., sickle cell disease or splenectomy [if elective splenectomy is planned, vaccinate at least 2 weeks before surgery]); immunocompromising conditions including chronic renal failure or nephrotic syndrome; and cochlear implants and cerebrospinal fluid leaks. Vaccinate as close to HIV diagnosis as possible.

Other: Residents of nursing homes or long-term care facilities and persons who smoke cigarettes. Routine use of PPSV is not recommended for American Indians/Alaska Natives or persons aged <65 years unless they have underlying medical conditions that are PPSV indications. However, public health authorities may consider recommending PPSV for American Indians/Alaska Natives and persons aged 50 through 64 years who are living in areas where the risk for invasive pneumococcal disease is increased.

8. Revaccination with PPSV

One-time revaccination after 5 years is recommended for persons with chronic renal failure or nephrotic syndrome; functional or anatomic asplenia (e.g., sickle cell disease or splenectomy); and for persons with immunocompromising conditions. For persons aged ≥65 years, one-time revaccination is recommended if they were vaccinated ≥5 years previously and were younger than age <65 years at the time of the primary vaccination.

9. Hepatitis A vaccination

Vaccinate persons with any of the following indications and any person seeking protection from hepatitis A virus (HAV) infection.

Behavioral: Men who have sex with men and persons who use injection drugs.

Occupational: Persons working with HAV–infected primates or with HAV in a research laboratory setting.

Medical: Persons with chronic liver disease and persons who receive clotting factor concentrates.

Other: Persons travelling to or working in countries that have high or intermediate endemicity of hepatitis A (a list of countries is available at wwwn.cdc.gov/travel/contentdiseases.aspx).

Unvaccinated persons who anticipate close personal contact (e.g., household contact or regular babysitting) with an international adoptee from a country of high or intermediate endemicity during the first 60 days after arrival of the adoptee in the United States should consider vaccination. The first dose of the 2-dose hepatitis A vaccine series should be administered as soon as adoption is planned, ideally ≥2 weeks before the arrival of the adoptee.

Single-antigen vaccine formulations should be administered in a 2-dose schedule at either 0 and 6–12 months (Havrix), or 0 and 6–18 months (Vaqta). If the combined hepatitis A and hepatitis B vaccine (Twinrix) is used, administer 3 doses at 0, 1, and 6 months; alternatively, a 4-dose schedule, administered on days 0, 7, and 21–30 followed by a booster dose at month 12 may be used.

10. Hepatitis B vaccination

Vaccinate persons with any of the following indications and any person seeking protection from hepatitis B virus (HBV) infection.

Behavioral: Sexually active persons who are not in a long-term, mutually monogamous relationship (e.g., persons with more than one sex partner during the previous 6 months); persons seeking evaluation or treatment for a sexually transmitted disease (STD); current or recent injection-drug users; and men who have sex with men.

Occupational: Health-care personnel and public-safety workers who are exposed to blood or other potentially infectious body fluids.

Medical: Persons with end-stage renal disease, including patients receiving hemodialysis; persons with HIV infection; and persons with chronic liver disease.

Other: Household contacts and sex partners of persons with chronic HBV infection; clients and staff members of institutions for persons with developmental disabilities; and international travelers to countries with high or intermediate prevalence of chronic HBV infection (a list of countries is available at wwwn.cdc.gov/travel/contentdiseases.aspx).

Hepatitis B vaccination is recommended for all adults in the following settings: STD treatment facilities; HIV testing and treatment facilities; facilities providing drug-abuse treatment and prevention services; health-care settings targeting services to injection-drug users or men who have sex with men; correctional facilities; end-stage renal disease programs and facilities for persons with hemodialysis patients; and institutions and nonresidential daycare facilities for persons with developmental disabilities.

Administer or complete a 3-dose series of HepB to those persons not previously vaccinated. The second dose should be administered 1 month after the first dose; the third dose should be administered at least 2 months after the second dose (and at least 4 months after the first dose). If the combined hepatitis A and hepatitis B vaccine (Twinrix) is used, administer 3 doses at 0, 1, and 6 months; alternatively, a 4-dose schedule, administered on days 0, 7, and 21–30 followed by a booster dose at month 12 may be used.

Adult patients receiving hemodialysis or with other immunocompromising conditions should receive 1 dose of 40 μg/mL (Recombivax HB) administered on a 3-dose schedule or 2 doses of 20 μg/mL (Engerix-B) administered simultaneously on a 4-dose schedule at 0, 1, 2 and 6 months.

FIGURE 14. *(CONT.)*

11. Meningococcal vaccination

Meningococcal vaccine should be administered to persons with the following indications.

Medical: Adults with anatomic or functional asplenia, or persistent complement component deficiencies.

Other: First-year college students living in dormitories; microbiologists routinely exposed to isolates of *Neisseria meningitidis*; military recruits; and persons who travel to or live in countries in which meningococcal disease is hyperendemic or epidemic (e.g., the "meningitis belt" of sub-Saharan Africa during the dry season [December through June]), particularly if their contact with local populations will be prolonged. Vaccination is required by the government of Saudi Arabia for all travelers to Mecca during the annual Hajj.

Meningococcal conjugate vaccine (MCV4) is preferred for adults with any of the preceding indications who are aged ≤55 years; meningococcal polysaccharide vaccine (MPSV4) is preferred for adults aged ≥56 years. Revaccination with MCV4 after 5 years is recommended for adults previously vaccinated with MCV4 or MPSV4 who remain at increased risk for infection (e.g., adults with anatomic or functional asplenia). Persons whose only risk factor is living in on-campus housing are not recommended to receive an additional dose.

12. Selected conditions for which *Haemophilus influenzae* type b (Hib) vaccine may be used

Hib vaccine generally is not recommended for persons aged ≥5 years. No efficacy data are available on which to base a recommendation concerning use of Hib vaccine for older children and adults. However, studies suggest good immunogenicity in patients who have sickle cell disease, leukemia, or HIV infection or who have had a splenectomy. Administering 1 dose of Hib vaccine to these high-risk persons who have not previously received Hib vaccine is not contraindicated.

13. Immunocompromising conditions

Inactivated vaccines generally are acceptable (e.g., pneumococcal, meningococcal, influenza [inactivated influenza vaccine]) and live vaccines generally are avoided in persons with immune deficiencies or immunocompromising conditions. Information on specific conditions is available at www.cdc.gov/vaccines/pubs/acip-list.htm.

TABLE 15. LEGIONELLA

	Legionnaires' Disease	Pontiac Fever
Site	Pneumonia	Flu-like illness without pneumonia
Incubation period	2–10 days	24–48 hrs
Sx	Chills, fever, dyspnea	Chills, fever, headache, myalgias
Diagnosis	Culture, resp. secretion, urine antigen, serology	Serology, culture common source
Epidemiology	Sporadic and epidemic	Epidemic
Risk	Predisposed—age >40 yrs, smokers, compromised CMI	Attach >90% including young and healthy
Outcome	Mortality 15–25%	Recovery ≤1 wk

Note: *Legionella pneumophila* serogroup 1 is predominant cause of both Legionnaires' Disease and Pontiac Fever.

TABLE 16. MALARIA PROPHYLAXIS

Provide antimalarial drug dosages, schedules, and warnings			

Advise pts that antimalarial drugs are most effective if take exactly on schedule without skipping doses and that their drug should be continued post-travel for the most complete protection. Antimalarial drugs should be purchased before travel; drugs purchased overseas may not be manufactured according to U.S. standards and may not be effective. They may also be dangerous, contain the wrong drug or an incorrect amount of active drug, or be contaminated.

Halofantrine (marketed as Halfan) is widely used overseas to treat malaria. CDC does not recommend the use of Halfan because of serious cardiac complications, including death. Travelers should be advised to avoid Halfan unless they have been diagnosed with life-threatening malaria and no other options are immediately available.

Overdosage of antimalarial drugs can be fatal. Parents should be advised to keep drugs in childproof containers out of the reach of children.

		Drugs used in the prophylaxis of malaria	
Drug	**Usage**	**Adult Dose**	**Pediatric Dose**	**Adverse Reactions, Contraindications, and Comments**
---	---	---	---	---
Atovaquone/proguanil (Malarone®)	Primary prophylaxis* in areas with chloroquine-resistant or mefloquine-resistant *Plasmodium falciparum*	Adult tablets contain 250 mg atovaquone and 100 mg proguanil hydrochloride. 1 adult tab PO daily	Pediatric tablets contain 62.5 mg atovaquone and 25 mg proguanil hydrochloride. Daily dose by weight: 5–8 kg: ½ tab >8–10 kg: ¾ tab 11–20 kg: 1 tab 21–30 kg: 2 tabs 31–40 kg: 3 tabs >40 kg: 1 adult tab	Contraindicated in persons with severe renal impairment (creatinine clearance <30 mL/min). Atovaquone/proguanil should be taken with food or a milky drink. Not recommended for children under <5 kg, pregnant women, and women breastfeeding infants <5 kg. Begin 1–2 days before travel and for 7 days after leaving malarious area.
Chloroquine phosphate (Aralen® and generic)	Primary prophylaxis* only in areas with chloroquine-sensitive *P. falciparum*	300 mg base (500 mg salt) orally, once per wk	5 mg/kg base (8.3 mg/kg salt) orally once per wk, up to maximum adult dose of 300 mg base	May exacerbate psoriasis. Begin 1–2 wks before travel and for 4 wks after leaving malarious area.
Doxycycline (many brand names and generic)	Primary prophylaxis* in areas with chloroquine-resistant or mefloquine-resistant *P. falciparum*	100 mg PO daily	≥8 yrs of age: 2 mg/kg up to adult dose of 100 mg/day	Contraindicated in children <8 yrs of age and pregnant women Begin 1–2 days before travel and for 4 wks after leaving malarious area.

DIAGNOSES AND PATHOGENS

TABLE 16. [CONT.]

<table>
<tr><th rowspan="2">Drug</th><th colspan="4">Drugs used in the prophylaxis of malaria</th></tr>
<tr><th>Usage</th><th>Adult Dose</th><th>Pediatric Dose</th><th>Adverse Reactions, Contraindications, and Comments</th></tr>
<tr>
<td>Hydroxychloroquine sulfate (Plaquenil®)</td>
<td>An alternative to chloroquine for primary prophylaxis* only in areas with chloroquine-sensitive P. falciparum</td>
<td>310 mg base (400 mg salt) PO once per wk</td>
<td>5 mg/kg base (6.5 mg/kg salt) PO once per wk up to maximum adult dose of 310 mg base</td>
<td>May exacerbate psoriasis. Begin 1–2 wks before travel and for 4 wks after leaving malarious area.</td>
</tr>
<tr>
<td>Mefloquine (Lariam® and generic)</td>
<td>Primary prophylaxis* in areas with chloroquine-resistant P. falciparum</td>
<td>228 mg base (250 mg salt) PO once per wk</td>
<td>Dosing by weight: ≤9 kg:
4.6 mg/kg base, once per wk
9–19 kg: 1/4 tab PO qwk
>19–30 kg: 1/2 tab qwk
>31–45 kg: 3/4 tab PO qwk
>45 kg: 1 tab qwk</td>
<td>Contraindicated in persons allergic to mefloquine and in persons with active depression or a previous history of depression, generalized anxiety disorder, psychosis, schizophrenia, other major psychiatric disorders, or seizures. Not recommended for persons with conduction abnormalities.
Begin 1–2 wks before travel and for 4 wks after leaving malarious area.</td>
</tr>
<tr>
<td>Primaquine</td>
<td>An option for primary prophylaxis* in special circumstances. Call Malaria Hotline (770-488-7788) for additional information. Used for terminal prophylaxis† to decrease risk of relapses of P. vivax and P. ovale or both. Indicated for persons who have had prolonged exposure to P. vivax and P. ovale or both.</td>
<td>30 mg base (52.6 mg salt) PO once daily for 7 days after departure from the malarious area. Note: the recommended dose of primaquine for terminal prophylaxis† has been increased from 15 mg to 30 mg for adults. Terminal is T4d.</td>
<td>0.5 mg/kg base (0.8 mg/kg salt) up to adult dose PO once daily for 7 days after departure from the malarious area. Note: the recommended dose of primaquine for terminal prophylaxis† has been increased from 0.3 mg/kg to 0.6 mg/kg for children. Terminal is T4d.</td>
<td>Contraindicated in persons with G6PD deficiency. Also contraindicated during pregnancy and lactation unless the infant being breastfed has a documented normal G6PD level. Use in consultation with malaria experts.
Begin 1–2 days before travel and for 7 days after leaving malarious area.</td>
</tr>
</table>

*Primary prophylaxis refers to the use of antimalarial drugs to prevent symptoms associated with the blood stage infections; these drugs are taken before, during and for a period of time after travel in the malaria-risk area.

†Terminal prophylaxis refers to the use of primaquine to lower the risk of relapses from liver stage infection with Plasmodium vivax or P. ovale. Primaquine is taken after departure from the malaria-risk area.

APPENDIX II
GENERAL THERAPEUTIC TABLES

TABLE 1. TYPICAL DURATION OF ANTIBIOTIC THERAPY

Site of Infection	Diagnosis/Pathogen	Duration	Referenced within this guide (page#)
Actinomycosis	Cervicofacial	4–6 wk IV, then PO × 6–12 mos	223
Arthritis (septic)	Septic arthritis—S. aureus	4–6 wks	7, 15, 327
	Septic arthritis—GNB	4–6 wks	7, 15
	Septic arthritis—streptococci	2 wks	7, 15
	Septic arthritis—H. influenzae	2 wks	15, 271
	Septic arthritis—N. gonorrhoeae	1 wk	15
Bacteremia	Gram-negative bacteremia	10–14 days*	314
	S. aureus, portal of entry known	2 wks (post source control; consider ECHO)	327
	S. aureus, unknown source	4–6 wks (should r/o endocarditis)	327
	Line sepsis: S. aureus	14 days (post-removal)	180, 327
	Line sepsis: Coagulase-negative Staphylococci	5–7 days (post-removal) or 14 days (catheter salvage)	180
	Line sepsis: E. faecalis	10–14 days (post-removal)	
	Line sepsis: GNB	10–14 days (post-removal)	180
	Line sepsis: Fungal	14 days (post-removal and after first negative culture). Consider ECHO.	180
	Vascular graft	4 wk (post-removal)	214
Bone	Osteomyelitis (acute)	4–6 wk IV (consider 2 wks IV, then 4–6 wks PO)	11
	Osteomyelitis (chronic)	≥3 mos or until ESR/CRP normal	13
Bronchi	Acute Exacerbation of Chronic Bronchitis	7–10 days	160
Brucella	Brucellosis	6 wk	236
Bursitis	S. aureus	10–14 days or until clinical improvement	327
Central Nervous System	Cerebral abscess	Minimum 4–6 wk IV	144
	Meningitis—Listeria	≥21 days	141, 280
	Meningitis—N. meningitidis	7 days	141, 304
	Meningits—S. pneumonia	10–14 days	141, 332
Ear	Acute Otitis Media	5–10 days	127
Gastrointestinal	Diarrhea: C. difficile colitis	10–14 days	91, 251
	C. jejuni	7 days	91, 240

Site of Infection	Diagnosis/Pathogen	Duration	Referenced within this guide (page#)
Gastrointestinal	*E. histolytica*	5–10 days	91, 383
	Giardia	5–7 days	91, 385
	Salmonella	14 days (consider longer treatment duration pts with comorbidities or immunosuppression)	91, 320
	Shigella	3–5 days or single dose	91, 324
	Traveler's diarrhea	3 days	95
	H. pylori gastritis	10–14 days	99
	Typhoid fever	5–14 days	320
	Tropical Sprue	6 mos	
	Whipple's disease	1 yr	342
Heart	Endocarditis: PCN-sensitive (MIC ≤0.12) Viridan strep	14 days (PCN in combination with gentamicin in uncomplicated cases OR 28 days PCN monotherapy)	19 19
	Endocarditis: PCN-Intermediate sensitivity (MIC >0.12 – ≤0.5) Viridan strep, Group B, C, G strep	28 days (gentamicin in combination with PCN for the first 2 wks)	19
	Endocarditis: PCN Viridan strep (MIC >0.5) OR Enterococci	4–6 wks (gentamicin in combination with PCN or ampicillin)	19
	Endocarditis: *S. aureus*	6 wks	19, 327
	Endocarditis: HACEK organism	4 wks	19
	Prosthetic valve endocarditis	6 wks (from clearance of blood culture)	22
	Pericarditis (pyogenic)	14–42 days (usually 1 mo post-source control)	27
Intra-abdominal	Cholecystitis (complicated)	5–14 days for complicated cholecystitis +/− sepsis. Can stop abx once obstruction has been relieved or post-cholecystectomy once pt stable.	197
	Cholangitis	7–14 days (biliary drainage if obstructed)	195
	Diverticulitis	7–14 days	97
	Primary peritonitis	10–14 days	203

TABLE 1. *(cont.)*

Site of Infection	Diagnosis/Pathogen	Duration	Referenced within this guide (page#)
Intra-abdominal	Secondary Peritonitis (secondary to Peritoneal Dialysis)	10–14 days	203
	Secondary Peritonitis	5–7 days for complicated cases after adequate source control or clinical resolution, whichever is earlier	203
	Intra-abdominal abscess	≤7 days after surgery	201
	Infected pancreatic necrosis	2 wks (with adequate source control)	102, 202
Joint	Septic arthritis, gonococcal	7 days (purulent arthritis may require 2 wks)	15
	Pyogenic, non-gonococcal	3–4 wks (after washout)	15
	Prosthetic joint	Abx duration depends on replacement arthroplasty and virulence of organism.	7
Liver	Pyogenic liver abscess	4–16 wk or 2 wks post-drainage	199
	Amebic	10 days (tissue agent) followed by 7–20 days (luminal agent)	199
Lung	Pneumonia: *C. pneumoniae*	10–14 days	168, 246
	Legionella	7–10 days (14–21 days if immunosuppressed or critically ill)	168, 278
	Mycoplasma	10–14 days	168, 300
	Nocardia	6–12 mos. Consider secondary prophylaxis in pts with continued immunosuppression	305
	Pneumococcal	5–7 days or until afebrile × 48–72 hrs and clinically stable	168, 332
	Pneumocystis	21 days	
	Staphylococcal	≥14 days (a minimum of 14 days for necrotizing PNA and/ or bacteremia).	327
	Tuberculosis	6–9 mos (9 mos if cavitary disease and + culture after 2 mos of Tx)	172
	Lung abscess	Until x-ray clear or until small stable residual lesion; usually >3 mos	165
	HAP/VAP	8 days*	170

Site of Infection	Diagnosis/Pathogen	Duration	Referenced within this guide (page#)
Nocardia	Nocardiosis	6–12 mos. Consider secondary prophylaxis in pts with continued immunosuppression.	305
Pharynx	Pharyngitis-group A strep	10 days (PCN)	130
	Pharyngitis, gonococcal	1 dose	130
	Diphtheria	14 days	130
Prostate	Prostatitis, acute	4 wk	71
	Prostatitis, chronic	3 wks–4 mos (unclear if treatment duration >1 mo is more effective)	73
Soft tissue	Cellulitis	7–10 days	33
	Bite Wound	7 days	182
	Gas gangrene	Duration based on surgical margins post-surgery.	183
	Lymphangitis	10–14 days	334
	Necrotizing fasciitis	Duration variable	184
	Pyomyositis	14–28 days (post-debridement/drainage)	186
STDs	Chancroid	7 days (erythromycin) or 1 dose (azithromycin or ceftriaxone)	269
	Chlamydia	7 days (doxycycline) or 1 dose (azithromycin)	243
	Gonococcal infection (disseminated)	>7 days	301
	Gonococcal (cervicitis)	1 dose	105, 301
	Gonococcal (urethritis)	1 dose	82, 301
	H. simplex (excluding CNS disease)	7–14 days (14 days in severe disease and immunosuppressed)	416
	Lymphogranuloma venereum	21 days	282
	Pelvic inflammatory disease	14 days	109
	Syphilis (primary, secondary, or early latent)	1 dose (benzathine PCN) or 14 days (doxycycline)	338
	Syphilis (late latent)	3 doses (benzathine PCN 1 wk apart) or 28 days (doxycycline)	338
	Syphilis (neurosyphilis or ocular syphilis)	10–14 days	338
Sinus	Sinusitis, acute	10–14 days	133
	Sinusitis, chronic	Duration variable	

GENERAL THERAPEUTIC

TABLE 1. *(cont.)*

Site of Infection	Diagnosis/Pathogen	Duration	Referenced within this guide (page#)
Systemic	Brucellosis	≥6 wks	236
	Listeria: immunosuppressed host	3–6 wks	280
	Late Lyme arthritis	28 days	9
	Meningococcemia	7–10 days	304
	Rocky Mountain spotted fever	7 days or 3 days after afebrile	258
	Salmonellosis	10–14 days	320
	Bacteremia	≥3–4 wk	
	AIDS patients	4–6 wk	
	Carrier state	6–9 mos	
	Tuberculosis— Extrapulmonary	9 mos	
	Tularemia	10 days (gentamicin). Longer duration with second line agent	268
Urinary tract	Cystitis	3 days	69
	Pyelonephritis	14 days	80
Vaginitis	Bacterial vaginosis	7 days	112
	Candida albicans	Single dose fluconazole	353
	Trichomoniasis	7 days or 1 dose metronidazole	395

*Most experts recommend a minimum of 14 days for Serratia, Pseudomonas, Acinetobacter, Citrobacter, and Enterobacter.

Figure 2. Pathogen Classification: Gram-Negative

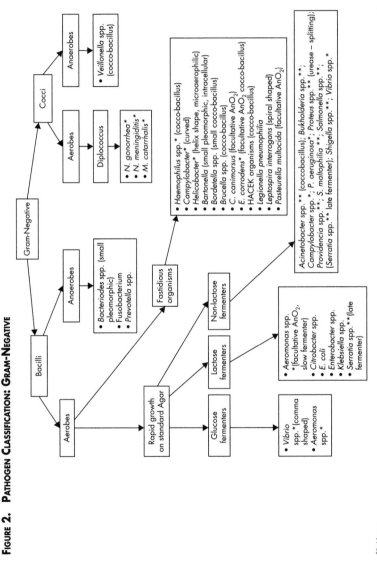

*Oxidase +
**Oxidase −

FIGURE 3. PATHOGEN CLASSIFICATION: GRAM-POSITIVE

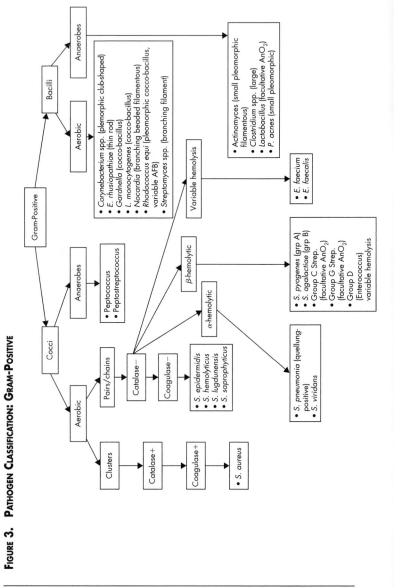

FIGURE 4. FUNGAL CLASSIFICATION

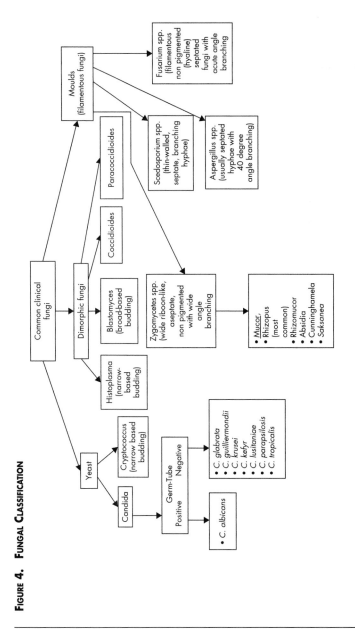

TABLE 7.   APACHE II SCORING SYSTEM

APACHE II Score (sum of A + B + C)

		Points
A	APS points	_____
B	Age points	_____
C	Chronic health points	_____
Total APACHE II Score		_____

Interpretation of Score

0 to 4 = ~4% death rate	20 to 24 = ~40% death rate
5 to 9 = ~8% death rate	25 to 29 = ~55% death rate
10 to 14 = ~15% death rate	30 to 34 = ~75% death rate
15 to 19 = ~25% death rate	>34 = ~85% death rate

A. Total Acute Physiology Score (APS)

Refer to Acute Physiology Score (Table 8)

Glasgow Coma Scale
(circle appropriate response)

Eyes open

4—Spontaneously

3—To verbal

2—To painful stimuli

1—No response

Verbal—*nonintubated*

5—Oriented and controversed

4—Disoriented and talks

3—Inappropriate words

2—Incomprehensive sounds

1—No response

Motor response

6—To verbal command

5—Localize to pain

4—Withdraws to pain

3—Decorticate

2—Decerebrate

1—No response

Verbal—*intubated*

5—Seems able to talk

3—Questionable ability to talk

1—Generally unresponsive

B. Age Points

Assign points to age as follows	*Points*
≤44 yrs	0
45–54 yrs	2
55–64 yrs	3
65–74 yrs	5
≥75 yrs	6

C. Chronic Health Points

If the pt has a hx of severe organ system insufficiency or is immunocompromised, assign points as follows:

    a. for nonoperative or emergency postoperative pts—5 points, OR

    b. for elective postoperative pts—2 points

Definitions

Organ insufficiency or immunocompromised state must have been evident prior to this hospital admission and conform to the following criteria:

    Liver. Biopsy-proven cirrhosis and documented portal hypertension, episodes of past upper GI bleeding attributed to portal hypertension, or prior episodes of hepatic failure/encephalopathy/coma

    Cardiovascular. New York Heart Association Class IV

    Respiratory. Chronic restrictive, obstructive, or vascular disease resulting in severe exercise restriction, i.e., unable to climb stairs or perform household duties; or documented chronic hypoxia, hypercapnia, secondary polycythemia, severe pulmonary hypertension (>40 mm Hg), or respirator dependency

    Renal. Receiving chronic dialysis

    Immunocompromised. The pt has received therapy that suppresses resistance to infection, e.g., immunosuppression, chemotherapy, radiation, long-term recent high-dose steroids; or has a disease that is sufficiently advanced to suppress resistance to infections, e.g., leukemia, lymphoma, AIDS

Chronic Health Points = _____

Source: Knaus WA, Draper EA, Wagner DP, et al, "APACHE II: A Severity of Disease Classification System," *Crit Care Med.* 1985;13(10):818–829. Reprinted with permission.

TABLE 8. APACHE II APS POINTS

Physiologic Value	Total Acute Physiology Score (APS) (Choose the worst value in the past 24 hrs)								
	High Range				0	Low Abnormal Range			
	+4	+3	+2	+1		+1	+2	+3	+4
Temperature, rectal (°C)	≥41	39–40.9	—	38.5–38.9	36–38.4	34–35.9	32–33.9	30–31.9	≤29.9
Mean arterial pressure (mm Hg)	≥160	130–159	110–129	—	70–109	—	50–69	—	≤49
Heart rate (ventricular response)	≥180	140–179	110–139	—	70–109	—	55–69	40–54	≤39
Respiratory rate (nonventilated or ventilated)	≥50	35–49	—	25–34	12–24	10–11	6–9	—	≤5
Oxygenation: A-aDO$_2$ or PaO$_2$ (mm Hg)									
a. FiO$_2$ ≥0.5: record A-aDO$_2$	≥500	350–499	200–349	—	<200	—	—	—	—
b. FiO$_2$ <0.5: record only PaO$_2$	—	—	—	—	PO$_2$ >70	PO$_2$ = 61–70	—	PO$_2$ = 55–60	PO$_2$ <55
Arterial pH* (if no ABGs record serum HCO$_3$ below)	≥7.7	7.6–7.69	—	7.5–7.59	7.33–7.49	—	7.25–7.32	7.15–7.24	<7.15
Serum sodium (mmol/L)	≥180	160–179	155–159	150–154	130–149	—	120–129	111–119	≤110
Serum potassium (mmol/L)	≥7	6–6.9	—	5.5–5.9	3.5–5.4	3–3.4	2.5–2.9	—	<2.5
Serum creatinine (mmol/L)(double point score for acute renal failure)	≥3.5	2–3.4	1.5–1.9	—	0.6–1.4	—	<0.6	—	—
Hematocrit (%)	≥60	—	50–59.9	46–49.9	30–45.9	—	20–29.9	—	<20
White blood count (total/mm$_3$) (in 1,000s)	≥40	—	20–39.9	15–19.9	3–14.9	—	1–2.9	—	<1
Glasgow Coma Score (GCS)	15 minus actual GCS (See Table 7)								
Total Acute Physiology Score (APS)	Sum of the 12 individual variable points (See Table 7)								
*Serum HCO$_3$ (venouse-mmol/L) (not preferred, use if no ABGs)	≥52	41–51.9	32–40.9	—	22–31.9	18–21.9	—	15–17.9	<15

Source: Knaus WA, Draper EA, Wagner DP, et al, "APACHE II: A Severity of Disease Classification System," *Crit Care Med.* 1985;13(10):818–829. Reprinted with permission.

TABLE 9. GFR AND MDRD CALCULATIONS

IBW	Men	$50.0 + (2.3 \times \text{height in inches over 5 feet})$
	Women	$45.5 + (2.3 \times \text{height in inches over 5 feet})$
CrCl	Men	$\dfrac{(140 - \text{age}) \times \text{IBW (kg)}}{\text{Scr (mg/dL)} \times 72}$
	Women	Estimated CrCl male $\times 0.85$
BSA		$0.007187 \times \text{height (cm)}^{0.725} \times \text{weight (kg)}^{0.425}$
GFR		$0.81 \times \text{CrCl} \times 1.73/(\text{BSA})$
MDRD		$186 \times \text{Scr (mg/dL)}^{1.154} \times \text{age (yrs)}^{-0.203} \times 1.212 \text{ (if Black)} \times 0.742 \text{ (if female)} \times 1.73/\text{BSA}$

IBW: ideal body weight; CrCl: creatinine clearance; BSA: body surface area; GFR: glomerular filtration rate; MDRD: modification of diet in renal disease.

TABLE 10. Aa GRADIENT

$\text{Aa} = (\text{BP} - \text{pH}_2\text{O}) \times \text{FiO}_2 - (1.25 \times \text{PaCO}_2) - \text{PaO}_2$

At sea level and room air: $\text{Aa} = 150 - (1.25 \times \text{PaCO}_2) - \text{PaO}_2$

BP: barometric pressure; pH_2O: partial pressure of water at body temperature (47 mm Hg at 37°C); FiO_2: fraction of inspired oxygen.

TABLE 11. ABX SENSITIVITY: CARBAPENEMS/MONOBACTAMS

	Aztreonam	Ertapenem	Imipenem/Cilastatin	Meropenem
Acinetobacter baumannii	3		1	1
Actinomyces			2	2
Aeromonas hydrophila	2	3	2	2
Bacillus anthracis				
Bacteroides fragilis		1	1	1
Bartonella henselae				
Bordetella species		3	3	3
Burkholderia cepacia		3	3	2
Campylobacter jejuni		3	3	3
Chlamydia pneumoniae				
Chlamydia trachomatis				
Citrobacter species	2	1	1	1
Clostridium difficile				
Clostridium species		2	2	2
Coxiella burnetii				

TABLE 11. *(cont.)*

	Aztreonam	Ertapenem	Imipenem/ Cilastatin	Meropenem
Ehrlichia/Anaplasma species				
Enterobacter species	2	2	1	1
Enterococcus faecalis		3	2	3
Enterococcus faecium			3	
Enterococcus faecium (VRE)				
Escherichia coli	2	2	2	2
Francisella tularensis				
Haemophilus influenza	2	2	2	2
Klebsiella species	2	2	2	2
Legionella species				
Leptospira interrogans				
Listeria monocytogenes			3	3
Moraxella catarrhalis	2	2	2	2
Morganella morganii	2	2	2	2
Mycobacterium avium MAI (non-HIV)				
Mycoplasm pneumoniae				
Neisseria gonorrhoeae	3		3	3
Neisseria meningitidis	2		2	2
Nocardia			2	
Pasteurella multocida			2	2
Proteus mirabilis	2	2	2	2
Proteus vulgaris	2	2	2	2
Providencia staurtii	2	2	2	2
Pseudomonas aeruginosa	1		1	1
Rickettsia species				
Salmonella species	2	2	2	2
Serratia species	2	2	2	2
Shigella species	2	2	2	2
Staphylococcus aureus (MRSA)				
Staphylococcus aureus (MSSA)		2	2	2
Staphylococcus epidermis		2	2	2

	Aztreonam	Ertapenem	Imipenem/ Cilastatin	Meropenem
Staphylococcus epidermis (MRSE)				
Stenotrophomonas maltophilia				
Streptococcus pneumoniae[†]		2	2	2
Streptococcus pneumoniae[§]		2	2	2
Streptococcus (Group A, B, C, E, F, G)		2	2	2
Streptococcus species		2	2	2
Treponema pallidum (syphilis)				
Vibrio vulnificus				
Yersinia enterocolitica	2			
Yersinia pestis				

1—first-line recommendation; 2—second-line recommendation; 3—acceptable *in vitro* data suggesting some isolates may be sensitive; blank—no or insufficient activity, or unknown.
[†]PCN sensitive; MIC ≤ 1.0 mcg/mL.
[§]PCN resistant; MIC ≥ 2.0 mcg/mL.

GENERAL THERAPEUTIC

TABLE 12. ABX SENSITIVITY: CEPHALOSPORINS

	Cefaclor	Cefadroxil	Cefazolin	Cefdinir	Cefepime	Cefixime	Cefotaxime
A. baumannii					2		3
Actinomyces							3
A. hydrophila					2	2	2
B. anthracis							
B. fragilis							
B. henselae							
Bordetella species							
B. cepacia					3		
C. jejuni					3		3
C. pneumoniae							
C. trachomatis							
Citrobacter species					1		2
C. difficile							
Clostridium species	3		3		3		3
C. burnetii							
Ehrlichia/Anaplasma species							
Enterobacter species					1		3
E. faecalis							
E. faecium							
E. faecium (VRE)							
E. coli	2	1	1	2	2	2	1
F. tularensis							
H. influenza	2			1	2	2	1
Klebsiella species	3	2	2	2	2	2	1
Legionella species							
L. interrogans							
L. monocytogenes							
M. catarrhalis	1	3	3	1	2	2	1
M. morganii					2		1
M. avium MAI (non-HIV)							
M. pneumoniae							
N. gonorrhoeae	3				2	1	2
N. meningitidis					2	3	2
Nocardia							2
P. multocida			3	2	2	2	2
P. mirabilis	2	2	2	1	2	2	1
P. vulgaris					2	2	1
P. stuartii					1		1
P. aeruginosa					1		
Rickettsia species							
Salmonella species							1††

Cefotetan	Cefoxitin	Cefpodoxime Proxetil	Cefprozil	Ceftazidime	Ceftibuten	Ceftizoxime	Ceftriaxone	Cefuroxime axetil	Cephalexin
				2	3	3	3		
						3	3		
2	3			2		2	2	3	
3	2					3			
				2		3			
							3		
3				2		2	2	3	
2	2		3	3		3	3	3	
3				2		2	2		
2	2	2	1	2	2	2	1	2	1
2	2	1	2	2	2	1	1	2	
2	2	2	2	2	2	1	1	2	2
							2		
2	3	1	1	3	1	1	1	2	3
3	3			2	2	1	1	3	
3	2	2	3	3	2	2	1	2	
3	3			3		2	2	2	
							2	3	
		2		2	2	2	2	2	3
2	2	1	1	2	1	1	1	1	2
3	3	3			3	1	1	2	
3	3	3		1	3	1	1	3	
				1					
							1		

TABLE 12. *(cont.)*

	Cefaclor	Cefadroxil	Cefazolin	Cefdinir	Cefepime	Cefixime	Cefotaxime	Cefotetan
Serratia species				3	1	3	1	3
Shigella species				3	2		2	3
S. aureus (MRSA)								
S. aureus (MSSA)	3	1	1	2	2		2	3
S. epidermis	3	2			3		3	3
S. epidermis (MRSE)								
S. maltophilia								
S. pneumoniae†	2	2	2	2	2	2	2	3
S. pneumoniae§					3		1	
Streptococcus (Group A, B, C, E, F, G)	2	2	2	2	2	2	2	3
Streptococcus species	2	2	2	2	2	2	2	3
T. pallidum (syphilis)							2	
V. vulnificus							2	
Y. enterocolitica				2	2	2	2	3
Y. pestis							3	

	Cefoxitin	Cefpodoxime Proxetil	Cefprozil	Ceftazidime	Ceftibuten	Ceftizoxime	Ceftriaxone	Cefuroxime axetil	Cephalexin
Serratia species	3	3		2		1	1		
Shigella species	3	2	3	2	3	2	2	2	
S. aureus (MRSA)									
S. aureus (MSSA)	3	2	3	3	3	2	2	2	2
S. epidermis	3	3	2			3	3	2	2
S. epidermis (MRSE)									
S. maltophilia				3					
S. pneumoniae†	3	2	2	3	3	2	2	2	2
S. pneumoniae§		3				2	1		
Streptococcus (Group A, B, C, E, F, G)	3	2	2	3	3	2	2	2	2
Streptococcus species	3	2	2	3	3	3	2	2	2
T. pallidum (syphilis)						3	2		
V. vulnificus				1					
Y. enterocolitica	3	2		2	2	2	2	3	
Y. pestis							3		

1—first-line recommendation; 2—second-line recommendation; 3—acceptable *in vitro* data suggesting some isolates may be sensitive; blank—no or insufficient activity, or unknown.
†PCN sensitive; MIC ≤ 1.0 mcg/mL.
§PCN resistant; MIC ≥ 2.0 mcg/mL.
††Second line against *S. typhi*.

TABLE 13. ABX SENSITIVITY: PENICILLINS

	Amoxicillin	Amoxicillin + Clavulanate	Ampicillin	Ampicillin + Sulbactam	Dicloxacillin	Nafcillin/Oxacillin	Penicillin	Piperacillin	Piperacillin + Tazobactam	Ticarcillin	Ticarcillin + Clavulanate
Acinetobacter baumannii				2				3	2	3	2
Actinomyces	1	2	1	2			1				
Aeromonas hydrophila								3	3	3	3
Bacillus anthracis	2	3	2	3			2				
Bacteroides fragilis		1		1				3	1		1
Bartonella henselae											
Bordetella species											
Burkholderia cepacia									3		3
Campylobacter jejuni	2	3									3
Chlamydia pneumoniae											
Chlamydia trachomatis											
Citrobacter species								2	2	2	2
Clostridium difficile											
Clostridium species	2	2	2	2			1	2	2	2	2
Coxiella burnetii											
Ehrlichia/Anaplasma species											
Enterobacter species								2	2	2	2
Enterococcus faecalis	1	2	1	2			1	2	2		
Enterococcus faecium	3	3	3	3			3	3	3		
Enterococcus faecium (VRE)											
Escherichia coli	1	2	1	2				2	2	2	2
Francisella tularensis											
Haemophilus influenza	3	1	3	2					2		2
Klebsiella species		2		2				2	2		2
Legionella species											
Leptospira interrogans	2		1				1				
Listeria monocytogenes	1	2	1	2			2	2	2	2	2
Moraxella catarrhalis		1		2					2		2
Morganella morganii								2	2	2	2
Mycobacterium avium MAI (non-HIV)											
Mycoplasm pneumoniae											
Neisseria gonorrhoeae		2		2					2		2

GENERAL THERAPEUTIC

	Amoxicillin	Amoxicillin + Clavulanate	Ampicillin	Ampicillin + Sulbactam	Dicloxacillin	Nafcillin/Oxacillin	Penicillin	Piperacillin	Piperacillin + Tazobactam	Ticarcillin	Ticarcillin + Clavulanate
Neisseria meningitidis	3	2	2	2			1	2		2	
Nocardia	3	2	3	2							
Pasteurella multocida	2	1	2	2			1	2	2	2	2
Proteus mirabilis	1	2	1	2				2	2	2	2
Proteus vulgaris								2	2	2	2
Providencia stuartii								2	2	2	2
Pseudomonas aeruginosa								1	1	3	
Rickettsia species											
Salmonella species	3	2	3	2				2	2	2	2
Serratia species								2	2	2	2
Shigella species	2	2	2	3				3	3	3	3
Staphylococcus aureus (MRSA)											
Staphylococcus aureus (MSSA)		2		2	1	1		2			2
Staphylococcus epidermis		2		2	1	1		2			2
Staphylococcus epidermis (MRSE)											
Stenotrophomonas maltophilia								3	3	3	2
Streptococcus pneumoniae[†]	1	2	2	2	3	3	1	2	2	2	2
Streptococcus pneumoniae[§]	2	2	2	2			2	3	3	3	3
Streptococcus (Group A, B, C, E, F, G)	1	3	1	3	3	3	1	3	3	3	3
Streptococcus species	1	3	2	3	3	3	1	2	3	2	3
Treponema pallidum (syphilis)	2		2				1				
Vibrio vulnificus				2					2		
Yersinia enterocolitica				2				2	2	3	2
Yersinia pestis	3	3	3								

1—first-line recommendation; 2—second-line recommendation; 3—acceptable *in vitro* data suggesting some isolates may be sensitive; blank—no or insufficient activity, or unknown.

[†] PCN sensitive; MIC ≤ 1.0 mcg/mL.

[§] PCN resistant; MIC ≥ 2.0 mcg/mL.

[††] Second line against S. *typhi*.

TABLE 14. ABX SENSITIVITY: AMINOGLYCOSIDES

	Amikacin	Gentamicin	Streptomycin	Tobramycin
Acinetobacter baumannii	2	3		2
Actinomyces				
Aeromonas hydrophila	2	2		2
Bacillus anthracis				
Bacteroides fragilis				
Bartonella henselae		2		
Bordetella species				
Burkholderia cepacia				
Campylobacter jejuni		3		
Chlamydia pneumoniae				
Chlamydia trachomatis				
Citrobacter species	2	2		1
Clostridium difficile				
Clostridium species				
Coxiella burnetii				
Ehrlichia/Anaplasma species				
Enterobacter species	1	1		1
Enterococcus faecalis		2	2	
Enterococcus faecium		3	3	
Enterococcus faecium (VRE)		3	3	
Escherichia coli	3	2		2
Francisella tularensis		1	1	3
Haemophilus influenza	3	3		3
Klebsiella species	2	2		2
Legionella species				
Leptospira interrogans				
Listeria monocytogenes	3	3		3
Moraxella catarrhalis	3	3		3
Morganella morganii	2	2		2
Mycobacterium avium MAI (non-HIV)	2		3	
Mycoplasm pneumoniae				
Neisseria gonorrhoeae				
Neisseria meningitidis				
Nocardia	2			
Pasteurella multocida				
Proteus mirabilis	2	1		2
Proteus vulgaris	2	1		2
Providencia stuartii	2	2		2

	Amikacin	Gentamicin	Streptomycin	Tobramycin
Pseudomonas aeruginosa	1	1		1
Rickettsia species				
Salmonella species				
Serratia species	2	2		2
Shigella species	3	3		3
Staphylococcus aureus (MRSA)				
Staphylococcus aureus (MSSA)				
Staphylococcus epidermis			3	
Staphylococcus epidermis (MRSE)			3	
Stenotrophomonas maltophilia				
Streptococcus pneumoniae[†]				
Streptococcus pneumoniae[§]				
Streptococcus (Group A, B, C, E, F, G)				
Streptococcus species		3		
Treponema pallidum (syphilis)				
Vibrio vulnificus				
Yersinia enterocolitica	2	2		2
Yersinia pestis		2	1	3

1—first-line recommendation; 2—second-line recommendation; 3—acceptable *in vitro* data suggesting some isolates may be sensitive; blank—no or insufficient activity, or unknown.

[†] PCN sensitive; MIC ≤ 1.0 mcg/mL.

[§] PCN resistant; MIC ≥ 2.0 mcg/mL.

[††] Second line against *S. typhi.*

Table 15. ABX Sensitivity: Fluoroquinolones

	Ciprofloxacin	Gemifloxacin	Levofloxacin	Moxifloxacin	Norfloxacin	Ofloxacin
Acinetobacter baumannii	2		2	3		3
Actinomyces				3		
Aeromonas hydrophila	1		1	1	3	1
Bacillus anthracis	1		2	2		2
Bacteroides fragilis				3		
Bartonella henselae	3					
Bordetella species	3		3	3		
Burkholderia cepacia	2		3	3		
Campylobacter jejuni	1		2	1	2	2

TABLE 15. *(cont.)*

	Ciprofloxacin	Gemifloxacin	Levofloxacin	Moxifloxacin	Norfloxacin	Ofloxacin
Chlamydia pneumoniae	2	2	2	2		2
Chlamydia trachomatis			2	2		2
Citrobacter species	2		2	3	3	3
Clostridium difficile						
Clostridium species				3		
Coxiella burnetii	2		2			2
Ehrlichia/Anaplasma species	3		3			3
Enterobacter species	2		2	2	2	2
Enterococcus faecalis	3		2	2	3	3
Enterococcus faecium	3		3	3		3
Enterococcus faecium (VRE)						
Escherichia coli	2		2	2	1	2
Francisella tularensis	2					
Haemophilus influenza	2	2	2	2		2
Klebsiella species	2	3	2	2	2	2
Legionella species	1	2	1	1		1
Leptospira interrogans						
Listeria monocytogenes						
Moraxella catarrhalis	2	2	2	2		2
Morganella morganii	2		2	3	2	3
Mycobacterium avium MAI (non-HIV)	2		2	2		2
Mycoplasm pneumoniae	2	2	2	2		2
Neisseria gonorrhoeae	1		1	2	3	1
Neisseria meningitidis	2		2	2		2
Nocardia						
Pasteurella multocida	2		3			3
Proteus mirabilis	2		2	2	1	2
Proteus vulgaris	2		2	2	1	2
Providencia stuartii	2		2	3	2	3
Pseudomonas aeruginosa	1		1	1	2	2
Rickettsia species	2		2	3		2
Salmonella species	1	2††	1	3		1
Serratia species	1		1	2	2	2
Shigella species	1		1	1	1	1
Staphylococcus aureus (MRSA)						
Staphylococcus aureus (MSSA)	3	2	2	2	3	3

	Ciprofloxacin	Gemifloxacin	Levofloxacin	Moxifloxacin	Norfloxacin	Ofloxacin
Staphylococcus epidermis	3		3	3	3	3
Staphylococcus epidermis (MRSE)	3		3	3		3
Stenotrophomonas maltophilia	3		3	2	3	3
Streptococcus pneumoniae†	3	2	2	2		3
Streptococcus pneumoniae§	3	1	1	1		3
Streptococcus (Group A, B, C, E, F, G)	3	3	3	3		3
Streptococcus species	3	2	2	2	3	3
Treponema pallidum (syphilis)						
Vibrio vulnificus	3		3	3		
Yersinia enterocolitica	2		2	2	2	2
Yersinia pestis	3		3			

1—first-line recommendation; 2—second-line recommendation; 3—acceptable *in vitro* data suggesting some isolates may be sensitive; blank—no or insufficient activity, or unknown.

† PCN sensitive; MIC ≤ 1.0 mcg/mL.

§ PCN resistant; MIC ≥ 2.0 mcg/mL.

†† Second line against *S. typhi*.

TABLE 16.   ABX SENSITIVITY: MACROLIDES & CLINDAMYCIN

	Azithromycin	Clarithromycin	Clindamycin	Erythromycin	Telithromycin
Acinetobacter baumannii					
Actinomyces	2	2	2	2	
Aeromonas hydrophila					
Bacillus anthracis		3	2	3	
Bacteroides fragilis			2		
Bartonella henselae	1	1		1	
Bordetella species	1	1		1	2
Burkholderia cepacia					
Campylobacter jejuni	1	1	2	1	
Chlamydia pneumoniae	1	1		1	2
Chlamydia trachomatis	1	2	2	2	
Citrobacter species					
Clostridium difficile					
Clostridium species			2		

TABLE 16. (cont.)

	Azithromycin	Clarithromycin	Clindamycin	Erythromycin	Telithromycin
Coxiella burnetii				3	
Ehrlichia/Anaplasma species					
Enterobacter species					
Enterococcus faecalis					
Enterococcus faecium					
Enterococcus faecium (VRE)					
Escherichia coli					
Francisella tularensis					
Haemophilus influenza	2	2		3	2
Klebsiella species					
Legionella species	1	1		2	2
Leptospira interrogans				2	
Listeria monocytogenes				2	
Moraxella catarrhalis	1	1		2	2
Morganella morganii					
Mycobacterium avium MAI (non-HIV)	2	1			
Mycoplasm pneumoniae	1	1		1	2
Neisseria gonorrhoeae	2			3	
Neisseria meningitidis					
Nocardia					
Pasteurella multocida	3				
Proteus mirabilis					
Proteus vulgaris					
Providencia stuartii					
Pseudomonas aeruginosa					
Rickettsia species				3	3
Salmonella species	2				
Serratia species					
Shigella species	3				
Staphylococcus aureus (MRSA)			2		
Staphylococcus aureus (MSSA)	2	2	2	3	2
Staphylococcus epidermis	3	3	2	3	
Staphylococcus epidermis (MRSE)	3	3	2	3	
Stenotrophomonas maltophilia					
Streptococcus pneumoniae[†]	2	2	2	2	2
Streptococcus pneumoniae[§]			2		1

	Azithromycin	Clarithromycin	Clindamycin	Erythromycin	Telithromycin
Streptococcus (Group A, B, C, E, F, G)	2	2	2	2	2
Streptococcus species	2	2	2	2	
Treponema pallidum (syphilis)	3			3	
Vibrio vulnificus					
Yersinia enterocolitica					
Yersinia pestis					

1—first-line recommendation; 2—second-line recommendation; 3—acceptable *in vitro* data suggesting some isolates may be sensitive; blank—no or insufficient activity, or unknown.
† PCN sensitive; MIC ≤ 1.0 mcg/mL.
§ PCN resistant; MIC ≥ 2.0 mcg/mL.
†† Second line against *S. typhi.*

TABLE 17.   ABX SENSITIVITY: SULFANOMIDES AND TETRACYCLINES

	Sulfanomides	Tetracyclines		
	TMP/SMX	Doxycycline	Minocycline	Tetracycline
Acinetobacter baumannii	3	2	2	2
Actinomyces		2	2	2
Aeromonas hydrophila	2	2	2	2
Bacillus anthracis		2		2
Bacteroides fragilis		3		3
Bartonella henselae		1	2	2
Bordetella species	2	3		3
Burkholderia cepacia	1		2	
Campylobacter jejuni		2	2	2
Chlamydia pneumoniae		1	1	1
Chlamydia trachomatis		1	1	1
Citrobacter species	3			
Clostridium difficile	2			
Clostridium species		3		3
Coxiella burnetii		1	1	1
Ehrlichia/Anaplasma species		1		1
Enterobacter species	2			
Enterococcus faecalis		3	3	3
Enterococcus faecium				
Enterococcus faecium (VRE)		3	3	3
Escherichia coli	1	3	3	3

TABLE 17. *(cont.)*

	Sulfanomides	Tetracyclines		
	TMP/SMX	Doxycycline	Minocycline	Tetracycline
Francisella tularensis		2	2	2
Haemophilus influenza	1	2	2	2
Klebsiella species	1**	3	3	3
Legionella species	2	2	2	2
Leptospira interrogans		2	2	2
Listeria monocytogenes	2	3	3	3
Moraxella catarrhalis	2	2	2	2
Morganella morganii		2	2	2
Mycobacterium avium MAI (non-HIV)				
Mycoplasm pneumoniae		2	2	2
Neisseria gonorrhoeae		3	3	3
Neisseria meningitides		3	3	3
Nocardia	1	2	2	3
Pasteurella multocida	2	2		2
Proteus mirabilis	2	3	3	3
Proteus vulgaris	2	3	3	3
Providencia stuartii	2			
Pseudomonas aeruginosa				
Rickettsia species		1	1	1
Salmonella species	2	3	3	3
Serratia species	3			
Shigella species	2	3	3	3
Staphylococcus aureus (MRSA)	2	2	2	3
Staphylococcus aureus (MSSA)	2	2	2	3
Staphylococcus epidermis	2	2	2	3
Staphylococcus epidermis (MRSE)	2	2	2	2
Stenotrophomonas maltophilia	1		3	
Streptococcus pneumoniae†	2	2	2	2
Streptococcus pneumoniae§		3	3	3
Streptococcus (Group A, B, C, E, F, G)	2	3	3	3
Streptococcus species	2	3	3	3
Treponema pallidum (syphilis)		2	2	2
Vibrio vulnificus		1	1	1

GENERAL THERAPEUTIC

| | Sulfanomides | Tetracyclines | | |
	TMP/SMX	Doxycycline	Minocycline	Tetracycline
Yersinia enterocolitica	1			
Yersinia pestis	3	2	2	2

1—first-line recommendation; 2—second-line recommendation; 3—acceptable *in vitro* data suggesting some isolates may be sensitive; blank—no or insufficient activity, or unknown.

† PCN sensitive; MIC ≤1.0 mcg/mL.

§ PCN resistant; MIC ≥2.0 mcg/mL.

†† Second line against *S. typhi*.

TABLE 18. ABX SENSITIVITY: MISCELLANEOUS

	Chloramphenicol	Colistin	Daptomycin	Fosfomycin	Linezolid	Metronidazole	Nitrofurantoin	Quinupristin + Dalfopristin	Rifampin	Vancomycin
Acinetobacter baumannii		2							3	
Actinomyces								3		3
Aeromonas hydrophila	3									
Bacillus anthracis	2								2	2
Bacteroides fragilis	2					1	3			
Bartonella henselae	3								2	
Bordetella species	3								3	
Burkholderia cepacia	2								3	
Campylobacter jejuni	2									
Chlamydia pneumoniae								3	3	
Chlamydia trachomatis							3		3	
Citrobacter species	3	3		3			2			
Clostridium difficile					3	1			3	2
Clostridium species	2					3	2	3		3
Coxiella burnetii	3								2	
Ehrlichia/Anaplasma species	2								2	
Enterobacter species		3		3						
Enterococcus faecalis	3			2	2		2		3	2
Enterococcus faecium	2		2	2	1		2	2	3	1
Enterococcus faecium (VRE)	2		2	3	1		2	1	3	
Escherichia coli	3	3		2			2		3	

TABLE 18. *(cont.)*

	Chloramphenicol	Colistin	Daptomycin	Fosfomycin	Linezolid	Metronidazole	Nitrofurantoin	Quinupristin + Dalfopristin	Rifampin	Vancomycin
Francisella tularensis	2									
Haemophilus influenza	2							3	3	
Klebsiella species	3	3		3						
Legionella species								3	2	
Leptospira interrogans										
Listeria monocytogenes	2				3			3	2	3
Moraxella catarrhalis	2							3	3	
Morganella morganii				3			3			
Mycobacterium avium MAI (non-HIV)						3			2	
Mycoplasm pneumoniae								3		
Neisseria gonorrhoeae					3			3	2	
Neisseria meningitidis	2							3	2	
Nocardia						3				
Pasteurella multocida									3	
Proteus mirabilis				2			2		3	
Proteus vulgaris				3			3		3	
Providencia stuartii	3			3			2			
Pseudomonas aeruginosa		2								
Rickettsia species	2								3	
Salmonella species	2	3								
Serratia species	3			3			3		3	
Shigella species	2	3								
Staphylococcus aureus (MRSA)	3		2		2		3	2	2	1
Staphylococcus aureus (MSSA)	3		2		2		2	2	2	2
Staphylococcus epidermis	3		2		2		2	2	2	1
Staphylococcus epidermis (MRSE)	3		2		2		3	2		1
Stenotrophomonas maltophilia	3									
Streptococcus pneumoniae[†]	3		2		2			2	2	2
Streptococcus pneumoniae[§]	3		2		2			2	2	1
Streptococcus (Group A, B, C, E, F, G)	3		3		2			2	3	2
Streptococcus species	3		3		2			3	3	2
Treponema pallidum (syphilis)	2									

GENERAL THERAPEUTIC

	Chloramphenicol	Colistin	Daptomycin	Fosfomycin	Linezolid	Metronidazole	Nitrofurantoin	Quinupristin + Dalfopristin	Rifampin	Vancomycin
Vibrio vulnificus										
Yersinia enterocolitica	2									
Yersinia pestis	2									

1—first-line recommendation; 2—second-line recommendation; 3—acceptable *in vitro* data suggesting some isolates may be sensitive; blank—no or insufficient activity, or unknown.

[†] PCN sensitive; MIC ≤1.0 mcg/mL.

[§] PCN resistant; MIC ≥2.0 mcg/mL.

[††] Second line against *S. typhi*.

APPENDIX III
DRUG-TO-DRUG INTERACTION TABLES

DRUG-TO-DRUG INTERACTION – AZITHROMYCIN

Drug	Effect of Interaction	Recommendations/Comments
Cyclosporin	May increase cyclosporin serum concentrations (low likelihood).	Close monitoring of cyclosporine concentrations recommended. Azithromycin did not affect cyclosporine in report of 6 pts (*Nephron*,1996;73:724).
Pimozide	Pimozide concentrations may be increased (low likelihood).	Avoid concurrent administration due to potential for QTc prolongation and cardiac arrhythmia.
Tacrolimus	May increase tacrolimus serum concentrations (low likelihood).	Case report of increased tacrolimus serum concentrations with azithromycin co-administration (*Transpl Int.*, 2005;18:757–8).
Theophylline	Serum concentrations of theophylline may be increased.	Monitor theophylline levels with co-administration.
Warfarin	INR may be increased with co-administration.	Monitor INR closely.

DRUG-TO-DRUG INTERACTION – CIPROFLOXACIN

Drug	Effect of Interaction	Recommendations/Comments
Antacids (magnesium, aluminum, calcium, Al-Mg contained in buffered ddI), vitamins, and minerals	Cations bind to ciprofloxacin resulting in decreased absorption and loss therapeutic efficacy.	Avoid co-administration. Administer ciprofloxacin at least 2 hrs before cations.
Didanosine (buffered suspension)	Antacid buffer bind to ciprofloxacin resulting in decreased absorption and loss therapeutic efficacy.	Avoid co-administration. Administer ciprofloxacin at least 2 hrs before cations. No interaction with ddI EC.
Glyburide	May cause hyper-or hypo-glycemia.	Monitor glucose levels closely.
Methotrexate	May increase methotrexate serum concentrations.	Monitor for methotrexate toxicity.
Mexiletine	Ciprofloxacin may inhibit CYP1A2 resulting in increased mexiletine concentrations.	Monitor mexiletine serum concentrations with co-administration.
NSAIDs	May increase risk of seizure.	Avoid co-administration in pts with seizure history.
Probenecid	Probenecid interferes with renal tubular secretion of ciprofloxacin, this may result in 50% increase in serum levels of ciprofloxacin.	No dose adjustment.
Sevelamer	Ciprofloxacin absorption significantly decreased.	Avoid co-administration. Administer ciprofloxacin 2 hrs before sevelamer.

Drug	Effect of Interaction	Recommendations/Comments
Sucralfate	Decreased absorption of cipro-floxacin.	Do not co-administer. Administer cipro-floxacin at least 2 hrs before sucralfate.
Theophylline	Increases theophylline concen-trations by 17–257%.	Monitor theophylline serum concentra-tions with co-administration.
Warfarin	Ciprofloxacin inhibit R-warfarin metabolism. Case reports of ciprofloxacin enhancing anti-coagulation effect of warfarin.	Monitor INR with co-administration.

DRUG-TO DRUG-INTERACTION – CLARITHROMYCIN

Drug	Effect of Interaction	Recommendations/Comments
Alfuzosin	May significantly increase Alfuzosin serum concentrations.	Contraindicated.
Alprazolam	May increase serum concentra-tions of alprazolam.	Use alternative benzodiazepines (i.e., lorazepam, oxazepam, temaze-pam).
Amiodarone	May increase amiodarone serum concentrations.	Monitor closely with proper dose adjustment.
Astemizole	May significantly increase astemizole serum concentrations.	Contraindicated.
Atazanavir (ATV)	Clarithromycin AUC increased by 94%. QTc prolongation observed with co-administration.	50% of clarithromycin dose recom-mended when co-administered with ata-zanavir. Consider using Azithromycin. Further dose adjustment needed with moderate to severe renal insufficiency and ESRD, no specific dosing guidelines consider: Cr clearance 30–60 ml/min = 250 mg once daily. Cr clearance <30 ml/min = 250 mg once every other day.
Carbamazepine	Carbamazepine AUC increased by 60%. Clarithromycin serum con-centrations may be decreased.	Avoid or use with close monitoring of carbamazepine levels with appropriate dose adjustment. Monitor of clarithro-mycin's therapeutic efficacy.
Cisapride	May significantly increase cisap-ride serum concentrations.	Contraindicated.
Cyclosporine	May increase cyclosporine serum levels.	Monitor cyclosporine serum concentra-tions closely with co-administration.
Diazepam	May increase serum concentra-tions of alprazolam.	Use alternative benzodiazepines (i.e., lorazepam, oxazepam, temazepam).
Disopyramide	May increase QTc.	Monitor Closely.
Digoxin	Case reports of digoxin toxicity.	Monitor closely with co-administration.
Efavirenz (EFV)	Clarithromycin AUC decreased with co-administration.	Consider azithromycin.
Ergot alkaloids	May significantly increase ergot serum concentrations.	Avoid co-administration.

CLARITHROMYCIN (cont.)

Drug	Effect of Interaction	Recommendations/Comments
ETR	Clarithromycin AUC decreased 39%, but active OH-clarithromycin increased 21%. ETR AUC increased 42%.	Consider azithromycin when clarithromycin is used for MAC infections.
Fentanyl	May significantly increase fentanyl serum concentrations.	Avoid co-administration. Consider morphine.
HIV protease inhibitors.	Clarithromycin concentrations may significantly increase. With indinavir (IDV), clarithromycin AUC increased 53% and IDV AUC increased 29%.	Reduce clarithromycin dose by 50% in end stage renal disease. Consider using azithromycin.
Lovastatin	May significantly increase lovastatin serum concentrations.	Consider pravastatin or rosuvastatin with clarithromycin co-administration.
Maraviroc (MVC)	Clarithromycin serum concentrations not affected. MVC may be increased.	Dose: MVC 150 mg twice daily.
Midazolam	May increase serum concentrations of midazolam.	Use alternative benzodiazepines (i.e., lorazepam, oxazepam, temazepam).
NVP	Clarithromycin AUC may be decreased with co-administration.	Consider azithromycin.
Pimozide	May significantly increase Pimozide serum concentrations. May increase QTc.	Contraindicated.
Quinidine	May increase QTc.	Monitor closely.
Raltegravir	Interaction unlikely.	Use standard doses.
Ranolazine	May significantly increase Ranolazine serum concentrations.	Contraindicated.
Rifabutin	Clarithromycin AUC decreased by 44% and 14-hydroxy-clarithromycin increased by 57%.	14-hydroxy metabolite has less activity against MAC. Rifabutin AUC increased by 56%. Consider using azithromycin.
Rifampin	May significantly decrease clarithromycin serum concentration.	Contraindicated.
Simvastatin	May significantly increase simvastatin serum concentrations.	Consider pravastatin or rosuvastatin with clarithromycin co-administration.
Sirolimus	May significantly increase sirolimus serum concentrations.	Monitor closely with dose adjustments.
Tacrolimus	May significantly increase tacrolimus serum concentrations.	Monitor closely with dose adjustments.
Terfenadine	May significantly increase terfenadine serum concentrations.	Contraindicated.
Theophylline	May increase theophylline serum concentrations.	Monitor serum level with dose adjustment.

Drug	Effect of Interaction	Recommendations/Comments
Triazolam	May increase serum concentrations of triazolam.	Use alternative benzodiazepines (i.e., lorazepam, oxazepam, temazepam).
Warfarin	May increase anticoagulant effect of warfarin.	Monitor INR closely.

DRUG-TO-DRUG INTERACTION – DAPSONE

Drug	Effect of Interaction	Recommendations/Comments
Bismuth	Dapsone absorption may be decreased.	Avoid co-administration. Administer dapsone 2 hrs before bismuth.
Cimetidine	Dapsone absorption may be decreased.	Avoid co-administration. Administer dapsone 2 hrs before H-2 blockers.
ddI (buffered suspension)	Dapsone solubility may be decreased and result in decreased absorption.	Clinical significance unknown (a PK study did not find interaction). Use ddI (enteric-coated).
Esomeprazole	Dapsone absorption may be decreased.	Avoid co-administration.
Famotidine	Dapsone absorption may be decreased.	Avoid co-administration. Administer dapsone 2 hrs before H-2 blockers.
Lansoprazole	Dapsone absorption may be decreased.	Avoid co-administration.
Nizatidine	Dapsone absorption may be decreased.	Avoid co-administration. Administer dapsone 2 hrs before H-2 blockers.
Omeprazole	Dapsone absorption may be decreased.	Avoid co-administration.
Pantoprazole	Dapsone absorption may be decreased.	Avoid co-administration.
Primaquine	Risk of hemolysis may be increased, particularly in G6PD deficiency.	Avoid or monitor closely with co-administration.
Probenecid	Dapsone serum concentrations may be increased.	Monitor for anemia with co-administration.
Pyrimethamine	Risk of anemia may be increased.	Monitor.
Rabeprazole	Dapsone absorption may be decreased.	Avoid co-administration.
Ranitidine	Dapsone absorption may be decreased.	Avoid co-administration. Administer dapsone 2 hrs before H-2 blockers.
Ribavirin	Risk of hemolysis may be increased.	Avoid or monitor closely with co-administration.
Rifampin	Dapsone serum levels decreased by 85–90%.	Avoid co-administration.
Sucralfate	Dapsone absorption may be decreased.	Avoid co-administration. Administer dapsone 2 hrs before sucralfate.

DAPSONE *(cont.)*

Drug	Effect of Interaction	Recommendations/Comments
Trimethoprim	Trimethoprim serum levels increased by 48%. Dapsone serum levels increased by 40%. Methemoglobinemia has been reported with co-administration.	Clinical significance unknown, but cases of methemoglobinemia reported with TMP + dapsone in pts who tolerated dapsone alone.
Zidovudine	Risk of anemia may be increased.	Monitor.

DRUG-TO-DRUG INTERACTION – DOXYCYCLINE

Drug	Effect of Interaction	Recommendations/Comments
Acitretin	May increase intracranial pressure.	Contraindicated.
Bismuth salts (bismuth subsalicylate-pepto-bismol)	Bismuth salts chelate tetracyclines resulting in a decreased absorption of tetracycline.	Administer bismuth 2 hrs after tetracycline.
Carbamazepine	Co-administration may decrease tetracyclines serum concentrations.	Avoid carbamazepine co-administration. Monitor closely for tetracycline therapy failure.
Cholestyramine	Co-administration may significantly reduce tetracyclines absorption.	Avoid co-administration.
Colestipol	Co-administration significantly reduce tetracyclines absorption.	Avoid co-administration.
ddI (buffer in peds formulation) contains cations	Polyvalent metal cations form an insoluble chelate with tetracyclines resulting in decreased absorption and serum levels of tetracyclines.	Separate administration by 4 hrs.
Digoxin	Co-administration may result in increased digoxin concentration (in about 10% of pts).	Monitor serum level with sign and symptoms of digoxin toxicity.
Methoxyflurane	Case reports of renal failure with co-administration with tetracycline.	Avoid co-administration.
Non-depolarizing neuromuscular blocker (e.g., vecuronium, pancuronium, rocuronium)	May potentiate non-depolarizing neuromuscular blocker.	Use with close monitoring.
Oral contraceptives	Tetracyclines may decrease the efficacy of oral contraceptives.	Consider an additional form of contraception.
Penicillins	*In vitro* antagonism when co-administered. Bacteriocidal effect of penicillins may be diminished *in vivo*.	Avoid co-administration.

Drug	Effect of Interaction	Recommendations/Comments
Phenobarbital	Co-administration may decrease tetracyclines serum concentrations.	Avoid phenobarbital co-administration. Monitor closely tetracycline for therapy failure.
Phenytoin	Co-administration may decrease tetracyclines serum concentrations.	Avoid phenytoin co-administration. Monitor closely for tetracycline therapy failure.
Polyvalent metal cations (aluminum, zinc, magnesium, iron, calcium [milk])	Polyvalent metal cations form an insoluble chelate with tetracyclines resulting in decreased absorption.	Separate administration by 4 hrs.
Quinapril	Magnesium excipient may reduce tetracyclines absorption.	Avoid co-administration.
Rifabutin	Co-administration may decrease tetracyclines serum concentrations.	Avoid rifabutin co-administration. Monitor closely for tetracycline therapy failure.
Rifampin	Co-administration may decrease tetracyclines serum concentrations.	Avoid rifampin co-administration. Monitor closely for tetracycline therapy failure.
Urinary alkalinizers (sodium lactate, sodium bicarbonate)	Co-administration results in increased urinary excretion of tetracyclines by 24–65%.	Avoid co-administration.
Warfarin	Co-administration may increase INR.	Monitor INR closely.

DRUG-TO-DRUG INTERACTION – ERYTHROMYCIN

Drug	Effect of Interaction	Recommendations/Comments
Alprazolam	Alprazolam serum levels may be increased.	Consider lorazepam, oxazepam, or temazepam.
Amiodarone	Amiodarone serum levels may be increased.	Avoid co-administration. May increase risk of QTc prolongation.
Amitriptyline	Risk of QTc prolongation may be increased.	Avoid co-administration.
Amoxapine	Risk of QTc prolongation may be increased.	Avoid co-administration.
Astemizole	Risk of QTc prolongation increased.	Contraindicated.
Atazanavir (ATV)	Erythromycin AUC may be increased. Risk of QTc prolongation may be increased.	Avoid co-administration.
Bretylium	Risk of QTc prolongation may be increased.	Avoid co-administration.
Budesonide	Budesonide serum levels may be increased.	Monitor.
Carbamazepine	Carbamazepine serum levels may be increased. Erythromycin serum levels may be decreased.	Avoid co-administration or monitor serum level.

ERYTHROMYCIN *(cont.)*

Drug	Effect of Interaction	Recommendations/Comments
Cisapride	Risk of QTc prolongation increased.	Contraindicated.
Cyclosporine	Cyclosporine serum levels may be increased.	Monitor.
Desipramine	Risk of QTc prolongation may be increased.	Avoid co-administration.
Diazepam	Diazepam serum levels may be increased.	Consider lorazepam, oxazepam, or temazepam.
Digoxin	Digoxin serum levels may be increased.	Monitor.
Diltiazem	Diltiazem serum levels may be increased. Erythromycin serum levels may be increased. May increase risk of sudden cardiac death.	Avoid co-administration. Consider azithromycin.
Disopyramide	Risk of QTc prolongation may be increased.	Avoid co-administration.
Dofetilide	Dofetilide serum levels may be increased. Risk of QTc prolongation may be increased.	Avoid co-administration.
Doxepin	Risk of QTc prolongation may be increased.	Avoid co-administration.
Darunavir (DRV/r)	Erythromycin AUC may be increased. Risk of QTc prolongation may be increased.	Avoid co-administration.
Efavirenz (EFV)	Erythromycin serum levels may be decreased.	Consider azithromycin.
Ergot alkaloids	Risk of ergotism increased.	Avoid co-administration.
Fentanyl	Fentanyl serum levels may be increased.	Consider morphine.
Fluticasone	Systemic exposure of fluticasone may be increased.	Consider beclomethasone inhaler
Fosamprenavir (FPV)	Erythromycin AUC may be increased. Risk of QTc prolongation may be increased.	Avoid co-administration.
Ibutilide	Risk of QTc prolongation may be increased.	Avoid co-administration.
Indinavir (IDV)	Erythromycin AUC may be increased. Risk of QTc prolongation may be increased.	Avoid co-administration.
Imipramine	Risk of QTc prolongation may be increased.	Avoid co-administration.
Irinotecan	Irinotecan serum levels may be increased.	Avoid co-administration.
Itraconazole	Itraconazole serum levels may be increased. Erythromycin serum levels may be increased. May increase risk of sudden cardiac death.	Avoid co-administration. Consider azithromycin.

Drug	Effect of Interaction	Recommendations/Comments
Ketoconazole	Ketoconazole serum levels may be increased. Erythromycin serum levels may be increased. May increase risk of sudden cardiac death.	Avoid co-administration. Consider azithromycin.
Lovastatin	Lovastatin serum levels may be increased.	Consider pravastatin.
Lopinavir (LPV/r)	Erythromycin AUC may be increased. Risk of QTc prolongation may be increased.	Avoid co-administration.
Methadone	Methadone serum concentrations may be increased. Increased QTc prolongation	Monitor for increased sedation. Methadone dose reduction may be needed.
Methylprednisolone	Methylprednisolone serum levels may be increased.	Monitor.
Midazolam	Midazolam serum levels may be increased.	Consider lorazepam, oxazepam, or temazepam.
Nelfinavir (NFV)	Erythromycin AUC may be increased. Risk of QTc prolongation may be increased.	Avoid co-administration.
Nortriptyline	Risk of QTc prolongation may be increased.	Avoid co-administration.
Nevirapine (NVP)	Erythromycin serum levels may be decreased.	Consider azithromycin.
Olanzapine	Olanzapine serum levels may be increased.	Monitor.
Phenobarbital	Erythromycin serum levels may be decreased.	Consider azithromycin.
Phenytoin	Erythromycin serum levels may be decreased.	Consider azithromycin.
Pimozide	Risk of QTc prolongation increased.	Contraindicated.
Posaconazole	Posaconazole serum levels may be increased. Erythromycin serum levels may be increased. May increase risk of sudden cardiac death.	Avoid co-administration. Consider azithromycin. Monitor posaconazole serum concentrations.
Prednisone	Prednisone serum concentrations may be increase.	Monitor.
Protriptyline	Risk of QTc prolongation may be increased.	Avoid co-administration.
Procainamide	Risk of QTc prolongation may be increased.	Avoid co-administration.
Quinidine	Quinidine serum levels may be increased. Risk of QTc prolongation may be increased.	Avoid co-administration.
Rifabutin	Rifabutin serum levels may be increased. Erythromycin serum levels may be decreased.	Consider azithromycin.

DRUG INTERACTIONS

ERYTHROMYCIN *(cont.)*

Drug	Effect of Interaction	Recommendations/Comments
Rifampin	Rifampin AUC may be increased. Erythromycin AUC may be decreased.	Avoid co-administration. Consider azithromycin.
Rifapentine	Erythromycin serum levels may be decreased.	Consider azithromycin.
Rilonavir (RTV)	Erythromycin AUC may be increased. Risk of QTc prolongation may be increased.	Avoid co-administration.
Sildenafil	Sildenafil serum levels may be increased.	Monitor. Sildenafil dose needs to be decreased.
Simvastatin	Simvastatin serum levels may be increased.	Consider pravastatin.
Sirolimus	Sirolimus serum levels may be significantly increased.	Monitor.
Sotalol	Risk of QTc prolongation may be increased.	Avoid co-administration.
Saquinavir (SQV)	Erythromycin AUC may be increased. Risk of QTc prolongation may be increased.	Avoid co-administration.
Tacrolimus	Tacrolimus serum levels may be significantly increased.	Monitor.
Tadalafil	Tadalafil serum levels may be increased.	Monitor. Tadalafil dose needs to be decreased.
Terfenadine	Risk of QTc prolongation increased.	Contraindicated.
Theophylline	Theophylline serum levels may be increased.	Monitor serum level.
Tipranavir (TPV/r)	Erythromycin AUC may be increased. Risk of QTc prolongation may be increased.	Avoid co-administration.
Triazolam	Triazolam serum levels may be increased.	Consider lorazepam, oxazepam, or temazepam.
Trimipramine	Risk of QTc prolongation may be increased.	Avoid co-administration.
Troleandomycin	May increase erythromycin serum concentrations and increase risk of sudden cardiac death.	Avoid co-administration.
Vardenafil	Vardenafil serum levels may be increased.	Monitor. Vardenafil dose needs to be decreased.
Verapamil	Verapamil serum levels may be increased. Erythromycin serum levels may be increased. May increase risk of sudden cardiac death.	Avoid co-administration. Consider azithromycin.
Voriconazole	Voriconazole serum levels may be increased. Erythromycin serum levels may be increased. May increase risk of sudden cardiac death.	Avoid co-administration. Consider azithromycin. Monitor voriconazole serum concentrations.
Warfarin	Anticoagulation may be increased.	Monitor INR.

DRUG-TO-DRUG INTERACTION – FLUCONAZOLE

Drug	Effect of Interaction	Recommendations/Comments
Astemizole	May increase astemizole serum concentrations.	Contraindicated.
Benzodiazepines (alprazolam, diazepam, midazolam, triazolam)	May increase benzodiazepine serum concentrations.	Use with caution. Benzodiazepine dose may need to be decreased. Consider lorazepam.
Cisapride	May increase cisapride serum concentrations.	Contraindicated.
Cyclosporine	Cyclosporine concentrations may be significantly increased.	Monitor cyclosporine concentrations closely. Cyclosporine dose may need to be decreased.
Efavirenz (EFV)	No significant interaction.	Usual dose.
Etravirine (ETR)	May increase ETR serum concentrations.	No data. Monitor for LFTs and rash with co-administration.
Fentanyl	Fentanyl serum concentrations may be significantly increased.	Use with caution. Fentanyl dose may need to be decreased.
Lovastatin	May increase lovastatin serum concentrations.	Consider pravastatin or rosuvastatin.
Maraviroc	May increase MVC serum concentrations.	No data. Use standard dose.
Nevirapine (NVP)	NVP clearance decreased by 2-fold.	Monitor LFTs closely with co-administration.
Oral hypoglycemics	Risk of hypoglycemia may be increased.	Monitor closely.
Phenytoin	Phenytoin AUC was increased by 88%.	Monitor phenytoin concentrations closely with co-administration.
Raltegravir	Interaction unlikely.	Use standard dose.
Rifabutin	No effect on fluconazole, but rifabutin serum concentrations increased by 80%.	Monitor for rifabutin-associated toxicity (i.e., uveitis). Rifabutin dose may need to be decreased.
Rifampin	May significantly decrease fluconazole serum concentrations.	Avoid co-administration. Consider rifabutin.
Simvastatin	May increase simvastatin serum concentrations.	Consider pravastatin or rosuvastatin
Sirolimus	Sirolimus concentrations may be significantly increased.	Monitor sirolimus concentrations closely. Sirolimus dose may need to be significantly decreased.
Tacrolimus	Tacrolimus levels may be significantly increased.	Monitor tacrolimus concentrations closely. Tacrolimus dose may need to be significantly decreased.
Terfenadine	May increase terfenadine serum concentrations.	Contraindicated.
Warfarin	INR may be significantly increased.	Monitor INR closely with co-administration.
Zidovudine (AZT)	AZT AUC increased by 74%.	Monitor for AZT-associated toxicity.

DRUG INTERACTIONS

DRUG-TO-DRUG INTERACTION – ITRACONAZOLE

Drug	Effect of Interaction	Recommendations/Comments
Alfuzosin	May significantly increase alfuzosin serum concentrations resulting in hypotension.	Avoid co-administration. Consider doxazosin and terazosin for BPH (with close monitoring).
Alprazolam	Alprazolam serum concentrations may be increased.	Avoid co-administration. Consider lorazepam, oxazepam, or temazepam.
Antacid	Itraconazole serum concentrations decreased.	Avoid co-administration.
Astemizole	Risk of QTc prolongation may be increased.	Contraindicated.
Bismuth	Itraconazole absorption decreased.	Avoid co-administration.
Carbamazepine	Itraconazole serum concentrations may be decreased.	Monitor itraconazole concentrations closely with co-administration. Consider valproic acid or levetiracetam.
Cimetidine	Itraconazole absorption decreased.	Avoid co-administration.
Cisapride	Risk of QTc prolongation may be increased.	Contraindicated.
Cyclosporine	Cyclosporine serum concentrations may be increased.	Monitor cyclosporine concentrations closely with co-administration.
ddI (buffered)	Itraconazole absorption decreased.	Consider fluconazole or separate >2 hrs apart. No interaction with ddI EC.
Diazepam	Diazepam serum concentrations may be increased.	Avoid co-administration. Consider lorazepam, oxazepam, or temazepam.
Digoxin	Digoxin serum concentrations may be increased.	Monitor digoxin serum concentrations with co-administration.
Diltiazem	Diltiazem serum concentrations may be increased.	Monitor.
Darunavir (DRV/r)	Itraconazole serum concentrations may be increased.	Itraconazole dose >200 mg is not recommended by some; consider monitoring itraconazole serum concentrations to guide dosing PIs serum concentrations may be increased (clinical significance unknown).
Dofetilide	Increased QTc.	Contraindicated.
Efavirenz (EFV)	Itraconazole serum concentrations may be decreased.	Monitor itraconazole concentrations closely with co-administration.
Ergot alkaloids	Ergot alkaloid serum concentrations may be increased.	Avoid co-administration. Contraindicated.
Esomeprazole	Itraconazole absorption decreased.	Avoid co-administration.

Drug	Effect of Interaction	Recommendations/Comments
Etravirine	Itraconazole serum concentrations may be decreased.	Monitor itraconazole serum concentrations with co-administration.
Famotidine	Itraconazole absorption decreased.	Avoid co-administration.
Fosamprenavir (FPV/r)	Itraconazole serum concentrations may be increased.	Itraconazole dose >200 mg is not recommended by some; consider monitoring itraconazole serum concentrations to guide dosing. PIs serum concentrations may be increased (clinical significance unknown).
Glimepiride	Risk of hypoglycemia may be increased.	Monitor.
Glipizide	Risk of hypoglycemia may be increased.	Monitor.
Glyburide	Risk of hypoglycemia may be increased.	Monitor.
Indinavir (IDV)	IDV serum concentrations may be increased. Itraconazole may be increased.	Itraconazole dose >200 mg is not recommended by some; consider monitoring itraconazole serum concentrations to guide dosing. PIs serum concentrations may be increased and increase risk for IDV stones.
Isoniazid	Itraconazole serum concentrations may be decreased.	Avoid co-administration.
Lansoprazole	Itraconazole absorption decreased.	Avoid co-administration.
Levacetylmethadol	Increased QTc.	Contraindicated.
Lopinavir (LPV/r)	Itraconazole serum concentrations may be increased.	Itraconazole dose >200 mg is not recommended by some; consider monitoring itraconazole serum concentrations to guide dosing PIs serum concentrations may be increased (clinical significance unknown).
Lovastatin	May increase lovastatin.	Avoid co-administration.
Maraviroc	MVC serum concentrations may be significantly increased.	Dose: MVC 150 mg twice-daily.
Midazolam	Midazolam serum concentrations may be increased.	Avoid co-administration. Consider lorazepam, oxazepam, or temazepam.
Nizatidine	Itraconazole absorption decreased.	Avoid co-administration.
NVP	Itraconazole serum concentrations may be decreased. NVP serum concentrations may be increased.	Monitor itraconazole concentrations closely with co-administration.
Omeprazole	Itraconazole absorption decreased.	Avoid co-administration.

ITRACONAZOLE *(cont.)*

Drug	Effect of Interaction	Recommendations/Comments
Pantoprazole	Itraconazole absorption decreased.	Avoid co-administration.
Pimozide	Risk of QTc prolongation may be increased.	Contraindicated.
Phenobarbital	Itraconazole serum concentrations may be decreased.	Monitor itraconazole concentrations closely with co-administration. Consider valproic acid or levetiracetam.
Phenytoin	Itraconazole serum concentrations may be decreased.	Monitor itraconazole concentrations closely with co-administration. Consider valproic acid or levetiracetam.
Quinidine	Risk of QTc prolongation may be increased.	Contraindicated.
Rabeprazole	Itraconazole absorption decreased.	Avoid co-administration.
Raltegravir	Interaction unlikely.	Usual dose.
Ranitidine	Itraconazole absorption decreased.	Avoid co-administration.
Ranolazine	May significantly increase ranolazine serum concentrations.	Avoid co-administration.
Rifabutin	Rifabutin serum concentrations may be increased. Itraconazole AUC decreased by 70%.	Avoid co-administration.
Rifampin	Itraconazole serum concentrations may be significantly decreased.	Avoid co-administration.
Ritonavir (RTV)	Itraconazole serum concentrations may be increased.	Itraconazole dose >200 mg is not recommended by some; consider monitoring itraconazole serum concentrations to guide dosing PIs serum concentrations may be increased (clinical significance unknown).
Sildenafil	Sildenafil serum concentrations may be increased.	Use with close monitoring. Do not exceed 25 mg in 48-hrs recommended by some.
Sirolimus	Sirolimus serum concentrations may be increased.	Monitor sirolimus concentrations closely with co-administration.
Saquinavir (SQV/r)	Itraconazole serum concentrations may be increased.	Itraconazole dose >200 mg is not recommended by some; consider monitoring itraconazole serum concentrations to guide dosing. PIs serum concentrations may be increased (clinical significance unknown).
Simvastatin	May increase simvastatin.	Avoid co-administration.
Tacrolimus	Tacrolimus serum concentrations may be increased.	Monitor tacrolimus concentrations closely with co-administration.

Drug	Effect of Interaction	Recommendations/Comments
Tadalafil	Tadalafil serum concentrations may be increased.	Use with close monitoring Start with 5 mg. Do not exceed 10 mg in 72 hrs recommended by some.
Terfenadine	Risk of QTc prolongation may be increased.	Contraindicated. Alternative: fexofenadine.
Triazolam	Triazolam serum concentrations may be increased.	Avoid co-administration. Consider lorazepam, oxazepam, or temazepam.
Tolbutamide	Risk of hypoglycemia may be increased.	Monitor.
Tipranavir (TPV/r)	Itraconazole serum concentrations may be increased.	Itraconazole dose >200 mg is not recommended by some; consider monitoring itraconazole serum concentrations to guide dosing PIs serum concentrations may be increased (clinical significance unknown).
Vardenafil	Vardenafil serum concentrations may be increased.	Use with close monitoring. Do not exceed 2.5 mg in 24 hrs recommended by some.
Verapamil	Verapamil serum concentrations may be increased.	Monitor.
Warfarin	Anticoagulation may be increased.	Monitor INR closely with co-administration.

DRUG-TO-DRUG INTERACTION – KETOCONAZOLE

Drug	Effect of Interaction	Recommendations/Comments
Alprazolam	Alprazolam serum levels may be increased .	May increase risk of sedation. Consider lorazepam, oxazepam, or temazepam.
Astemizole	Risk of QTc prolongation may be increased.	Contraindicated.
Amprenavir (APV)	Ketoconazole AUC increased by 44%.	Ketoconazole dose > or = 400 mg/day is not recommended.
Atazanavir (ATV)	No significant interaction.	No dose adjustment necessary.
Alcohol	Disulfiram-type reaction may occur.	Avoid co-administration.
Antacid	May significantly decrease ketoconazole serum concentrations.	Separate administration time by >2 hrs.
Bismuth	Ketoconazole serum concentrations may be decreased.	Avoid co-administration.
Carbamazepine	Ketoconazole serum concentrations may be decreased.	Monitor for therapeutic effect; ketoconazole dose may need to be increased.
Cimetidine	Ketoconazole serum concentrations may be decreased.	Avoid co-administration.
Cisapride	Risk of QTc prolongation may be increased.	Contraindicated.
Clarithromycin	Clarithromycin and ketoconazole serum concentrations may be increased.	Consider clarithromycin dose adjustment with CrCl <30 mL/min. Consider Azithromycin with ketoconazole co-administration.

KETOCONAZOLE *(cont.)*

Drug	Effect of Interaction	Recommendations/Comments
Cyclosporine	Cyclosporine serum concentrations may be significantly increased.	Monitor cyclosporine serum concentrations closely with dose adjustment.
Diazepam	Diazepam serum levels may be increased.	May increase risk of sedation. Consider lorazepam, oxazepam, or temazepam.
ddI (buffered suspension)	Ketoconazole serum concentrations may be decreased.	Use ddI (enteric-coated) Consider fluconazole or separate >2 hrs apart.
Dofetilide	Increased QTc.	Avoid.
DLV	DLV Cmin increased by 50%.	Clinical significance unknown. Use standard dose.
DRV/r	DRV AUC increased by 42%. Ketoconazole AUC increased by 300%.	Ketoconazole dose >200 mg is not recommended.
EFV	EFV serum concentrations may be increased. Ketoconazole serum concentrations may be decreased.	Monitor for therapeutic efficacy and EFV CNS side effects.
Ergot alkaloids	Ergot alkaloid serum concentrations may be increased.	Avoid co-administration.
Esomeprazole	Ketoconazole serum concentrations may be decreased.	Avoid co-administration.
Etravirine	Ketoconazole serum concentrations may be decreased.	Monitor for therapeutic efficacy.
Famotidine	Ketoconazole serum concentrations may be decreased.	Avoid co-administration.
FPV	Ketoconazole AUC increased by 44% (studied with APV).	Ketoconazole dose > or = 400 mg/day is not recommended.
IDV	IDV AUC increased by 68%.	IDV 600 mg q8h.
Isoniazid	Ketoconazole serum concentrations may be decreased.	Monitor for therapeutic effect; ketoconazole dose may need to be increased.
Lansoprazole	Ketoconazole serum concentrations may be decreased.	Avoid co-administration.
Levacetylmethadol	Increased QTc.	Avoid co-administration.
Lovastatin	Significantly increased lovastatin.	Avoid co-administration.
LPV/r	Ketoconazole AUC increased by 300%.	Ketoconazole dose >200 mg is not recommended.
Maraviroc	Maraviroc serum concentrations may be increased.	Dose: MVC 150 mg twice daily.
Methylprednisolone	Methylprednisolone metabolism decreased by 50%.	Methylprednisolone dose adjustment may be required when co-administration is expected to exceed 7 days.
Midazolam	Midazolam serum levels may be increased.	Contraindicated. Consider lorazepam, oxazepam, or temazepam.
NFV	NFV AUC increased by 36%.	No dose adjustment necessary.

Drug	Effect of Interaction	Recommendations/Comments
Nizatidine	Ketoconazole serum concentrations may be decreased.	Avoid co-administration.
NVP	Ketoconazole AUC decreased by 63%.	Avoid co-administration.
Omeprazole	Ketoconazole serum concentrations may be decreased.	Avoid co-administration.
Pantoprazole	Ketoconazole serum concentrations may be decreased.	Avoid co-administration.
Phenobarbital	Ketoconazole serum concentrations may be decreased.	Monitor.
Phenytoin	Ketoconazole serum concentrations may be decreased.	Monitor for therapeutic effect; ketoconazole dose may need to be increased.
Pimozide	Risk of QTc prolongation may be increased.	Contraindicated.
Quinidine	May significantly increase quinidine serum concentrations.	Contraindicated.
Rabeprazole	Ketoconazole serum concentrations may be decreased.	Avoid co-administration.
Raltegravir	Interaction unlikely.	Use standard dose.
Ranitidine	Ketoconazole serum concentrations may be decreased.	Avoid co-administration.
Rifabutin	Rifabutin serum concentrations may be increased. Ketoconazole serum concentrations may be decreased.	Monitor for therapeutic efficacy of ketoconazole and rifabutin toxicity (e.g., uveitis).
Rifampin	Ketoconazole serum concentrations decreased by 50%.	Avoid co-administration. Consider rifabutin.
RTV	Ketoconazole AUC increased by 300%.	Ketoconazole dose >200 mg is not recommended.
Simvastatin	Significantly increased simvastatin.	Avoid co-administration.
Sirolimus	Sirolimus serum concentrations may be significantly increased.	Monitor sirolimus serum concentrations closely with dose adjustment.
SQV	SQV AUC increased by 300%.	No dose adjustment necessary.
Tacrolimus	Tacrolimus serum concentrations may be significantly increased.	Monitor tacrolimus serum concentrations closely with dose adjustment.
Terfenadine	Risk of QTc prolongation may be increased.	Contraindicated.
Triazolam	Triazolam serum levels may be increased.	Contraindicated. Consider lorazepam, oxazepam, or temazepam.
Theophylline	Theophylline serum concentrations may be increased.	Monitor theophylline serum concentrations with dose adjustment.

DRUG INTERACTIONS

KETOCONAZOLE *(cont.)*

Drug	Effect of Interaction	Recommendations/Comments
TPV/r	Ketoconazole serum concentrations may be increased.	Ketoconazole dose >200 mg is not recommended.
Warfarin	Anticoagulation may be increased.	Monitor INR closely.

DRUG-TO-DRUG INTERACTION – LAMIVUDINE

Drug	Effect of Interaction	Recommendations/Comments
Abacavir	3TC AUC decreased by 15%; Cmax decreased by 35%.	Not clinically significant. Use standard dose.
Methadone	3TC: No reported interaction. Methadone: No change.	Not clinically significant. Use standard dose.
Nelfinavir	No effect on 3TC AUC.	Not clinically significant. Use standard doses of both.
Trimethoprim/ Sulfamethoxazole	3TC AUC increased by 44%.	Not clinically significant. Use standard dose.

DRUG-TO-DRUG INTERACTION – MINOCYCLINE

Drug	Effect of Interaction	Recommendations/Comments
Acitretin	May increase intracranial pressure.	Contraindicated.
Bismuth salts (bismuth subsalicylate-pepto-bismol)	Bismuth salts chelate tetracyclines resulting in a decreased absorption of tetracycline.	Administer bismuth 2 hrs after tetracycline.
Carbamazepine	Co-administration may decrease tetracyclines serum concentrations.	Avoid carbamazepine co-administration. Monitor closely for tetracycline therapy failure.
Cholestyramine	Co-administration may significantly reduce tetracyclines absorption.	Avoid co-administration.
Colestipol	Co-administration significantly reduce tetracyclines absorption.	Avoid co-administration.
ddI (buffer in peds formulation) contains cations	Polyvalent metal cations form an insoluble chelate with tetracyclines resulting in decreased absorption and serum levels of tetracyclines.	Separate administration by 4 hrs.
Digoxin	Co-administration may result in increased digoxin concentration (in about 10% of pts).	Monitor serum level with sign and symptoms of digoxin toxicity.
Methoxyflurane	Case reports of renal failure with co-administration with tetracycline.	Avoid co-administration.
Non-depolarizing neuromuscular blocker (e.g., vecuronium, pancuronium, rocuronium)	May potentiate non-depolarizing neuromuscular blocker.	Use with close monitoring.

Drug	Effect of Interaction	Recommendations/Comments
Oral contraceptives	Tetracyclines may decrease the efficacy of oral contraceptives.	Consider an additional form of contraception.
Penicillins	*In vitro* antagonism when co-administered. Bacteriocidal effect of penicillins may be diminished *in vivo*.	Avoid co-administration.
Phenobarbital	Co-administration may decrease tetracyclines serum concentrations.	Avoid phenobarbital co-administration. Monitor closely tetracycline for therapy failure.
Phenytoin	Co-administration may decrease tetracyclines serum concentrations.	Avoid phenytoin co-administration. Monitor closely for tetracycline therapy failure.
Polyvalent metal cations (aluminum, zinc, magnesium, iron, calcium [milk])	Polyvalent metal cations form an insoluble chelate with tetracyclines resulting in decreased absorption.	Separate administration by 4 hrs.
Quinapril	Magnesium excipient may reduce tetracyclines absorption.	Avoid co-administration.
Rifabutin	Co-administration may decrease tetracyclines serum concentrations.	Avoid rifabutin co-administration. Monitor closely for tetracycline therapy failure.
Rifampin	Co-administration may decrease tetracyclines serum concentrations.	Avoid rifampin co-administration. Monitor closely for tetracycline therapy failure.
Urinary alkalinizers (sodium lactate, sodium bicarbonate)	Co-administration results in increased urinary excretion of tetracyclines by 24–65%.	Avoid co-administration.
Warfarin	Co-administration may increase INR.	Monitor INR closely.

DRUG-TO-DRUG INTERACTION – POSACONAZOLE

Drug	Effect of Interaction	Recommendations/Comments
Alprazolam	Alprazolam serum concentrations may be increased.	Consider lorazepam, oxazepam, or temazepam.
Amiodarone	Amiodarone serum concentrations may be increased.	Avoid or use with close monitoring.
Amlodipine	Amlodipine serum concentrations may be increased.	Avoid or use with close monitoring.
Astemizole	Risk of QTc prolongation may be increased.	Contraindicated.
Atazanavir	May increase posaconazole serum concentrations.	Clinical significance unclear; use standard doses.
Bismuth	No significant interaction.	No dose adjustment necessary.
Carbamazepine	Carbamazepine serum concentrations may be increased.	Monitor carbamazepine serum concentrations closely with co-administration.

POSACONAZOLE *(cont.)*

Drug	Effect of Interaction	Recommendations/Comments
Cimetidine	Posaconazole AUC decreased by 39%.	Avoid co-administration. Use an alternative H₂ blocker.
Cisapride	Risk of QTc prolongation may be increased.	Contraindicated.
Cyclosporine	Cyclosporine serum levels concentrations may be increased.	Reduce cyclosporine dose by 25% with TDM.
Diazepam	Diazepam serum concentrations may be increased.	Consider lorazepam, oxazepam, or temazepam.
Digoxin	May increase digoxin serum concentrations.	Monitor digoxin serum concentrations with co-administration.
Diltiazem	Diltiazem serum concentrations may be increased.	Avoid or use with close monitoring.
Dofetilide	Dofetilide serum concentrations may be increased.	Avoid or use with close monitoring.
EFV	May increase EFV serum concentrations. Posaconazole AUC decreased 50%.	Avoid concomitant use unless the benefit outweighs the risks.
Ergot alkaloids	Ergot alkaloid serum levels may be increased.	Contraindicated.
Esomeprazole	Posaconazole decreased 32%.	Avoid co-administration.
ETR	May decrease posaconazole serum concentrations.	Use with close monitoring for therapeutic efficacy.
Famotidine	No significant interaction.	No dose adjustment necessary.
Felodipine	Felodipine serum concentrations may be increased.	Avoid or use with close monitoring.
Glimepiride	No significant interaction.	No dose adjustment necessary.
Glipizide	No significant interaction.	No dose adjustment necessary.
Glyburide	No significant interaction.	No dose adjustment necessary.
Halofantrine	Risk of QTc prolongation may be increased.	Contraindicated.
Indinavir	May increase posaconazole serum concentrations.	Clinical significance unclear; use standard doses.
Irinotecan	Irinotecan serum concentrations may be increased.	Avoid or use with close monitoring.
Lansoprazole	May decrease posaconazole.	Use with caution.
Lovastatin	Lovastatin serum concentrations may be increased.	Consider pravastatin, atorvastatin, and rosuvastatin.
LPV/r	Posaconazole serum concentrations may be decreased.	Use with close monitoring for therapeutic efficacy.
Midazolam	Midazolam AUC increased by 83%.	Consider lorazepam, oxazepam, or temazepam.
MVC	May increase MVC serum concentrations.	Consider MVC 150–300 mg twice daily.

Drug	Effect of Interaction	Recommendations/Comments
NFV	Posaconazole serum concentrations may be decreased.	Use with close monitoring for therapeutic efficacy.
Nifedipine	Nifedipine serum concentrations may be increased.	Avoid or use with close monitoring.
Nisoldipine	Nisoldipine serum concentrations may be increased.	Avoid or use with close monitoring.
Nizatidine	No significant interaction.	No dose adjustment necessary.
Omeprazole	May decrease posaconazole.	Use with caution.
Pantoprazole	May decrease posaconazole.	Use with caution.
Phenytoin	Posaconazole AUC decreased by 50%.	Avoid co-administration unless the benefit outweighs the risks.
Pimozide	Risk of QTc prolongation may be increased.	Contraindicated.
Quinidine	Risk of QTc prolongation may be increased.	Contraindicated.
Rabeprazole	May decrease posaconazole.	Use with caution.
RAL	Interaction unlikely.	Use standard doses.
Ranitidine	No significant interaction.	No dose adjustment necessary.
Rifabutin	Rifabutin AUC increased by 72%. Posaconazole AUC decreased by 49%.	Avoid co-administration unless the benefit outweighs the risks. Monitor for sign and symptoms of uveitis.
Rifampin	May significantly decrease posaconazole serum concentrations.	Avoid co-administration.
RTV	May increase RTV serum concentrations.	No dose adjustment necessary when RTV dose is 100–200 mg/day.
Sildenafil	Sildenafil serum concentrations may be increased.	Avoid or use with close monitoring.
Simvastatin	Simvastatin serum concentrations may be increased.	Consider pravastatin, atorvastatin, and rosuvastatin.
Sirolimus	Sirolimus serum concentrations may be increased.	Contraindicated. Consider tacrolimus with co-administration.
Tacrolimus	Tacrolimus serum concentrations may be increased.	Reduce tacrolimus dose to 1/3 of original dose with TDM.
Tadalafil	Tadalafil serum concentrations may be increased.	Avoid or use with close monitoring.
Terfenadine	Risk of QTc prolongation may be increased.	Contraindicated.
TPV/r	Posaconazole serum concentrations may be decreased.	Use with close monitoring for therapeutic efficacy.
Triazolam	Triazolam serum concentrations may be increased.	Consider lorazepam, oxazepam, or temazepam.
Vardenafil	Vardenafil serum concentrations may be increased.	Avoid or use with close monitoring.
Verapamil	Verapamil serum concentrations may be increased.	Avoid or use with close monitoring.

POSACONAZOLE *(cont.)*

Drug	Effect of Interaction	Recommendations/Comments
Vinblastine	Vinblastine serum concentrations may be increased.	Avoid or use with close monitoring for neuropathy. Consider dose adjustment.
Vincristine	Vincristine serum concentrations may be increased.	Avoid or use with close monitoring for neuropathy. Consider dose adjustment.
Warfarin	May increase INR.	Monitor INR closely.

DRUG-TO-DRUG INTERACTION – RIFABUTIN

Drug	Effect of Interaction	Recommendations/Comments
Atazanavir (ATV)	Rifabutin AUC increased by 110% and Cmin increased by 243% with rifabutin 150 mg every day co-administration. ATV AUC increased by 191%.	Recommended dosing: ATV 400 mg once-daily **or** ATV 300 mg + RTV100 mg once daily with rifabutin 150 mg 3 × /wk.
Bisoprolol	Rifabutin may decrease serum concentrations of co-administered drug.	Titrate to effect.
Clarithromycin	Rifabutin AUC increased by 56% and clarithromycin AUC decreased by 50%.	Clinical significance unknown since clarithromycin intracellular level is likely to be higher. Monitor for uveitis. Consider switching to azithromycin.
Corticosteroids	Rifabutin may decrease serum concentrations of co-administered drug.	Corticosteroid dose may need to be increased.
Cyclosporine	Rifabutin may decrease serum concentrations of co-administered drug.	Monitor cyclosporine serum concentrations closely with co-administration. Cyclosporine dose will likely need to be increased.
Darunavir (DRV)	Rifabutin serum concentrations may be increased. The rifabutin PK parameters are comparable between rifabutin 150 mg every other day plus DRV/r 600/100 mg twice daily and rifabutin 300 mg once daily.	Dose: rifabutin dose reduction (rifabutin 150 mg every other day with DRV/r co-administration).
Delavirdine (DLV)	Rifabutin AUC increased by 100% and DLV AUC decreased by 80%.	Contraindicated.
Diazepam	Rifabutin may decrease serum concentrations of co-administered drug.	Titrate to effect.
Digoxin	Rifabutin may decrease co-administered drug.	Monitor digoxin serum concentrations with co-administration.
Disopyramide	Rifabutin may decrease co-administered drug.	Monitor for therapeutic efficacy.

Drug	Effect of Interaction	Recommendations/Comments
Doxycycline	Rifabutin may decrease serum concentrations of co-administered drug.	Consider an alternative antibiotic.
Efavirenz (EFV)	Rifabutin AUC decreased by 38%. No change in EFV AUC.	Recommended dosing: increase rifabutin to 450 mg/day **or** 600 mg 3 ×/wk with standard dose EFV 600 mg qhs.
Etravirine (ETR)	ETR AUC and Cmin decreased 37% and 35%, respectively. Rifabutin AUC decreased 17%.	Clinical significance unclear. Dose: ETR 200 mg twice daily plus rifabutin 300 mg once daily. Avoid co-administration of DRV/r or SQV/r with rifabutin and ETR due to potential additive decrease in etravirine exposure.
Fluconazole	Fluconazole increases rifabutin AUC by 80%. Fluconazole AUC not affected.	Monitor for uveitis.
Indinavir (IDV)	Rifabutin AUC increased by 204% and IDV AUC decreased by 32%.	Recommended dosing: rifabutin 150 mg every other day (**or** 150 mg 3 ×/wk) with IDV 800 mg + RTV 100 mg twice daily (recommended but no data) **or** rifabutin 150 mg once daily (**or** 300 mg 3 ×/wk) with IDV 1000 mg q8h (bid dosing with RTV boosting preferred).
Itraconazole	Rifabutin may decrease co-administered drug.	Monitor itraconazole serum concentrations and signs and symptoms of uveitis with co-administration.
Ketoconazole	Rifabutin may decrease ketoconazole. Ketoconazole may increase rifabutin.	Monitor for uveitis with co-administration.
Levothyroxine	Rifabutin may decrease serum concentrations of co-administered drug.	Monitor T3/T4 with co-administration.
Lopinavir (LPV/r)	Rifabutin AUC increased by 203%. LPV serum level increased by 20% (NS).	Recommended dosing: LPV/r 2 tabs (400/100 mg) twice daily with rifabutin 150 mg every other day (**or** 150 mg 3 ×/wk).
Maraviroc (MVC)	MVC serum concentrations may be decreased.	No data. Dose: MVC 600 mg twice daily.
Methadone	No significant interactions.	Use standard dose.
Metoprolol	Rifabutin may decrease serum concentrations of co-administered drug.	Titrate to effect.
Mexiletine	Rifabutin may decrease co-administered drug.	Monitor for therapeutic efficacy.
Midazolam	Rifabutin may decrease serum concentrations of co-administered drug.	Titrate to effect.
Nelfinavir	NFV AUC decreased by 32%. Rifabutin concentrations increased by 207%.	Recommended dosing NFV 1000 mg three times daily with rifabutin 150 mg once daily (**or** 300 mg 3 ×/wk).

RIFABUTIN *(cont.)*

Drug	Effect of Interaction	Recommendations/Comments
Nevirapine (NVP)	Rifabutin AUC increased by 16% (NS). NVP AUC unchanged.	Unlikely to be clinically significant. Recommended dosing: rifabutin 300 mg/day (**or** 300 mg 3 × /wk).
Oral contraceptives and estrogens	Rifabutin may decrease serum concentrations of co-administered drug.	Consider an alternative barrier form of contraception with co-administration.
Posaconazole	Rifabutin AUC increased by 72%. Posaconazole AUC decreased by 49%.	Avoid co-administration.
Propranolol	Rifabutin may decrease serum concentrations of co-administered drug.	Titrate to effect.
Quinidine	Rifabutin may decrease serum concentrations of co-administered drug.	Monitor for therapeutic efficacy.
Quinine	Rifabutin may decrease serum concentrations of co-administered drug.	Monitor for therapeutic efficacy.
Raltegravir	No significant interaction.	Use standard dose.
Ritonavir (RTV)	Rifabutin AUC increased by 400%.	Recommended dose: rifabutin 150 mg every other day (**or** 150 mg 3 × /wk) with standard dose of RTV.
Saquinavir (SQV)	SQV AUC decreased by 43%.	Do not co-administer SQV with rifabutin as sole PI. Recommended dosing: consider RTV + SQV 400 mg + 400 mg with rifabutin 150 mg every other day (**or** 3 × /wk) **or** SQV 1000 mg + RTV 100 mg twice daily with rifabutin 150 mg every other day (no data, but likely to attain adequate serum concentrations).
Sirolimus	Rifabutin may significantly decrease sirolimus serum concentrations.	Monitor sirolimus serum concentrations closely with co-administration. Sirolimus dose will need to be increased.
Tacrolimus	Rifabutin may significantly decrease tacrolimus serum concentrations.	Monitor tacrolimus serum concentrations closely with co-administration. Tacrolimus dose will likely need to be increased.
Theophylline	Rifabutin may decrease serum concentrations of co-administered drug.	Monitor theophylline serum concentrations with co-administration.
Tipranavir (TPV)	Rifabutin AUC increased 190%. No significant change in TPV.	Dose reduce rifabutin to 150 mg every other day.
Tocainide	Rifabutin may decrease serum concentrations of co-administered drug.	Monitor for therapeutic efficacy.

Drug	Effect of Interaction	Recommendations/Comments
Triazolam	Rifabutin may decrease serum concentrations of co-administered drug.	Titrate to effect.
Verapamil	Rifabutin may decrease co-administered drug.	Titrate to effect.
Voriconazole	May significantly decrease voriconazole serum concentrations.	Contraindicated.
Warfarin	Rifabutin may decrease serum concentrations of co-administered drug.	Monitor INR closely with co-administration. Warfarin dose may need to be increase.

DRUG-TO-DRUG INTERACTION – RIFAPENTINE

Drug	Effect of Interaction	Recommendations/Comments
Aluminum containing antacids	Controversial but may decrease oral absorption of RIF; some studies found no effect.	Consider separate oral administration by 4 hrs.
Aminosalicylic acid granules	Absorption of RIF may be impaired by the bentonite excipient.	Separate administration by 8–12 hrs intervals.
Amiodarone	Amiodarone serum concentrations may be significantly decreased.	Monitor EKG with co-administration. Amiodarone dose may need to be increased.
Amlodipine	Amlodipine serum concentrations may be significantly decreased.	Titrate to effect.
Aprepitant	Aprepitant serum concentrations may be decreased.	Apretitant dose may need to be increased.
Atazanavir	Atazanavir Cmin decreased 60%–93%.	Contraindicated. Use rifabutin with co-administration.
Atorvastatin	Atorvastatin decreased by 80%.	Titrate to effect. Pravastatin or rosuvastatin are less likely to interact with rifampin.
Atovaquone	Atovaquone AUC decreased by approximately 50%.	Avoid co-administration. Consider Aerosolized pentamidine for PCP prophylaxis.
Bisoprolol	Bisoprolol serum concentrations may be significantly decreased.	Bisoprolol dose may need to be increased.
Bosentan	Bosentan AUC decreased 60%.	May need to increase bosentan dose.
Buprenorphine	Buprenorphine serum concentrations may be decreased.	Titrate buprenorphine to effect.
Caspofungin	Caspofungin trough concentrations decreased 30%.	Use caspofungin 70 mg with rifampin co-administration.
Chlorpropamide	Chlorpropamide serum concentrations decreased by up to 50%.	Monitor blood glucose control with co-administration. Consider a shorter acting hypoglycemic agent.
Clarithromycin	Clarithromycin serum concentrations may be significantly decreased.	Consider azithromycin.
Cyclosporine	Cyclosporine serum concentrations may be significantly decreased.	Monitor cyclosporine serum concentrations closely with co-administration. Cyclosporine dose may need to be increased.

DRUG INTERACTIONS

RIFAPENTINE *(cont.)*

Drug	Effect of Interaction	Recommendations/Comments
Dapsone	Dapsone serum concentrations may be decreased.	For PCP prophylaxis, if unable to tolerate TMP/SMX, consider using aerosolized pentamidine.
Darunavir/ ritonavir	DRV serum concentrations may be significantly decreased.	Contraindicated. Use rifabutin with co-administration.
Dasatinib	Dasatinib AUC decreased 82%.	Higher dasatinib dose is recommended at steady-state (2 wks).
Delavirdine	Delavirdine area under the curve decreased 96%.	Contraindicated.
Dexamethasone	Dexamethasone serum concentrations may be significantly decreased.	Dexamethasone dose may need to be increased.
Diazepam	Diazepam serum concentrations may be significantly decreased.	Titrate to effect.
Digoxin	Digoxin serum concentrations may be decreased by 30% to 60%.	Monitor digoxin serum concentrations with co-administration.
Diltiazem	Diltiazem serum concentrations may be significantly decreased.	Titrate to effect.
Disopyramide	Disopyramide half-life decreased by 40%.	Monitor EKG with co-administration. Disopyramide dose may need to be increased.
Doxycycline	Doxycycline serum concentrations may be decreased.	Clinical significance unclear.
Efavirenz	Efavirenz area under the curve decreased 26%. No change in rifampin area under the curve.	Recommended dosing: efavirenz 600–800 mg/day with rifampin 600 mg once daily (monitor for efavirenz central nervous system side effects). May decrease to efavirenz 600 mg/day if 800 mg dose not easily tolerated.
Erlotinib	Erlotinib AUC decreased by approximately 67% to 80%.	Higher dose of Erlotinib may be needed.
Etravirine	ETR serum concentrations may be significantly decreased.	Avoid co-administration until more data becomes available.
Everolimus	Everolimus AUC decreased by 58%.	Monitor everolimus serum concentrations closely with co-administration. Dose may need to be increased.
Fluconazole	Fluconazole serum concentrations decreased by 23–56%.	Consider switching to rifabutin with co-administration.
Fosamprenavir	No data, but significant decrease in amprenavir serum concentrations expected. When studied with Amprenavir, AUC decreased 82%; Cmin decreased 92%.	Contraindicated. Use rifabutin with co-administration.
Glimepiride	Glimepiride serum concentrations may be significantly decreased.	Monitor glucose control with co-administration.
Glyburide	Glyburide serum concentrations may be significantly decreased.	Monitor glucose control with co-administration.

Drug	Effect of Interaction	Recommendations/Comments
Indinavir	Indinavir area under the curve decreased 89%.	Contraindicated. Use rifabutin with co-administration.
Itraconazole	Itraconazole serum concentrations may be significantly decreased.	Avoid co-administration. Consider rifabutin with monitoring of itraconazole serum concentrations and monitor for uveitis.
Ketoconazole	Ketoconazole serum concentrations decreased by 50%.	Avoid co-administration. Consider rifabutin.
Lamotrigine	Lamotrigine AUC decreased by approximately 40%.	Titrate to effect.
Levothyroxine	Levothyroxine serum concentrations may be significantly decreased.	Monitor TSH. May need higher levothyroxine dose with co-administration.
Linezolid	Case reports of significant decrease in linezolid serum concentrations with co-administration.	Avoid or use with caution.
Lopinavir/ ritonavir	Lopinavir AUC decreased 75%, and Cmin decreased 99%.	Co-administration not recommended. Although studies used lopinavir/ritonavir 400/100 mg twice daily (3 capsules) plus ritonavir 300 mg twice daily or LPV/r 3 to 4 tablets twice daily to overcome this interaction, high incidence of nausea, vomiting, and grade 4 LFTs elevation were common. Consider rifabutin with LPV/r co-administration.
Lovastatin	Lovastatin serum concentrations may be significantly decreased.	Titrate to effect. Pravastatin or rosuvastatin are less likely to interact with rifampin.
Maraviroc	Maraviroc AUC decreased by 63%.	Increase maraviroc's dose to 600 mg BID with rifampin co-administration.
Mefloquine	Mefloquine AUC decreased 68%.	Consider an alternative anti-malarial drug.
Methadone and other opiate agonists	Opiate serum concentrations may be significantly decreased. Methadone AUC decreased 30–65%.	Monitor for signs and symptoms of withdrawal and titrate opiate to effect.
Metoprolol	Metoprolol serum concentrations decreased by 33%.	Titrate to effect.
Mexiletine	Mexiletine half-life decreased by 5–9 hrs.	Monitor EKG with co-administration. Mexiletine dose may need to be increased.
Midazolam	Midazolam serum concentrations may be significantly decreased.	Titrate to effect.
Montelukast	Montelukast AUC decreased by 40%.	Dose of montelukast may need to be increased.
Morphine	Morphine AUC decreased by 45%.	Titrate to effect.
Moxifloxacin	Moxifloxacin serum concentrations decreased by approximately 30%.	Monitor for therapeutic efficacy. Consider levofloxacin.
Mycopheno-late Mofetil	Mycophenolate AUC decreased 67%.	Mycophenolate dose may need to be increased.
Nelfinavir	Nelfinavir area under the curve decreased 82%.	Contraindicated. Use rifabutin with co-administration.

RIFAPENTINE *(cont.)*

Drug	Effect of Interaction	Recommendations/Comments
Nevirapine	Nevirapine Cmin decreased 37%–68%. Nevirapine area under the curve decreased 37%–58%. Rifampin area under the curve increased 11% (not significant).	Avoid co-administration.
Nifedipine	Nifedipine serum concentrations may be decreased up to 70%.	Titrate to effect.
Nilotinib	Nilotinib AUC decreased by 80%.	Avoid co-administration.
Oral contra-ceptives	Ethinyl estradiol Cmin decreased by 79%. Norethindrone Cmin decreased by 89%.	Use an alternative or additional barrier form of contraception. Despite these PK interactions, all subjects remained anovulatory as indicated by undetectable progesterone levels.
Phenytoin	Phenytoin serum concentrations may be decreased.	Monitor phenytoin serum concentrations closely with co-administration.
Pioglitazone	Pioglitazone AUC decreased 54%.	Monitor glucose control with co-administration. Pioglitazone dose may need to be increased.
Posaconazole	Posaconazole serum concentrations may be significantly decreased.	Contraindicated. Rifabutin may be considered if benefit outweighs the risks. Use with close monitoring of posaconazole serum concentrations and monitor for sign and symptoms of uveitis.
Praziquantel	Praziquantel serum concentrations may be significantly decreased.	Avoid co-administration.
Prednisone	Prednisone serum concentrations decreased by up to 60%.	Prednisone dose may need to be increased.
Propafenone	Propafenone serum concentrations may be significantly decreased.	Monitor EKG with co-administration. Propafenone dose may need to be increased.
Propranolol	Propranolol serum concentrations may be significantly decreased.	Titrate to effect.
Quinidine	Quinidine serum concentrations may be significantly decreased.	Monitor quinidine serum concentrations. May need to increase quinidine dose.
Quinine	Quinine serum concentrations may be significantly decreased.	Quinine dose may need to increased.
Raltegravir	RAL AUC and Cmin decreased by 40% and 61%, respectively. Increasing raltegravir to 800 mg twice daily resulted in adequate area under the curve but Cmin was decreased by 53%.	Increase raltegravir dose to 800 mg BID with close monitoring of virologic efficacy. Consider using rifabutin with co-administration.
Ranolazine	Ranolazine AUC decreased 95%.	Contraindicated.
Repaglinide	Repaglinide AUC decreased 57%.	Titrate to effect.
Ritonavir	Ritonavir area under the curve decreased 35%.	Ritonavir standard dosage recommended by manufacturer, but co-administration with rifampin should be avoided.

Drug	Effect of Interaction	Recommendations/Comments
Rosiglitazone	Rosiglitazone AUC decreased by 54%	Monitor glucose control with co-administration.
Saquinavir	Saquinavir area under the curve decreased 70% (saquinavir soft gel capsules without ritonavir-boosting).	Contraindicated due to the high incidence of hepatitis with saquinavir 1000 mg + ritonavir 100 mg twice daily.
Simvastatin	Simvastatin serum concentrations decreased by 56% to 94%.	Titrate to effect. Pravastatin or rosuvastatin are less likely to interact with rifampin.
Sirolimus	Sirolimus serum concentrations decreased 82%.	Monitor sirolimus serum concentrations closely with co-administration. Sirolimus dose may need to be increased.
Tacrolimus	Tacrolimus serum concentrations may be significantly decreased.	Monitor tacrolimus serum concentrations closely with co-administration. Tacrolimus dose may need to be increased.
Tamoxifen	Tamoxifen AUC decreased 86%.	Higher dose may be needed.
Telithromycin	Telithromycin AUC decreased 79%.	Avoid co-administration.
Temsirolimus	Temsirolimus AUC decreased up to 56%.	Monitor temsirolimus serum concentration with dose titration.
Theophylline	Theophylline serum concentrations decreased 18%.	Monitor Theophylline serum concentrations. Theophylline dose may need to be increased.
Tipranavir/ritonavir	May significantly decrease tipranavir serum concentrations.	Contraindicated. Use rifabutin with co-administration.
Tocainide	Tocainide AUC decreased 28%.	Tocainide dose may need to be increased.
Tolbutamide	Tolbutamide serum concentrations may be significantly decreased.	Monitor blood glucose control with co-administration.
Triazolam	Triazolam serum concentrations may be significantly decreased.	Titrate to effect.
Verapamil	Verapamil serum concentrations may be significantly decreased.	Titrate to effect.
Voriconazole	Voriconazole serum concentrations decreased.	Contraindicated.
Warfarin	Warfarin serum concentrations may be significantly decreased.	Monitor INR closely. May need higher warfarin dose.
Zidovudine	Zidovudine area under the curve decreased 47%. Intracellular concentrations not measured.	Consider switching to rifabutin.

DRUG-TO-DRUG INTERACTION – TELITHROMYCIN

Drug	Effect of Interaction	Recommendations/Comments
Amiodarone	May significantly increase amiodarone serum concentrations.	Use with caution. Consider an alternative antimicrobial.
Atazanavir	May significantly increase telithromycin serum concentrations.	Use with caution. Monitor closely for hepatitis.

TELITHROMYCIN *(cont.)*

Drug	Effect of Interaction	Recommendations/Comments
Atorvastatin	Significant increase in atorvastatin serum concentrations.	Should be avoided, if telithromycin used, hold statins for duration of therapy. Pravastatin and fluvastatin (and perhaps rosuvastatin) may be considered.
Carbamezapine	May significantly decrease telithromycin serum concentrations.	Avoid or use with caution.
Cisapride	Increase risk of QTc prolongation.	Contraindicated.
Cyclosporine	May significantly increase cyclosporine serum concentrations.	Monitor cyclosporine serum concentrations closely.
Delavirdine	May significantly increase telithromycin serum concentrations.	Use with caution. Monitor closely for hepatitis.
Darunavir	May significantly increase telithromycin serum concentrations.	Use with caution. Monitor closely for hepatitis.
Digoxin	Digoxin Cmax was increased by 73% with co-administration.	Use with close monitoring.
Dofetilide	Significant increase in dofetilide serum concentrations.	Contraindicated.
Efavirenz	May significantly decrease telithromycin serum concentrations.	Avoid or use with caution.
Ergotamine	Significant increase in ergotamine serum concentrations.	Contraindicated.
Etravirine	May decrease telithromycin serum concentrations.	Avoid or use with caution.
Fentanyl	May significantly increase fentanyl serum concentrations.	Avoid co-administration. Consider morphine.
Fluconazole	May increase QTc.	Use with caution.
Fosamprenavir	May significantly increase telithromycin serum concentrations.	Use with caution. Monitor closely for hepatitis.
Indinavir	May significantly increase telithromycin serum concentrations.	Use with caution. Monitor closely for hepatitis.
Itraconazole	May significantly increase telithromycin serum concentrations.	Use with caution. Monitor closely for hepatitis.
Ketoconazole	May increase telithromycin serum concentrations. Use with caution.	Use with caution. Monitor closely for hepatitis.
Lopinavir	May significantly increase telithromycin serum concentrations.	Use with caution. Monitor closely for hepatitis.
Lovastatin	Significant increase in lovastatin serum concentrations.	Should be avoided, if telithromycin used, hold statins for duration of therapy. Pravastatin and fluvastatin (and perhaps rosuvastatin) may be considered.
Metoprolol	Metoprolol Cmax increased by 38%.	Use with caution in pts with CHF.
Midazolam	May significantly increase midazolam serum concentrations.	Avoid co-administration. Consider lorazepam.

Drug	Effect of Interaction	Recommendations/Comments
Nelfinavir	May significantly increase telithromycin serum concentrations.	Use with caution. Monitor closely for hepatitis.
Nevirapine	May significantly decrease telithromycin serum concentrations.	Avoid or use with caution.
Oral contraceptive	Levonorgestrel was increased by 50% with co-administration, but no effect on ethinyl estradiol was observed.	Monitor for increased levonorgestrel associated adverse events.
Phenobarbital	May significantly decrease telithromycin serum concentrations.	Avoid or use with caution.
Phenytoin	May significantly decrease telithromycin serum concentrations.	Avoid or use with caution.
Pimozide	Increase risk of QTc prolongation.	Contraindicated.
Posaconazole	May significantly increase telithromycin serum concentrations.	Use with caution. Monitor closely for hepatitis.
Procainamide	Significant increase in procainamide serum concentrations.	Contraindicated.
Quinidine	Significant increase in quinidine serum concentrations.	Contraindicated.
Ranolazine	May significantly increase ranolazine serum concentrations.	Avoid co-administration.
Rifabutin	May decrease telithromycin serum concentrations.	Use with close monitoring for therapeutic efficacy. Consider alternative antimicrobial.
Rifampin	Significant decrease in telithromycin serum concentrations.	Contraindicated.
Ritonavir	May significantly increase telithromycin serum concentrations.	Use with caution. Monitor closely for hepatitis.
Saquinavir	May significantly increase telithromycin serum concentrations.	Use with caution. Monitor closely for hepatitis.
Sildenafil	May significantly increase sildenafil serum concentrations.	Use with caution. Do not exceed sildenafil 25 mg in 48 hrs.
Simvastatin	Significant increase in simvastatin serum concentrations.	Should be avoided, if telithromycin used, hold statins for duration of therapy. Pravastatin and fluvastatin (and perhaps rosuvastatin) may be considered.
Sirolimus	May significantly increase sirolimus serum concentrations.	Monitor sirolimus serum concentrations closely.
St Johns Wort	May significantly decrease telithromycin serum concentrations.	Avoid.
Tacrolimus	May significantly increase tacrolimus serum concentrations.	Monitor tacrolimus serum concentrations closely.
Tadalafil	May significantly increase tadalafil serum concentrations.	Use with caution. Do not exceed tadalafil 10 mg in 72 hrs.
Triazolam	May significantly increase triazolam serum concentrations.	Avoid co-administration. Consider lorazepam.

DRUG INTERACTIONS

TELITHROMYCIN *(cont.)*

Drug	Effect of Interaction	Recommendations/Comments
Vardenafil	May significantly increase vardenafil serum concentrations.	Use with caution. Do not exceed vardenafil 2.5 mg in 24 hrs.
Voriconazole	May significantly increase telithromycin serum concentrations.	Use with caution. Monitor closely for hepatitis.
Warfarin	Telithromycin may increase INR with co-administration.	Monitor closely with co-administration.

DRUG-TO-DRUG INTERACTION – TENOFOVIR DF

Drug	Effect of Interaction	Recommendations/Comments
ABC	No evidence of drug-drug interactions.	ABC + TDF + 3TC once daily associated with suboptimal viral suppression. Effect probably due to increased selection for resistance (K65R) rather than drug interaction. Preliminary analysis of AZT/ABC/3TC + TDF as a twice daily regimen showed more favorable results, though unclear whether better than AZT/3TC/ABC alone. Do not co-administer ABC/TDF/3TC without a PI or thymidine analog.
ATV	ATV: AUC decreased by 25%; Cmin decreased by 26% (with RTV); tenofovir not measured. ATV AUC decreased by 25% and Cmin decreased by 40% (without RTV); tenofovir AUC: increased by 24%.	With co-administration use RTV-boosted ATV (ATV 300 mg + RTV 100 mg once-daily). Avoid unboosted ATV.
ddI	ddI EC AUC: increased by 48% (fasted); ddI EC AUC: increased by 60% (fed state). Tenofovir: No change.	Dose adjust ddI EC to 250 mg once daily (for >60 kg) or 200 mg once daily (for <60 kg) with TDF co-administration. Suboptimal virologic response in 91% of pts treated with ddI + TDF + 3TC once daily. Do not use ddI + TDF + 3TC as a triple-NRTI regimen.
Etravirine	ETR AUC decreased by 19%, TDF AUC increased by 15%.	Use standard dose.
Food	Increased bioavailability with food (AUC increased 60%), especially high-fat meals, but levels adequate in fasting state.	Take with or without food.
FTC	No significant drug interaction.	Use standard dose, usually in coformulated version (TDF/FTC or TDF/FTC/EFV).
LPV/r	Tenofovir AUC increased by 34%.	Unlikely to be clinically significant. Use standard dose of both TDF and LPV/r.

Drug	Effect of Interaction	Recommendations/Comments
Norgestimate/ ethinyl estradiol	No significant drug interaction.	Use standard dose.
Probenecid	Tenofovir levels may be increased due to probenecid-induced inhibition of the renal tubular secretion.	Clinical significance unknown.

DRUG-TO-DRUG INTERACTION – TETRACYCLINE

Drug	Effect of Interaction	Recommendations/Comments
Acitretin	May increase intracranial pressure.	Contraindicated.
Bismuth salts (bismuth subsalicylate-pepto-bismol)	Bismuth salts chelate tetracyclines resulting in a decreased absorption of tetracycline.	Administer bismuth 2 hrs after tetracycline.
Carbamazepine	Co-administration may decrease tetracyclines serum concentrations.	Avoid carbamazepine co-administration. Monitor closely for tetracycline therapy failure.
Cholestyramine	Co-administration may significantly reduce tetracyclines absorption.	Avoid co-administration.
Colestipol	Co-administration significantly reduce tetracyclines absorption.	Avoid co-administration.
ddI (buffer in peds formulation) contains cations:	Polyvalent metal cations form an insoluble chelate with tetracyclines resulting in decreased absorption and serum levels of tetracyclines.	Separate administration by 4 hrs.
Digoxin	Co-administration may result in increased digoxin concentration (in about 10% of pts).	Monitor serum level with sign and symptoms of digoxin toxicity.
Methoxyflurane	Case reports of renal failure with co-administration with tetracycline.	Avoid co-administration.
Non-depolarizing neuromuscular blocker (e.g., vecuronium, pancuronium, rocuronium)	May potentiate non-depolarizing neuromuscular blocker.	Use with close monitoring.
Oral contraceptives	Tetracyclines may decrease the efficacy of oral contraceptives.	Consider an additional form of contraception.
Penicillins	*In vitro* antagonism when co-administered. Bacteriocidal effect of penicillins may be diminished *in vivo*.	Avoid co-administration.
Phenobarbital	Co-administration may decrease tetracyclines serum concentrations.	Avoid phenobarbital co-administration. Monitor closely tetracycline for therapy failure.

TETRACYCLINE *(cont.)*

Drug	Effect of Interaction	Recommendations/Comments
Phenytoin	Co-administration may decrease tetracyclines serum concentrations.	Avoid phenytoin co-administration. Monitor closely for tetracycline therapy failure.
Polyvalent metal cations (aluminum, zinc, magnesium, iron, calcium [milk])	Polyvalent metal cations form an insoluble chelate with tetracyclines resulting in decreased absorption.	Separate administration by 4 hrs.
Quinapril	Magnesium excipient may reduce tetracyclines absorption.	Avoid co-administration.
Rifabutin	Co-administration may decrease tetracyclines serum concentrations.	Avoid rifabutin co-administration. Monitor closely for tetracycline therapy failure.
Rifampin	Co-administration may decrease tetracyclines serum concentrations.	Avoid rifampin co-administration. Monitor closely for tetracycline therapy failure.
Urinary alkalinizers (sodium lactate, sodium bicarbonate)	Co-administration results in increased urinary excretion of tetracyclines by 24–65%	Avoid co-administration.
Warfarin	Co-administration may increase INR.	Monitor INR closely.

DRUG-TO-DRUG INTERACTION – TINIDAZOLE

Drug	Effect of Interaction	Recommendations/Comments
Alcohol and propylene glycol	Potential for disulfiram reaction.	Avoid co-administration.
Cholestyramine	May decrease the absorption of tinidazole.	Avoid co-administration or administer tinidazole 2 hrs before cholestyramine.
Cyclosporine	Tinidazole may increase serum level of cyclosporine (based on case reports).	Monitor cyclosporine serum concentration closely.
CYP3A4 Inducers (e.g., rifampin, nevirapine, efavirenz, phenytoin, phenobarbital, carbamezapine.)	May decrease tinidazole serum concentrations.	Monitor for tinidazole therapeutic efficacy.
CYP3A4 Inhibitors (e.g., macrolides, azole anti-fungals, HIV-protease inhibitors...)	May increase tinidazole serum concentrations.	Usual dose likely with single dose administration.
Fluorouracil	Tinidazole may increase serum level and toxicity of fluorouracil.	Monitor for fluorouracil toxicity with co-administration.
Fosphenytoin	Tinidazole may prolong the t½ of fosphenytoin. Fosphenytoin may decrease tinidazole serum concentrations.	Monitor phenytoin serum concentrations and therapeutic effect of tinidazole.

Drug	Effect of Interaction	Recommendations/Comments
Lithium	Tinidazole may increase lithium serum level.	Monitor lithium serum concentration and sign/symptoms of toxicity.
Tacrolimus	Tinidazole may increase serum level of tacrolimus (based on case reports).	Monitor tacrolimus closely with co-administration
Warfarin	Tinidazole may enhance the anticoagulant effect of warfarin.	Monitor INR closely with co-administration.

DRUG-TO-DRUG INTERACTION – TRIMETHOPRIM + SULFAMETHOXAZOLE

Drug	Effect of Interaction	Recommendations/Comments
Cyclosporine	May decrease cyclosporine serum concentrations.	Monitor cyclosporine serum concentrations.
Folinic acid	Possible antagonism.	Avoid co-administration.
Para-aminobenzoic acid (PABA) and derivatives (such as benzocaine, procaine, tetracaine):	theoretical antagonism.	Avoid co-administration.
Phenytoin	May increase phenytoin serum concentrations.	Monitor free phenytoin concentrations with co-administration.
Porfimer	May increase the risk of photosensitivity reaction.	Avoid co-administration.
Sulfonylurea	May increase hypoglycemia.	Monitor closely with co-administration.
Warfarin	May increase INR.	Monitor closely with co-administration.

DRUG-TO-DRUG INTERACTION – VORICONAZOLE

Drug	Effect of Interaction	Recommendations/Comments
Alprazolam	Alprazolam serum levels concentrations may be increased.	Consider lorazepam, oxazepam, or temazepam.
Amlodipine	Amlodipine serum concentrations may be increased.	Monitor.
Astemizole	Risk of QTc prolongation may be increased.	Contraindicated.
Atazanavir	Interaction unlikely with unboosted ATV. Voriconazole AUC may be decreased with ATV/r	Consider voriconazole TDM (target Cmin >2.05 mcg/mL) with ATV/r co-administration.
Azithromycin	No significant interaction.	No dose adjustment necessary.
Carbamazepine	Voriconazole serum concentrations may be decreased.	Contraindicated.
Cimetidine	No significant interaction.	No dose adjustment necessary.
Cisapride	Risk of QTc prolongation may be increased.	Contraindicated.

VORICONAZOLE *(cont.)*

Drug	Effect of Interaction	Recommendations/Comments
Cyclosporine	Cyclosporine AUC increased by 70%.	Reduce cyclosporine dose by 50% with close TDM.
Delavirdine	Voriconazole serum concentrations may be increased.	Consider voriconazole TDM (target Cmin >2.05 mcg/mL and Cmax <6 mcg/mL) with DLV co-administration.
Diazepam	Diazepam serum concentrations may be increased.	Consider lorazepam, oxazepam, or temazepam.
Digoxin	No significant interaction.	No dose adjustment necessary.
Diltiazem	Diltiazem serum concentrations may be increased.	Avoid or use with caution.
DRV/r	Voriconazole serum concentrations may be decreased.	Avoid co-administration. Consider voriconazole TDM (target Cmin >2.05 mcg/mL) with DRV/r co-administration.
Efavirenz	EFV AUC increased by 44%. Voriconazole steady state serum levels decreased by 77%.	Avoid co-administration at standard doses. Voriconazole 400 mg twice-daily plus EFV 300 mg qhs recommended with co-administration.
Ergot alkaloids	Ergot alkaloid serum concentrations may be increased.	Contraindicated.
Erythromycin	No significant PK interaction.	No dose adjustment necessary, but monitor QTc
Etravirine	May increase voriconazole serum concentrations.	Consider voriconazole TDM (target Cmin >2.05 mcg/mL and Cmax <6 mcg/mL) with ETR co-administration.
Felodipine	Felodipine serum concentrations may be increased.	Monitor.
Fosamprenavir	May decrease voriconazole serum concentrations.	Avoid co-administration. Consider voriconazole TDM (target Cmin >2.05 mcg/mL) with FPV/r co-administration.
Glimepiride	Glimepiride serum concentrations may be increased.	Monitor glucose closely with co-administration.
Glipizide	Glipizide serum concentrations may be increased.	Monitor glucose closely with co-administration.
Glyburide	Glyburide serum concentrations may be increased.	Monitor glucose closely with co-administration.
Indinavir	No significant interaction with unboosted IDV.	No dose adjustment necessary with unboosted IDV. Consider voriconazole TDM with IDV/r co-administration.
Lovastatin	Lovastatin serum concentrations may be increased.	Consider pravastatin, atorvastatin, or rosuvastatin.
LPV/r	Voriconazole serum concentrations may be decreased.	Avoid co-administration. Consider voriconazole TDM (target Cmin >2.05 mcg/mL) with LPV/r co-administration.
Maraviroc	May increase MVC serum concentrations.	No data; consider MVC 150 or 300 mg twice daily with co-administration.

Drug	Effect of Interaction	Recommendations/Comments
Methadone	R-methadone AUC increased by 47%.	Monitor for increased sedation May need to dose adjust methadone with co-administration.
Methylpredni-solone	No significant interaction.	No dose adjustment necessary.
Midazolam	Midazolam serum concentrations may be increased.	Consider lorazepam, oxazepam, or temazepam.
Mycophenolic acid	No significant interaction.	No dose adjustment necessary.
Nevirapine	Voriconazole serum concentrations may be decreased.	Consider voriconazole TDM (target Cmin >2.05 mcg/mL) with NVP co-administration.
Nifedipine	Nifedipine serum concentrations may be increased.	Monitor.
Nisoldipine	Nisoldipine serum concentrations may be increased.	Monitor.
Omeprazole	Omeprazole AUC increased by 400%. VORI AUC increased 40%.	Reduce omeprazole dose by 50%. Consider VORI TDM.
Pentobarbital	Voriconazole serum concentrations may be decreased.	Contraindicated.
Phenobarbital	Voriconazole serum concentrations may be decreased.	Contraindicated.
Phenytoin	Phenytoin AUC increased by 80%. Voriconazole AUC decreased by 70%.	Voriconazole 400 mg PO q12h or 5 mg/kg IV q12h.
Pimozide	Risk of QTc prolongation may be increased.	Contraindicated.
Quinidine	Risk of QTc prolongation may be increased.	Contraindicated.
Raltegravir	Interaction unlikely	Use standard dose.
Ranitidine	No significant interaction.	No dose adjustment necessary.
Ranolazine	May significantly increase ranolazine serum concentrations.	Avoid co-administration.
Rifabutin	Rifabutin serum concentrations may be increased. Voriconazole serum level concentrations may be decreased.	Contraindicated.
Rifampin	Voriconazole serum concentrations may be decreased.	Contraindicated.
Ritonavir	RTV 400 mg q12h: Voriconazole AUC decreased by 82%. RTV 100 mg q12h: Voriconazole AUC decreased by 39%.	With RTV 400 mg q12h: Contraindicated. With RTV 100 mg q12h: Avoid or use with close monitoring of voriconazole Cmin (target Cmin >2 mcg/mL). Consider voriconazole 400 mg twice daily for invasive disease.
Secobarbital	Voriconazole serum concentrations may be decreased.	Contraindicated.

VORICONAZOLE *(cont.)*

Drug	Effect of Interaction	Recommendations/Comments
Simvastatin	Simvastatin serum concentrations may be increased.	Consider pravastatin, atorvastatin, or rosuvastatin.
Sirolimus	Sirolimus serum concentrations may be increased.	Contraindicated. Use tacrolimus with close TDM.
Tacrolimus	Tacrolimus AUC increased by 300%.	Reduce tacrolimus dose to 1/3 of original dose with close TDM.
Terfenadine	Risk of QTc prolongation may be increased.	Contraindicated.
TPV/r	Voriconazole serum concentrations may be decreased.	Avoid co-administration. Consider voriconazole TDM (target Cmin >2.05 mcg/mL) with TPV/r co-administration.
Triazolam	Triazolam serum concentrations may be increased.	Consider lorazepam, oxazepam, or temazepam.
Verapamil	Verapamil serum concentrations may be increased.	Monitor.
Vinblastine	Vinblastine serum concentrations may be increased.	Monitor closely for ADR and consider dose adjustment.
Vincristine	Vincristine serum concentrations may be increased.	Monitor closely for ADR and consider dose adjustment.
Warfarin	Anticoagulation may be increased.	Monitor INR closely.

Index